Sexually Transmitted Diseases and HIV/AIDS

Sexually Transmitted Diseases and HIV/AIDS

Editor-in-Chief
Vinod K Sharma, MD, FAMS
Professor and Head,
Department of Dermatology and Venereology,
All India Institute of Medical Sciences,
New Delhi, India

A Textbook of Indian Association for the Study of Sexually Transmitted Diseases and AIDS

Viva Books

New Delhi | Mumbai | Chennai | Kolkata | Bangalore | Hyderabad | Kochi | Guwahati

Cover Design: Vinod K Sharma

First Published in 2003
Reprinted 2006
Second Edition 2009, Reprinted 2011, 2012, 2014, 2015, 2018, 2019, 2020, 2022, 2023

VIVA BOOKS PRIVATE LIMITED

- 4737/23 Ansari Road, Daryaganj, New Delhi 110 002
  E-mail: vivadelhi@vivagroupindia.in Tel. 42242200
- 76, Service Industries, Shirvane, Sector 1, Nerul, Navi Mumbai 400 706
  E-mail: vivamumbai@vivagroupindia.in, Tel. 27721273, 27721274
- Megh Towers, Old No. 307, New No. 165, Poonamallee High Road, Maduravoyal
  Chennai - 600 095 E-mail: vivachennai@vivagroupindia.in, Tel. 23780991, 23780992
- B-103, Jindal Towers, 21/1A/3 Darga Road, Kolkata 700 017
  E-mail: vivakolkata@vivagroupindia.in, Tel. 22836381, 22816713
- 7, Sovereign Park Apartments, 56-58, K. R. Road, Basavanagudi, Bengaluru 560 004
  E-mail: vivabangalore@vivagroupindia.in, Tel. 26607409, 26607410
- 101-102 Mughal Marc Apartments, 3-4-637 to 641, Narayanguda, Hyderabad 500 029
  E-mail: vivahyderabad@vivagroupindia.in, Tel. 27564481, 27564482
- Beevi Towers, First Floor, SRM Road, Kaloor, Kochi 682 018, Kerala
  E-mail: vivakochi@vivagroupindia.in, Tel: 0484-2403055, 2403056
- 232, GNB Road, Beside UCO Bank, Silpukhuri, Guwahati 781 003
  E-mail: vivaguwahati@vivagroupindia.in, Tel: 0361-2666386

www.vivagroupindia.com

ISBN : 978-81-309-1204-2

Published by Viva Books Private Limited, 4737/23, Ansari Road, Daryaganj, New Delhi - 110 002.

Printed and bound in India.

Dedicated

to

Dr CN Sowmini

Patron, IASSTD & AIDS

Former Director

Institute of Venereology

Chennai

Editorial Board

PREFACE FOR THE SECOND EDITION

The first edition of text book of "Sexually Transmitted Diseases and HIV/AIDS" commissioned by Indian Association for the Study of Sexually Transmitted Diseases & AIDS (IASSTD & AIDS) was a great success. In the second edition, all chapters have been updated and new chapters on Historical Aspects, Vaccines against STIs and Erectile Dysfunction have been added. HIV/AIDS in Pregnancy and Children have been dealt in detail as separate chapters. The chapter on Miscellaneous Viral and Bacterial STDs, has been expanded. The treatment guidelines for STDs by National AIDS Control Organisation (NACO 2007) and Centre for Disease Control (CDC 2006) have been incorporated. The main target for the book remains postgraduates in dermatology and venereology and general practitioners involved in care of STDs & HIV/AIDS. The clinical and syndromic approach for the treatment of STDs has been highlighted and syndromic treatment charts have been included in the appendix.

Finally, keeping up with changing times, the book is produced in four colour print with photographs included along with the text for easy readability. The book would be useful to all physicians and health care givers dealing with the Sexually Transmitted Diseases and HIV/AIDS in Indian subcontinent and Asia.

Vinod K Sharma
Editor-in-Chief

ACKNOWLEDGEMENTS

I am grateful to Dr N Usman, President and Dr K Venkateswaran, Secretary, Indian Association for the Study of Sexually Transmitted Diseases and AIDS for their support in preparing the second edition of the textbook of Sexually Transmitted Diseases and HIV/AIDS. I am also grateful to Dr Devinder M Thappa, Past President, IASSTD and AIDS and Dr YS Marfatia, Chief Editor, Indian Journal of Sexually Transmitted Diseses and AIDS for constant help and encouragement in completing this difficult task. I acknowledge all the authors who have contributed and revised their chapters and did their best to improve the second edition. I am grateful to all residents of department of Dermatology, AIIMS, New Delhi who were of immense help in cross-checking & updating the information and proof reading. I am also grateful to contributors of photographs for the second edition. I also thank the National AIDS Control Organisation (NACO) and Centres for Diseases Control (CDC), USA and World Health Organisation (WHO) for preparing update guidelines and flow charts for treatment of STDs and HIV/AIDS and same have been included in the book.

I also acknowledge my family who accepted my frequent late return from the office and non availability at times.

Finally, I acknowledge my publisher, Viva Books Private Limited, for preparing excellent four colour edition of the text book.

Vinod K Sharma

PREFACE FOR THE FIRST EDITION

Sexually transmitted diseases (STD) have great impact on health of the individual and community. They can cause genital infection, infertility, abortion, still birth, pneumonia, neonatal deaths, and are associated with cervical cancer; death during and after childbirth, birth defects, impaired vision, blindness; shortened life span and death especially in AIDS. The study and knowledge of STD is essential for improving the health of the community. This book was conceived keeping these aspects in view and an effort was made to address all aspects. STD are more dynamic than other infections and their prevalence and clinical profile varies especially in developing countries like India where syphilis, chancroid and donovanosis are prevalent. However, the picture is undergoing change at fast pace and bacterial STD are becoming less common and viral STD are increasing. The advent of AIDS has caused a sea change in the attitude of all concerned. The STD were a trivial nuisance and now with arrival of AIDS they have become a matter of national concern. We have accorded a high priority to AIDS and STD prevalent in developing countries in this book. STD have a special impact on women and children and this subject has been extensively covered. The prevention of STD especially in viral infections is the only remedy available and special chapters on sexual behaviour, condoms and STD have been included. The NACO is making unprecedented efforts in control of STD and implementing syndromic approach which has been incorporated. The book is meant for postgraduates in dermatology & venereology and general practitioner involved in the care of STD and AIDS. The book has included not only international guidelines of treatment recommended by CDC and WHO but also NACO guidelines for treatment.

The book also includes an Atlas on STD and AIDS along with chapters on clinical approach to a patient with genital ulcer disease, urethral and vaginal discharge. This would help general practitioners and general duty medical officers in the management of STD.

Vinod Kumar Sharma

CONTRIBUTORS

Dr. Vinod K Sharma, MD, FAMS
Professor & Head
Department of Dermatology and Venereology
All India Institute of Medical Sciences, New Delhi 110029
vksaiims@yahoo.co.in

Dr. S. Khandpur, MD, DNB, MNAMS
Associate Professor
Department of Dermatology and Venereology
All India Institute of Medical Sciences, New Delhi 110029
sujaykhandpur@yahoo.co.in

Dr. H R Jerajani, MD
Professor & Head
Department of Dermatology
LTM Medical College and LTM General Hospital
Sion, Mumbai 400022
jerajani@rediffmail.com

Shubha Melkote, MD
Senior Resident
Department of Dermatology
LTM Medical College and LTM General Hospital
Sion, Mumbai-400022

Dr. Devinder M Thappa, MD, DHA, MNAMS
Professor and Head
Department of Dermatology and STD
JIPMER, Pondicherry 605006
dmthappa@satyam.net.in

Dr. H K Kar, MD, MNAMS
Senior Consultant and Head
Department of Dermatology
Dr. Ram Manohar Lohia Hospital, New Delhi
hkkar_2000@yahoo.com

Dr. J K Maniar, MD DVD, DDV
Former Professor of Dermatovenereology and AIDS Medicine
Grant Medical College, Mumbai
Consulting AIDS Physician
Jaslok Hospital and Research Centre
The Bhatia General Hospital and Masina Hospital
Mumbai
jkmaniar@vsnl.com

Dr. R R Kamath, MD
Lecturer
Department of Dermatovenereology
J J Group of Hospitals
Grant Medical College, Mumbai, India
ratnakar.kamath@gmail.com

Dr. Pradeep Seth, MD
Fomer Professor and Head
Department of Microbiology
AIIMS, New Delhi 110029
dr.pradeepseth@gmail.com

Dr. S. Sujatha
Professor
Department of Microbiology
JIPMER, Pondicherry 605 006
sujathasistla@gmail.com

Dr. Praveen Aggarwal MD, DNB, MAMS, FRCP
Professor
Division of Emergency Medicine
AIIMS, New Delhi
peekay_124@hotmail.com

Dr. Jyoti Prakash Wali MD, MAMS, FRCP,
FIMSA, FIACH
Formerly Professor
Department of Medicine
AIIMS, New Delhi
jyotiwali@yahoo.com

Dr. Rohini Handa MD, DNB, FAMS, FRCP, FRCS
Division of Rheumatology
Department of Medicine
AIIMS, New Delhi
rohinihanda@hotmial.com

Dr. Suneeta Mittal, MD, FRCOG, FICOG, FAMS, FICMCH, FIMSA
Professor and Head
Deapartment of Obstetrics & Gynaecology
Director-in Charge, WHO-CCR in Human Reproduction
Chief, ART Centre & IVF Facility
AIIMS, New Delhi 110029
suneeta.mittal@gmail.com

Dr. Pakhee Aggarwal, MD
Senior Resident
Deapartment of Obstetrics & Gynaecology
AIIMS, New Delhi 110029
drpakhee@gmail.com

K Neeladri Raju, MD
Former Professor of STD
Gandhi Hospital
Secunderabad, Andhra Pradesh
neeladri_k7@yahoo.co.in

Dr. Dinesh Mahur, MD (Skin), MD (Medicine)
Professor and Head
Department of Skin and STD
SMS Medical College and Hospital, Jaipur
drdineshmathur@yahoo.com

Dr. Veena Acharya, MS, Diploma in STD
Professor
Department of Gynaecology and Obstetrics
Zanana Hospital
SMS Medical College, Jaipur

Dr. Gurvinder P Thami, MD
Professor and Head
Department of Dermatology, Venereology and Leprology
Govt. Medical College and Hospital,
Sector 32, Chandigarh 160 031
drgurvinder@mantraonline.com

Dr. G. Sethuraman, MD
Associate Professor
Department of Dermatology and Venereology
All India Institute of Medical Sciences
New Delhi 110029
kgsethu@yahoo.com

Dr. R S Misra, MD
Senior Consultant Dermato-Venereologist
Sir Ganga Ram Hospital
Rajinder Nagar, New Delhi 110061
drrsm@usa.net

Dr. Joginder Kumar, MD
Consultant
Department of Dermatology, Venereology & Leprology
Regional STD Teaching, Training and Research Centre
Safdarjung Hospital
New Delhi 110029

Dr. Sanjeev Handa, MD, MNAMS
Professor
Department of Dermatology, Venereology and Leprology
PGIMER, Chandigarh 160012
handa_sanjeev@yahoo.com

Dr. Madhu Vajpayee, MD
Associate Professor
Incharge, HIV & Immunology Division
Department of Microbiology
AIIMS, New Delhi 110029
mvajpayee@hotmail.com

Dr. Purva Mathur, MD
Assistant Professor
Department of Laboratory Medicine
JPNA Trauma Centre
AIIMS
New Delhi
purvamathur@yahoo.co.in

Dr. Yogesh S Marfatia, MD
Professor and Head
Department of Skin and VD
Medical College, SSG Hospital,
Vadodara 390001
ym11256@yahoo.com

Dr. Archana Sharma, MD
Assistant Professor
Department of Skin & VD
Medical College
Vadodara
archanakangra@gmail.com

Dr. C Balachandran, MD
Professor and Head
Department of Skin and STD
Kasturba Medical College and Hospital
Manipal 576119
drbalannair@yahoo.com

Dr. Satish Pai B, MD
Professor
Department of Skin and STD
Kasturba Medical College and Hospital
Manipal 576104
drsbpai@yahoo.co.in

Dr. R. Ganesh, MD, DV
Profesor and Head
Department of STD
Tirunelveli Medical College and Hospital
Palayamkottai
Tirunelveli 627002, Tamil Nadu
ganeshsharma@sancharnet.in

Dr. V S Dorairaj, MD, DV
Director and Professor
Institute of Venereology
Govt. General Hospital, Chennai 600003
dorairaj1950@yahoo.co.in

Dr. K Venkateswaran, MD, DV
Assistant Professor
Institute of Venereology
Madras Medical College
Chennai 600003, Tamil Nadu
drkvt@yahoo.co.in

Dr. Usha Gupta, MD (Skin, VD & Leprosy),
PhD (Skin)
MD (Pathology & Microbiology), DGO
Professor and Head
Department of Dermatology, STD and Leprosy
NSCB Medical College
Jabalpur, Madhya Pradesh
ushaguptadr@hotmail.com

Dr. D K Gupta, MD (Medicine), ZDV, PhD (Skin)
Former Professor & Head
Department of Dermatology, STD and Leprosy
NSCB Medical College
Jabalpur, Mahya Pradesh

Dr. A K Bajaj, MD, FICAI
Former Professor & Head
Department of Dermatology
MLN Medicial College
Allahabad
Uttar Pradesh
bajajak1945@yahoo.co.in

Dr. Rajeev Sharma, MD
Consultant Dermatologist
Bishen Skin Centre
M-69, Marris Road, Aligarh 202001
skindoc_alg@dataone.in

Balaji Adityan, MBBS
Junior Resident
Department of Dermatology and STD
JIPMER, Pondicherry 605006
balajiderm@gmail.com

Dr. Joseph A Sundharam, MD
Sundharam's Dermatology and Pediatric Centre
Office No. 1, KD Market, Pitampura, Delhi 110034
jsundharam@gmail.com

Dr. N. Usman, MD, DV, PhD
Former Professor and Head
Department of STD
Kilpak Medical College and Govt.
Royapettah
Hospital, Chennai 600014
atharusman786@hotmail.com

Dr. P N Arora, MD, SFCP
Former Professor and Head
Department of Dermatovenereology
Armed Forces Medical College, Pune
Visiting consultant
Indraprastha Apollo Hospitals, New Delhi
pranarora18@yahoo.co.in

Dr. S Arora, MD
Dermatologist
Base Hospital, New Delhi 110010
sarora@vsnl.com

Dr. Manish Bansal, MD
Assistant Professor
Department of Dermatology
Banaras Hindu University
Varanasi
manishdoc@rediffmail.com

Dr. Jyoti Dhawan, MD
Senior Resident
Department of Dermatology and Venereology
All India Institute of Medical Sciences
New Delhi
jyotiderma@gmail.com

Trilokraj Tejasvi, MD
Post doc Research Fellow,
Psoriasis Genetics Laboratory
Department of Dermatology
University of Michigan
Ann Arbor, MI, 48105
trilokraj_a@yahoo.com, ttejasvi@umich.edu

Dr. Sowmya Kaimal, MBBS
Junior Resident
Dermatology and STD Department
JIPMER, Pondicherry 605 006
sowmyakaimal@hotmail.com

Dr. Nitin S Walia, MD, DNB
Classified specialist
(Dermatology & STD)
Military Hospital, Secunderabad
Trimulghery, Secunderabad, Andhra Pradesh
slg_nitin@sancharnet.in

Dr. (Maj-Gen) A K Jaiswal, MD
Additional DGAFMS (EXS)
Office of the DGAFMS
Ministry of Defence
M Block, Room No. 50
New Delhi 110001
ashokjaiswal48@yahoo.co.in

Dr. Ashok Kumar, MD
Professor and Head
Division of Rheumatology
Department of Medicine, AIIMS,
New Delhi 110029
ashok_145@hotmail.com

Dr. S. Murugan, MD, DV
Former Professor and Head
Department of STD
Govt. Mohan Kumara Mangalam Medical College
Salem, Tamil Nadu
malamurugan@yahoo.com

Dr. Amit K Malhotra, MD
Assistant Professor
SMS Medical College
Jaipur, Rajasthan
dramitmalhotra@rediffmail.com

Dr. R K Sharma, MD
Additional Professor
Department of Forensic Medicine
AIIMS, New Delhi 110 029
rksharma1@hotmail.com

Dr. Meera Sharma, MD
Professor and Head
Department of Medical Microbiology
PGIMER, Chandigarh 160 012
meerasharma48@rediffmail.com

Dr. Sunil Sethi, MD
Associate Professor
Department of Medical Microbiology
PGIMER, Chandigarh 160012
sunilsethi10@hotmail.com

Dr. Neena Khanna, MD
Professor
Department of Dermatology and Venereology
All India Institute of Medical Sciences
New Delhi
neena_aiims@yahoo.co.in

Dr. Ajay Khera, MD
Joint Director (Basic Services Division)
NACO
Ministry of Health & Family Welfare
New Delhi
kheranaco@gmail.com

Dr. R D Mehta, MD
Associate Professor
Department of Skin and VD
SP Medical College, Bikaner 334 003
mehtard@datainfosys.net

Dr. Alison Blume MRCP, Dip GUM, Dip HIV Med
Southampton City PCT
Southampton
United Kingdom
adblume@yahoo.com

Dr. Rajul Patel FRCP
University of Southampton
Southampton
United Kingdom
prj466@aol.com

Dr. Binod K Khaitan, MD
Associate Professor
Department of Dermatology and Venereology
All India Institute of Medical Sciences
New Delhi
binodkhaitan@hotmail.com

Dr. M Ramam, MD
Additional Professor
Department of Dermatology and Venereology
All India Institute of Medical Sciences
New Delhi
mramam@hotmail.com

Dr. B M Tripathi, MD, MRCPS psych
Professor
Department of Psychiatry& National Drug Dependence Treatment Center
AIIMS, New Delhi 110 029
bmt_54@yahoo.com

Dr. Atul Ambekar, MD
Assistant Professor
Department of Psychiatry & National Drug Dependence Treatment Center
AIIMS, New Delhi 110029
atul.ambekar@gmail.com

Dr, Sameer Malhotra, MD, MNAMS, CCST, FIPS, FIASP, FIACAMH
Head, Department of Psychiatry
Fortis Hospital, Ex-Consultant Psychiatrist
Senior Psychiatrist & Psychotherapist
AIIMS, New Delhi
sameersankalp2003@yahoo.com

Dr. Prem Nath Dogra, MS, MCh
Professor
Department of Urology
AIIMS, New Delhi
dograpn@rerdiffmail.com

Dr. Anup Kumar, M S, MCh
Senior Research Associate
Department of Urology
AIIMS, New Delhi110029
anup_14k@yahoo.com

Dr. Uttam Kumar, MD
Senior Resident
Department of Dermatology and Venereology
AIIMS, New Delhi 110 029
uttamderma@gmail.com

Dr. A J Kanwar, MD
Professor & Head
Department of Dermatology, Venereology and Leprology
PGIMER, Chandigarh 160 012
ajkanwar@sify.com

Dr. Megha Modi, MBBS
Junior Resident
Department of Skin and VD
Medical college and SSG Hospital
Vadodra, Gujarat
dr.meghamodi@gmail.com

Dr. K P Narendar, MD
Former Director
Institute of Venereology
Madras Medical College
Chennai 600002
Tamil Nadu

Dr. Komal Aggarwal, MD
Senior Reseach Fellow
Department of Dermatology and Venereology
AIIMS, New Delhi 110029
komal_aiims@yahoo.com

Dr. Sushruta Dash, MD
Senior Resident
Department of Dermatology, Venereology and Leprology
Safdarjung Hospital
New Delhi
drsushruta@gmail.com

CONTRIBUTORS OF THE PHOTOGRAPHS

Dr. Vinod K Sharma, MD, FAMS
Professor & Head
Department of Dermatology and Venereology
All India Institute of Medical Sciences,
New Delhi 110029
vksaiims@yahoo.co.in

Dr. Amit K Malhotra, MD
Assistant Professor
SMS Medical College
Jaipur
Rajasthan
dramitmalhortra@rediffmail.com

Dr. J K Maniar, MD, DVD, DDV
Former Professor of Dermatovenereology and AIDS Medicine
Grant Medical College, Mumbai
Consulting AIDS Physician
Jaslok Hospital and Research Centre
The Bhatia General Hospital and Masina Hospital
Mumbai
jkmaniar@vsnl.com

Dr. O P Singh, MD
Former Associate Professor
Department of Dermatology and Venereology
AIIMS, New Delhi 110029

Dr. P N Arora, MD, SFCP
Former Professor and Head
Department of Dermatovenereology,
Armed Forces Medical College, Pune
Visiting consultant
Indraprastha Apollo Hospitals, New Delhi
pranarora18@yahoo.co.in

Dr. R S Misra, MD
Senior Consultant Dermato-Venereologist
Sir Ganga Ram Hospital
Rajinder Nagar, New Delhi 110061
drrsm@usa.net

Dr. R. Ganesh, MD, DV
Profesor and Head
Department of STD
Tirunelveli Medical College and Hospital
Palayamkottai
Tirunelveli 627002, Tamil Nadu
ganeshsharma@sancharnet.in

Dr. M Ramam, MD
Additional Professor
Department of Dermatology and Venereology
All India Institute of Medical Sciences
New Delhi
mramam@hotmail.com

Dr. Binod K Khaitan, MD
Associate Professor
Department of Dermatology and Venereology
All India Institute of Medical Sciences
New Delhi
binodkhaitan@hotmail.com

Dr. Sanjeev Handa, MD, MNAMS
Professor
Department of Dermatology, Venereology and Leprology
PGIMER, Chandigarh 160012
handa_sanjeev@yahoo.com

Dr. G. Sethuraman, MD
Associate Professor
Department of Dermatology and Venereology
All India Institute of Medical Sciences
New Delhi 110029
kgsethu@yahoo.com

Dr. Manoj K Singh, MD
Professor
Department of Pathology
AIIMS, New Delhi 110029

Dr. H K Kar, MD, MNAMS
Professor and Head
Department of Dermatology
Dr. Ram Manohar Lohia Hospital, New Delhi
hkkar_2000@yahoo.com

Dr. Devinder M Thappa, MD, DHA, MNAMS
Professor and Head
Department of Dermatology and STD
JIPMER, Pondicherry 605 006
dmthappa@satyam.net.in

Dr. N. Usman, MD, DV, PhD
Former Professor and Head
Department of STD
Lolpak Medical College and Govt. Royapettah
Hospital, Chennai 600014
atharusman786@hotmail.com

Dr. T S Chandra Gupta
Professor and Head
Department of STD,
Government General Hospital,
Kakinada – 533001, Andhra Pradesh
drchandragupta_ts@radiffmail.com

Dr. Pradeep Sethy, MD
Junior Resident
Department of Dermatology & Venereology
AIIMS, New Delhi 110029
pksethybdk@gmail.com

Dr. Somesh Gupta, MD
Assistant Professor
Department of Dermatology & Venereology
AIIMS, New Delhi 110029
someshgupta@hotmail.com

Dr. Prem Nath Dogra, MS, MCh
Professor
Department of Urology
AIIMS, New Delhi
dograpn@rediffmail.com

Dr. Kavita N Singh
Associate Professor
Department of Obstetrics and Gynaecolosy
NSCB Medical College, Jabalpur
Madhya Pradesh

ACKNOWLEDGEMENT OF THE PHOTOGRAPHS

Vinod K Sharma
Figures 5.3, 5.4, 5.13, 5.14, 5.16, 5.17, 5.18, 14.1, 14.7, 14.9, 14.11, 14.13, 14.15, 14.16, 19.2, 19.3, 19.6, 20.5, 21.2, 21.3, 21.5, 23.3, 23.4, 25.1, 25.3, 25.5, 26.2, 26.3, 26.6, 26.10, 27.1, 27.3, 27.4, 27.6, 28.1, 28.2, 28.3, 28.4, 28.6, 28.8, 28.9, 32.1, 32.2, 40.1, 40.2, 40.5, 40.6, 40.7, 40.10, 41.4, 41.8

Vinod K Sharma/Amit Malhotra
Figures 27.2, 27.5, 27.8, 28.10, 28.11, 35.5, 40.11, 40.13, 41.1, 41.2, 41.5, 41.6, 41.7

J K Maniar
Figures 5.2, 5.5, 5.6, 5.7, 5.8, 5.9, 5.10, 5.11, 5.12, 5.15, 5.19, 5.26

O P Singh
Figures 14.19, 14.20, 15.2, 15.3, 15.4, 19.4, 21.4, 21.6, 21.7, 23.1, 23.2

P N Arora
Figures 14.14, 14.21, 20.3, 25.2, 27.7, 40.4, 40.8, 44.3, 44.4

R S Misra
Figures 14.2, 14.4, 14.5, 4.6, 14.18, 14.22, 19.1, 20.4, 23.5

R Ganesh
Figures 20.6, 20.7, 33.1, 33.2

M Ramam
Figures 13.4, 14.3, 14.10, 20.1, 40.9, 41.3, 41.9

Binod K Khaitan
Figures 14.8, 14.12, 20.2

Sanjeev Handa
Figures 14.17, 15.1, 19.5

G Sethuraman/M K Singh
Figures 13.1, 13.3, 25.6

H K Kar
Figures 25.4, 26.5, 28.5

P N Dogra
Figures 44.1, 44.2

T S Chandra Gupta
Figures 20.8, 20.9, 20.10

N Usman
Figures 26.4, 33.3, 33.4, 33.6

Davinder M Thappa
Figure 13.2

Vinod K Sharma/Pradeep Sethy
Figure 27.9

G Sethuraman
Figure 28.7

Somesh Gupta
Figure 40.3

Amit K Malhotra
Figure 40.12

Kavita N Singh
Figure 22.2

CONTENTS

PART 1

General

1 EPIDEMIOLOGY OF SEXUALLY TRANSMITTED INFECTIONS

Vinod K Sharma, Sujay Khandpur

In this chapter

- Risk Factors and Risk Behaviours in STIs
- High-risk Groups
- Addictions
- High-risk Sexual Practices
- Other Sexual Practices
- Health Care Behaviour
- STIs in Special Age-Groups
- Demographic and Social Correlates of STIs
- Modes of Transmission of STIs
- Epidemiology of Individual STIs

INTRODUCTION

Sexually transmitted infections (STIs) include diseases that are transmitted by sexual intercourse. Sexual transmission requires the agent to be present in one partner, the other partner to be susceptible to infection with that agent, and that the sex partners engage in sexual practices so as to be able to transmit the pathogen.

STI differs from a sexually transmitted disease (STD) in that STDs conventionally include infections that result in clinical diseases involving the genitalia and other parts of the body in sexual interaction. Syphilis, gonorrhoea, chancroid, donovanosis, nongonococcal urethritis, genital warts, and herpes genitalis are STDs. STI also includes infections that may not cause clinical diseases of the genitals but are transmitted by sexual interaction, e.g. all STDs, hepatitis B, HIV, and HTLV-1. Nowadays, the term STI is preferred since it covers all the diseases transmitted by sexual intercourse. **However, for all practical purposes, both STD and STI are used synonymously.**

STIs have been known to exist since time immemorial. Medical descriptions date back to the 15th century in Europe where syphilis and gonorrhoea were primarily responsible for the abandonment of public baths. The golden era of microbiology in the late 19th and early 20th centuries identified microbes responsible for five traditional venereal diseases, namely gonorrhoea, syphilis, chancroid, lymphogranuloma venereum and donovanosis. After World War II, new diagnostic techniques and defined clinical and epidemiological studies in North America and Europe established that many 'non-traditional' microbes could also produce infections when transmitted sexually (Table 1.1).

Table 1.1 Sexually Transmitted Agents and Diseases

S.No.	Agents	Disease or Syndrome	Complications
1.	**Bacteriae**		
	Neisseria gonorrhoeae	Urethritis, epididymitis, bartholinitis, cervicitis, endometritis, salpingitis, proctitis, pharyngitis	Infertility, ectopic pregnancy, chorioamnionitis, premature rupture of membranes, premature delivery, conjunctivitis, PID, disseminated gonococcal infection (DGI)
	Chlamydia trachomatis D-K	Urethritis, epididymitis, bartholinitis, cervicitis, endometritis, salpingitis, proctitis, pharyngitis	Same as gonorhoea except DGI, and including Reiter's syndrome, pneumonia
	Chlamydia trachomatis L1,L2,L3	Lymphogranuloma venereum	Esthiomene, anorectogenital syndrome, proctocolitis, skin rashes, pneumonia, hepatitis, meningoencephalitis
	Treponema pallidum	Syphilis - primary, secondary, latent	Benigh tertiary syphilis, neurosyphilis, cardiovascular
	Haemophilus ducreyi	Chancroid	Phimosis, sclerosis, meatal stenosis
	Calymmatobacterium granulomatis	Donovanosis	Phimosis, sclerosis, SCC

(*Contd.*)

S.No.	Agents	Disease or Syndrome	Complications
	Mycoplasma hominis	Nongonococcal urethritis, cervicitis, salpingitis	PID, postpartum fever
	Ureaplasma urealyticum	Nongonococcal urethritis, cervicitis, salpingitis	Chorioamnionitis, low birth weight
	Gardnerella vaginalis and others	Bacterial vaginosis	
	Group B β-hemolytic streptococcus		Neonatal sepsis, neonatal meningitis
2.	**Viruses**		
	Herpes simplex virus 1,2	Primary and recurrent genital herpes	Aseptic meningitis, neonatal herpes and associated mortality or neurological sequelae, spontaneous abortion, premature delivery
	Human papilloma virus	Condyloma acuminata	Laryngeal papilloma in infants, squamous epithelial neoplasia of cervix, anus, vagina, vulva, penis
	Hepatitis B virus	Acute, chronic and fulminant hepatitis B	Cirrhosis, hepatocellular carcinoma
	Cytomegalovirus	Infectious mononucleosis	Congenital infection, birth defects, infant mortality, cognitive impairment (mental retardation, sensorineural deafness),
	Molluscum contagiosum virus	Genital molluscum contagiosum	protean manifestations in immunocompromized hosts
	HIV (Human immunodeficiency virus)	AIDS and related conditions	Infection, eczematoid dermatitis, erythema annulare centrifugum
	Human T-lymphotropic virus (HTLV-10)	T-cell leukemia, lymphoma, tropical spastic paraparesis	Opportunistic infections, death
3.	**Protozoan**		
	Trichomonas vaginalis	Urethritis, balanitis, vaginitis	
4.	**Fungus**		
	Candida albicans	Vulvovaginitis, balanitis, balanoposthitis	
5.	**Ectoparasites**		
	Pthirus pubis	Pubic lice infestation	
	Sarcoptes scabiei	Scabies	Norwegian scabies in immunocompromised host

In the United States, five of the top 11 reportable diseases in 1996 were transmitted sexually (gonorrhoea, chlamydial infection, syphilis, hepatitis B and AIDS). STIs rank among the five leading health problems in developing countries.[1] During 1995 WHO estimated 400 million cases including 333 million new cases of curable STIs in adults globally, of which 150 million were in South and South-East Asia, including 50 million in India.[2] In 1999, there were 340 million new cases. These diseases are endemic in the tropics, and the morbidity and mortality caused by them now rivals that by Plasmodium falciparum malaria in several African and Asian nations. STIs and HIV may be responsible for up to 17% of productive years lost in certain regions.

STIs have a tremendous impact on national health. They are responsible for a significant proportion of maternal morbidity, ectopic pregnancy, infant illness and death, malignancies, infertility and increased susceptibility to HIV infection. They are one of the major causes of infertility in both women and men. STIs are also one of the significant contributors of fetal death, abortions and low birth weight (Table 1.2). HIV infection is the most significant STI that has resulted in widespread deaths and considerable impact on social and economic survival of countries especially in Africa. It is also responsible for renewed interest in STIs and their control.

The epidemiology of STIs results from the interaction between STI pathogens, the behaviours that help transmit them and the effectiveness of prevention and control interventions. Their epidemiological patterns are very distinct and differ from other diseases since their incubation periods are highly variable, the genetic structure of most STI pathogens is so diverse that researchers have been unable to design a vaccine against them, and these diseases are primarily spread by a class of behaviours which is inherently resistant to change because it is highly motivated and varies considerably within and between social and ethnic groups.

A variety of demographic and medical factor contributes to the high prevalence of STIs, especially in developing countries where a large percentage of population belongs to the sexually active agegroup.[3] Rural-to-urban migration in these countries has led to family separation and unbalanced sex ratios in both rural and urban areas, loss of traditional values of sexual behaviour and increased sexual promiscuity. In most traditional societies, the stigma associated with STIs is still strong, and embarrassment may prevent infected persons from seeking medical treatment, thereby increasing the reservoir of infections. The incidence and distribution of these diseases is also influenced by factors such as lifestyle and susceptibility of the individual, pathogenicity of the microbes, prevailing therapy and disease control measures. A complex set of behavioural factors also determines the risk of acquiring STIs (Table 1.3). Moreover, cure by appropriate antibiotic therapy is no longer certain for some infections such as gonorrhoea and chancroid because of growing antibiotic resistance.

In the era of HIV infections, there is a resurgence of interest in STIs amongst both researchers and health policy makers. The control of STIs to prevent the transmission of HIV infections is now considered a public health priority. This recognition has also led to an increased focus on STI cases being managed at the primary health care level using the syndromic approach thereby reducing their global burden.

The epidemiological profile of STIs is more dynamic than any other diseases. Most published data are based on surveillance systems that rely heavily on reports from STI and gynecology clinics and family planning centers. Surveillance data provide valuable information, especially, regarding long-term trends, but they represent a biased sample derived from limited subpopulations which are subject to change over time. Mostly the STI rates, especially those obtained from the developing countries, are unreliable due to delay in presentation to a health care facility, lower rate of self-reported STI, lack of recognition of small or asymptomatic lesions as an STI problem and non-availability of skilled personnel and specific diagnostic tests in most of the centers. The current trend is that experts undertake large population-based surveys, supported by necessary diagnostic tests.

In developed countries, there has been a steady increase in STI rates, especially the viral STIs and genital chlamydia infection, since the development of sophisticated diagnostic tests has helped in the recognition of widespread reservoirs of sub-clinical infections. In the STI clinics in UK, a 9% increase in the incidence of acute STIs was observed between 1996 and 1997.[4] The annual number of genital herpes has almost tripled during the past 15 years in England. This has forced a reappraisal of the importance of sexual and health care behaviours and use of contraceptive devices, since the control of incurable viral STIs depends to a great extent on societal efforts at

Table 1.2 **Morbidity Due to Sexually Transmitted Infections**

S.No.	*Disease*	*Morbidity*
1.	Gonorrhoea	Reproductive morbidity in men and women (infertility), impaired vision, blindness
2.	Chlamydial infection	Infertility in adults, neonatal death, impaired vision and blindness
3.	Lymphogranuloma venereum	Genital deformity, obstruction during delivery, carcinoma
4.	Syphilis	Involvement of heart and brain, impaired vision and blindness, abortions, fetal and infant deaths
5.	Chancroid	Destruction of genitalia
6.	Donovanosis	Genital destruction, carcinoma, bone involvement (rarely)
7.	Mycoplasma infection	Infertility
8.	Ureaplasma infection	Infertility, fetal morbidity, low birth weight
9.	Bacterial vaginosis	Female genital tract infection
10.	Group B β-hemolytic streptococcus	Septicaemia, multiorgan failure
11.	Genital herpes	Severe neonatal infection and death, female genital tract cancer (implicated)
12.	Human papillomavirus infection	Respiratory tract obstruction, premalignant and malignant disease of genitalia
13.	Hepatitis B infection	Chronic liver disease, hepatic carcinoma, death
14.	Cytomegalovirus infection	Severe neonatal multiorgan involvement, birth defects
15.	Molluscum contagiosum virus infection	Spread of infection to partner and family members
16.	HIV	Multisystemic involvement, death
17.	Trichomoniasis	Reproductive tract infection in men and women
18.	Candida infection	Genital involvement, neonatal complications
19.	Pthriasis	Infection, spread to partner and community
20.	Scabies	Severe skin infection, septicaemia, spread to household and community

Table 1.3 Determinants of Sexually Transmitted Infections

Behavioural Risk Factors	**High-risk Groups**
Age at first intercourse	CSWs
Marital status	Drivers
Frequency of sexual intercourse	Restaurant workers
Number of lifetime partners	Prison inmates
Rate and type of partners recruited	Transsexuals
Age difference between partners	
Addictions - crack cocaine, IV drug use, alcohol, smoking	
High-risk Sex Practices	**Health Care Behaviour**
Receptive and insertive anogenital intercourse	Contraception: barrier, OCPs, IUDs
Oro-anal intercourse	Circumcision
Oro-genital intercourse	
Receptive manual-anal intercourse	
Dry sex	
Sex during menstruation	
Vaginal douching	
Demographic and Social Correlates	
Age	
Gender	
Education	
Socioeconomic status	
Ethnicity	

primary prevention through health education and counselling of the infected carrier rather than early diagnosis and treatment of the disease, which is an effective strategy for curable bacterial STIs. A rapid decline in the incidence of syphilis has been observed in the White communities with stable or even increasing rates among the Blacks.[5] This rise has occurred among the urban, poor and minority populations, particularly adolescents, with the highest rates recorded among adolescent females. Prostitution has emerged as an STI multiplier, and the phenomenon of sex in exchange for drugs has contributed to epidemic spread of syphilis, gonorrhoea and chancroid in North America. There has been a constant decline in the incidence of gonorrhoea especially among heterosexual men and all women.[6] However, it has been on the increase in homosexual men.[7,8]

In the developing world, 10-20% of adult patients attend government health facilities because of STIs.[9] In Delhi, between 1954 and 1994, the number of STI cases increased eight times. However, these figures are most certainly an underestimate, since these infections are rarely treated in the official health sector, and patients prefer to visit traditional healers, quacks, pharmacists or private practitioners who are more accessible and less judgemental in their attitudes. In 1970s and early 1980s, syphilis and chancroid were the main causes of the genital ulcer disease (GUD), while the viral GUDs such as genital herpes were so rare that they even merited publication as case reports.[10] In India, it was recorded under 'other minor STIs'. The spread of HIV since the late 1980s with subsequent behavioural change has resulted in significant alterations in STI epidemic patterns, and similar to developed countries, there has been a significant rise in viral STIs and a relative fall in the incidence of traditional infections. In 1980s, herpes infection accounted for 17% of genital ulcers in Singapore and 12% in Bangkok. The incidence of gonorrhoea is still very high in African and Asian countries. In early 1990s, the incidence of gonococcal urethritis in Africa was estimated to be approximately 10% annually.[11] Numerous surveys conducted in recent years have shown that gonorrhoea is the commonest cause of male urethritis accounting for approximately 53-80% of the cases.[12] In India also, gonorrhoea is a major health problem. At a regional STI center in North India, a comparison of incidences of STIs during four periods, i.e. between 1990-1993, 1994-1997, 1998-2001 and 2002-2004, showed that in 1990-93, genital discharges predominated, while in other periods, GUDs were predominant. Syphilis was the commonest STI. There was a significant rise in the cases of syphilis, herpes progenitalis and genital warts and a reduction in the cases of chancroid, LGV, donovanosis, candidiasis, trichomoniasis and bacterial vaginosis. The number of cases with primary syphilis diminished significantly ($P<0.001$), with a concomitant rise in secondary and early latent syphilis.[13]

RISK FACTORS AND RISK BEHAVIOURS IN STIs[1-3]

The determinants of risk of STIs, including HIV infection, and STI distribution patterns include a complex set of ecological and behavioural factors. In industrialized countries, behavioural surveys have provided important insights to help guide public health intervention in preventing STIs.

Behavioural Risk Factors

Sexual behaviour is largely a private activity, subject to varying degrees of social, cultural, religious, moral and legal norms and constraints. Behavioural risk factors are related to a greater probability of acquiring the disease and a higher risk of developing complications. They play a key role in acquiring incurable viral STDs. Behavioural determinants include age at first intercourse or 'coitarche', marital status of the individual, frequency of sexual intercourse, number of lifetime partners, rate and type of sexual partners recruited, rate of partner change, number of current relationships, age difference between partners, sexual mixing with high-risk groups such as commercial sex workers (CSWs), truck drivers, mine workers, etc., addictions such as drug abuse, alcoholism and smoking, and types of sexual practices (vaginal, anal or oral intercourse).

Age at First Intercourse

There is a strong association between acquisition of STIs and young age at first intercourse. Early sexual debut leads to higher rates of partner exchange and greater chances of STI transmission. It also has a bearing on the development of a specific disease. It has been associated with cervical cancer owing to the biological development of cervix during teenage. In a survey conducted in South Africa, the median age at first sex of HIV-positive individuals was 16.6 years for men and 17.2 years for women.[14] The tremendous rise in STIs and HIV in this region was possibly due to the rise in the proportion of sexually active women aged 15 to 19 years (from 57% in 1994 to 67.5% in 1999). In two sub-Saharan urban population groups, women with STIs were found to have had their sexual debut before age 15.[15] In a survey in Peru, 51% of men with STIs have had their first intercourse between 15 and 17 years.[16] Moreover, a greater percentage of women who initiated sexual activity before 18 years of age had antibodies to *Chlamydia trachomatis* than women who indulged in sex after 18 years (23% vs 9%). In a study from Sweden, women attaining sexual debut at mean of 15.3 years had a greater frequency of genital signs including abnormal vaginal discharge, erythema of vaginal mucosa, and lower genital tract infections as compared to women with sexual debut at mean age of 20.7 years.[17] Similarly, a higher incidence of gonorrhoea, chlamydial infection and genital warts was observed among the teenage population in a study from Thames, England.[4] A strong correlation between early age of first intercourse and acquisition of HPV infection has been observed, which may be explained by frequent visits to prostitutes by husbands of cases with early sexual debut.[18] In several Indian studies, the average age of sexual debut in STI clinic attendees has been observed to be between 15 and 20 years.[19-22]

Marital Status

Several studies from India and abroad have shown that married individuals especially women are at a higher risk of acquiring STIs and HIV.[14,15,19-24] This can be explained by the fact that women who acquire an additional sex partner after marriage, are more likely to be infected than having casual partners before marriage. In addition, a higher frequency of unprotected sex within marriage could result in a higher probability of disease transmission as compared with casual partnerships where sexual intercourse is less frequent. In two studies from Delhi, a majority (54.5% and 62.4% respectively) of STD patients were married, in that 91.2% of men had acquired the diesease outside marriage while 88.1% of women acquired it from their spouses.[19,25]

Number of Lifetime Sex Partners

The risk of exposure to an STI and the development of cervical and other genital cancers is directly associated with the number of lifetime sex partners, and the rate of partner recruitment and partner change. However, this correlation is complicated by differences in patterns with respect to the choice of partner, partners' own sexual behaviour and the degree of his infectiousness.

In a Peruvian study, a direct correlation was noted between STI seropositivity and presence of more than 20 sex partners.[16] In South Africa, HSV-2 seropositivity was also related to the number of partners, the mean number in men being 4.7, and in women 2.6.[14] In an American study, patients with cervical HPV infections had a mean of 4.8 sex partners as compared to 2.6 for controls.[18] This correlation has been demonstrated in Indian studies as well.[19-25] In 1996, in Delhi/Haryana, the proportion of sexually active persons having at least one sex partner other than a regular partner in the last 12 months was 2.5; in Maharashtra 3.2; in Tamil Nadu 4.2; and in West Bengal 2.7. This has been one of the major causes of the rise in STI prevalence in India.[26]

Age Difference Between Sex Partners

Few studies have shown that a greater age difference (>11 years) between sex partners was found to increase the risk of STIs and HIV, especially in women.[15]

HIGH-RISK GROUPS

Commercial Sex Workers (CSWs)

A CSW or prostitute is a person who provides sexual service for money or other material gains. They could be identified in brothels, night clubs, massage parlors and bars or are casual freelance sex workers. Sexual exposure with CSWs has been implicated as an important risk factor for STI transmission, because they experience a higher rate of partner change, longer exposure to infection, and poorer access to health care facilities. The role of prostitutes has been assessed by monitoring the incidence of STIs in this group and the proportion of male STI patients who acknowledge recent sex with a prostitute. The incidence of STIs is directly related to early age of commencement of sex work, longer duration of prostitution and the current age of the CSW. In Mexico in 1999, a higher HSV-2 seroprevalence (60.8%) was recorded among prostitutes.[27] Infection with high-risk and multiple HPV types was also high with the highest rates recorded among younger women. In Japan, CSWs showed a greater prevalence of HPV, *C. trachomatis* and gonococcal infections than the control group.[28] In France also, a higher seroprevalence of anti-HPV type 16, 18, 31 and 58 antibodies was detected in CSWs (25%) than in general population (3%), indicating that this group is at increased risk of oncogenic infections and that the number of sex partners is a major determinant in the acquisition of oncogenic HPV.[29] Numerous epidemiological studies in developing countries have shown that GUDs are most common among CSWs. In a cross-sectional survey undertaken among female CSWs in Nigeria, a high seroprevalence of chancroid and syphilis was observed.[30] Low-class CSWs were significantly more likely than upper-class CSWs to be seropositive for syphilis and *Haemophilus ducreyi*. In women who saught primary care for genital discharge syndrome in Madagascar, the highest seroprevalence of bacterial vaginosis (85%), trichomoniasis (16%), cervical infection (49%) and syphilis (16%) was found in prostitutes, followed by occasional sex traders and general population, with syphilis being associated with low education, young age at coital debut and more than one partner in the previous 3 months.[31] An etiological study conducted among CSWs in Dhaka, Bangladesh, revealed 84% of workers to be positive for STI pathogen, 35.5% for gonorrhoea, 25% for chlamydial infection, 45.5% for trichomoniasis, 32.6% for syphilis and 62.5% for HSV-2 infection.[32]

Several studies conducted in India show that the majority of male patients (74.5% to 89%) give history of contact with CSWs.[19-25] In Kolkata, in 1994, a high prevalence of STIs (80.6%) was observed among CSWs.[33] Oral infection with HSV-1 and 2 and HPV 16/18 was detected in prostitutes in 24.6%, 11.6% and 29%, respectively, and cervical infections in 0%, 44% and 63% of cases, indicating a high prevalence of oral sex in this group. In a survey of the clients visiting a red-light area in Kolkata, seropositivity of HCV was found in 15.1% cases, while syphilis occurred in 40.9% and HbsAg in 20.4% of clients.[34] In Pune, 81.5% of CSWs were found to be suffering from STIs, thus posing a potential risk of transmitting these diseases to their clients.[35] Syphilis was the commonest STI (36.8%) followed by chancroid (31.3%). CSWs differed from women engaged in other works in being of older age group, illiterate, unmarried and staying away from home. Forty-seven percent of CSWs were HIV positive as compared to 14% positivity recorded in the control group. A survey from Tirupati, Andhra Pradesh, demonstrated HIV seropositivity in 25% of CSWs, primary chancre in 15%, gonorrhoea in 15%, LGV in 10%, donovanosis in 5%, seropositivity for syphilis in 70% and HbsAg in 50%.

Unless prevention strategies are enforced in this high-risk group, it was estimated that HIV infection among CSWs in India would increase from the 1999 level of 2.49 million to 3.93 million in a favourable scenario and to 6.87 million in a worse scenario by 2005.[37] Hence, continuous surveillance, early diagnosis, appropriate treatment and rigorous follow-up are of utmost importance in limiting the transmission of STIs. Moreover, the focus is on the prevention of CSWs from acquiring an STI by using barrier contraceptives.

Transport Workers (Drivers)

Drivers have been identified as a male occupational group at a high risk of STI and AIDS acquisition, who may play an important role in the dissemination of these infections because of their geographical mobility. They often come in contact with various types of sex workers such as homosexuals and prostitutes while they are away from their families for long periods. They get enough chance to visit CSWs during the time their trucks are being loaded and unloaded. Poverty, illiteracy, low level of awareness about STDs and HIV and lack of healthy recreation facilities are other contributing factors. In a study conducted in Pondicherry between 1997 and 1999, truck drivers were found to have the highest rates of HbsAg (23.8%) and HIV (47.6%) and the second highest rate of hepatitis C positivity (42.8%).[38] In another survey from the same city between 1993 and 1997, 51.4% of truck drivers reacted seropositive for HIV antibodies.[39] In Nagpur, 43.7% of long-distance truck drivers were found to have one or more STIs with HIV infection detected in 15.2% cases, syphilis in 21.9%, gonorrhoea in 6.7% and hepatitis B in 5.1% cases.[40] In Delhi, 1% of truck drivers were found to be HIV positive.[41] The risk behaviours include sex with CSWs, homosexuality, illiteracy and non-usage of condoms. In a cross-section study conducted among long-distance truck drivers in Kenya, seroprevalence for syphilis was 4.6%, 26.5% for chancroid and 18% for HIV.[42] In sub-Saharan Africa, rates of HIV infection among truck drivers as high as 26-35% have been reported.[42] STIs detected in Bangladesh's trucking industry were HSV-2 (25.8%), serological syphilis (5.7%), gonorrhoea (2.1%) and chlamydia (0.8%).[43] The significant risk factors were sex with CSWs and lower rates of condom use (in 11.8% drivers only).

Restaurant Workers

They are another high-risk group for STIs. In a survey undertaken among restaurant workers along a highway in Assam, over one-third had sexual contact with multiple partners or CSWs and 2% were engaged in homosexual activity. Majority of them were illiterates, 30% were alcoholic and smokers, and 3% were addicted to cannabis.[44] GUD was present in 25.7% of workers, 11.8% had gonorrhoea while 5.1% were VDRL reactive.

Transsexuals

In the Indian subcontinent, male sex workers are predominantly transvestites and transsexuals, popularly known as 'Hijras'. Many centuries ago Hijras believed themselves to be the incarnation of Lord Krishna. This community now engages in commercial sex and is at high risk for STIs and HIV. They indulge mainly in insertive anogenital intercourse with men. A survey from Karachi, Pakistan, in 1999 documented syphilis in 37%, urethritis in 70%, genital warts in 54% and HbsAg positivity in 3.4% of transvestite sex workers.[45] Fifty-seven percent of them reported sexual abuse in childhood, the average age of first intercourse with consent was 12 years, condom use by their sex partners was minimal, almost 50% took drugs while 63% consumed alcohol. Hence, intervention strategies can have a great impact on STI and HIV prevention for this community.

Prison Inmates

STIs tend to cluster even in socially excluded populations of the prisons. Consequently, numerous studies have found high STI rates among prison inmates. Moreover, the increasing imprisonment rate of drug users is linked to the spread of HIV and hepatitis B and C. A study conducted among female prisoners in Brazil revealed a high prevalence of STIs including syphilis in 16% cases, gonorrhoea in 7.6%, chlamydial infection in 11%, HPV infection in 9.3%, trichomoniasis in 30% and bacterial vaginosis in 15% of prison inmates.[46] The fourth Australian National HIV/AIDS Strategy has given priority to prisons as potential environments for the spread of STIs. In a New South Wales prison in Australia, 2% of male and 1% of female inmates had confirmed evidence of syphilis.[47] An outbreak of syphilis was reported in Alabama prisons in 1999 as a result of mixing of prisoners with unscreened jail populations, transfer of infected inmates between prisons and multiple concurrent sexual partnerships.[48] A high risk of urethritis (20.8%) was reported amongst prisoners in Sindh, Pakistan, due to a high prevalence of homosexuality and multiple sex partners.[49] An epidemiological study conducted among prison inmates in a district jail around Delhi showed that 4.6% of inmates had primary syphilis, 33.33% were positive for HbsAg, 5% were reactive for HCV infection and 1.3% were Western blot confirmed HIV-1 positive cases.[50] Moreover, 28.8 percent of the inmates were homo/bisexuals, 54.2% had multiple sexual partners, 83% had contact with CSWs and 80.6% indulged in unprotected sex. Sixty-eight percent of inmates were alcoholics, 24% consumed smack while 4.8% were IV drug abusers.

ADDICTIONS

Populations of drug abusers have been associated with epidemics of STIs especially HIV infection.

Crack Cocaine Users

The drug most often associated with STIs is smokable freebase (crack) cocaine. Ethnographic research suggests that crack addiction forces young women to sell sex directly for money to buy crack. Also, sex workers under the influence of the drug may be less careful when choosing sexual practices or partners. Epidemiological data indicate that 'crack for sex' exchange differs from other types of prostitution because of the high proportion of adolescent population involved in drug abuse, and oral sex is the predominant type of sexual activity and crack users often indulge in unprotected sex.[51] In a study of female drug abusers, use of crack was the most significant predictor of syphilis, and more than one-third of the subjects had an STI.[52] In a 1997 survey in Houston, USA, a high prevalence of STI markers was associated with crack smoking - 13% positivity for syphilis, 61% for HSV-2, 11% for HIV, 53% for hepatitis B and 42% for hepatitis C infection.[53] Statistics from Atlanta revealed 25% seropositivity for HIV infection, 37.5% for syphilis and 66.8% for HSV-2 infection among crack-smoking sex workers.[54] Interestingly, a study from Bahamas showed an outbreak of lymphogranuloma venereum (LGV) associated with the epidemic of crack use.[55]

Intravenous Drug Abuse

Epidemiological studies of intravenous drug abusers have shown a high frequency of blood-borne STIs including HIV, HBV, HCV infection and syphilis. In Bangladesh, syphilis, HBV and HIV rates were found to be 23%, 66.5% and 1.4% respectively among IV drug abusers.[56] In Manipur, in the year 2000, the prevalence of HIV among IV drug abusers was 80% and vaginal discharge was strongly associated with HIV positivity.[57] A study of sexual behaviours among drug abusers in Delhi showed greater number of sex partners, higher rate of anal intercourse (25.7%), greater frequency of visits to CSWs and hence a significantly higher prevalence of STIs in this group.[58]

Alcoholism and Smoking

Smoking has been shown to be strongly associated with the persistence of oncogenic HPV cervical infection. Moreover, adolescent females with alcohol use disorder in the United States appeared to be at a substantially high risk of HSV-2 infection, with seroprevalence of 19% as compared to 10% in those without this disorder.[59]

HIGH-RISK SEX PRACTICES

Certain sex practices are associated with a higher risk of acquiring STIs. For a specific sex practice, the number and type of partners and the setting in which the practice occurs significantly affects the actual risk associated with that practice. High-risk sex practices include a) receptive anogenital intercourse, which increases the risk of STIs such as anorectal gonorrhoea, condyloma acuminata, herpes simplex infection, LGV, chancroid etc., b) oro-anal intercourse, which may lead to oral gonorrhoea, syphilis, chancroid, warts or amoebiasis, c) insertive anogenital intercourse, which may cause gonococcal or non-gonococcal urethritis, herpes genitalis, condyloma acuminata, LGV or donovanosis, d) receptive manual-anal intercourse and e) rectal douching in association with receptive anogenital intercourse. The higher risk of STIs in these groups is also related to the fact that these individuals also engage in other high-risk activities. In San Francisco, both homosexual and bisexual men reporting a high prevalence of HSV-2 antibody were associated with increased use of alcohol, ecstasy and heroin and unprotected anal intercourse.[60] A resurgence in syphilis was reported from Washington (from 6 cases reported in 1995 to 46 cases in 1999) among men who have sex with men (MSM).[61] A similar outbreak of syphilis in this population was reported in South California, where the number of cases increased from 26% in 1999 to 51% in 2000.[62] Homosexual men are at increased risk of infection with HPV, as manifested by anal warts and anal carcinoma. In 1987, in the United States, the incidence of anal carcinoma among homosexual men was estimated to be 35/100,000. In HIV seropositive men especially those with CD4 counts < 500/ml, there is an increased risk of high-grade anal squamous intraepithelial lesions.[63] In San Francisco, in 1994, anal HPV DNA was detected in 93% of HIV-positive and 61% of HIV-negative homosexual and bisexual men, with infection due to multiple HPV types in 73% of HIV-positive and 23% of HIV-negative men.[64] In Amsterdam, the Netherlands, a considerable increase in the incidence of rectal gonorrhoea (from 4% in 1994 to 5.4% in 1999) and syphilis (from 0.5% to 0.8%) was reported in MSM after the introduction of HAART, possibly because of an increase in unprotected anal intercourse due to treatment optimism.[65] In India, STI prevalence among the homosexuals has been shown to vary from 2.2% to 6.16%, confirming that frequent mucosal damage caused by intercourse through the unnatural route poses a high risk for STI transmission in this group.[19,39]

In women having sex with women (WSW), in Australia, a significantly high incidence of bacterial vaginosis, hepatitis C and HIV was reported as compared to the control group.[66] This group showed a higher frequency of IV drug abuse and previous contact with homo/bisexual men. This study corroborated with another report from England in which a higher incidence of bacterial vaginosis, cervical HPV infection and trichomoniasis in WSW as compared to heterosexual women was observed.[67] The possibility of sexual transmission via exchange of vaginal secretions or orogenital contact was suggested. The higher incidence of genital warts in this group may be explained by the fact that the infection can also be transmitted through non-penetrative intercourse between women. The transmission of *Trichomonas vaginalis* via fomites or inoculation with infected vaginal secretions may have been responsible for a high incidence in this group. WSW have been reported to have a high incidence of HPV infection. A very high incidence of HPV infection and cervical dysplasia has been reported from USA and UK.[67-69] Sexual practices between female partners that could account for a high rate of HPV transmission include digital-vaginal sex, oral sex and use of insertive sex toys. A recent study demonstrated genital HPV on the fingertips of subjects, substantiating the hypothesis that HPV could be introduced intravaginally with digital vaginal contact between female partners.[70]

The population groups engaged in high-risk sex practices should be identified and given specialized attention including individualized risk-reduction counselling, assistance with partner notification and follow-up on treatment referrals.

OTHER SEX PRACTICES

There are also less well-characterized health behaviours and sexual practices that may influence the risk of acquiring or transmitting STIs. These include dry sex, sex during menses and vaginal douching.

'Dry sex', or the practice of removing vaginal secretions with astringent preparations before engaging in vaginal intercourse, has been documented in many sub-Saharan African countries. The most commonly stated reason for engaging in such acts is pleasure for the male partner because of the drying effect. This practice has been followed by 86% of women in Zambia, 93% women in Zimbabwe and 13% in Malawi.[71,72] The risk of STI acquisition is higher due to abrasions and ulcers that result from such practice.

Sex during menses has been linked with increased risk among women of acquiring gonorrhoea, trichomoniasis and HIV.[73] This practice has been often found in educated White women. According to a National Survey of Women in the United States, 26% of the female population indulge in this practice.[74]

Vaginal douching, a method used to remove vaginal secretions as a preliminary to dry sex or sex during menses, has in the recent National Survey of Family Growth in the United States been found to be practiced by 55% of Black and 21% of White women.[75] It is associated with increased risk of pelvic inflammatory disease (PID), cervicitis and endometritis, tubal pregnancy and infertility due to alteration of the vaginal microflora. In Kenya, regular douching was reported by 72% of women, and it was found to be significantly associated with bacterial vaginosis.[76]

HEALTH CARE BEHAVIOURS

Contraception

The transmission and sequelae of STIs is markedly influenced by the pattern of contraception. There has been a recent resurgence of interest in the pattern of contraceptive use as a result of the rising incidence of STIs and HIV infection.

Condoms

Condoms offer strong protection against organisms like *Chlamydia trachomatis* and *Neisseria gonorrheae* and partial protection against those such as herpes simplex and human papilloma viruses which commonly infect the stratified squamous epithelium. In developed countries, rates of condom use range from 3% to 50%.[77] In developing countries, condom use has been reported by less than 1% of couples, the lowest rates being reported from sub-Saharan Africa, which led to a high prevalence of HIV infection in these countries. Several STI clinics in India have reported condom use in less than 2% of attendees.[39] An interesting study undertaken in Ghana, Africa, showed a significant decline in the prevalence of gonorrhoea (from 33 to 11%), genital ulcers (from 21 to 4%), syphilis (from 21 to 2%), trichomoniasis (from 26 to 11%) and HIV infection (from 89 to 32%) between 1992 and 1998 owing mainly to increase in condom use through social marketing programmes.[78]

The use of diaphragm with spermicide offers protection to women against organisms transmitted mainly between columnar or transitional epithelia including *Chlamydia trachomatis* and *Neisseria gonorrheae*.

Oral Contraceptives

Oral contraceptives have been associated with a lower risk of PID and a higher risk of cervical infections with *Chlamydia trachomatis*, HPV, *Neisseria gonorrheae* and candidal vulvovaginitis.[77] High-estrogen-containing oral contraceptives have shown a strong correlation with the risk of hepatitis B and HPV-induced cervical cancers.[79]

Intrauterine Devices

There is a strong correlation between use of intrauterine devices (IUDs) and PID. Two reports from the 'Women's Health Study' in the United States showed that the use of IUDs increased the risk of PID by 60%.[80] Similarly, 'The Oxford Family Planning Association Contraceptive Study' attributed the risk by a factor of 10.[81] However, recent WHO reports have shown the risk of PID in IUD users to be less than 2 episodes per 1000 years of use, which is consistent with the risk in general population.[82] A meta-analysis of 36 studies has suggested that the risk of PID is related only to the process of inserting the device, and that after the first month of use, it is not significantly higher than non-IUD users. In a study from Mumbai, India, the prevalence of genital chlamydial infection among Cu-T users (14%) was found to be significantly lower than that of non-users (20%) with no greater risk of developing PID.[83]

Circumcision

This practice is strongly connected with specific religions, ethnicity, culture and socio-economic status. Circumcision has been implicated as a major defense against STIs including syphilis, chancroid, genital herpes, gonorrhoea, genital warts, candidal and non-specific balanitis and HIV infection.[84] The hypothesis is that the non-keratinized recesses of the preputial sac are predisposable to physical trauma and microbial invasion. The preputial sac serves as a reservoir of STD pathogens acquired during intercourse from where the entire genitalia may get involved.

STIs IN SPECIAL AGE GROUPS

Individuals of age between 15 and 45 years fall into the sexually active age group, and STIs are commonly associated with this group. However, other age groups have also been found to be at a high risk for STIs.

Adolescents and Teenagers

Adolescence, which corresponds to the age group of 10 to 15 years, and teenage (13 to 19 years) is a stage of psychosocial development when individuals are intensely aware of their physical changes and are emotionally vulnerable. Their psychosocial maturity does not usually correspond with their physical maturity. This group is at a high risk of STIs, and a number of behavioural, social and biological factors have been implicated. In the United States, an estimated 15.3 million new STI cases occur each year, one-quarter of them being teenagers.[85] The higher incidence in this group has been related to greater number of sex partners, inconsistent and incorrect use of barrier contraceptives, sex with older partners and excessive use of alcohol and drugs. Moreover, this group shows excessive neglect towards genital hygiene. Individuals in this age group who suspect an STI are frightened or embarrassed to seek prompt medical attention, thus acting as reservoirs of infection. A high frequency of asymptomatic carrier state and the adolescent practice of partial treatment with self-prescribed antibiotics are other risk factors. The biological developments occurring in the genitalia of this age group make them more susceptible to certain STIs such as gonorrhoea, chlamydial infection and trichomoniasis.

A study conducted in Atlanta, USA, to assess the prevalence of STIs in the homeless adolescent population revealed a higher incidence among females (16.7%) than males (9.8%), the prevalence of *C. trachomatis* infection being 10.5%, 18.2% for HSV-2, 3.6% for HBV, 5% for HCV and 0.3% for HIV infection.[86] The HPV infection rates in sexually active adolescent and teenage girls in the United States have been reported to range from 19% to 30%.[87] In a study from Agra, India, in 1987, syphilis among teenagers was observed in 44% of cases, chancroid in 18%, genital warts in 14%, gonorrhoea in 10%, herpes simplex infection in 8% and LGV, donovanosis and non-specific urethritis in 2% cases each.[88]

Elderly

Elderly individuals have traditionally not been considered at risk for acquiring STIs. However, several factors may put them at risk. Older persons are not necessarily monogamous, and they use condoms infrequently as they link it with contraception only. Safe sex practices are less well-developed in this population. The aging process is also accompanied by increased susceptibility to STIs. In older women, the increased friability of the vaginal mucosa can result in tears and microabrasions during sexual intercourse, thus facilitating disease transmission. The newly available oral medications (Sildenafil citrate) for erectile dysfunction has also precipitated a rise in the incidence of STIs. The Washington State STDs surveillance data of 1992-1998 reported a prevalence rate of 1.3% in the elderly population.[89] The STIs included chlamydial infection (0.4%), gonorrhoea (1.4%), herpes genitalis (3.5%), syphilis (4.1%) and NGU (3.1%). In a retrospective study from Singapore in 1996, 43 cases (41 males and 2 females) of HIV infection in the population aged 50 years and above at first presentation were observed.[90] The proportion of older individuals among HIV-seropositive patients significantly increased from 4.8% in 1991 to 16.7% by mid-1996. They were mainly heterosexuals (93%); majority (79.1%) were previously or currently married and had multiple sexual exposures to CSWs (83.7%). More than half (58%) of the patients had acquired immunodeficiency virus (AIDS) at the time of first presentation with a low median CD4 count of 17 cells/mm^3.

DEMOGRAPHIC AND SOCIAL CORRELATES OF STIs

Demographic and social factors including age group, gender, educational and socio-economic status also determine the epidemiological profile of STIs in different regions.

Age

The highest proportion of STI clinic attendees is composed of population in the age group of 20-30 years. Being adventurous and immature with considerable inquisitiveness for sex and lack of healthy recreation, individuals in this age group may indulge in high-risk sexual practices. In various STI clinics in India, majority of the attendees (42 to 78.6%) were found to belong to this age group.[19-25,91-103] In other Asian and African countries also, the highest incidence of STIs has been reported in the 20 to 30 years age group.[3]

Gender

Several surveys conducted in developing countries including India have shown a significantly high male-to-female sex ratio among STI clinic attendees (ranging from 1.3:1 to 11:1).[3,19-25,91-103]

This difference in presentation may probably be due to the asymptomatic nature of infections in the female sex, lesser degree of freedom to women to go outdoors, lower awareness amongst women of the need for availing medical facilities or their frequent consultation in gynecological clinics instead of STI clinics.

Educational and Socio-economic Status

The correlation between the incidence of STIs and socio-economic indicators is epidemiologically very useful, since it helps in predicting the nature of practices which lead to its transmission, informs policy makers about its effects on the society and helps in the efforts of intervention. In India, illiterates and those with primary level of education and lower income levels form a major proportion of STI clinic attendees.[19-25,91-103] This may be due to lack of general awareness about safe sex practices, paucity of healthy recreation facilities and high-risk sexual behaviour in this group. Contrastingly, in sub-Saharan Africa, the higher prevalence rates among the richer class have been observed, in view of the relatively greater access of the rich to sex tourism and higher rates of sex partner change among high-income adults.[104]

Ethnicity

A strong correlation between ethnicity and STI risk has been observed. Several population-based cross-sectional studies in the United States have demonstrated increased rates of gonorrhoea, chlamydial infection and genital herpes in African-American populations.[105] In the United Kingdom, gonorrhoea and chlamydial infection rates are substantially higher among Black residents.[106,107] Remote aboriginal communities in northern and central Australia experience high rates of gonorrhoea, chlamydial infection and syphilis. Higher prevalence rates of HPV infection have been reported among African-American women than in Whites or Hispanics.[108] Donovanosis is endemic in the South Indian Dravidian population.[109] Thirty percent of the tribals of Gadchiroli district in Maharashtra in 1998 were found to be engaged in sex trade, with VDRL positivity recorded in 8% of individuals during this period.[110]

These ethnic variations may be explained by differences in educational and socio-economic status, housing, recreational facilities, rates of drug abuse, geographical variations, genetic predisposition towards greater susceptibility to acquisition and persistence of infections, endogenous hormonal factors or differences in sexual behaviours among the ethnic groups.

MODES OF TRANSMISSION OF STIs (Tables 1.4 and 1.5)

A common biological feature of many micro-organisms that cause STIs is their unique and often exclusive adaptation to humans, the main mode of transmission being genital-mucosal contact, i.e. sexual intercourse. However, there is enough evidence to support non-venereal transmission of these infections via perinatal transmission, parenteral transmission or by fomites, although the relative risk is different for different diseases.

Gonorrhoea

The risk of sexual transmission of gonorrhoea depends on the anatomic site infected or exposed and the frequency of exposures. The risk of acquiring the infection from male-to-female is 50% to 90% as against 20% from female-to-male, because of the retention of infected ejaculate within the vagina.[111] The acquisition of rectal gonorrhoea by insertive or receptive anal intercourse or pharyngeal gonorrhoea by fellatio or cunnilingus is also well documented.[112] The possibility of sexual transmission in lesbians through exchange of vaginal secretions has also been suggested.[67] Genital infection via contaminated fingers has also been observed.[113]

Non-venereal transmission of gonorrhoea is rare. The organism can survive for upto 24 hours on clothings although periodically rinsed with warm, physiological saline.[113] Since gonococci have been recovered from a variety of hard and soft materials such as utensils for up to 3 days after contamination, infection through contaminated food or utensils is theoretically possible. There are interesting reports of spread of pharyngeal gonorrhoea between two sisters[114] via sweets passed by mouth in the absence of direct oral contact. Similar transmission from an inflatable doll has also been reported.[115] Moreover, the spread of infection in children by sharing of beds, towels and flannels with infected parents has also been documented, but is rare.[113] There are occasional reports of outbreaks of gonococcal infection in the children wards by sharing of inadequately sterilized thermometers or toilet articles.[113] Perinatal transmission to neonates causing pharyngeal gonorrhoea or urethritis is also documented.

Chlamydia Infection

Chlamydia trachomatis is transmitted sexually, although its transmissibility is less common than *Neisseria gonorrhoeae*, since male partners with dual infection are found to be more often affected with gonorrhoea than chlamydial infection.[116] Initial studies using less specific diagnostic techniques showed higher infection rates among female partners of infected males than among male partners of infected women, attributing this to more efficient male-to-female transmission. However, using PCR studies, the frequency of transmission has been found to be equal.[117] Chlamydial proctitis occurs in homosexual men who practice receptive anal intercourse.[118] Pharyngeal infection via orogenital contact has also been documented.[119] The possibility of sexual transmission in lesbians through exchange of vaginal secretions has also been suggested.[67] Perinatal transmission in neonates is reported in 5% of cases.[120] Chlamydial infection of the pharynx, conjunctiva and middle ear in neonates during perinatal transmission is well documented.

Table 1.4 **Infections Transmitted Predominantly by Sexual Intercourse**

Bacteriae	*Viruses*	*Others*
Neisseria gonorrhoeae	HIV-1,2	Trichomoniasis
Treponema pallidum	HSV-2	Pthrus pubis
Haemophilus ducreyi	HPV	
Chlamydia trachomatis	HBV	
Calymmatobacterium granulomatis	CMV	
Ureaplasma urealyticum	MCV*	

* Molluscum contagiosum virus

Table 1.5 **Sexually Transmitted Infections in Which Fomites are Implicated**

- Gonorrhoea
- Syphilis - extragenital chancre
- Chancroid - extragenital ulcers
- HSV infection - rare
- HPV infection
- Trichomoniasis
- Molluscum contagiosum infection
- Genital scabies

Syphilis

Syphilis is acquired via sexual exposure to moist mucosal-or cutaneous lesions through micro or macroscopic breaks in the squamous or columnar epithelium. The chance of acquisition from an infected sex partner has been estimated to be up to 60%.[121] The incubation period depends upon the size of the treponemal inoculum.

Extragenital syphilitic chancres have been found on lips, tongue, tonsils, fingers, eyelids or nipples as a result of inoculation with contaminated fingers or fomites.[122]

Transplacental transmission of *Treponema pallidum* into the foetal circulation occurs in congenital syphilis, especially in the first four months of gestation. The risk of transmission is higher when the mother is suffering from early syphilis (primary or secondary) than when she has late syphilis.[123] The risk of infecting the foetus declines gradually during the course of untreated syphilis to become inconspicuous after 8 years of untreated infection.

The transmission of syphilis by blood transfusion, referred to as 'syphilis d'emblee', is well documented. The primary stage is usually absent with this mode of transmission, The risk of transmission is greater by fresh blood components rather than transfusion of refrigerated products, although treponema can survive for up to 120 hours in blood stored at 4°C.[124,125] In India and other parts of the world, the prevalence of HIV infection and syphilis among blood donors is on the rise. A survey undertaken in Vellore, Tamil Nadu, showed that the seroprevalence of syphilis among blood donors fell between 1990 and 1995 and then rose for the next 3 years.[125] In Tanzania, in 1999, syphilis antibodies were detected in 12.7% of blood donors.[126] The HIV-seropositive donors had a high risk for being positive for syphilis antibodies. In Bangladesh, in 2000, a high prevalence of syphilis (23%) was found among IV drug users.[127]

Chancroid

The disease is highly contagious, with the likelihood of male-to-female spread of 63% during a single act of unprotected exposure.[128] However, studies have shown that the risk of acquiring the disease from an infected partner with visible lesions is significantly higher than that without them. In women, the ulcers may often be subclinical.[129] In such situations, they act as reservoirs of infection, thus transmitting the disease to their sexually promiscuous clients or spouses. However, in men, the urethra has not been shown to be a reservoir of infections. Extragenital chancroidal ulcers on the hands or breasts are also documented.[130,131]

Herpes Simplex Infection

The transmission occurs between individuals who shed the virus at a peripheral site, mucosal surface or secretion.[132] Infection occurs via inoculation of the virus onto susceptible mucosal surfaces (oropharynx, cervix, conjunctiva) through microabrasions. The transmission is more frequent in women from men than in men from women. In one study, the risk of acquisition of HSV-2 infection was found to be 32% in HSV seronegative women, while it was 6% in seronegative men.[133] The higher rate of asymptomatic infection in men may be responsible for the greater male-to-female transmission. Since HSV is readily inactivated at room temperature and by drying, transmission via aerosols or fomites is unusual.[134] However, there is some evidence that non-venereal transmission of HSV-2 occurs in humid environment, particularly when children sleep with infected parents or share towel or clothing.[134] Neonatal herpes by perinatal transmission is well documented. However, there are no reports to show transplacental spread of infection.

Donovanosis

The disease is mildly contagious, and multiple and repeated sexual exposures are required for its transmission. Anal intercourse leads to rectal lesions in homosexuals and penile lesions in their partners.[135] The infection can spread from the genitalia by direct contact with the adjoining areas of the thigh, lower abdomen, scrotum or buttocks. Non-venereal transmission to children can occur when they sit on the laps of infected adult patients.[136]

Lymphogranuloma Venereum

Sexual transmission is common, but LGV is not as contagious as gonorrhoea. Perinatal transmission is documented, although transplacental transmission does not occur.[137]

Human Papilloma Virus Infection

Penile or vulvar warts occurring as a result of heterosexual transmission can spread to contiguous sites including the anal canal. Approximately 8% of men and 20% of women with genital warts have concomitant anal warts.[138] Receptive homosexual contact is the commonest cause of anal warts.[139] Sexual transmission amongst lesbians has also been reported, since the transmission of HPV requires mere skin-to-skin contact rather than penetrative intercourse.[68] Sex practices that could account for the infection in WSW include digital-vaginal sex, oral sex and use of insertive sex toys.

A recent study reported the detection of genital HPV on the fingertips of subjects, substantiating the hypothesis that HPV could be introduced intravaginally by digital-vaginal contact.[70] Condyloma acuminata of the lips, tongue or palate can occur by the inoculation of the pathogen by contaminated fingers or by oral sex with an infected partner.[140]

In neonates, perinatal transmission of HPV causing infection to the genitalia or buccal and laryngeal mucosa is frequently reported. The detection rate of HPV DNA in oral swabs of newborn babies varies from 4 to 87%.[141] There is evidence that transmission is possible in-utero, either by hematogenous route, by semen at the time of fertilization or as an ascending infection. HPV can also be transmitted non-venereally via fomites.[142] In children, the commonest cause of genital warts is sexual abuse, which has been documented in 30 to 80% of cases.[143]

Trichomoniasis

Trichomoniasis is most prevalent among sexual partners of patients with documented infection. The organism can be isolated in 70% of men who had sexual contact with infected women within the previous 48 hours, and in only 33% cases if their last contact was 2 weeks previously.[144] The infection could be documented in 85% of female partners of infected men.[145] Asymptomatic men act as reservoirs and are principal vectors of the disease. Symptomatic infection in men, presenting as urethral irritation and a thin milky-white urethral discharge, is responsible for the higher risk of transmission. In Zimbabwe, in 1983-1984, 99.4% of men with trichomonal urethritis were symptomatic and were more responsible than asymptomatic men[146] for significantly greater transmission of the infection to their sexual partners. The detection of the infection in prepubertal children indicates sexual abuse.[147]

Perinatal transmission in 5% of female babies has been reported.[148] Non-venereal transmission from contaminated lavatory seats, towels or clothings, douche nozzles, rubber gloves or unsterile instruments is possible.[145]

Hepatitis B Infection

The infection is commonly acquired via blood transfusion, needle stick injuries, body secretions including saliva, vaginal fluids, menstrual blood, semen, sweat, urine and faeces and by homosexual contact. There is a direct correlation between the duration of homosexual activity, number of partners practicing anorectal intercourse and the risk of acquiring the infection.[134] This risk increases with increase in the number of sex partners engaged in anal intercourse and the duration of homosexuality. There is considerable evidence to support transmission by heterosexual contact as well.[149] In one study, HbsAg was detected in 27% of the spouses of HbsAg carriers, and in only 11% of spouses of non-carrier controls. Approximatety 20% of the reported cases of hepatitis B infection in the United States occur by heterosexual contact, and 30% cases from India have been contracted through homo/heterosexual route.[150,151] In a study from Mumbai in 1995, HBV prevalence was found to be 8.8%.[152] A quarter of these individuals were seropositive for syphilis and HIV, confirming the definite role of sexual transmission in the spread of HBV. This was also proved by another study from Pondicherry in 1999, in which HbsAg positivity was found in 10% of STI clinic attendees, predominantly drivers, bisexuals, patients with infected spouse, sex partners of CSWs and those with concomitent presence of another STI.[38]

Regular blood donors and IV drug abusers are also at high risk of acquiring the infection. In Tanzania, HbsAg and anti-HBs antibody were detected in 22% and 11% of blood donors, respectively.[126] In a recent study from Bangladesh, 12% of IV drug users were positive for HBV infection.[56]

Perinatal transmission in neonates via infected vaginal secretions has also been documented.[153]

EPIDEMIOLOGY OF STIs

In this chapter, we discuss the epidemiological aspects of major STIs (Tables 1.6 and 1.7). The epidemiology of HIV infection is dealt with in a separate chapter.

Table 1.6 **Pattern of STIs Among STI Clinic Attendees in Major Hospitals in India**

S.No	Region	Syphilis	Chancroid	LGV	Donovanosis	HSV	HPV	Gonorrhoea	NGU
1	Chandigarh[99] 1977-1985	10.4	12.2	0.6	6.3	11.4	21.4	16.9	4.1
2	Chandigarh[98] 1985-1992	8.7	8.1	0.9	1.6	19.7	25.2	5.3	4.1
3	Chandigarh[91] 1995-1996	2	3	6	0.5	21	7	3	6
4.	Delhi[100] 1955-61	7.3	22.5	0.6	0.25	–	–	15.9	4.9
5.	Delhi[25] 1965-1978	54.9	5.9	0.9	1.2	2.5	2	1.9	–
6.	Delhi[101] 1989-1995	14.3	23.9	1.6	1.4	11.8	9.2	12.2	3.7
7.	Delhi[19] 1995-1999	15.6	11	0.45	0.48	11.8	9.3	11.6	7.4
8.	Patiala[95] 1983-1988	29.6	8.8	0.2	0.2	11.6	12	10	5.2
9.	Patiala[94] 1990-1998	17.2	1.6	0.15	0.28	9.4	5.1	4.2	10.8
10.	Rohtak[97] 1992-1994	30.2	22.1	0.97	1.45	10.6	18.1	12.9	4.7

(*Contd.*)

S.No	Region	Syphilis	Chancroid	LGV	Donovanosis	HSV	HPV	Gonorrhoea	NGU
11.	Rohtak[96] 1995-1996	7.4- P 17.5- S	14.5	0.67	0.8	11.1	21.5	12.6	6.7
12.	Rohtak[102] 1995-2000	24	10.9	0.2	0.86	16.9	19.4	16.2	4.8
13.	Ahmedabad[92] 1993-1994	22.2- P 28.7- S	7.6	0.58	2	8.2	7.2	5.05	–
14.	Ahmedabad[22] 1998-1999	28.9	9.6	–	1	27.9	9.1	12.7	1.5
15.	Kolkata[93] 1997	23.9	30.8	5.07	0.55	11.3	–	15.3	12.4
16.	Kurnool[24] 1992-1996	14.4	2.8	9.7	–	14	11.3	11.7	19.1
17.	Pondicherry[103] 1982-1990	18	10.6	8	8.2	14.1	11.9	11.9	0.8
18.	North East[342] 1980-90	14.6	35				9.17	17.8	3.33
19.	North East[342] 1995-99	9.26	25.7	9.98			19.6	4.72	13.97
20.	Udaipur[343] 1988	32.4	37.7	0.39	1.1			24.7	
21.	Cuttack[344] 1993-94	16.27	11.82	0.58	7.55	21.8	3.87	3.87	
22.	Vadodara[345] 1995-96				0.43	28.8	8.9	8.26	

Table 1.7 **Pattern of STIs Among STI Clinic Attendees in District Hospitals in India**

S.No	Region	Syphilis	Chancroid	LGV	Donovanosis	HSV	HPV	Gonorrhoea	NGU
1	Srinagar[21] 1986-1994	20.8	28.8	9.7	0.2	4.1	11.25	11.7	2.6
2.	Port Blair[23] 1992-1993	25.4	21.1	–	–	7.7	9.2	19	7.04
3.	Port Blair*	12.4	10.7	2.4	–	57.4	4.1	4.1	8.5
4.	Tezpur[20] 1986-1990	14.6	35	10	0.013	5	9.2	17.1	3.3

* Data presented in 26th National Conference of IASSTDs and AIDS at New Delhi, October 19–20, 2002.

Syphilis

Syphilis is caused by the bacterium *Treponema pallidum*. It is a major cause of GUD and an important risk factor in transmission of HIV infection. In developed countries, the prevalence of syphilis has fallen steeply, except for few focal outbreaks, due to improved access to health care, effective control programmes and efficacious treatment. However, in some developing countries, it still remains a major public health problem with an estimated 12 million cases occurring worldwide annually, of which 4 million occur in Africa.[2]

In the United States, syphilis is characteri-zed by spontaneous epidemics rather than persistent endemicity. An estimated 70,000 cases of syphilis occur annually.[85] In 1986-1990, an epidemic of syphilis occurred throughout the country. The incidence of primary and secondary syphilis in 1984-1994 ranged from 0 to 87 per 100,000 population, and in 1990 alone, the rate was 20.3 cases per 100,000 persons.[154,155] The rates began to decline since 1991 to touch 2.5 per 100,000 population in 1999 and 2.2 per 100,000 in 2000.[156-158] **(Fig. 1.1)**. The incidence among the Blacks (12.8 per 100,000) was 21 times greater than in Whites (0.6 per 100,000). Focal outbreaks have occurred from time to time in different cities including Seattle, Atlanta and Guilford County.[159,160] The factors associated with these outbreaks include missed opportunities for syphilis screening and treatment in high-risk settings, substantial rates of co-infection with HIV, sex with multiple partners, exchange of sex for drugs especially crack cocaine, and unprotected sex. Syphilis is re-emerging among MSM. Focal outbreaks during the periods 1997-1998 and 1999-2000, especially in Chicago, New York, Boston, Miami, Seattle and San Francisco, were among this group (comprising 68% of syphilis cases), of which two-thirds were HIV-positive.[159] Higher rates occurred among African-Americans living in poverty in the metropolitan areas in southeastern United States. The city of Baltimore had the highest number of syphilis cases in the country with an incidence of 270 per 100,000 live births for congenital syphilis and 99.3 per 100,000 population for early syphilis, with 96% of cases occurring in the Black population.[161] Since last 5 years, syphilis has been on the rise, especially among MSM.[162] Between 2004 and 2005, the national syphilis rate increased 11.1%, from 2.7 to 3.0 cases per 100,000 population. The rates are 6 times higher in men than in women; there is narrowing of racial gaps in syphilis rates and the rates in women also are on the rise (increase of 12.5% from 2004 to 2005). Syphilis elimination at the national level may be defined as the absence of sustained transmission of the disease within 90 days of the report of an imported case. The national goal of syphilis elimination is to reduce primary and secondary syphilis to < 1000 cases, i.e. 0.4 per 100,000 population.[157]

In England and Wales, after almost two decades of consistent decline, infectious syphilis is again on the rise.[163] Since 1997, when the Bristol outbreak heralded the resurgence of the disease, outbreaks

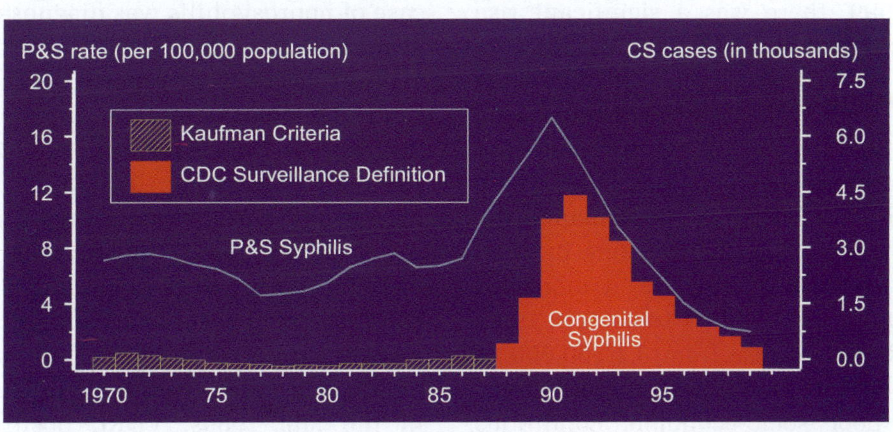

Fig. 1.1 Congenital syphilis (cs)—reported cases for infants <1 year of age and rates of primary (p) and secondary (s) syphilis among women: United States, 1970–1999 (CDC, Atlanta).

have been reported in the north-west, south-east and London, such that, by 2000, nearly two-thirds of the nationally reported cases were diagnosed in these areas. In 1999-2000, the infection rose by 160% in males (from 153 to 248 cases) and 130% in females (from 55 to 73 cases), and in MSM, it rose from 52 to 113 cases. These outbreaks were associated with high rates of partner exchange, travel or migration from endemic areas, predominance of homosexuality and a high proportion of HIV co-infection.

Resurgence of syphilis has also been reported from other European countries. In the STI clinics in Amsterdam, the Netherlands, in 1999, 76 new cases of infectious syphilis were reported, an increase of 111% from 1998, with the largest increase seen among MSM (from 9 cases in 1998 to 40 in 1999).[164] This rise was attributed to unsafe sex practices due to treatment optimism after the introduction of HAART for HIV infection. In Rotterdam, syphilis cases increased dramatically in 1995-1997, with the highest rates reported among CSWs.[165] However, with the introduction of prophylactic treatment, the prevalence rate dopped to 1.3% in 1998. A significant increase in the incidence has been noticed in Czech Republic during the past 10 years.[166] From 1992 to 1998, the number of early syphilis cases doubled, while the number of stillbirths due to syphilis increased three times. In Belgrade, Yugoslavia, early syphilis incidence rates showed a decreasing trend between 1985 and 1992 (2.53/100,000 in 1985 to 0.8/100,000 in 1992) as a result of change in sexual behaviour, in response to the AIDS epidemic.[167] However, from 1993 to 1999, there was a significant rise in the incidence from 1.67/100,000 in 1993 to 3.65/100,000 in 1999. It was highest in men aged 30-39 years and 40-49 years, and in women aged 20-29 years and 30-39 years. An alarming increase in the incidence has been reported in many eastern European countries.[168-170] In Romania, the incidence rose from 7.1/100,000 persons in 1986 to 34.7/100,000 in 1998; in Bulgaria, it increased from 14.4/100,000 in 1994 to 27.3/100,000 in 1996; and in central Russia, it rose from 3.2/100,000 in 1990 to 300/100,000 in 1997. In all these regions, low education, poor socio-economic conditions and migration were the main causes of resurgence of infectious syphilis.

Syphilis is an important cause of morbidity in sub-Saharan Africa. In Tanzania, seroprevalence of syphilis in the 1990s was unacceptably high, with rates ranging from 5.9 to 12.8%.[171] Higher rates were reported in illiterate individuals with early sexual debut and multiple partners, in individuals with self-perceived high risk of STIs and among uncircumcised males. However, in Madagascar, the rates decreased from 56% in 1995 to 29% in 1997 after the introduction of syndromic management of GUD.[172] In Nairobi, Kenya, a marked decline in seroprevalence was observed among pregnant women (7.2% in 1994 to 3.8% in 1997) after the development of a specific syphilis control programme.[173]

In many Asian countries, especially India, syphilis continues to be a major health problem. However, a constant decline in its prevalence has been observed in recent years. In a retrospective analysis of data obtained from STI clinic attendees in a tertiary hospital of Delhi between 1954 and 1994, although the STD cases increased eight times from 1954 to 1984, with prevalence increasing from 5.5% in 1964 to 14.7% in 1994, the syphilis load declined from 61.2% in 1954 to 9.1% in 1994.[174] Males outnumbered females in the ratio of 2.8:1, probably because women report for investigations and treatment much later than their male counterparts due in part to the asymptomatic nature of the disease in the female sex. In this analysis, it was also observed that the prevalence in adult males increased until 1984 in contrast to children under 14 years, in whom it decreased from 12.6% in 1954 to 0.5% in 1994. No case of neurosyphilis was diagnosed during the 40-year study period, while 10 cases of cardiovascular syphilis were last reported in 1954. In other Delhi hospitals also, the incidence was shown to decrease from 54.9% in 1965-78 to 15.56% in 1995-99.[19,25] During 1965-78, two cases each of neuro- and cardiovascular syphilis in the female sex were reported.[25] In Madurai, in 1992, 17.5% men presenting with neurological manifestations and associated past history of multiple sex partners were diagnosed with neurosyphilis, predominantly meningovascular syphilis.[175] In Himachal Pradesh, in the late 1980s, VDRL positivity among the high-risk groups was reported in 9% of cases.[176] A significant decline in syphilis trends has been observed in Chandigarh, with incidence rates reducing from 10.4% in 1977-85 to 2% in 1995-96[98,99]; in Rohtak from 30.2% in 1992-93 to 24% in 1995-2000[96,97,102]; and in Patiala from 29.6% in 1983-88 to 17.2% in 1990-98.[94,95] This reduction may be attributed to regular supply and consistent use of effective drugs. A cross-sectional survey of women in the reproductive age group in an urban slum community in Mumbai in 1995 reported a VDRL seropositivity of 0.5%, while a study from a similar population in Delhi in 1996-2000 showed seropositivity in 4% of cases.[177,178]

Blood donors are a high-risk group for acquiring and transmitting syphilis (Table 1.8). In A.I.I.M.S., New Delhi, between 1989 and 1995, among voluntary and replacement blood donors, VDRL reactivity increased from 0.23 to 0.52%.[179] In other parts of India, sero-prevalence of syphilis in this group has been shown to vary from 0% in Lucknow, 2.8% in Delhi, 3.62% in Tirunelvelli to 7% in Bihar.[180-183]

Table 1.8 **VDRL Positivity Among Blood Donors in India**

A.I.I.M.S., New Delhi[179]	1989	0.23%
	1995	0.52%
Lucknow[180]	1996	0%
Delhi[181]	1987	2.8%
Tirunelvelli[182]	1985	3.62%
Bihar[183]	1993	7%

Congenital syphilis (CS) is the most dreaded consequence of untreated syphilis in pregnant women, and estimated to occur in 25-75% of exposed infants.[104] It has been suggested that approximately 10 to 12% of infants born to mothers with positive syphilis serology would die if untreated, yielding a mortality of 1-3% among the under-fours. In the United States, chronic drug abuse and inadequate prenatal care has been suggested as the main causes of CS. From 1990 to 1993, in the state of Georgia, 438 deliveries were classified as CS, a prevalence of 0.9%.[184] It was 5 times higher in the Black population (9.6 cases per 1000 live births) than among Whites (1.7/1000 live births). The CS rates in the united States have declined significantly between 1997 and 2000, being 27.8 per 100,000 live births in 1997, 14.5 in 1999 and 13.4 in 2000 (Fig. 1.1).[185] In Bolivia, in 1996, 4.3% of live-born and 26% of stillborn infants were found to have syphilis at delivery.[186] In Asian and African countries, including India, only sporadic reports of CS have been published. In Delhi, between 1965 and 1978, 82 cases of CS were reported, with a higher female-to-male ratio (1.73:1).[25] In Kurnool, Andhra Pradesh, 7 cases of CS were observed from 1980 to 1990.[187]

The surveys conducted among antenatal women in Africa have shown VDRL seropositivity in 3.6% of cases in Malawi, 9.3% in Gambia and 14% in Zimbabwe, with an average of 10% in Africa.[188-190] In India, it has ranged from 1.8% in Chandigarh to 2.9% in Aligarh and 3.4% in Delhi (1996).[191-193] The seroprevalence of syphilis among pregnant women attending an antenatal clinic in another tertiary level hospital in Delhi in 1998 was found to be 2.5%, with 10% of cases being HIV-positive.[194] (Table 1.9)

Table 1.9 **VDRL Positivity Among Antenatal Women**

	Africa	
Malawi[188]	1993	3.6%
Gambia[189]	1992	9.3%
Zimbabwe[188]	1993	14%
	India	
Chandigarh[189]	1986	1.8%
Aligarh[190]	1987	2.9%
Delhi[193]	1996	3.4%
Delhi[194]	1998	2.53%

Chancroid

Chancroid is a bacterial GUD caused by *Haemophilus ducreyi*, and predominantly transmitted through heterosexual contact. The epidemiological data for chancroid may be inaccurate in view of the difficulty in diagnosing the condition on clinical grounds alone. Recently, chancroid received greater attention because of the strong association with HIV transmission. In industrialized countries, it is an uncommon cause of GUD. In the United States, 9515 cases were reported in 1947, which steadily declined to fewer than 1000 cases in the late 1970s, when the number of cases reported annually was 646.[195] However, chancroid oubreaks occurred in 1980s. Between 1981 and 1983, 15% of GUD cases in California were caused by chancroid. Between 1986 and 1988, in the New York city, the number of reported cases increased from 556 to 1140, and in 1987, 4986 cases were reported to the Center for Disease Control (CDC) from USA. Subsequently, from 1993 to 1999, the annual number of cases has constantly declined from 1399 in 1993 to approximately 250 cases in 1999 (Fig. 1.2). However, in 1997, in New York, chancroid was the third major cause of GUD, observed in 33% of patients.[196] Two outbreaks of chancroid were identified from the inner cities in USA, one in New Orleans (1990-1992), where *H. ducreyi* was isolated by culture in 39% of GUD patients and the other in Jackson, Mississippi (1994-1995), where it was identified from another 39% of GUD cases by polymerase chain reaction.[197,198] The disease was most prevalent among the urban African-Americans and Hispanics with a high male-to-female ratio. It was significantly associated with alcohol (44%) and cocaine abuse (25%), sex with prostitutes (17%), multiple sex partners, trading drugs for sex (16%) and infrequent use of condoms. Besides, the behavioural factors, and improvement in diagnostic techniques for isolation and detection of *H. ducreyi* may have been responsible for the higher incidence. In Paris, France, 673 cases were diagnosed between 1973 and 1979.[199] It is a rare disease in Australia and the Scandinavian countries, mainly seen in travelers returning from South-East Asia or in the aboriginal population.[104]

Chancroid is the leading cause of GUDs in developing countries, particularly in sub-Saharan Africa and South-East Asia. In African countries, the prevalence varies from 9.8% to 68%.[200] The risk factors include early age at first coitus, first coitus before menarche, longer duration of marriage (>20 years), greater number of lifetime sex partners, serological evidence of exposure to another STI and lower socio-economic status, and is highest among divorcees and CSWs. In India, the incidence rates range from 1.6% in Patiala to as high as 51.9% in Mumbai.[94,201] On comparing the rates from the same region during different periods, a significant decrease in the incidence may be observed. This may be due to the availability of newer antibiotics, their indiscriminate use at the primary care due to free availability, prophylactic use before or after sexual exposure, greater awareness regarding early diagnosis and treatment among the masses, and the immense success of the syndromic approach and condom promotion campaigns.

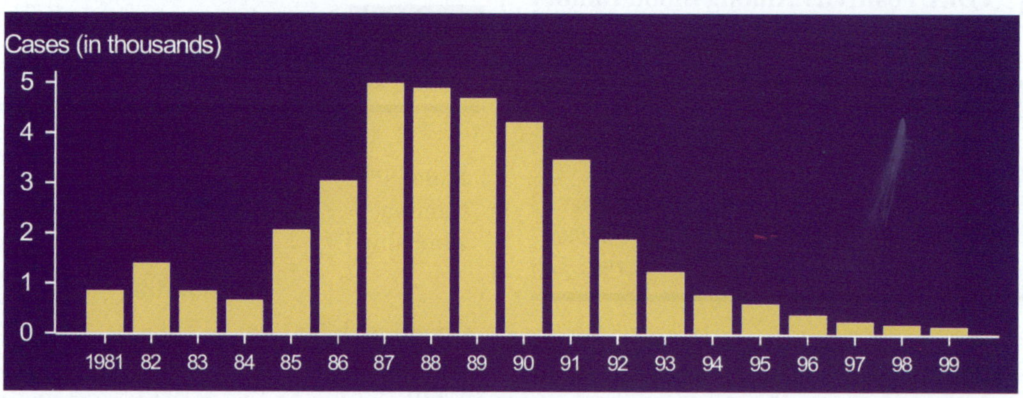

Fig. 1.2 Chancroid—Reported cases: United States, 1981–1999. (CDC, Atlanta)

Donovanosis

Donovanosis is a chronic, mildly contagious STI characterized by granulomatous ulceration of the genitalia and neighbouring sites caused by *Calymmatobacterium granulomatis*. It has been unknown as a cause of GUD for many years due to the non-availability of specific diagnostic facilities. However, during the past decade, there has been renewed interest in the disease, owing to the emergence of HIV infection and consequent increase in the number of donovanosis cases. Although donovanosis has a world-wide distribution, it is endemic in tropical and sub-tropical countries, especially in India, Papua New Guinea, aborigines of Australia, South Africa and Brazil. Racial and ethnic predispositions have been associated with the disease since it is more common among the local natives than the Europeans staying in Papua New Guinea, in Negroes than the poor Whites in the United States, in Dravidians in South India and in Pahari dwellers of Himachal Pradesh.[109] In Durban, South Africa, following the introduction of a rapid test (PCR) for its diagnosis, the number of reported cases has increased substantially from 312 in 1988 to 2385 in 1995, 2733 in 1996 and 3153 in 1997.[202] Sixty-one women, predominantly pregnant individuals (88.5%), were diagnosed with this condition between 1990 and 1993.[203] In a Brazilian city, between 1954 and 1990, 259 cases of donovanosis were reported, of which only 56 cases occurred between 1954 and 1974, while 133 cases were reported in the last five years.[204] Greater sexual liberty, poor socio-economic conditions and increasing homosexual behaviour were implicated for this augmented disease incidence. In Papua New Guinea, although the disease has been endemic for the past 80 years with a prevalence of 54.4%, the incidence has recently increased, particularly in the urban areas, and is associated with low socio-economic status and poor personal hygiene.[205]

The disease is very common in some parts of India, especially in Tamil Nadu, Pondicherry, Andhra Pradesh, Orissa and Himachal Pradesh. It has an uneven geographical distribution, with incidence varying from 0.013% in Tezpur[21] to 8.2% in Pondicherry[103] and 10% in Mumbai among STI clinic attendees.[206] It has been speculated that specific climatic factors such as moderate relative humidity and persistent high temperature have influenced the geographical distribution of the disease. A strong association with HLAB57 has also been observed.[207] Two epidemics of donovanosis occurred in Delhi in 1983, when the reported incidence was 6.38%, and another in 1985, when the incidence was 8.33%.[208] The disease mainly affected young unmarried men during extramarital heterosexual intercourse with prostitutes, illiterates and low socio-economic groups. In Chandigarh, the incidence declined significantly from 6.3% in 1977-85[99] to 0.5% in 1995-96.[91] This may be due to the availability of broad-spectrum antibiotics and the changing sexual behaviours in the era of HIV infection. However, in Delhi, the incidence increased from 0.25% in 1955-61[100] to 1.4% in 1989-95[102] and then declined to 0.48% in 1995-99.[19] The increase in incidence in Delhi may be attributed to large-scale immigration of high-risk individuals from endemic areas.

Lymphogranuloma Venereum

LGV is a less commonly encountered STD in industrialized countries, with only sporadic cases reported from North America, Europe and Australia, especially in immigrants and travelers returning from endemic areas.[209] The rate of reported disease has been declining since 1972 in the United States, with only 113 cases recorded in 1997.[210] In the United Kingdom, only 91 cases of chancroid, granuloma inguinale and LGV were reported in 1995 from genitourinary clinics.[211] Since 2003, LGV has emerged as a significant problem among MSM in Europe.[212] In 2003, an outbreak occurred in Rotterdam, the Netherlands, with over 100 cases, most of whom were HIV-positive and many had concomitant STIs including hepatitis C infection. Unprotected anal sex, fisting and sharing of sex toys appeared as possible routes of transmission. In 2005, by mid-February, 34 cases of LGV were detected in the United Kingdom.

LGV is endemic in several tropical and sub-tropical countries including West, Central and East Africa, India, Malaysia, Korea, Vietnam, South America, Papua New Guinea and the Caribbean Islands.[213-218] The proportion of genital ulcers that can be attributed to LGV in these areas varies from 1 to 10%.

In India, the incidence ranges between 0.15 and 9.74% in different parts of the country.[19-25,91-103] Perhaps the lack of specific diagnostic criteria in these studies and the relatively poor degree of clinical suspicion of the condition may have biased these estimates.

In two cross-sectional surveys undertaken in Jamaica in 1982-83 and 1990-91, the disease prevalence of 4.1% and 3.9%, respectively, was reported, and in 1996, the incidence decreased to 2.63%.[219] In Madagascar, in 1997, 8% of genital ulcer patients were clinically diagnosed as LGV, with only 0.5% accounting for confirmed cases by micro-IF test.[220] In Hong Kong, the disease accounted for only 0.001% of all the new STD cases in 1995.[221] An incidence of 1% was recorded in Singapore in 1995.[222] In Nairobi, Kenya, 0.6% of genital ulcer cases were attributed to LGV in 1996.[213] A prospective study of inguinal buboes conducted on Thai men between 1987 and 1989 revealed LGV-*C. trachomatis* by immunofluorescent microscopy in 3.9% of cases.[217]

LGV is diagnosed six times more frequently in men than in women, because of the asymptomatic nature of early lesions in females.[223] However, late complications such as ulceration, rectal strictures or esthiomene are more frequently reported in women.[224]

The disease has a peak incidence during the second and third decade of life with peak sexual activity. It is more common in urban population, among the sexually promiscuous and lower socio-economic classes.[225] CSWs play a major role in disease transmission, as documented during an outbreak in Florida in late 1980s.[226]

Gonorrhoea

Gonorrhoea is a well-recognized public health problem. It is still one of the commonest bacterial STDs in the world. Approximately 62 million new *Neisseria gonorrhoeae* cases occur annually worldwide, making it a major public health problem.[227] The importance of this disease is not only limited to its high incidence and acute manifestations but also to the complications and disturbing sequelae it causes besides constituting an important risk factor for the transmission of HIV infection.

In developed countries, there has been a constant decline in the incidence of gonorrhoea. In Europe, a peak incidence of gonorrhoea occurred during World Wars I and II and of late during 1960s and early 1970s following the liberation in sexual values.[228] Thereafter, there has been a sharp decline especially in north European countries such as Sweden, England, Denmark and Germany. In Sweden, the incidence decreased from 487 per 100,000 in 1970 to 3 per 100,000 in 1995. It reached an all-time low of 2.4 cases per 100,000 in 1996; however, the incidence has been increasing since 1997.[229] Heterosexual teenagers and homosexual men were identified as core groups infected by different serovars of *N. gonorrhoeae*. In England, it declined from 210 per 100,000 population in 1970 to approximately 34.1 per 100,000 in 1995. In the United States, the peak incidence occurred around 1975 with approximately 473 per 100,000. This was followed by a plateau till 1982, a decrease until 1984 and a slight increase till 1986. Thereafter, the incidence has been declining steadily. It was approximately 149.5 per 100,000 in 1995 and 133.2 per 100,000 in 1999.[230-232] This decline may be related largely to behavioural changes in response to the AIDS ally and treatment of asymptomatic infected persons and their sex partners to interrupt disease transmission. With a 74% decline in the rate of reported gonorrhoea from 1975 through 1997, the overall gonorrhoea rates have plateaued in the recent years. In 2004, the gonorrhoea rate was 112.4 cases per 100,000 population, while in 2005 it was 115.6 (Fig. 1.3). Between 1999 and 2002, in the age group of 14-39 years, 0.24% cases had gonorrhoea while 2.2% had chlamydia infection.[233] Adolescents had the highest disease burden. Almost half the people with gonorrhoea infection also had chlamydia infection. The characteristics associated with higher infection rates were younger age, previous infection with gonorrhoea or chlamydia, and non-Hispanic Black race or ethnicity. Healthy People 2010 in USA set a target of 19 per 100,000 cases. The incidence of gonorrhoea in the United States has been seasonal, with the highest rates observed in late summer and the lowest in late winters and early spring.[234] In Canada also, a similar trend in epidemiology has been observed. The incidence of gonorrhoea

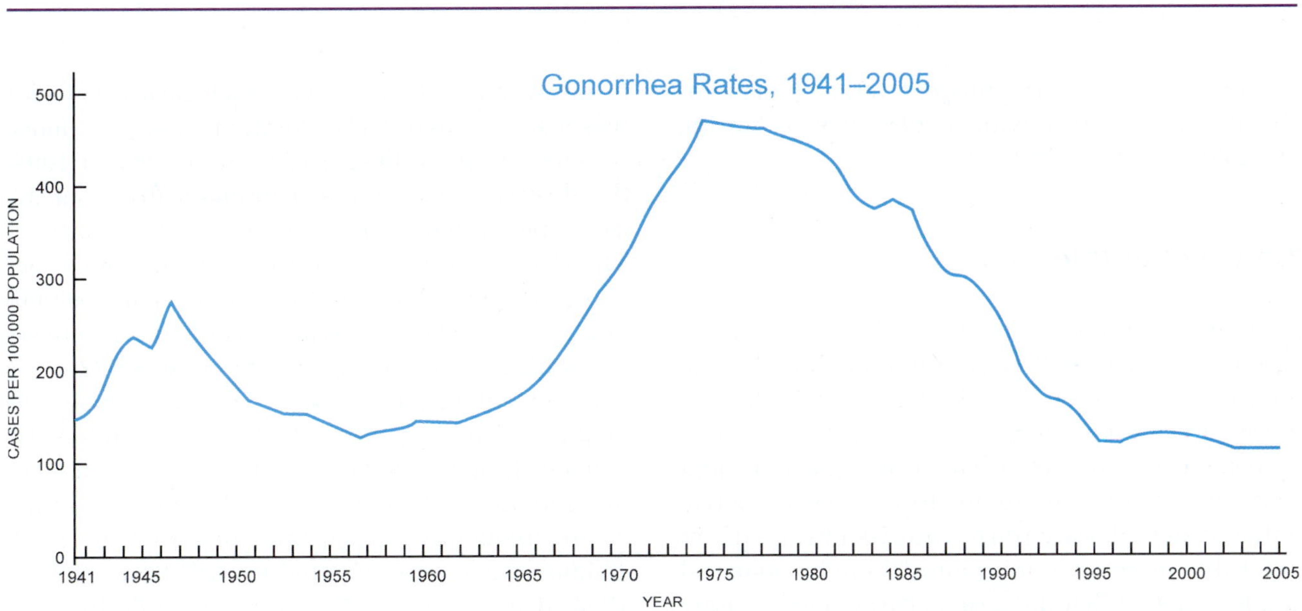

Fig. 1.3 Gonorrhea - Reported Rates: United States, 1941-2005 (CDC, Atlanta).

declined from 223 per 100,000 in 1980 to 18.6 per 100,000 in 1995.[227]

In developed countries, a declining trend has been observed among heterosexual men and all women. However, it has been on the increase in homosexual men. In 1996, in England, the incidence was much higher in homosexual men (812 per 100,000 population) as compared to heterosexual men (27 per 100,000 population).[235] In 1999, in USA, 13.1% of the participants in the Gonococcal Isolate Surveillance Project (GISP) were homosexuals as compared to 4% homosexuals in 1988.[231] In Stockholm, a sharp increase was seen among MSM in 2000s, and the proportion of pharyngeal infections increased significantly (P <0.001) from 15% to 38% during the last 7 years.[236] The male-to-female ratio of the disease is also decreasing steadily. In England and USA, the male-to-female ratio has fallen from 3:1 in 1965 to 1.5:1 in 1990s, with fewer than 1% infected men citing prostitutes as the source of infection. From 1985 to 1995 and 1999, the peak incidence in men was observed in the 20-24 years age group. However, a shift in the age structure was obsarved in women from 20-24 years age group in 1985 to 15-19 years in 1995 and 1999.[237]

In developing countries, the incidence of gonorrhoea is very high. In Africa, in early 1990s, the incidence of gonococcal urethritis was estimated to be approximately 10% annually.[238] Numerous surveys conducted in the past have shown that gonorrhoea is the commonest cause of male urethritis, accounting for approximately 53-80% of all cases. The prevalence of gonococcal infection in African women is also very high, ranging from 20 to 40% among prostitutes and 3-10% among pregnant women. A study from Bangladesh has shown disease positivity in 35.5% of female sex workers.[239] In India also, gonorrhoea is a major health problem with incidence varying from 3 to 19% among STI clinic attendees in different regions.[19-25,91-103] The majority of reported cases are in the 20-24 years age group. However, over the years, there has been a steady decline in its incidence, which may be attributed to the availability of medical facilities at primary health care, indiscriminate use of over-the-counter drugs for unrelated illnesses, prophylactic use of antibiotics after sexual exposure, and growing awareness about AIDS in the Indian population. A steady decline in the incidence was observed in Chandigarh, Delhi and Patiala, while a marginal increase was reported from Rohtak and Ahmedabad (Table 1.3). In a survey of women attending an STI clinic in Mumbai in 1996, 9.7% were positive for gonorrhoea.[240] This rate was much higher than that reported from gynaecological OPDs in Amritsar (1995) and Chandigarh (1986), i.e. 0.8% and 1.8%

respectively.[241,242] The apparent ratio of male-to-female cases is 10:1 with 80-90% men acquiring the infection from CSWs.[243]

Chlamydial Infection

Genital *Chlamydia trachomatis* infection is an STI of epidemic nature. It causes upto half of all acute nongonococcal urethritis (NGU) and atleast one-third of acute epididymitis in men. In women, it is responsible for up to half of all mucopurulent cervicitis cases and 20 to 40% cases of pelvic inflammatory disease (PID) with risk of subsequent infertility or ectopic pregnancy.[104] Epidemiological studies suggest that these sequelae are more closely linked to second or subsequent infection than to the initial infection. Eighty-five percent of women with chlamydial infection are asymtomatic while 40% of infected men report no symptoms. Perinatal transmission may cause neonatal conjunctivitis and pneumonia.[244]

WHO estimates that the global frequency of infection has risen to 50 million cases per year. In 1997, 89 million new cases and in 1999, 92 million new cases were detected.[2,244] In developed countries, including the United States, it is the most commonly reported STI and the commonest notifiable infectious disease, with 3 million cases occurring annually.[85] The prevalence of this infection among women screened in family planning and prenatal clinics, where most of the cases do not seek care for genital symptoms, has been reported to be over 5%. In men who seek health care for reasons other than STD symptoms, the prevalence is generally more than 5%.[245] From 1984 to 1994, the disease rates increased dramatically from 3.2 cases per 100,000 population to 188.4 cases.[246] These rates were higher for women (265.3 per 100,000 population) than men (46.2 per 100,000) (Fig 1.4). In 1995 alone, state-specific rates were six times higher for women than men (46.4-622 cases per 100,000 versus 52.1).[247] This difference was mainly due to increased detection of asymptomatic women through regular screening. The lower rates in men suggest that they are either not diagnosed or are frequently treated but not tested. In 1994, 448,984 cases were reported to CDC from USA; in 1995, it increased to 477,638 cases while in 1997, it was 526,653. In a study conducted as part of the National Health and Nutrition Survey between 1989 and 1994 to determine the prevalence of chlamydial infection using the ligase chain reaction assay on urine samples, the prevalence of 7% was found among non-Hispanic Black population, 3% in Mexican Americans and 2% in non-Hispanic Whites.[245] The prevalence rate was greater among women than men, with the highest rates in the 15-19 years age group. In another study conducted in Washington between 1994 and 1996 using the same method among the adolescent population, the prevalence among female participants was 8.6% which declined with increasing age, while among the male attendees it was 5.4% which increased with age.[248] Disease positivity among women screened at family planning clinics in 1995 ranged

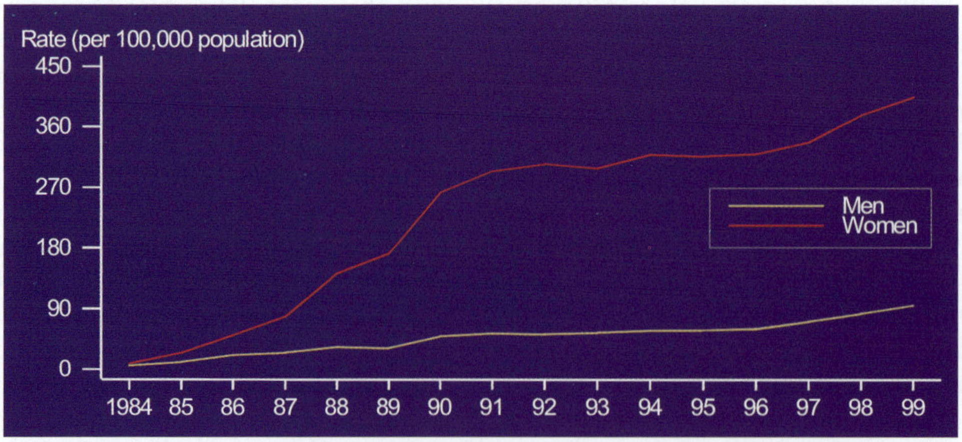

Fig. 1.4 Chlamydia—Rates by Gender: United States, 1984–1999 (CDC, Atlanta).

from 2.8% to 9.4%.[247] In HIV infected women, a prevalence rate of 4% was found. Approximately 1 million cases of PID occur annually in the United States, and 15% of infertility cases are secondary to tubal damage resulting from PID.[8] In 2004, 929,462 cases of chlamydia infection were diagnosed, while in 2005 there were 976,445. The increase in reported cases and rates likely reflects the continued expansion of screening efforts and increased use of more sensitive diagnostic tests; however, this trend may also reflect an actual increase in the rate of infection.

In Europe, chlamydial infection is a major bacterial STI with prevalence rates varying from 2.6 to 51.5% among women attending a variety of health centers, including STI, family planning, antenatal and abortion clinics.[249] It has been shown to be higher among abortion and STI clinic attendees than family planning (prevalence rates of 3 to 4% in UK) and general clinic attendees (3 to 7% in UK).[250] The prevalence rates also depend upon the modality used for *C. trachomatis* isolation. In men, the prevalence rates of 4.1 to 11.3% have been reported from different parts of Europe.[251] In London, among MSM, a prevalence of 11% was found.[252] The attendance is highest among women aged 16 to 19, while in men it peaks in the 20-24 years age group.

In Australia, the notification for chlamydial infection has been reported to be the highest among STIs and the third highest for all notifiable diseases, predominantly among the female gender and heterosexual adolescent population.[253] In a survey of heterosexual patients attending an urban sexual health service in Sydney between 1994 and 2000, the prevalence rate doubled from 1.8 to 3.5% among women and tripled from 2.1 to 6.6% among men.[254] Among the non-trachoma acute conjunctivitis cases seen in Melbourne in 1991, 2% were due to chlamydial infection, of which 83% had a concomitant genital infection.[255]

In sub-Saharan Africa, the prevalence is very high ranging from 47 to 52%, predominantly in women in the age group of 21-25 years.[256,257] The estimated incidence is 0.4 to 1.5% for PID, 0.3 to 1.5% for bilateral tubal occlusion, 0.01 to 0.04% for ectopic pregnancy and 0.04 to 0.2% for maternal mortality cases resulting from postpartum chlamydial infection complications.[104] In China, the reported prevalence ranges from 9 to 37.6%, with the highest rates recorded among women with high abortion rates, low education, multiple sex partners and non-use of condoms.[258] Seroprevalence of chlamydial infection in China in 1993 was shown to be 20.8% in CSWs, 10% in STI clinic attendees, 3% among antenatal clinic visitors and 1.3% among sexually active men (Fig. 1.5). In Manila, Phillipines, in 1994, chlamydial antibodies were detected in 17.3% of female sex workers and 5.6% of antenatal attenders (Fig. 1.6). In rural Thai women attending antenatal, postpartum and family planning clinics, the prevalences of *C. trachomatis* infection were 6.8%, 5.2% and 6.7% respectively.[259] In Bangladesh, a lower prevalence of 1.9% has been reported. In 1999, in South and South-East Asia, 43 million new cases were detected.

The majority of epidemiological studies conducted in India have used the criteria of

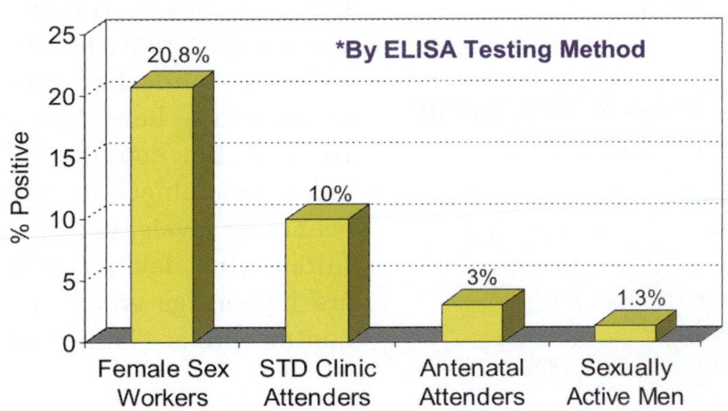

Fig. 1.5 Prevalence of Chlamydial Infection in High- and Low-risk Groups, Nanjing, China, 1993 (WHO Initiative on HIV/AIDS and Sexually Transmitted Infections).

demonstration of >5 neutrophils in urethral smears or endocervical specimens to establish the diagnosis of NGU without isolating the causative organism. The incidence rates using this criteria have been reported to vary from 1.5 to 19% among STI clinic attendees from different parts of the country.[19-25,91-103] There are only few studies in which prevalence rates have been established by utilizing specific diagnostic modalities for genital chlamydial infection. Among STD clinic attendees in Delhi in 1998-99, 50% positivity for *C. trachomatis* was found using the plasmid-based PCR assay, 26% positivity using enzyme immunoassay for antigen detection and 52% positivity using ELISA for antibody detection.[261]

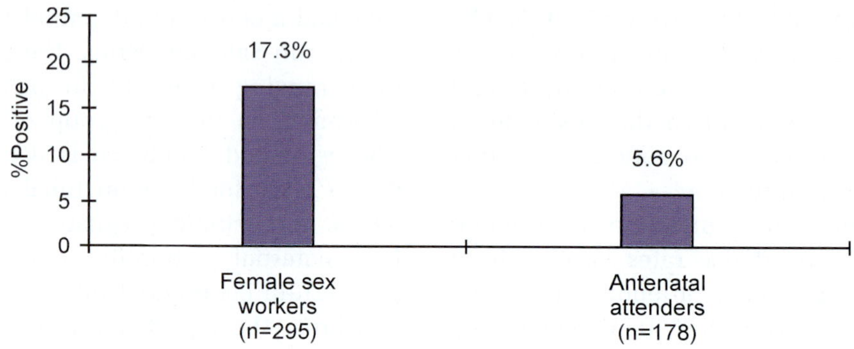

Fig. 1.6 Prevalence of Chlamydial Infection in High- and Low-risk Groups, Manila, Philippines, 1994 (UNAIDS/WHO Working Group on Global HIV/AIDS and STI Surveillance).

Among antenatal clinic attendees in Delhi in 1999, 21.3% were found to be infected with *C. trachomatis* with a significantly higher incidence of still-births, prematurity and low birth weight in this group.[262] Another study from the same city published in 1999 showed the prevalence of 17 and 18.6% during mid-pregnancy and labour, with however no difference in neonatal complications except for purulent conjunctivitis as compared to the control group.[263] (Table 1.10)

Table 1.10 Prevalence of Chlamydia Trachomatis Infection in Antenatal Clinics

USA[245]	1990s	5%
UK[250]	1990s	3 - 4%
China[258]	1993	3%
Phillipines (Fig.6)	1994	5.6%
Thailand[259]	1999	6.8%
India		
Delhi[262]	1999	21.3%
Delhi[263]	1999	17 - 18.6%

In women who attended the gynaec OPD in a Delhi hospital between 1990 and 1992 with symptoms of lower genital tract infection and infertility, the prevalence of 41 and 36% respectively was found.[264] In young women undergoing routine gynaecological check-ups in Mumbai in 1994, genital chlamydial infection was diagnosed in 15% cases with 53% cases showing clinical signs suggestive of cervicitis and only 2% cases suffering from PID.[265] The contribution of *C. trachomatis* in the etiology of PID in this study was much lower than that from Nagpur, in which it was found to be responsible for 33% cases of PID.[266] This infection was detected in 23.3% of gynaec OPD attendees of Delhi in 1994.[267] Among women seeking medical service for reproductive health complications, chlamydial infection rates varying from 0.3-3.2% to 23.3-33% have been reported from different parts of the country.[268,269] High risk factors for chlamydial infection in India include low socio-economic levels, multiple sex partners and use of intrauterine devices, while the protective factors are higher age group and use of oral and barrier contraceptives (Table 1.11).

Table 1.11 Prevalence of Chlamydia Trachomatis Infection in Gynaec Clinic Attendees in India

Delhi[264]	1990-92	36–41%
Delhi[267]	1994	23.3%
Mumbai[265]	1994	15%
Mumbai[268]	2000	14.3–20%
Chandigarh[269]	1989	33%

Genital Herpes Infection

Genital herpes is the second most prevalent STI worldwide and the commonest cause of GUD in developed world.[270] The seroprevalence of antibodies to HSV-2 is 22% in general population. This infection has important public health implications since undiagnosed cases (asymptomatic shedding or atypical, unrecognized lesions) contribute to population reservoir and transmission of the virus; perinatal transmission to the neonate may result in disseminated disease, neurological damage and high mortality; and herpetic ulcers facilitate HIV transmission. Approximately 60% of seropositive persons are able to identify symptoms of genital herpes after receiving symptom-recognition counselling, while more than 80% of asymptomatic seropositive women shed HSV intermittantly from the genital tract. In heterosexual couples, the risk of acquisition of HSV-2 infection from a sex partner with genital herpes is lowest in men (less than 5%), higher in HSV-1 seropositive women (less than 10%), and highest (about 30%) in women without antibody to HSV-1 or HSV-2.[271] The risk of transmission to infants exposed to asymptomatic shedding at delivery is low (about 3%) from women with or without a history of genital herpes if HSV antibody of the same type is present in cord blood.

The outbreak of HIV since 1980s and subsequent behavioural changes have resulted in considerable alteration in STI patterns in which the relative importance of genital herpes has increased significantly. In 1990s, HSV-2 seroprevalence from different parts of the world in population-based studies has been found to be 3.4 to 23.4%. Among specific target groups such as STD clinic attendees, CSWs, factory workers, army recruits and blood donors, it has ranged from 12 to 80%.[272]

Genital herpes is one of the three most prevalent STIs in the United States (with chlamydial and HPV infections) and probably of greatest concern to sexually active people, apart from HIV infection.[273] In USA, one in five persons over age 12 (i.e. approximately 45 million people) is infected with HSV-2 infection with up to one million new HSV-2 infections transmitted annually. There has been a constant increase both in the incidence and prevalence of genital herpes. From 1970 to 1985, the annual incidence of HSV-2 infection increased by 82% from 4.6 per 1000 to 8.4 per 1000. The incidence in 1985 was higher in women, Black population and in the age group of 20-29 years. The age-adjusted seroprevalence of HSV-2 has also increased by 30% from the National Health and Nutrition Examination Survey II (NHANES II) 1976-1980 figures of 16.7% to NHANES III (1988-1994) rates of 21.9%.[273,274] (Fig. 1.7) In the third survey, the seroprevalence was higher among women (25.6%) than men (17.8%) and greater among Black population (45.9%) than Whites (17.6%). These surveys have also shown increased HSV-2 seroprevalence in Hispanic (25%) and Black women (55%) as compared to White women of child-bearing age (21%). It quintupled among White teenagers and doubled among the white population in their twenties. The other risk factors include older age, female gender, male homosexuality, history of previous STI, illiteracy, poverty, cocaine use and greater number of lifetime sex partners. Among STI clinic attendees in USA, the seroprevalence is even higher, varying from 30 to 70%.[275] In California, among young women in the lowincome group, HSV-2 seropositivity was detected in 34.8% individuals in 1999-2000.[276]

In Australia, HSV-2 infection is a major cause of STI, although its prevalence in pregnant women is less than that in USA. Between 1995 and 1998, 12.5% of antenatal clinic attendees were found to be positive for HSV-2, while 79.3% were positive for HSV-1 antibodies.[277]

In Europe, HSV-2 prevalence has been reported to range from 8% in pregnant women to 50% in homosexual men, while that for HSV-1 ranges from

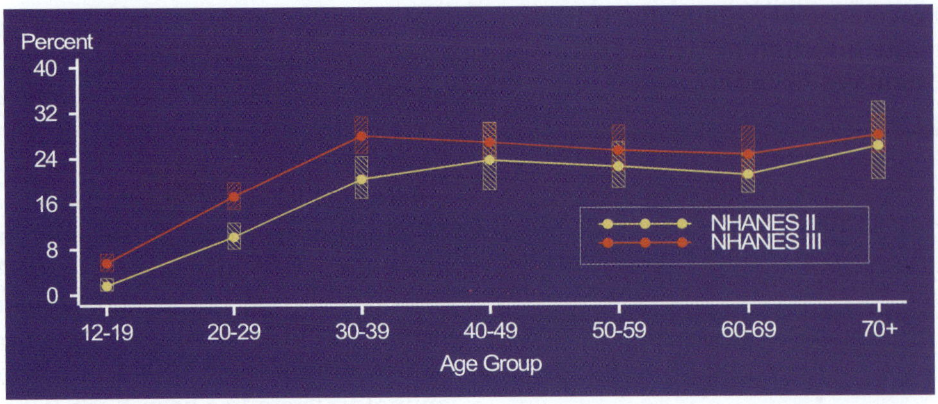

Fig. 1.7 Genital Herpes Simplex Virus Type 2—Percent Seroprevalence According to Age in NHANES II (1976–1980) and NHANES III (1988–1994). (From Division of STD Prevention, National Center for HIV, STD and TB Prevention, CDC, Atlanta)

60 to 90%.[278,279] In 1999-2000, the seroprevalence of HSV-1 and 2 among HIV infected women in Europe was found to be 76 and 42% respectively.[279] The majority of genital herpes cases are caused by HSV-2. HSV-1 has been reported in an increasing number of genital ulcer cases in UK. Among STI clinic attendees from 1995 to 1999, 62% of males and 77% of females were found to have HSV-1 isolate in their genital lesions. Among general population groups in UK, HSV-2 seroprevalence was found to be low (3.3% in men and 5.1% in women) as compared to HSV-1 positivity observed in 24-54% individuals during 1994-95.[280]

In Rotterdam, the Netherlands, the seroprevalence of both HSV-1 and 2 was found to decrease from 68% and 59% to 30% and 22%, respectively, between 1993 and 1998 among STI clinic attendees.[281] In Amsterdam also, HSV-2 seroprevalence was found to decrease from 32% in 1986 to 22% in 1998.[282] The decreasing trend in the Netherlands could be due to the ongoing national public health campaigns promoting safer sex practices.

In Scandinavia, the seroprevalence of HSV-2 infection among pregnant women has nearly doubled over the past two decades, from 19% to 33%.[283] Studies from Scandinavia also indicate that HSV-1 is also responsible for a significant proportion of genital herpes in women. This was identified in a study from Norway in 1990s, in which HSV-1 was identified in 70-90% of suspected female genital herpes cases.[284] In 1992-94, in Norway, the seroprevalence of HSV-2 among pregnant women was 27%, which increased with age, since 17% of the 20-24-year-olds and 34% of the 35-year-olds and above were infected with this disease.[285] Twenty-five percent of STI clinic attendees in UK, 14 to 90% of the STI population in Sweden and 5 to 40% in other European populations are infected with HSV-2.[286]

Genital herpes is a significant problem in Central and South America. In 1990s, HSV-2 type-specific antibodies were detected in 61% of CSWs in the Mexico city, 53% of STI patients in Brazil and 39% of women in Costa Rica.[272,287,288] In a seroepidemiological survey undertaken in Brazil in 1994 among voluntary blood donors, HIV-positive homo/heterosexual men and CSWs, HSV-2 seropositivity was detected in 72% of cases.[289]

In sub-Saharan Africa, the proportion of herpes-culture positive GUD has increased from 3-11% in 1980s to 21-48% in 1990s.[290] In rural populations, HSV-2 antibodies were detected in 75% of women >25 years and 60% of men >30 years. According to the data published in 2001, in four urban African populations, HSV-2 seroprevalence was 50% among women and 25% among men.[291] The significant increase in HSV-2 as a cause of GUD may be explained by the fact that immunosuppression during the advanced stages of HIV disease can increase the duration, severity and incidence of herpetic recurrences, leading to increased herpes ulcer load. The decrease in the prevalence of bacterial STIs, especially chancroid, may induce a relative increase in HSV-2 as a cause of GUD. The apparent increase in genital herpes may also reflect changes in the detection rates rather than a true shift in the GUD etiology. The higher HSV-2 detection could result from increased awareness among clinicians and patients as well as improved diagnostic choices including viral culture, specific serologic tests and PCR.

In Asia, a considerable shift in the pattern of GUDs has occurred since early 1980s when syphilis and chancroid were the primary causes of genital ulcers. In Singapore, the seroprevalence of herpes infection changed from 17% in 1980 to 72% in 1993.[292] In Kuala Lumpur, Malaysia, in the 1990s, HSV-2 was identified by culture and immunofluorescence in 19% of GUD cases.[293] Similarly, in Papua New Guinea, genital herpes was identified as the commonest cause of GUD.[294] In Dhaka, Bangladesh, the seroprevalence among married women was found to be 12%.[260] In young men recruited in the armed forces in Thailand, HSV-2 seroprevalence was 41%. Among STI clinic attendees with GUDs, using the multiplex-PCR technique, the prevalence of HSV-2 was found to be 82%.[295] In another study among female STI clinic attendees with clinical symptoms of genital herpes between 1994 and 1996, HSV-1 was isolated by culture in 18.7% and HSV-2 in 81.3% of cases in Thailand.[296]

In India, there has been a significant increase in the proportion of viral STIs especially HSV infection, with incidence rates varying from 4.11 to 27.9% among STI clinic attendees in different regions of the country.[19-25,91-103] In Pune, in 1994, 26% of GUD patients were diagnosed with herpes etiology using the multiplex-PCR technique.[297] In a study published from Nagpur in 1998, the seroprevalence of HSV-2 was shown to be 40.22% among GUDs.[298] It was higher among sexually active, unmarried men. During 1983-86, genital herpes was diagnosed in 19% of STI clinic attendees in south India, with culture positivity in 38.7% cases with primary infection and 38.2% cases with recurrent disease.[299] The wide variation in incidence rates may be attributed to differences in the patterns of sexual behaviours, frequency of contact, abstinence during the period of viral replication, or variations in the use of barrier contraceptives. The exact prevalence is difficult to ascertain because of the large percentage of subclinical cases and limitations of serologic assays for HSV-2 antibody detection. In Chandigarh, a fourfold increase in genital herpes was observed among STD clinic attendees from 1977 to late 1990s. The incidence rose from 11.4% in 1977-85 to 21% in 1995-96.[98,99] In Ahmedabad, the incidence increased from 8.23% in 1993-94 to 27.9% in 1998-99.[22,92] In Delhi also, a significant increase in the proportion of herpes genitalis was observed, with the incidence rising from 2.5% in 1965-78 to 11.8% in 1995-99.[19,25] In a cross-sectional study of gynaecological clinic attendees in a Delhi hospital in 1994, IgA antibodies to HSV were detected in 20.6% of women.[267] The increasing incidence of genital herpes infection may be attributed to a decrease in the incidence of bacterial STIs owing to their treatment at the primary level with large number of newly available over-the-counter antibiotics and changes in the pattern of sexual behaviours.

Seroepidemiological studies have established that HSV is among the most common viral coinfection in AIDS patients, with 95% of MSM and 40.5 to 60% of IV drug users demonstrating serum antibodies to HSV-1, 2 or both.[300] In 1998, in the United States, anogenital HSV-2 cultures were found to be positive in 9.7% of HIV-positive men as compared to 3.1% in HIV-negative individuals.[301] The risk factors for increased viral shedding included low CD4 counts and antibodies to both HSV-1 and 2. Similarly, in an Indian study, herpes genitalis was diagnosed in 7.7% of HIV-positive individuals.[302]

The prevalence of HSV-1 varies between 50% and 90% across various study populations.[279-281] Although HSV-1 is associated with orolabial disease, upto 50% of new genital ulcers in some developed countries are caused by this virus.

The most serious consequence of genital HSV infection is neonatal herpes, which results from perinatal transmission from mother to infant. The transmission is greatly influenced by the mother's serological status. If the infection was recently acquired and the mother is seronegative, 15 to 50% of vaginally delivered infants acquire the infection. However, the risk is lower among women with long-standing infection.[303]

The incidence of culture-proven cases of neonatal herpes in the Netherlands from 1992 to 1998 was 2.4 per 100,000 livebirths, and HSV-1 was the primary cause (73%) of neonatal herpes infection.[304] In the British Isles, during 1986-1991, 76 infants with neonatal herpes were reported, an incidence of 1.65 per 100,000 live births.[305] In a majority of cases, the infection was caused by HSV-1, with 25% fatalities occurring in the neonatal period and a further 33% showing long-term sequalae. The reported incidence of neonatal HSV infection in the United States is approximately 11-33 cases per 100,000 live births During 1985, 1990 and 1995, 11.7, 11.3 and 11.4 infants per 100,000 live births were diagnosed to have HSV infection.[306] British Columbia in Canada records 1-3 cases of neonatal herpes per 45000 live births.[307]

Human Papilloma Virus Infection

Genital HPVs infect the epithelial lining of the anogenital tract. Of the 100 HPV types identified so far, approximately 30 have affinity for the anogenital tract. The low-risk HPVs (6 and 11) are causative agents of genital warts, and the high-risk types (16, 18, 31, 33, 45), which exhibit oncogenicity, have been implicated in penile, vulval, vaginal and cervical cancers. Recent advances in laboratory techniques have made large-scale epidemiological investigations of HPV more feasible.

Genital HPV infection is the commonest viral STI in developed world, with an estimated 30 million new cases diagnosed annually worldwide.[308] Approximately 15% of general population harbour subclinical infection.[309] Epidemiological studies indicate that 50% of sexually active women contract a genital HPV infection within 2 years.[310] The lifetime risk of a genital HPV infection is estimated to be 80%, but very few of these women develop cervical cancer.

In the United States, genital HPV infection is the third most commonly diagnosed STI, besides chlamydial infection and trichomoniasis, and the most frequently reported viral STI.[311] Ninety-nine percent of all cervical cancers and over 50% of other anogenital cancers are due to oncogenic HPV infection.[312] CDC estimates that 24 million Americans are infected with HPV and 7,50,000 new cases are diagnosed annually.[311] The incidence of genital warts increased over the past four decades (from 13/100,000 population in 1950 to 106/100,000 in 1978 in Minnesota) with a fivefold increase in the number of visits to physicians for its diagnosis and treatment.[313] The number of visits increased significantly from 60,000 in 1966 to 3,40,000 in 1988, after which it declined marginally to 2,00,000 visits in 1996 and then increased to 2,40,000 in 1999.[311] (Fig. 1.8) In a seroepidemiological study of HPV infection in a male cohort of STI clinic attendees in Louisiana between 1993 and 1995, the seroprevalence of HPV-6/11 and HPV-16 was 31.6% and 36.1% respectively.[314] The significant predictors for HPV-6/11 antibodies include history of syphilis, NGU or genital warts, presence of concomitant HSV-2 antibodies and use of multiple partners in the previous one year. History of trichomoniasis, syphilis and presence of HSV-2 antibodies, more than 10 years of sexual activity, older age, exchanging drugs or money for sex, and cocaine or IV drug abuse were strongly associated with oncogenic HPV infection. Condoms were shown to have no protective effect against HPV-6/11 acquisition and only marginally protective against HPV-16 infection, since they do not prevent exposure to external genital warts which are predisposed to infect keratinized epithelia.

In the United States-Mexico border, in 1997-1998, the overall HPV prevalence among women attending gynaecological care centers was 14.4%, with HPV-16 being the commonest type detected.[315] The prevalence declined linearly with age from 25% among 15-19-year-olds to 5.3% among 56-65 years age group. Other risk factors include multiple sex partners, concurrent chlamydial infection and current use of injectable contraceptives.

Mexico and Central America have the highest incidence of cervival cancer with age-adjusted incidence of 44.4 cases per 100,000 women.[316] In a study conducted during 1996-1999 among Mexican women with normal cervical cytology, an overall prevalence of cervical HPV DNA was found to be 14.5%, with the highest rate of 16.7% observed under 25 years of age, which declined to 3.7% in the age group of 35-44 years and then increased progressively among women of 65 years and older.

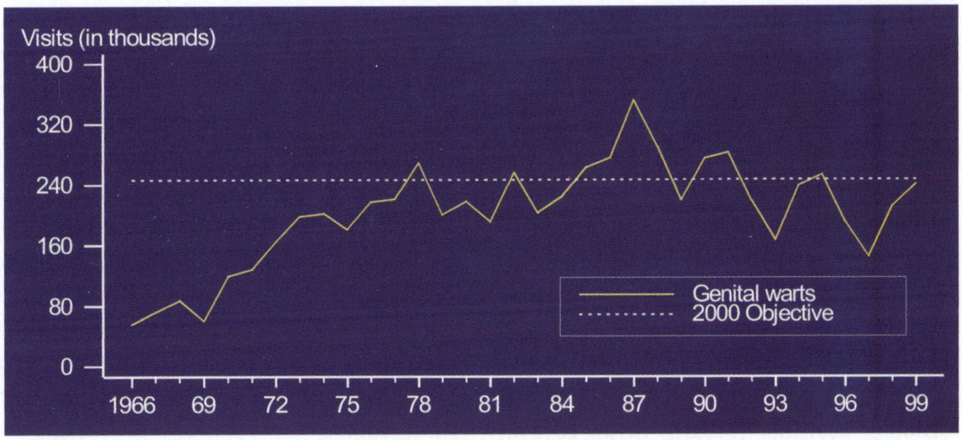

Fig. 1.8 Human Papillomavirus (Genital Warts)—Initial Visits to Physicians' Offices: United States, 1966–1999 and the Healthy People Year 2000 Objective.

Low education was associated with high-risk HPV, while low socio-economic status correlated with low-risk HPV. In Brazilian women with abnormal cervical cytology, HPV prevalence ranged from 85.6% in low-grade squamous intraepithelial lesions to 55.2% in frank squamous cell carcinoma.[317] History of another STI mainly syphilis, but not oral contraceptive use or smoking, was associated with progression to malignancy. Among women prison inmates in Sao Paulo, in 1997-1998, the prevalence of 16.3% for high-risk HPV and 4.8% for low-risk HPV was reported.[318]

In the United Kingdom, the incidence of HPV infection is on the rise. It increased 2.5-fold in both the sexes between 1971 and 1982.[319] Among asymptomatic women in Hungary, HPV prevalence was 17%.[320] The risk factors include young age, unmarried status, unemployment and smoking. The lowest prevalence rates in cytologically normal women have been reported among Spanish (4.7%) and Colombian (10.5%) women.[321] The prevalence of HPV infection among indigenous women attending various health centers in Australia in 1996 was low (0.42%).[322] The rates decreased with increasing age.

In sub-Saharan Africa, cervical cancer is the commonest malignancy in women, with incidence rates being fourfold higher than in United States or Europe.[323] In Tanzania, in 1994, among antenatal clinic attendees, HPV prevalence was found to be 34%, with high-risk HPV DNA detected in 83% of women.[324] The infection was strongly associated with short duration of relationship, single marital status, non-usage of condoms and gonorrhoea.

In the last 5 years, a high incidence of HPV infection has been reported from the United Kingdom and the Russian Federation (20-70/100,000), and in the year 2000, the highest incidence was recorded from the United Kingdom (80-120/100,000) and Ireland (100/100,000).[325]

In India, the incidence of genital warts ranges from 2 to 25.2% in STI clinic attendees.[19-25,91-103] The data collected from STI clinics show contradictory trends in different regions. In Delhi, in 1955-61, no case was reported;[100] the incidence in 1965-78 was 2%,[25] which increased to 9.3% in 1995-99.[19] In women attending gynaec OPDs in Delhi in 1994, HPV was found to be the leading infection, affecting 49.4% of women.[267] In Rohtak, during 1990s, it marginally increased from 18.1 to 21.54% and then declined to 19.35%.[96,97,102] Similarly, in Ahmedabad, a slight increase in the incidence of HPV infection was observed from 7.17% in 1993-94 to 9.1% in 1998-99.[22,92] However, in Chandigarh and Patiala, the incidence of genital warts has been declining (Table 1.3). These studies are based on clinical diagnosis only, rather than detection of HPV DNA or serological diagnosis. The subclinical and asymptomatic nature of HPV infection, especially in women, may have been responsible for the wide disparity in incidence rates.

Infection with oncogenic HPV is the leading cause of cervical cancer in India (Table 1.12). In a study from Delhi during late 1990s among women STI clinic attendees, HPV-16 DNA was detected in 30% of cases, which increased to 52 and 72% among women with precancerous and cancerous cervical lesions.[261] In Mumbai, using the method of Southern Hybridization of the HPV PCR product using HPV-16/18 probes, HPV-16/18 was detected in 77% of cervical cancer patients, 38% of low-grade squamous intraepithelial squamous neoplasia lesions (LSIL), 80% of high-grade intraepithelial squamous neoplasia lesions (HSIL) and 15.2% of healthy women.[326] In the same city, using the non-isotopic in-situ hybridization technique, HPV DNA was detected in 76.4% of cervical cancer lesions, with HPV-16/18 found in 29.4% cases with squamous cell carcinoma, and HPV 18 in all cases with adenocarcinoma and neuroendocrine carcinoma of the cervix.[327] HPV-16 was isolated in 29.1% and HPV-18 in 8.3% of SIL lesions. In Kolkata, HPV DNA was detected in 50% of biopsy specimens and none of the exfoliative cervical cell specimens of carcinoma cervix patients, with HPV-16/18 isolated in 56% of positive biopsy materials.[328]

Table 1.12 Prevalence of Oncogenic HPV Types in Cervical Disease in India

Delhi[261]	HPV-16	Healthy women	30%
		SIL*	52%
		Carcinoma cervix	72%
Mumbai[326]	HPV-16/18	Healthy women	15.2%
		LSIL**	38%
		HSIL***	80%
		Carcinoma cervix	77%
Mumbai[327]	HPV-16/18	SIL	37.4%
		Carcinoma cervix	76.4%
Kolkata[328]	HPV-16/18	Carcinoma cervix	37%

*squamous intraepithelial neoplastic lesion

**low-grade squamous intraepithelial neoplastic lesion

***high-grade squamous intraepithelial neoplastic lesion

In the majority of studies cited above, it has been observed that the risk of acquiring HPV infection, especially among cytologically normal women, is inversely associated with age and directly with the number of sex partners, poor socio-economic status, low education, use of oral contraceptives, reproductive characteristics, concomitant presence of other STIs, smoking and dietary factors. Some of the highest prevalence rates have been found among adolescent population, ranging from 15.6 to 46% in early 1990s.[329] The inverse association with age may be explained by the fact that immunological or hormonal changes occurring in old age may clear or suppress the existing infection. Moreover, lesser number of sex partners in older women may reduce the rate of infection. In a study from Japan, it was observed that the risk of acquiring premalignant and malignant cervical lesions with HPV-16 was 8 times higher in women 44 years of age or younger than in women 45 years of age or older.[330] Use of oral contraceptives may influence the transcription and translation of the HPV genome, hence playing an important role in the causation of cervical neoplasia. Ethnographic variations have also been observed in the epidemiology of HPV infection.[331] Higher prevalence rates have been reported among African-American women than in Whites or Hispanics. This may be due to differences in the probability of encountering HPV-positive partners, genetic predisposition towards greater susceptibility to acquisition and persistence of infection, endogenous hormonal factors or differences in sexual behaviours among ethnic groups.

Several studies have demonstrated a higher risk of cervical cancer in HIV-positive women especially with lower CD4 counts as compared to HIV-negative women or HIV-positive cases with higher CD4 counts. This may be due to the persistence of greater HPV load in this group of women. The prevalence of oncogenic HPV types in HIV-positive patients varies from 14.4 to 93%, depending upon the circulating CD4 levels.[332,333] Combinations of several HPV types have been found simultaneously in most of the studied groups. In a study from Atlanta, it was shown that HIV-positive women with CD4 counts less than 200/mm^3 were 1.8, 2.1 and 2.7 times more likely to have high-, intermediate- and low-risk HPV infection respectively as compared with HIV-negative women.[334] Also, the cumulative prevalence of HPV infection after 3 years of follow-up was 90.2% in the former group as compared to 54.6% in the latter. In Mexico, HPV DNA was detected by PCR in 69% of HIV-positive women and only 29% of healthy controls.[335] In a survey conducted in 12 European countries between 1993 and 1998 among HIV infected women, individuals with CD4 counts <200/mm^3 had a twofold increase in the prevalence of squamous intraepithelial lesions (SIL) and non-regression from low-grade SIL as compared to women with CD4 count >500/mm^3.[336]

A strong causal association exists between HPV infection and anal and vulvar carcinoma. The incidence of anal cancer is increasing in the United States among both men and women, being twice more common in women.[337] Since 1960, the incidence of anal cancer in Connecticut increased twofold among men and 2.3-fold among women, being the highest among African-American women (0.74/100,000 between 1973 and 1989) and lowest among White men (0.41/100,000).[338] In men, anal cancer is common among those indulging in receptive anal intercourse, with an incidence of 36/100,000 population.[339] The incidence of anal cancer in this group of men is 5 times higher than the incidence of cervical cancer among women in the United States. With the advent of HIV infection, the incidence has increased twofold from the pre-AIDS era. In a study conducted in San Francisco during 1995-1997, 76% of HIV positive and 42% of HIV-negative women were found to have anal HPV DNA.[333] In HIV-positive women, lower CD4 counts and concomitant cervical HPV infection were strongly associated with anal infection. Younger White women were at increased risk as compared to older African-American women. Al-Ghamdi et al[340] detected HPV DNA in 85% cases of vulvar carcinoma reported between 1970 and 1998 in Canada.

Table 1.13 **Community Prevalence of Sexually Transmitted Infections in Tamil Nadu[341]**

Genital Symptoms (47.3%)	
Genital discharge	52.5% women 1.7% men
Vaginal discharge, abdominal pain, dyspaurenia	60% women
Asymptomatic infection	32% women 72% men
STI Syndromes	
GUD (men)	0.1%
GUD (women)	2.7%
Vaginal discharge	41.5%
Urethral discharge (men)	0.2%
Bubo (men)	0.02%
Scrotal swelling	2.5%
PID	0.6%
Pattern of STIs	
Any STI	15.8%
Classical STI	9.7%
Gonorrhoea	3.7%
Syphilis	0.3%
Chlamydia infection	3.9%
Trichomoniasis	5.1%
HbsAg	5.3%
HIV	1.8%

The epidemiology of STIs depends upon several distinct and complex yet interrelated behavioural, socio-demographic, economic, geographical and ethnic factors. A comprehensive knowledge of the various epidemiological parameters is extremely essential in order to design preventive and control strategies against these infections which are responsible for significant morbidity and mortality throughout the world.

REFERENCES

1. Centers for Disease Control and prevention. Summary of notifiable diseases in the United States, 1996. MMW R 1997; 45: 1-103.
2. World Health Organization. World Health Report 1998. Geneva: WHO, 1998.
3. Mabey D. Sexually transmitted diseases in developing countries. Trans R Soc Trop Med Hyg 1996; 90: 97-9.
4. Hughes G, SimmsI, Rogers PA, et al. New cases seen at genitourinary medicine clinics: England 1997. Commun Dis Rep CDR Suppl 1998; 8: S1-11.
5. Panchaud C, Singh S, Fievelson D, et al. Sexually transmitted diseases among adolescents in developed countries. Fam Plann Perspect 2000; 32: 24-32.
6. Fox KK. Gonorrhoea in the United States, 1981-1996. Sex Transm Infect 2000; 76910; 18-24.
7. Hughes G. Investigation of the increased incidence of gonorrhoea diagnosed in genitourinary medicine clinics in England, 1994-1996. Sex Transm Infect 2000; 76: 18-24.
8. Eng TR, Butler WT. Reported rates of gonorrhea in selected developed countries. In: The hidden epidemic: Confronting sexually transmitted diseaes. Washington DC, National Academy Press, 1997, p. 29.
9. Arya OP, Lawson JB. Sexually transmitted diseases in the tropics. Epidemiological, diagnostic, therapeutic and control aspects. Tropical Doctor 1977; 7: 51-6.
10. O'Farrell N. Increasing prevalence of genital herpes in developing countries: implications for heterosexual HIV transmission and STI control programme. Sex Transm Infect 1999; 75: 377-84.
11. Perine PL. Sexually transmitted diseases in the tropics. Med J Australia 1994; 160: 360-4.
12. De Schryver A, Meheus A. Epidemiology of sexually transmitted diseases: The global picture. Bull World Health Org 1990; 68: 639-54.
13. Ray K , Bala M , Gupta SM, et al. Changing trends in sexually transmitted infections at a Regional STDs Centre in north India. th Indian J Med Res 2006; 124: 559-68.
14. Auvert B, Ballard R, Campbell C, et al. HIV infection among youth in a South African mining town is associated with herpes simplex virus-2 seropositivity and sexual behaviour. AIDS 2001; 15: 885-98.
15. Auvert B, Buve A, Ferry B, et al. Ecological and individual level analysis of risk factors for HIV infection in four urban populations in sub-Saharan Africa with different levels of HIV infection. AIDS 2001; 15(Suppl 4): S15-30.
16. Sanchez J, Gotuzzo E, Escamilla J, et al. Gender differences in sexual practices and sexually transmitted infections among adults in Lima, Peru. Am J Public Health 1996; 86: 1098-1107.
17. Mardh PA, Creatsas G, Guaschino S, et al. Correlation between an early sexual debut and reproductive health and behavioural factors: a multinational European study. Eur J Contracept Reprod Health Care 2000; 5: 177-82.
18. Melissa S, Becker TM, Masuk M, et al. Risk factors for cervical intraepithelial neoplasia in Southwestern American Indian women. Am J Epidemiol 2000; 152: 716-26.
19. Khandpur S, Agarwal S, Kumar S, et al. Clinico-epidemiological profile and HIV seropositivity of STDs patients. Indian J Sex Transm Dis 2001; 22: 62-5.
20. Jaiswal AK, Bhushan B. Pattern of sexually transmitted diseases in North-Eastern India. Indian J Sex Transm Dis 1994; 15: 19-20.
21. Jaiswal AK, Singh G. Pattern of sexually transmitted diseases in Jammu & Kashmir region of India. Indian J Sex Transm Dis 1998; 19: 113-5.
22. Parmar J, Raval RC, Bilimoria FE. Clinical profile of STDs at Civil Hospital Ahmedabad. Indian J Sex Transm Dis 2001; 22: 14-6.
23. Sharma PK. A profile of sexually transmitted diseases at Port Blair. Indian J Sex Transm Dis 1994; 15: 21-2.
24. Ranganayakulu B, RaviKumar GP, Bhaskar GV. Pattern of STDs at Kurnool. Indian J Sex Transm Dis 1998; 19: 117-21.
25. Reddy BSN, Jaitley V. Profile of sexually transmitted diseases: A 14-year-study. Indian J Sex Transm Dis 1985; 6: 37-40.

26. UNAIDS/WHO Epidemiological fact sheet (India) on HIV/AIDS and sexually transmitted infections. 2000 Update (revised).
27. Conde-Glez CJ, Juarez- Figueroa L, Uribe-Salas F, et al. Analysis of herpes simplex virus 1 and 2 infection in women with high risk sexual behaviour in Mexico. Int J Epidemiol 1999; 28: 571-6.
28. Ishi K, Suzuki F, Saito A, et al. Prevalence of human papilloma virus, *Chlamydia trachomatis* and *Neisseria gonorrhoeae* in commercial sex workers in Japan. Infect Dis Obstet Gynecol 2000; 8: 235-9.
29. Touze A, de Sanjose S, Coursaget P, et al. Prevalence of anti-human papilloma virus types 16, 18, 31 and 58 virus-like particles in women in the general population and in prostitutes. J Clin Microbiol 2001; 39: 4344-8.
30. Dada AJ, Ajayi AO, Diamond stone L, et al. A serosurvey of Haemophilus ducreyi, syphilis and herpes simplex virus type 2 and their association with human immunodeficiency virus among female sex workers in Lagos, Nigeria. Sex Transm Dis 1998; 25: 237-42.
31. Behets F, Andriamiadana J, Rasamilalao D, et al. Sexually transmitted infections and associated socio-demographic and behavioural factors in women seeking primary care suggest Madagascar's vulnerability to rapid HIV spread. Trop Med Int Health 2001; 6: 202-11.
32. Rahman M, Alam A, Nessa K, et al. Etiology of sexually transmitted infections among street-based female sex workers in Dhaka, Bangladesh. J Clin Microbiol 2000, 38: 1244-6.
33. Chatterjee R, Mukhopadhyay D, Murmu N, et al. Prevalence of human papilloma virus infection among prostitutes in Calcutta. J Environ Pathol Toxicol Oncol 2001; 20: 113-7.
34. Thawani G, Singh US, Jana S. Prevalence of antibodies to hepatitis-C virus among visitors of red light areas in Calcutta. Indian J Sex Transm Dis 1998; 19: 105-8.
35. Urmil AC, Dutta PK, Basappa K, et al. A study of morbidity pattern among prostitutes attending a municipal clinic in Pune. J Indian Med Assoc 1989; 87: 29-31.
36. Lakshmi N, Kumar AG. HIV infection among commercial sex workers. Indian J Sex Transm Dis 1994; 15: 11-2.
37. Venketaramana CB, Sarada PV. Extent and speed of spread of HIV infection in India through the commercial sex network: a perspective. Trop Med Int Health 2001; 6: 1040-61.
38. Singh S, Thappa DM, Jaisankar TJ, et al. Risk factors in transmission of HIV, hepatitis B, C in STDs clinic attenders. Indian J Sex Transm Dis 2001; 22: 17-23.
39. Singh S, Jaisankar TJ, Thappa DM, et al. Risk factors for transmission of HIV infection among STDs clinic attenders at Pondicherry. Indian J Sex Transm Dis 2001; 22: 27-30.
40. Gawande AV, Vasudeo ND, Zodpey SP, et al. Sexually transmitted infections in long distance truck drivers. J Commun Dis 2000; 32: 212-5.
41. Singh YN, Malviya AN. Long distance truck drivers in India: HIV infection and their possible role in disseminating HIV into rural areas. Int J STDs AIDS 1994; 5: 137-8.
42. Bwayo JJ, Omari AM, Mutere AN, et al. Long distance truck-drivers: 1. Prevalence of sexually transmitted diseases (STDs). East Afr Med J 1991; 68: 425-9.
43. Gibney L, Saquib N, Macaluso M, et al. STDs in Bangladesh's trucking industry: prevalence and risk factors. Sex Transm Infect 2002; 78: 31-6.
44. Biswas D, Hazarika NC, Hazarika D, et al. Prevalence of communicable disease among restaurant workers along a highway in Assam, India. Southeast Asian J Trop Med Public Health 1999; 30: 539-41.
45. Baqi S, Shah SA, Baig MA, et al. Seroprevalence of HIV, HBV and syphilis and associated risk behaviours in male transvestites (Hijras) in Karachi, Pakistan. Int J STDs AIDS 1999; 10: 300-4.
46. Miranda AE, Vargas PM, St Louis ME, et al. Sexually transmitted diseases among female prisoners in Brazil: prevalence and risk factors. Sex Transm Dis 2000; 27: 491-5.
47. Butler T, Robertson P, Kaldor J, et al. Syphilis in New South Wales (Australia) prisons. Int J STDs AIDS 2001; 12: 376-9.
48. Wolfe MI, Xu F, Patel P, et al. An outbreak of syphilis in Alabama prisons: correctional health policy and communicable disease control. Am J Public Health 2001; 91: 1220-5.

49. Akhtar S, Luby SP, Rahbar MH. Risk behaviours associated with urethritis in prison inmates, Sindh. J Pak Med Assoc 1999; 49: 268-73.
50. Singh S, Prasad R, Mohanty A. High-prevalence of sexually-transmitted and blood-borne infections among the inmates of a district jail in Northern India. Int J STDs AIDS 1999; 10: 475-8.
51. Ratner M, ed. Crack pipe as pimp: An ethnographic investigation of sex for crack exchanges. New York: Lexington Books, 1993: 1-35.
52. De Hovitz JA, Kelly P, Feldman J, et al. Sexually transmitted diseases, sexual behaviour and cocaine use in inner city women. Am J Epidemiol 1994; 140: 1125-34.
53. Ross MW, Hwang LY, Leonard L, et al. Sexual behaviour, STDs and drug use in a cocaine house population. Int J STDs AIDS 2000; 10: 224-30.
54. Jones DL, Irwin KL, Inciardi J, et al. The high-risk sexual practices of crack-smoking in sex workers recruited from the streets of three American cities. Sex Transm Dis 1998; 25: 187-93.
55. Baumens JE, Orlanders H, Gomez MP, et al. Epidemic lymphogranuloma venereum during epidemics of crack cocaine use and HIV infection in the Bahamas. Sex Transm Dis 2002; 29: 253-8.
56. Azim T, Bogaerts J, Yirrell DL, et al. Injecting drug users in Bangladesh: prevalence of syphilis, hepatitis, HIV and HIV subtypes. AIDS 2002; 16: 121-5.
57. Agarwal AK, Singh GB, Khundom KC, et al. The prevalence of HIV in female sex workers in Manipur, India. J Commun Dis 1999; 31: 23-8.
58. Sharma AK, Aggarwal OP, Dubey KK. Sexual behaviour of drug-users: Is it different? Prev Med 2002; 34: 512-5.
59. Cook RL, Pollock NK, Rao AK, et al. Increased prevalence of herpes simplex virus type 2 among adolescent women with alcohol use disorders. J Adolesc Health 2002; 30: 169-74.
60. Waldo CR, McFarland W, Katz MH, et al. Very young gay and bisexual men are at risk for HIV infection: The San Francisco Bay Area Young Men's Survey II. J Acquir Immune Defic Syndr 2000; 24: 168-74.
61. Resurgent bacterial sexually transmitted diseases among men who have sex with men- King county, Washington, 1997-1999. MMWR Morb Mortal Wkly Rep 1999; 48: 773-7.
62. Outbreak of syphilis among men who have sex with men- Southern California, 2000. MMWR Morb Mortal Wkly Rep 2001; 50: 117-20.
63. Daling JR, Weiss NS, Hislop TG, et al. Sexual practices, sexually transmitted diseases and the incidence of anal cancer. N Engl J Med 1987; 317: 973-7.
64. Palefsky JM, Holly EA, Ralston ML, et al. High incidence of anal high-grade squamous intraepithelial lesions among HIV-positive and HIV-negative homosexual and bisexual men. AIDS 1998; 12: 495-503.
65. Stolte IG, Dukers NHTM, deWit JBF, et al. Increase in sexually transmitted infections among homosexual men in Amsterdam in relation to HAART. Sex Transm Infect 2001; 77: 184-6.
66. Fethers K, Marks C, Minder A, et al. Sexually transmitted infections and risk behaviours in women who have sex with women. Sex Transm Infect 2000; 76(5): 345-9.
67. Skinner CJ, Stokes J, Kirlew Y, et al. A case-controlled study of the sexual health needs of lesbians. Genitourin Med 1996; 72: 272-80.
68. Edwards A, Thin RN. Sexually transmitted diseases in lesbians. Int J STDs AIDS 1990; 1: 178-81.
69. Robertson P, Schachter J. Failure to identify venereal disease in a lesbian population. Sex Transm Dis 1981; 8: 75-6.
70. Sonnex C, Strauss S, Gray JJ. Detection of human papilloma virus DNA on the fingers of patients with genital warts. Sex Transm Infect 1999; 75: 317-9.
71. Nyirenda MJ. A study of the behavioural aspects of dry sex practice in urban Lusaka. Int Conf AIDS 1992; 8: D101.
72. Runganga A, Pitts M, McMaster J. The use of herbal and other agents to enhance sexual experience. Soc Sci Med 1992; 35: 1037-42.
73. Tanfer K, Aral SO. Sexual intercourse during menstruation and self-reported sexually

transmitted disease history among women. Sex Transm Dis 1996; 23: 395-401.

74. Foxman B, Aral SO, Holmes KK. Interrelationships among douching practices, risky sexual practices and history of self-reported sexually transmitted diseases in an urban population. Sex Transm Dis 1998; 25: 90-9.
75. National Survey of Family Growth. From Vital and Health Statistics. Data from the National Survey of Family Growth. Hyattsville, MD: U.S. Department of Health and human Services, Public Health Service, National Center for Health Statistics, 1995.
76. Fonck K, Kaul R, Keli F, et al. Sexually transmitted infections and vaginal douching in a population of female sex workers in Nairobi, Kenya. Sex Transm Infect 2001; 77: 271-5.
77. Aral SO, Holmes KK. Epidemiology of sexual behaviour and sexually transmitted diseases. In; Holmes KK, Mardh PA, Sparling PF, eds, Sexually Transmitted Diseases, 2nd ed, 1990, New York: McGraw-Hill, pp19-36.
78. Ghys PD, Diallo MO, Ettiegne-Traore V, et al. Increase in condom use and decline in HIV and sexually transmitted diseases among female sex workers in Abidjan, Cote d' Ivoire, 1991-1998. AIDS 2002; 16: 251-8.
79. Daling JR, Madeleine MM, McKnight B, et al. The relationship of human papillomavirus-related cervical tumours to cigarette smoking, oral contraceptives use and prior herpes simplex virus type 2 infection. Cancer Epidemiol Biomarkers Prev 1996; 5: 541-8.
80. Kramer RL. The intrauterine device and pelvic inflammatory disease revisited: new results from The Women's Health Study. Obstet Gynecol 1989; 73: 300-1.
81. Vessey M, Doll R, Peto R, et al. A long-term follow-up study of women using different methods of contraception- an interim report. J Biosoc Sci 1976; 8: 373-427.
82. Farley TM, Rosenberg MJ, Rowe PJ, et al. Intrauterine devices and pelvic inflammatory disease: an international perspective. Lancet 1992; 339: 785-88.
83. Palayekar V, Joshi JV, Hazari KT, et al. *Chlamydia trachomatis* detected in cervical smears from Copper-T users by DFA test. Adv Contracept 1996; 12: 145-52.
84. Fink AJ. Circumcision: A parent's decision for life. Mountain view, CA, Kavanah Publishing Co., 1988.
85. American Social Health Association. Sexually transmitted diseases in America: How many cases and at what cost? Menlo Park, CA: Kaiser Family foundation, 1998.
86. Noell J, Rohde P, Ochs L, et al. Incidence and prevalence of chlamydia, herpes and viral hepatitis in a homeless adolescent population. Sex Transm Dis 2001; 28: 4-10.
87. Moscicki AB, Palefsky J, Gonzales J, et al. Human papillomavirus infection in sexually active females: prevalence and risk factors. Pediatr Res 1990; 28: 507-13.
88. Sharma RP, Dhir GG. Sexually transmitted diseases in teenagers in Agra. Indian J Sex Transm Dis 1987; 8: 51-2.
89. Xu F, Schillinger JA, Aubin MR, et al. Sexually transmitted diseases of older persons in Washington state. Sex Transm Dis 2001; 28: 287-91.
90. Lee CC, Leo YS, Snodgrass L, et al. The demography, clinical manifestations and natural history of HIV infection in an older population in Singapore. Ann Acad Med Singapore 1997; 26: 731-5.
91. Mehta Swami D, Jaswal R, Bedi GK, et al. Pattern of sexually transmitted diseases in a new Northern Indian Hospital. Indian J Sex Transm Dis 1998; 19: 109-12.
92. Raval RC, Desai N, Bilimoria FE. Clinical profile of STDs at B.J. Medical college and Civil Hospital, Ahmedabad. Indian J Sex Transm Dis 1995; 16: 54-5.
93. Majumdar S, Saha SS. Epidemiological survey of chancroid in Calcutta area. Indian J Sex Transm Dis 1997; 18: 9-11.
94. Chopra A, Dhaliwal RS, Chopra D. Pattern of changing trends of STDs at Patiala. Indian J Sex Transm Dis 1999; 20: 22-5.
95. Chopra A, Mittal RR, Singh P, et al. Pattern of sexually transmitted diseases in Patiala. Indian J Sex Transm Dis 1990; 11: 43-5.

96. Gupta SK, Jain VK, Aggarwal K. Trends of sexually transmitted diseases at Rohtak. Indian J Sex Transm Dis1997; 18: 2-3.
97. Gupta SK, Jain VK. Pattern of sexually transmitted diseases in Rohtak. Indian J Sex Transm Dis 1995; 16: 28-9.
98. Kumar B, Handa S, Malhotra S. Changing trends in sexually transmitted diseases. Indian J Sex Transm Dis 1995; 16: 24-7.
99. Kumar B, Sharma VK, Malhotra S. et al. Pattern of sexually transmitted diseases in Chandigarh. Indian J Sex Transm Dis 1987; 53: 286-91.
100. Singh R. Pattern of VDs as seen at VD training demonstration center, Safdarjung Hospital, New Delhi. Ind J Dermatol Venereol leprol 1962; 28: 62-7.
101. Narayan R, Kar HK. Pattern of STDs in a Delhi Hospital. Indian J Sex Transm Dis 1996; 17: 14-6.
102. Aggarwal K, Jain VK, Brahma D. Trend of STDs at Rohtak. Indian J Sex Transm Dis 2002; 23: 19-21.
103. Reddy BSN, Garg BR, Rao MV. An appraisal of trends in sexually transmitted diseases. Indian J Sex Transm Dis 1993; 14: 1-4.
104. Over M, Piot P. HIV infection and sexually transmitted diseases. In: Jamison DT, et al eds., Disease control priorities in developing countries. 1993, New York: Oxford University Press, pp. 455-67.
105. Laumann EO, Youm Y. Racial/ethnic group differences in the prevalence of sexually transmitted diseases in the United States: a network explanation. Sex Transm Dis 1999; 26: 250-61.
106. Shahmanesh M, Gayed S, Ashcroft M, et al. Geomapping of chlamydia and gonorrhea in Birmingham. Sex Transm Infect 2000; 76: 268-72.
107. Miller PJ, Law M, Torzillo PJ, et al. Incident sexually transmitted infections and their risk factors in an Aboriginal community in Australia: a population based cohort study. Sex Transm Infect 2001; 77: 21-5.
108. Ley C, Bauer HM, Reingold A, et al. Determinants of genital human papilloma virus infection in young women. J Natl Cancer Inst 1991; 83: 997-1003.
109. Reddy BSN, Rao MV, Gharami RC, et al. Clinico-epidemiological study of donovanosis in Pondicherry. JIPMER Bulletin 1994; 13: 14-7.
110. Aswar NR, Wahab SN, Kale KM. Prevalence and some epidemiologic factors of syphilis in Madia tribes of Gadchiroli district. Indian J Sex Transm Dis 1998; 19: 53-8.
111. Holmes KK. An estimate of the risk of men acquiring gonorrhoea by sexual contact with infected females. Am J Epidemiol 1970; 91: 170.
112. Tice RW, Rodriguez VL. Pharyngeal gonorrhoea. JAMA 1981; 246: 2717.
113. King A, Nicol C, Rodin P, eds. Gonorrhoea: Mode of infection; Diagnostic methods; Pathology; The Incubation period. In: Venereal Diseases, 4th ed, 1980, ELBS, Great Britain, pp. 189-99.
114. David IM. Acquisition of pharyngeal gonorrhoea via sweets passed by mouth. Genitourin Med 1997; 73: 146.
115. Kleist E, Mei H. Transmission of gonorrhoea through an inflatable doll. Genitourin Med 1993; 69: 321-5.
116. Lycke E. The risk of genital *Chlamydia trachomatis* infection is less than that of *Neisseria gonorrhoeae* infection. Sex Transm Dis 1980; 7: 6.
117. Quinn TC, Gaydos C, Shepherd M, et al. Epidemiologic and microbiologic correlates of *Chlamydia trachomatis* infection in sexual partnerships. JAMA 1996; 276: 1737-42.
118. Goldmeier D, Darougar S. Isolation of chlamydia trachomatos from the throat and rectum of homosexual men. Br J Vener Dis 177; 53: 184.
119. Jones RB. *Chlamydia trachomatis* in the pharynx and rectum of heterosexual patients at risk of genital infection. Ann Intern Med 1985; 102: 757.
120. Hammerschlag MR. Prospective study of maternal and infantile infection with *Chlamydia trachomatis*. Pediatrics 1979; 64: 142.
121. Schroeter AL. Therapy for incubating syphilis.: Effectiveness of gonorrhoea treatment. JAMA 1971; 218: 711.
122. King A, Nicol C, Rodin P, eds. Early acquired syphilis. In: Venereal Diseases, 4th ed, 1980, ELBS, Great Britain, pp. 15-43.

123. Harter CA, Benirschke K. Fetal syphilis in the first trimester. Am J Obstet Gynecol 1976; 124: 705.
124. Chambers RW, Foley HT, Schmidt PJ. Transmission of syphilis by fresh blood components. Transfusion 1969; 9: 32-4.
125. Harris VK, Nair SC, Das PK, et al. Prevalence of syphilis and parasitic infection among blood donors in a tertiary-care centre in southern India. Ann Trop Med Parasitol 1999; 93: 763-5.
126. Matee MI, Lyamuya EF, Mbena EC, et al. Prevalence of transfusion-associated viral infections and syphilis among blood donors in Muhimbili Medical Centre, Dar es Salaam, Tanzania. East Afr Med J 1999; 76: 167-71.
127. Azim T, Islam MN, Bogaerts J, et al. Prevalence of HIV and syphilis among high-risk groups in Bangladesh. AIDS 2000; 14: 210-1.
128. Plummer FA, D'Costa LJ, Nsanze H, et al. Epidemiology of chancroid and Haemophilus ducreyi in Nairobi, Kenya. Lancet 1983; 2: 1293-5.
129. Plummer FA. Clinical and microbiological studies of genital ulcers in Kenyan women. Sex Transm Dis 1985; 12: 193.
130. Diaz-Mitoma F. Etiology of non-vesicular genital ulcers in Winnipeg. Sex Transm Dis 1987; 14: 33.
131. King A, Nicol C, Rodin P, eds. Chancroid. In: Venereal Diseases, 4th ed, 1980, ELBS, Great Britain, pp. 251-7.
132. Cesario TC. Six years' experience with herpes simplex virus in a chidren's home. Am J epidemiol 1969; 90: 416.
133. Stanberry L, Cunningham A, Mertz G, et al. New developments in the epidemiology, natural history and management of genital herpes. Antiviral Res 1999; 42: 1-14.
134. King A, Nicol C, Rodin P, eds. Herpes genitalis and Hepatitis B infection. In: Venereal Diseases, 4th ed, 1980, ELBS, Great Britain, pp. 325-32.
135. Marmell M. Donovanosis of the anus in the male: An epidemiologic consideration. Br J Vener Dis 1958; 34: 213.
136. King A, Nicol C, Rodin P, eds. Granuloma inguinale.. In: Venereal Diseases, 4th ed, 1980, ELBS, Great Britain, pp. 268-73.
137. Perine PL, Osoba AO. Lymphogranuloma venereum. In: Holmes KK, Mardh PA, Sparling PF, et al, Sexually Transmitted Diseases, 2nd ed, 1990, New York: Mcgraw-Hill, pp. 195-204.
138. Oriel JD. Natural history of genital warts. Br J Vener Dis 1971; 47: 1.
139. Oriel JD. Anal warts and anal coitus. Br J Vener Dis 1971; 47: 373.
140. Judson FN. Condyloma acuminatum of the oral cavity: A case report. Sex Transm Dis 1981; 8: 218.
141. Puranen M, Yliskoski M, Saarikoski S, et al. Vertical transmission of human papillomavirus from infected mothers to their newborn babies and persistence of the virus in childhood. Am J Obstet Gynecol 1996; 174: 694-9.
142. Tang CK. Congenital condylomata acuminata. Am J Obstet Gynecol 1978; 131: 912.
143. De Jong AR. Condylomata acuminata in children. Am J Dis Child 1982; 136: 704.
144. Weston TET, Nicol CS. Natural history of trichomonal infection in males. Br J Vener Dis 1963; 39: 251.
145. Honigberg B. Trichomonads of importance in human medicine. In: Kreier JP ed., Parasitic protozoa, 1978, vol 2, New York, Academic, pp. 275.
146. Latif AS, Mason PR, Marowa E. Urethral tricomoniasis in men. Sex Transm Dis 1987; 14: 9-11.
147. Jones JG. Trichomonas vaginalis infestation in sexually abused girls. Am J Dis Child 1985; 139: 846.
148. Al-Sahili FL. Neonatal Trichomonas vaginalis: Report of 3 cases and review of literature. Pediatrics 1974; 53: 196.
149. Szmuness W. On the role of sexual behaviour in the spread of hepatitis B infection. Ann Intern Med 1975; 83: 489.
150. Center for Disease Control. Changing patterns of groups at high risk for hepatitis B in the United States. MMWR 1988; 37: 429.
151. Mehendale SM, et al. Evidence of high prevalence and rapid transmission of HIV among individuals attending STDs clinics in Pune. Ind J Med Res 1996; 104: 327-35.
152. Kura KM, Hira S, Kohli M, et al. High occurrence of HBV among STDs clinic attenders in Bombay, India. Int J SYD AIDS 1998; 9: 231-3.

153. Villarejos V. Role of saliva, urine and faeces in transmission of type B hepatitis. N Engl J Med 1974; 291: 1375.
154. Koumans EH, Sternberg M, Gwinn M, et al. Geographic variation of HIV infection in childbearing women with syphilis in the United States. AIDS 2000; 14: 279-87.
155. Cook RL, Royce RA, Thomas JC, et al. What's driving an epidemic/ The spread of syphilis along an interstate highway in rural North Carolina. Am J Public Health. 1999; 89: 369-73.
156. Finelli L, Levine WC, Valentine J, et al. Syphilis outbreak assessment. Sex Transm Dis 2001; 28: 131-5.
157. Primary and secondary syphilis- United States, 1999. MMWR Morb Mortal Wkly Rep 2001; 50: 113-7.
158. Division of STDs Prevention. Sexually Transmitted Disease Prevention, 2000. Atlanta, Centers for Disease Control and Prevention, US Department of Health and Human Services, Public Health Service, 2001.
159. Kahn RH, Heffelfinger JD, Berman SM. Syphilis outbreaks among men who have sex with men. A public health trend of concern. Sex Transm Dis 2002; 29: 285-7.
160. Outbreak of primary and secondary syphilis-Guilford County, North Carolina, 1996-1997. MMWR Morb Mortal Wkly Rep 1998; 47: 1070-3.
161. Williams PB, Ekundayo O. Study of distribution and factors affecting syphilis epidemic among inner-city minorities of Baltimore. Public Health 2001; 115: 387-93.
162. Centers for Disease Control and Prevention (homepage on the Internet). Trends in reportable sexually transmitted diseases in the United States, 2005. Available from: http://www.cdc.gov/STDs/stats/trends2005.htm. [Last accessed on 2007 Feb 19].
163. Fenton KA, Nicoll A, Kinghorn G. Resurgence of syphilis in England: time for more radical and nationally coordinated approaches. Sex Transm Infect 2001; 77: 309-10.
164. Fennema JS, Cairo I, Coutinho RA. Substantial increase in gonorrhea and syphilis among clients of Amsterdam sexually transmitted diseases clinic. Ned Tijdschr Geneeskd 2000; 144: 602-3.
165. Bosman A, de Zwart O, Schop WA, et al. Increase of early syphilis in a red light district of Rotterdam (1995-1997) and preventive treatment. Ned Tijdschr Geneeskd 1999; 143: 2324-8.
166. Machovcova A, Konkolova R, Schmiedbergerova R, et al. Syphilis in the third millenium. Cas Lek Cesk 2002; 141: 96-100.
167. Bjekic M, Vlajinac H, Sipetic S, et al. Trends of gonorrhea and early syphilis in Belgrade, 1985-99. Sex Transm Infect 2001; 77: 387-9.
168. Diaconu JD, Benea V, Muresian D, et al. Incidence of sexually transmitted disease in Romania in the transition period. JEADV 1999; 12 (Suppl 2): 342.
169. Dencheva R, Spirov G, Gilina K, et al. Syphilis in Bulgaria-epidemiological survey 1990-1999. CEEDVA, Bulletin 2000; 2: 10-13.
170. Karieva MT, Umanov TM. Incidence of syphilis in the Republic of Uzbekistan: epidemiological aspects. JEADV 1997; 9 (Suppl 1): 228.
171. Todd J, Munguti K, Grosskurth H, et al. Risk factors for active syphilis and TPHA seroconversion in a rural African population. Sex Transm Infect 2001; 77: 37-45.
172. Behets F M-T, Andriamiadana J, Randrianasolo D, et al. Chancroid, primary syphilis, genital herpes and lymphogranuloma venereum in Antananarivo, Madagascar. J Infect Dis 1999; 180: 1382-5.
173. Temmerman M, Fonck K, Bashir F, et al. Declining syphilis prevalence in pregnant women in Nairobi since 1995: another success story in the STDs field? Int J STDs AIDS 1999; 10: 405-8.
174. Rathore AS, Ray K, Ramesh V, et al. Periodic syphilis profile in a New Delhi hospital. J Commun Dis 1999; 30: 153-7.
175. Ganesh R, Stanley A, Ganesh N, et al. Prevalence of neurosyphilis at Government Rajaji Hospital, Madurai, India. Int J STDs AIDS 1994; 5: 290-2.
176. Thakur TS, Sharma V, Goyal A, et al. Seroprevalence of HIV antibodies, Australia antigen and VDRL reactivity in Himachal Pradesh. Indian J Med Sci 1991; 45: 332-5.

177. Pandit DD, Angadi SA, Chavan MK, et al. Prevalence of VDRL sero-positivity in women in reproductive age group in an urban slum community in Bombay. Indian J Public Health 1995; 39(1): 4-7.
178. Garg S, Sharma N, Bhalla P, et al. Reproductive morbidity in an Indian urban slum: need for health action. Sex Transm Infect 2002; 78: 68-69.
179. Nanu A, Sharma SP, Chatterjee K, et al. Markers of transfusion-transmissible infections in north Indian voluntary and replacement blood donors: prevalence and trends 1989-1996. Vox Sang 1997; 73: 70-5.
180. Choudhary N, Ramesh V, Saraswat S, et al. Effectiveness of mandatory transmissible diseases screening in Indian blood donors. Indian J Med Res 1995; 101: 229-32.
181. Bhargava NC, Ray K, Kumari S, et al. Incidence of HIV versus VDRL antibody positivity in a major STDs clinic in Delhi. Indian J Sex Transm Dis 1987; 8: 44-6.
182. Murugan S, Srinivasan G, Kaleellulah MCA. Screening of blood donors for syphilis. Indian J Sex Transm Dis 1991; 12: 45-6.
183. Gupta AK, Saran R. Detection of antibodies to HIV-infection among high risk group in Bihar, India. Indian J Public Health 1993; 37: 54-6.
184. Warner L, Rochat RW, Fichtner RR, et al. Missed opportunities for congenital syphilis prevention in an urban Southeastern Hospital. Sex Transm Dis 2001; 28: 92-8.
185. Congenital syphilis- United States, 2000. MMWR 2001; 50: 573-7.
186. Southwick KL, Blanco S, Santander A, et al. Maternal and congenital syphilis in Bolivia, 1996: prevalence and risk factors. Bull World Health Organization 2001; 79: 33-42.
187. Anandam K, Seethamma R. Variegated presentation of congenital syphilis. Indian J Sex Transm Dis 1999; 20: 57-9.
188. McDermott J, Steketee R, Larsen S, et al. Syphilis associated perinatal and infant mortality in rural Malawi. Bull World Health Organization 1993; 71: 773-80.
189. Greenwood AM, D'Alessandro U, Sisay F, et al. Traponemal infection and the outcome of pregnancy in a rural area of The Gambia, West Africa. J Infect Dis 1992; 166: 842.
190. Rutger S. Syphilis in pregnancy: a medical audit in a rural district. Cent Afr J Med 1993; 39: 248-53.
191. Sharma M, Kumar B, Sharma SK, et al. Blood VDRL reactivity in STDs and antenatal clinics in Chandigarh. Indian J Sex Transm Dis 1986; 7: 14-5.
192. Rattan A, Maheshwari N, Sharma R, et al. Significance of low titre VDRL reactions. Indian J Sex Transm Dis 1987; 8: 5-6.
193. Nair D, Bhalla P, Mathur MD. A study of antenatal screening for syphilis. Indian J Sex Transm Dis 1996; 17: 54-6.
194. Vajpayee M, Seth P, Malhotra N. HIV and syphilis in pregnant women at a tertiary care hospital. Tropical Doctor 2001; 31: 56.
195. Schmid GP, Sanders Jr LL, Blount JH, et al. Chancroid in the United States- Reestablishment of an old disease. JAMA 1987; 258: 3265-68.
196. Dillon SM, Cummings M, Rajagopalan M, et al. Prospective analysis of genital ulcer disease in Brooklyn, New York. Clin Infect Dis 1997; 24: 945-50.
197. DiCarlo RP, Armentor BS, Martin DH. Chancroid epidemiology in New Orleans men. J Infect Dis 1995; 172: 446-52.
198. Mertz KJ, Weiss JB, Webb RM, et al. An investigation of genital ulcers in Jackson, Mississippi, with use of multiplex polymerase chain reaction assay: High prevalence of chancroid and human immunodeficiency virus infection. J Infect Dis 1998; 178: 1060-6.
199. Morel P, Casin I, Gandiol C, et al. An epidemic of chancroid. 587 cases. Nouv Presse Med 1982; 11: 655-6.
200. Kamali A, Nunn AJ, Mulder DW, et al. Seroprevalence and incidence of genital ulcer infections in a rural Ugandan population. Sex Transm Infect 1999; 75: 98-102.
201. Hira SK. Sexually transmitted diseases in the era of AIDS. AIDS watch. WHO South-East Asia Region Newletter 1997; 2: 1-2.
202. Annual Reports of the Medical Officer of Health for Durban 1996, 1997.
203. Bassa AG, Hoosen AA, Moodley J, et al. Granuloma inguinale (Donovanosis) in women. An analysis of 61 cases from Durban, South Africa. Sex Transm Dis 1993; 20: 164-7.

204. Siva D, Salgado U, Macedo C, et al. Donovanosis in Para. Rev Soc Bras Med Trop 1991; 24: 251-2.
205. Kuberski T, Philips P, Tabua TW. Status of granuloma inguinale in Papua New Guinea. P N G Med J 1979; 22: 5-12.
206. Jamkhedkar PP, Hira SK, Shroff HJ, et al. Clinico-epidemiologic features of granuloma inguinale in the era of acquired immune deficiency syndrome. Sex Transm Dis 1998; 25: 196-200.
207. O'Farrell N, Hammond M. HLA antigens in donovanosis (granuloma inguinale). Genitourin Med 1991; 67: 400-02.
208. Sehgal VN, Jain MK. Pattern of epidemics of Donovanosis in the nonendemic region. Int J Dermatol 1988; 27: 396-9.
209. Abrams AJ. Lymphogranuloma venereum. JAMA 1968; 205: 199.
210. Division of STDs Prevention. Sexually Transmitted Disease Surveillance, 1997. U.S. Department of Health and Human Services, Public Heaith Service. Atlanta, Center for Disease Control, September 1998.
211. Department of Health. New cases of genitourinary medicine clinics in England. Annual figures 1995, Summary information from KC 60. London, 1996.
212. French P, Ison CA, Macdonald N. Lymphogranuloma venereum in the United Kingdom. Sex Transm Infect 2005; 81: 97-8.
213. Ndinya-Achola JO. Presumptive specific clinical diagnosis of genital ulcer disease in a primary health care setting in Nairobi. Int J STDs AIDS 1996; 7: 201-5.
214. Mabey DCW. Aetiology of genital ulceration in the Gambia. Genitourin Med 1987; 63: 312-5.
215. O'Farrel. Genital ulcer disease: accuracy of clinical diagnosis and strategies to improve control in Durban, South Africa. Genitourin Med 1994; 70: 7-11.
216. Ray K. Usefulness of immunoperoxidase for serodiagnosis of genital chlamydial infections. Ind J Med Res 1993; 97: 67-71.
217. Viravan C. A prospective clinical and bacteriological study of inguinal buboes in Thai men. Clin Infect Dis 1996; 22: 233-9.
218. Piot P. Sexually Transmitted Disease. In: Warren KS, Mahmoud AAF, eds. Tropical and geographical medicine. 2nd ed. New York: McGraw-Hill, 1990: 894-910.
219. Brathwaite AR. A comparison of prevalence rates of genital ulcers among persons attending a sexually transmitted disease clinic in Jamaica. West Indian Med J 1997; 46: 67-71.
220. Frieda MT. Chancroid, primary syphilis, genital herpes and lymphogranuloma venereum in Antananarivo, Madagascar. J Infect Dis 1999; 180: 1382-5.
221. Luk NM. Lymphogranuloma venereum. In: Social Hygiene Handbook, Handbook of Dermatology and Venereology, 2nd ed, 1996: 1-14.
222. Chua SH. Genital ulcer disease in patients attending a public sexually transmitted disease clinic in Singapore: an epidemiological study. Ann Acad Med Singapore 1995; 24: 510-4.
223. Schachter J. Lymphogranuloma venereum and other non ocular *Chlamydia trachomatis* infections. Hobson D, Holmes KK, eds. Washington, American Society of Microbiology, 1977: 91-7.
224. Koteen H. Lymphogranuloma venereum. Medicine 1945; 24: 1.
225. Annamuthoda H. Rectal Lymphogranuloma venereum in Jamaica. Ann R Coll Surg Engl 1961; 29: 141.
226. Chamber'S Infectious Diseases: Bacterial and Chlamydial. In: Lawrence M, Tierney Jr, eds. Current Medical Diagnosis and Treatment, 1998, Stamford, CT: Appleton and Lange, 1997.
227. Tapsall JW. Surveillance of antibiotic susceptibility of *Neisseria gonorrhoeae* in the WHO western pacific region 1992-1994. Genitourin Med 1997; 73: 355-61
228. Cates W Jr. Sexually transmitted diseases, pelvic inflammatory disease and infertility - an epidemiologic update. Epidemiol Rev 1990; 12: 199-220.
229. Berglund T, Fredlund H, Giesecke J. Epidemiology of the re-emergence of gonorrhea in Sweden. Sex Transm Dis 2001; 28: 111-4.
230. Low N. Success and failure in gonorrhea control. Dermatologic Clinics 1998; 16: 713-20.
231. Eng TR. Reported rates of gonorrhea in selected developed countries. In: The hidden epidemic: Confronting sexually transmitted diseases. Washington DC, National Academy Press, 1997, p. 29.

232. Division of STDs Prevention. Sexually transmitted disease surveillance, 1999. US Department of Health and Human Services, Public Health Service. Atlanta: Centers for Disease Control and Prevention, October 2000: 1-112.
233. Datta SD, Sternberg M, Johnson RE, et al. Gonorrhea and Chlamydia in the United States among Persons 14 to 39 Years of Age, 1999 to 2002. Annals Intern Med 2007; 147: 89-96.
234. Wright PA. Relative and seasonal incidences of the sexually transmitted diseases: A two-year statistical review. Br J Vener Dis 1978; 54: 433.
235. Hughes G. Investigation of the increased incidence of gonorrhea diagnosed in genitourinary medicine clinics in England, 1994-1996. Sex Transm Infect 2000; 76: 18-24.
236. Berglund T, Asikainen T, Grützmeier S,et al. The epidemiology of gonorrhea among men who have sex with men in Stockholm, Sweden, 1990-2004. Sex Transm Dis. 2007 Mar; 34: 174-9.
237. Fox KK. Gonorrhoea in the United States, 1981-1996: Demographic and Geographic trends. Sex Transm Dis 1998; 25: 386-93.
238. Cates W Jr. Sexually transmitted diseases, pelvic inflammatory disease and infertility - an epidemiologic update. Epidemiol Rev 1990; 12: 199-220.
239. Rahman M. Etiology of sexually transmitted infections among street-based female sex workers in Dhaka, Bangladesh. J Clin Microbiol 2000; 38: 1244-6.
240. Divekar AA, Gogate AS, Shivkar LK, et al. Disease prevalence in women attending the STDs clinic in Mumbai, India. Int J STDs AIDS 2000; 11: 45-8.
241. Kaur H, Saini JS, Jasmeen. Prevalence of gonorrhoea in Punjabi women. J Obstet Gynecol India 1995; 45: 100-5.
242. Kaur S, Kumar B, Malhotra S, et al. Screening for gonococal infection in patients attending gynaecological clinics. Indian J Sex Transm Dis 1986; 7: 44-6.
243. Hook EW. Gonococcal Infections. Ann Int Med 1985; 102: 229-43.
244. Tchoudomirova K, Nuhov Ph, Tchapanova A. Prevalence, epidemiological and clinical correlates of genital *Chlamydia trachomatis* infection. JEADV 1998; 11: 214-20.
245. Mertz KJ, McQuillan GM, Levine WC, et al. A pilot study of the prevalence of chlamydial infection in a national household survey. Sex Transm Dis 1998; 25: 225-8.
246. Center for Disease Control. Ten leadind nationally notifiable infectious diseases- United States, 1995. MMWR 1996; 45: 883-4.
247. *Chlamydia trachomatis* genital infections- United States, 1995. JAMA 1997; 277: 952-3.
248. Marrazzo JM, White CL, Krekeler B, et al. Community-based urine screening for *Chlamydia trachomatis* with a ligase chain reaction assay. Ann Intern Med 1997; 127: 796-803.
249. Oakeshott P, Hay P. General practice update.: chlamydia infection in women Br J Gen Pract 1995; 45: 615-20.
250. Stokes T. Screening for chlamydia in general practice: a literature review and summary of the evidence. J Public Health Med 1997; 19: 222-32.
251. Shafer MA, Schachter J, Moncada J, et al. Evaluation of urine-based screening strategies to detect *Chlamydia trachomatis* among sexually active asymptomatic young males. JAMA 1993; 270: 2065-70.
252. Benn PD, Rooney G, Carder C,et al.*Chlamydia trachomatis* and *Neisseria gonorrhoeae* infection and the sexual behaviour of men who have sex with men. Sex Transm Infect. 2007; 83: 106-12.
253. Thompson J, Lin M, Halliday L. Australia's notifiable disease status, 1998. Annual report of the National Notifiable Diseases Surveillance System. Commun Dis Intell 1999; 23: 277-305.
254. Donova B. Rising prevalence of genital *Chlamydia trachomatis* infection in heterosexual patients at the Sydney Sexual Health Center, 1994 to 2000. Commun Dis Intell 2002; 26: 51-5.
255. Garland SM, Malatt A, Tabrizi S, et al. *Chlamydia trachomatis* conjunctivitis. Prevalence and association with genital tract infection. Med J Aust 1995; 162: 363-6.

256. Harms G, Matull R, Randrianasolo D, et al. Pattern of sexually transmitted diseases in a Malagasy population. Sex Transm Dis 1994; 21: 315-20.
257. Azenabor AA, Eghafona NO. Association of *Chlamydia trachomatis* antibodies with genital contact disease in Benin City, Nigeria. Trop Med Int Health 1997; 2: 389-92.
258. Bai H, Bo N, Huan Li, et al. Prevalence of genital *Chlamydia trachomatis* infection in selected populations in China. Sex Transm Dis 1995; 383-4.
259. Thongkrajai P, Thongkrajai E, Pengsaa P, et al. The prevalence of *Chlamydia trachomatis* infection in rural Thai women. Southeast Asian J Trop Med Public Health 1999; 30: 52-7.
260. Bogaerts J, Ahmed J, Akhter N, et al. Sexually transmitted infections among married women in Dhaka, Bangladesh: unexpected high prevalence of herpes simplex type 2 infection. Sex Transm Infect 2001; 77: 114-9.
261. Gopalkrishna V, Aggarwal N, Malhotra VL, et al. *Chlamydia trachomatis* and human papillomavirus infection in Indian women with sexually transmitted diseases and cervical precancerous and cancerous lesions. Clin Microbiol Infect 2000; 6: 88-93.
262. Rastogi S, Kapur S, Salhan S, et al. *Chlamydia trachomatis* infection in pregnancy: risk factors for an adverse outcome. Br J Biomed Sci 1999; 56: 94-8.
263. Paul VK, Singh M, Gupta U, et al. *Chlamydia trachomatis* infection among pregnant women: prevalence and prenatal importance. Natl Med J India 1999; 12: 11-4.
264. Mittal A, Kapur S, Gupta S. Screening for genital chlamydial infection in symptomatic women. Indian J Med Res 1993; 98: 119-23.
265. Joshi JV, Palayekar S, Hazari KT, et al. The prevalence of *Chlamydia trachomatis* in young women. Natl Med J India 1994; 7: 57-9.
266. Shrikhande SN, Joshi SG, Zodpey SP, et al. *Chlamydia trachomatis* in pelvic inflammatory disease. Indian J Pathol Microbiol 1995; 38: 181-4.
267. Singh V, Sehgal A, Satyanarayana L, et al. Clinical presentation of gynaecologic infections among Indian women. Obstet Gynecol 1995; 85: 215-9.
268. Brabin L, Gogate A, Gogate S, et al. Reproductive tract infections, gynaecological morbidity and HIV seroprevalence among women in Mumbai, India. Bull World Health Organization 1998; 76: 277-87.
269. Sharma M, Nayak N, Malhotra S, et al. Chlamydiazyme test for rapid detection of *Chlamydia trachomatis*. Indian J Med Res 1989; 89: 87-91.
270. Brugha R, Keersmaeker K, Renton A, et al. Genital herpes infection: a review. Int J Epidemiol 1997; 26: 698-709.
271. Mertz GJ. Epidemiology of genital herpes infections. Infect Dis Clin North Am. 1993; 7: 825-39.
272. Corey L, Hansfield HH. Genital herpes and Public Health. Addressing a global problem. JAMA 2000; 283: 791-4.
273. Fleming DT, Mcquillan GM, Johnson RE, et al. Herpes simplex virus type 2 in the United States, 1976 to 1994. N Engl J Med 1997; 337: 1105-11.
274. Johnson RE, Nahmias AJ, Magder LS, et al. A seroepidemiologic survey of the prevalence of herpes simplex virus type 2 infection in the United States. N Engl J Med 1990; 321: 8-12.
275. Koutsky L, Stevens CE, Holmes KK, et al. Underdiagnosis of genital herpes by current clinical and viral isolation procedures. N Engl J Med 1992; 326: 1533-9.
276. Buchacz K, McFarland W, Hernandez M, et al. Prevalence and correlates of herpes simplex virus type 2 infection in a population-based survey of young women in low-income neighbourhoods of North California. The Young Women's survey team. Sex Transm Dis 2000; 27: 393-400.
277. Mindel A, Taylor J, Tideman RL, et al. Neonatal herpes prevention: a minor public health problem in some communities. Sex Transm Infect 2000; 76: 287-91.
278. Nahmias AJ, Lee FK, Beckman-Nahmias S. Seroepidemiological and sociological patterns of herpes simplex virus infection in the world. Scand J Infect Dis Suppl 1990; 69: 19-36.
279. Van Benthem BHB, Spaargaren J, van den Hoek JAR, et al. Prevalence and risk factors of HSV-1 and HSV-2 antibodies in European HIV infected women. Sex Transm Infect 2001; 77: 120-4.

280. Vyse AJ, Gay NJ, Slomka MJ, et al. The burden of infection with HSV-1 and HSV-2 in England and Wales: implications for the changing epidemiology of genital herpes. Sex Transm Infect 2000; 76: 183-7.
281. Roest RW, van der Meijden WI, van Dijk G, et al. Prevalence and association between herpes simplex virus types 1 and 2-specific antibodies in atendees at a sexually transmitted disease clinic. Int J Epidemiol 2001; 30: 580-8.
282. Van der Laar MJW, Termorshuizen F, Slomka MJ, et al. Prevalence and correlates of herpes simplex virus type 2 infection: evaluation of behavioural risk factors. Int J Epidemiol 1998; 27: 127-34.
283. Forsgren M. Genital herpes simplex virus infections and incidence of neonatal disease in Sweden. Scand J Infect Dis 1990; 69(Suppl 1): 37-41.
284. Nilsen A, Myrmel H. Changing trends in genital herpes simplex virus infection in Bergen, Norway. Acta Obstet Gynecol Scand 2000; 79: 693-6.
285. Eskild A, Jeansson S, Jenum PA. Antibodies against herpes simplex virus type 2 among pregnant women in Norway. Tidsskr Nor Laegeforen 1999; 119: 2323-6.
286. International Herpes Management forum. Report from the sixth Annual meeting of the IHMF. Herpes 1999; 6: 1-27.
287. Uribe-Salas F, Hernandez-Avila M, Juarez-Figueroa L, et al. Risk factors for herpes simplex virus type 2 among female commercial sex workers in Mexico city. Int J STDs AIDS 1999; 10: 105-11.
288. Carvalho M, de Carvalho S, Pannuti CS, et al. Prevalence of herpes simplex type 2 antibodies and a clinical history of herpes in three different populations in Campinas city, Brazil. Int J Infect Dis 1998-99; 3: 94-8.
289. Da Rosa-Santos OL, Goncalves Da Silva A, Pereira AC Jr. Herpes simplex virus type 2 in Brazil: seroepidemiologic survey. Int J Dermatol 1996; 35: 794-6.
290. Korenromp EL, Bakker R, De Vlas SJ, et al. Can behaviour change explain increase in the proportion of genital ulcers attributable to herpes in sub-Saharan Africa. A simulation modeling study. Sex Transm Dis 2001; 29: 228-30.
291. Weiss HA, Buve A, Robinson NJ, et al. The epidemiology of HSV-2 infection and its asociation with HIV infection in four urban African populations. AIDS 2001; 15(Suppl 4): S 97-108.
292. Chua SH, Cheong WK. Genital ulcer disease in patients attending a public sexually transmitted disease clinic in Singapore: an epidemiologic study. Ann Acad Med Singapore 1995; 24: 510-4.
293. Zainah S, Sinniah M, Cheong YM, et al. A microbiological study of genital ulcers in Kuala Lumpur. Med J Malaysia 1991; 46: 274-82.
294. Hudson BJ, van der Mehden W, Lupiwa T, et al. A survey of sexually transmitted diseases in five STDs clinics in Papua New Guinea. PNG Med J 1994; 37: 152-60.
295. Beyrer C, Jitwatcharanan K, Natpratan C, et al. Molecular methods for the diagnosis of genital ulcer disease in a sexually transmitted disease clinic population in Northern Thailand: predominance of herpes simplex virus infection. J Infect Dis 1998; 178: 243-6.
296. Puthavathana P, Kanyok R, Horthongkham N, et al. Prevalence of herpes simplex virus infection in patients suspected of genital herpes; a virus typing by type specific fluorescent monoclonal antibodies. J Med Assoc Thai 1998; 81: 260-4.
297. Risbud A, Chan-Tack K, Gadkari D, et al. The etiology of genital ulcer disease by multiplex polymerase chain reaction and relationship to HIV infection among patients attending sexually transmitted disease clinics in Pune, India. Sex Transm Dis 1999; 26: 55-61.
298. Ambhore NA, Thakar YS, Gaval SR, et al. Seroprevalence of herpes simplex virus type-2 in STDs patients with genital ulcers. Indian J Sex Transm Dis 1998; 19: 81-4.
299. Jacob M, Rao PS, Sridharan G, et al. Epidemiology and clinical profile of genital herpes. Indian J Med Res 1989; 89: 4-11.
300. Enzensberger R, Braun W, July C, et al. Prevalence of antibodies to human herpesviruses and hepatitis B virus in patients at different stages of HIV infection. Infection 1991; 19: 140-5.

301. Schacker T, Zeh J, Hu HL, et al. Frequency of symptomatic and asymptomatic herpes simplex virus type 2 reactivations among human immunodeficiency virus-infected men. J Infect Dis 1998; 178: 1616-22.
302. Kumarasamy N, Soloman S, Madhivanan P, et al. Dermatologic manifestations among human immunodeficiency virus patients in south India. Int J Dermatol 2000; 39: 192-95.
303. Whitley RJ. Neonatal herpes simplex virus infections. J Med Virol 1993; Suppl 1: 13-21.
304. Gaytant MA, Steegers EA, van Cromvoirt PL, et al. Incidence of herpes neonatorum in Netherlands. Ned Tijdschr Geneeskd 2000; 144: 1832-36.
305. Tookey P, Peckham CS. Neonatal herpes simplex virus infection in the British Isles. Pediatr Perinat Epidemiol 1996; 10: 432-42.
306. Gutierrez KM, Meira S, Halpern F, et al. The epidemiology of neonatal herpes simplex virus infections in California from 1895 to 1995. J Infect Dis 1999; 180: 199-202.
307. Patrick DM, Dawar M, Cook DA, et al. Antenatal seroprevalence of Herpes simplex virus type 2 (HSV-2) in Canadian women. Sex Transm Dis 2001; 28: 424-8.
308. Khanna J, Van Look PFA, Griffin PD. Reproductive health: a key to a brighter future.: Biennial report 1990-91, Geneva, World Health Organization, 1992.
309. Koutsky L. Epidemiology of genital human papillomavirus infection. Am J Med 1997; 102: 3-8.
310. Bekkers RL, Massuger LF, Bulten J, et al. Epidemiological and clinical aspects of human papillomavirus detection in the prevention of cervical cancer. Rev Med Virol. 2004; 14: 95-105.
311. Centers for Disease Control and Prevention: The challenge of STDs prevention in the United States. Atlanta, Centers for Disease Control and Prevention, Division of STDs Prevention, 1996.
312. Severson J, Evans TY, Lee P, et al. Human papillomavirus infections: epidemiology, pathogenesis and therapy. J Cutan Med Surg 2001; 5: 43-60.
313. Chuang TY, HO P, Kurland LT, et al. Condyloma acuminatum in Rochester, Minnesota, 1950-1978. I. Epidemiology and clinical features. Arch Dermatol 1984; 120: 469-75.
314. Slavinsky J, Kissinger P, Burger L, et al. Seroepidemiology of low and high oncogenic risk types of human papillomavirus in a predominantly male cohort of STDs clinic patients. Int J STDs AIDS 2001; 12: 516-23.
315. Giuliano AR, Papenfuss M, Abrahamsen M, et al. Human papillomavirus infection at the United States- Mexico border: implications for cervical cancer prevention and control. Cancer Epidemiol Biomarkers Prev 2001; 10: 129-36.
316. Lazcano-Ponce E, Herrero R, Musoz N, et al. Epidemiology of HPV infection among Mexican women with normal cervical cytology. Int J Cancer 2001; 91: 412-20.
317. Cavalcanti SM, Zardo LG, Passos MR, et al. Epidemiological aspects of human papillomavirus infection and cervical cancer in Brazil. J Infect 2000; 40: 80-87.
318. Lopes F, Latorre MR, Campos Pignatari AC, et al. HIV, HPV and syphilis prevalence in a women's penitentiary in the city of Sao Paulo, 1997-1998. Cad Saude Publica 2001; 17: 1473-80.
319. Koutsky LA, Galloway DA, Holmes KK. Epidemiology of genital human papillomavirus infection. Epidemiol Rev 1988; 10: 122-63.
320. Nyari T, Cseh I, Woodwart M, et al. Screening for human papillomavirus infection in asymptomatic women in Hungary. Human Reprod 2001; 16: 2235-37.
321. Bosch FX, Munoz N, de Sanjose S, et al. Human papillomavirus and cervical intraepithelial neoplasia grade III/ carcinoma in situ: A case-control study in Spain and Columbia. Cancer Epidemiol Biomarkers Prev 1993; 2: 415-22.
322. Bowden FJ, Paterson BA, Mein J, et al. Estimating the prevalence of *Trichomonas vaginalis*, *Chlamydia trachomatis*, *Neisseria gonorrhoeae* and human papillomavirus infection in indigenous women in northern Australia. Sex Transm Infect 1999; 75: 431-4.
323. Parkin DM, Pisani P, Ferlay J. Estimates of the worldwide incidence of 25 major cancers in 1990. Int J Cancer 1999; 80: 827-41.

324. Mayaud P, Gill DK, Weiss HA, et al. The interrelation of HIV, cervical human papillomavirus and neoplasia among antenatal clinic attenders in Tanzania. Sex Transm Infect 2001; 77: 248-54.
325. World Health Organization (homepage on the internet). Trends in sexually transmitted infections and HIV in the European region, 1980-2005. Technical briefing document 01B/06 Copenhagen; 12 September 2006. Available from: http://www.euro.who.int/Document/RC56/etb01b.pdf.
326. Saranath D, Khan Z, Tandle AT, et al. HPV 16/18 prevalence in cervical lesions/cancers and p53 genotypes in cervical cancer patients from India. Gynecol Oncol 2002; 86: 157-62.
327. Menon MM, Sinha MR, Doctor VM, Detection of human papillomavirus types in precancerous and cancerous lesions of cervix in Indian women: a preliminary report. Indian J Cancer 1995; 32: 154-9.
328. Chatterjee R, Roy A, Basu S, et al. Detection of type specific human papillomavirus DNA in cervical cancers of Indian women. Indian J Pathol Microbiol 1995: 38: 33-42.
329. Jamison JH, Kaplan DW, Hamman R, et al. Spectrum of genital human papillomavirus infection in a female adolescent population. Sex Transm Dis 1995; 22: 236-43.
330. Tanaka H, Karube A, Tanaka T, et al. Much higher risk of premalignant and malignant cervical diseases in younger women positive for HPV 16 than in older women positive for HPV 16. Microbiol Immunol 2001; 45: 323-6.
331. Tortolero-Luna G. Epidemiology of genital human papillomavirus. Haematol Oncol Clin North Am 1999; 13: 245-56.
332. Palefsky JM, Holly EA, Ralston ML, et al. Prevalence and risk factors for anal human papillomavirus infection in human immunodeficiency virus-positive and high-risk HIV-negative women. J Infect Dis 2001; 183: 383-91.
333. Palefsky JM, Holly EA, Ralston ML, et al. Prevalence and risk factors for human papillomavirus infection in human immunodeficiency virus-positive and HIV-negative homosexual men. J Infect Dis 1998; 177: 361-67.
334. Ahdieh L, Klein RS, Burk R, et al. Prevalence, incidence and type-specific persistence of human papillomavirus in human immunodeficiency virus-positive and HIV-negative women. J Infect Dis 2001; 184: 682-90.
335. Volkow P, Rubi S, Lizano M, et al. High prevalence of oncogenic human papillomavirus in the genital tract of women with human immunodeficiency virus. Gynecol Oncol 2001; 82(1): 27-31.
336. Delmas MC, Larsen C, van Benthem B, et al. Cervical squamous intraepithelial lesions in HIV-infected women: prevalence, incidence and regression. AIDS 2000; 14: 1775-84.
337. Holmes F, Borek D, Owen-Kummer M, et al. Anal cancer in women. Gastroenterology 1988; 95: 107-11.
338. Melbye M, Rabkin C, Frisch M, et al. Changing patterns of anal cancer incidence in the United States, 1940-1989. Am J Epidemiol 1994; 139: 772-80.
339. Daling JR, Weiss NS, Hislop TG, et al. Sexual practices, sexually transmitted diseases and the incidence of anal cancer. N Engl J Med 1987; 317: 973-77.
340. Al-Ghamdi A, Freedman D, Miller D, et al. Vulvar squamous cell carcinoma in young women: a clinicopathologic study of 21 cases. Gynecol Oncol 2002; 84(1): 94-101.
341. Thomas K, Thyagarajan SP, jeyaseelan l, et al. Community prevalence of sexually transmitted diseases and human immunodeficiency virus infection in Tamil Nadu, India: A probability proportional to size cluster survey. Natl Med J India 2002; 15: 135-40.
342. Jaiswal AK, Banerjee S, Matety AR, Grover S. Changing trends in sexually transmitted diseases in North Eastern India. Indian J Dermatol Venereol Leprol 2002;68:65-66
343. Bansal KN, Khare KA, Upadhyay PO. Pattern of sexually transmitted diseases in and Around Udaipur. Indian J Dermatol Venereol Leprol 1988; 54: 90-2.

344. Mohanty J, Das KB, Mishra C. Clinical profile of sexually transmitted diseases in Cuttack. Indian J Dermatol Venereol Leprol 1995; 61: 143-4.

345. Mishra M, Mishra S, Singh PC, et al. Pattern of sexually transmitted diseases at VSS Medical College. Indian J Dermatol Venereol Leprol 1998; 64: 231-2.

2 SEXUALLY TRANSMITTED DISEASES IN WOMEN AND REPRODUCTIVE HEALTH

H R Jerajani, Shubha Melkote

In this chapter

INTRODUCTION

It is difficult to predict the true incidence and prevalence of sexually transmitted diseases (STDs), especially in the Indian context. A compilation of reported prevalence rates of STDs among men and women in hospitals and community-based studies is given in chapter 1 (Tables 1.6, 1.7, 1.13). The figures suggest that the prevalence of RTIs/STIs in both men and women is high not only among high-risk population groups but also among low-risk groups in many parts of the country, including rural areas.[1]

Sexually Transmitted Diseases in Women

There are principal differences in clinical manifestations, disease susceptibility and transmission and long-term reproductive health consequences of STDs between men and women. These are due to the inherent differences between both sexes in their anatomy and physiology of reproductive organs, sexual behaviours and health care utilization and compliance.

CLINICAL MANIFESTATIONS

STD in women more or less follow the same clinical course as in men. However, there are some differences. Women infected with STDs are more likely to be either completely asymptomatic or minimally symptomatic as compared to men. Even when symptoms do occur, for anatomical reasons, either painless lesions may go unnoticed, like primary chancre which is most commonly located on the cervix, or abnormal discharge may be attributed to other infectious processes like urinary tract or vaginal infections rather than to STDs. These factors in turn delay diagnosis and treatment, thus increasing disease transmission and morbidity. Traditionally painful conditions like chancroid are less painful in women, but genital herpes infection in women tends to be associated with a greater number of lesions and systemic symptoms than in men. These differences have to be borne in mind during the management of STDs in women.

SUSCEPTIBILITY TO STIs[2]

The susceptibility and the outcome of various STDs are modulated by changes in the anatomy, physiology, and cellular morphology of the genital tract that begins at puberty, and continues through monthly menstrual cycles, pregnancy and also follows menopause. In the neonatal period, due to the effect of maternal estrogens, the vagina is lined by stratified squamous epithelium. Until puberty it gets replaced by thin atrophic columnar epithelium. Estrogen stimulation at puberty restores the thicker, glycogen-laden stratified squamous epithelium while columnar epithelium is limited to the cervix. These evolving changes influence STD acquisition. Chlamydia and gonococci infect columnar and cuboidal epithelial cells whereas HPV, HSV, trichomonas and candida are associated with stratified squamous epithelial cells. From infancy to adolescence,s vaginal ecology shifts from flora dominated by enteric organisms to lactobacilli. Lactobacilli make the vaginal fluid more acidic and also elaborate antibacterial substances like H_2O_2 that are inhibitory to other pathogens and perhaps have a protective effect on HIV transmission.

Cervical mucus acts as a functional barrier both to the attachment of pathogens to epithelial surfaces and also to their ascent to the uterus and fallopian tubes. High levels of estrogen stimulate copious mucus secretion which is high during neonatal period, at puberty, and during periovulatory phase. Hence PID is commoner in older adolescents and adult women.

The opening of the endocervical canal occurs the at nine or ten years of age and could explain the increased risk of PID in peripubertal girls as compared to their younger counterparts.

Menstrual cycle influences the risk of upper genital tract infections in women; symptomatic gonococcal and chlamydial PID are more common in the first week of cycle.

Contraceptives are also important factors. While condoms and diaphragms act as mechanical barriers, spermicides like nanoxynol are capable of killing gonococci, chlamydia, treponemes, trichomonads, HSV and HIV. Users of intrauterine devices are at a 1.5 to 2 times increased risk of PID. Hormonal oral contraceptives increase the risk of chlamydial infection by increasing the size of zone of ectopy. However, they decrease the severity and frequency of PID.

TRANSMISSION OF STIs

Sexual behaviours greatly influence disease transmission. Due to the early age of marriage, women in India initiate sexual activity at an early age. The risk of STDs is determined by partner number, rate of partner change and sexual practice, which are in turn determined by education, religion and cultural practices.

The available data, though not definite, suggest that the transmission of STD pathogens like HIV, HBV, gonococci and chlamydiae have a more efficient male-to-female than female-to-male transmission due to the extended period of contact with pathogens after sexual exposure.[3]

Consequences on Reproductive Health

The most threatening aspect of an STI in women is the adverse effect it can have on fertility. Diseases like gonorrhoea and chlamydia are implicated in pelvic inflammatory diseases cause significant morbidity and long-term changes that may result in infertility, ectopic pregnancy or recurrent abortions. STIs in pregnancy pose a greater problem due to following reasons[4]:

Effect of pregnancy on infection: Immunological and anatomical changes and changes in the microbial flora of the lower genital tract can alter the natural course of many of the sexually acquired infections. For example, there is accelerated progression or expression of HPV, augmented frequency of severity and recurrence of genital herpes.

Effect of infection on pregnancy: STIs, even the asymptomatic ones, can adversely a effect the outcome of pregnancy as they increase the chances of spontan-eous abortions, chorioamnionitis, preterm labour, premature rupture of membranes and pre-erm births, low birth weight, still births and postpartum infections.

Transmission from mother to child: This can occur in utero, intrapartum or postpartum, and its prevention is a great public health challenge.

Problems in diagnosis and management: Many first-line therapies in the management of STIs may be contraindicated in pregnancy. In our society, the stigma associated with acquiring STDs is especially more in women. This greatly limits the already poor healthcare-seeking behaviour. Even when they seek medical attention, the detection of STDs is more difficult in women as vaginitis and cervicitis are the most commonly encountered syndromes. Clinical criteria alone lack sensitivity and specificity for diagnosis of non-ulcerative STDs in women. Due to the large number of normally resident flora in the lower genital tract, simple diagnostic methods like gram stain, culture and fluorescent monoclonal antibody staining for pathogens are less likely to yield any conclusive results. On the other hand, accurate diagnosis of STDs in men can be made on clinical grounds and simple inexpensive investigative methods.

The vulnerability to acquiring STDs as well as its long-term adverse effects is disproportionately more in women than men. Therefore, it is essential that interventions for reduction of risk factors, transmission and treatment be tailored and targeted with regard to these differences in gender perspectives, so as to have the greatest impact.

REPRODUCTIVE HEALTH

The International Conference on Population and Development held in Cairo in 1994 defined reproductive health as a state of physical, mental, and social well-being in all matters relating to the reproductive system and to its functions and processes at all stages of life. Reproductive health implies that people are able to have a satisfying and safe sex life, and that they have the capability to reproduce and the freedom to decide if, when, and how often to do so. Implicit in this are the rights of men and women to be informed and to have access to safe, effective, affordable and acceptable methods of family planning of their choice, and the right to appropriate healthcare services that enable women to safely go through pregnancy and childbirth.[5] Key concerns of reproductive health include the treatment and control of STIs that not only cause significant morbidity but also increase vulnerability to HIV infection and mother-to-child transmission. Another important focus is or adolescents, whose lack of awareness, information and skills during their initiation of sexual relationships make them especially vulnerable to acquiring and transmitting STDs and also to unwanted pregnancies.

Reproductive health is an important part of general health. It is crucial during adolescence and adulthood, sets the stage for health beyond reproductive years for both women and men, and affects the health of the next generation as the health of the newborn is largely a function of the mother's health and nutrition status and of her access to health care. Failure to deal with reproductive health problems at any stage in life sets the scene for later health and developmental problems.

As a result of the above understanding, India has moved to a "target-free" dispensation of reproductive health services through a demand-driven, decentralized, client-centered, participatory planning approach. There has been a paradigm shift whereby the hitherto segregated programmes were converged under the common Reproductive and Child Health (RCH) programme.[6]

The RCH programme also incorporates the com-ponents covered under the Child Survival & Safe Motherhood Programme and additional compo-nents for management of RTIs and STIs, family welfare, adolescent health care and family life education. This programme commenced in 1997 and the first phase was implemented by June 2004. The RCH programmes Phase-II was launched with effect from April 1, 2005 for a period of 5 years.[7]

In many countries, the HIV/AIDS pandemic has compelled the fields of sexual and reproductive health (SRH) and HIV/AIDS to better leverage their strengths and address missed opportunities. the Convergence of HIV and SRH services can mean just mutual referrals. It can also mean providing HIV behaviour change communication (BCC) within an SRH setting, and vice versa, or sharing training and training resources.

Convergence of activities or interventions, amd convergence of management, administrative, and support functions may result in more efficient infrastructure[8] as well.

CHLAMYDIAL INFECTION

Approximately 75% of infected women and 50% of men have no symptoms.[9] In women it causes bartholinitis, cervicitis, urethritis, salpingitis, and endometritis similar to that of gonococcal infection, but the majority of them remain asymptomatic and without any visible signs of infection. As they harbour the infection for longer periods of time, they are at a risk of the infection colonizing the endometrial mucosa and the fallopian tubes, leading to pelvic inflammatory disease (PID). Chlamydial PID can cause tubal occlusion and subsequent infertility, or partial occlusion with an increased risk of ectopic pregnancy.[10,11] If the infection remains undetected and therefore untreated, 40% will develop PID, 20% will become infertile, 18% will experience debilitating, chronic pelvic pain, and 9% will have a life-threatening tubal pregnancy.[9]

Chlamydia is known to cause conjugal infection. When female partners of *C. trachomatis* positive and *C. trachomatis*-negative men with non-gonoccocal urethritis were examined, 60-70% of the former and 0-10% of the latter group were found to have *C.trachomatis*-induced cervicitis.[12] Chlamydia infection may also result in adverse outcomes of pregnancy, neonatal conjunctivitis and pneumonia. In addition, recent research has shown that women infected with chlamydia have a 3–5-fold increased risk of acquiring HIV.

Untreated chlamydia in men typically causes urethral infection, but may also result in epididymitis, prostatitis, proctitis and may be implicated in Reiter's syndrome.

Strong evidence is now available that chlamydia screening and treatment not only reduces the prevalence of lower genital tract infection, but also decreases the incidence of dreaded complications like PID. CDC has developed recommendations for the prevention and management of chlamydia infection.[13] Annual screening of all sexually active women aged <25 years is recommended (as is screening of older women with risk factors (e.g. those who have a new sex partner or multiple sex partners). All women with infection of the cervix and all pregnant women should also be tested for chlamydia.

Lymphogranuloma venereum (LGV) is caused by *Chlamydia trachomatis* serovar L1, L2, and L3. Acute LGV is more common in males while late lesions such as esthiomene and rectal strictures are more common in women.[14]

The most common sites of appearance of the primary lesion (papule, ulcer, herpetiform lesion) in women are posterior vaginal wall, fourchette, posterior lip of cervix and vulva. It can also manifest as urethritis and cervicitis. The latter can presumably extend locally and cause perimetritis or salpingitis. It was found that only 20 to 30% of women present with inguinal syndrome, which is the most common manifestation of the secondary stage of LGV in men. However due to the involvement of deep pelvic and lumbar lymphnodes, they present with lower abdominal and back pain. Numerous adhesions fixing the pelvic organs together (frozen pelvis) can occur, which will result in infertility.

In anogenitorectal syndrome, there is proctocolitis and hyperplasa of perirectal lymphatic tissues. The dire late manifestations inwhich rectovaginal and anal fistulas, rectal and vaginal strictures, and stenosis.

Esthiomene, a primary infection affecting the lymphatics of the vulva, can cause progressive lymphangitis, long standing oedema, and sclerosing fibrosis of subcutaneous tissues. Accompanying ulcers are superficial and later become more invasive and destructive. These painful chronic ulcers are commonly situated on labia majora, at genitocrural folds and perineum in later stages. Urethral and vaginal fistulas and vaginal stenosis are added complications.[14] All these changes can interfere with normal sexual functions and also obstruct normal vaginal delivery.

Penoscrotal elephantiasis (saxophone penis), which appears after 1 to 20 years of infection, causes severe oedema and induration of the area involved.[15] These changes are long-standing in nature and interfere with sexual functions due to deformities and erectile dysfunction.

CHANCROID

Women can also present with dysuria, rectal bleeding, dyspareunia or vaginal discharge. Multiple ulcers are a rule in women in contrast to solitary ulcers seen in more than 50% of men. However, the bubo formation in women is rarer than in men.

The epidemiology of chancroid has a striking gender difference, with more than 90% of cases being reported in men. In women the lesions are either overlooked or they have an inapparent carrier state. CSWS are an important aspect in the epidemiology of chancroid and are capable of infecting many male partners. It has been observed that women are less likely to progress from the papule stage to the pustule stage when inoculated experimentally, and this could explain the different epidemiology in women.[16]

GONORRHOEA

Endocervical canal is the primary site of urogenital gonococcal infection in women. After hysterectomy, urethra is the usual site. Periurethral (Skene glands), Bartholin's gland too may be involved. Non specific signs and symptoms like vaginal discharge, dysuria, menorrhagia and other menstrual irregularities can occur either in isolation or in combination. These can occur with other STDs also. Acute salpingitis or acute PID is the most common complication of gonorrhoea in women, occurring in about 10 to 20% of with acute gonococcal infection. This is of immense concern due to its acute manifestations of fever, lower abdominal pain, dyspareunia, and abnormal menses as well as due to its long-term sequelae of chronic pelvic pain, infertility and ectopic pregnancy. Younger females (15%) are particularly at risk of developing salpingitis following vaginitis (prepubertal age) and are also prone to developing PID. Younger age of acquisition of gonorrhoea, multiple sex partners and use of intrauterine devices for contraception are the major risk factors for PID. Puerperal infection and infection following dilatation and curettage of the infected cervix, douching, sexual intercourse and menstruation are added risk factors. The risk for ectopic pregnancy is ten-folds following an attack of acute salpingitis. The prevalence of disseminated gonococcal infections ranges from 0.1 to 0.3of the total cases, with females outnumbering males (4 to 1)[17,18]

SYPHILIS

Syphilis continues to be one of the most common sexually acquired infections in women in India, especially among pregnant women. Primary syphilitic chancre frequently occurs on labia, fourchette, urethra, perineum or cervix. Extra-genital sites include anus, mouth, oropharynx and nipple. Since painless chancre in the cervix is not visible, syphilis is rarely diagnosed clinically in women until it progresses to the secondary stage. Recent studies have shown no difference in the prevalence of primary and secondary syphilis in men and women.[19] Benign tertiary syphilis is more common in women and late complications like cardiovascular and neurosyphilis are twice as common in men than in women.[20]

Morbid reproductive health sequelae of syphilis are found in pregnant women. Syphilis is a common cause of stillbirth Especially in developing countries. Syphilis has benign effect on mother due to the prevalent immunosuppressive state during pregnancy; however, it has disastrous effect on the foetus.

In males, gummatous syphilis may cause localized or generalized infiltration of the testis, usually unilaterally; however, epididymis remains unaffected. If left untreated, interstitial fibrosis ensues. There are no reports suggesting sterility following gummatous syphilis of testis.

GRANULOMA INGUINALE

Clinical variants of this STD include ulcerogranulomatous, hypertrophic, necrotic, and cicatrical. The usual sites involved in women are labia minora and fourchette, rarely extending to cervix uteri. Lesions on cervix may mimic carcinoma. Donovanosis has a higher aggressive course in pregnancy. Disseminated disease is usually associated with pregnancy and cervical lesions.[21,22]

Occasionally, phagedena supervenes to cause severe destruction of the genitals. The eventual scarring could be keloidal in some cases. Scarring results in elephantine enlargement of the genitals in both genders with resultant impact on the reproductive health. Malignant transformation is known to occur in long-standing cases. Rajam and Rangiah found 0.25% of 2000 cases of donovanosis developing squamous cell carcinoma.[23] It is often difficult to differentiate carcinomatous changes from pseudoepitheliomatous changes. General health too deteriorates due to accompanying anaemia, anorexia and cachexia. Urethral, vaginal and anal orifices develop sclerosis and stenosis with resultant complications such as dysparaeunia and difficulty in defaecation.

BACTERIAL VAGINOSIS

Bacterial vaginosis (BV) is the most common disease affecting females and often coexists with trichomoniasis and candidiasis. *Gardernella vaginalis*, mycoplasma, bacteroid species,and anaerobic organisms such as peptostreptococci, mobiluncus and prevotella are the main causative organisms of BV. Multiple sex partners, douching and presence of intrauterine devices are the risk factors. It is seldom found in women who have never had sexual intercourse.[24]

BV is generally more commonly seen in women attending STD clinics than in those attending family planning or prenatal clinics.[25]

Many studies have reported adverse pregnancy outcomes like preterm labour and delivery, premature rupture of membranes, low birth weight, post-partum endometritis[24,25] Post and abortal infections and post-caesarean wound infections too have been reported. A study reported that women with BV in second trimester had 50% more chance developing fever during labour as compared to women with lactobacillus predominant flora. *G. Vaginalis* has infrequently caused neonatal bacteremia, cutaneous abscess and congenital pneumonia.

Vaginal cuff cellulitis occurs when vaginal bacteria contaminate the operative field during hysterectomy. It is known to occur four times more commonly in patients with BV those with normal flora. BV also has a strong association with PID especially in the post-abortal phase. In a study, 174 women with BV underwent double-blind randomization to a placebo or metronidazole prior to abortion. Placebo treated women had higher rates of post-abortal PID. Spontaneous PID is also strongly linked with BV. A study by Paavonen et al reported 29% of 31 patients who have histological to have evidence of endometritis BV, while none of the 14 controls without endometritis had BV. PID can cause infertility or damage the fallopian tubes enough to increase the future risk of ectopic pregnancy and infertility. BV can increase a woman's susceptibility to HIV infection when exposed to the virus. Having BV increases the chances that an HIV infected woman pass HIV to her sex partner and also increases a woman's susceptibility to other STD such as chlamydia and gonorrhoea.

TRICHOMONAS VAGINALIS (TV) INFECTION

T. vaginalis is specific to the genitourinary tract and has been isolated from virtually all genitourinary structures. However, many women diagnosed with trichomoniasis are asymptomatic. It has been associated with vaginitis, cervicitis, urethritis and PID. Trichomoniasis also impacts upon birth outcomes and is a cofactor in HIV transmission and acquisition. *T. vaginalis* infection in women can have postcoital bleeding due to cervicitis, and 12% of women are reported to have abdominal pain perhaps due to salpingitis or endometritis. Pregnant women with *T. vaginalis* infection are reported to have reproductive complications such as post-caesarian infection, premature rupture of membranes and preterm birth. Approximately 2-17% female infants of mothers infected with TV are reported to have developed vaginal infections. This infection may not be overt in all cases. Within 3 to 4 weeks, the maternal estrogens, which cause the neonatal vaginal epithelium to predispose to TV infection, are now in low levels and thus the neonatal vagina reverts to the prepubertal stage and resists the TV infection.

In males, besides urethritis, TV has been detected in cases of prostatitis (9-100%), especially in long-standing cases not responding to antimicrobials.[27] Balanoposthitis with phimosis, chronic sinus formation along the median raphe,[28] urethral stricture formation, epididymitis and infertility are some of the sequelae in males. *T. vaginalis* has adverse effects on the sperm motility and is considered to contribute to male infertility. *T. vaginalis* has been reported in 4% of 1131 semen specimens of infertile males. Further, abnormality of sperm morphology and motility along with abnormal seminal fluid viscosity and increased particulate debris were reported more in the group with *T. vaginalis* infection than the non-infected group. There are some reports linking *T. vaginalis* infection with erectile dysfunction and premature ejaculation.

MYCOPLASMA INFECTION

Mycoplasma hominis has a role in the development of non-specific vaginosis and usually coexists with *T. vaginalis* and anaerobic Gram-negative rods in the vagina. *M. hominis* could be recovered from 63% of bacterial vaginitis and 10% of normal controls. The role of *Ureaplasma urealyticum* in bacterial vaginosis is not well defined. The mycoplasmas are copathogens to *N. gonorrhoeae* and *C. trachomatis* in causing PID. Mardh and Westrom in their study reported the isolation of *M. hominis* from 8% of 50 women with salpingitis but not from women without salpingitis.[29] The direct yield of mycoplasma by laparoscopy has been achieved in 11% of women with salpingitis.[29] *Mycoplasma genitalium* has been implicated in PID especially in women the infection with *N. gonorrhoeae* and *C. trachomatis*.

There exists an association between colonization of vagina with mycoplasma and post-abortal and postpartum fever due to endometritis, especi-ally where there is evidence of early rupture of membranes and prolonged labour.[30] The mycoplasma associates itself virulent bacteria and have symbiotic relation with these bacteria to cause endometritis. In one study, *M. hominis* was isolated from blood of out of 125 febrile postpartum women,as compared to none of 60 afebrile postpartum women ($P < 0.005$).[31]

Ureaplasmas have profound effect on the motility of sperm and can cause oligospermia (low sperm count).[32] The Elimination of these offending agents has improved sperm motility, quantity and appearance. Ureaplasmas have been recovered more frequently from infertile couples than fertile ones.[43] Conception rate from 23% to 84% has been recorded among ureaplasma colonised infertile couples. But later studies have not substantiated these claims. Thus, to date role of mycoplasma in infertility remains. Similarly despite their isolation from lower genital tract in women with habitual abortions and still-birth, mycoplasma is not the predominant organism in these cases. Low birth weight is associated with the isolation of *U. urealyticum* in the infants. Mycoplasma colonization in vagina of women with bacterial vaginosis and the resultant effect on the pregnancy in terms of preterm delivery or low birth weight of the foetus have to be taken with due consideration as these effects may be due to organisms coexisting with mycoplasma.

GENITAL HERPES SIMPLEX VIRUS 2 (HSV 2) INFECTION

There is tremendous increase in genital HSV-2 infection worldwide. HSV-2 infection predisposes the infected individual to acquisition of HIV infection. The frequency of HSV 2 antibody is higher in STD clinic attendees and homosexual men. It is linked to age of initiation of sexual activities, multiple sex partners in lifetime, history of present and past STDs, advancing age and low socio-economic status. Conjugal infection transmission rate is about 12% per year.[33] Women and seronegative individuals have more chances for acquisition of HSV.

Many times the primary and secondary episodes remain asymptomatic. Subclinical shedding from various mucosal surfaces such as oral, genital and anorectal canal is an important issue. candidial vaginitis is frequently encountered with active HSV infection. A study recorded 14% of women who have had primary genital HSV infection also had candidal vaginitis.[33] Bacterial superinfection may add to severe discomfort and pain of the primary infection. HSV cervicitis can be found without infection on the external genitals and often could be asymptomatic. HSV infection of pregnant women is linked to age, past sexual activities and poor socio-economic status. The clinical course of infection, both primary and recurrent, does not change during pregnancy. The frequency and severity of episodes may increase during pregnancy.

CYTOMEGALOVIRUS (CMV) INFECTION

CMV infection occurs as compare to in developing countries takes place in early age group developed countries especially in low socioeconomic group. Recently many indications that have emerged which point to CMV infection as a STD. A significant correlation was found with seropositivity to CMV and increased number of sex partners and past or current infection with chlamydia and history of STDs. Increased seroprevalence of CMV and shedding of virus is observed in women attending STD clinics among and young group of homosexuals. Virus shedding is noted in semen, cervical secretions and saliva and these sites form a potential source of infection and sexual transmission of CMV. Viral shedding takes place from multiple sites following primary or recurrent secondary infection. Pregnancy has marginal impact on viral shedding; however, the rate of shedding is lowest in the first trimester. Maternal infection and perinatal infection often are subclinical.

As CMV is secreted in breast milk, perinatal infection could be attributed due to breast feeding practices. Maternal primary CMV infection could be acquired during pregnancy with resultant congenital perinatal CMV infection and variable outcomes.

HUMAN PAPILLOMA VIRUS

The subtypes most commonly associated with genital warts are HPV6 and 11. Types 16, 18, 31,

33, 35 which also affect the anogenital region, are strongly associated with cervical neoplasias. In addition to external genitalia, these warts are also seen in cervix, vagina, urethra, anus and mouth. Approximately 50% of sexually active young women are infected with some type of HPV, and of these, 5to 10% are estimated to be persistently infected with oncogenic HPV types that could progress to cervical cancer.

Few reports have suggested an association with first trimester abortions but these need to be confirmed.[34] A higher prevalence of high-risk HPV infection is reported in pregnant women. HPV frequency increases with gestational age, it being more common in the third trimester as compared to the first and the second.

High progesterone levels may activate transcriptional HPV replication or change an immune response activating latent HPV infection. Worsening of cervical intraepithelial neoplasia can also occur in pregnancy.[35,36]

Genital warts tend to increase in size and become more vascular during pregnancy and regress after delivery. They may mechanically obstruct the birth canal or cause torrential bleeding. Since HPV infection can be sub-clinical multifocal vulvar and cervical lesions can occur concomitantly.

HPV6 and 11 account for the majority of laryngeal papillomas ,which is the most frequent form of recurrent respiratory papillomatoses seen in children. A maternal history of genital condyloma at the time of delivery or during pregnancy among RRP patients has been reported to vary from 54 to 67%.[37] Neonatal exposure probably occurs at the time of delivery by aspiration of contaminated cervical, vaginal or vulvar materials Contamination of child's mouth with genital HPV from the mother's cervix appears to occur commonly at birth or during the perinatal period. Such acquired HPV DNA or infection may persist for at least 6 weeks. Caesarean section does not decrease the neonatal affection.[38]

Theoretically, in utero transmission of HPV can occur hematogenously, by semen at fertilization, or as an ascendant infection of the mother. A proper understanding of viral transmission routes is of crucial importance, particularly because several vaccination programmes are ongoing worldwide.

INFERTILITY DUE TO STIs

Infertility is defined as lack of conception after one year of regular sexual (penovaginal) intercourse without the use of any contraception.

Exceptionally, STDs in male results in infertility. Bilateral epididymitis and blocking of vas deferens due to *N. gonorrhoeae* and *C. trachomatis* could result in obstruction to the passage of sperm. *T. vaginalis* and genital mycoplasma are known to affect motility, quantity and morphology of spermatozoa. However, these changes are reversible following antimicrobial therapy. The DNA of STIpathogens have been detected in semen from a high percentage of asymptomatic male patients with infertility, and was associated with poor semen quality.[40] However, this needs to be investigated further.

T. pallidum infection of testis could result in orchitis, which is usually unilateral and therefore less likely to cause infertility.

The greater impact of STDs on fertility is seen in women. The common-cause of STDest related infertility is PID. Salpingitis is the most common preceding event, and tubal infertility is generally perceived as the direct result of acute salpingitis. There is inflammation of the epithelial surfaces of the fallopian tubes due to one or more active organisms, which have ascended from the lower genital tract. The local peritonitic, tuboovarian adnexal masses contribute to tubal occlusion.

However, most women with tubal factor infertility have no prior history of symptomatic PID. But several retrospective studies have demonstrated strong associations between tubal infertility and previous chlamydial and gonococcal infections among women without a prior history of acute symptomatic PID. These data suggest that damage to the fallopian tubes may be due to an inflammatory process that is clinically inapparent, a condition termed subclinical, unrecognized or silent PID.

N. gonorrhoeae and *C. trachomatis* are the two most important causative agents of PID and STD related infertility. However, other organisms like *Mycoplasma genitalium* responsible for bacterial vaginosis too have been implicated.[41]

A WHO multicentric study was undertaken to compare STD related infertility in five different regions of the world.[42] Out of the 8000 infertile couples, 71% completed evaluation of the fallopian tubes. In Africa, approximately 66% infertility was due to infection. Bilateral tubal occlusion accounted for 49% and pelvic adhesions for 24% of infertility.[43] Developed countries had far less prevalence of tubal occlusion (11%) as the cause of infertility. The non-African developing countries had higher rates of tubal occlusion than in developed countries, but certainly less than that of African countries. The risk factors for tubal infertility are shown in Table 2.1.

Table 2.1 Risk Factors for Tubal Infertility

1. Number of episodes of pelvic inflammatory disease
2. Severity of pelvic inflammation
3. Delay in access to treatment
4. Type of contraceptives used
5. Smoking

Acute salpingitis due to *N. gonorrhoeae* or *C. trachomatis* results in varying degree of inflammation. The proportion of women who become infertile after the first episode of inflammation is 0.6% after mild, 6.2% after moderate and 21% after severe inflammation of the fallopian tubes.

Morbidity and risk of infertility increases with each episode of PID. A single episode of PID would be responsible for 8%, two episodes for 19% and three or more for 40% of infertility. The necrosis of ciliated epithelium gives rise to permanent damage, and therefore, despite surgical correction of adhesions and assuring tubal patency, conception does not take place. Women taking steroidal contraceptives have milder impact and suffer from less severe types of PID.[44] As compared to gonoccocal infection, chlamydial infection has more chances to cause PID and tubal infertility. In larger studies, 70% women with tubal infertility had chlamydia antibodies as compared to 26% of control women.[45] Persistent, untreated chlamydial infection causes chronic stimulation of the host immune system against immunogenic antigens such as chlamydial heat shock proteins (cHSP) 60 and 10. A special antigen called HSP 60, which is now available in recombinant form, has facilitated many studies related to PID and infertility.[46] It has been possible to detect antibodies to cHSP 60 by microimmunofluorescence. It is observed that 16-25% of normal fertile women have these antibodies as compared to 44% cases of cervicitis, 48-60% of PID and 81-90% cases of fallopian tube obstruction caused by *C.trachomatis*.[61] Women with cHSP 60 antibodies have more damaging inflammation than those without it, suggesting the role of cHSP 60 in inciting inflammation. The type of contraceptive choice has definite impact on the degree of inflammation of PID. Intrauterine devices (IUCD) are associated with increased risk of tubal infertility.[47] Condoms and spermicides provide significant protection against tubal infertility. Oral contraceptives mask the degree of inflammation and therefore reduce the signs and symptoms of PID ,but do not reduce the potential of tubal obstruction.[48] Smoking has direct suppressive effect on the immune mechanisms, which prevent the upward, ascent of organisms from the lower genital tract.[49,50] Women who smoke and also use an IUCD have a greater risk of developing tubal infertility.

Infertility is a medical problem having a significant psychological and social impact. Early detection,and prompt and appropriate treatment of STDs will help in preventing its long-term complications. However, the dismally low health-seeking behaviour of women especially in rural India, and lack of awareness of and poor access to family planning methods, antenatal and gynaecological clinics pose a big hurdle.

STIs IN WOMEN IN INDIA

Vaginal discharge occurs in 22-50% patients visiting gynaecology outpatient in different parts of India (Table 2.2) and various etiological agents as depicted in Table 2.3. The occurrence of different STIs in various settings is summarized in Table 2.4. It is concluded from above that STIs have major adverse effect on sexual and general health and fertility potential of an individual.

Table 2.2 **Prevalence of Clinically Detectable Gynaecological Morbidity**

Study	*Total women*	*Vaginal discharge (%)*	*Lower backache (%)*	*Lower abdominal pain (%)*
Bombay (urban slum)	1001	30.8	39.3	21.5
Baroda (urban slum)	840	22.4	24.1	9.3
West Bengal (rural)	875	50.1	5.3	17.5
South Gujarat (rural)	835	57.0	29.7	—
Ambala (urban slum)	2325	45.1	47.9	—
Chandigarh (urban slum)	576	42.4	30.4	39.3

Source: Kumar B, Sharma NM. Ind J Sex Transm Dis 2000: 21; 4-7

Table 2.3 **Correlation of Gynaecologic Conditions with Aetiological Agents**

Total %	*Clinical condition*	*Candida*	*T. vaginalis*	*G.vaginalis*	*N.gon*	*C. trachom*	*M. hom*	*U. urealyt*
43.18	Vaginitis	27.97	23.31	20.98	1.29	1.81	10.88	32.53
32.21	Cervicitis	15.28	10.42	9.37	2.08	7.29	5.21	24.31
15.21	Infertility	11.02	3.67	6.62	2.94	15.44	9.55	19.83
5.26	PID	6.38	2.12	4.25	6.38	21.27	12.76	31.91
4.14	Miscellaneous	13.51	10.81	5.40	8.10	8.10	18.91	4.14
100	Total	19.57	14.54	13.42	2.24	6.94	8.84	27.18
100	Control	9.06	5.14	4.9	0.0	1.22	1.47	12.5

Aetiological agents in %

N. gon - N. gonorrhoeae, C. trachom - C. trachomatis, M. hom - M. hominis, U. urealyt - U. urealyticum

Source: Gogate A. Reproductive tract infections (RTI) in women of childbearing age from Dharavi slums of Mumbai. Ind J Sex Transm Dis 1999: 20; 11-15

Table 2.4 STI Rates Among Women in India[1]

Study population	Prevalence rangeaa (%)							
	GC	CT	Syphilis	TV	HSV	HPV (clinical diagnosis)	HBV	HIV
Community-based								
Ever/currently married women	0.0-4.2	0.5-28.7	0.2-8.8	4.3-27.4	–	11.8	–	–
Unmarried & married women	0.3-3.9	1.4-5.2	0.2-10.5	0.8-14.0	1.4	–	4.8	2.0-2.1
Symptomatic women	0.3	4.3	1.2-11.0	16.8	–	–	–	–
Pregnant women	–	–	–	10.0	–	–	–	–
Facility-based and convenience samples								
STDs clinic patients	1.3-20.0	20.3	29.3-43.3	3.3	4.0-15.4	6.7-15.6	–	1.2-13.6
Wives of STDs patients	2.4	4.6-22.9	7.4	8.8-54.1	–	–	–	–
Commercial Sex Workers	0.5-19.1	0.2-31.3	4.3-63.0	0.4-26.0	7.5-20.0	0.5	2.0-12.0	2.6-49.9
Gynaecological OPD patients	0.0-5.5	2.3	4.4-17.0	17.8	0.3-25.0	0.6-42.4	–	0.0
Antenatal patients	–	2.6-20.0	0.9-6.2	1.6-17.6	–	–	–	–
Gynaecological patients with vaginitis complaint	0.0-2.6	3.0	2.2	–	12.0	–	–	–
Gynaecological patients with 'cervical erosion'	0.1-11.0	0.5-24.2	–	0.5	–	–	–	–
Infertility and PID patients	–	18.8	0.5	–	–	–	–	–
Women with obstetric complications	0.1-2.2	0.0-0.2	–	0.9	–	–	–	–
Acceptors of tubal ligation	–	–	0.5-7.0	–	–	–	–	–

REFERENCES

1. Reproductive Tract and Sexually Transmitted Infections In: searo.who.int/LinkFiles/Reporductive_Health_Profile_reproductive.pdf.
2. Erhardt AA, Bolan G, Wasserheit J, et al. Gender perspectives and STDs In: Holmes KK, Sparling PF, Mardh PA, eds. Sexually Transmitted Diseases. 3rd edition. New York: McGraw-Hill; 1999. p. 117-29.
3. Padian NS: The heterosexual transmission of Human Immunodefeciency Virus in nothern California: Results from a ten year study. Am J Epidemiol 1997; 146: 350-7.
4. Watts DH, Brunhan RC. Sexually transmitted diseases including HIV in pregnancy In: Holmes KK, Sparling PF, Mardh PA, eds. Sexually Transmitted Diseases. 3rd edition. New York: McGraw-Hill; 1999. p. 1089-113.
5. Menken J, Rahman OM. Reproductive health In: Merson MH, Black RE, Mills A, eds International Public Health: Diseases, Programmes, Systems,

and Policies. 2nd edition. London: Jones & Bartlett; 2006. p. 71-126.
6. Training Module of medical health personnel on RCH, Study fellowship on reproductive and child health, 1999-2000, Family Welfare training and research Centre, Mumbai. Sponsored by Department of Family Welfare, Government of India and World Health Organization (WHO).
7. Reproductive & Child Health Programme Phase II 3rd Joint Review Mission, January 15 – February 8, 2007 AIDE MEMOIRE March 2007. Donor coordination division. Ministry of Health and Family Welfare. Govt. of India.
8. Options and challenges for converging HIV and Sexual Reproductive Health Services in India. Findings from an assessment in Andhra Pradesh, Bihar, Maharashtra and Uttar Pradesh. June 2007. http://www.path.org/files/CP_India_cnvg_rpt.pdf
9. Chlamydial infections In: WHO/HIV-AIDS/2001.02, 2001 http://www.who.int/HIV_AIDS/STDsGlobalReport/index.htm
10. Honey E, Templeton A. Prevention of pelvic inflammatory disease by the control of *C. trachomatis* infection. Intern J Gynecol Obstet 2002; 78: 257-61.
11. Machado AC, Guimara EM, Sakurai E, et al. High titers of *Chlamydia trachomatis* antibodies in Brazilian women with tubal occlusion or previous ectopic pregnancy. Infect Dis Obstet Gynecol 2007; 2007: 24816.
12. Stamm W. *Chlamydia trachomatis* infections of the adults. In: Holmes KK, Sparling PF, Mardh PA, eds. Sexually Transmitted Diseases. 3rd edition. New York: McGraw-Hill; 1999. p. 407-22.
13. Chlamydia infection. In:CDC. MMWR 2006; 55(No. RR-11): 38.
14. Hopsu-Havu VK, Sonck CE. Infiltrative, ulcerative and fistular lesions of the penis due to Lymphogranuloma venereum. Br J Vener Dis 1973; 49: 193-202.
15. Willcox RR, Willcox JR. Lymphogranuloma venereum. In: Willcox RR, Willcox JR, eds. Pocket consultant of venereological Medicine. 1st edition. Bombay: Oxford University Press; 1992. p. 248-55.
16. Bong CT, Harezlak J, Katz BP et al. Men are more susceptible than women to pustule formation in the experimental model of Haemophilus ducreyi infection. Sex Trans Inf 2002; 29: 114-8.
17. Sweet RL, Gibbs RS. Infectious diseases of the female genital tract. 2nd ed. Baltimore, MD: Williams & Wilkins; 1990.
18. Al-Suleiman SA, Grimes EM, Jonas HS. Disseminated gonococcal infections. Obstet Gynecol 1983; 61: 48-51.
19. Hahn RA, Magder LS, Aral SO et al. Race and the prevalence of syphilis seroreactivity in the United States population: a national sero-epidemiologic study. Am J Public Health 1989; 79: 467-70.
20. Gjestland T. The Oslo study of untreated syphilis; an epidemiologic investigation of the natural course of the syphilitic infection based upon a re-study of the Boeck-Bruusgaard material. Acta Derm Venereol Suppl (Stockh) 1955; 35 (Suppl 34): 3-368.
21. O'Farrell N. Donovanosis (granuloma inguinale) in pregnancy. Int J STDs AIDS 1991; 2: 447-8.
22. Cherny WB, Jones CP, Peete CH Jr. Disseminated granuloma inguinale and its relationship to granuloma of the cervix and pregnancy. Am J Obstet Gynecol. 1957; 74: 597-605.
23. Rajam RV, Rangiah PN. Donovanosis (Granuloma Inguinale, Granuloma Venereum). Geneva, World Health Organization, WHO Monograph Series No 24, 1954: 1-72.
24. Jacobsson B, Pernevi P, Chidekel L, et al. Bacterial vaginosis in early pregnancy may predispose for preterm birth and postpartum endometritis. Acta Obstet Gynecol Scand 2002; 81: 1006-10.
25. Svare JA, Schmidt H, Hansen BB, et al. Bacterial vaginosis in a cohort of Danish pregnant women: prevalence and relationship with preterm delivery, low birthweight and perinatal infections. BJOG. 2006 Dec; 113: 1419-25.
26. Paavonen J, Tejsala K, Heinonen PK, et al. Microbiological and histopathological findings in acute pelvic inflammatory disease.Br J Obstet Gynaecol 1987; 94: 454-60.
27. Sowmini CN, Vijayalakshmi K, Chellamuthiah C, et al. Infection of the median raphe of the penis: report of three cases. Br J Vener Dis 1973; 49: 469-74.

28. Pavithran K. Trichomonal abscess of the median raphe of the penis. Int J Dermatol 1993; 32: 820-1.
29. Mardh PA, Westrom L. Tubal and cervical cultures in acute salpingitis with special reference to *Mycoplasma hominis* and T-strain mycoplasmas Brit J Vener Dis 1970; 46: 179-85.
30. Harwik HJ. *Mycoplasma hominis* and abortion. J Infect Dis 1970; 121: 260-6.
31. Wallace RJ. Isolation of mycoplasma hominis from blood cultures in patients with post partum fever. Obstet Gynecol 1978; 51: 181-5.
32. Toth A. Light microscopy as an aid in predicting ureaplasma infection in human semen. Fertil Steril 1978; 42: 586-93.
33. Bryson Y. Risks of acquisition of genital herpes simplex virus type 2 in sex partners of persons with genital herpes: a prospective couple study. J infect Dis 1993; 167: 942-6.
34. Hermonat PL Kechelava S, Lowery CL, et al. Trophoblasts are the preferential target for human papilloma virus infection in spontaneously aborted products of conception. Hum Pathol 1998; 29: 170-4.
35. Hernández-Girón C, Smith JS.High-risk human papillomavirus detection and related risk factors among pregnant and nonpregnant women in Mexico. Sex Transm Dis 2005; 32: 613-8.
36. Smith EM, Johnson SR. The association between pregnancy and human papilloma virus prevalence. Cancer Detect Prev 1991; 15: 397-402.
37. Hallden C, Majmudar B. The relationship between juvenile laryngeal papillomatosis and maternal condylomata. J Reprod Med 1986; 31: 804-87.
38. Cook TA, Cohn AM, Brunschwig JP, et al. Laryngeal papilloma: etiologic and therapeutic considerations. Ann Otol Rhinol Laryngol 1993; 82: 649-55.
39. Bandyopadhyay S, Sen S .Human papillomavirus infection among Indian mothers and their infants. Asian Pac J Cancer Prev 2003; 4: 179-84.
40. Bezold G, Politch JA, Kiviat NB et al.Prevalence of sexually transmissible pathogens in semen from asymptomatic male infertility patients with and without leukocytospermia. Fertil Steril 2007; 87: 1087-97.
41. Clausen HF, Fedder J, Drasbek M, et al. Serological investigation of Mycoplasma genitalium in infertile women. Hum Reprod 2001; 16: 1866-74.
42. World Health Organization Task Force on the prevention and management of infertility: Tubal infertility: serological relationship to past chlamydial and gonococcal infection. Sex Transm Dis 1995; 22: 71-7.
43. Westrom L. Pelvic inflammatory disease and fertility. A cohort study of 1,844 women with laparoscopically verified diseases and 657 control women with normal laparoscopic results. Sex Transm Dis 1992; 19: 185-92.
44. Svensson L Mardh PA, Westrom L. Infertility after acute salpingitis with special reference to *Chlamydia trachomatis*. Fertil Steril 1983; 40: 322-9.
45. Cates W Jr. Genital chlamydia infections: Epidemiology and reproductive sequelae. Am J Obstet Gynecol 1991; 164: 1777-81.
46. Cerrone MC. Cloning and sequence of the gene for heat shock protein 60 from *Chlamydia trachomatis* and immunological reactivity of protein. Infect Immun 1991; 59: 79-90.
47. Darling JR, Weiss NS, Metch BJ et al. Primary tubal infertility in relation to intrauterine device. N Eng J Med 1985; 312: 937-41.
48. Cramer DW. The relationship of tubal infertility to barrier method and oral contraceptive use. JAMA 1987; 257: 2446-50
49. Phipps WR, Cramer DW, Schiff Z, et al. The association between smoking and female infertility as influenced by cause of the infertility. Fertil Steril 1987; 48: 377-82.
50. Hershey P, Prendergast B, Edwards A. Effects of cigarette smoking on the immune system. Follow-up studies in normal subjects after cessation of smoking. Med J Aust 1983; 2: 425-9.

3 HISTORICAL ASPECTS OF SEXUALLY TRANSMITTED DISEASES AND AIDS

Devinder M Thappa

In this chapter

- Sources of STDs
- Prostitution
- Homosexuality
- Origin of STDs
- Syphilis
- Gonorrhoea
- Chancroid
- Donovanosis
- Lymphogranuloma venereum
- Other STDs
- British India and STDs control measures
- Independent India and STDs Control Measures
- Advent of AIDS in India
- HIV epidemic in India
- Academic developments
- Emerging STIs scenario
- Future directions

INTRODUCTION

The older terminology of 'venereal diseases' (VDs) has largely been superseded in the past 50 years by 'sexually transmitted diseases' (STDs) and more recently by 'sexually transmitted infections' (STIs).[1-3] Venereology (the study of venereal diseases) today encompasses more than five classical venereal diseases (syphilis, gonorrhoea, chancroid, donovanosis and lymphogranuloma venereum).[4] A growing number of other diseases are being identified, which might be considered the new generation of STDs. Their importance is newly recognized due to the development of laboratory techniques of diagnosis and increasing awareness of the consequences of STDs on the health of society.

SOURCES OF STDs

In India, a majority of patients with STDs give history of having visited prostitutes. There is a widespread belief that prostitutes are primarily responsible for the origin and spread of AIDS, and it could be mostly controlled by testing all of them for HIV and isolating those who are found positive.[5] This belief was partly based on the highly publicized initial detection of HIV infection among a few prostitutes in Chennai in 1986 and also on subsequent publicity about the phenomenal rise of HIV infection among prostitutes in the red-light areas of Mumbai and other cities. Hijras and male prostitutes also play a significant role in the spread of STDs and AIDS.

PROSTITUTION

Prostitution describes sexual intercourse in exchange for a remuneration.[5] The legal status of prostitution varies across countries, from punishable by death to complete legality.[5] The greater degree of social stigma associated with prostitution, of both buyers and sellers, has lead to new terminology such as 'commercial sex trade', 'commercial sex worker' (CSW), female sex worker (FSW) or sex trade worker. Organizers of prostitution are typically known as pimps (if male) and madams (if female).

Brothels are establishments specifically dedicated to prostitution, often confined to special red-light districts in big cities.[5] Sonagachi in Kolkata, Kamathipura in Mumbai, G.B. Road in New Delhi and Budhwar Peth in Pune host thousands of sex workers. Sex tourism refers to travelling to poorer countries such as Thailand in search of sexual services that may be unavailable in one's own country, or simply too expensive there.

Prostitutes are stigmatized in most societies and religions; their customers are typically stigmatized to a lesser degree.[5,6] Prostitutes have more abortions and venereal diseases and hence become more easily sterile, but still many sex workers complete their term of pregnancy and give birth to children.

History: Prostitution as a profession has a long history in India. A whole chapter was devoted to it in Kautilya's *Arthashastra* written circa 300 BC and Vatsayana's *Kama Sutra* written between the first and fourth centuries AD.[7] Vedic texts give account of a mythic empire builder, Bharata, and prove that people were acquainted with prostitution through references to "loose" women, female "vagabonds" and sexually active unmarried girls.[6] The Vedic word "sadbarani" refers to a woman who offers sex for payment. In Vedic times, most prostitutes were dressed in red, even their gold jewelry was reddened as this hue was believed to scare away demons and give protection to those who chose to live in a moral gray zone.[6]

The devadasi (handmaiden of God) system of dedicating unmarried young girls to Gods in Hindu temples, which often made them objects of sexual pleasure of temple priests and pilgrims, was an established custom in India by 300 AD.[7] There are reasonably good records of prostitution in large Indian cities during the eighteenth and the first half of the nineteenth centuries of British rule; prostitution was not considered a degrading profession until second half of the nineteenth century. A Calcutta Corporation publication of 1806 reports there were 2540 women in 593 brothels in 82 streets of Calcutta and that they were tax-payers of about 6% of Calcutta's property.[8] During Lord Robert's return to England in May 1893, the 7500 military prostitutes in the Lal Bazaars made up barely a couple of percent of the whole sex industry. Indian prostitution was completely independent of the British and other foreigners.[6] Temple dancers, aristocratic courtesans, independent village girls and big brothels could be found in every corner of India.

Because of the clandestine nature of the sex industry and also because of their wide geographical distribution, it is impossible to have an accurate estimate of their number in contemporary India. Some guesses are, however, available. Gilada's estimates of 100,000 in Mumbai, 100,000 in Kolkata, 40000 in Delhi, 40000 in Pune and 13000 in Nagpur are considered overestimates by some critics and underestimates by others.[9]

Empirical data on the way of life and sexual practices of prostitutes in contemporary India are scarce.[7] The advent of AIDS has generated a few empirical studies along with intervention programmes in red-light areas of a few large cities. The findings of these studies corroborate the common knowledge that prostitutes, in general, lead a poor standard of life in dilapidated and unhygienic environments.[8,10] A major portion of what their clients pay is shared by pimps, landlords, madams, financiers and policemen. They do not get nutritional food and they are exploited by local traders who sell them essential goods. A large proportion of them suffer intermittently from various kinds of STDs. Most of them are forced to enter this occupation under adverse circumstances.[8] Life events and reactions to these events that led them to become prostitutes belong to two categories: 1) women were either widowed or abused by husbands and in-laws, leaving them with no social or economic support and 2) women choosing prostitution as an easy means to support themselves or because they had sexual urge or were curious.[11]

Devadasi System: The devadasi system still prevails in contemporary India as an institution in few Hindu temples, mostly in Karnataka and Andhra Pradesh.[7] Its operations are, however, clandestine because laws prohibit it. Gilada and Thakur[12] report that every year about 10000 young girls of poor families are offered as devadasis to the Goddess Yallama in a small temple of northern Karnataka.[12,13] They speculate that most prostitutes in the border districts of Maharashtra and Karnataka are devadasis.

The devadasi tradition in India extends as far back as the twelfth century. In brief, the devadasi tradition involves a religious rite in which girls and women are offered, through marriage, to different Gods and Goddesses, where they become wives or servants of deities and perform various temple duties. Over time, these duties have come to include the provision of sexual services to priests and patrons of the temples, and owing to the sacred setting and the view that Devadasi women embody a form of divinity, it has been referred to by some as "sacred prostitution".

A recently published study gives the extent of devadasi tradition in Karnataka sex industry.[13] Of 1588 female sex workers (FSWs) interviewed in Karnataka, 414 (26%) reported they entered sex work through the devadasi tradition. Devadasi FSWs had initiated sex work at a much younger age (mean, 15.7 vs. 21.8 years), were more likely to be home-based (68.6% vs. 14.9%), had more clients in the past week (average, 9.0 vs. 6.4), and were less likely to migrate for work within the state (4.6% vs. 18.6%) but more likely to have worked outside the state (19.6% vs. 13.1%).

Early age at entry: An estimated 85% of prostitutes in Kolkatta and Delhi entered sex work at an early age.[14] Their numbers are rising. The promotion of tourism has given impetus and thrust to this. These prostitutes are primarily located in low-middle income areas and business districts and are known to government officials. Brothel keepers regularly recruit young girls. An estimated 33% of prostitutes are young girls. In Bangalore, Kolkata, Delhi, and Hyderabad, there are an estimated 10000 girl prostitutes. UNICEF estimates about 300,000 child prostitutes. Girl prostitutes are classified as common prostitutes, singers and dancers, call girls, religious prostitutes or devadasis, and caged brothel prostitutes. Caged ones are found in Mumbai. A little over 50% of prostitutes have come from other countries such as Nepal and Bangladesh. Most girls have come from urban slums and poor rural areas. High supply regions include Andhra Pradesh, Karnataka,

Maharashtra, Uttar Pradesh, Tamil Nadu and West Bengal. About 85% are Hindus, and about 66% are from backward castes. Bangalore and Mumbai have a higher proportion of girl prostitutes. The causes of prostitution include illtreatment by parents, bad company, family prostitutes, social customs, inability to get into marriage, lack of sex education, media, prior incest and rape, early marriage and desertion, lack of recreational facilities, ignorance, and acceptance to prostitution. Most of them enter involuntarily and become part of the system of exploitation.

Call-girls and high-class escort girls: Prostitutes who are known as call-girls are usually more educated and attractive than those living in brothels, and are often engaged in some other occupation.[7] They earn higher incomes and have some freedom in choosing their clients who mostly belong to the middle and upper classes. In a study of 150 call-girls, 20 clients and 10 madams in Delhi, Mumbai and Kolkatta in 1970s, Kapur found that the earning of call-girls ranged from Rs. 50 to 100 per hour and Rs. 400 to 10,000 per night.[15] Eighty percent of their clients were married. Many of them had suffered from STDs at one time or other and experienced induced abortion, but in general, they take good care of their health by visiting physicians whenever necessary. Many of them wanted their clients to use condoms, but most clients did not comply. A high proportion of their clients preferred oral sex to vaginal intercourse. In a subsequent study of nine call-girls belonging to the upper middle class in Delhi in 1993, Kapur found that some of them were aware of AIDS and rejected clients who refused to use condoms.[16]

At the other end of the spectrum operate high-class escort girls recruited from women's colleges and the vast cadres of India's fashion and film industries.[5] They command large sums of money. These services usually operate by way of introduction. However, a recent trend has seen the emergence of several snazzy websites openly advertising their services.

Clients of Prostitutes

A few hundred thousand men have sexual relations with prostitutes every day in India.[7] Insights derived by health practitioners and social workers from their experience of working in red-light areas suggest that the following categories of men are frequent visitors to prostitutes: low-level workers in manufacturing and transport industries; other workers living away from their families for a length of time; traders and customers in transitory markets; visitors to fairs, festivals and pilgrim centres; defence personnel living away from families; students; pimps and others who have some control over prostitutes; traders and service providers in red-light areas; and professional blood donors.[3] Marriage, festivals and fairs are considered 'peak' seasons, while winter, summer and rainy seasons are considered 'lean'.[17,18]

Joardar reported that married men comprise two-thirds to three-quarters of the clients. Employees and white-collar workers constitute 29% of the clientele.[19] A multistate Indian study conducted in 1996 found that 0.9-3.2% of the urban and 0.7-4.2% of the rural population had high-risk sexual behaviours[20] A study in Delhi indicated that 30% of urban men had premarital sex, while in Tirupati, South India, it was 37%.[21]

As in many other countries, Indian truck drivers and their helpers are generally known to visit many prostitutes during their stopovers. In-depth interviews with 79 truck drivers and 21 helpers in a check-post near Kolkatta in 1993 showed that a majority of them reported visits to between three and seven prostitutes in a week and that the number visited by each trucker ranged from 50 to 100 in a year.[22] Also, most of them reported never having used condoms. Blood tests in a sample of truckers in the same place in 1993-1994 showed that 5.6% were already HIV-positive.

Legal provisions: Legislation passed in India regarding prostitution in 1956 and 1986 did not have the objective of abolishing prostitution; the stated objectives of the legislation were 'suppression' and 'prevention' of prostitution.[7] The 1956 Act (SITA) assumed that prostitution was a 'necessary evil', and prohibited a prostitute from soliciting clients in public places and forced her to work in certain areas known as red-light areas, thereby exposing her to exploitation by pimps and others. Though the SITA did not aim to punish prostitutes unless they solicited, it gave enough powers to police and other government agencies to terrorize, harass and financially exploit a prostitute. The 1986 Act (IPTA) provides marginal benefits to prostitutes by prohibiting male police officers from arresting them unless accompanied by two female police officers; and seeks to draw women away from prostitution through rehabilitation in Protective Homes.

Legislation regarding AIDS was introduced in the Rajya Sabha in 1989, which gave some government agencies sweeping powers to infringe the liberties of certain categories of people, but owing to strong opposition by a few activist groups, it was withdrawn in 1992.[7]

The commercial sex industry is a multibillion dollar Indian and global market which now includes strip clubs, massage brothels, phone sex, adult and child pornography, street brothels and escort prostitution.[5] For a vast majority of the world's prostituted women, prostitution is the experience of being hunted, dominated, harassed, assaulted and battered. In prostitution, it is the demand that creates supply. The key factors for these women adopting prostitution in India are lack of family support and inability to provide for themselves due to poverty and illiteracy. As long as these factors remain operative, the supply chain will remain intact. Moreover, so long as men want to buy sex, prostitution is assumed to be inevitable.

HOMOSEXUALITY

Homosexuality can be described as the orientation and inclination of a person to have sexual relations with a person of his or her own sex.[7] It is difficult, however, to identify a person as a homosexual, heterosexual or bisexual because the behavioural expression of sexual inclination of a person may take a multitude of forms and change in one's life cycle. This is why in their analysis of sexual behaviour data of White males and females in USA, Kinsey et al. developed a six-point scale to identify a person's position in the heterosexual-homosexual scale from his or her history of sexual behaviour.[23,24] Because of lack of any such behavioural survey data, such identification is not possible for the Indian population. In India, people are commonly identified as homosexuals if they have experienced as adults any kind of explicit sexual act with any person of their own sex.

The clustering of AIDS cases among male homosexuals in the initial phase of HIV epidemic in USA and a few other Western countries led to a misleading notion that the disease afflicted only 'reckless' male homosexuals, and it was often referred to as the 'gay plague' or 'gay cancer', 'gay' being the current vogue word for homosexuals.[7] Recent studies have shown that HIV is spreading everywhere more through heterosexual relations than through any other mode of transmission. It is, however, true that the risk of HIV infection is greater for persons who practise anal intercourse, and this type of intercourse is more common between homosexual partners than between heterosexual partners.

Historical Evidence of Homosexuality in India

Vatsayana's *Kama Sutra* refers to the practice of eunuchs and male servants giving oral sex to their male patrons and masters.[7] Some erotic sculptures of medieval Hindu temples depict lesbian acts. The Muslim rulers in India were reported to have maintained harems of young boys. During the British rule, sodomy (anal intercourse) was made illegal under Section 377 of the Indian Penal Code enacted in 1861; this legislation is still in force. Indian homosexual activists think that male homosexuals are often subjected to undue harassment and blackmailing.[25]

Current Situation of Homosexuality in India

Very little is known about the practice of homosexuality in contemporary India. According to Ashok Row-Kavi, a self-acclaimed homosexual activist, the number of exclusively or predominantly homosexual men in India may be over 50 million.[26] His estimate was, however, based on the prevalence of homosexual behaviour Kinsey et al. found for White American males in 1938-1947.[23,24] But recent surveys have shown that Kinsey et al. overestimated the number of homosexuals in USA.[23,24]

A vast majority of homosexuals are already married and living with their partners, reflecting the cultural obligation in South Asian countries that all men and women marry members of the opposite sex, whatever may be their sexual orientation.[7] The most common locations of first homosexual experience were parks and toilets. Relatives, mostly male cousins and uncles, were the second most common category of first homosexual partner, strangers being the most common category. Mutual masturbation was the most common type of homosexual act.

Strong prejudices against homosexuality in India, coupled with continuing neglect of the government to inclue homosexuals in AIDS prevention programmes prompted homosexuals to organize into formal groups for social and political purposes.[7] The Government of India has already recognized the need for intervention programmes among homosexuals and has taken the initiative to collect information necessary for the purpose.

Hijras and Male Prostitutes

A culturally identifiable group known by the Urdu term "hijra" lives in most parts of India, and are known to depend at least partly on working as male prostitutes for their livelihood. Most hijras are castrated males and dressed as females. A few are hermaphrodites who are born with ambiguously male-like genitals.[7] The total population of hijras in India is not known; in censuses, many of them reported themselves as females. An unofficial estimate of their population in India varies from 50000 to 500,000.

They adopt some aspects of female behaviour. Hijras traditionally earn their living by collecting alms and receiving payment for performances at weddings, births and festivals.[7,27] In reality, many hijras are male prostitutes and serve as passive partners for anal intercourse without use of condoms and are at high risk of STDs and AIDS. The central feature of their culture is their devotion to Bahuchara Mata, one of the many Mother Goddesses worshipped all over India, for whom emasculation is performed. The hijras are commonly believed by many to be intersexed impotent men, who undergo emasculation in which the whole or part of the genitals are removed. Castration is usually performed by a hijra called dai-ma under crude insanitary conditions. It is illegal but reported to be performed secretly in large numbers. This identification with the Mother Goddess is the source of the hijras' claim for both their special place in the society and the traditional belief in their power to curse or confer blessings on male infants.

Hijras live predominantly in the cities of North India, but small groups of hijras are found all over India. Seven "houses", or subgroups, comprise the hijra community; each house has a guru or leader, all of whom live in Mumbai.[27] All houses have equal status, but one, Laskarwallah, has the special function of mediating disputes which arise among others. Each house has its own history, as well as rules particular to it. For example, members of a particular house are not allowed to wear certain colours. Hijra houses appear to be patterned after the *gharanas* (literally houses), or family lineages among classical musicians, each of which is identified with its own particular musical style. Though the culturally distinct features of hijra houses have almost vanished, the structural feature remains.

The most significant relationship in the hijra community is that between the guru (master) and *chela* (disciple).[27] When an individual decides to (formally) join the hijra community, he is taken to one of the seven major gurus, usually the guru of the person who has brought him there. At the initiation ritual, the guru gives the novice a new, female name. The novice vows to obey the guru and the rules of the community. The guru then presents the new *chela* with some gifts. The *chela*, or more likely someone on her behalf, pays a fee and the guru writes the chela's name in her record book. This guru-chela relationship is a lifelong bond of reciprocity in which the guru is obliged to help the chela and the chela is obliged to be loyal and obedient to the guru.

Hijras live together in communes generally of about 5 to 15 members, and the heads of these local groups are also called guru.[27] Hijras make no distinctions based on caste, origin or religion, although in some parts of India, Gujarat for example, Muslim and Hindu hijras reportedly live apart. In Mumbai, Delhi, Chandigarh and Bangalore, hijras of Muslim, Christian, and Hindu origin live in the same houses.

In addition to the hierarchical guru-chela relationship, there is fictive kinship by which hijras relate to each other.[27] Rituals exist for "taking a daughter" and "daughters" of one "mother" consider themselves "sisters" and relate on a reciprocal, affectionate basis. Other fictive kinship relations such as "grandmother" or "mother's sister" (aunt) are the basis of warm and reciprocal regard. Fictive kins exchange small amounts of money, clothing, jewelry and sweets to formalize their relationship. Such relationships connect hijras all over India, and there is a constant movement of individuals to visit their gurus and fictive kins in different cities. Various annual gatherings, both religious and secular, attract thousands of hijras from all over India.

Hijras with strong feminine identity are involved in relatively long-term relationships with men who may be known as their 'husbands'. Having a 'husband' in an economically reciprocal and emotionally satisfying relationship is a preferred alternative for hijras who openly engage in sexual relations with men.

Male Prostitutes

In addition to a large section of the hijra community, there are many full-time or part-time male prostitutes in India.[7] Some of them live in the red-light areas of metropolitan cities; many seek male clients by offering massage services in parks, beaches, hotels and houses. Thousands of homeless and poor boys and young men employed in various establishments and firms are compelled to provide sexual services to their male bosses in return for their job security. Young men who work as helpers to highway provide such services truck drivers in their long trips.

Male prostitution is increasingly visible in India.[28] In Delhi, there are as many as twenty "agencies" offering "handsome masseurs" in the classifieds of newspapers (*Hindustan Times*). They offer in and out services, although the facilities are usually very basic. Most western clients are visited at hotels. Local middle-class citizens are also now using these services. Fees are discussed over the phone, typically between Rs 1000 and 3000.

ORIGINS OF STDs

The origins of venereal (sexually transmitted) diseases are obscure.[2] Medical scientists and other historians have often suggested that well-known diseases such as syphilis, gonorrhoea, chancroid and lympho-granuloma venereum have existed since earliest times. In fact, some of these individuals have drawn conclusions from ancient texts and manuscripts that may not be accurate. While the infections certainly exist in *Homo sapiens*, did they occur in the preceding species *Homo erectus* prior to 150,000 BC? No one knows, but the French philosopher Voltaire summed it up well when he declared in his *Dictionnaire philosophique* that venereal diseases are like fine arts - it is pointless to ask who invented them.[2]

Among uninformed people in India, we often hear remarks to the effect that the occurrence of a venereal disease is a 'visitation from God,' 'a sign of growing adolescence,' 'a sign of maturity,' 'the result of eating nettle leaves' and 'from sexual intercourse with menstruating woman'.[29] Such fallacious ideas about the causation of venereal diseases are still prevalent all over the world with varying emphasis.

Vedic researchers had carried their researches farther than any of their contemporaries.[30] The *Upanishads* contain the most convincing evidence of their passion for enquiry into the nature of things. Padmini, or the Lotus woman, is the symbol of woman beauty in Hindu mythology.[30] According to Hindu philosophy, the Lord of Beings (Brahma) created men and women and laid down rules for regulating their existence with regard to *Dharma* (acquisition of religious merit), *Artha* (acquisition of wealth, property, etc.) and *Kama* (love, pleasure and sensual gratification).[30] The commandments related to Kama were expounded by Nandi, the follower of Mahadeva. This document written by Nandi, known as *Kama Sutra* (aphorisms on love), was transformed into a small volume of Sanskrit literature by Vatsayana between the 1st and 6th centuries of the Christian era. This manuscript was known by name *Vatsayana Kama Sutra*. This document was withheld from public gaze as sex was considered a taboo amongst Hindus. This Sanskrit literature was later translated into English by Sir Richard Burton and F. F. Arbuthanot and published in England in 1883. There was no mention of venereology in the days of *Kama Sutra*.[30]

SYPHILIS

Some attempts have been made in the past to identify syphilis and gonorrhoea in ancient Ayurvedic texts, but evidence strongly suggests that syphilis, at least, was unknown in India before the early 16th century.[31] So explosive was the nature of the epidemic in this region during that time and so deep was the cultural impact that various religious/cultural communities started blaming each other as the source.[29,32] A careful examination of available records shows that Charaka and Sushruta, two ancient ayurvedic physicians, did not know anything about syphilis.[29] However, Bloomfield, Hirsch, Hessler and other Orientalists suggested that syphilis was prevalent in ancient India.[5] Some of the first references to the disease and its treatment are found in the *Bhavaprakasa*, a mid-sixteenth-century text, reputedly the work of Bhavamisra, an Ayurvedic physician at Benares. During that period and subsequently for a long time, syphilis was known in India as the Portuguese disease, or *firanga* or *firangi roga*, terms that identified the disease with the *firangis* ('Franks'), or Europeans.[29,31] According to historians, the disease was first recognized in India in 1498 after the arrival of Vasco de Gama, who left Portugal in 1497. It seems probable that the Portuguese introduced the disease to India in the early 16th century.[29] The researches of Okamura in Japan, Susuki in China and Jolly and others in India show that syphilis was introduced into this country from Europe.[29] By the early 19th century, when the British had gained ascendancy over a large part of the subcontinent, syphilis was already widely disseminated, although the extent of its incidence can only be guessed at.[31]

GONORRHOEA

During British Raj, in the official statistics of the army, venereal diseases like syphilis, gonorrhoea and soft chancre (now called chancroid) figured.[33] In the regiments of the British army stationed in India, the number of cases admitted to hospital with venereal diseases (identified in almost equal proportion as primary syphilis and gonorrhoea) rose to 205 per 1000 in 1875 and peaked at 522 per 1000 in 1895.[31] For unknown reasons, syphilis was relatively more common than gonorrhoea in the army personnel of Indian origin than in the British Army in India.[33]

CHANCROID

Chancroid, one of the five classic venereal diseases, was first described by Brassereau in 1852 in France.[34] Venereal diseases in the British Army comprised of syphilis, gonorrhoea and soft chancre, but it was decided to eliminate the latter one as not of public health importance in the run-up to the Royal Commission indian of 1916.[35] In the Army Indian (71001 men), the venereal disease rate in 1912 was 55.5 per 1000 (10.1% of all admissions). In the army at home, in India, the total venereal disease rate of 56.5 per 1000 consisted of 18.7 for primary and secondary syphilis, 29.5 for gonorrhoea and 8.3 for soft sore.[35]

DONOVANOSIS

Historically, donovanosis, formerly called granuloma inguinale, was first recognized and described in India. It was first identified in 1881 in Madras, India, by name 'serpiginous ulcer' by Kenneth MacLeod, a Scot who joined the Indian Medical Service and became professor of surgery in Kolkatta.[36] The causative organism was identified by Colonel Charles Donovan.[35] In 1905, he described the intracellular bodies, and was also the co-discoverer of the etiological agent in kala-azar.[37,38] The so-called 'Donovan bodies' were found in the exudate from an oral lesion in a ward boy of the General Hospital in Madras. The nature of the organism was disputed from the beginning. Donovan himself thought that they were protozoa. It was not until 1943 that the 'Donovan bodies' were proved to be bacterial in nature.[39] The natural history of donovanosis and its probable venereal nature was subsequently elucidated by others.[38,40]

LYMPHOGRANULOMA VENEREUM

In 1902, Caddy first recorded cases of lymphogranuloma venereum (LGV) in India under the title 'Climatic bubo'.[41] At the Institute of Venereology in Madras, 3884 cases of LGV were diagnosed between 1968 and 1977, accounting for 6% of STD cases seen in the same period.[42] Towards the end of the 19th century, most authors in India held the opinion that the disease was due to climatic influences (mainly tropical), and consequently, many textbooks today still refer to LGV as 'Climatic bubo'.[43,44]

OTHER STDs

No description of genital warts, herpes genitalis and trichomoniasis was found in the modern Indian literature of the early 20th century.[4] Despite considerable doubt raised by most observers, by 1920s and 1930s, many venereologists had concluded that genital warts is a sexually transmitted disease.[2] Genital herpes was rarely considered in the differential diagnosis of genital ulcers prior to 1965.[45] It was only in 1966 that herpes genitalis was recognized as a venereal disease. At present, it is the most common presentation in some of the STD clinics in India.[4] Donne first described the protozoal organism *Trichomonas vaginalis* in 1836,[46] which he observed in purulent genital secretions from both men and women. Microbiological investigations of chlamydial infection began in 1907 when Halberstaedter and Prowazek detected intracytoplasmic chlamydial inclusions in the conjunctival scrapings of nonhuman primates that were experimentally infected with materials collected from the conjunctiva of patients with active trachoma. Similar inclusions were later demonstrated in conjunctival cells of trachomatous patients, in scrapings from the conjunctiva of the eyes of babies with ophthalmia neonatorum, from the endocervix of mothers of these babies and from the urethra of patients with bacterial urethritis. In a study published in 2000, among 319 women with vaginal discharge attending a reproductive health clinic in New Delhi, the most common infection was bacterial vaginosis (26%).[47] At least one sexually transmitted infection was detected in 21.9% of women. The prevalence of *C. trachomatis* infection was 12.2%, trichomoniasis 10% and syphilis 2.2%.[47]

BRITISH INDIA AND STD CONTROL MEASURES

The British military authori-ties did not rely solely upon mercury to deal with STDs, especially syphilis, in the army (mainly contracted from prostitutes).[31] Around 1780s, lock hospitals were used to confine and treat prostitutes associated with the army and found suffering from STDs.[33] There was no specialist venereologist in India before 1910, but there was an army adviser who laid down treatment schedules and special wards were provided for complicated cases in the military hospitals in Britain.[33]

During the 19th century, attempts to control STDs centered on the control of prostitutes.[33] The Contagious Diseases Acts were promulgated between 1864 and 1869.[33] They ensured that, in garrison towns and major ports, women named to the police as prostitutes had to undergo regular medical examination. If found infected, they were confined to a lock hospital for up to 3 months for treatment, after which they were regarded as cured. The sole object was to protect soldiers. Indian prostitutes were segregated in special enclosures called '*chaklas*' within the cantonments where there was usually a lock hospital. A prostitute wishing to take up residence in a '*chakla*' had to apply for permission to be placed on the register of prostitutes. Registered prostitutes in '*chaklas*' were called '*Lal Kurti*', 'queen's ladies'. The *chaklas* were supervised by '*mahaldarnis*' appointed by the government. They were required to act as pimps and provide women for soldiers at the request of their commanding officers.[33] There were scanty data on the extent of STDs in the civilian population.[31] A report on Jafer Suleman Dispensary for women and children in Bombay by the pioneer lady doctor Edith Pechey recorded that among 2817 patients examined in the second half of 1884, 74 women and 23 children were suffering from syphilis; 55 had gonorrhoea.[48]

As a result of public agitation, particularly from women's groups in Britain, the Indian Contagious Diseases Acts were repealed in 1888.[33] Traditionally, the military authorities had accepted that reinstituting the system was essential. The army was not prepared to abandon all controls over army prostitution, and through a series of cantonment acts from 1889 onwards, it retained many of the formally renounced measures (like registration and licensing of prostitutes, the old rigid lock hospital system).[31,33] The provision of registered and inspected women was seen as a preferable alternative to masturbation or homosexuality, which was dreaded.[33] However, the women had to be presentable.

M. I. Balfour, a leading member of the Women's Medical Service, remarked in 1924 on the basis of 30 years' work in India that STDs were responsible for 'much of the gynecological disease which fills our women's hospitals and also no doubt for much of the high rate of infant mortality and the many miscarriages and stillbirths'.[49] The extent of STDs just before independence could be gauged from the report of Sir John Megaw, Director-General of the Indian Medical Services.[50] His survey in 1933 recorded 37 cases of syphilis and gonorrhoea for every 1000 cases attending the hospitals and clinics; it was also estimated that there were as many as 5.5 million cases of syphilis and 7.5 million of gonorrhoea in India at that time.

INDEPENDENT INDIA AND STD CONTROL MEASURES

Until 1949 there were practically no control measures adopted either on a limited or a large scale in India.[29] At the request of the Government of India, the World Health Organization (WHO) sent a venereal disease demonstration team in 1949 to work with a national matching team to establish a center for survey and mass treatment of syphilis in Himachal Pradesh in India. The Venereal Disease Main Clinic and Laboratory at Shimla in Himachal Pradesh was established in May 1949. It was one of the first states to have a full-time venereologist in control of a state VD organization. Subsequently, more VD clinics were established in Himachal Pradesh in the next 2-3 years. As a result, the percentage of seropositivity for syphilis was brought down from 40-45% in 1949-1951 to 18% by 1959.[29]

The WHO VD demonstration team in Himachal Pradesh trained medical and paramedical personnel from different states in India and South-East Asian region.[29] The team was withdrawn in December 1951, but as a result of the efforts of trained personnel in other states in India, in 1953 alone, about 100,000 new cases of syphilis were identified and treated. In view of the prevailing high incidence of VDs in the country, the Directorate General of Health Services (DGHS) in the Ministry of Health of Government of India included certain measures for VD control in the first Five Year Plan.[5,7] A full-scale VD organization came into existence in Himachal Pradesh. A VD training and demonstration center was established in New Delhi. The VD department of the Government General Hospital, Madras, was upgraded to a postgraduate training center in 1952. Measures were taken to make India self-sufficient in the production of cardiolipin antigen and penicillin.[29]

In the second Five Year Plan, greater emphasis was laid on the problem of venereal diseases.[29] On the advice of the health panel of the Planning Commission, the central and state governments made provision for a central VD organization, strengthening of state VD organizations, setting up 8 VD clinics and laboratories at the headquarters of states, 75 clinics at district headquarters, mass survey and treatment, free supply of penicillin and training of health personnel. A VD section was formed in November 1957 in the DGHS and some planned operations were set in progress. Training facilities for intensive refresher courses for all types of VD workers were offered in the VD training and demonstration center, Safdarjang Hospital, New Delhi, and for short-term refresher courses and a university diploma in VD at the upgraded VD department of Madras General Hospital.[29]

In the third Five Year Plan, it was envisaged to expand the existing facilities by providing additional VD clinics, stepping up epidemiological and health education programmes, case finding, routine testing of pregnant women for syphilis and further integration of VD control within the existing public health services.[29]

During 1949 to 1958, a consolidated report from different states in India showed syphilis to be the most common STD, followed by gonorrhoea, chancroid and other VDs.[29] The total number of VD cases was 867,268 in 1949 (syphilis - 345,219, gonorrhoea - 243,696, chancroid - 87306, other VDs - 27702); and in 1958, it was 484,602.[29] It has been estimated that for every single patient seeking help at a VD clinic, 20 such patients go elsewhere.[51] In 1970, a modest estimate of the incidence of VDs in India was around 8-10% of the population.[51]

During the first three Five Year Plans, although there was stress on opening one clinic in each state headquarters and at least one clinic in each district, only 261 VD clinics were established in the whole of India.[51] In the fourth Five Year Plan, only Rs. 1.5 crores was earmarked for VD control programmes, which included the establishment of five state headquarter VD clinics, 78 district clinics and a central VD organization, besides four mobile units. However, the VD control programmes remained far from satisfactory.[51]

VDs are higher in the urban and industrial areas in India.[51] They are also higher in the sub-Himalayan areas and in some southern states. The continuing population shift to urban areas from rural areas is also a cause for prostitution. There are plenty of commercial and individual prostitution centers in spite of the suppression of immoral traffic by law.[51] The scale of prostitution in Mumbai today remains a crude human index of the extent of poverty in India, as well as of the continuing humiliation and exploitation of women.[7] Health education, sex education, propaganda and publicity were practically nonexistent in independent India and so also epidemiological investigations. Thus, there was persistent complacency among medical and public health administrators in India.[51]

ADVENT OF AIDS INTO INDIA

The first reported cases of HIV infection in India were among Madras sex workers in May 1986.[52] The epidemic of HIV in India was similar in many ways to the experience in sub-Saharan Africa and Thailand. The advent of AIDS in India in 1980s was not at first regarded as a serious threat, with probable thinking that it is a White man's disease and is due to Western immorality.[31] In 1988, AIDS began to spread rapidly in India, thus awakening the health authorities.

- Sir William Osler once coined a dictum that "Physician who knew syphilis in all its manifestations knew medicine".
- The same is true for HIV/AIDS today.
- Dr. Jonathan M. Mann (former director, Global Programme for AIDS) once said, "Knowing AIDS is to know medicine".

To formulate a strategy and plan for the prevention and control of HIV/AIDS in the country, the Ministry of Health and Family Welfare constituted a National AIDS Committee in 1986 under the chairmanship of the Union Ministry of Health and Family Welfare with representatives from various sectors.[53] The committee was formed with a view to bring together various ministries, non-government organizations (NGOs) and private institutions for effective coordination in implementing the programme. The National AIDS Control Programme (NACP) was launched in 1987. In the initial years, it focussed on the generation of public awareness through more communication programmes, introduction of blood screening for transfusion and conducting surveillance activities in the epicenters of the epidemic.[53]

In 1989, with the support of the WHO, a medium-term plan for HIV/AIDS control was developed with a US$10 million budget provided from external sources.[53] However, activities like implementation of an education and awareness programme, blood safety measures, control of hospital infections, condom promotion to prevent HIV/AIDS and strengthening of clinical services for both STDs and HIV/AIDS gained momentum only in 1992. State AIDS cells were created in all the 32 states and union territories for effective implementation and management of NACP.[53]

The NACP (Phase I) was the first in India to develop a national public health programme in HIV/AIDS prevention and control, and was implemented between 1992 and 1999.[53] In order to assess the prevalence of HIV, it conducted anonymous unlinked surveys on CSWs, STD clinics, and antenatal clinics. The ultimate objective of the project was to control the spread of HIV to reduce future morbidity and mortality.

The Phase II of the NACP became effective from 9 November 1999.[53] This 100% federal sponsored scheme is being implemented in 32 states/union territories and 3 municipal corporations, namely Ahmedabad, Chennai and Mumbai, through AIDS control societies. In this effort, NGOs and voluntary agencies are helping to a great extent.

HIV EPIDEMIC IN INDIA

HIV/AIDS is a major health problem in India.[4] The higher HIV prevalence in the various states reflects the wide societal differences within India.[54] Evidence indicates multiple points of entry of the HIV epidemic into India, dating back to 1984. This led to a heterogeneous pattern of spread, including rapid intravenous drug use-related transmission in Manipur and predominant sexual transmission in Tamil Nadu, Maharashtra and neighboring states (associated with commercial sex). By 2003, an estimated 5.1 million people were living with HIV/AIDS in India, second only to South Africa in absolute numbers.[54] In 2007, the government claimed that the actual number of estimated HIV cases in India is just 2.5 million. Most infections have been acquired through sexual transmission (80.8%), with 5.1% through injecting drug use, 5.5% associated with blood or blood products, and less than 1% of cases infected through mother-to-child transmission.[53]

Government Nodal Agencies in Independent India

India has been plagued by many life-threatening diseases, and as in most other countries, STD services were a low priority.[33] Even before the country achieved independence, a National STD Control Programme was set up in 1946.[4] A Venereal Disease section was formed in November 1957 in the Directorate General of Health Services.[29] With the arrival of HIV infection in the country and because of its strong relation with STDs, the programme was brought under the purview of National AIDS Control Organization in 1992.[4] The National AIDS Control Programme existed from 1987, but NACO was set up in 1992. This programme had emphasis on health-seeking behaviour of individuals having STDs and removal of the social stigma attached to the disease.[4]

ACADEMIC DEVELOPMENTS

Europeans introduced modern medicine to India. At the time of independence, there were already 19 medical colleges in undivided India (including two in the princely states of Mysore and Hyderabad).[55] The total number of students admitted each year was about 1200. Calcutta Medical College and Madras Medical College were founded in 1835.[55,56] Madras Medical College actually started on 16 November 1664 as a small hospital at Fort St. George to treat sick soldiers of the East India Company. Other well-known colleges of colonial India are Grant Medical College, Mumbai (founded in 1845, it gave native citizens the presidency to study western medicine from some outstanding teachers), King George Medical College, Lucknow (1911), and Lady Hardinge Medical College (exclusively for women), Delhi (1916).[55,57] The Institute of Venereology in Madras Medical College was founded in 1952 to be the oldest venereology department in India.[4] In the early formative years, the strength and solidity to this institute was given by Col. Vasudeva Rao. Dr. R. V. Rajam was the founder director, an international figure for his research on venereal diseases. The successors to Dr. Rajam were Dr. P. N. Rangiah and Dr. C. N. Sowmini. After independence, venereology developed along with dermatology in most parts of India.[4]

In 1935, Dr. U. B. Narayan Rao started a private publication, the *Indian Journal of Venereology* from Mumbai.[58,59] In 1940, the journal was renamed *Indian Journal of Venereal Diseases and Dermatology* and it was published quarterly. This journal subsequently merged with the *Indian Journal of Dermatology and Venereology* in 1947. On 31 March 1955, the journal became the official publication of the Association. It had three editors: Dr. G. Panja, Dermatology Section; Dr. R. V. Rajam, Venereology Section; and Dr. U. B. Narayan Rao, Managing Editor. After the death of Dr. Narayan Rao in 1960, Dr. T. K. Mehta took over as the Managing Editor. Dr. U. B. Narayan Rao also gets the credit for the creation of an association of dermatologists and venereologists in Mumbai in 1947. Subsequent to the event of its inauguration on 1 July 1947, it organized an All-India Conference of Dermatologists and Venereologists on December 27 and 28, 1947, at J. J. Hospital, Mumbai.[58,59] In 1973, at a conference held in Udaipur, the Indian Association of Dermatologists and Venereologists merged with other dermatology associations to form the Indian Association of Dermatologists, Venereologists and Leprologists. The name *Indian Journal of Dermatology and Venereology* was changed to *Indian Journal of Dermatology, Venereology and Leprology* (*IJDVL*). Since then, Dr. S. C. Desai, Dr. Bhaktavizam, Dr. (Mrs.) Rachel Mathai, Dr. J. S. Pasricha, Dr. S. G. Deshpande, Dr. Gurmohan Singh, Dr. K. Pavithran and Dr. Uday Khopkar had been the chief editors of *IJDVL*.

The Indian Association for the Study of Sexually Transmitted Diseases (IASSTDs) came into existence in 1975 with its founder members being Dr. K. N. Gopalan, Dr. G. Chandrashekhar Rao, Dr. K. Vijaylaksmi, Dr. P. K. Dharmalingam and Dr. M. K. Venkataraman.[4] Dr. Sowmini was its president and Dr. C. C. Mohan Ram was its secretary then. After the advent of AIDS in India, its name was changed to Indian Association for the Study of Sexually Transmitted Diseases and AIDS (1993). Since its formation, this association has been organizing several annual conferences. In 1980, the Indian Association for the Study of Sexually Transmitted Diseases started its own exclusive journal, the *Indian Journal of Sexually Transmitted Diseases*.[4] The late Dr. Sardari Lal was its founder editor and guiding force, who had already made a mark in donovanosis research.[60] Dr. R. C. Sharma, Dr. Rishi Bhargava and Dr. Y. S. Marfatia were successors to Dr. Sardari Lal (Table 3.1).[4]

In 2003, the textbook and atlas of 'Sexually transmitted diseases and AIDS' was published by IASSTDs with Dr. V. K. Sharma as editor-in-chief. However, venereology did not prosper, even though it led dermatology and leprology to academic recognition, probably due to lack of interest and government commitment in the specialty.[4] The academic interest for venereology in India could be judged from the report of Webster in 1966.[61] The average time spent in the teaching of venereology as a separate subject in 437 schools was 17.1 hours. The average number of hours devoted to teaching venereology in India was 61.2 as compared to 137 in USSR, 106 in Bulgaria, 105 in Iran, 104 in Jamaica, 100.7 in Poland, 90 in Greece, 84 in Malta, 76.8 in Yugoslavia and 66.3 in Mexico. The current teaching on the subject provides adequate exposure. The monograph by Dr. Rajam and Dr. Rangiah on donovanosis (granuloma inguinale, granuloma venereum) is a testimony of teaching and research standards set by these two giants at the Institute of Venereology, Madras.[38] In 1942, Bombay University appointed a committee to frame rules and regulations for starting a diploma course in dermatology and venereology (DVD). It was a course of 1-year duration, and the first DVD examination was held in October 1945. In 1947, the College of Physicians and Surgeons (Bombay) encouraged candidates to appear for their fellowship examination in dermatology and venereology. Since then, many medical colleges have been recognized for training of postgraduates in this specialty.[59]

Venereology has been combined with dermatology in most universities in India.[4,51] At Grant Medical College and Sir J. J. Group of Hospitals,

Mumbai, skin and STDs were two different units, which were later merged. Diploma and degree courses have been offered by many universities, but the scope of research in venereology is extremely poor and inadequate due to poorly equipped STD clinics in terms of manpower and infrastructure. Throughout the world, experts in STIs have come from a variety of medical specialties over the course of the 20th century.[1] During the first 50 years and owing to medical importance of syphilis and its dermatologic manifestations, a specialty of dermato-venereology emerged in Europe and North America. However, with the near eradication of syphilis and gonorrhoea in the Western world in 1950s, many dermatology training programmes lost interest in venereology and journals of syphilology and dermato-venereology ceased to publish.

Table 3.1 **Profile of Select Distinguished Venereologists of India**

Dr. RV Rajam

- Founder director of Institute of Venereology in Madras (now Chennai)
- The first president of Indian Association of Venereologists and Dermatologists in 1947
- Served as member and chairman of the expert committee of venereal diseases of ICMR from 1948 to 1966
- Perpared a monograph on granuloma inguinale for WHO along with Dr. PN Rangiah

Dr. CW Chacko

- First to set up Treponema Immoblization test for syphilis
- Also had to his credit the discovery of Chacko strain of Yaws and Chacko-Nair culture media for gonococcal culture

Dr. CN Sowmini

- Director of Institute of Venereology, Madras Medical College, Madras, after Dr. PN Rangiah
- Instrumental in starting the 'Indian Association for the Study of Sexually Transmitted Diseases' (IASSTDs) in 1975, which was later renamed 'IASSTDs & AIDS' and served as President of the Association for 8 years

Dr. Sardari Lal

- Founder editor of *Indian Journal of Sexually Transmitted Diseases* (*IJSTD*)
- Research interest in donovanosis

EMERGING STI SCENARIO

With regard to India, most STIs are managed in informal and private medical sectors or are self-treated. STI survey data are limited in India, but these surveys indicate a very diverse picture.[62] In community-based surveys of married and unmarried women in India, chlamydia prevalence ranged between 0.5 and 28.7%, gonorrhoea between 0 and 4.2%, and syphilis between 0.2 and 10.5%.[63] Sharma and Khandpur reviewed the changing patterns of different STIs (excluding HIV infection) in India and their various risk factors.[64] It was observed that most published data are institution-based. There is paucity of community-based data, except for information obtained from high-risk groups such as CSWs, truck drivers, hotel workers and drug abusers. From the literature search undertaken, it may be observed that, during 1960s and 1970s, bacterial infections including syphilis, chancroid and gonorrhoea were the major STIs, while viral infections caused by herpes simplex virus and human papilloma virus were so rare that they merited publication as case reports. As in developed countries, there has been a rise in viral and chlamydial infections and a relative fall in the incidence of traditional infections. In a recently published retrospective study of the pattern of STDs during the 10-year period from 1990 at Kottayam, GUDs accounted for the maximum number of STDs (73.5%), followed by condyloma acuminatum (17.5%) and gonorrhoea (10.1%).[65] Amongst GUDs, syphilis was the most common disease, accounting for 57.3% of cases. Granuloma inguinale and lymphogranuloma venereum were found rare. The overall trend of STDs was declining, with the total number of patients during the first year of study being 129, while it was 41 during the last year of study. Bacterial STDs showed a striking reduction in numbers. The decline was less marked in the case of viral STDs. In a recent review of the current status of STDs in India in 2007, Thappa and Kaimal[66] summarized the emerging Indian scenario as under. Bacterial STDs like chancroid and gonorrhoea are showing a declining trend, but viral STDs like herpes genitalis and condyloma acuminatum are showing an upward trend. There is a decline in the number of patients with STDs attending the hospitals. Whether it is due to an actual decrease in the incidence of STDs or due to other factors is uncertain. The increased availability of facilities for treatment of STDs at peripheral centers might be a factor leading to a decline in the number of patients with STDs approaching medical college where various studies are undertaken. The emphasis on the syndromic approach to the management of STDs might have increased the accessibility to health care for patients with STDs. Awareness about HIV and fear of contracting STDs are likely to have influenced the risk-taking behaviour of people, thereby reducing the likelihood of being infected with STDs. Another factor to be considered is the widespread use of antibacterials, including quinolones and the new macrolides, for the treatment of other diseases. This could result in partial treatment or modified course of bacterial STDs, thereby leading to apparent reduction in the total number of cases of STDs attending STD clinics as well as a decrease in the proportion of bacterial to viral STDs. The evident decline of bacterial STDs with an apparent increase of viral STDs is the trend worth noting.

During the last 10-15 years, the rates of gonorrhoea, syphilis, hepatitis B infection and HIV have declined by 80-95% or more in USA.[1] For the past 7-9 years, STI rates in homosexual men are rising modestly. Globally, the HIV incidence is still rising in some areas of Africa, Asia and eastern Europe and declining in others.[1]

In India, the main strategy aimed at achieving effective management of people with established infections has been to integrate STD services into the existing health care system, with special emphasis on the integration at the primary health care (PHC) level. The National AIDS Control Organization (NACO)[67] recommends syndromic management for case management at this level. Effectiveness of syndromic management in women is currently under debate.[63] The NACO is now also focusing on women reproductive health issues involving gynecologists.

FUTURE DIRECTIONS

Donovanosis will soon be eradicated from several nations, but syphilis eradication will be successful only around 2020.[68] Gonorrhoea, chlamydial infection, chancroid and trichomoniasis may also persist despite their curability. With the exception of hepatitis B and HIV, other blood-borne pathogens will continue to flourish until blood supplies and medical injections, as well as illicit drug use and tattooing, are made safe. Anogenital warts and herpes will also persist and possibly increase, as may candidiasis, vulvovaginitis, bacterial vaginosis, balanitis, and prostatitis. The problems of spreading HIV epidemic, drug resistance, poor health facilities and financial constraints are a great hindrance in achieving a reduction in the incidence and prevalence of STIs. A worthy vision for 2020 is a world with universal sexual health as well as a world free of sexual illhealth. Our task for the future, therefore, is to work together to make this vision a reality.[68] Vast numbers of people in India are severely disadvantaged in terms of income, education, power structures and gender.[63] Addressing these basic issues of human rights lies at the core of achieving better health outcomes[69] (including reproductive and infectious diseases) in India. Such a challenge is formidable in terms of its required scope and coverage but lies at the heart of improving sexual health for the greatest number of people in India.

REFERENCES

1. Thappa DM. Evolution of venereology in India. Indian J Dermatol Venereol Leprol 2006; 72: 187-96.
2. Bingham JS. Historical aspects of sexually transmitted infections. *In*: Kumar B, Gupta S, editors, Sexually Transmitted Infections, 1st ed. Elsevier: New Delhi; 2005. p. 5-17.
3. Sharma VK, Khandpur S. Epidemiology of sexually transmitted diseases. *In*: Sharma VK, editor. Sexually Transmitted Diseases and AIDS. Viva Books Pvt Ltd: New Delhi; 2003. p. 1-41.
4. Thappa DM. History of venereal diseases and venereology in India. Indian J Sex Transm Dis 2002; 23: 67-79.
5. Thappa DM, Singh N, Kaimal S. Prostitution in India and its role in the spread of HIV infection. Indian J Sex Transm Dis 2007; 28: 69-75.
6. Ringdals NJ. Love for sale: A world history of prostitution, Grove Press 2004.
7. Nag M. Sexual behaviour in India with risk of HIV/AIDS transmission. Health Transition Review, 1995; 5 (Supplement): 293-305.
8. Ghosh M, Das NK. Anonder Opekshay: Chondalika Ekdal Khokkosh [Report on prostitution in Calcutta, in Bengali]. Calcutta: Calcutta Development Dialogue, 1990.
9. Gilada IS. Women in prostitution in urban centres: study perspectives and positional problems for social interventions. Paper presented to the NGO Forum of World Conference to Review and Appraise the Achievements of the United Nations Decade for Women, Nairobi, 5-26 July, 1985.
10. Gilada, I.S. No date. Prostitution in India: causes, extent, prevention, rehabilitation. Indian Health Organization, Bombay (manuscript).
11. Chattopadhyay M, Bandyopadhyay S, Duttagupta C. Biosocial factors influencing women to become prostitutes in India. Soc Biol. 1994; 41: 252-9.
12. Gilada IS, Thakur V. Devadasis: In Exploitation of Women and Children: Its Causes and Effects. Proceedings of the Asian Regional Conference, Delhi, 17-19 November 1988. Delhi: International Abolitionist Federation, 1988.
13. Blanchard JF, O'Neil J, Ramesh BM, et al. Understanding the social and cultural contexts of female sex workers in Karnataka, India: Implications for prevention of HIV infection. JID 2005; 191: S139–46.
14. Mukhopadhyay KK. Girl prostitution in India. Soc Change. 1995; 25: 143-53.
15. Kapur P. The Life and World of Call Girls in India. New Delhi: Vikas Publishing House, 1978.
16. Kapur P. A study of changes in the sexual behaviour of call-girls and their clients in India. Paper presented at Workshop on Sexual Aspects of AIDS/STDs Prevention in India, Tata Institute of Social Science, Bombay, 23-6 November 1993.
17. Joardar B. Prostitution in Historical and Modern Perspectives. Inter-India Publications, New Delhi, 1984: 153.
18. Mukherjee KK. Flesh Trade: a Report. Gram Niyojan Kendra, Ghajiabad, 1989: 44, 45, 81.

19. Joardar B. A sociological study of prostitution in Calcutta. Journal of the Anthropological Society 1973: 8.
20. Kar HK, Satpathy SK, Van Padmana P, et al. Evaluation of National AIDS Control Programme using prevention indicators: a case study in India. International Conference on AIDS 1998 (Abstract # 44317). Geneva, Switzerland, 1998.
21. Kumar A, Mehra M, Badhan SK, et al. Heterosexual behaviour and condom use in an urban population of Delhi, India. AIDS Care 1997; 9: 311-8.
22. Rao A, Nag M, Mishra K, et al. Sexual behaviour pattern of truck drivers and their helpers in relation to female sex workers. Indian Journal of Social Work 1994; 55: 603-16.
23. Kinsey AC, Pomeroy WB, Martin CE. Sexual Behaviour in the Human Male. Philadelphia: W.B. Saunders, 1948.
24. Kinsey AC, Pomeroy WB, Martin CE, Gebhard PH. Sexual Behaviour in the Human Female. Philadelphia: W.B. Saunders, 1953.
25. AIDS Bhedhav Virodhi Andolan (ABVA). Less than Gay: A Citizens' Report on the Status of Homosexuality in India. New Delhi, 1991.
26. Row-Kavi A. HIV/AIDS awareness in the self-identified gay community and its implications. Paper presented at Workshop on Sexual Aspects of AIDS/STDs Prevention in India, Tata Institute of Social Sciences, Bombay, 23-26 November, 1993.
27. Nanda S. The Hijras of India: cultural and individual dimensions of an institutionalized third gender role. In: Blackwood E, editor, Anthropology and homosexual behaviour, Binghampton: Haworth Press.1985: 35-54.
28. Prostitution. From Wikipedia, the free encyclopedia. http://en.wikipedia.org/wiki/Prostitution.
29. Tampi RB. Venereal diseases in India. Central Health Education Bureau, New Delhi: DGHS, Ministry of Health, Government of India, 1962. p. 1-27.
30. The Kama Sutra of Vatsyayana-The classic Hindu treatise on love and social conduct, translated by Sir Richard F Burton and FF Arbuthnot, 15th Jaico Impression. Jaico Publishing House: Mumbai; 2005.
31. Arnold D. Sexually transmitted diseases in nineteenth and twentieth century India. Genitourin Med 1993; 69: 3-8.
32. Kumar B, Gupta S, Muralidhar S. Mucocutaneous manifestations of secondary syphilis in North Indian patients: A changing scenario. J Dermatol 2001; 28: 137-44.
33. Roy RB. Sexually transmitted diseases and the Raj. Sex Transm Infect 1998; 74:20-6.
34. Ronald AR, Plummer FA. Chancroid and Haemophilus ducreyi. Ann Intern Med 1985; 102: 705-7.
35. Willcox RR. Fifty years since the conception of an organized venereal diseases service in Great Britain: The Royal commission of 1916. Br J Venereal Dis 1967; 43: 1-9.
36. MacLeod K. Precis of operations performed in the wards of First Surgeon, Medical College Hospital during the year 1881. Indian Med Gazette 1882; 17: 112-23.
37. Donovan C. Medical cases from Madras General Hospital: ulcerating granuloma of the pudenda. Indian Med Gazette 1905; 40: 414.
38. Rajam RV, Rangiah PN. Donovanosis. (Granuloma inguinale, Granuloma venereum) World Health Organization: Geneva; 1954. p. 10.
39. Goldberg J. Studies on granuloma inguinale VII. Some epidemiologic considerations of the disease. Br J Vener Dis 1964; 40: 140-5.
40. Ramachandra Rao MG. A case of granuloma inguinale. Indian Med Gazette 1931; 66: 21.
41. Caddy A. Climatic buboes-twelve cases in Calcutta. Indian Med Gazette 1902; 27: 27.
42. Sowmini CN. Late manifestations of LGV. Paper presented at the 29th General Assembly of International Union against Venereal Diseases and Treponematoses, Leeds: 1978.
43. Rangiah PN, Vijayalakshmi K, Siddapppa K. Lymphogranuloma venereum. *In*: Valia RG, Valia AR, editors. IADVL Textbook and Atlas of Dermatology. 1st ed. Bhalani Publishing House: Mumbai; 1994. p. 1225-33.

44. Rajam RV, Rangiah PN. Lymphogranuloma venereum. Indian J Dermatol Venereol 1955; 21: 4.

45. Ramana Rao RV, Bose YS, Kumar BS. Viral STDs. *In* : Valia RG, Valia AR, editors. IADVL Textbook and Atlas of Dermatology, 1st ed. Bhalani Publishing House: Mumbai; 1994. p. 1234-50.

46. King A, Nicol C, Rodin P. Venereal diseases. 4th ed. The English Language Book Society and Bailliere Tindall: London; 1980. p. 309-20.

47. Vishwanath S, Talwar V, Prasad R, et al. Syndromic management of vaginal discharge among women in a reproductive health clinic in India. Sex Transm Infect 2000; 76: 303-6.

48. First annual report of the Medical Women for India Fund, 1884 in Home Medical, 32, Sept. National Archives of India: New Delhi; 1886.

49. Balfour MI. 'Venereal disease in India'. J Assoc Med Women India 1924; 12: 15.

50. Report of the Health Survey and Development Committee 1. Manager of Publications: Delhi; 1946. p. 123.

51. Banerjee BN. Venereology-Conditions in India. JIMA 1971; 56: 139-40.

52. Simoes EA, Babu PG, John TJ, et al . Evidence for HTLV-III infection in prostitutes in Tamil Nadu (India). Indian J Med Res 1987; 85: 335-8.

53. National AIDS Control Organization. National AIDS Control Programme and Indian Scenario. National AIDS Control Organization (NACO). http://www.naco.nic.in/ Accessed 8th December, 2003.

54. Donovan B, Kaldor JM. The epidemiology of HIV infection and AIDS in Asia and the Pacific: Global perspective. In: Kumar B, Gupta S, editors. Sexually Transmitted Infections, 1st ed. Elsevier: New Delhi; 2005. p. 57-66.

55. IQRA Society for Career Guidance [Course Guide-Chapter 43: Medicine and Dentistry] Hyderabad, Andhra Pradesh, India: IQRA Society for Career Guidance [updated 2002 IQRA; cited 2004 Feb 19]. http://iqra-careers.com/c43.html Accessed 19th February, 2004.

56. Madras Medical College [History of MMC] Chennai, Tamil Nadu, India: Madras Medical College. http://mmcindia.edu/ Accessed 19th February, 2004.

57. King Edward VII Memorial Hospital and Seth Gordhandas Sunderdas Medical College [Seth Gordhandas Sunderdas Medical College and King Edward VII Memorial Hospital, Bombay: Sunil. K. Pandya], Mumbai: King Edward VII Memorial Hospital and Seth Gordhandas Sunderdas Medical College, http://www.kem.edu/college/history.htm Accessed 19th February, 2004.

58. Sehgal VN. Indian Dermatology. Int J Dermatol 1993; 32: 838-44.

59. Thappa DM. History of Dermatology, Venereology and Leprology in India. J Postgrad Med 2002; 48: 160-5.

60. Sharma RC. Obituary. Dr Sardari Lal. Indian J Sex Transm Dis 1993; 14: 72.

61. Webster B. Teaching of venereal diseases in medical schools throughout the world: Preliminary report. Br J Venereal Dis 1966; 42: 132-3.

62. Bourne C, Donovan B. The epidemiology of sexually transmitted infections in Asia and the Pacific. In: Kumar B, Gupta S, editors. Sexually Transmitted Infections, 1st ed. Elsevier: New Delhi; 2005. p. 44-56.

63. Hawks S, Santhya KG. Diverse realities: sexually transmitted infections and HIV in India. Sex Transm Infect 2002; 78: 131-9.

64. Sharma VK, Khandpur S. Changing patterns of sexually transmitted infections in India. Natl Med J India 2004; 17: 310-9.

65. Narayanan B. A retrospective study of the pattern of sexually transmitted diseases during a ten-year period. Indian J Dermatol Venereol Leprol 2005; 71: 333-7.

66. Thappa DM, Kaimal S. Sexually transmitted infections in India: Current status (Except human immunodeficiency virus/acquired im-

munodeficiency syndrome). Indian J Dermatol 2007; 52: 78-82.

67. National AIDS Control Organisation. Country scenario 1997-98. Ministry of Health and Family Welfare: New Delhi; 1998.

68. Philipot R. Future directions for STIs and sexual health in Asia-Pacific region: 2002-2020. *In:* Kumar B, Gupta S, editors, Sexually Transmitted Infections. 1st ed. Elsevier: New Delhi; 2005. p. 18-26.

69. Aral SO, Mann JM. Commercial sex work and STDs: the need for policy interventions to change societal patterns. Sex Transm Dis 1998; 25: 455-6.

PART 2

HIV/AIDS

4 GLOBAL AND NATIONAL OVERVIEW OF HIV/AIDS EPIDEMIC

H K Kar

In this chapter

- Historical Milestones
- An Overview of the Epidemic
- Focusing on Risk
- HIV Epidemic: Indian Scenario
- Basic Epidemiology
- HIV Prevalence in Risk Groups in India
- The Interplay of Factors Driving Sexual Transmission
- Survival Time After Diagnosis of AIDS and Advent of Anti-HIV Treatment

INTRODUCTION

AIDS represents the late clinical stage of infection with HIV. The syndrome was first recognized in 1981, but probably existed at a low endemic level in Central Africa before it spread to several regions of the world during 1980s.[1]

After two and a half decades into the epidemic, there is still no vaccine and no "cure" for AIDS. There is considerable information now avail-able on how the HIV leads to AIDS, its spread, and a wealth of "lessons learned" in implementing prevention strategies and increased understanding of what constitutes effective management of HIV/AIDS patients. The social and economic conditions that facilitate the spread of HIV are also well understood. Despite all that, risk behaviour and risk environments persist and HIV continues to spread among individuals and across national and regional borders, the latest frontier being Asia.

Due to the association of HIV/AIDS with commercial sex, drugs and men having sex with men, the disease has also acquired a stigma that is difficult to overcome. Those infected and affected by HIV and AIDS face discrimination and alienation. The early uncertainity of the mode of HIV spread, and knowledge that it is a fatal illness with no cure currently available, created considerable fear and consequent alienation of people living with HIV and AIDS as well as their close family members. Stigma is one of the most crucial impediments in breaking the chain of transmission of HIV in the community. It is time to cross the boundaries laid by misinformation, fear and stigma and break the barriers in taking proactive, sensible and effective measures to contain the spread of HIV/AIDS in the country.

HISTORICAL MILESTONES

The first indication that the disease is caused by a retrovirus came in 1983 from French scientists, when Prof. Montagnier and his coworkers isolated the causative viral agent, which was later named HIV.[2] Enzyme-inked immunosorbent assay (ELISA) was developed in 1984 to detect the presence of antibodies in blood against HIV technique.The CD4 molecule was identified as the major receptor for HIV. HIV was isolated from semen[3] and the central nervous system[4]. Thus, by 1984, it became apparent that the virus is lymphocytotrophic and also has neurotropism. The viral isolation in semen explains the reason why the epidemic is being observed in gay groups. In 1986, Montagnier's team discovered a new type of HIV in West Africa and labeled it HIV-2.[5] In 1987, zidovudine was reported to be useful in managing the patients with HIV infection.[6] Later came the combination therapy in vogue, which became more popular after the discovery of protease inhibitors. The "Call to Action" on HIV/AIDS at the UN General Assembly Special Session (June 2001) pushed forward a new global consensus on the need of antiretroviral therapy (ART). The WHO guidelines for "Antiretroviral use in resource-constrained settings" were revised in December 2003 and in August 2006. A subsequent amendment on the dose of stavudine (d4T) was issued by WHO in April 2007.

OVERVIEW OF THE EPIDEMIC

HIV/AIDS Pandemic (Global Scenario)[7]

Promising developments have been seen in the recent years in the global efforts to address the AIDS epidemic, including increased access to effective treatment and prevention programmes. However, the number of people living with HIV continues to grow, as does the number of deaths due to AIDS. A total of 39.5 million (34.1–47.1 million) people were living with HIV in 2006—which was 2.6 million more than that in 2004. This figure includes the estimated 4.3 million (3.6–6.6 million) adults and children who were newly infected with HIV in 2006, which is about 400,000 more than that in 2004.

In many regions of the world, new HIV infections are heavily concentrated among young people (15–24 years of age), which accounted for 40% of new HIV infections in 2006.

a. **Number of people living with HIV in 2006**
Total 39.5 million (34.1–47.1 million)
Adults 37.2 million (32.1–44.5 million)
Women 17.7 million (15.1–20.9 million)
Children under 15 years 2.3 million (1.7–3.5 million)

b. **People newly infected with HIV in 2006**
Total 4.3 million (3.6–6.6 million)
Adults 3.8 million (3.2–5.7 million)
Children under 15 years 530,000 (410,000–660,000)

c. **Death due to AIDS in 2006**
Total 2.9 million (2.5–3.5 million)
Adults 2.6 million (2.2–3.0 million)
Children under 15 years 380,000 (290,000–500,000)

Globally, more adult women (15 years or older) than ever before are now living with HIV. The 17.7 million (15.1–20.9 million) women living with HIV in 2006 represented an increase of over one million as compared with 2004. In sub-Saharan Africa, for every ten adult men living with HIV, there are about 14 adult women infected with the virus. Across all age groups, 59% of people living with HIV in sub-Saharan Africa in 2006 were women. In the Caribbean, the Middle East and North Africa, and Oceania, nearly one in every two adults with HIV is female. Meanwhile, in many countries of Asia, eastern Europe and Latin America, the proportions of women living with HIV continue to grow.

Access to treatment and care has greatly increased in the recent years, albeit from a very low starting level in many countries. Nevertheless, the benefits are dramatic. Through the expanded provision of ART, an estimated two million life-years were gained since 2002 in low- and middle-income countries. In sub-Saharan Africa alone, some 790,000 life-years have been gained, the vast majority of them in the past two years of ART scale-up. In Latin America, where wide-scale treatment provisions began earlier, some 834,000 life-years have been gained since 2002.

Latest Regional Developments

Almost 25 million people are living with HIV in sub-Saharan Africa—63% of all persons with HIV globally. Considerable efforts have been made towards improving access to ART in the recent years. Nonetheless, 2.1 million (1.8-2.4 million) Africans died of AIDS in 2006-almost three quarters (72%) of all AIDS deaths globally.

Southern Africa was the hardest hit where Zimbabwe remains the only country where national adult HIV prevalence has declined. The declining trend appears to be partly associated with behaviour changes in the mid- to late-1990s.

Meanwhile, the HIV epidemic in Mozambique, South Africa and Swaziland continues to grow. An estimated one in three (33%) adults in Swaziland was living with HIV in 2005—the most intense epidemic in the world. In South Africa, which has one of the world's largest HIV epidemics, the prevalence of HIV among women attending public antenatal clinics was more than one-third (35%) higher in 2005 than it had been in 1999. While HIV infection levels among young pregnant women appear to be stabilizing, they continue to increase among older women. The epidemic is having a significant impact. Death rates from natural causes for women aged 25–34 years increased fivefold between 1997 and 2004, and for males aged 30–44, it has more than doubled. A large part of it was due to the AIDS epidemic.

In East Africa, where HIV infection levels have been lower than that in the south, the general trend of stabilizing or declining HIV prevalence appears to be continuing. National HIV prevalence among pregnant women has declined in Kenya, as it has in Tanzania and, to a lesser extent, in Rwanda. In many other countries though, discrepant trends are often being found at local levels. Meanwhile, new research indicates a possible erosion of the gains Uganda made against AIDS in 1990s, and HIV prevalence has again been rising in some rural areas. A sudden increase in infection levels among pregnant women in 2005 in Burundi's capital, Bujumbura, could reverse the post-2000 decline in HIV prevalence in that country.

West and Central Africa's lower epidemics show divergent trends. There are signs of declining HIV prevalence in the urban parts of Burkina Faso, Côte d'Ivoire and Ghana, but in Mali, the HIV epidemic appears to be growing. A recent development in sub-Saharan Africa is the emergence of injecting drug use as a potential factor in HIV epidemics, notably in Kenya and Tanzania (as well as Nigeria and South Africa).

In Asia, national HIV infection levels are highest in South-East Asia, where combinations of unprotected paid sex and unprotected sex between men, along with unsafe injecting drug use, are the largest risk factors. HIV outbreaks among men who have sex with men are now becoming evident in Cambodia, China, India, Nepal, Pakistan, Thailand and Vietnam. In very few of these countries, national AIDS programmes adequately address the role of sex between men in the epidemics. HIV outbreaks are reported in Afghanistan and Pakistan, particularly among injecting drug users. High levels of use of non-sterile injecting equipment and other risk behaviours offer considerable scope for HIV epidemics in these two countries.

The HIV epidemic in India may be best described as a series of epidemics, widely varying with respect to prevalence levels, risk factors for infection and transmission patterns. Some of these epidemics appear to be stable or diminishing in parts of the south, while others are growing at a modest rate elsewhere, especially in the north-east (details below). In China, HIV is spreading gradually from most-at-risk populations (especially injecting drug users, and commercial sex workers and clients) to the general population, and the number of HIV infections in women is growing.

Latin America's epidemics remain generally stable, with Brazil, in particular, providing proof that a dual emphasis on prevention and treatment can keep an HIV epidemic under control. Outbreaks of the virus continue among injecting drug users and men who have sex with men in most countries of South America. Although largely a hidden behaviour, sex between men likely accounts for as much as one-tenth of reported HIV cases in the Caribbean. In that region, HIV prevalence remains stable in Dominican Republic, and has declined in the urban parts of Haiti, but there are indications that epidemics in both countries could show if prevention efforts are not enhanced.

In most countries with repeated surveys, there are some positive trends in young people's sexual behaviours. The future course of the world's HIV epidemics hinges in many respects on behaviours young people adopt or maintain, and contextual factors that affect those choices.

Racial and ethnic minorities in the United States continue to be disproportionately affected by HIV epidemic, while aboriginal people are over-represented in Canada's epidemic. As in Western and Central Europe, the main risk factor for HIV remains unprotected sex between men. HIV prevalence ranges between 10 and 20% among men who have sex with men in several countries of Western Europe, due to increased casual and unprotected sex in this population group. At the same time, approximately three-quarters of heterosexually acquired HIV infections in Western and Central Europe are among immigrants. This fact underlines the need to reach prevention, treatment and care services to these populations.

HIV epidemics in eastern Europe and Central Asia are still relatively small, but they continue to grow—most strikingly in Ukraine, which has the highest HIV prevalence in all of Europe. With regard to the Russian Federation's expanding epidemic and the smaller but growing epidemics of Tajikistan and Uzbekistan, the use of non-sterile injecting drug equipment remains the main mode of HIV transmission. HIV epidemics in these regions are greatly affecting the young people; in the Russian Federation, for example, some 80% of people with HIV are younger than 30 years of age. In the Russian Federation and Ukraine, women (many of them less than 25 years old) bear a growing proportion of the HIV burden, accounting for more than 40% of new HIV diagnoses in 2005.

Inadequate HIV surveillance remains a hindrance in many countries, including Europe, the Caribbean, Central America, the Middle East and North Africa. It is thus difficult to discern precisely the patterns and trends of some HIV epidemics, and design and implement potentially effective responses. However, there are exceptions, notably Iran. However, which has acted on improved HIV information gathering by expanding AIDS response among at-risk populations.

As per WHO and UNAIDS estimation, the following figures (Figs 4.1-4.4) show the estimated global, sub-Saharan Africa and regional figures of HIV burden by 2005.

Although children represented only 6% of all people infected with HIV/AIDS as of December 2005, they accounted for 18% of the 3.1 million AIDS deaths in 2005.

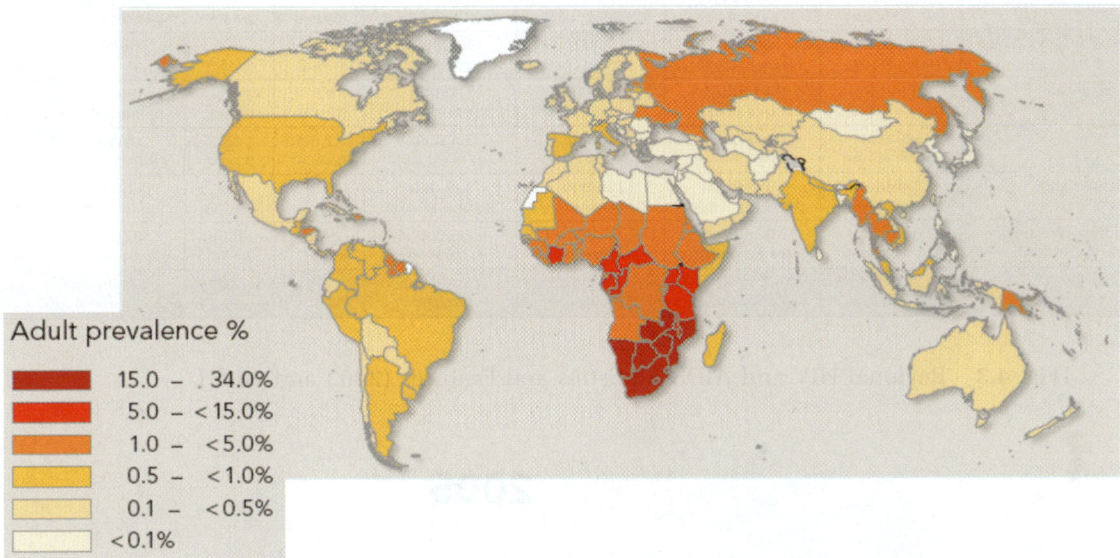

Fig. 4.1 A Global View of HIV Infection. 38.6 Million People (33.4–46.0 million) Living with HIV by (2005)

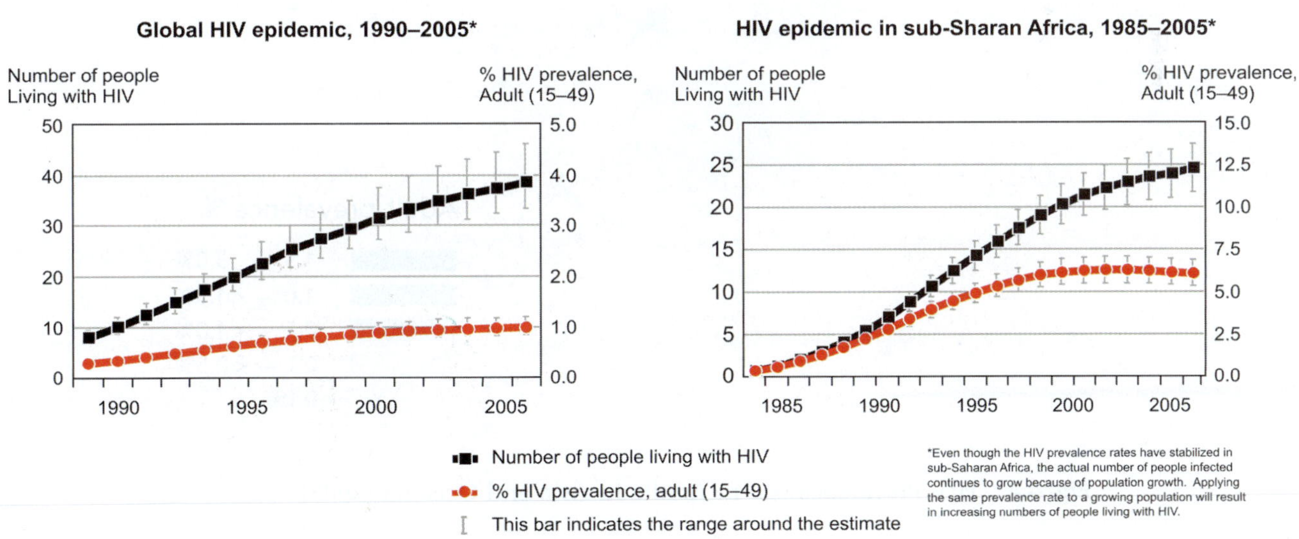

Fig. 4.2 Estimated Number of People Living with HIV

REGION	Adults (15+) and children living with HIV		Adults (15+) and children Newly infected with HIV		Adult (15-49) prevalence (%)		Adult (15+) and child deaths due to AIDS	
	2005	2003	2005	2003	2005	2003	2005	2003
Sub-Saharan Africa	24.5 million [21.6–27.4 million]	23.5 million [20.8–26.3 million]	2.7 million [2.3–3.1 million]	2.6 million [2.3–3.0 million]	6.1 [5.4–6.8]	6.2 [5.5–7.0]	2.0 million [1.7–2.3 million]	1.9 million [1.7–2.3 million]
North Africa and Middle East	440 000 [250 000–720 000]	380 000 [220 000–620 000]	64 000 [38 000–210 000]	54 000 [31 000–150 000]	0.2 [0.1–0.4]	0.2 [0.1–0.3]	37 000 [20 000–62 000]	34 000 [18 000–57 000]
Asia	8.3 million [5.7–12.5 million]	7.6 million [5.2–11.3 million]	930 000 [620 000–2.4 million]	860 000 [560 000–2.3 million]	0.4 [0.3–0.6]	0.4 [0.2–0.6]	600 000 [400 000–850 000]	500 000 [340 000–710 000]
Oceania	78 000 [48 000–170 000]	66 000 [41 000–140 000]	7200 [3500–55 000]	9000 [4300-69 000]	0.3 [0.2–0.8]	0.3 [0.2–0.7]	3400 [1900–5500]	2300 [1300–3600]
Latin America	1.6 million [1.2–2.4 million]	1.4 million [1.1–2.0 million]	140 000 [100 000–420 000]	130 000 [95 000–310 000]	0.5 [0.4–1.2]	0.5 [0.4–0.7]	59 000 [47 000–76 000]	51 000 [40 000–67 000]
Caribbean	330 000 [240 000–420 000]	310 000 [230 000–400 000]	37 000 [26 000–54 000]	34 000 [24 000–47 000]	1.6 [1.1–2.2]	1.5 [1.1–2.0]	27 000 [19 000–36 000]	28 000 [19 000–38 000]
Eastern Europe and Central Asia	1.5 million [1.0–2.3 million]	1.1 million [790 000–1.7 million]	220 000 [150 000–650 000]	160 000 [110 000–440 000]	0.8 [0.6–1.4]	0.6 [0.4–1.0]	53 000 [36 000–75 000]	28 000 [19 000–39 000]
North America, Western and Central Europe	2.0 million [1.4–2.9 million]	1.8 million [1.3–2.7 million]	65 000 [52 000–98 000]	65 000 [52 000–98 000]	0.5 [0.4–0.7]	0.5 [0.3–0.6]	30 000 [24 000–45 000]	30 000 [24 000–45 000]
TOTAL	38.6 million [33.4–46.0 million]	36.2 million [31.4–42.9 million]	4.1 million [3.4–6.2 million]	3.9 million [3.3–5.8 million]	1.0 [0.9–1.2]	1.0 [0.8–1.2]	2.8 million [2.4–3.3 million]	2.6 million [2.2–3.1 million]

Fig. 4.3 Regional HIV and AIDS Statistics and Features (2003 and 2005)

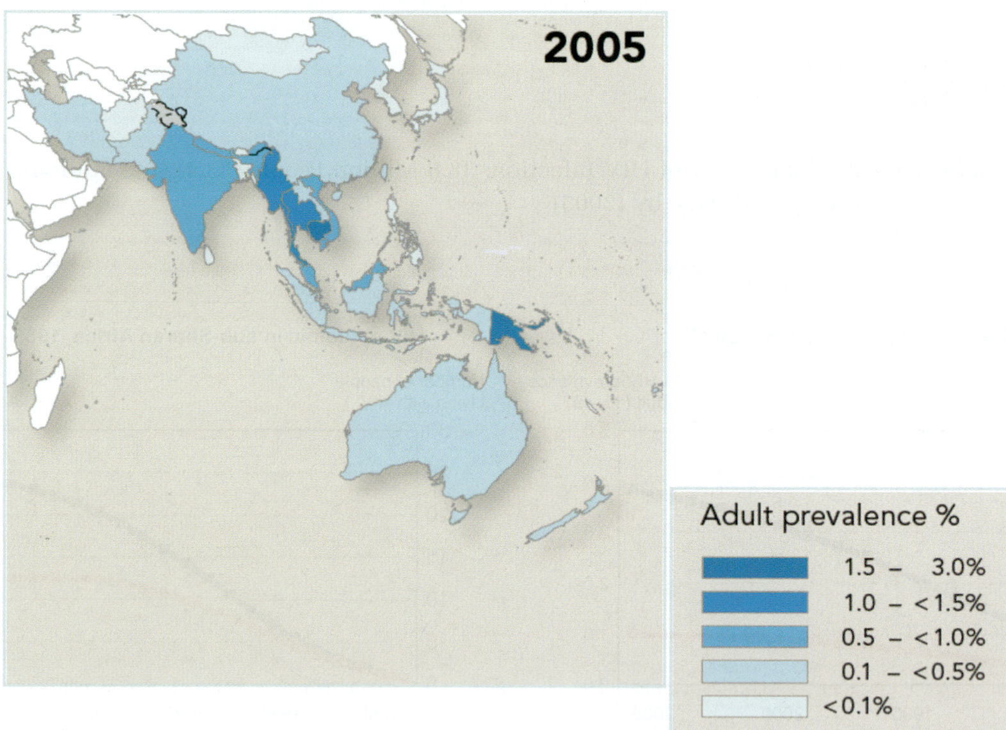

Fig. 4.4 HIV Prevalence (%) in Adults in Asia and Oceania (2005)

FOCUSING ON RISK

High-risk behaviours (such as injecting drug use, unprotected paid sex and unprotected sex between men) are especially evident in the HIV epidemics of Asia, eastern Europe and Latin America. In eastern europe and Central Asia, for example, two in three (67%) prevalent HIV infections in 2005 were due to the use of non-sterile durg injecting

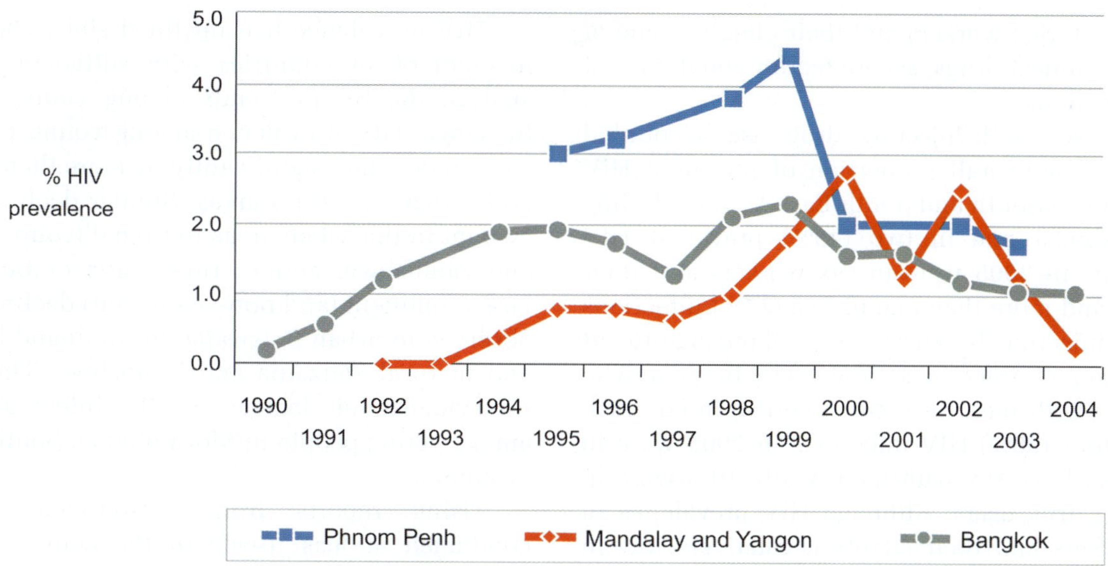

Sources: Cambodia National Center for HIV/AIDS, Dermatology and STDs (Phnom Penh); Myanmar Ministry of Health (Mandalay and Yangon); Thailand Ministry of Public Health (Bangkok), 2005.

Fig. 4.5 HIV Prevalence Among Pregnant Women in Major Cities in Cambodia, Myanmar and Thailand (1990–2004)

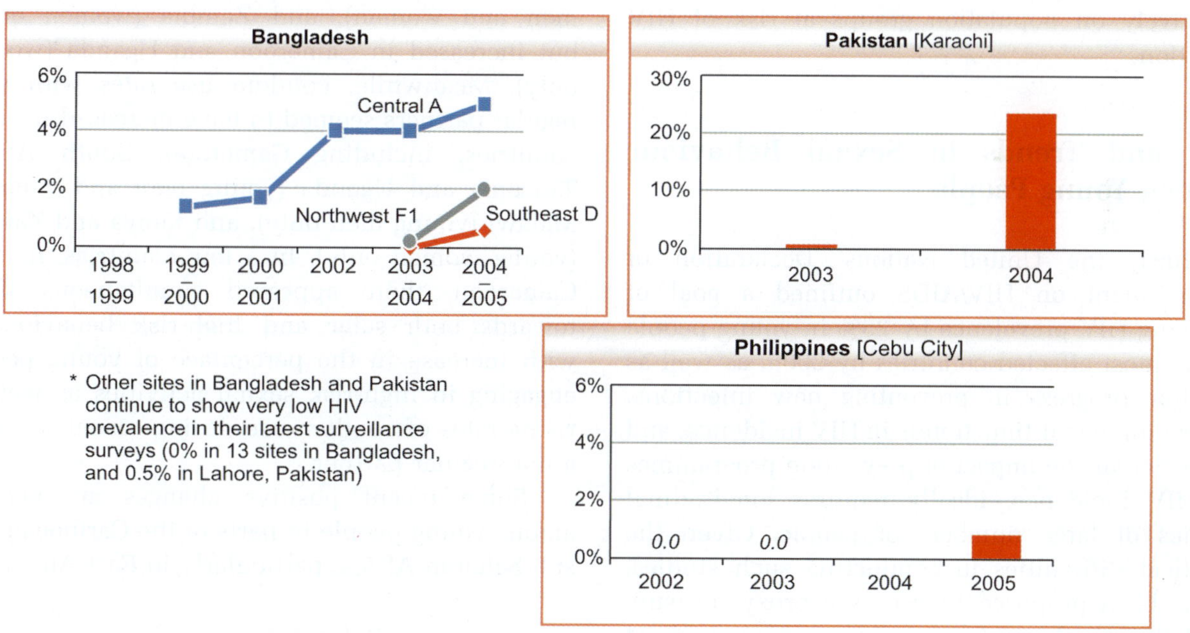

Sources: 2005 Integrated HIV Behavioral and Serologic Surveillance Findings, Summary Report. National Epidemiology Center, Department of Health (Philippines); National HIV Serological Surveillance, 2004-2005, 6th Round Technical Report. Natonal AIDS/STD Programme, Ministry of Health and Family Welfare (Bangladesh); National Study of Reproductive Tract and Sexually Transmitted Infections, Survey of High Risk Groups in Lahore and Karachi, 2005. National AIDS Control Program, Ministry of Health (Pakistan)

Fig. 4.6 HIV Prevalence (%) Among Injecting Drug Users in Bangladesh, Pakistan and the Philippines (1998–2005)*.

equipment. Sex workers and their clients, some of them also inject drugs, accounted for about 12% of HIV infections.

Paid sex and injecting drug use accounted for a similar overall proportion of prevalent HIV infections in South and South-East Asia. Excluding India, almost one in two (49%) prevalent HIV infections in 2005 were in sex workers and their clients, and more than one in five (22%) infections were in injecting drug users. A small but significant proportion of infections (5%) were in men who have sex with men. In Latin America, in contrast, one in four (26%) HIV infections in 2005 were in men who have sex with men, while 19% were in injecting drug users. Although HIV prevalence in sex workers and their clients is relatively low in this region, they accounted for almost one in six (17%) HIV infections.

Although the epidemics extend into the general population of countries in those regions, they remain highly concentrated around specific population groups. This highlights the need to focus prevention, treatment and care strategies effectively on population groups at risk of HIV infection.

HIV and Trends in Sexual Behaviour Among Young People

In 2001, the United Nations' Declaration of Commitment on HIV/AIDS outlined a goal of reducing HIV prevalence by 25% in young people in the most affected countries by 2005, as well as monitor progress in preventing new infections. Determining real-time trends in HIV incidence, and in particular the impact of prevention programmes on HIV incidence, ideally requires longitudinal studies of large numbers of people. Given the practical difficulties in conducting such studies, it has been proposed to use as a proxy measure the HIV prevalence in young women aged 15–24 attending antenatal clinics.

The objective of the WHO/UNAIDS Working Group on Global HIV/AIDS and STI Surveillance was to motivate countries where the national prevalence exceeds 3% to participate in this endeavour.

HIV prevalence had declined since 2000/2001 in eight of 11 countries with sufficient data to analyze the recent trends among young people. In Kenya, HIV prevalence among young pregnant women declined significantly by more than 25% in both urban and rural areas. Similar declines were evident in the urban areas in Côte d'Ivoire, Malawi and Zimbabwe, and in rural parts of Botswana. Less prominent (and non-significant) declines were observed in urban Botswana, Burundi and Rwanda and in rural Tanzania and Zimbabwe. There was no evidence of decreasing HIV infection levels among young people in Mozambique, South Africa or Zambia.

Using reports from nation-wide surveys conducted at least twice in the country during 1994–2005, the trends in behaviours among young people were assessed. In Kenya, behaviour trend data point to a significant reduction in such kinds of sexual behaviour that place people at risk of HIV infection. The proportion of young persons having sex with non-regular partners decreased in Haiti (men only), Kenya and Malawi (young men and women), and Zambia (women only), but increased in Cameroon and Uganda (women only). Meanwhile, condom use rates with non-regular partners seemed to have increased in some countries, including Cameroon, South Africa, Tanzania and Uganda (young men and women), Malawi (young men only), and Kenya and Zambia (young women only). In a few countries, notably Cameroon, there appeared simultaneous shifts towards both safer and high-risk behaviours—with increase in the percentage of young people engaging in high-risk sexual activities as well as rising rates of condom use during casual sex with a non-regular partner.

Some recent positive changes are evident among young people in parts of the Caribbean and sub-Saharan Africa, particularly in East Africa.

HIV EPIDEMIC: THE INDIAN SCENARIO[8]

HIV epidemic has been evolving in the country since the first case was detected in Tamil Nadu in 1986. Based on sentinel surveillance data, the estimated number of HIV infected persons has gone up from 3.5 million in 1998 to over 5.206 million in 2005, accounting for one-eighth of all infections in the world. According to NFHS-III and Behavioural Surveillance Survey (BSS), there were 2–3.1 million (2.47 million) people living with HIV/AIDS at the end of 2006. Out of these, 0.97 million (39.3%) are women and 0.09 million (3.8%) are children. The estimated adult prevalence in the country is 0.36% (0.27-0.47%). These estimates no dramatic upsurge in the spread of HIV infection across the country since 1998. However, state-specific variations in the profile of the epidemic have been observed. Several states in southern India and north-eastern part of the country have shown a higher HIV prevalence and diversity in predominant patterns of HIV transmission. Even states with low HIV prevalence are characterized as being potential for increased spread of the epidemic. The higher incidence of HIV infection in the past two decades reflects an increase in the number of AIDS patients and consequent medical, economic and social implications.

Categories of States Based on Prevalence and Vulnerability

Based on antenatal prevalence (ANC), six states in India have been identified as high prevalence states (having more than 1.0% HIV prevalence in general population), three states as moderate prevalence states (concentrated epidemic with more than 5% HIV prevalence in high-risk population) and the rest as low prevalence states. However, on the basis of vulnerability factors such as migration, size of the population and weak health infrastructure, the low prevalence states/UTs have been further classified as "highly vulnerable" and "vulnerable" (see Table 4.1).

Table 4.1 Categories of States

High Prevalence	*Moderate Prevalence*	*Low Prevalence*	
		Highly Vulnerable	*Vulnerable*
Tamil Nadu Andhra Pradesh Maharashtra Karnataka Nagaland Manipur	Gujarat Goa Pondicherry	Assam Bihar Delhi Himachal Pradesh Kerala Madhya Pradesh Punjab Rajasthan Uttar Pradesh West Bengal Chhattisgarh Jharkhand Orissa Uttaranchal	Arunachal Pradesh Haryana J & K Meghalaya Mizoram Sikkim Tripura A & N Islands Chandigarh D & N Haveli Daman & Diu Lakshadweep

Heterogeneity of HIV Epidemic

The epidemic in India is very heterogeneous due to its diverse modes of infection, particularly in southern and western states, namely Tamil Nadu, Karnataka, Andhra Pradesh, Maharashtra, and two north-eastern states, namely Nagaland and Manipur. Even within a state, there may be a wide variance in HIV prevalence between districts and intra-districts as evidenced by the data from HIV sentinel surveillance centres and Voluntary Counselling and Testing Centres (VCTCs).

Categories of Districts

Based on the HIV surveillance data, epidemiological profile, risk and vulnerability, NACO has classified the 611 districts in the country into 4 categories (Table 4.2 and Figure 4.7), many of them located in low prevalence states.

Table 4.2 **Categories of Districts**

	Description	*Category*
1.	More than 1% ANC/PPTCT prevalence in the district in any time in any of the sites in the last 3 years	A
2.	Less than 1% ANC/PPTCT prevalence in all the sites during the last 3 years associated with more than 5% prevalence in any HRG group (STDs/CSW/MSM/IDU)	B
3.	Less than 1% ANC prevalence in all sites during the last 3 years with less than 5% in all STD clinic attendees or any HRG with known hot spots (migrants, truckers, large aggregation of factory workers, tourist, etc.)	C
4.	Less than 1% ANC prevalence in all sites during the last 3 years with less than 5% in all STD clinic attendees or any HRG or no or poor HIV data with no known hot spots	D

Routes of Transmission

Information from AIDS case-reporting indicates that sex continues to be the main route (86%) of transmission. Blood products, intravenous drug use and perinatal transmission are the other routes (see Figure 4.8). Intravenous drug use is the predominant route of transmission in the north-eastern states.

Demographic Pattern of Vulnerable Population in India

Since 2001, more than two million clients have been tested in the VCTC units, nearly 800,000 people in 2005 alone. Of these, nearly 13% were tested HIV-positive in 2005 (see Table 4.3).

Table 4.3 **Test Results from VCTC - All India**

	2003	2004	2005
People tested for HIV/AIDS at VCTC	673,698	784,040	807,109
Number of HIV-positives receiving test results	82,848	105,840	105,118
% of HIV-positives receiving test results	12.3	13.5	13.0

Source: CMIS Data 2003-2005, NACO

According to the VCTC data (CMIS 2005), 16 and 26% of those who access VCTC are below 25 years and 30 years respectively. These two groups represent 9% and 20% respectively of cases being identified as positive. It is important to note that. in the age groups of 15-19 and 20-24 years, the majority were women, 60 and 63% respectively (see Figure 4.9).

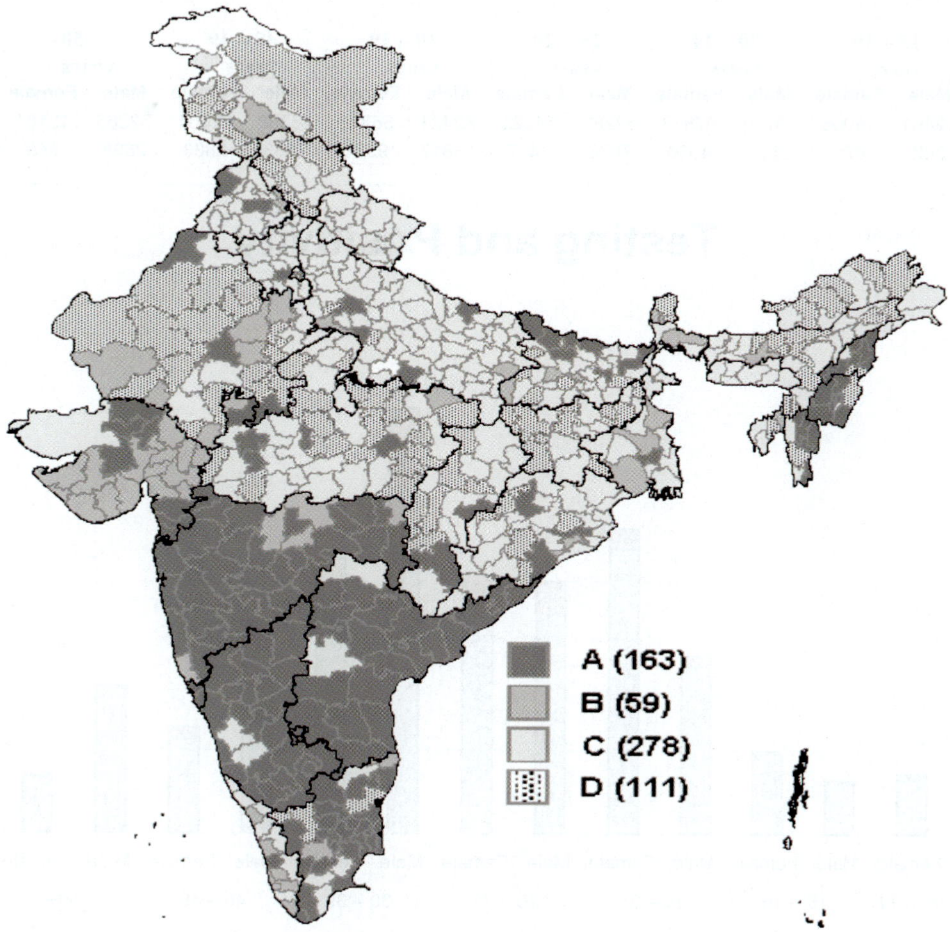

Fig. 4.7 Classification of Districts Based on Epidemiology, Risk and Vulnerability

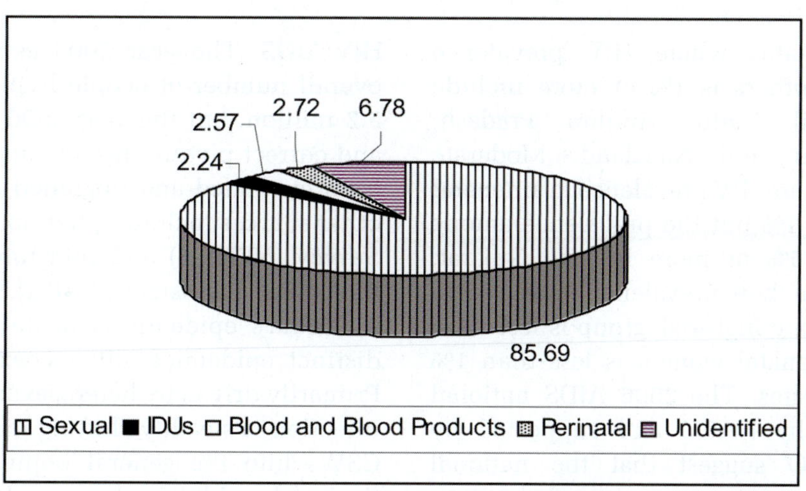

Fig. 4.8 Routes of HIV Transmission

Less than 14 years		15 – 19 years		20 – 24 years		25 – 29 years		30 – 39 years		40 – 49 years		>50 years		Age not Specified	
Male	Female	Male	Female	Male	Female	Male	Female	Male	Female	Male	Female	Male	Female	Male	Female
16962	12971	12461	19005	39717	67852	52283	54221	82421	56320	43388	22601	32365	13181	1839	1197
2142	1577	302	670	2623	4806	7876	7417	18817	9321	7663	2883	2698	855	158	91

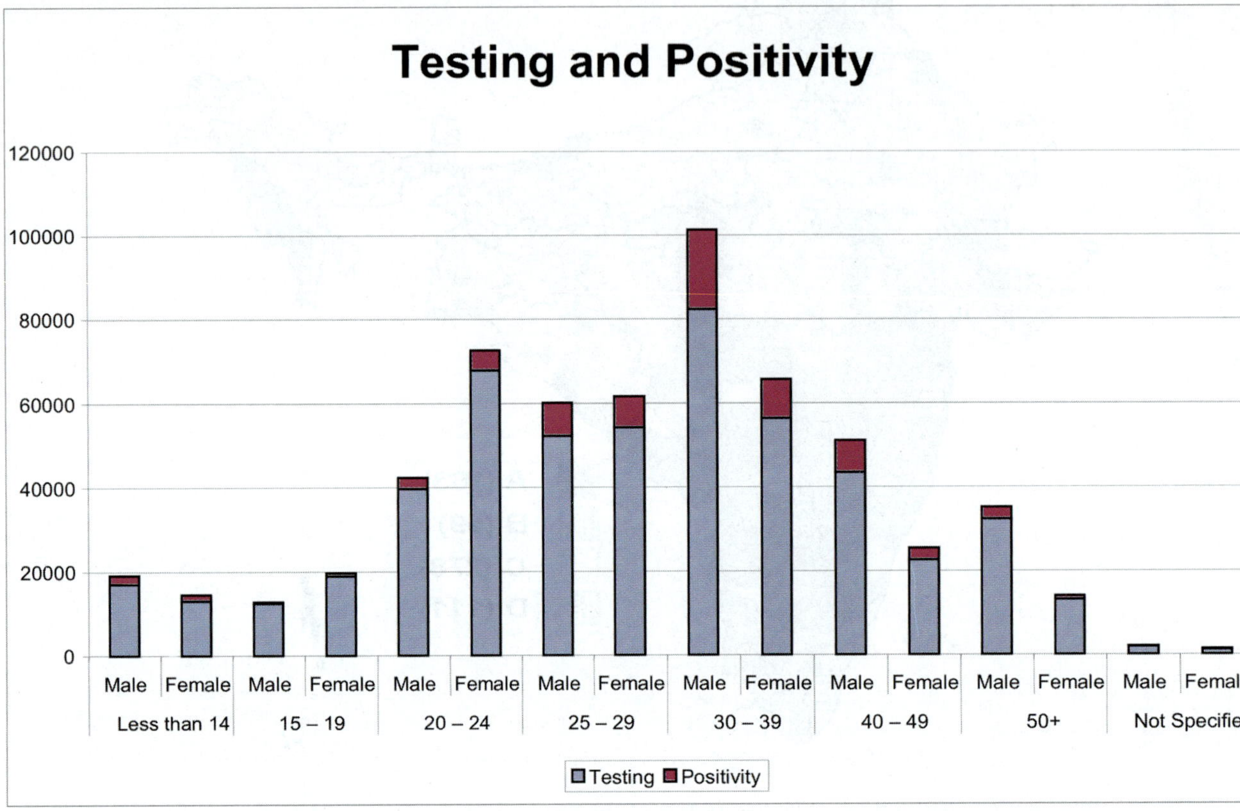

Fig. 4.9 Age and Sex Distribution of Testing and Positivity at VCTC

High prevalence states where HIV prevalence among antenatal mothers is 1% or more include Maharashtra, Tamil Nadu, Andhra Pradesh, Karnataka, Manipur and Nagaland. Moderate prevalence states where HIV prevalence in antenatal women is less than 1% but the prevalence among high-risk group is 5% or more include Gujarat, Pondicherry and Goa. Low prevalence states where HIV prevalence among high-risk group is less than 5% and among antenatal women is less than 1% include all other states. The 2006 AIDS national estimates collated by NACO and supported by UNAIDS and WHO suggest that the national adult HIV prevalence is approximately 0.36%, amounting to between 2 and 3.1 million people. Thus an average 2.5 million people live with HIV/AIDS. The year 2005 estimates had put the overall number of people living with HIV/AIDS at 5.2 million, but the year 2006 NACO had a better and correct picture through analysis of robust data from expanded and upgraded sentinel survey and other sources including National Family and Health Survey (NFHS-3) and Integrated Behavioural and Biological Assessment (IBBA).[9]

India's epidemic is made up of a number of distinct epidemics, often coexisting in one state. Primarily driven by heterosexual transmission, HIV infection is steadily shifting its initial focus among CSWs into the general population. At the same time, sub-epidemics have evolved with potentially explosive spread among groups of IDUs. There has been a increasing trend of the epidemic in the southern, western and a few northeast states of India. In other parts of the country, the overall levels of HIV are still low.

High levels of STDs, evidence of sexual networks and presence of migration indicate significant vulnerability. The epide-mic continues to shift towards women and young people with an expected accompanying increase in vertical transmission and pediatric HIV. Migration within and between states is a source of transmission of HIV between urban and rural populations, but remains poorly studied. Gender bias, unequal power in decision-making, and women's inability to negotiate safer sex remain major obstacles. In the case of drug users, indications are there for a shift from "inhaling" to over-the-counter injecting drugs. Harm minimization approach is followed in areas with high drug use, notably Manipur and the metropolises of Mumbai, Chennai and Delhi.

Pattern of Spread

India's epidemic seems to be following the so-called Type 4 pattern, first described in Thailand. The epidemic shifts from the highest risk groups (CSWs, drug users) to bridge populations (clients of sex workers, STD patients, partners of drug users) and then to the general population. The shift usually occurs when the prevalence in the first group reaches 5%.There is a time lag of 2-3 years between shift from one group to the next. Forecasting an epidemic is so complex. Important new elements are entering into the picture. The burden of AIDS cases will soon be felt in states affected early in the epidemic, like Tamil Nadu, Maharashtra and Manipur.

BASIC EPIDEMIOLOGY

Human Immunodeficiency Virus

HIV is a retrovirus belonging to the subfamily of lentiviruses. It contains a genome comprising of two single-stranded RNA molecules. HIV gets integrated into the chromosomal DNA of the host cell by using reverse transcriptase enzyme to produce a double-stranded proviral DNA. Majority of the proviral particles may go into latency for a variable period of time. Upon activation, it reproduces RNA transcripts and proteins which are used to synthesize new HIV virions. There are two main types of HIV: HIV 1 and HIV 2. HIV 1 and 2 have originated from the simian immunodeficiency virus (SIV), probably from the ones found in chimpanzees (SIVcpz) and in sooty mangabey monkeys (SIVsm). HIV is a lymphocytotropic and neurotropic virus. Therefore, it may be found in almost all the body fluids and organs. It is present in infective dosages in semen, vaginal and cervical secretions and blood. Exchange of these body fluids from an infected individual can lead to the transmission of HIV infection to another person. Semen contains about fifty times higher concentration of the virus as compared to vaginal and cervical secretions and blood. The central nervous system, testis, lymph nodes, etc., act as reservoirs of HIV. The highest concentration of HIV is found in the cerebrospinal fluid.[5]

Molecular Epidemiology

The transmission efficiency of HIV 2 infection through sexual route is lower than that of HIV 1. The efficiency of mother-to-child transmission (MTCT) of HIV 2 is reported to be 1.2% as compared to 24.7% of HIV 1.[10] Moreover, the incubation period of HIV 2 infection is reported to be longer than that of HIV 1. Of persons infected with HIV in India, 1.7-4.6% has been reported to be due to HIV 2 alone and 3.3-20.1% due to HIV 1 and 2. The presence of dual infection of HIV 1 and 2 and not of HIV 2 alone has been also reported among IDUs from Manipur.

Genetic mutations are very frequent in most RNA viruses, especially in HIV. Therefore, every patient is likely to have swarm virus variants (quasi-species). The development of recombinant HIV has also been well reported. Such mutations can theoretically confer some selective advantage to HIV. It can theoretically lead to the evolution of a species that may have a higher sexual transmission efficiency and slower disease progression. The identification of mutations and their sub-types is important in HIV vaccine development.

The strains of HIV 1 are divided into two groups as Major and Outlier, designated as M and O groups, respectively. Recently a new HIV 1, group N, has been discovered in Cameroon. The viruses belonging to group M are more closely related to one another, which is not the case with the viruses belonging to group O. The M group has ten subtypes, named alphabetically from A to K.[11]

The predominant HIV 1 subtype in the United States and Europe is subtype B. In Thailand, HIV 1 subtype E and subtype B are commonly seen. However, with increasing international tourism and migration, more and more subtypes are being seen in a specified geographic area. A distribution profile of the subtypes of HIV 1 viruses prevalent in India has emerged as a result of a few studies. These strains are closely related to those isolated from South Africa. According to phylogenetic analysis, most of the Indian HIV 1 strains belong to the subtype C.

Reports from the National AIDS Research Institute reveal that of the 46 samples studied, 44 were identified as subtype C and one each of subtype A and B. Of the samples belonging to subtype C, 15 were most homologous to the C2 reference strain from Zambia, and others to the Indian reference strain C3. The predominance of HIV 1 subtype C was also shown in samples collected from Punjab, Delhi and Vellore. Surprisingly, a study has shown that all the four isolates from Hyderabad belonged to subtype B. Additionally, a recombinant HIV between subtype C and A has been reported from Pune.[12]

Waves of HIV Epidemic

The predominant route of transmission of HIV is sexual. HIV epidemic spreads classically in three waves. In the first wave, HIV infection is seen amongst sex workers or IDUs who are the *core transmitters* or *core groups*. In its second wave, HIV infection reaches the clients of sex workers or partners of IDUs. When evidences suggest the affection of spouses and children of the clients of sex workers, the HIV epidemic is understood to have reached its third wave. HIV infection is brought into the low-risk population from *core transmitters* through the *bridge population*, a term used to connote mobile population such as truck drivers, single male migrants, etc. Some scientists consider that IDUs constitute the first wave followed by sex workers and so on. Recently, a fourth wave comprising of adolescents has also been proposed to indicate the severity of the epidemic.

Estimating the Magnitude

Estimating the number of affected cases in any disease outbreak is essential for undertaking advocacy, planning the extension of health care services, control strategies including budgetary allocation, and evolving research priorities.

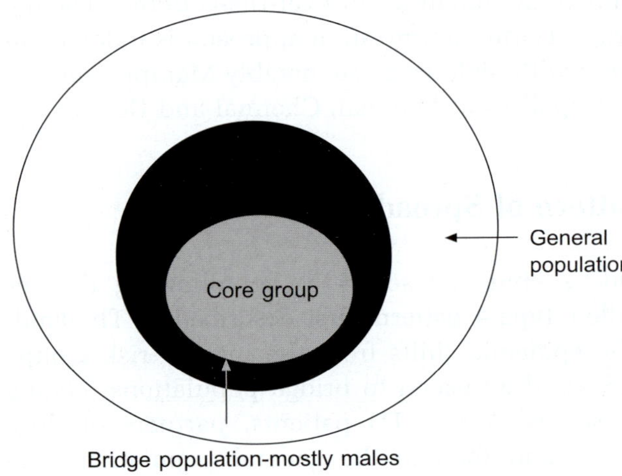

Fig. 4.10 A Schematic Model of Waves in the Spread of HIV Epidemic

Such estimations could be made by initiating surveillance among the most vulnerable population groups. The proportion of people found infected at any given point of time is called the prevalence rate. However, such a rate may not be very useful in chronic diseases. In these circumstances, one needs to estimate the rate of occurrence of new cases in the community every year. This rate is called the incidence. However, the estimation of incidence requires the establishment of a cohort of susceptible population group(s). It is costly and a time-consuming activity. Hence a rough estimate is made through surveillance at periodic intervals on various vulnerable groups. Such studies are often carried out from the clinics or hospital settings from both rural and urban areas. Thus the generalizability of the findings is limited. However, the estimates of cases could be made using different statistical models and data.

HIV Incidence and Prevalence, and AIDS Mortality

The rate of spread of HIV and the current levels of infection are measured by incidence and prevalence. The incidence of HIV is the number of new cases, i.e., the number of people who become infected during a specified period of time, usually over a twelve-month interval.

The prevalence of HIV is the number of people infected at a given point of time. Because there is no cure for HIV/AIDS, HIV prevalence reflects the cumulative number of infections from the past and the mortality rate of those infected.

Incidence and prevalence of HIV/AIDS are often expressed in terms of the number of infections per 1000 adults. At the beginning of the epidemic, HIV prevalence grew rapidly and AIDS mortality was not evident because of the long asymptomatic period of infection. Years later, when the first few cases of AIDS appeared, large numbers of people were already infected with HIV. The incidence may still be climbing but growth in prevalence may be slow because of rising HIV/AIDS mortality or saturation of the population. As long as incidence exceeds mortality, the prevalence of HIV will continue to rise. The prevalence will be at a peak in the year in which the incidence exactly equals the rising mortality rate. Whether prevalence then levels off, declines or resumes climbing toward a new peak will depend on whether the number of new infections is equal to, less than, or greater than the number of deaths of people with HIV/AIDS. In the absence of a cure, the key to reducing future HIV prevalence is by preventing new cases, i.e. by lowering the incidence.

Stable or declining prevalence does not necessarily signal the end of the epidemic. Eventually HIV prevalence will level off in all populations; in some it will stabilize at a high level, and in others at a low level. However, a plateau simply indicates that there is an equilibrium, in which the number of new infections exactly offsets AIDS mortality. In populations where the prevalence is declining, mortality is occurring at a faster rate than new infections. The number of new infections may still be quite high, coexisting with high mortality.

The relationship between HIV incidence and prevalence and the lag in the appearance of AIDS cases has important implications for public policy:

- ⇑ Early intervention is critical to prevent an AIDS epidemic that may persist for decades. Only a fraction of those infected with HIV are showing symptoms of AIDS at any given point of time. By the time AIDS morbidity becomes a significant health issue, HIV may have spread widely in the population, making prevention efforts very difficult. Countries with few reported AIDS cases should not be complacent about launching prevention campaigns.
- ⇑ The full impact of infection levels on mortality is delayed. Even if all HIV infections could be prevented, in the absence of a cure, AIDS deaths would continue because of the population having been already infected and the long asymptomatic period between HIV infection and AIDS. Countries where HIV prevalence is high are only beginning to experience the profound mortality impact of the epidemic, which will last for decades even with the best prevention efforts.
- ⇑ Biology and behaviour affect the spread of HIV. Not all infectious agents introduced into a population will be self-sustaining. If each infected person were to transmit the infection, on an average to less than one other person over his or her life time, then the infection would possibly disappear. The reproductive rate of a sexually transmitted disease is the average number of susceptible people infected by an infected person over his or her life time. If each person infected with the disease transmits it to exactly one other person, then the reproduction rate is one[1].

In population with a reproductive rate of less than 1, the epidemic will not be self-sustained. Thus, the greater the reproductive rate of HIV, the more rapidly the epidemic will spread. Three main factors have a large influence on the reproductive rate of all STDs, including HIV:

- ⥣ The amount of time a person remains infectious
- ⥣ The risk of transmission per sexual contact
- ⥣ The rate of acquisition of new partners

These factors are common for transmission through contaminated injecting equipment, except for the risk per injection, and the number of partners should refer to the number of people with whom injecting equipment is shared.

Each of the three factors is in turn influenced by the biology of the virus and individual behaviour.

Duration of Infectiousness

Lack of cure and long duration of infectiousness are characteristics that distinguish HIV from most other STDs. The long duration of infectiousness increases the likelihood that an infected individual pass the infection to others. Further more, because an infected person typically remains asymptomatic for years together, they or their sexual (or injecting) partners are often unaware of the risk of transmission. Thus, the long duration of asymptomatic HIV infection potentially puts many partners at risk than is the case for other STDs.

Risk of Infection per Contact

The average risk of infection per sexual exposure is much smaller than that for other STDs; however, because of the long period of infectiousness and numerous cofactors that enhance HIV transmission, the chance of an HIV-positive person who is not precautious infecting others can be quite high.

Most extensive studies on the risk of HIV transmission have been conducted in industrial countries. Because of the generally superior health levels and the ready availability of treatment for other STDs, the average risk of HIV infection per sexual contact in industrial countries is quite small. For example, the average chance that an infected male transmit HIV to an uninfected female partner by unprotected vaginal sex is estimated at between 1 and 2 per 1000 exposure. The risk of transmission from an infected female to an uninfected male partner through unprotected vaginal sex is one-third to one-half.[10]

Anal sex carries the highest risk, especially for the receptive partner. However, all these figures very likely underestimate the average transmission probability of HIV infection per exposure.

The probability of HIV-1 infection per exposure is shown in Table 4.4.

The probability of HIV infection per sexual act is generally based on the studies of transmission within discordant couples of whom one partner is HIV-positive and other is HIV-negative. The "per contact" risk of HIV transmission with a commercial or casual partner is likely to be substantially less than that for other STDs. In the case of gonorrhoea, for example, the probability that an infected woman transmit the disease to an uninfected male partner during intercourse is 20-30% per exposure, while the probability that an infected male transmit the disease to his female partner is 50-70%.

The risk of infection per contact is not constant; it may be influenced by a variety of factors, some of

Table 4.4 Probability of HIV 1 Infection per Exposure

Mode of transmission	*Infection per 100 exposures*
Male to female, unprotected vaginal sex	0.1 to 0.2
Female to male, unprotected vaginal sex	0.033 to 0.1
Male to male, unprotected anal sex	0.5 to 3.0
Needle stick	0.3
Mother to child	13 to 48
Exposure to contaminated blood products	90 to 100

which may exacerbate the epidemic. Some of these include stage of HIV infection, untreated STDs, use of latex condoms, male circumcision, etc.

Role of Partner Change

The average rate of partner change in a population and the variation in the rate across individuals have an impact on the spread of HIV. Other factors being constant, the higher the average rate of partner change, the higher the reproductive rate of HIV. However, in a population in which a few people have very high rates of partner change, HIV and other STDs will spread more quickly than if the average number of partners were distributed more equally across the entire population.

Mixing Patterns

The extent of the epidemic within the overall population depends on the patterns of mixing among people with high-risk behaviour and mixing between people with high- and low-risk behaviours. By high-risk behaviour, we mean unprotected sexual intercourse with multiple partners or sharing of unsterilized injecting equipment. People with low-risk behaviour, who have few partners, who consistently use condoms, who do not inject drugs, or (if they do) do not share injecting equipment, are less likely to pass HIV to others. The speed at which HIV spreads from people with large number of partners to those with very few partners depends on the extent of mixing between people with different levels of sexual activity. If persons with large numbers of partners have intercourse only with those who are similarly active (known as assortative sexual mixing), then HIV will tend to rise rapidly within those groups, but only very slowly and to a limited extent to the rest of the population. As a result, the epidemic will achieve lower peak levels of infection in the entire population than in the case of random or disassortative mixing (people with large number of partners also have sex with those who have fewer partners).

The mixing patterns explain why HIV spread through a population is not at a uniform rate. Rather it spreads in a series of smaller epidemics that race through overlapping subpopulations whose behaviours put them at various degrees of risk than those with less risky behaviours.

HIV PREVALENCE IN RISK GROUPS

Core Groups

HIV infections have been reported from all the states in India, and heterosexual contact is the predominant mode of transmission. In contrast, intravenous drug use was recognized as an important risk behaviour among the youth in the north-eastern Indian state of Manipur. A high HIV prevalence rate among the IDUs was observed along the national highway linking India and Myanmar. The HIV seroprevalence of almost 50% in IDUs in 1991 has increased to about 87% in 1996, highlighting the explosive HIV epidemic faced in the north-eastern states. However, the HIV prevalence rate among IDUs in Kolkata was reported to be about 1%.[13]

In Vellore, the prevalence of HIV 1 antibodies among CSWs increased from 1.8% in 1986 to 28.6% in 1990, while in the western cities of Pune and Mumbai, the HIV sero-prevalence among female sex workers has greatly increased to 47 and 70%, respectively. An alarming high HIV incidence of 20.2 per 100 person-years among CSWs was observed in a HIV incidence study in Pune. Surprisingly, a slow rise in HIV prevalence among sex workers in Kolkata from 0.53% (1991) to 5.5% (1998) was observed.[14]

STD Patients

The prevalence of HIV infection in STD patients increased from 0.19% in 1986 to 3.9% in 1992 in South India[14]. However, the reported HIV seroprevalence in Mumbai was as high as 14-26% in 1992-93 and that in Pune was 19.9% in 1998. An HIV incidence of 9.7 per 100 person-years and 5.6 per 100 person-years was observed among males who had recent exposure to sex workers and those who did not have, respectively, in Pune.[16] Factors like number of sex partners, lack of condom use and history of previous or present STDs were found to be important predictors of prevalent and incident HIV infections. Recent increases in condom use have reduced the risk of HIV acquisition by almost half. A high HIV prevalence of about 14% was found amongst women attending STD clinics but denied any history of sex work[16]. Surprisingly, the small difference in HIV prevalence rates between male STD patients who reported multipartner sex and those married to monogamous women suggests that the epidemic has established its roots in the low-risk population.

STI prevalence is a good indicator for HIV as both share common modes of transmission; in fact STI multiplies the probability of exposure to HIV infection. Over 5% of the adult population in India suffers from STDs, and most regions of the country show relatively high levels of STDs. HIV prevalence rates among STD patients also remain high: 22.8% in Andhra Pradesh, 15.2% in Maharashtra, 12.2% in Manipur and 7.47% in Delhi. Among women, 14% of those attending STD clinics were found to be HIV-positive in some states.

A community-based prevalence study conducted by NACO substantiated the findings of regional studies undertaken in some southern states of India. Vulnerability of the rural and urban regions to HIV is evident from the community-level data (Table 4.5).

'Bridge' Population

A high HIV prevalence of 5.2% was found amongst 500 truck drivers and helpers in West Bengal in 1994, which provides epidemiological support to the findings of other studies that little or no awareness about AIDS and higher practice of risk behaviour is seen among the bridge population groups.[18]

Table 4.5 Summary Results of STD/RTI Community Prevalence Study (NACO 2003)

Diseases	*Low-Moderate*		*High*	
	Urban	*Rural*	*Urban*	*Rural*
No STD/RTI	83.9	86.0	84.8	82.0
Normal, excluding candidiasis and *B. vaginosis*	94.2	95.3	94.0	88.3
Trichomoniasis	2.7	1.8	1.5	0.3
Candidiasis	6.6	5.5	6.6	8.1
Bacterial vaginosis	7.2	6.4	4.0	6.5
Chancroid	0	0.1	0	0.1
Herpes simplex virus 2	0.6	0.7	1.6	1.9
Syphilis	0.4	1.0	0.8	1.2
HPV	1.6	0.8	0.4	0.3
HIV	0.1	0.3	1.4	1.1
Gonorrhoea	0.2	0.1	0.2	0.6
Chlamydia	0.1	0	0.4	0.2
Multiple infection, excluding candidiasis	0.4	0.2	0.2	0.3
STI prevalence	**5.8**	**4.7**	**6.0**	**6.2**

Blood Donors and Recipients

HIV prevalence among voluntary blood donors in the metropolitan cities of India during 1990-93 was reported to be 0.3 to 0.9%. Vellore showed a statistically significant increasing trend from 1.5 per 1000 in 1988-89 to 3.1 per 1000 in 1992-93[19] and similar rates were observed in Mumbai and Pune.

Mandatory testing of blood and blood products for HIV antibodies was initiated in July 1989. Consequent to the reports stating high HIV prevalence in commercial blood donors and HIV reactivity among some commercially available blood products[20], a ban on these in India was enforced. The ban was subsequently lifted following improvements in the manufacturing process and quality control procedures. However, no HIV seroconversions were observed among women receiving Anti-D immunoglobulin during pregnancy.

Several studies among thalassemic and other children who received multiple transfusions reported a high HIV seroprevalence between 8.9 and 30.4%[21], mostly due to transfusions of commercially available cryoprecipitates. Multitransfused thalassemic children showed no evidence of HIV 2 infection in New Delhi.

Pregnant Women

HIV seroprevalence among pregnant women primarily attending the public hospitals has been reported to be between 0.5 and 3.3% in various parts of the country. The HIV sentinel surveillance data amongst pregnant women show that six states in India, namely Maharashtra, Tamilnadu, Andhra Pradesh, Karnataka, Manipur and Nagaland, have a HIV prevalence of more than 1%[22]. Most of these states are highly industrialized or are affected due to internal strife.

Mother-to-Child Transmission (MTCT)

The risk of transmission from a pregnant mother to her baby is reported to be between 21 and 43% in developing countries.[23] A prospective study involving 143 tribal pregnant women and their infants followed until 18 months of age reported an overall MTCT efficiency of 48%.[24] Almost 30-50%

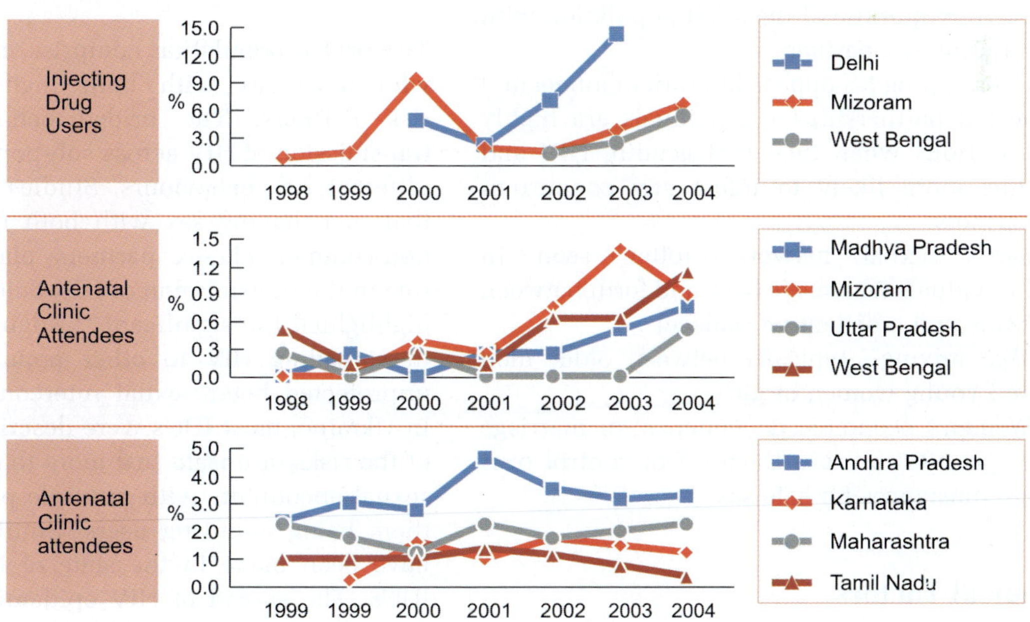

*Data from consistent surveillance sites only.

Fig. 4.11 HIV Prevalence (%) Trends in India Among Injecting Drug Users and Pregnant Women (1998–2004)*

of neonates acquire HIV infection during antenatal period, and about 50-70% during delivery. The risk of acquiring HIV infection through breast milk is 14-29%, according to a study based on the meta-analysis of other studies.[25] The only observation study conducted in Malawi has reported that HIV incidence amongst infants who are breastfed between 1 and 5 months is higher (0.7% per month) when compared to that between 6 and 11 months (0.6% per month) and between 12 and 17 months (0.3% per month).[26] However, exclusive breastfeeding has now been shown to be better than mixed feeding.[27]

INTERPLAY OF FACTORS DRIVING SEXUAL TRANSMISSION

Evidence from around the world suggest that many factors play a role in kick-starting a sexually transmitted HIV epidemic or driving it to higher levels.

Behavioural and Social Factors

- ⥣ Little or no condom use
- ⥣ Large proportion of the adult population with multiple sex partners
- ⥣ Overlapping (as opposed to serial monogamy) sexual partnerships - individuals are highly infectious when they first acquire HIV and thus more likely to infect any concurrent partners
- ⥣ Large sexual networks (often seen in individuals who move back and forth between home and a distant workplace)
- ⥣ "Age mixing", typically between older men and young women or girls
- ⥣ Women's economic dependence on marriage or prostitution robs them off of control over circumstances for safe sex

Biological Factors

- ⥣ High rates of STDs, especially those causing genital ulcers, and low rates of male circumcision
- ⥣ High viral load - HIV levels in the bloodstream are typically high when a person is first infected and again in the late stages of illness

Men Who Have Sex with Men (MSM)

In many countries around the world, open gay communities are rare or non-existent. Male homosexual behaviour, on the other hand, exists in every country. It often involves penetrative anal sex, an act that carries a high risk of HIV infection. Sex is one of the major factors behind the spread of HIV epidemic in many high-income countries and in some parts of Latin America. In Asia, the contribution of male homosexuality to HIV epidemic has been recorded regularly but has rarely been quantified. In India, HIV transmission among men has been reported from Mumbai and Chennai. In most developing countries including India, male homosexuality is far more likely to be secretive, and they are less likely to have access to prevention, information and care services.

Bridge Population—the Key for Further HIV Spread

The bridge population comprise men and women who have sex with both high-risk and low-risk partners. The bridge behaviour involves transmission of HIV across sub-populations having different risk behaviours. Studies have suggested that men having sex with both commercial and non-commercial sex partners play a significant role in the transmission of HIV. Scientists have also highlighted the significant "bridging role of IDUs" in spreading HIV to other populations through unprotected heterosexual intercourse in Ukraine. In Ukraine, most IDUs were described as unaware of the risks of unsafe sex; more than 50% reported sexual encounters with multiple partners, most of them being non-drug users. Similar observations have been made in the state of Manipur among IDUs. The spread of HIV epidemic in the region depends on the extent of localized IDU epidemic to the so-called general population through sexual contacts. Widespread HIV transmission among sex partners of IDUs is likely to occur due to their low level of protected sex, as reported by some behaviour surveillance.

Vulnerability of Women to HIV

Women are biologically more susceptible than men to HIV infection. Male-to-female transmission of HIV is 2-4 times more efficient than female-to-male. This is because women have a larger mucosal surface exposed during sexual intercourse. Another reason is that a much higher concentration of HIV could be found in semen than in vaginal fluids. Women are also disproportionately represented among those who receive blood or blood products as a consequence of their childbearing role, which exposes them to the risk of yet another mode of transmission. The fact that young women are inclined to have sex with or marry older men also increases the risk of infection. This is because age or delayed marriage in men is associated with a higher likelihood of premarital sex with more than one partner, including CSWs, thereby creating a greater likelihood of infection.

Poverty, lack of education and poor earning opportunities often propel women into commercial sex, thus significantly increasing their risk of infection. There was a sharp increase in HIV prevalence rates among CSWs in Mumbai from 1 to 51% between 1987 and 1993. The risk of HIV transmission is known to increase with the number of male partners a sex worker has had intercourse within the course of a day. For many women, high-risk activity could simply mean being married. Social norms which accept extra-marital and premarital sexual relationships in men, and women's inability to negotiate safe sex practices with their partners, are factors that make women vulnerable to HIV infection.

Men's unwillingness to use condoms further accentuates women's risk. For example, in a study of the prevalence of and risk factors for HIV infections in Tamil Nadu (1994-95) covering a population of about 97000, less than 2% of married men were found to be condom users. Negotiating condom use with male partners becomes especially difficult in contexts where a vast majority of women using contraception have undergone sterilization, as is the case in India and Sri Lanka.

The presence of untreated STDs, especially if ulcerative, multiplies the risk of HIV infection by 300-400%. Women with STDs face a higher risk of HIV infection than men for a number of reasons. To begin with, more women than men in the developing world have STDs. Secondly, many STDs in women are asymptomatic and, therefore, less likely to be recognized. Above all, the stigma attached to visiting an STD clinic, together with other barriers such as lack of time, money and decision-making power, discourages women from seeking treatment.

For all the above reasons, the prevalence of HIV infection is increasing among women who have traditionally been considered low-risk populations. Perinatal transmission is bound to increase under these conditions, leaving behind more and more infants and children infected with HIV. A holistic approach needs to be taken into consideration in the prevention of mother-to-child transmission of HIV.

Barriers in Access to Reproductive Health Services

Studies from India on gynaecological morbidity mention "shame and guilt" as important reasons why most women do not seek medical treatment. A study from Karnataka (1995) found that the proportion of women reporting untreated reproductive mor-bidity ranged from 44 to 57% across different socio-demographic groups. In a study (1989) of gynaecological morbidity in rural Maharashtra, 92% of women with a self-reported problem had not sought treatment prior to the screening camp conducted as a part of the study.

The National Family Health Survey, 1992-93, enquired women for reasons why they did not seek antenatal care. Almost 60% of women, 66% in urban and 58% in rural areas, felt that antenatal care was unnecessary. The higher proportion of women in urban areas stating antenatal care was not necessary must be interpreted in the context of a much smaller proportion in urban (18%) than in rural areas (43%) having no provision of antenatal services. Thirteen percent of women did not know about the existence of antenatal services; about 7% could not afford the cost involved; and a little over 5% did not have time or had not been given permission to go. In India, just over 30% of births are attended by trained persons. The proportion of institutional deliveries is approximately one-fourth of the total annual deliveries.

For an effective prevention of perinatal transmission, it is essential that maternity and child health services and facilities for STDs/RTIs and HIV/AIDS prevention, screening and management be incorporated in the MCH package.

SURVIVAL AFTER DIAGNOSING AIDS AND ADVENT OF ANTI-HIV TREATMENT

Survival with severe characteristic illness is also variable, but the average survival time was about 2-4 years in most developed countries and about 6 months or less in developing regions which was most likely due to diagnosis at a later stage of the disease and limited access to good supportive medical care. The case fatality rate attributable to HIV is among the highest of any human infectious agent.

The proportion of HIV infected persons who, in the absence of anti-HIV treatment, will ultimately develop AIDS has been estimated to be over 90%. Less than 5% of HIV infected persons who have been followed with detailed clinical and laboratory studies for 10 years or longer have been classified as possible non-progressors. Most (80-90%) patients in developed countries die within 2-4 years after the diagnosis. However, in the United States and most developed countries. The routine use of prophylactic drugs for the prevention of *P. carinii* pneumonia and other opportunistic infections was able to delay the development of AIDS and death significantly. In Hong Kong triple anti-HIV drug therapy is provided to all residents, where as in the poorer Asian countries, such as Cambodia and Myanmar, anti-HIV drug treatment is virtually unavailable.

National Response

Refer to Chapter 37 "Control of Sexually Transmitted Diseases and AIDS" for details.

REFERENCES

1. HIV/AIDS in Asia and Pacific Region, World Health Organization, 2001.
2. Barre Sinoussi F, Chermann JC, Rey F, et al. Isolation of a T-lymphotropic retro virus from a patient at risk for acquired immune deficiency syndrome (AIDS). Science 1983; 220: 868-71.
3. Zagury D, Bernard J, Leibowitch J, et al. HTLV III in cells cultured from semen of two patients with AIDS. Science 1984; 226: 449-51.
4. Levy JA, Shimabukuro J, Hollander H, et al. Isolation of AIDS associated retroviruses from cerebrospinal fluid and brain of patients with neurological symptoms. Lancet 1985; 2: 586-8.
5. Clavel F, Guetard D, Brun-Vezilnet F, et al. Isolation of human retrovirus from west African patients with AIDS. Science 1986; 233: 343-6.
6. Fischi MA, Richman DD, Gricco MH, et al. The efficacy of 3'-azido-3' deoxythymidine (azidothymidine) in the treatment of patients with AIDS and AIDS related complex: a double blind, placebo controlled trial. N Eng J Med 1987; 317: 185-91.
7. Report on the global HIV/AIDS epidemic, UNAIDS & WHO: 2006.
8. National AIDS Control Programme Phase III (2006-2011), Strategy and Implementation Plan, November 30, 2006, National AIDS Control Organization, Ministry of Health and Family Welfare, Government of India.
9. NACO NEWS, Ministry of Health & Family Welfare, Government of India. Vol. III Issue 3, Jul-Sep 2007.

10. Haverkos HW, Battjes RJ. "Female to male transmission of HIV. JAMA 1992; 268: 1855-6.
11. HIV/AIDS Round Table Conference Series Number-6, April 2000. Ranbaxy Science, Foundation, New Delhi, India.
12. Lole KS, Bollinger RC, Paranjape RS, et al. Full length human immunodeficiency virus type-1 genome from subtype C-infected seroconvert in India; with evidence of intersub type recombination. J Virol 1999; 73: 152-60.
13. Panda S, Chatterjee A, Bhattacharjee S, et al. HIV, hepatitis B and sexual practices in the street-recruited injecting drug users of Kolkatta: risks perception versus observed risk. Int J STDs AIDS 1998; 9: 214-8.
14. Jana S. Intervention through peer-based approach–A lesson from Sonagachi, AIDS Res Rev 1999; 2: 58-63.
15. Jacob M, John TJ, George S, et al. Increasing prevalence of human immunodeficiency virus infection among patients attending a clinic for sexually transmitted diseases. Indian J Med Res 1995; 101: 6-9.
16. Mehendale SM. HIV infection amongst persons with high risk behaviour in Pune city: Update on findings from a prospective cohort study. AIDS Res Rev 1998; 1: 2-9.
17. Gangakhedkar RR, Bentley ME, Divekar AD, et al. Spread of HIV infection in married monogamous women in India. JAMA 1997; 278: 2090-2.
18. Mistry S, Misra K, Rao A, et al. An HIV point prevalence study among truck driver at Uluberia, West Bengal. Abstract no. Pub.C. 1111 published in XI International Conference on AIDS, Vancouver, July 7-12, 1996.
19. Bhushan N, Pulimood BR, Babu PG, et al. Rising trend in the prevalence of HIV infection among blood donors. Indian J Med Res 1994; 99: 195-7.
20. Banerjee K, Rodrigues J, Israel Z, et al. Outbreak of HIV seropositivity among commercial plasma donors in Pune, India. Lancet 1989; 2: 166.
21. Sen S, Mishra NM, Giri T, et al. Acquired immunodeficiency syndrome (AIDS) in multi-transfused children with thalassemia. Indian Pediatr 1993; 30: 455-60.
22. Joshi PL, Rao P. Changing epidemiology of HIV/AIDS in India. AIDS Res Rev 1999; 2: 7-9.
23. Working Group on Mother-to-Child Transmission of HIV. Rates of mother-to-child transmission of HIV 1 in Africa, America and Europe; results from 13 perinatal studies. J Acquir Immune Defic Syndr Retroviral 1995; 8: 506-10.
24. Kumar RM, Uduman SA, Khurana AK. A prospective study of mother-to-infant HIV transmission in tribal women from India. J Acquired Immune Defic Syndr Hum Retroviral 1995; 19: 238-42.
25. Dunn DT, Newell ML, Ades AE, et al. Risk of human immunodeficiency virus type 1 transmission through breastfeeding. Lancet 1992; 340: 585-8.
26. Miotti PG, Taha ET, Kumwenda NI, et al. HIV transmission through breastfeeding a study in Malawi. JAMA 1999; 282: 744-9.
27. Coutsoudis A, Pillay K, Spooner E, et al. Influence of infant-feeding patterns on early mother-to-child transmission of HIV 1 in Durban, South Africa: a prospective cohort study. Lancet 1999; 354: 471-6.

5 | CLINICAL PRESENTATION OF HIV INFECTION

J K Maniar, R R Kamath

In this chapter

- Natural History of HIV Infection
- Acute Retroviral Syndrome/Primary HIV Infection
- Asymptomatic HIV Infection
- Early Symptomatic HIV Disease
- Late Symptomatic HIV Disease
- Advanced HIV Disease
- Dermatological Manifestations of HIV Infection
- Sexually Transmitted Infections (STI) and HIV/AIDS
- Systemic Involvement in HIV Infection
- Opportunistic Infection in AIDS
- Immune Reconstitution Inflammatory Syndrome (IRIS)
- Clinical Manifestation of HIV Disease in India

INTRODUCTION

The clinical presentation of HIV infection in India is largely similar as elsewhere, except for minor variations depending on the local microbial, socio-economic and environmental factors.[1–4] HIV 1 is responsible for most of the disease globally. HIV 2 is mostly confined to West Africa, but has been detected in Asia and India. HIV 1 is classified into three groups: M (major), N (new) and O (outlier). The M group is further divided into subtypes A-J. In India, HIV 1 subtypes C and E the most common. Unfortunately, there are no consolidated indigenous data on the natural history of HIV 1, HIV 2 or dual infection from India.[5] HIV/AIDS medicine is now increasingly been recognized as a distinct specialty, as in this era of matured HIV epidemic in India good clinical acumen is required to recognize the symptoms and signs of HIV/AIDS-related diseases in clinical practice. HIV/AIDS should be considered as a possible etiological factor while managing common clinical problems like pyrexia of unknown origin (PUO), chronic cough, chronic diarrhoea, weight loss, lymphadenopathy, anemia and idiopathic thrombocytopenic purpura (ITP).

Also, the clinical spectra of both HIV 1 and HIV 2 diseases are almost similar except that HIV 2 infection has a slower progression with longer incubation period.[6] The infectivity of HIV 2 is much lower than that of HIV 1. The laboratory diagnosis needs careful consideration using appropriate Western Blot kits specific for HIV 2 detection. Currently, HIV 2 viral load measuring kits are not available in India. Even in markedly immunosuppressed HIV 2 infected individuals, with an absolute CD4 count below 200 cells/mm^3, the HIV 2 viral load is likely undetectable. Importantly, the efficacy of available antiretroviral drugs is poor against HIV 2, with only nucleoside molecules and selected protease enzyme inhibitors being viricidal.

NATURAL HISTORY OF HIV INFECTION[7]

The following description is related solely to HIV 1 infection, since the natural course of HIV 2 infection has not been completely characterized. Within 2-4 weeks of viral transmission, acute retroviral syndrome (seroconversion illness) develops lasting for about 2-3 weeks. It is followed by early asymptomatic HIV disease that lasts for 2-10 years (average 8 years), after which the patient develops late symptomatic HIV disease. This is indicative of advancing immunosuppression and increased likelihood of opportunistic infections **(Fig. 5.1).** Lastly, the patient develops advanced HIV disease or full-blown AIDS. In India, death may occur after a mean period of 1.3 years, in the absence of ART.

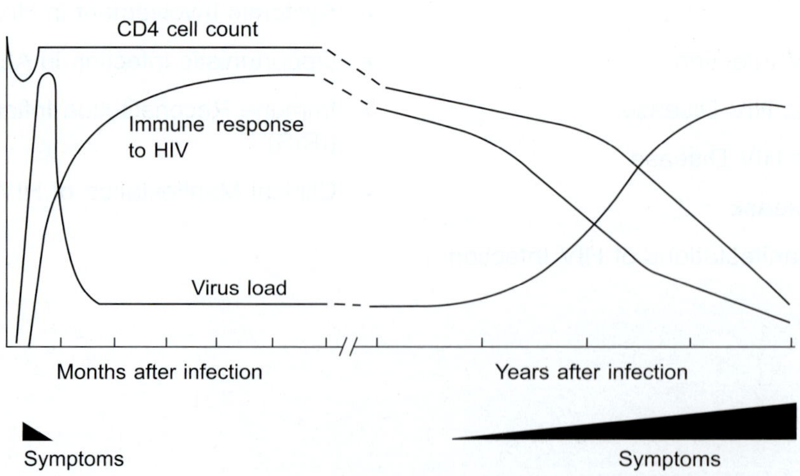

Fig. 5.1 Natural History of Untreated HIV Infection.

The World Health Organization (WHO) has divided the course of the disease from the time of initial infection to the development of full-blown AIDS into four stages **(Table 5.1)**.

Table 5.1 WHO Clinical Staging of HIV/AIDS for Adults and Adolescents (Interim Definitions)

Primary HIV Infection
Asymptomatic Acute retroviral syndrome
Clinical Stage 1
Asymptomatic Persistent generalized lymphadenopathy
Clinical Stage 2
Moderate unexplained weight loss (<10% of presumed or measured body weight) Recurrent respiratory infections (respiratory tract infections, upper respiratory infections, sinusitis, bronchitis, otitis media, pharyngitis) Herpes zoster Minor mucocutaneous manifestations (angular cheilitis, recurrent oral ulcerations, seborrheic dermatitis, prurigo, papular pruritic eruptions, fungal fingernail infections)
Clinical Stage 3
Conditions for which presumptive diagnosis could be made on the basis of clinical signs or simple investigations:
Severe weight loss (>10% of presumed or measured body weight) Unexplained chronic diarrhoea for >1 month Unexplained persistent fever for >1 month (intermittent or constant) Oral candidiasis (thrush) Oral hairy leukoplakia Pulmonary tuberculosis within the last 2 years Severe presumed bacterial infections (e.g., pneumonia, empyema, pyomyositis, bone or joint infection, meningitis, bacteremia) Acute necrotizing ulcerative stomatitis, gingivitis or periodontitis
Conditions for which confirmatory diagnostic testing is necessary:
Unexplained anemia (haemoglobin <8 g/dL) Neutropenia (neutrophils <500 cells/μL) Thrombocytopenia (platelets <50,000 cells/μL)
Clinical Stage 4
Conditions for which presumptive diagnosis could be made on the basis of clinical signs or simple investigations:
HIV wasting syndrome, as defined by the CDC (see Table 5.3) *Pneumocystis jiroveci* (formerly *carinii*) pneumonia Recurrent severe or radiologic bacterial pneumonia Chronic herpes simplex infection (oral or genital, or anorectal site) for >1 month Esophageal candidiasis Extrapulmonary tuberculosis Kaposi sarcoma

(*Contd.*)

Central nervous system toxoplasmosis
HIV encephalopathy

Conditions for which confirmatory diagnostic testing is necessary:

Cryptococcosis, extrapulmonary
Disseminated non-tuberculous Mycobacteria infection
Progressive multifocal leukoencephalopathy
Candida of the trachea, bronchi or lungs
Cryptosporidiosis
Isosporiasis
Visceral herpes simplex infection, cytomegalovirus infection (retinitis or organs other than liver, spleen or lymph node)
Any disseminated mycosis (e.g., histoplasmosis, coccidioidomycosis, penicilliosis)
Recurrent non-typhoidal Salmonella septicemia
Lymphoma (cerebral or B-cell non-Hodgkin)
Invasive cervical carcinoma
Visceral leishmaniasis

World Health Organization. *Interim WHO Clinical Staging of HIV/AIDS and HIV/AIDS Case Definitions for Surveillance*. 2005. Accessed March 23, 2006. Available online at www.who.int/hiv/pub/guidelines/casedefinitions/en/index.html.

Refined Clinical Staging System

A further refinement of the WHO clinical staging system includes a laboratory axis. The laboratory axis divides each category into three strata (A, B, C) depending on the number of CD4 cells. If this is not available, the total lymphocytes is used as an alternative marker.

Laboratory axis		*Clinical axis*			
Lymphocytes	CD4	Stage 1: Asymptomatic PGL	Stage II: Early HIV	Stage III: Intermediate (ARC)	Stage IV: Late AIDS
A > 2000	> 500	1A	2A	3A	4A
B 1000-2000	200-500	1B	2B	3B	4B
C <1000	< 200	1C	2C	3C	4C

ACUTE RETROVIRAL SYNDROME/ PRIMARY HIV INFECTION[8–13]

Acute retroviral syndrome is a complex symptom that follows viral transmission and is experienced by 50-90% of HIV infected patients. Most symptomatic patients seek medical consultation, but this diagnosis is rarely recognized, and an extremely high index of suspicion and a detailed clinical and sexual history is essential.[13] The time lag for the onset of symptoms is usually 2-4 weeks of the initial exposure, but the incubation period may be as long as 10 months in rare cases. The clinical symptoms include an 'infectious mononucleosis-like' illness with fever, lymphadenopathy, pharyngitis, erythematous maculopapular rash, arthralgia, myalgia, diarrhoea, nausea, vomiting, headache, mucocutaneous ulceration involving the mouth, oesophagus or genitals, hepatosplenomegaly and oral thrush. The neurological features include menin-goencephalitis, peripheral neuropathy, facial palsy, Guillain-Barre syndrome, brachial neuritis, radi-culopathy, cognitive impairment and psychosis. The laboratory findings include an initial CD4 T cell lymphopenia followed by CD8 T cell lymphocytosis, and often atypical lymphocytes, and elevated hepatic transaminase levels. The diagnosis is established by the demonstration of quantitative plasma HIV RNA or qualitative HIV DNA along with negative or indeterminate HIV serology, but should always be confirmed by HIV ELISA at 12 weeks. Complete clinical recovery with a reduction in plasma levels of HIV RNA is the norm. The cytotoxic T lymphocyte (CTL) response occurs first and precedes detectable humoral responses. Preliminary studies indicate that aggressive ART during acute retroviral illness protects activated HIV-specific CD4 cells from HIV infection to preserve a response analogous to the response seen in non-progressors. This observation emphasizes the importance of early initiation of aggressive ART. Seroconversion to positive HIV serology generally takes place at an average of six weeks after transmission with the standard third-generation enzyme immunoassay (EIA), and it now appears that more than 95% of patients seroconvert within 12 weeks following transmission.

ASYMPTOMATIC HIV INFECTION[8,11]

During this stage the patient is asymptomatic and generally has no findings on physical examination except for persistent generalized lymphadenopathy (PGL) in some cases. PGL is defined as enlarged lymph nodes (>1 cm) involving at least two non-contiguous sites, other than inguinal nodes, in the absence of an obvious cause. Quite often, such patients are first detected incidentally following the screening tests before blood or organ donation and emigration or during tests done at a voluntary counselling and testing centre (VCTC). Post-test counselling is a priority in such individuals. Detailed history-taking followed by a thorough clinical examination is necessary. Incidental findings could be scars on genitalia from previous genital ulcer disease, lymphadenopathy and even asymptomatic dermatological manifestations. HIV screening of the conjugal partner or offspring at risk after informed consent is essential. The baseline investigations to be undertaken include complete haemogram (including platelet count), ESR, serological tests for syphilis, hepatitis B and C serology, liver and renal function tests, urine examination, chest X-ray, sonography of abdomen/pelvis and Mantoux test. The evaluation of CD4/CD8 lymphocytes as well as the estimation of HIV 1 viral load is optional in resource-limited settings. It may only help to decide the initiation of chemoprophylaxis against opportunistic infections. Counselling should emphasize on maintaining food and water hygiene, life style modification such as practicing safer sex, and refraining from organ donation (viz. blood, semen, kidney, etc.). Periodic follow-up is very essential (every three to six months), and should include sexual history-taking, clinical examination, baseline investigations and counselling.

EARLY SYMPTOMATIC HIV DISEASE[8,11]

During symptomatic HIV infection, the skin and mucous membranes are predominantly involved. Constitutional symptoms include unexplained weight loss, recurrent diarrhoea, fatigue, headache, malaise and fever. Widespread seborrhoeic dermatitis, folliculitis, recurrent vulvovaginal or oral candidiasis, recurrent herpes simplex infection, oral hairy leukoplakia (OHL) and herpes zoster are the most common presentations. Other features include molluscum contagiosum, pruritic papular dermatitis, dermatophytic infection (especially fingernails) and recurrent upper and lower respiratory tract infections caused by *Streptococcus pneumoniae*, *Haemophilus influenzae* and *Mycoplasma pneumonia*. Idiopathic thrombocytopenic purpura (ITP) and pulmonary or lymph node tuberculosis (TB) have also been described.

LATE SYMPTOMATIC HIV DISEASE[8,11]

A decrease in CD4 counts to below 200 cells/mm^3 indicates the risk of developing opportunistic infections. Common conditions are *Pneumocystis carinii* pneumonia (PCP), toxoplasmosis, disseminated *Mycobacterium avium* complex infection, oesophageal candidiasis and related malignancies. These are described in detail later in the chapter. Other features include persistent and progressive constitutional symptoms, AIDS-related wasting disease and neurological disease (peripheral neuropathy and AIDS dementia complex).

ADVANCED HIV DISEASE[8,11]

This stage is also characterized by AIDS-defining opportunistic infections and malignancy. Some more frequently seen infections are *M. avium* complex, CMV, cryptococcal meningitis, histoplasmosis, slow virus disease and cervical dysplasia. CNS involvement is very prominent: AIDS dementia complex, CNS lymphoma and CMV infection. AIDS wasting syndrome or 'Slim disease' with a weight loss of >10% of ideal body weight is common.

Centers for Disease Control and Prevention (CDC) have proposed the clinical classification of HIV infection in adults and adolescents. It is based on three ranges of CD4 cell counts and three clinical categories (Table 5.2).[14] The AIDS case definition as given by WHO and NACO is shown in Table 5.3. The management of HIV infection includes diagnosing the disease and secondary/opportunistic infections, as well as classifying the patient on the basis of CD4 T cell counts so as to determine exactly the level of immunosuppression and to facilitate decision-making regarding the initiation of ART. For these purposes, the CDC categorization of HIV/AIDS is based on the lowest documented CD4 cell count and on previously diagnosed HIV-related conditions (Tables 5.2 and 5.3). For example, if a patient had a condition that once met the criteria for Category B but is now asymptomatic, the patient would remain in Category B. Additionally, the categorization is also based on specific conditions. Patients in categories A3, B3 and C1-C3 are considered to have AIDS.

Table 5.2 **CDC Classification System for HIV Infection**

CD4 cell count	*A*	*B*	*C*
>500/mm^3 (>29%)	A1	B1	C1
200 - 499/mm^3 (14 - 28%)	A2	B2	C2
<200/mm^3 (<14%)	A3	B3	C3

Category A
- Asymptomatic HIV infection
- Persistent generalized lymphadenopathy
- Acute retroviral syndrome

Category B
- Bacillary angiomatosis
- Oral or recurrent vulvovaginal candidiasis
- Cervical dysplasia
- Constitutional symptoms (fever of 38.5°C, diarrhoea >1 month)
- Oral hairy leukoplakia
- Herpes zoster
- Idiopathic thrombocytopenic purpura
- Listeriosis
- Pelvic inflammatory disease
- Peripheral neuropathy

(Contd.)

Category C (AIDS-defining Conditions)
Candidiasis of oesophagus, pulmonary
Cervical cancer, invasive
Coccidioidomycosis, disseminated or extrapulmonary
Cryptococcosis, extrapulmonary
Cryptosporidosis, chronic intestinal (>1 month)
Cytomegalovirus infection, other than liver, spleen or nodes
Herpes simplex with oesophageal, pulmonary or mucocutaneous involvement of >l month
Histoplasmosis, disseminated or extrapulmonary
HIV encephalopathy
Isosporiasis, chronic intestinal (>1 month)
Kaposi's sarcoma
Lymphoma, Burkitt's
Mycobacterium avium complex or *M. kansasii*, disseminated or extrapulmonary
Mycobacterium tuberculosis, any site (pulmonary or extrapulmonary)
Pneumocystis carinii pneumonia
Pneumonia, recurrent with more than two episodes in 12 months
Progressive multifocal encephalopathy
Salmonella septicemia, recurrent
Toxoplasmosis of brain

Centers for Disease Control and Prevention. 1993 revised classification system for HIV infection and expanded surveillance case definition for AIDS among adolescents and adults. MMWR Recomm Rep. 1992 Dec 18;41 (RR-17):1-19. Available online at www.cdc.gov/mmwr/preview/mmwrhtml/00018871.htm

Table 5.3 Case Definition of AIDS

Expanded WHO Definition for AIDS (1994) for Suveillance
If the HIV antibody test gives a positive result and one or more of the following conditions, the individual is considered to have AIDS. • > 10% body weight loss or cachexia, with diarrhoea or fever, or both, intermittent or constant for at least 1 month, not known to be due to a condition unrelated to HIV infection • Cryptococcal meningitis • Pulmonary or extrapulmonary tuberculosis • Kaposi's sarcoma • Neurological impairment that is sufficient to prevent independent daily activities, not known to be due to a condition unrelated to HIV infection (for example, trauma or cerebrovascular accident) • Candidiasis of the oesophagus (which may be presumptively diagnosed based on the presence of oral candidiasis accompanied by dysphagia • Clinically diagnosed life-threatening or recurrent episodes of pneumonia, with or without etiological confirmation • Invasive cervical cancer
NACO Guidelines for Case Definition of AIDS
Case definition of AIDS in adults (for persons above 12 years of age) 1. Two positive results for HIV infection by ERS test (ELISA/RAPID/SIMPLE) and

(*Contd.*)

2. Any one of the following criteria:
   a) Significant weight loss (>10% of body weight) within last one month/cachexia (not known to be due to a condition other than HIV infection) and
   Chronic diarrhoea (intermittent or continuous) > 1 month duration, or prolonged fever (intermittent or continuous)>1 month duration
   b) Tuberculosis: extensive pulmonary, disseminated, miliary, extrapulmonary
   c) Neurologic impairment preventing independent daily activities, not known to be due to conditions unrelated to HIV infections (e.g. trauma)
   d) Candidiasis of oesophagus (diagnosable by oral candidiasis with odynophagia)
   e) Clinically diagnosed life-threatning or recurrent episodes of pneumonia, with or without etiological confirmation
   f) Kaposi's sarcoma
   g) Other conditions:
   Cryptococcal meningitis
   Neurotoxoplasmosis
   CMV retinitis

DERMATOLOGICAL MANIFESTATIONS OF HIV INFECTION[8,15–17]

The dermatological manifestations of HIV infection are summarized in Table 5.4 and mucocutaneous indicators for HIV serotesting in Table 5.5.

Table 5.4 Dermatological Manifestations of HIV and AIDS

Infectious	
Pyomyositis	It is an AIDS-defining illness, and may be localized or extensive. It is associated with severe constitutional symptoms. Various bacteria have been implicated, and culture/sensitivity testing is essential to decide appropriate antibiotics. Surgical intervention may be required.
Bacillary angiomatosis	It is caused by *B. henselae* and *B. quintana.* Three kinds of cutaneous lesions may develop: pyogenic granuloma-like lesions subcutaneous nodules and hyperpigmented indurated plaques. It can also involve liver in the form of bacillary peliosis besides affecting spleen, bone, soft tissues, CNS, respiratory and gastrointestinal system.
Herpes zoster (Fig. 5.2)	Painful rash of small fluid-filled haemorrhagic blisters in distribution on a erythematous background, and not crossing midline, occurring currently or in the last two years. Ophthalmic division of trigeminal nerve is commonly involved. Eye complications are common as are multisegmental or bilateral, necrotic, haemorrhagic, generalized eruptions. Severe or recurrent herpes zoster is usually associated with more advanced HIV disease. The rash may become chronic or there may be recurrent episodes.

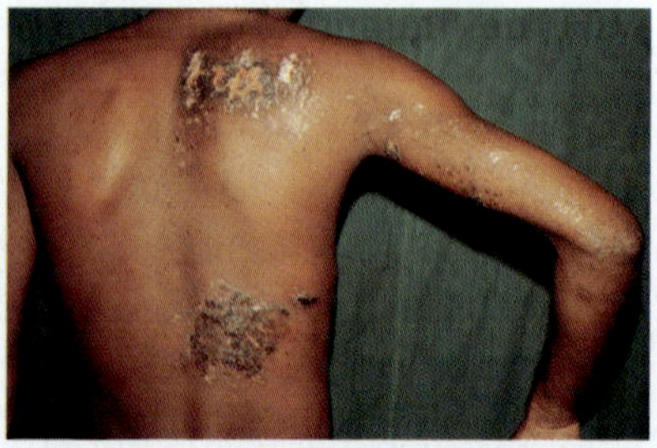

Fig. 5.2 Multidermatomal herpes zoster in a HIV-positive patient

Herpes simplex infection (Fig. 5.3, 5.4)

It is usually a reactivation of latent HSV, and the disease may be recurrent, aggressive and extensive. Bilateral, lumbar or perianal lesions are common. Response to acyclovir is variable, with a high degree of resistance. Severe and progressive, chronic orolabial, genital or anorectal ulcers can occur. History of previous episodes may be present and scarring may be evident. The presence of active disease increases the likelihood of transmission, unless safe sex is practiced.

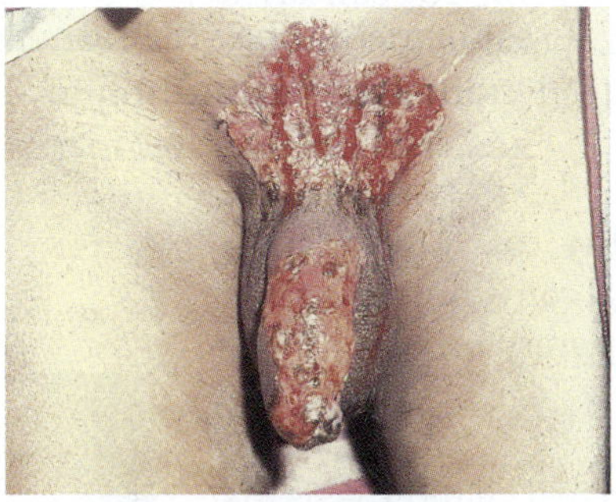

Fig. 5.3 Genital herpes in a HIV-positive patient

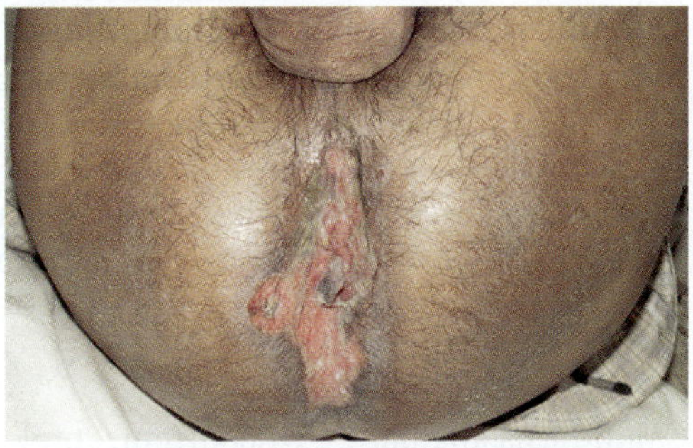

Fig. 5.4 Anogenital herpes in a HIV-positive patient

Oral hairy leukoplakia (OHL) (Fig. 5.5)

OHL is characterized by fine, small, linear patches on lateral borders of the tongue, generally bilateral, and do not get scraped off. It is a marker of HIV infection, and is sometimes difficult to distinguish from oral candidiasis. It is caused by Epstein-Barr virus (EBV) and is asymptomatic.

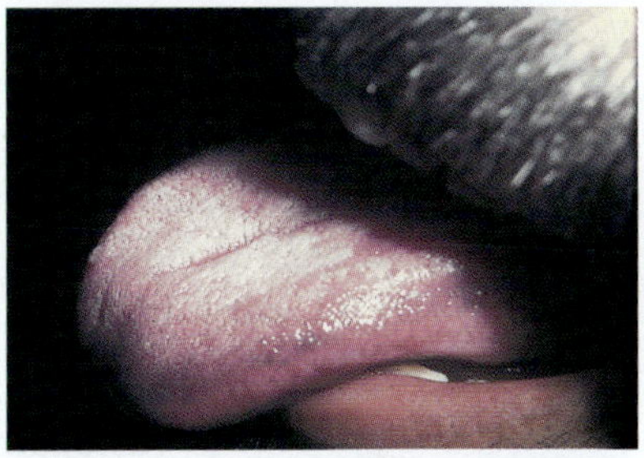

Fig. 5.5 Oral hairy leukoplakia in a HIV-positive patient

Molluscum contagiosum (Fig. 5.6)

In HIV infection, disease severity varies with widespread and atypical lesions, as well as extragenital locations. Giant, multiple and inflamed lesions are common. Treatment is difficult.

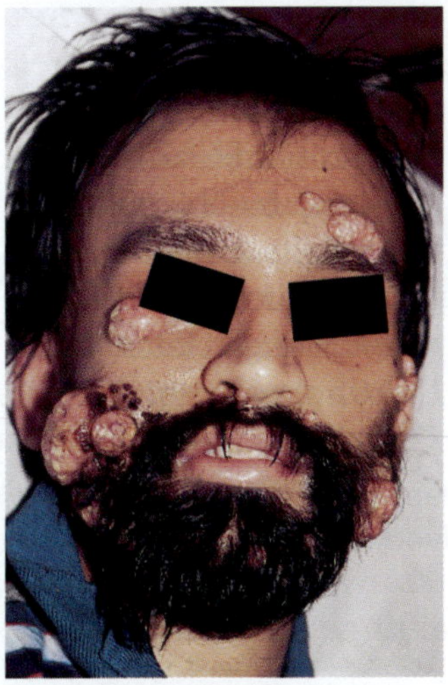

Fig. 5.6 Giant molluscum contagiosum in a HIV-positive patient

Viral wart (Fig. 5.7)

In advanced HIV infection, verrucae can enlarge, become confluent and become unresponsive to treatment. HPV type 5 can cause an unusal pattern of extensive verruca plana and pityriasis versicolour-like warts, similar to the pattern seen in epidermodysplasia verruciformis. With advanced immunodeficiency, low-grade SIL or high-grade SIL (caused by HPV 16, 18) can arise on cervix, external genitalia, perianal/perineum, anus, oropharynx or keratinzed skin, especially nail bed.

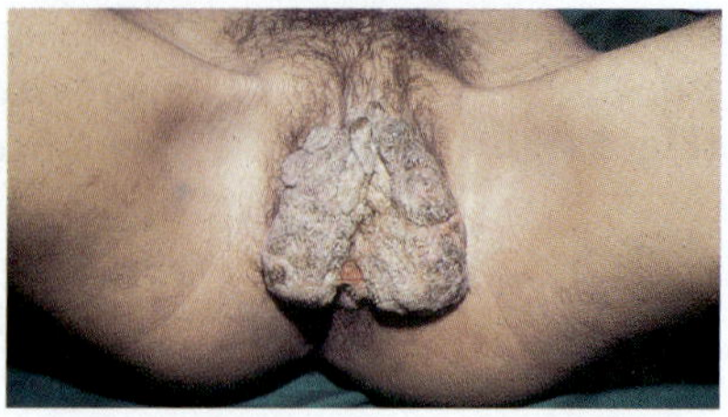

Fig. 5.7 Exuberant genital warts in a HIV-positive patient

Dermatophytoses

The severity and variability of presentation increases. Proximal subungal onychomycosis is pathogenomic of immunosuppression.

Candidiasis/angular cheilitis (Fig. 5.8)

Recurrent, oral or oesophageal candidiasis is common, with varied morphological appearance (erosive, membranous, vegetative, angular cheilitis). Systemic fluconazole is required for treatment and resistance is increasingly observed. Newer molecules such as voriconazle may be required in resistant cases.

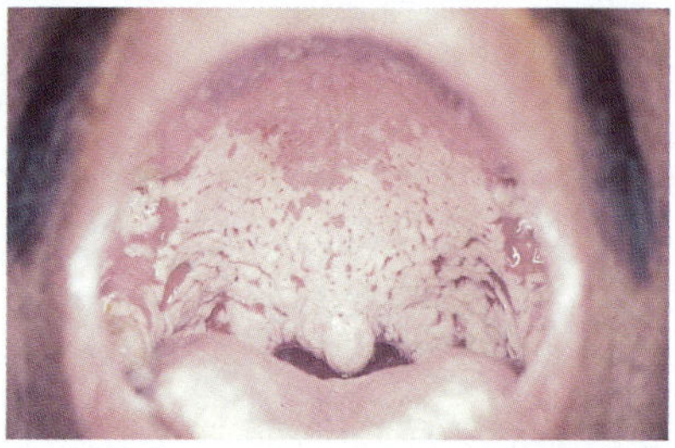

Fig. 5.8 Oropharyngeal candidiasis in a HIV-positive patient

Cutaneous cryptococcosis (Fig. 5.9)

Usually associated with systemic disease such as meningitis or pneumonitis. The skin lesions mimic molluscum contagiosum, and diagnosis requires histopathological evidence. Treatment consists of systemic antifungals such as Amphotericin B, 5-Flucytosine and fluconazole.

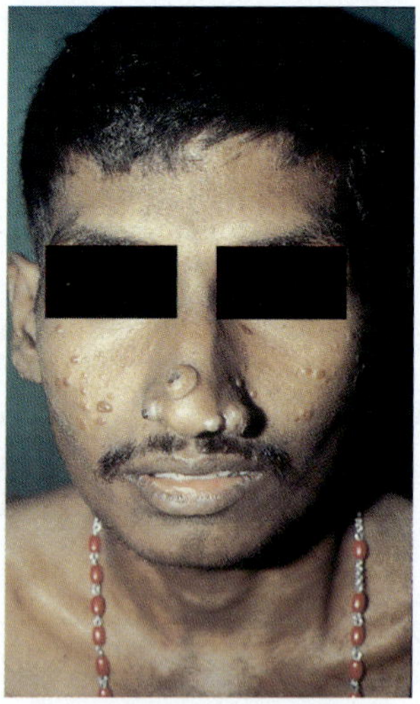

Fig. 5.9 Cutaneous cryptoccosis in a HIV-positive patient

Deep fungal infections

Deep fungal infections occur more frequently and may be disseminated.

Norwegian (crusted) scabies (Fig. 5.10)	In advanced disease, crusted and hyperkeratotic lesions involving unusual sites such as palms, soles, face, scalp and trunk may be seen. These house millions of mites. Erythroderma may occur. The condition is chronic, and itching may be almost absent. Treatment is similar to HIV uninfected individuals, but is to be continued for a longer duration.

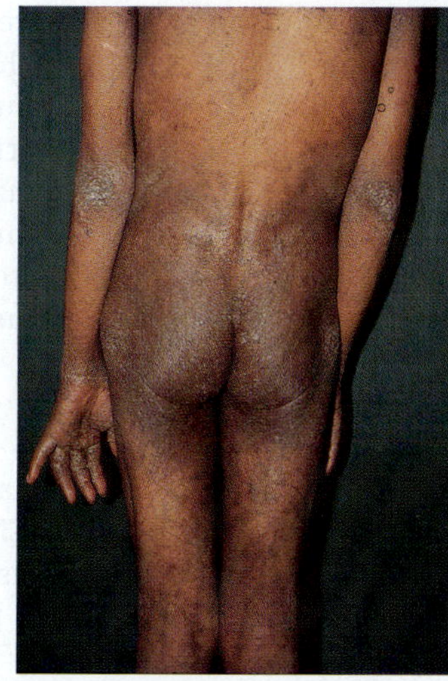

Fig. 5.10 Norwegian scabies in a HIV-positive patient

Non-infectious

Seborrhoeic dermatitis	Chronic, itchy, scaly skin condition, particularly affecting scalp, face, upper trunk and perineum. It may progress to erythroderma. It is quite often the presenting feature of HIV. Its severity correlates inversely with CD4 counts.
Psoriasis	There seems to be a strong correlation between initial onset of psoriasis and HIV infection, such that eruptive disease or sudden exacerbation of pre-existing disease may be seen in a person at risk. Severe disease with widespread lesions, erythroderma, palmoplantar keratoderma, psoriatic arthritis and pustular psoriasis are more common in HIV infected individuals. Phototherapy, retinoids and ART containing Zidovudine (AZT) are effective.
Reiter's syndrome	Presents with migratory arthritis and erythematous papules and plaques with "limpet"-like scales. Circinate balanitis and plantar fascitis are common, but urethritis and uveitis may or may not be present. Higher prevalence in HIV infection may be considered almost as an AIDS-defining illness. Disease is persistent and varies in severity. Oral retinoids are the drugs of choice.
Pruritic papular eruptions (Fig. 5.11)	Pruritic papulovesicular lesions present on face, exposed surfaces of the extremities and trunk are common, more than in uninfected adults. Scabies and obvious insect bites should be excluded. The disease is chronic, recurrent or persistent with intense itching and is difficult to treat.
Aphthae	Recurrent, occurring twice or more in 6 months, and difficult to treat.

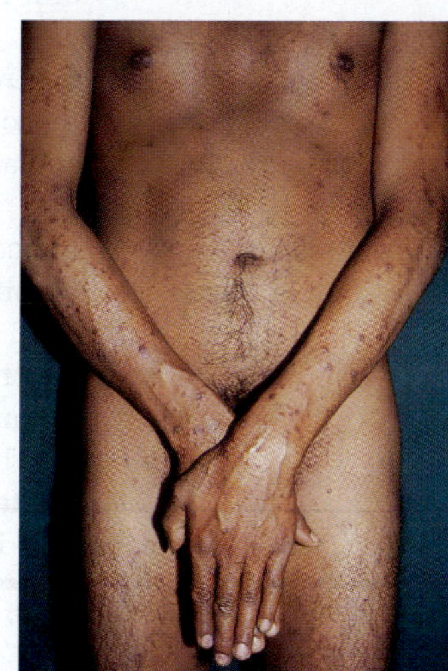

Fig. 5.11 Pruritic papular eruptions in a HIV-positive patient

Stevens-Johnson syndrome (Fig. 5.12)

Adverse drug reactions (ADRs) are more common in HIV infection than in uninfected adults. Commonly implicated drugs are sulphonamides (cotrimoxazole), nevirapine, abacavir, dilantin, pyrazinamide, rifampicin and carbamazepine. Complications including toxic epidermal necrolysis, sepsis, electrolyte imbalance, renal failure, etc., are common and death may result.

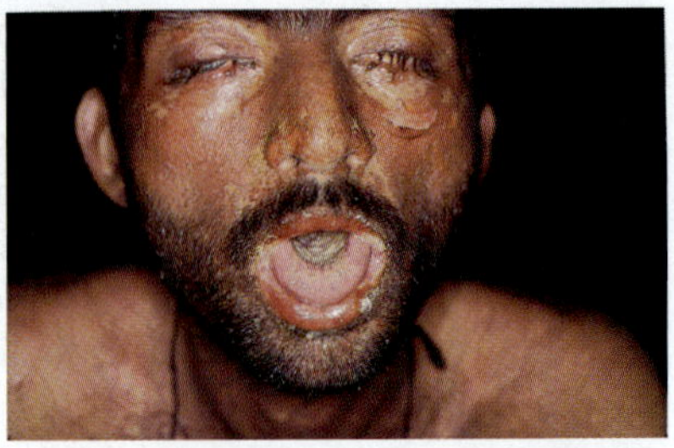

Fig. 5.12 Stevens-Johnson syndrome in a HIV-positive patient

Addisonian pigmentation

It may occur without adrenal dysfunction or as a consequence of adrenalitis due to TB or CMV infection. Diffuse melanotic pigmentation of skin on the face, photoexposed areas, skin creases and buccal mucosa, with longitudinal melanonychia, is common and progressive. The condition is cosmetically stigmatizing. Reversible pigmentation may occur with HAART as well.

Erythroderma

It can be a usual presenting feature of the disease. Mostly it is primary HIV-related erythroderma, but it may also occur due to exacerbation of pre-existing dermatoses described above. It responds well to HAART.

Tuberculides

Papulonecrotic tuberculides or lichen scrofulosorum lesions are common, and most often associated with detectable tuberculous focus. It is a hypersensitive state to the mycobacterial antigen and responds well to antituberculous therapy (ATT).

ITP

It is chronic, of varied severity, and is difficult to correct.

Ichthyosis/xerosis (Fig. 5.13)

It is acquired and quite often marked and extensive. Disease severity correlates with CD4 counts. It is pruritic, and responsive to ART.

Acne conglobata

Disease is severe and extensive, and responds to oral retinoids or HAART.

Hair changes

Lustreless hair, thin hair, various types of alopecia, discoloration of hair, premature graying and long eyelashes have been described.

Nail changes

Leuconychia, pigmentation, half and half nail, clubbing, onychomycosis, paronychia and yellow nail syndrome have been described. Fungal paronychia (painful red and swollen nail bed) or onycholysis (separation of the nail from the nail bed) of the fingernails are common. Proximal white/subungual onychomycosis is a marker of HIV infection.

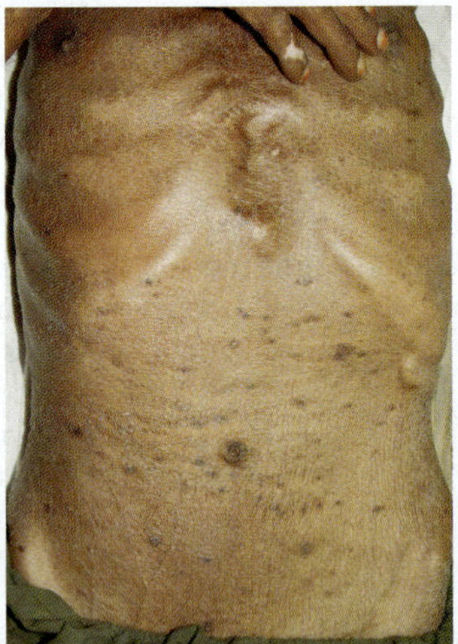

Fig. 5.13 Acquired ichthyosis in a HIV-positive patient

Table 5.5 **Mucocutaneous Disorders as Indicators for HIV Serotesting**

Highly indicative of HIV infection
Exanthem of acute retroviral syndrome
Proximal subungual onchycomycosis
Chronic herpetic ulcers **(Fig. 5.3, 5.4, 5.14)**
Oral hairy leukoplakia **(Fig. 5.5)**
Kaposi's sarcoma **(Fig. 5.15)**
Eosinophilic folliculitis **(Fig. 5.16)**
Multiple facial molluscum contagiosum (in adults) **(Fig. 5.6)**

Strongly associated with HIV infection
Any STDs **(Fig. 5.17, 5.18)**
Herpes zoster **(Fig. 5.2)**
Signs of injected drug use
Candidiasis: oropharyngeal **(Fig. 5.8)** or recurrent vulvovaginal

May be associated with HIV infection
Generalized lymphadenopathy
Seborrhoeic dermatitis (extensive, refractory to therapy)
Aphthous ulcer (recurrent, refractory to therapy)

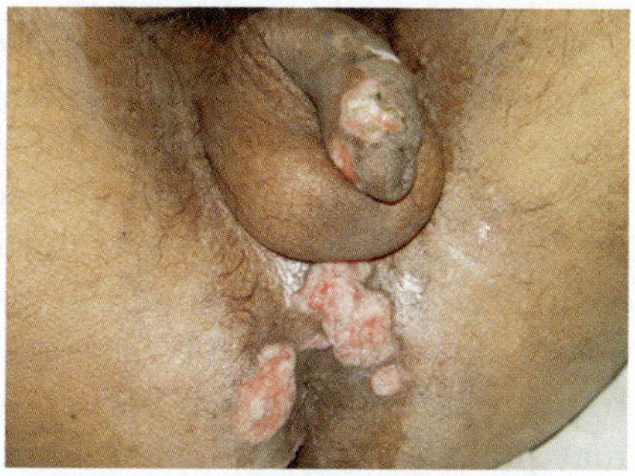

Fig. 5.14 Extensive anogenital herpes infection in a HIV-positive patient

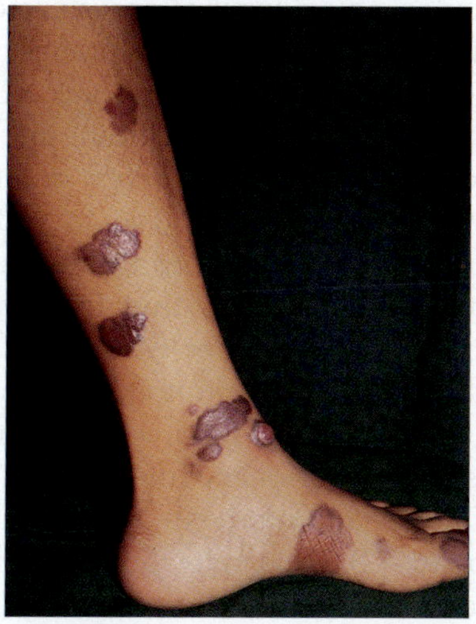

Fig. 5.15 Kaposi's sarcoma on the leg in a HIV-positive patient

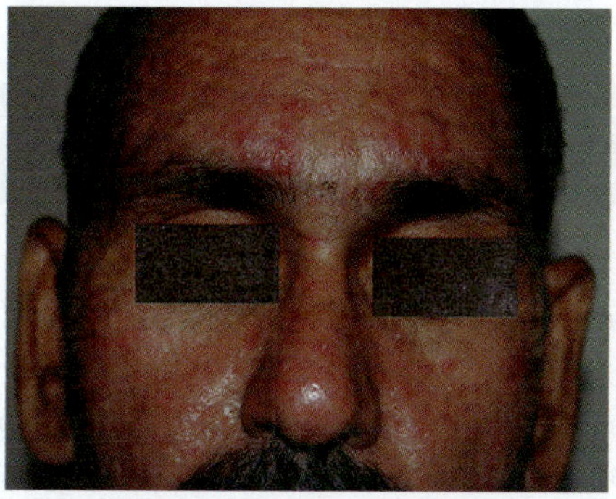

Fig. 5.16 Eosinophilic folliculitis: erythematous papules and plaques on the forehead in a HIV-positive patient

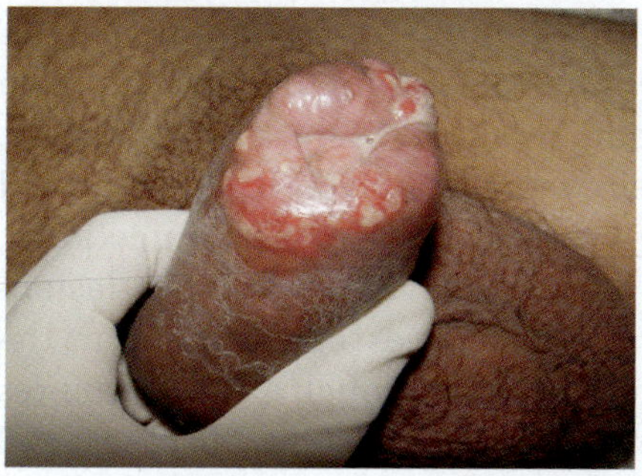

Fig. 5.17 Mixed infection in a HIV-positive patient – genital herpes with gonorrhoea

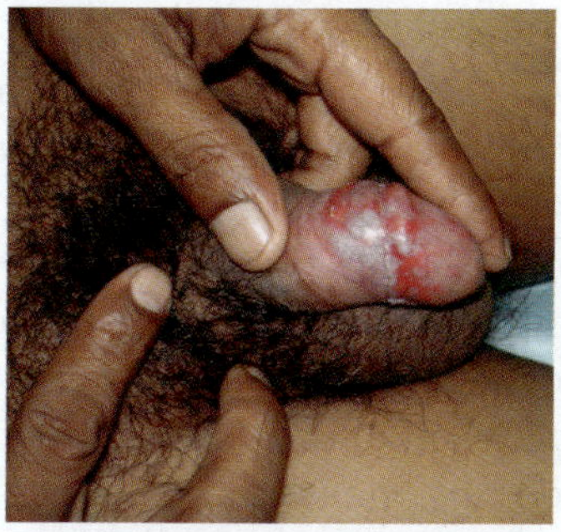

Fig. 5.18 Mixed infection in a HIV-positive patient – genital herpes with warts

SEXUALLY TRANSMITTED INFECTIONS AND HIV/AIDS

There is a well-known synergistic relationship between STDs and HIV infection. It is known that the presence of STI's such as genital ulcer disease, urethritis, vaginitis or cervicitis favours the transmission of HIV during unprotected sexual intercourse. Therefore, prompt diagnosis and treatment of the STI reduces the risk of HIV transmission. Besides, HIV infected individuals may present with atypical or severe manifestations of common STIs. Depending upon the severity of immunosuppression, the clinical features of various STIs show varying degrees of aggressiveness. The recommended therapy for a particular case may need modification depending upon the severity of the disease and extent of immunosuppression. Besides, the occurrence of more than one STI at a given time carries higher positive predictive value for HIV/AIDS. For details refer to the chapter on interaction of STDs and HIV.

SYSTEMIC INVOLVEMENT IN HIV INFECTION

Diseases of the Respiratory System[8]

The lung is the most frequent site of opportunistic infection in AIDS, because, along with the gastrointestinal tract, it serves as an interface with all potential pathogens in the environment. The clinical profile depends on the stage of the disease and CD4 counts. At higher counts (>250 cells/mm^3), recurrent bacterial URTI, sinusitis, bronchitis and otitis media are more common. As the disease progresses, other manifestations appear. In the Western world, *Pneumocystis carinii* pneumonia (PCP) is the commonest respiratory complaint. In the developing world, however, tuberculosis remains the most common infection. Pulmonary involvement in HIV infection may have infective, neoplastic or inflammatory causes. Infective agents implicated in pneumonitis/pneumonia in HIV infection include bacteria inclusive of mycobacteria, viruses, fungi and protozoa. The various pathogens described include:

- Bacteria: *Streptococcus pneumoniae, Haemophilus influenzae, Pseudomonas aeruginosa, Staphylococcus aureus, Moraxella catarrhalis, Rhodococcus equi, Nocardia asteroides, Mycobacterium tuberculosis* and *Mycobacterium avium* complex
- Viruses: Cytomegalovirus, Adenovirus, Herpes simplex.
- Fungi: *Cryptococcus neoformans, Histoplasma capsulatum, Aspergillus fumigatus, Coccidioides immitis, Blastomyces dermatitidis, Pneumocystis jirovecii* and *Penicillium marneffei*
- Protozoa: *Toxoplasma gondii*
- Metazoa: *Strongyloides stercoralis*

Tuberculosis: In the tropics, the almost ubiquitous presence of *Mycobacterium tuberculosis* leads to the flaring-up of hitherto quiescent lesions into active foci of infection as a result of immunosuppression. Tuberculosis may occur at any stage of the disease, and is therefore the commonest presentation of HIV disease in the tropics. Over 15% of tuberculosis patients in India are likely to be HIV-positive. Approximately one-third of all AIDS-related deaths are due to tuberculosis. TB also hastens the onset and progression of other opportunistic infections, thus increasing morbidity and mortality. At higher CD4 counts, the disease resembles that in immunocompetent individuals, while atypical presentation is common at lower counts. Extrapulmonary infections (Figs 5.19, 5.20) occur more commonly in advanced HIV disease. Pulmonary TB tends to be more occult, and patients with advanced AIDS form poor granulomas and have a large number of AFB in their sputum. They may be clinically and radiologically normal. However, radiologic evidence of diffuse, bilateral lower lobe infiltrates is commoner than the upper lobe lesions seen in immunocompetent patients. Patients with HIV are also highly prone to the development of active TB. Thus, TB in HIV patients may be as a result of new infections, rather than just the reactivation of previous lesions. Treatment of TB in HIV does not differ from that in normal individuals, although multidrug-resistant and extensive drug-resistant diseases (MDR-TB/XDR-TB) are commoner in HIV infected individuals.

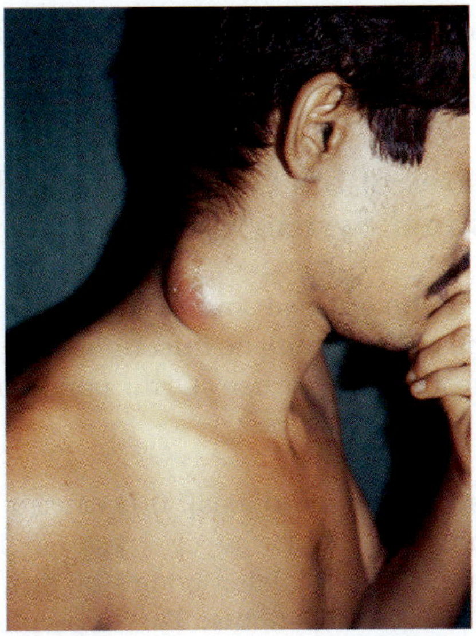

Fig. 5.19 Tuberculosis of lymph nodes in a HIV-positive patient

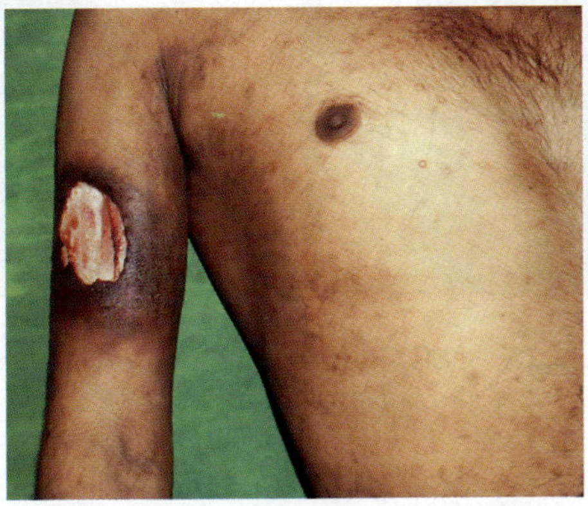

Fig. 5.20 Tuberculous gumma with molluscum contagiosum in a HIV-positive patient

Other respiratory tract infections: Acute bronchitis and maxillary sinusitis are quite common, and recurrent respiratory tract infections (sinusitis, pneumonitis, otitis media, etc.) are markers of HIV infection. The most common manifestation of pulmonary disease is pneumonia. Both bacterial (pyogenic) and *P. carinii* pneumonia (PCP) occur in AIDS.

Pneumocystis carinii **pneumonia (PCP):** *Pneumocystis jirovecii* (formerly *P. carinii*) is the organism that causes the most common life-threatening opportunistic infections in most developed countries. The usual presentation is subacute (over 2-4 weeks), with malaise, fatigue, weight loss, characteristic retrosternal chest pain that is typically worse on inspiration, and non-productive cough. The patient may be breathless, but auscultation reveals no adventitious sounds. Chest radiograph may be normal or may show the classical finding of dense perihilar infiltrate. (Fig. 5.21, 5.22) Arterial oxygen tension is usually low, and serum LDH (fraction LDH-3) is elevated. An LDH > 450 IU/L is strongly predictive of PCP, and higher levels are associated with poorer prognosis. The diagnosis is usually confirmed by direct demonstration of trophozoite or cyst in sputum induced with hypertonic saline or in bronchial lavage (BAL) obtained by fibre-optic bronchoscopy. A gallium scan may be contributory. Cotrimoxazole is the drug of choice. Pentamidine isethionate, trimetrexate with leucovorin, dapsone with trimethoprim, clindamycin, primaquine and atovaquone are second-line drugs. Adjunctive corticosteroids are indicated in patients with moderate and severe disease.

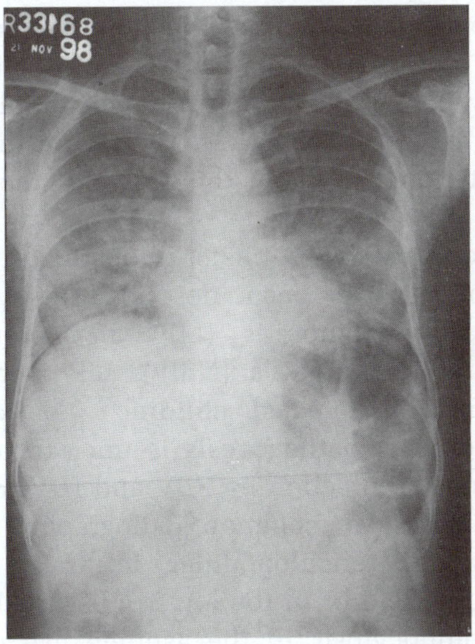

Fig. 5.21 X-ray chest showing soap bubble appearance - *Pneumocystis carinii* pneumonia

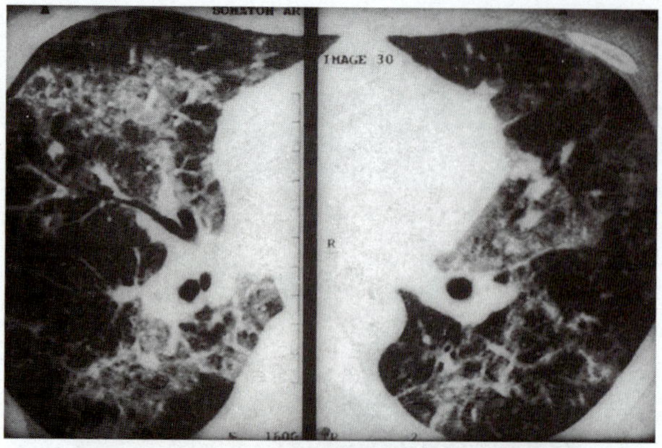

Fig. 5.22 CECT chest showing *Pneumocystis carinii* pneumonia

Atypical mycobacterial infections: These are also seen in AIDS patients, especially with *M. avium* complex (MAC). MAC infection is usually a late occurrence when the CD4+ T cell count is <50 cells/mm^3. The most common presentation is disseminated disease with fever, weight loss and night sweats. Other findings include abdominal pain, diarrhoea, lower lobe infiltrates suggestive of miliary spread, and sometimes alveolar, nodular, hilar or mediastinal adenopathy.

Fungal infections: Pulmonary fungal infections such as histoplasmosis, coccidioidomycosis, penicilliosis and aspergillosis have been described, mostly in endemic areas. These infections are rare, and present with pneumonia and severe constitutional and respiratory symptoms. Demonstration of the fungus may be necessary to achieve a diagnosis. Amphotericin B remains the drug of choice.

Miscellaneous: Two forms of idiopathic interstitial pneumonia have been described – lymphoid interstitial pneumonitis (LIP) and nonspecific interstitial pneumonitis (NSIP). LIP is common in perinatally infected children <13 years of age. The exact pathogenesis is unclear, although simultaneous infection by EBV and HIV may play a role. The most common radiographic features are bilateral reticulonodular infiltrates in the entire lung field or in the lower lobes. BAL shows CD8 lymphocytosis in the aspirate. No effective treatment is known. NSIP is similar to LIP, but commoner in adults. It is a diagnosis of exclusion. Primary pulmonary hypertension, emphysema and bronchiectasis have also been reported.

Diseases of the Oropharynx and Gastro-intestinal System[8]

Most oropharyngeal and gastrointestinal diseases are due to opportunistic infections. The oral lesions manifest due to thrush, OHL, periodontal disease and aphthous ulcers.

Thrush (oral candidiasis): It is caused by *Candida albicans* and rarely by *C. krusei*. It is the most common HIV-associated condition and is reported in upto 70% of patients. The hyperplastic variant is more common, and appears as a white, cheesy exudate often on erythematous mucosa in the posterior oropharynx. (Fig. 5.8) Buccal mucosa and soft palate are the commonest sites, but early lesions are seen along the gingival border. Other clinical variants include the acute erythematous/atrophic variant, angular cheilitis (perleche) and median rhomboid glossitis. The disease is suggestive of advanced immunosuppression and is an indicator for introducing cotrimoxazole prophylaxis in affected individuals. Fluconazole is the drug of choice, although resistance has been reported.

Oral hairy leukoplakia (OHL): It is caused by Epstein-Barr virus (EBV), and presents as white frond-like lesions along the lateral borders of the tongue (Fig. 5.5) but sometimes involving the buccal mucosa. The condition is asymptomatic, and treatment may be unnecessary, although high-dose aciclovir, topical podophyllotoxin and retinoic acid could be tried. Thrush and OHL usually occur in patients with CD4+ T cell counts <250/cm^3.

Periodontal disease: Three characteristic presentations have been described – necrotizing periodontal disease, linear gingival erythema (LGE) and exacerbated attachment loss. LGE is characterized by rapid bone and soft tissue destruction in patients with good oral hygiene, without any plaque or calculus. It has a high predictive value for immunosuppression.

Aphthous stomatitis: Recurrent oral ulcers, with a characteristic erythematous halo occurring at least twice over six months, are a marker of HIV infection. Their cause is obscure, although a vasculitic process has been suggested as in herpes simplex virus infection. The disease is refractory to therapy, and thalidomide may be prescribed in severe cases.

Gastrointestinal tract involvement in HIV usually consists of oesophagitis and diarrheal diseases.

Oesophagitis: It presents with dysphagia and odynophagia and is usually caused by candida, cytomegalovirus (CMV) or herpes simplex virus (HSV). CMV infection is associated with a single large ulcer, whereas herpetic infection presents with multiple small ulcers. Oesophagitis is a sign of worsening immunosuppression.

Diarrhoea: Diarrhoea is the most common GI complaint in HIV infection. Infections of the small and large intestines with various bacteria, protozoa and viruses can cause diarrhoea and abdominal pain. Also, drug-associated diarrhoea, especially with protease inhibitors, is also reported. In one-fifth of cases, no pathogen or cause could be detected. These cases are considered idiopathic or HIV-associated enteropathy. The small intestine or the colon may be involved. Small intestine involvement is associated with large-volume diarrhoea, and associated dehydration and electrolyte anomalies. Abdominal pain, nausea and vomiting are present, while large bowel disease is associated with low-volume diarrhoea, tenesmus, hematochezia and fecal leukocytosis. Bacteria, protozoa, parasites and viruses have been implicated. Salmonella, Shigella, Campylobacter and Clostridium difficile diarrhoea have been described.The disease is more severe in HIV infected individuals. MAC and *M. tuberculosis* are also implicated. *Cryptosporidia* spp., Microsporidia and *Isospora belli* are the most common opportunistic protozoa that infect the GIT causing non-inflammatory diarrhoea. *Giardia intestinalis* and *E. histolytica* infections are common in homosexual men. CMV colitis presents as non-bloody diarrhoea, abdominal pain, weight loss and anorexia. Endoscopic examination reveals multiple mucosal ulcerations, and the biopsy shows characteristic intranuclear inclusion bodies. In advanced disease, various systemic fungal infections like histoplasmosis, coccidioidomycosis, etc. may also cause diarrhoea. Nelfinavir causes diarrhoea in upto 20% individuals, and the disease may be severe enough to withhold therapy. Besides these secondary infections, HIV infection per se can cause AIDS enteropathy. The exact pathogenetic mechanism by which HIV causes diarrhoea is unknown. Analysis of stool samples with relevant special stains is required for diagnosis. Sigmoidoscopy, colonoscopy or upper GI endoscopy with biopsy may be indicated if stool analysis is inconclusive. The management of diarrhoea involves treatment of the cause with relevant anti-infective agents. The maintenance of fluid-electrolyte balance is essential. Oral rehydration is mandatory, and total parenteral nutrition may be required in unresponsive cases. Luminal agents such as dietary fibre supplements may be helpful, but may bind medication as well. Antimotility agents may be used judiciously, and octreotide may be required in intractable AIDS-associated secretory diarrhoea.

HIV and the Nervous System (Neuro–AIDS)[8]

Cerebral toxoplasmosis is the most frequent opportu-nistic infection of the central nervous system. It usually results from the reactivation of toxoplasma cyst in the brain, causing abscess formation. Abscess may be unifocal or multifocal. Clinically, it presents with features of a space-occupying lesion (SOL). CT scan shows ring-enhancing lesions with surrounding oedema. (Fig. 5.23)

Cryptococcal meningitis accounts for 5-10% of opportunistic infections in patients with HIV. Clinical presentation is subacute with headache, fever and cranial nerve palsies. Neck stiffness is relatively rare. CSF analysis will demonstrate yeast in 70% of cases (Fig. 5.24) and antigen detection is positive in 100% of patients.

Progressive multifocal leukoencephalopathy (PMFL) is a demyelinating disease (slow virus

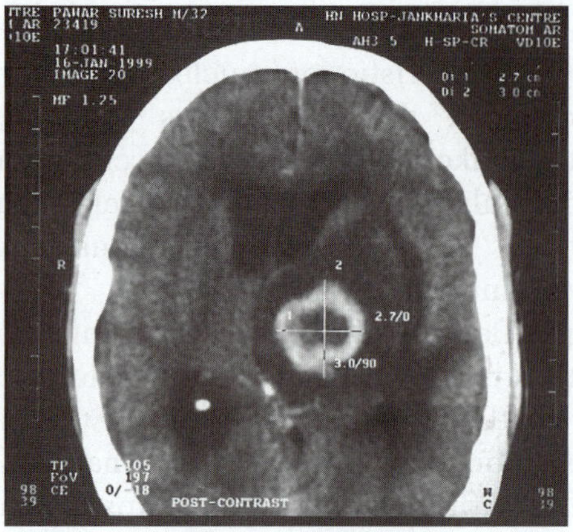

Fig. 5.23 Toxoplasmosis-CECT head, ring enhancing lesion

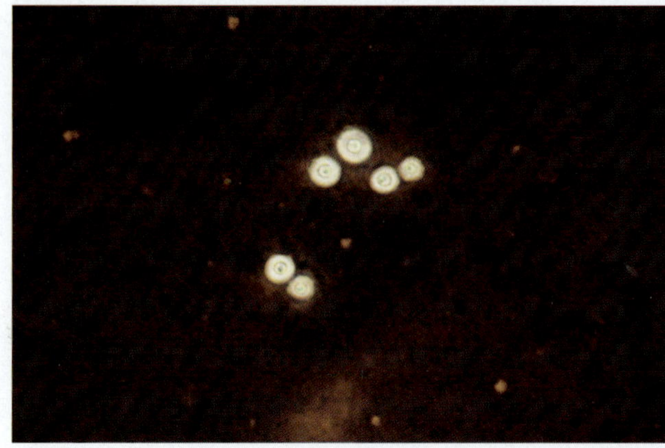

Fig. 5.24 Cryptococcosis-India ink preparation

disease) caused by JC virus. Clinically there may be focal neurological deficits, ataxia and personality changes.

Patients with HIV encephalopathy have a form of dementia known as AIDS-related cognitive-motor complex. In early stages, there is impairment of memory and concentration. Later, motor signs appear including hyper-reflexia, extensor plantar responses, incoordination and ataxia.

Other neurological features in HIV infection include progressive vacuolar myelopathy (with spastic paraplegia, ataxia and loss of sphincter control), transverse myelitis (due to VZV, HSV and CMV infections), peripheral neuropathy and psychiatric manifestations (acute psychosis, depression).

Diseases of the Liver, Gall Bladder and Pancreas[8]

Liver involvement is usually in the form of coinfection with HBV/HCV. Direct HIV infection of the liver may lead to functional defects, which may present as porphyria cutanea tarda (PCT). Liver is also affected as a result of drug administration, both HAART and therapy for opportunistic infections, especially antituberculous treatment.

Sclerosing cholangitis and papillary stenosis are reported in cryptosporidiosis, CMV infection and Kaposi's sarcoma. Pancreatitis usually occurs secondary to drug toxicity, mainly with didanosine.

HIV/AIDS and hepatitis coinfection is the current topic of interest globally. There is paucity of epidemiological data on HBV or HCV infection in India, including its incidence, genotyping study, natural history and incidence of HIV and HBV/HCV coinfection[21]. It is suggested that the effective mode of transmission for HBV or HCV in descending hierarchy would be transfusion > intravenous drug use > sexual > needle stick injury > unknown. According to Fauci, over 95% of HIV infected individuals have evidence of infection with HBV; 5-40% are coinfected with HCV, and co-infection with hepatitis D, E and/or G viruses is common. There was approximately a threefold increase in persistent hepatitis B surface antigenemia. Patients coinfected with HIV and HBV have a low incidence of inflammatory disease, presumably because of antecedent immunosuppression. Severe hepatitis may develop due to immune-reconstitution as a result of antiretroviral therapy. IFN-alpha may be less successful in the treatment of HBV, and Lamivudine is the drug of choice. Since it is also a potent antiretroviral drug, it should never be used as a single agent to prevent the development of resistant quasi-species.

In contrast, HCV infection is more severe in patients with HIV, and levels of HCV are 10-fold higher than in HIV-negative patients, as is also the incidence of liver failure. It has been recommended that those HIV-positive individuals without natural infection be immunized with Hepatitis A and/or Hepatitis B vaccines. End-stage liver disease (ESLD) is the commonest cause of mortality amongst such individuals, especially if not treated with HAART.

Diseases of the Kidney[8]

HIV-associated nephropathy (HIVAN) involves the kidneys in HIV infection, and the most common presentation is with nephrotic syndrome and renal failure. Focal segmental glomerulosclerosis and mesangial proliferative glomerulonephritis account for most of the cases of HIVAN. Renal disease can also occur as a side effect of therapy.

Diseases of the Eye[21]

The most common ophthalmic opportunistic infection in India is CMV retinitis, which almost always occurs in patients with CD4 counts <50 cells/mm^3. The second most common manifestation is HIV retinopathy. This is a non-infectious condition seen in 13-15% patients, presenting with cotton-wool spots on the fundus.

Other conditions include extensive blepharitis, spontaneous lid ulceration, molluscum contagiosum, herpes simplex keratitis, frosted branch angiitis due to CMV retinitis, subretinal cysticercosis, acute retinal necrosis syndrome, squamous cell carcinoma and immune recovery vitritis following treatment with protease inhibitors.

HIV and Tumours[8]

Kaposi's Sarcoma (KS)

Kaposi's Sarcoma has been the first neoplasm reported in HIV disease. It is usually seen in gay and bisexual men, and in women in Africa. The worldwide incidence of KS in patients with AIDS may approach 34%. KS occurs at all stages of HIV disease, and its severity is not strictly correlated with the degree of immunosuppression. KS is reportedly a proliferation of endothelial cells induced by human herpes virus-type 8 (HHV-8) acquired through sexual transmission.

About one-third of HIV infected cases have a preponderance of tumors on the legs and feet. However, lesions may develop also on the skin, including the scalp, lips, hard palate and gums. Lesions may occur singly or in groups. KS begins as pink, red, brown or purple macules that disseminate and progress to violaceous plaques or nodules (Fig. 5.15). They may easily be mistaken for bruises, purpura or nevi. Lesions may be symmetrical with smooth borders or asymmetrical with jagged edges. They darken and become scaly as they age. The involvement of internal organs and mucosa is common. As a rule, the patient has approximately one internal lesion for every five skin lesions. Gastrointestinal involvement is common and may result in haemorrhage or obstruction. The course of KS in HIV infected patients is more aggressive than in other clinical types of KS.

For limited infection, local therapy with liquid nitrogen, alitretinoin or intralesional vincristine may be effective. Surgery, radiotherapy and systemic single-agent chemotherapy, usually with vinblastine, vincristine, bleomycin, saclitaxel doxorubicin or etoposide, may be useful. However, systemic chemotherapy has not been shown to improve long-term survival rates. Immune-reconstitution after HAART may lead to the remission of KS. Interferon (IFN)-alpha and IFN-beta, photodynamic therapy and systemic hyperthermia have also been used. Cryotherapy, laser irradiation and electrodessication may be useful for localized solitary lesions of KS.

Non-Hodgkin's Lymphoma[22]

At least 6% of all AIDS patients develop lymphomas (Fig. 5.25, 5.26) at some point during their illness. The initiation of HAART has no effect on the incidence. Most tumours are extralymphatic and are histologically high-grade, large-cell immunoblastic or non-cleaved small-cell tumours. Burkitt's lymphoma has also been reported. Their pathogenesis may be related to EBV and also to HHV-8. CNS is the most common site. Clinically it presents with signs and symptoms of a space-occupying lesion (SOL).

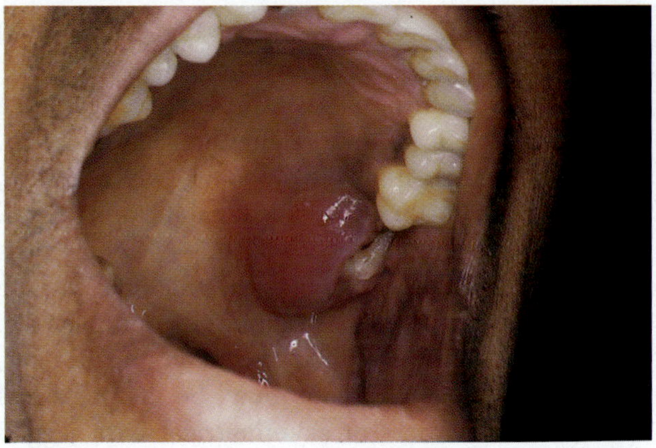

Fig. 5.25 B cell lymphoma in oral cavity of a HIV-positive patient

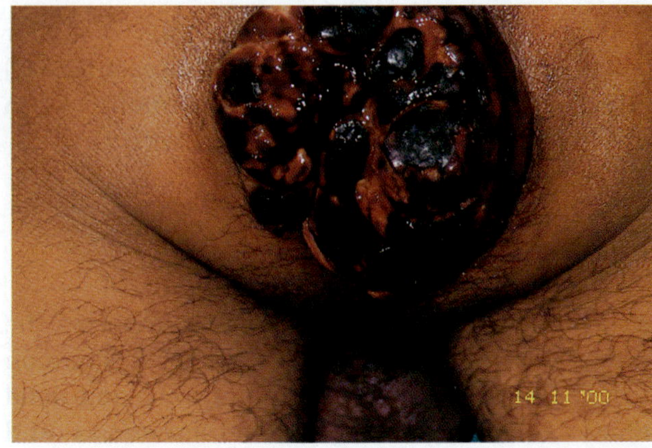

Fig. 5.26 Lymphoma in a HIV-positive patient

Systemic lymphoma is seen at an earlier stage of infection. In addition to lymph node involvement, the bone marrow (leading to pancytopenia), liver, lung and GIT (~ 25% patients) may be involved. Any site in the GIT may be involved. The patient may present with dysphagia and pain. Pulmonary disease may present as a mass lesion, multiple nodules or an interstitial infiltrate. A variant called primary effusion lymphoma or body cavity lymphoma has also been described. Lymphomatous pleural, pericardial and/or peritoneal effusions, in the absence of discreet nodal or extranodal masses, are seen.

Other tumors that can occur in AIDS are Hodgkin's lymphoma, squamous cell carcinoma (Ca) of the anus especially in homosexual men, cervical cancer, adenocarcinoma, renal cell Ca, teratoma and seminoma.

OPPORTUNISTIC INFECTIONS IN AIDS

Most opportunistic infections in AIDS occur when the CD4+ count falls below 200 cells/mm^3.

The various infections and their relation to CD4+ counts are depicted in **Fig. 5.27**.

IMMUNE-RECONSTITUTION INFLAMMATORY SYNDROME

The immune-reconstitution inflammatory syndrome (IRIS) in HIV infected patients who initiate ART results from restored immunity to specific infectious or non-infectious antigens. In these patients, clinical deterioration occurs despite increased CD4+ T-lymphocyte counts and decreased plasma HIV-1 viral loads. A paradoxical clinical worsening of a known condition or the appearance of a new condition after initiating the therapy characterizes the syndrome. Potential mechanisms for the syndrome include a partial recovery of the immune system or exuberant host immunological responses to antigenic stimuli. Possible infectious and non-infectious etiologies of IRIS are summarized in Table 5.6.

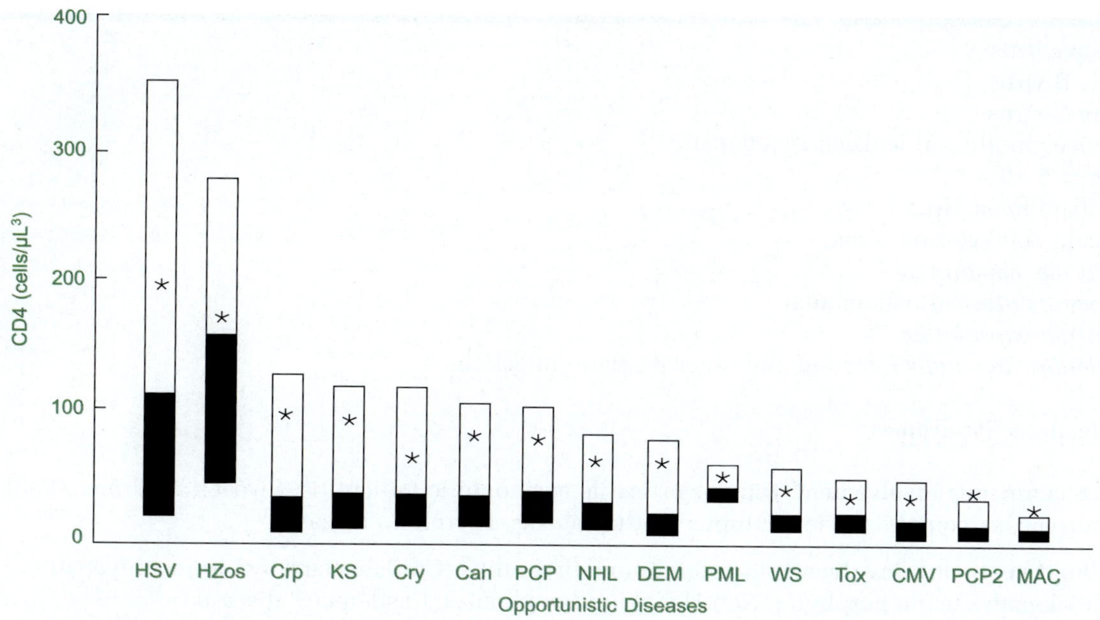

Fig. 5.27 Relationship Between CD4+ T cell Counts and Opportunistic Diseases

Boxplot of the median (line inside the box), first quartile (bottom of the box), third quartile (top of the box) and mean (asterix) CD4+ lymphocyte count at the time of the development of a opportunistic disease. Can, candidal oesophagitis; CMV, cytomegalovirus infection; Crp, cryptosporidiosis; Cyr, cryptococcal meningitis, DEM, AIDS dementia complex; HSV, herpes simplex virus infection; HZos, herpes zoster; KS, Kaposi's sarcoma; MAC, *Mycobacterium avium* complex bacteremia; PHL, Non-Hodgkin's lymphoma; PCP, primary *Pneumocystis carinii* pneumonia; PCP2, secondary *Pneumocystis carinii* pneumonia; PML, progressive multifocal leukoencephalopathy; Tox, *Toxoplasma gondii* encephalitis; WS, Wasting syndrome.

Table 5.6 **Infectious and Non-infectious Causes of IRIS in HIV Infected Patients**

Infectious EtiologiesZ
Bacterial infections
Mycobacteria
Mycobacterium tuberculosis
Mycobacterium avium complex
M. leprae
Other mycobacteria
Bartonella species
Viral infections
Herpes viruses
Herpes zoster virus
Herpes simplex virus
Herpes virus-associated Kaposi's sarcoma

(*Contd.*)

Cytomegalovirus
Hepatitis B virus
Hepatitis C virus
Progressivee multifocal leukoencephalopathy
Parvovirus B 19
Human papilloma virus
Molluscum contagiosum virus
Cryptococcus neoformans
Pneumocystis jirovecii pneumonia
Histoplasma capsulatum
Strongyloides stercoralis infection and other parasitic infections

Non-infectious Syndromes

(i) **With cutaneous involvement:** Papular urticaria, eosinophilic folliculitis, Sweet's syndrome, Reiter's syndrome, sarcoidosis, systemic lupus erythematosus, Peyronie's disease

(ii) **Without cutaneous involvement:** Autoimmune thyroiditis, Guillain-Barrt syndrome, myopathy, radiculopathy, acute porphyria, Non-Hodgkin's lymphomas, Castleman's disease

The risk factors identified for the development of IRIS in one cohort include male sex, a shorter interval between initiating treatment for opportunistic infections and starting ART, a rapid fall in HIV-1 RNA after ART, and being ART-naïve at the time of OI diagnosis. Other significant predictors include younger age, a lower baseline CD4 cell percentage, a lower CD4 cell count at ART initiation, and a lower CD4-to-CD8 cell ratio at baseline.

As of now, there are no standard guidelines for the treatment of IRIS, and the following interventions are mostly based on published case reports and other anecdotal clinical evidence. The treatment includes continuation of primary therapy against the offending pathogen in order to decrease the antigenic load, continuation of effective HAART and judicious use of anti-inflammatory agents.

1. Milder IRIS: Continue HAART, antimicrobial agents and non-steroidal anti-inflammatory drugs.
2. Severe life-threatening IRIS: Needs oral prednisolone, approximately 1-2 mg/kg. The exact duration and dose of the steroid is variable and depends upon clinical severity. Sometimes, the duration of the steroid therapy may extend to six months or one year. Consider discontinuation of HAART in case of severe life-threatening IRIS (e.g., encephalitis, ARDS, cerebritis and perilesional cerebral edema).

Patients with IRIS have almost invariably better outcomes than those who are HIV-positive with clinical progression of a given disease. The occurrence of IRIS does not require any modification in the treatment of OIs. Maintenance treatment for OIs should not be changed and previously completed OI treatment (e.g., for tuberculosis) should not be reinitiated. Similarly, the dosages of chronic suppressive treatment for an OI should not be increased.

The diagnosis of IRIS requires a high index of suspicion. Detailed clinical history should be taken in patients suspected to have IRIS, which includes a thorough physical examination based on syptoms and suspicion of systems involved. Ophthalmological examination should be included in all patients.

The following investigations should be considered before starting ART: complete blood count, ESR, serum electrolytes, liver function tests and renal function tests, CD4 count and HIV viral load, chest X-ray, Mantoux (tuberculin) test, sputum stain for AFB and culture, and ultrasonography of abdomen. In a suspected case, even an initially negative Mantoux test becoming positive could be suggestive of IRIS.

Patients who are started on ART having a CD4 count of less than 100 cells/μl require close clinical monitoring during the first weeks of ART. Similarly, they should be counseled about the risk of development of IRIS as well as to discourage defaulting on therapy as the development of IRIS suggests increase in immunity and is a good sign unless life-threatening.

CLINICAL MANIFESTATION OF HIV DISEASE IN INDIA[18, 19, 21]

In India, HIV infected individuals are being exposed to unfavorable conditions like malnutrition and poverty and also to a host of tropical infections which are peculiar to this region. Striking similarities and certain differences exist between clinical presentation of AIDS in Indian population and in other countries. Slim disease or the wasting syndrome is the most common mode of presentation in Africa. Similar presentation was seen in 62% patients in a series from South India. *P. carinii* pneumonia is the most common opportunistic infection in most developed countries. By contrast, PCP is unusual in Indian population, and the most common opportunistic infection is tuberculosis. The rarity of PCP among Indian patients may be due to the fact that they have many other tropical infectious diseases prior to reaching severe immunosuppressed state and consequent relatively early mortality due to these infections.

Among the tuberculosis group, *Mycobacterium avium intracellulare* is the most common of mycobacteria isolated from patients in US, whereas *M. tuberculosis* is more frequently isolated in patients from India.

Candidiasis (oropharyngeal and oesophageal) is the second commonest opportunistic infection in India. Toxoplasmosis, histoplasmosis, Kaposi's sarcoma and CNS lymphomas are uncommon in Indian population as compared to Western countries.

The dermatological manifestations of HIV infection from a major centre in India are given in **Table 5.7**. Many authors have correlated cutaneous manifestations with CD4 counts **(Table 5.8).**

The clinical comparison of HIV patients from Latin America, Africa, Asia and India is depicted in Table 5.9.

Table 5.7 Mucocutaneous Markers of HIV Infection (n = 20520)

Manifestation	*Percentage*
Candidiasis	92
Addisonian pigmentation	72
Herpes simplex infection	68
Hair changes	68
Oral hairy leukoplakia	68
Ichthyosis	65
Herpes zoster	52
Pruritic papular dermatosis	48
Molluscum contagiosum	42
Nail changes	28
Seborrhoeic dermatitis	25
Tinea incognito	21.5
Scabies	14.5
Pyoderma	14.5
Endogenous eczema	7
Drug reaction	4.5
Cutaneous tuberculosis	5.5
Photosensitivity	4.5
Oral aphthosis	3.5
Psoriasis	2.5
Reiter's syndrome	1.5
Cryptococcosis	1.5
Leg ulcer	1.0
Demodicidosis	1.0
Skin infarcts	0.5
Erythroderma	0.5
Eosinophilic folliculitis	0.5
Reactivation of leprosy	0.5
Kaposi's sarcoma	0.25
Histoplasmosis	0.12

Adapted from Maniar et al,[8] Mumbai, India

Table 5.8 **CD4 Cell Count and Dermatological Manifestations[16]**

	CD4 cells/µL		
Dermatological manifestation	***Mean***	***Standard deviation***	***Range (min–max)***
Herpes zoster (n = 35)	176.33	164.13	6–792
Papular pruritic dermatitis (n = 30)	149.23	171.65	6–624
Herpes simplex (n = 26)	196.92	209.10	9–730
Dermatophyte infections (n = 22)	178.41	189.45	9–755
Staphylococcal skin infection (n = 7)	410.00	487.32	33–1580
Genital warts (n = 6)	187.67	142.67	41–405
Molluscum contagiosum (n = 2)	277.00	280.01	79–475
Scabies (n = 1)	9.00	–	9
Oral candidiasis (n = 170)	196.52	233.18	6–1580

Table 5.9 **Spectrum of Clinical Diseases Among HIV Infected Adults in Africa, Latin America and Asia[23]**

Region/ Country	Sub-Saharan Africa, Cote d'Ivoire - Hospitalized HIV+ patients	Kenya - HIV+ medical ward admissions	Latin America, Brazil - Patients with AIDS, specialist clinics	Asia, India - AIDS cases, national surveillance	Thailand - Hospitalized patients with AIDS
No. of HIV+ patients	349	95	111	3551	1553
Tuberculosis	28%	18%	32%	62%	37%
Bacteremia	18%	26%	–	–	<1%
HIV wasting	11%	–	–	–	8%
Isosporiasis	7%	–	6%	–	0
Bacterial pneumonia	6%	16%	16%	–	<1%
Cerebral toxoplasmosis	6%	–	14%	3%	2%
Bacterial enteritis	5%	–	6%	–	–
Non-specific diarrhoea	5%	15%	–	–	–
Oesophageal candidiasis	3%	–	24%	57%	3%
Cryptoccosis	2%	1%	5%	4%	38%
Kaposi's sarcoma	1%	2%	5%	<1%	<1%
Cytomegalovirus	0	–	5%	1%	4%
PCP	0	–	22%	3%	5%
Cryptosporiodiosis	0	–	8%	4%	2%
Penicilliosis	0	–	–	–	3%
Histoplasmosis	0	–	–	–	2%

REFERENCES

1. Dietrich U, Maniar JK, Rubsamen- Walgmann H. The epidemiology of AIDS in India. Trend Microbiol 1995; 3: 17-21.
2. Maniar JK, Saple DG. The HIV/AIDS epidemic in India. HIV & AIDS current trends 1998; 4: 3-6.
3. Maniar JK. Health Care Systems in Transition III: The Indian Subcontinent. JPHM-2000; 22: 33-7.
4. Joshi PJ, Maniar JK, Bhave GG. Profile of HIV Infection in India. In: S. Jameel, L Villarreal, eds. Advances in animal virology. New Delhi: Oxford & IBH Publishing; 2000. p. 371-81.
5. Clarke JR, Sahi DK, Maniar JK, et al. Dual infection with HIV 1 and HIV 2. Thorax 1997; 52: 587-8.
6. Maniar J. The natural history of HIV 2 infection in India. HIV & AIDS. Current trends 2001; 7: 3-7.
7. Natural history and classification. In: Bartlett, edr. Medical Management of HIV infection. Baltimore: The Hopkins HIV report; 1999. p. 1-16.
8. Maniar J, Kamath R. HIV and HIV-associated Disorders. In: Tropical Dermatology. Tyring S, Lupi O, Hengge UR (eds.).London, Elsevier Health Sciences Publishers, pp. 93-124, 2005.
9. Acute HIV infection. In: Powderly WG, edr. Manual of HIV Therapeutics. 2nd edn. Philadelphia; Lippincott Williams; 2001. p. 6-13.
10. Schacker T, Collier AC, Hughes J, et al. Clinical and epidemiologic features of primary HIV infection. Ann Intern Med 1996; 125: 257-64.
11. Natural History. In: Powderly WG, edr. Manual of HIV Therapeutics. 2nd edn. Philadelphia. Lippincott Williams; 2001. p. 14-9.
12. Singh S, Singh N, Maniar JK. AIDS associated Toxoplasmosis in India and its correlation with serum tumour necrosis factor-alpha. J Parasit Dis 1996; 20: 49-52.
13. Epidemiology of communicable diseases. In: Park K, edr. Park's Text Book of Preventive and Social Medicine. 16th edn. Jabalpur: Banarsidas Bhanot; 2000. p. 257-66.
14. Centres for Disease Control and Prevention (CDC). 1993 Revised classification system for HIV infection. MMWR 1992; 41: 96.
15. Rajagopalan B, Jacob M, George S. Skin lesions in HIV-positive and HIV –negative in South India. Int J Dermatol 1996; 35: 489-92.
16. Kumarasamy N, Solomon S, Madhivanan P, et al. Dermatological manifestations among human immunodeficiency virus patients in South India. Int J Dermatol 2000; 39: 192-5.
17. Singh A, Thappa DM, Hamide A. The spectrum of mucocutaneous manifestations during the evolutionary phases of HIV disease: an emerging Indian scenario. J Dermatol 1999; 26: 294-304.
18. Chacko S, John TJ, Jacob M, et al. Clinical profile of AIDS in India: a review of 61 cases. JAPI 1995; 43: 535-8.
19. Maniar JK. The HIV/AIDS epidemic in India - real challenge for dermatovenereologists in the new millenium, 29th National Conference of IADVL, 1-4 February 2001, Agra.
20. Grant A. Clinical features of HIV disease in developing countries. Lepr Rev 2002; 73: 197-205.
21. Kumarasamy N, Vallabhaneni S, Flanigan TP, et al. Clinical profile of HIV in India. Ind J Med Res 2005;
22. Surjushe AU, Jindal SR, Kamath RR, et al. Immune reconstitution inflammatory syndrome. Indian J Dermatol Venerol Leprol. 2006; 72: 410-4.
23. Grant A. Clinical features of HIV disease in developing countries. Lepr Rev 2002; 73: 197-205.

6 LABORATORY DIAGNOSIS OF HIV INFECTION

Pradeep Seth, S Sujatha

In this chapter

- Biology of the HIV
- Natural History of HIV Infection
- Immune Response to HIV Infection
- Laboratory Tests
- Selection of HIV Antibody Test
- National HIV Testing Policy
- Strategy for Laboratory Diagnosis of HIV Infection

INTRODUCTION

The diagnosis of HIV infection can sometimes be intrigu-ing as the infected persons may present with a spectrum of illnesses ranging from acute to chronic infections in adults, children and even in newborns or neonates. These infections may be mistaken for other febrile illnesses; for example, acute infectious mononucleosis or constitutional symptoms which appear in chronically infected patients may mimic pulmonary tuberculosis. Therefore, it is necessary to make correct utilization of appropriate diagnostic tests to confirm HIV infection. Although standard serological techniques make the diagnosis of chronic asymptomatic or symptomatic disease relatively straightforward, the identification of HIV infection by these tests during the seroconversion period may be difficult.

It is, therefore, imperative that those who are involved in the laboratory diagnosis of HIV must provide accurate and reliable results. To accomplish this, a better understanding of the biology of the virus[1], the natural history of HIV infection, immune response of the host and various tests currently available for diagnosis including their principles, limitations and problems, performance characteristics and proper use is needed.

BIOLOGY OF THE HIV

The HIV is an enveloped, RNA-containing retro-virus that primarily infects CD4 receptor-bearing lymphocytes, or helper T cells. The virus has the ability to integrate its RNA genome into the host cell genome by first transcribing this genome into DNA (HIV-provirus) with the help of an enzyme called reverse transcriptase. The provirus is then transcribed and translated along with the host-cell DNA resulting in the synthesis of specific virus components which eventually assemble to produce complete virus particles.

The HIV is composed of an outer envelope and an inner core. The envelope consists of a bi-lipid membrane in which specific components of the virus are embedded. Each component is a mushroom-shaped glycosylated protein or glycoprotein and consists of an external portion (gp 120) and a transmembrane portion (gp 41). These two envelope glycoproteins together are involved in the process of attaching the virus to the CD4 receptor on the host cell and subsequent fusion of the virus envelope with the cell membrane. The inner core components are bound by a protein coat encompassing RNA genome and three viral enzymes, namely reverse transcriptase, integrase and protease.

There are two types of HIV: HIV 1 and HIV 2. HIV 1 infections are prevalent worldwide. In contrast, HIV 2 is endemic primarily in West Africa. However, HIV 2 infections are now making their presence felt all over the world. HIV 2 genome shares 40-45% homology with HIV 1 and it causes similar pathological consequences. Diagnostically, HIV 1 and HIV 2 can present problems. Laboratory tests designed to detect HIV 1 infections do not always detect HIV 2 infections and viceversa. Even then, the antibodies to HIV 1 may frequently cross-react with HIV 2 antigens and be detected in serological assays designed to detect the antibodies of HIV 2. Similarly, HIV 2 antibodies may cross-react in HIV 1 serological tests. All HIV serological assays available commercially detect both anti-HIV 1 and anti-HIV 2 antibodies.

NATURAL HISTORY OF HIV INFECTION

After 1 to 3 weeks of initial infection by any route, an infected individual may present with an acute infectious mononucleosis-like syndrome characterized by sore-throat, fever, lymphadenopathy, hepatosplenomegaly, rash and other constitutional symptoms[2]. Although some patients may be asymptomatic, majority (40-60%) develop a mild to moderate illness which generally lasts for 1-3 weeks. Clinical laboratory studies show that during the first week, such patients may have lymphopenia, thrombocytopenia and elevated transaminases. In the second week, the CD4+ lymphocytes are reduced and CD8+ lymphocytes rise in number, resulting in the inversion of CD4+/CD8+ cell ratio. At the same time, atypical lymphocytes are also seen in blood. After acute infection, over the following months, the CD4+ and CD8+ cell counts return to almost normal levels in most patients. These changes last for 1-3 weeks, and the recovery is complete. Generally speaking, the patients usually become asymptomatic for many months to years after primary HIV infection.

The infected individuals have high levels of infectious virus in the plasma in peripheral blood. This virus is relatively homogenous. Once the seroconversion takes place and the infected individual develops HIV-specific immune response, virus variants emerge which results in heterogeneity or quasi-species. During the asymptomatic phase, the plasma viremia is markedly reduced.

The duration of asymptomatic HIV infection may vary from 5 years to greater than 15 years, during which period most patients experience relatively good health. However, viral replication is highly dynamic and continues during this period of clinical latency. Evidently there is profound reduction in CD4+ lymphocytes. The infected individual may develop minor ailments related to immune deficiency, which has been referred to as AIDS-related complex. With continuous virus replication, there may be a further fall in CD4+ T cell counts and the individual becomes further immunocompromised. At this stage, the individual may develop a variety of opportunistic infections like *Pneumocystis jiroveci* pneumonia, generalized candidiasis, tuberculosis, cryptococcal meningitis, CMV retinitis, generalized herpes virus infection, toxoplasmosis, malignancies, etc. On the basis of CD4+ T cell count in peripheral blood and clinical conditions of the patient, the Centre for Disease Control and Prevention, Atlanta, USA, proposed a classification system for identifying HIV infected individuals with or without AIDS for clinical management and antiretroviral therapy[3] (Table 6.1). This classification has found universal acceptance.

Table 6.1 CDC Classification System for HIV Infection and Expanded AIDS Case Definitions

CD4+ T Cell Categories (cells/µl)	*Clinical Categories#*		
	A	B	C
500	A1	B1	C1
200-499	A2	B2	C2
<200	A3	B3	C3

A: asymptomatic including acute primary HIV infection and persistent generalized lymphadenopathy (PGL); B: symptomatic but no AIDS indicator conditions of group C; C: AIDS indicator conditions

IMMUNE RESPONSE TO HIV INFECTION

Following an HIV infection, both humoral and cellular immune responses develop. Although the initial antibody response is of IgM class, it is usually transient and not consistent. IgG antibodies to envelope and gag proteins first appear followed by antibodies to all other proteins of the virus. It is, therefore, important to understand the kinetics of the immune response in order to formulate a strategy for testing an individual infected with HIV. The antibodies are usually produced between 6 and 12 weeks following an infection. In rare instances, the antibodies may not be detected until 45 months after infection. Thus, any individual soon after acquiring an infection will test negative. Antibodies to envelope antigens (particularly gp 41) will persist throughout the infection, while antibodies to core antigen (p 24) will decrease once the clinical disease develops and the concentrations of viral core antigen p 24 increases in plasma.

HIV infection in the newborn is closely linked to maternal infection.[4] It occurs in the presence of maternally acquired antibodies. The risk of transmission is from 14.4 to 45% depending upon the severity of infection in pregnant mother. However, the diagnosis of congenital HIV infection presents enormous problems. Serodiagnostic tests are generally of not much help in the diagnosis of perinatal HIV infection especially in the presence of maternal IgG antibodies in cord blood, and IgM antibody production against HIV infection is very inconsistent and erratic. Maternal IgG has been reported to persist in infants for up to 18 months of age despite a reported half-life for IgG of only 23 to 26 days.

LABORATORY TESTS

Laboratory tests employed in the diagnosis of HIV infection may be classified into the following groups (Table 6.2).

Table 6.2 Laboratory Tests for the Diagnosis of HIV Infection

(I) Tests for HIV-specific antibodies in serum/plasma
- a. Screening tests
  - (i) ELISA
  - (ii) Rapid tests
- b. Supplemental tests
  - (i) Western blot assay
  - (ii) Immunofluorescence test
  - (iii) Line immunoassay

(II) Tests for HIV-specific antibodies in saliva

(III) Tests for HIV-specific antibodies in urine

(IV) Confirmatory tests
- a. Virus isolation
- b. Detection of HIV-specific core antigen (p24)
- c. Polymerase chain reaction (RT PCR/b-DNA)

Tests for HIV-specific Antibodies in Serum/Plasma

Screening Tests

Screening tests are rapid and inexpensive serological tests used for screening antibodies against HIV in infected individuals. These tests possess a high degree of sensitivity, but some false positive results do occur (i.e. some individuals will inevitably produce positive results even though they are not infected with the virus). Therefore, these tests are used as presumptive tests.

Since a positive result may be obtained due to technical error, it is imperative that repeat testing is done in duplicates before the sample is considered reactive by the screening assay. Furthermore, as these tests lack a sufficiently high degree of specificity, the positive results of these assays must be validated by supplemental tests. Screening tests include:

(a) Enzyme-linked immunosorbent assays (ELISA)

(b) Rapid tests

Enzyme-linked immunosorbent assays

These assays use enzymes as the indicator system for the detection and quantitation of analytes present in immune complexes formed as a result of reaction between solid surface-bound HIV antigen and circulating antibody. These tests are highly sensitive and specific and take 60 to 90 minutes for completion. Although these tests require an initial investment of expensive instruments like plate washer, spectrophotometers, etc., the running cost is rather low as compared to supplemental tests.

Rapid tests

These tests have a total reaction time of less than 30 minutes. They are more expensive per test than ELISA although they do not require complex equipment. The results are read with naked eyes. Some of these tests may be completed within a few minutes and, therefore, are best suited for emergency clinics, casualties and trauma clinics where immediate screening of a blood donor or a recipient may be required.

Several formats of rapid tests are available commercially but the most popular ones are the dot blot assays. In dot blot assay, the microscopic particles are coated with a synthetic peptide and then immobilized on a nitrocellulose membrane. To the patient's serum-containing antibodies, conjugate, developer and stop solutions are added in sequence with usual incubation and washing steps. Then colour develops in proportion to the amount of HIV antibodies bound to the peptide-coated microparticles.

Supplemental Tests

Supplemenal tests are also serological tests for the detection of antibodies against HIV. These tests are recommended for the validation of positive results of the screening assays. Three types of supplemental tests are commonly used:

(a) Western blot assay
(b) Immunofluorescence test
(c) Line immunoassay

Western blot assay

Western blot is a highly specific and equally sensitive assay. In this assay, specific viral proteins from the whole virus lysate are separated by polyacrylamide gel electrophoresis according to their molecular weight and then transferred onto a nitrocellulose membrane by a process called electroblotting. Following this transfer, the membrane is washed and cut into strips. A serum sample found positive by screening test is reacted with the HIV-proteins immobilized on the strip. An enzyme-conjugate and a substrate are added to generate a colorimetric reaction. If the sample has antibodies, coloured bands will appear to denote human IgG binding to the viral protein on the strip. In the absence of coloured bands, Western blot is interpreted as negative.

However, the interpretive criteria for HIV 1 Western blot remain a subject of much discussion. There is no unanimity on this subject. Another problem with this assay is its prohibitive cost.

Immunofluorescence test

An alternative but seldom used assay for HIV diagnosis is indirect immunofluorescence assay. In this test, the HIV infected cells are acetone-fixed onto glass slides and then reacted with test serum followed by fluorescein-conjugated anti-human antibody. A positive reaction appears as apple-green fluorescence on the membrane. This test is very inexpensive to perform but requires expertise to conduct as well as to interpret.

Line immunoassay

This test is based on the same principle as Western blot test but utilizes recombinant or synthetic peptides as antigens instead of virus lysate. It has comparable sensitivity and specificity to Western blot assay although it is used much less commonly.

Tests for HIV-specific Antibodies in Saliva

The immunoglobulins gain entry into the oral cavity by secretion from salivary glands and by transudation from blood capillaries beneath the gingival crevices. Since saliva contains low levels of IgG or IgM, sensitive and specific antibody assays with a class-specific antibody capture format have been designed for testing salivary specimens for the presence of anti-HIV antibodies. Although these kits are efficacious, there is some concern about how early the anti-HIV antibody could be detected in saliva during seroconversion as compared to serum/plasma following primary infection. In addition, it is important to determine the minimum concentration of IgG at which each kit can be relied on in order to not to give a false negative result. Finally, the role of supplementary/ confirmatory testing on saliva specimens is not known. Studies on these important features of sensitivity of anti-HIV assays are needed before they can be put into diagnostic use.

Tests for HIV-specific Antibodies in Urine

The use of urine as an alternative to serum has many advantages including ease of collection and lower danger posed in transmitting infections. Reports of detecting HIV antibodies in urine samples of patients have shown varied results. Some workers have suggested that the low sensitivity of some kits like the immunochromatography-based assays with potential to generate false negative reports limits its usefulness, while a few others have shown comparable sensitivity to serum-based tests. The apparently low sensitivity of urine may be because of its low pH or its low viscosity and faster migration, which may reduce antigen-antibody exposure times. Urine samples may be used in epidemiological studies in high-prevalence areas but not for individual diagnosis.[5]

Confirmatory Tests

These tests help confirm the presence of virus in an individual who is either seropositive or has equivocal results from various serological tests.

Virus Isolation

The most common method for the isolation of the virus from blood of infected individuals is by co-cultivating peripheral blood mononuclear cells (PBMC) with those from uninfected donors. It generally takes 4-8 weeks for isolation and identification of the virus. This assay is 100% specific but its sensitivity varies with the stage of HIV infection. Therefore, although virus isolation confirms the diagnosis, a negative result does not rule out HIV infection in an individual. Moreover, in both adults and children, the virus cannot be cultured from PBMC for approximately 6 weeks following the time of transmission. However, this procedure is labour-intensive and dangerous, which could be undertaken only by specialized laboratories.

Detection of HIV-specific Core Antigen (p24)

The antigen test detects HIV-free antigen (p24) in serum. HIV antigenemia occurs during "window period" and during late disease when the patient is usually symptomatic. It is also seen in HIV infected newborns. Therefore, an antigen test may be useful (a) during "window period" and late disease when the patient is symptomatic, (b) to detect HIV infection in a newborn because diagnosis is difficult due to the presence of maternal antibodies, (c) when HIV dementia and encephalopathy are suspected and the test is performed with cerebrospinal fluid. However, only 30% patients during window period, 50-60% of AIDS patients, 30-40% of patients with AIDS-related complex (ARC) and 10% of asymptomatic patients are antigen-positive.

Another important point to note is that this test detects soluble p24 antigen and does not specifically identify live virus. Therefore, an antigen-negative test sample may still be infectious. Similarly, the presence of antigen does not by itself confirm the sample is infectious.

This test employs indirect ELISA technology, in which a specific antibody is bound to the solid phase, and the serum containing free HIV antigen is made to react with this antibody. This is followed by the addition of conjugate (an antibody to the core antigen coupled to an enzyme), substrate and stop solutions in sequence with usual incubation and washing steps. In this format, the test is relatively insensitive, being able to detect 50-60 pg/ml of antigen. The reason for lack of sensitivity of this test is that the free antigen in serum may be complexed with anti-core antibody. However, incorporating a step of preliminary acid hydrolysis of the serum sample to dissociate immune complexes to free p24 antigen, which can then be measured, should improve its sensitivity.

Recently, an ultrasensitive p24 antigen detection test has become available, which utilizes a step of dissociation of immune complexes before the ELISA procedure. This has reportedly improved the sensitivity of the test to almost the same level as RT-PCR but is much less expensive and technically complex to perform. This test has been used for both diagnosis and prognosis of paediatric HIV.[6]

Polymerase Chain Reaction (PCR)

In this technique, the target HIV RNA or proviral DNA is amplified enzymatically in vitro by chemical reaction. It is an extremely sensitive assay because a single copy of proviral DNA can be amplified and then detected by the probe. This technique allows the detection of HIV prior to the detection by antibody assays. In our experience, PCR could detect infection even before viral culture becomes positive. Presently, it is the most sensitive known method for the identification of HIV infection. However, it is technically demanding and is expensive, and therefore it is not suitable for use in routine laboratories.

A modification of this assay, RT PCR, is employed for the quantitation of HIV present in plasma (plasma virus load). In this test, HIV-RNA from the circulating plasma virus is first reverse-transcribed to cDNA, which is then used as a template in PCR format for the quantitation of HIV in plasma. This test has now become an important marker in assessing the risk of disease progression and monitoring antiretroviral therapy. Three different techniques, namely RT PCR, NASBA (nucleic acid sequence-based amplification) and branched-DNA (b-DNA) assay, have been employed to develop commercial kits. RT PCR and NASBA reactions are template (plasma RNA) amplification assays, whereas b-DNA assay amplifies the signal from RNA-DNA hybridization reaction.

SELECTION OF HIV ANTIBODY TEST

The selection of the most appropriate test or a combination of tests for use depends on three criteria:

1. Objectives of the HIV antibody test
2. Sensitivity and specificity of the test(s) being used
3. Prevalence of HIV infection in the population under study

Objectives of the HIV Antibody Test

These are three main objectives of HIV antibody testing:

1. Transfusion/blood or organ donation safety: unlinked and anonymous screening of donated blood and blood products
2. Sero-surveillance: unlinked and anonymous testing of sera for the purpose of monitoring the prevalence and trends in HIV infection over time in a given population
3. Diagnosis of HIV 1 infection: voluntary testing of serum of asymptomatic persons or persons with clinical signs and symptoms suggestive of HIV infection/AIDS

Sensitivity and Specificity of Antibody Tests

Sensitivity and specificity are two major factors that determine the accuracy and reliability of an assay in distinguishing an infected from an uninfected person. A test with high sensitivity will have very few false negative results. Therefore, only those tests with highest possible sensitivity should be used when there is need to minimize the rate of false negative results (e.g. in transfusion/blood donation safety). On the other hand, a test with high specificity will have very few false positive results. Therefore, it may be used when there is need to minimize the rate of false positive results (e.g. in sero-surveillance and in the diagnosis of HIV infection in an individual).

Prevalence of HIV Infection

The probability that a test may determine the true infection status of a person accurately varies with the prevalence rate of HIV infection in the population. It is expressed as a predictive value. In general, the higher the prevalence of HIV infection in a population, the greater the probability a person testing positive is truly infected (i.e. the greater the positive predictive value, or PPV). Thus, with increasing prevalence, the proportion of serum samples testing false positive decreases.

The PPV of a test is very low when a population with low HIV prevalence is tested, although the specificity of the test is very high. For this reason, a supplemental test is necessary to enhance the PPV of HIV testing.

NATIONAL HIV TESTING POLICY

The most popular algorithm for HIV antibody testing uses a highly sensitive ELISA followed by the WB assay. This algorithm is expensive and produces indeterminate results of uncertain diagnostic significance quite often during early seroconversion. Studies have shown that combinations of EIAs (enzyme immunoassays) may provide results as reliable as and in some instances even more reliable than the ELISA/WB combination at a much lower cost.

On 10 September, 1993, the National AIDS Control Programme Technical Advisory Committee of Ministry of Health and Family Welfare, Government of India, recommended the implementation of the following HIV antibody testing policy:

Testing Algorithm I

For transfusion purposes, only one highly sensitive, reliable, economically feasible and technically easy EIA for both HIV 1 and HIV 2 antibodies should be carried out by the Zonal Blood Testing Centres/ Blood Banks, and if the results indicate the presence of antibodies, the blood should be discarded and no further test needed on this blood sample. The HIV screening is anonymous and unlinked. The EIA test selected should be of very high sensitivity and good specificity to ensure almost negligible false negative reports and considerably reduced number of wasted blood units respectively.

Testing Algorithm II

For sero-surveillance purposes, HIV 1 and HIV 2 combination kits conforming to the one used for blood safety purposes will be used by the surveillance centres. As in blood safety measures, the screening of blood samples is anonymous and unlinked. All sera are first tested with one EIA. Any serum found reactive on the first assay is retested with a second EIA based on a different antigen preparation or principle. If found reactive by the second assay also, it is considered antibody-positve. Any serum which is reactive on the first test but non-reactive on the second test is considered antibody-negative. The selection of EIA kits appropriate for sero-surveillance testing purposes is very critical for the predictive value of this algorithm. The first EIA should be of very high sensitivity and the second EIA should be of very high specificity. This algorithm will ensure almost negligible false negative reports and very few false positive reports.

Testing Algorithm III

HIV testing for diagnostic purposes depends on the clinical status of the patient. For asymptomatic persons, all samples are first tested with one EIA. Any reactive sample is further tested with a second EIA based on a different antigen preparation or principle. Samples found reactive by the second test are then subjected to a third EIA based on different antigen preparation or principle. The serum reactive on all three tests is considered HIV antibody-positive. Serum that is non-reactive either in the first test or in the second test is considered negative. The serum that is reactive in the first and second tests but non-reactive in the third test is considered equivocal/borderline-positive. Such serum samples should be subjected to retesting with the second and third EIA. In case of equivocal/borderline results on repeat testing, these sera should be tested with the Western blot assay. In many cases, a second blood sample from the same patient collected after 2 to 3 weeks may be helpful. All patients with clinical signs and symptoms of HIV infection/AIDS should be tested by the same strategy as used for sero-surveillance purposes, i.e. two EIA based on different antigens or based on different principles. The predictive value of this algorithm also depends on the selection of appropriate EIAs. The first EIA should be of very high sensitivity, the second EIA should be of very high specificity and the third EIA should be of good sensitivity and specificity to ensure negligible false negative as well as false positive reports.

STRATEGY FOR LABORATORY DIAGNOSIS OF HIV INFECTION

The choice of laboratory tests employed to establish HIV infection in an individual depends on the stage of infection (see Table 6.3). In acute HIV infection during the window period, in the absence of measurable antibody response, the diagnosis rests upon (i) demonstration of viral nucleic acid in PBMC by PCR, (ii) demonstration of HIV-specific P24 antigen in plasma/serum, and (iii) isolation of HIV from PBMC. On the other hand, during asymptomatic HIV infection, although the patients may be apparently healthy, they have detectable anti-HIV antibodies in their blood. Therefore, the diagnosis of HIV infection is straightforward by the demonstration of HIV-specific antibodies in blood.

Laboratory diagnosis of HIV infection (Table 6.4) in patients with clinical manifestations suggestive of AIDS includes (a) demonstratrion of HIV-specific antibodies in blood, (b) quantification of virus load in plasma and (c) demonstration of HIV-specific P24 antigen in plasma/serum.

Table 6.3 **NACO Guidelines for HIV Antibody Testing Strategies**

Objective of testing	*Prevalence of HIV Infection*	*Testing Algorithm*
Blood banks-transfusion safety	All prevalences	I
Sero-surveillance	< 10%	II
	> 10%	I
Clinical sign and symptoms suggestive HIV infection/AIDS	All prevalences	II
Diagnosis/identification of asymptomatic individuals	< 10%	III
	> 10%	II

Table 6.4 **Laboratory Tests Employed for the Diagnosis and Monitoring of HIV Infected Individuals**

Clinical Categories (Stages)	*HIV Serology*	*p24 Antigen Assay*	*PCR (Qualitative)*	*Plasma HIV Load (Quantitative)*	*Immunophenotyping*		
					CD4+	*CD8+*	*Ratio*
Asymptomatic (A1-A3)							
Window period	–	40%	+	++	↓↓/N	↑↑/N	Inv
With/without PGL	+	–/±	+	–/+	↓	↑	Inv
Symptomatic (B1-B3)	+	+/–	+	–/+	↓	↑	Inv
AIDS indicator *illnesses (C1-C3)*	+	++	+	++++	↓↓↓	↑↑	Inv
Paediatric HIV infection	+[a]	+	+	–/++	?[b]	?	?

Symbols used: +: positive; –: negative; +: borderline positive; ↓: counts low; ↑: counts high; N: counts normal; Inv: CD4+/CD+8 ratio inverted.

a: maternal antibodies may be present until 17 months after birth in newborn.

b: role unknown in the prediction or monitoring of HIV infection.

The diagnosis of HIV infection in newborns depends on the route of infection.[7] Conventional commercial assays for detecting anti-HIV antibodies may be unable to diagnose HIV infection in infants born to HIV-seropositive mothers owing to the inability of these tests to distinguish between maternal IgG and infants' own antibodies. Therefore, tests for the identification of virus or its constituents are the mainstay in the diagnosis of paediatric HIV infection. The isolation of virus by culture remains the 'gold standard' for diagnosis. In prenatal infections (that is, infants infected in utero), the presence of virus may be established either by detection of HIV genome by PCR or by isolation of the virus from cord blood lymphocytes within 48 hours of birth. In contrast, in perinatal infections (that is, intrapartum or infections acquired during passage through birthcanal), viremia could only be detected 7 to 90 days later either by PCR or by virus isolation. Therefore, a practical algorithm for the diagnosis of HIV in a range of clinical settings is to identify HIV by culture or PCR in infants born to HIV-seropositive mothers as close to birth as possible. If there is no evidence of virus at this time point, these tests should be repeated at the age of 3 and 6 months. The presence of virus by any of these tests should be interpreted as probable infection.

Estimating the incidence of HIV in various populations is important to understand the current status of transmission dynamics, identify high-risk groups and monitor prevention strategies. While estimating the prevalence of infection is simple using the routine diagnostic assays, it is relatively difficult to measure the incidence. Several statistical methods have been employed for this purpose, including cohort studies, but they may not give an accurate picture. Recently a few laboratory tests have been developed to detect new infections like the LS (less sensitive) ELISA, BED ELISA and line immunoassay. Most tests are based on the different properties of early as compared to late antibodies, specifically affinity/avidity. In the context of India, the estimation of the incidence of HIV will have an enormous impact on the ongoing surveillance activities and prevention strategies.[8]

REFERENCES

1. Seth P, Arora A. HIV applied virology and vaccine implications. J Int Med Sci Acad 1998; 11: 131-4.
2. Wali JP, Handa R, Aggarwal P. Acute HIV infection. J Int Med Sci Acad 1998; 11: 139-42.
3. Castro KG, Ward JW, Slutsker L, et al. 1993 revised classification system for HIV infection and expanded surveillance case definition for AIDS among adolescents and adults. MMWR 1992; 41: 1-19.
4. Kabra SK, Singh A, Jain Y. HIV/AIDS in children. J Int Med Sci Acad 1998; 11: 179-83.
5. Kagulire SC, Stamper PD, Opendi P, et al. Performance of two commercial immunochromatographic assays for rapid detection of antibodies specific to human immunodeficiency virus types 1 and 2 in serum and urine samples in a rural community-based research setting (Rakai, Uganda). Clin Vaccine Immunol, 2007; 14: 738-40.
6. Pattoni JC, Sherman GG, Coovadia AH, et al. Ultrasensitive Human Immunodeficiency Virus Type I p 24 antigen assay modified for use on dried whole blood spots as a reliable, affordable test for infant diagnosis. Clin Vaccine Immunol 2006; 13: 152-5.
7. Wara DW, Luzuriaga K, Martin NL, et al. Maternal transmission and diagnosis of human immunodeficiency virus during infancy. Ann N Y Acad Sci 1993; 693: 14-9.
8. Parekh BS, McDougal JS. Application of laboratory methods to estimate HIV-1 incidence. Indian J Med Res 2005; 121: 510-8.

7 ANTIRETROVIRAL THERAPY

Praveen Aggarwal, Jyoti Prakash Wali, Rohini Handa

In this chapter

INTRODUCTION

Nearly a decade ago, someone with HIV/AIDS had little hope. The years 1996-1998 were a turning point in the management of these patients due to three reasons: a new understanding of viral pathogenesis; development of more powerful tools for measuring HIV levels in blood, and most importantly, the introduction of new and effective antiretroviral treatment regimes. The measurement of HIV RNA using PCR techniques has shown that a patient with HIV infection could have 10,000 to 100,000 viral particles in 1 ml of blood during the latent period. HIV RNA allows interventions prior to the measurable evidence of immunosuppression as evidenced by CD4 counts, and is used in most studies to document the efficacy of antiretroviral strategies.

In this chapter, we shall first discuss the standard recommendations for treatment of HIV infection followed by a section on the treatment of HIV in a resource-poor country. Before putting down the details of the treatment, it is essential to learn the life cycle of HIV so as to understand the mode and site of action of antiretroviral drugs.

REPLICATION CYCLE OF HIV

The HIV is a retrovirus and is a single-stranded RNA virus. It can infect a number of different cells, including CD4-bearing macrophages and T-helper lymphocytes within the host. There are several steps in the viral replication cycle, which may be the target of antiretroviral therapies.

HIV attaches to the target cells through binding of surface glycoprotein (gp)120 to cell surface CD4 molecules. Following CD4 binding, a centre material change in the HIV gp120/gp41 complex is induced by the interaction of gp120 with chemokine receptors CCR5 or CXCR4. This change in conformation exposes gp41 to initiate fusion of the cell and viral membranes. T-cell tropic HIV strains mainly use CXCR4 as a co-receptor, and are called X4 strains, whereas macrophagetropic strains responsible for host-to-host transmission use CCR5 as a co-receptor, and are called R5 strains. The significant role of CCR5 in this process is borne out by the observation that individuals homozygous for mutations within CCR5 gene are resistant to infection by HIV1. Any agent which blocks this binding will inhibit viral replication. One of the most promising agents in this category, which has been approved for clinical use, is enfuvirtide (T-20). Other fusion inhibitors like T-1249 and AMD-3100 are under clinical trails.

Another site is the viral reverse transcriptase (RT) enzyme. After the virus invades a macrophage or T lymphocyte, the RT enzyme initiates copying of the viral RNA into DNA, which gets integrated into the host's DNA. Drugs like nucleoside RT inhibitors diffuse into infected cells and are converted to their active triphosphate forms by cellular kinases. These active nucleosides are incorporated into the growing viral DNA to cause premature chain termination. On the other hand, non-nucleoside RT inhibitors bind directly to the RT enzyme causing inhibition of its function.

The viral DNA migrates to and enters the host cell nucleus (a process facilitated by the HIV proteins vpr and MA) and becomes integrated into the cell DNA with the help of the enzyme integrase. The provirus can then remain latent or be active, generating products for the generation of new virions. A compound called S-1360, which targets integrase, is under trial.

Transcription and translation of viral DNA produces viral RNA. Drugs which act at the level of transcription are being tested. The HIV genes, gag and pol, produce large polypeptides. Before budding of the virus, these polypeptides undergo processing by the enzyme protease. The inhibition of protease using protease inhibitors results in the production of immature defective virus particles. The summary of HIV cycle and the action of antiretroviral drugs at different levels are shown in Figure 7.1. The antiretroviral drugs currently available are given in Table 7.1.

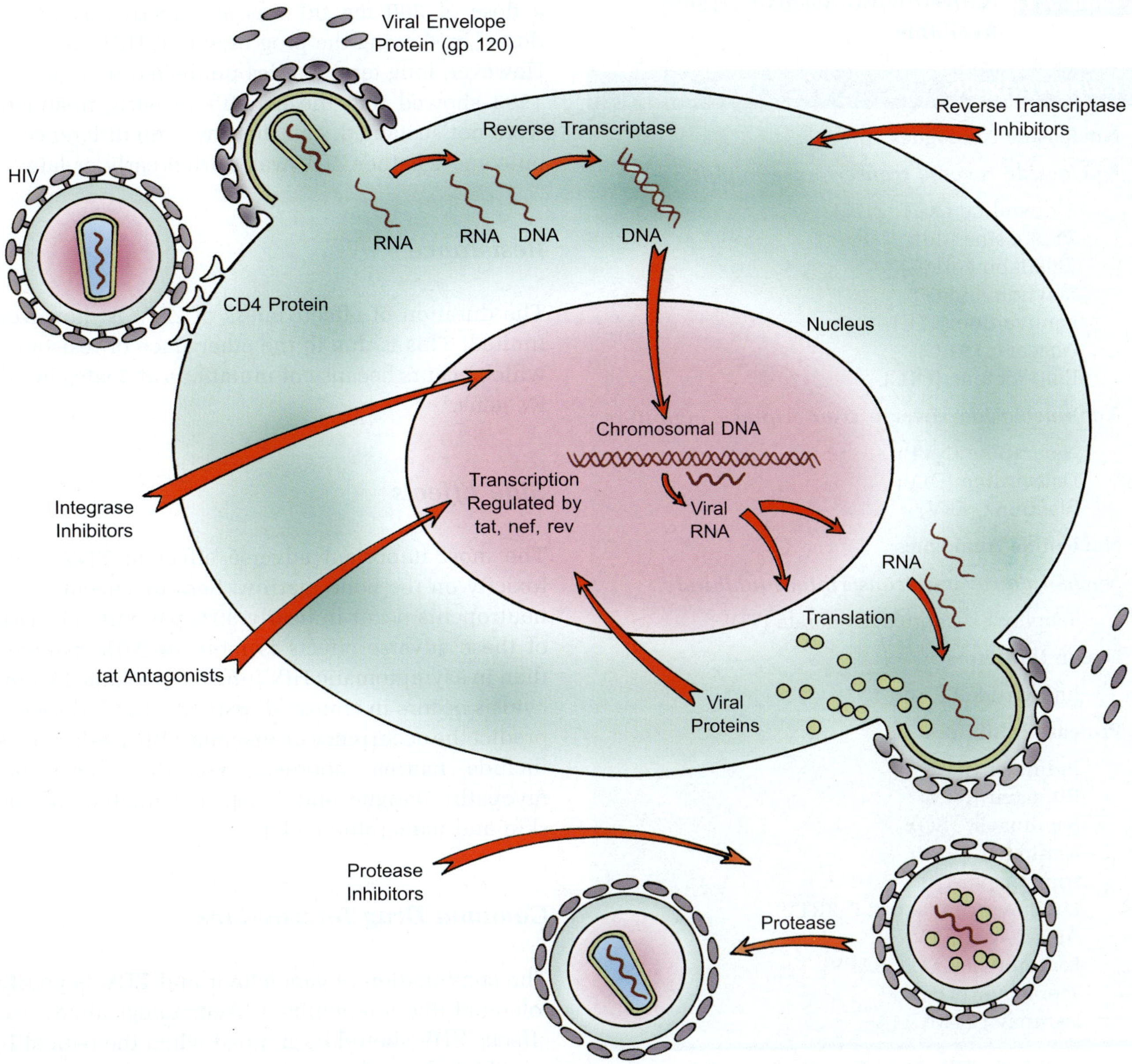

Fig. 7.1 Life Cycle of the Human Immunodeficiency Virus Type 1 Demonstrating Potential Points for Interference by Antiviral Agents. Adapted from JAMA HIV/AIDS Resource Centre www.ama.assn.org

Table 7.1 Antiretroviral Agents Currently Available

Category/Agents
Nucleoside Analogues
Nucleoside reverse transcriptase inhibitors
Zidovudine (AZT, ZDV)
Didanosine (ddI)
Zalcitabine (ddC)
Stavudine (d4T)
Lamivudine (3TC)
Abacavir (ABC)
Emtriciabine (FTC)
Non-nucleoside reverse transcriptase inhibitors
Nevirapine (NVP)
Delavirdine (DLV)
Efavirenz (EFV)
Nucleotide Analogues
Nucleotide reverse transcriptase inhibitors
Tenofovir disoproxil fumarate (TDF)
Fusion Inhibitors
Enfuvirtide (T20)
Protease Inhibitors
Indinavir (IDV)
Ritonavir (RTV)
Saquinavir/ (SQV)
Nelfinavir (NFV)
Amprenavir (APV)
Lopinavir/ritonavir (LPV/RTV)
Atazanavir (ATV)
Fosamprenavir (FOSAPV)
Tipranavir (TPV)
Darunavir (TMC114)

Adapted from 'The Hopkin's HIV Report' Sept. 2002. Life Cycle of HIV Infection [http://www.hopkins-aids.edu]

NUCLEOSIDE REVERSE TRANSCRIPTASE INHIBITORS (NRTIS)

Zidovudine

The first antiretroviral (ARV) drug licensed for use was zidovudine (ZDV). Studies reported by the AIDS Clinical Trial Group in 1990 showed that a dose of 200 mg tid was as effective as higher doses[2] in slowing the progression of HIV infection. However, long-term studies published in 1992 and 1993 showed that the benefits of early treatment were not sustained, and there was no difference in outcome whether ZDV was started early or late.[3]

Resistance

The duration of effectiveness of ZDV is, however, limited. This is due to the emergence of resistance which occurs because of mutations at 5 sites in the RT gene.[4]

Side Effects

The most important adverse effect of ZDV is its toxicity on the bone marrow. Serious anaemia and neutropenia occur in nearly 30% patients. The risk of these adverse effects is more in AIDS patients than in asymptomatic HIV infected patients. Macrocytosis occurs in almost all patients, but it does not predict the occurrence of anaemia. Other side effects include nausea, anorexia, vomiting, headache, myopathy, fatigue and hyperpigmentation of the skin and nails (blue nails).

Common Drug Interactions

The combination of ganciclovir and ZDV is poorly tolerated due to combined haematological adverse effects. ZDV should be stopped when the patient is on a high dose of ganciclovir, and may be restarted when the dose of ganciclovir is reduced during the maintenance phase. ZDV may decrease phenytoin levels, warranting monitoring.[5]

Other Nucleoside RT Inhibitors

Other nucleoside RT inhibitors include didanosine (ddI), zalcitabine (ddC), stavudine (d4T), abacavir (ABC), lamivudine (3TC) and emtricitabine (FTC).[6,7] There is little cross-resistance between these agents (except lamivudine and emtricitabine), and therefore these agents may be used in combination.

Didanosine is inactivated by the low pH of stomach; therefore, it is available in combination with a buffer which increases the gastric pH. ddC is less active clinically than ZDV. d4T and 3TC are well tolerated by most patients.

Emtricitabine is structurally similar to lamivudine. It has advantages in term of its longer half-life, higher oral bioavailability and greater in vitro activity against HIV. Emtricitabine is a component of a preferred initial combination regimen in adults, and can be used in place of lamivudine as part of dual NRTI backbone in combination with PI or NNRTI. Emtricitabine can be given once daily and without regard to food intake. Potential drug interaction is minimal because it neither inhibits nor is metabolized by the cytochrome P450 enzyme system.[7,8]

Side Effects

The most common side effect of these RT inhibitors is painful peripheral neuropathy.[7] This side effect is more common with ddC and d4T than with ddI. Therefore, these agents should be avoided in patients with pre-existing neuropathy. Hyperamylasemia and pancreatitis occur in 20 and 7% of patients treated with ddI. It is rare with other RT inhibitors. ddC may produce oral ulcers in as many as 10% of patients. NRTIs may cause fatty change in liver (hepatic steatosis) and lactic acidosis, a metabolic complication that is potentially fatal but rare.[9-11] These two adverse effects are due to the toxicity of NRTIs on cellular mitochondria. Lipodystrophy, which usually occurs with protease inhibitors (PI), has been described with the use of NRTIs. Due to the antiviral activity of emtricitabine against HBV, there have been cases of HBV exacerbation after its discontinuation; therefore, screening for HBV/HIV co-infection is recommended before starting treatment with emtricitabine.

Drug Interactions

In view of the possibility of pancreatitis, parenteral pentamidine should be avoided in patients on ddI. Ganciclovir increases the levels of ddI, and therefore the risk of pancreatitis is high if both are combined. Certain drugs like dapsone, ketoconazole, itraconazole, pyrimethamine and trimethoprim require acidic pH in stomach for their dissolution and absorption. Therefore, these drugs should be taken at least 2 hours before ddI. It has been hypothesized that zidovudine-5'-monophosphate (produced by the action of thymidylate kinase on ZDV) may inhibit the production of stavudine-5'-monophosphate, and therefore the combination of d4T and ZDV may be antagonistic.[5] Emtricitabine should not be combined with lamivudine.

NON-NUCLEOSIDE REVERSE TRANSCRIPTASE INHIBITORS (NNRTIs)

These analogues of RT inhibitors restrict the replication of the virus by binding to an active site of RT, which is different from that for nucleoside RT inhibitors. Members of this class are highly active against HIV 1 but not HIV 2. The development of resistance and cross-resistance is a major problem with these agents.[12] This group includes nevirapine (NVP), delavirdine (DLV) and efavirenz (EFV). Of these drugs, NVP is the most commonly used drug in India.

Nevirapine

It is the most commonly used NNRTI in India as it is cheap and relatively well tolerated. In combination with 2 NRTI, it provides an effective treatment for HIV infection. The recommended dosage is 200 mg once-a-day for the first two weeks and then 200 mg twice-a-day afterwards. This dosage schedule reduces the chance of adverse effects associated with this drug. The most common side effects associated with this class of drugs are skin rash, nausea, headache and hepatic enzyme elevation. Skin rash develops in about 25% of people taking the drug. If a patient develops rash during the lead-in (lower dose) period, the dose should not be increased. If rash is uncomfortable, the drug should be stopped. A rare side effect of NVP is Stevens-Johnson syndrome. Patients should be carefully monitored during the first two months for signs of skin or liver problems. Because of the risk of liver damage, NVP should not be used for post-exposure prophylaxis. NVP is metabolized by the liver, and can interact with other drugs with predominant hepatic metabolism. These drugs include antihistamines, sedatives and anti-fungal agents. NVP also increases the metabolism of PI and, therefore, should not be used in combination.[7,13]

Efavirenz

It is being increasingly used as the preferred NNRTI in the treatment of HIV infection. The usual adult dose is 600 mg once-a-day taken in empty stomach at bedtime. Efavirenz is metabolized by cytochrome P450 system in the liver, and possesses both inhibitory and inducing effects on it. Therefore, it may interact with other drugs metabolized in the liver, requiring either increased or decreased dosages. It lowers the blood levels of most protease inhibitors. Dosages of amprenavir, atazanavir and indinavir may need to be increased. The blood levels of saquinavir are dramatically lowered, and so the two drugs cannot be used simultaneously. Important adverse effects include psychiatric symptoms (insomnia, confusion, memory loss, depression), skin rash and headache. It is teratogenic and, therefore, should not be used in women who might become pregnant.[7,13]

NUCLEOTIDE REVERSE TRANSCRIPTASE INHIBITORS

Tenofovir, a nucleotide reverse transcriptase inhibitor, prevents HIV from entering the nucleus of healthy T cells. It is very similar to nucleoside analogues, but the difference is that tenofovir unlike the nucleoside analogues is chemically preactivated and requires less biochemical processing in the body. It must be used in combination with other drugs including a NRTI and at least one PI or NNRTI. The usual dosage is 300 mg once daily preferably with food. The most common side effects are nausea, vomiting, diarrhoea and flatulence. It appears less likely to cause mitochondrial toxicity when compared to other NRTIs. Similar to lamivudine and emtrictabine, tenofovir has an antiviral activity against hepatitis B virus; therefore, exacerbation of hepatitis B virus after discontinuation of tenofovir is possible, and patients should be screened for hepatitis B virus prior to the initiation of tenofovir.[7,8] It is not recommended in combination with lamivudine plus didanosine or lamivudine plus abacavir.

Adefovir is another nucleotide reverse transcriptase inhibitor. However, it has failed in the treatment of HIV infection.

FUSION INHIBITORS

Enfuvirtide (T-20) is the first agent of the newest antiretroviral class, fusion inhibitors. It binds to the gp41 subunit of the viral envelop glycoprotein; this interferes with the fusion of viral and human cellular membranes.[7,8] It does not have any activity against HIV-2. Currently, enfuvirtide is recommended for use in combination with other antiretroviral agents in treatment-experienced adults and in children older than 6 years of age with evidence of HIV-1 replication despite ongoing antiretroviral therapy. Enfuvirtide is not metabolized by cytochrome P450 enzymes, and hence there is no drug-drug interaction expected when co-administered with agents that are metabolized by the cytochrome P450 enzyme system. The most common side effect is an injection-site reaction (ISR). An increased incidence of pneumonia is also observed among patients receiving enfuvirtide. Other frequently observed adverse reactions are diarrhoea, nausea and fatigue. It is to be administered by subcutaneous injection. The recommended dose for adolescents and adults is 90 mg twice-a-day.

PROTEASE INHIBITORS (PIs)

Ten PIs, namely saquinavir (SQV), indinavir (IDV), ritonavir (RTV), nelfinavir (NFV), amprenavir (APV), lopinavir-plus/ritonavir (LPV/RTV), atazanavir (ATV), fosamprenavir (FOSAPV), tipranavir (TPV) and darunavir (TMC114), are in clinical use.[7,13] Tipranavir and darunavir are two new protease inhibitors approved for patients who are highly treatment-experienced or have HIV-1 strains resistant to multiple PIs based on its demonstrated activity against PI-resistant viruses.[8,14]

Resistance

The development of resistance is a major limitation, which is related to the dose. Therefore, these agents must be used in full therapeutic doses. Also, cross-resistance among these agents, particularly indinavir and ritonavir, is common.

Side Effects

The main side effects of PI are nausea and vomiting. Indinavir can produce transient increase in indirect bilirubin, and renal calculi can develop in 3–15% of patients. Hence, the patient should be asked to consume lot of fluids (48 ounces of water/day). Ritonavir has a bad taste and so produces more GI symptoms. Oral numbness is also seen in some patients. Two important side effects of atazanavir include hyperbilirubinemia and cardiac conduction abnormalities (prolonged PR interval and asymptomatic first-degree AV block).

PIs have been associated with body fat redistribution, which manifests physically as thinning of arms, legs and face and/or deposition of fat in the abdominal and shoulder regions along with lipomas (lipodystrophy). It occurs in 6 to 80% of patients and develops after several months of therapy. The effects on fat metabolism may lead to raised levels of serum cholesterol and triglycerides, insulin resistance and rarely elevated blood glucose levels.[11,15] The overall cumulative incidence of these metabolic disturbances may be high (30-60%) after 1 to 2 years of treatment.

Drug Interactions

Drugs like cisapride and metoclopramide, which are known to increase gut motility, reduce the absorption of saquinavir. If indinavir is used in combination with ddI, it should be administered at least one hour before ddI, as the buffer in latter increases gastric pH and thus reduces the absorption of indinavir. Ritonavir is available both in solution and capsule forms. Oral solution contains 43% alcohol, while capsules also contain small amounts of alcohol. Therefore, patients on ritonavir must avoid metronidazole and tinidazole. Saquinavir is available both as hard gel (less oral bioavailability) and soft gel (3 times more oral bioavailability than hard gel).[16]

Hepatic microsomal enzymes metabolize PIs, and therefore drug interactions are frequent. Enzyme-inducers like rifampicin, phenytoin, carbamazepine and phenobarbitone can reduce the concentration of PIs. Inhibitors of microsomal enzymes like ketoconazole and itraconazole increase serum levels of these agents. This is most significant with saquinavir whose concentration is increased by 80% when combined with ketoconazole. Co-administration of rifampicin with IDV is contraindicated because of 89% decrease in IDV's availability concentration (AUC).[13,16]

HMG-CoA reductase inhibitors (simvastatin and lovastatin) should not be used due to increased potential of myopathy and rhabdomyolysis. Atorvastatin in low doses can be used with caution.[13,16]

A summary of various antiretroviral drugs is given in Table 7.2. Lipoatrophy is seen with NRTI use and is most common with stavudine. On the other hand, fat accumulation at various sites is seen with PIs.

Table 7.2 Characteristics of Commonly Used Antiretroviral Drugs

Drug	Availability and Administration	Adverse Effects	Common Drug Interactions
Zidovudine (ZDV)	100 mg, 200 mg & 300 mg tab 200 mg tid or 300 mg bid Take without regard to food	Bone marrow suppression, GI intolerance, headache, lactic acidosis	Avoid ribavarin, ganciclovir
Didanosine (ddI)	100 mg buffered tab >60 kg: 200 mg bid <60 kg: 125 mg bid	Pancreatitis, peripheral neuropathy, GI intolerance, lactic acidosis	Avoid intravenous pentamidine and ganciclovir

(Contd.)

Drug	Availability and Administration	Adverse Effects	Common Drug Interactions
	Take 1/2 h before or 2 h after food		
Zalcitabine (ddC)	0.75 mg tab 0.75 mg tid Take without regard to food Avoid administration of antacids	Peripheral neuropathy, stomatitis, lactic acidosis	
Stavudine (D4T)	30 mg and 40 mg cap >60 kg: 40 mg bid <60 kg: 30 mg bid Take without regard to food	Pancreatitis, peripheral neuropathy, lactic acidosis stomatitis, lipoatrophy	Avoid combination with ZDV
Lamivudine (3TC)	150 mg tab 10 mg/ml solution 150 mg bid <50 kg: 2 mg/kg bid Take without regard to food	Well tolerated, lactic acidosis	No significant interactions
Abacavir (ABC)	300 mg tab 300 mg bid or 600 mg od Take without regard to food	Hypersensitivity reaction (features may include fever, rash, nausea, vomiting, fatigue, anorexia, malaise, cough, respiratory difficulty); may be fatal	No significant interactions
Emtrictabine (FTC)	200 mg cap 200 mg od Take without regard to food	Minimal toxicity, lactic acidosis and hepatic steatosis, hyperpigmentation of skin	No significant interactions
Nevirapine (NVP)	200 mg tab 200 mg od for 14 d and then 200 bid Take without regard to meals	Skin rash, hepatitis; do not restart after severe hepatitis or skin reaction	Avoid ketoconazole, rifampicin, oral contraceptives If used with IDV: IDV 1000 mg tid + NVP standard dose
Efavirenz (EFV)	200 mg cap 600 mg at night Avoid taking after high fat meals	Skin rash, CNS effects (dizziness, insomnia, abnormal dreams, confusion, agitation, hallucinations), hepatitis	Avoid astemizole, cisapride, midazolam If used with IDV: IDV 1000 mg tid + EFV standard dose If used with RTV: RTV 600 mg bid + EFV standard dose Not recommended with SQV
Tenofovir (TDF)	300 mg tab 300 mg od Take without regard to food	Asthenia, headache, nausea, vomiting, lactic acidosis, hepatic steatosis	Monitor for toxicity of cidofovir, ganciclovir
Enfuvirtide (T20)	108 mg/vial Store at room temperature Dissolve in 1.1 ml (90 mg/ml) subcutaneous injection 90 mg bid	Local injection site reaction (nearly 100%), increased rate of bacterial pneumonia, hypersensitivity reaction	No clinically significant interactions

(*Contd.*)

Drug	Availability and Administration	Adverse Effects	Common Drug Interactions
Indinavir (IDV)	400 mg cap 800 mg tid Separate dosing with ddI by 1 h Take 1 h before or 2 h after meals	Nephrolithiasis, GI intolerance, headache, asthenia, blurred vision, dizziness, hyperglycemia, redistribution of fat and lipid abnormalities	Avoid lovastatin, simvastatin, rifampicin, astemizole, cisapride, midazolam Use atorvastatin with caution Reduce dose to 600 mg tid if on ketoconazole
Ritonavir (RTV)	100 mg cap 600 mg/7.5 ml solution Day 1-2: 300 mg bid; Day 3-5: 400 mg bid; Day 6-13: 500 mg bid; Day 14 onwards: 600 mg bid Take with food Refrigerate capsules; do not refrigerate oral solution	GI intolerance, paraesthesias, hepatitis, hyperglycemia, redistribution of fat, lipid abnormalities, taste perversion	Avoid amiodarone, quinidine, lovastatin, simvastatin, astemizole, cisapride, midazolam, oral contraceptives Use atorvastatin with caution Ketoconazole dose 200 mg/day Monitor theophylline levels If used with IDV: IDV 400 mg bid + RTV 400 mg bid OR IDV 800 mg bid + RTV 100 or 200 mg bid
Nelfinavir (NFV) astemizole,	250 mg tab 750 mg tid Take with meal	Diarrhoea, hyperglycemia, redistribution of fat, lipid abnormalities, flatulence	Avoid lovastatin, simvastatin, rifampicin, rifabutin, cisapride, midazolam, oral contraceptives Use atorvastatin with caution If used with SQV: NFV standard dose + SQV 1200 mg bid
Saquinavir (SQV)	200 mg cap. Hard gel cap: 400 mg bid with ritonavir only. No effect of food 1200 mg tid/1800 mg bid Take with food Soft gel cap: store in refrigerator	GI intolerance, headache, hepatitis, hyperglycemia, redistribution of fat, lipid abnormalities, rhinitis	Avoid lovastatin, simvastatin rifampicin, rifabutin, astemizole, cisapride, midazolam Use atorvastatin with caution If used with RTV: SQV 400 mg bid + RTV 400 mg bid
Fosamprenavir	700 mg tab (combined with ritonavir) 1400 mg + 200 mg RTV od 700 mg + 100 mg RTV bid Take without regard to food	Skin rash, GI intolerance, headache, hyperglycemia, redistribution of fat, lipid abnormalities, hepatitis	Avoid lovastatin, simvastatin, rifampicin
Lopinavir + Ritonavir	400 mg lopinavir + 100 mg ritonavir bid Take with food abnormalities	GI intolerance, headache, hepatitis, hyperglycemia, redistribution of fat, lipid	Avoid lovastatin, simvastatin, rifampicin, astemizole, cisapride, midazolam Use atorvastatin with caution

GOALS OF ANTIRETROVIRAL THERAPY

The eradication of HIV infection is largely impossible due to the presence of latently infected CD4 T cells during the very early stages of acute HIV infection that persists with an extremely long half-life.

Clinical goal: Prolongation of life and improvement of quality of life

Virological goal: To achieve maximal and durable suppression of viral load (<50 copies/ml) so as to halt disease progression

Immunological goal: To achieve immune-reconstitution that is quantitative (CD4 count in normal range) and qualitative (pathogen-specific immune response)

Therapeutic goal: Rational sequencing of drugs in a fashion that not only achieves virological goals, but also (1) maintains therapeutic options; (2) is relatively free of side effects; (3) is realistic in terms of probability of adherence.

Epidemiological goal: To reduce HIV transmission

INDICATIONS FOR ANTIRETROVIRAL THERAPY[13]

Total eradication of HIV infection cannot be achieved with the currently available antiretroviral regimens. This is due to the establishment of a pool of latently infected CD4+ cells during the very early stages of acute HIV infection that persists with an extremely long-half life. However, the use of highly active antiretroviral therapy (HAART) or antiretroviral therapy (ART) has been successful in reducing morbidity in HIV patients and improving the quality of life. The term HAART or ART indicates the use of 2 NRTI along with one NNRTI or a PI in order to achieve the goals of maximal and durable suppression of the viral load, restoration and preservation of the immune function, improvement of the quality of life and reduction of HIV-related mortality and morbidity. CDC has formulated guidelines for the initiation of HAART in HIV infected patients (Table 7.3).[13] The role of ART in patients with acute HIV infection is controversial.

Table 7.3 Indications for Antiretroviral Therapy[13]

Clinical Category	*CD4+ Cell Count*	*Plasma HIV RNA**	*Recommendations*
Symptomatic HIV disease (wasting, unexplained fever for >2 weeks or thrush) including patients with AIDS	Any value	Any value	Start HAART
Asymptomatic	< 200/mm^3	Any value	Start HAART
Asymptomatic	200-350/mm^3	Any value	Offer HAART
Asymptomatic	> 350/mm^3	>100,000	Some experts recommend starting HAART
Asymptomatic	> 350/mm^3	<100,000	Defer HAART

*Using RT-PCR

HAART in Patients with CD4+ Cell Counts Above 200/mm^3

ART is recommended for all patients with symptomatic HIV disease, irrespective of CD4 cell counts. For patients without symptoms, therapy should be initiated at some point after the CD4 cell count declines below 350/μL but before reaching 200/μL. The closer the CD4 cell count to 200/μL, the stronger the recommendation, particularly if the plasma viral load is high (>100,000 HIV-1 RNA copies/mL) or if the CD4 cell count is declining rapidly (>100/μL per year).[17]

Evaluation Before Initiating HAART

Each patient should have a complete evaluation before initiating the treatment. The purpose is to confirm the presence of HIV infection, determine if HIV infection is acute, determine the presence of co-infections, and assess the overall health condition.[13] The evaluation includes the following:

- Complete history and physical examination
- Opthalmological examination
- Complete blood count, biochemistry profile, blood glucose and lipid profile
- CD4+ cell count
- Plasma HIV RNA measurement (load)
- Other tests including VDRL, Mantoux test, toxoplasma IgG serology, chest X-ray and serology for hepatitis C and B, urinalysis, stool routine and microscopy

ANTIRETROVIRAL REGIMENS[13]

Several regimens could be used while appreciating the fact that patient or provider preferences, or underlying comorbidities, may make an alternative regimen better in such instances. An initial regimen should contain two nucleoside/nucleotide reverse transcriptase inhibitors (NRTI) and either a non-nucleoside reverse transcriptase inhibitor (NNRTI) or a ritonavir-boosted or unboosted protease inhibitor (PI). A theoretical benefit of using a class-sparing regimen is to preserve one or more than one class of drugs for later use. Viral load suppression and CD4+ cell responses similar to those achieved with PI-containing regimens have been shown with selected PI-sparing regimens.

When initiating the therapy, one should begin with an effective regimen. Consideration should also be given to the number of pills per day, frequency of dosing, food requirements, toxicity, drug interactions and cost of antiretroviral drugs.

Ritonavir increases the plasma levels of other PI by inhibiting both gastrointestinal and hepatic cytochrome P450, thereby reducing the metabolism of other PIs. This effect of ritonavir is increasingly being used to elevate the plasma levels of other PIs. Standard doses of PI will result in trough drug levels that are only slightly higher than effective antiretroviral levels; this may allow the virus to replicate. Using ritonavir with other PIs (ritonavir-boosted) increases their trough levels, which markedly reduces the chances of viral multiplication and also enhances killing activity against viral strains that are moderately resistant to these PIs. Thus, ritonavir increases the levels of all PIs except nelfinavir. The major drawbacks associated with this strategy are the potential for increased risk of hyperlipidemia and a greater potential of drug-drug interactions from the addition of ritonavir. When starting ART, all drugs should be started simultaneously at full dose with the exception of ritonavir and nevirapine, where dose escalation is recommended.

Various combinations of drugs recommended are listed in Table 7.4.[13] One component (NNRTI or PI)

Table 7.4 Recommended Antiretroviral Agents for Initial Treatment of HIV infection (Choose One Each from Column A and Column B)

	Column A		*Column B*
	NNRTI	*PI*	*NRTI (two)*
Preferred	Efavirenz	Atazanavir + ritonavir Fosamprenavir + ritonavir Lopinavir/ritonavir	Tenofovir + emtricitabine Tenofovir + lamivudine Zidovudine + lamivudine Zidovudine + emtricitabine
Alternative	Nevirapine	Atazanavir Fosamprenavir Fosamprenavir + ritonavir Lopinavir/ritonavir	Abacavir + lamivudine Didanosine + lamivudine Didanosine + emtricitabine

is selected from column A and one from column B. Efavirenz can be used except during first trimester of pregnancy or in women expecting pregnancy. Nevirapine may be used as an alternative in adult females with CD4+ T cell counts <250 cells/mm^3 and adult males with CD4+ T cell counts <400 cells/mm^3. The risk of hepatitis is high if CD4 cell counts are higher than stated here for males and females.

Table 7.5 lists the agents or regimens which are acceptable if the preferred or alternative regimens cannot be used due to any reason. Agents or regimens not recommended for use are shown in Table 7.6.[13]

Table 7.5 Antiretroviral Components Acceptable as Initial Antiretroviral Components (Inferior to Preferred or Alternative Components)

Antiretroviral Agent or Regimen	*Special Indications*
Abacavir/lamivudine/zidovudine	When PI or NNRTI-based regimens cannot be used based on toxicities or concerns of significant drug-drug interactions
Nelfinavir	During pregnancy when others cannot be tolerated
Saquinavir (ritonavir-boosted)	When PI or NNRTI-based regimens cannot be used based on toxicities or concerns of significant drug-drug interactions
Stavudine + lamivudine	When preferred or alternative dual-NRTI combination cannot be used

Table 7.6 Agents/Regimens Not Recommended for Use as Initial Therapy

Saquinavir (hard gel capsules)	Darunavir
Stavudine + Zidovudine	Delavirdine
Stavudine + Didanosine	Enfuvirtide
Zalcitabine + Didanosine	Indinavir (unboosted)
Zalcitabine + Lamivudine	Ritonavir (as sole PI)
Zalcitabine + Stavudine	Tipranavir
Zalcitabine + Zidovudine	Saquinavir (unboosted)
Didanosine + Tenofovir	

Response to HAART

To maximize the benefits of ART, the following conditions should be ensured:

- ⥣ Adherence to the drug regimen
- ⥣ Adequate serum levels of antiretroviral drugs
- ⥣ Rational sequencing of antiretroviral drugs so as to preserve future treatment options for as long as possible.

Adherence to HAART[13]

The ability of a patient to adhere to HAART is essential for successful treatment. Numerous reports have shown an association between poor adherance and virological failure. In order to improve adherence to HAART, various strategies are listed in Table 7.7. In directly observed therapy, a health care worker observes the ingestion of medication by the patient. Te use of DOT in tuberculosis has shown highly encouraging results. In fact, both could be integrated in the same policy since both diseases are common in India. However, the treatment for HIV usually requires at least two doses per day and is a life-long therapy unlike tuberculosis where treatment is given on intermittent days and for a few months only. Modified DOT is being studied in which the morning dose is supervised while the evening and weekend doses are self-administered. The goal of this programme is to improve patient education and self-administration of medication over a period of about 3-6 months.

Table 7.7 Strategies to Improve Adherence to HAART

Educate the patient on utility of HAART, possible side effects and drug interactions
Reduce dose frequency and number of tablets to minimum possible
Simplify food requirements
Emphasize the need for strict compliance at every visit
Educate family members to support treatment plan
Use of modified DOT

Monitoring of Therapy[13]

Key decisions regarding initiation or change in ART should ideally be guided by monitoring plasma HIV RNA and CD4+ T cell counts, as well as clinical conditions of the patient. These laboratory parameters should be repeated every 3-6 months in patients who have not been initiated on ART. If the first values of HIV RNA and CD4+ cell counts indicate the requirement for ART, a repeat measurement of these parameters is recommended before initiating the treatment. After initiation of ART, HIV RNA should be measured at 4-8 weeks to assess the efficacy of the treatment, as there should be a large decline in viral load during this period. The viral load should continue to decline after that, and by 16-20 weeks, it should go undetectable (i.e., <50 RNA copies/mL). The rate of viral load decline is affected by the initial viral load, baseline CD4+ cell count, potency of regimen used and presence of any opportunistic infections and prior exposure to ART. However, the absence of decline of this magnitude should prompt the clinician to reassess the situation, including checking patient compliance with treatment, rule out intestinal malabsorption and confirm HIV RNA levels by repeating the tests. If compliance and absorption can be assured, a change in regimen should be considered. A minimally significant change in plasma HIV RNA is considered to be a threefold or 0.5 log10 increase or decrease. A significant decrease in CD4+ cell count is a decrease of >30% from baseline for absolute cell numbers and a decrease of >3% from baseline in percentage of cells.

Drug Resistance

Testing for viral resistance to antiretroviral drugs may help maximize the benefits of ART. Drug resistance can be identified by either genotypic or phenotypic assays. Genotypic assays detect drug resistance to mutations present in RT and protease genes of HIV, and the results may be reported within 1-2 weeks. Phenotypic assays measure the ability of HIV to grow in different concentrations of antiretroviral drugs, and the results are available in 2-3 weeks.[13] However, phenotypic assays are costlier and more difficult than genotypic assays.

Drug resistance assays are potentially useful in acute HIV infection and in selecting active drugs when changing ART in the context of treatment failure or in cases in which viral load suppression is suboptimal after the initiation of ART.[13,18]

Changing Antiretroviral Treatment

Change in ART may be required if there is suboptimal reduction in HIV RNA after initiation of the treatment, reappearance of viremia after initial suppression and decline in CD4 cell counts. Less than 0.5-0.75 $\log_{10}$ reduction in HIV RNA at 4 weeks or less than 1 $\log_{10}$ reduction at 8 weeks of therapy or failure to suppress HIV RNA to undetectable levels at 4-6 months of therapy indicate inadequate response and warrant change of therapy. If the patient is unable to tolerate one of the agents, it should be replaced with another agent while other agents should be continued. However, in case of failure of therapy, it is important to use at least two new drugs and preferably change all the drugs and use an entirely new regimen. Ritonavir should not be changed to indinavir and vice versa since a high level of cross-resistance is likely between these two drugs. Similarly, changing among NNRTIs is not recommended for the same reason.[13,19]

Interruption of HAART[13]

There has been a recent strategy of stopping HAART temporarily. This is called supervised or structured treatment interruption (STI). It encompasses three major strategies: salvage, auto-immunization and better immune control of HIV, and for reducing total time on HAART. *Salvage* indicates stopping HAART in patients who do not respond to ART. The idea is to allow replication of sensitive strains of HIV so that HAART can be restarted. *Auto-immunization* is directed to patients who have maintained viral suppression below the detection limit for a long time. The theoretical goal is to allow several short bursts of viral replication to augment HIV-specific immune responses. However, at present, none of these strate-gies are recommended.

IMMUNE-RECONSTITUTION INFLAMMATORY SYNDROME

During the treatment of HIV, immunity starts getting restored and the body begins to fight aggressively against coexisting infections, thereby causing atypical manifestations of opportunistic infections. The constellation of clinical symptoms, signs or investigational parameters resulting from such an inflammatory response is called immune-reconstitution inflammatory syndrome (IRIS) or immune-restoration disease (IRD). Thus, IRIS may be defined as occurrence or worsening of clinical and/or laboratory parameters despite favorable outcomes in CD4 cell count and plasma viral loads.[20] Both infective (clinical or subclinical) and non-infective conditions can act as triggering factors for precipitating IRIS.

The risk factors for IRIS include CD4 count <50 cells/mm^3, a high viral load, undetected presence of antigens of nonviable microorganisms (e.g., cryptococci and CMV), active or subclinical infection by opportunistic pathogens, and initiation of HAART in close proximity to the diagnosis and initiation of treatment for an opportunistic infection.[20]

The clinical features of IRIS differ according to the inflammatory or infective pathology that is responsible for causing it. Non-infectious IRIS may present with cutaneous involvement (papular urticaria, eosinophilic folliculitis, Sweet's syndrome, Reiter's syndrome, sarcoidosis and systemic lupus erythematosus) or without cutaneous involvement (autoimmune thyroiditis, Guillain-Barre syndrome, myopathy, radiculopathy, acute porphyria, Non-Hodgkin's lymphomas and Castleman's disease). The infectious syndromes occur with various opportunistic infections, with tuberculosis being the most common. IRIS in tuberculosis typically occurs one to six weeks after the patient begins ART. The signs and symptoms of tuberculous IRIS may include high fever, new or worsening lymphadenopathy (mediastinal or peripheral), worsening of pulmonary symptoms and infiltrates, and new or increasing pleural effusion.[21] Lymph node abscesses usually occur during the first weeks on HAART. Extrapulmonary presentations may occur, including expanding central nervous system lesions, skin or visceral abscesses, osteomyelitis, nephritis, meningitis, hypercalcemia, hepatosplenomegaly, epididymo-orchitis, psoas abscess and bowel perforation.

Failure of ART or toxicity, active opportunistic infections and failure of antimicrobial therapy are considered in differential diagnosis. Treatment includes continuation of primary therapy against the offending pathogen in order to decrease the antigenic load, continuation of effective HAART and judicious use of anti-inflammatory agents

HAART AND ANTITUBERCULAR DRUGS

PI and NNRTI are antiretroviral agents known to inhibit or induce cytochrome P450 isoenzymes (CYP450). Rifampicin induces CYP450 and may substantially decrease the blood levels of antiretroviral drugs. The pharmacological interactions are "drug-drug" because, in addition to the effect, rifampicin has on PI and NNRTI, the antiretroviral agents may affect the blood levels of rifampicin. The other class of antiretroviral agents, NRTIs, is not metabolized by CYP450. Concurrent use of NRTI and rifampicin is not contraindicated and does not require dose adjustments. Rifampicin can be used to treat active TB in three situations: (1) in a patient whose antiretroviral regimen includes efavirenz and two NRTI; (2) in a patient whose antiretroviral regimen includes ritonavir and one or more NRTI; or (3) in a patient whose antiretroviral regimen includes a combination of two PI (ritonavir and saquinavir).[13]

Rifabutin may be used in a dose of 300 mg/day in a selected group of patients on HAART, i.e. those taking NRTI, NVP and SQV alone. However, its dose should be reduced to 150 mg two or three times per week when administered to patients taking ritonavir or ritonavir/lopinavir, and to 150 mg once-a-day when used with IDV or NFV (dose of IDV and NFV is increased to 1000 mg tid). On the other hand, its dose should be increased to either 450 mg or 600 mg daily or 600 mg two or three times per week when used concurrently with efavirenz.

For patients who have not received ART, the simultaneous initiation of treatment for both conditions has been associated with a high rate of side effects and paradoxical reactions.[22] It is recommended that simultaneous initiation for tuberculosis and HIV should be avoided, with the possible exception of patients who have CD4+ T cell count <50 cells/mm^3. The optimal time to delay initiation of ART is not known, but many authorities suggest a delay of 4-8 weeks. The British HIV Association (BHIVA) recommends that if CD4+ counts are >200/mm^3, HAART can be started after the completion of antituberculous treatment, if indicated; if CD4+ counts are 100-200/mm^3, HAART can be started after 2 months of TB treatment, and if CD4+ counts are <100/mm^3, HAART has to be initiated as soon as possible after starting antituberculous treatment.[23]

The management of HIV/AIDS in pregnancy is discussed in Chapter 7.

ANTIRETROVIRAL THERAPY IN RESOURCE-POOR NATIONS

In resource-limited settings, most people with HIV infection have poor access to diagnosis and treatment. The decision to initiate ART often relies on clinical assessment due to the high cost for performing HIV RNA and CD4 cell counts. Drug access for the millions of poor people can be improved not only by guidance on rational selection or use of antiretroviral drugs, but also by providing accessibility to competent health services and cheaper drugs. Fortunately, at present, most ARV drugs are available whose costs have reduced remarkably over the past 5 years. Important strategies for increasing the accessibility of antiretroviral agents in resource-limited settings include:

1. Scaling up of antiretroviral treatment programmes to meet the needs of people living with HIV
2. Standardization and simplification of ART regimens to support efficient implementation of treatment programmes
3. Ensuring ART based on scientific evidence in order to avoid substandard treatment and emergence of drug-resistant virus

Indications for Initiating ART

The WHO recommends[24] that HIV infected people in resource-poor settings should be offered treatment when they have:

1. WHO stage IV disease (clinical AIDS), regardless of CD4+ cell counts
2. WHO stage I, II or III of HIV disease with a CD4+ cell count below 200/mm^3
3. WHO stage II or III of HIV disease with total lymphocyte count <1200/mm^3

Clinical staging is intended for use where HIV infection has been confirmed by HIV antibody testing. Clinics are encouraged to use CD4+ cell counts instead of HIV RNA levels in monitoring the patients. If facilities to detect CD4+ cell counts are not available, total lymphocyte count (TLC) may be used to make decision regarding the initiation of ART. However, TLC correlates poorly with CD4 count in asymptomatic patients. It is only useful in deciding when to initiate ART in symptomatic patients with WHO clinical stage 2 or 3 disease. It is suggested to use TLC below 1200/cells/mm^3 as a surrogate marker for CD4 count below 200 when CD4 count is not available. It is not useful for monitoring the response to ART or for deciding whether ART is failing.

First-Line Regimens

Antiretroviral treatment should be standardized in a clinical setting. It has been suggested to select a single first-line ART and a limited number of second-line regimens so that a large number of patients can be treated. Considerations in the selection of a regimen should carefully evaluate its potency, side effects, anticipated adherence, effects of coexisting conditions in the population (e.g., tuberculosis), potential drug interactions, cost and availability of health care facilities. Based on these considerations, an NNRTI-based regimen is recommended as the first-line treatment. The recommendations are as follows[24]:

1. Choose NVP or EFV as the primary NNRTI; both should be available for mutual substitution for toxicity and for issues related to drug choice in pregnancy and TB.
2. Choose either 3TC or FTC. It is not necessary to stock both.
3. Choose one companion NRTI to combine with 3TC or FTC in order to have two NRTI components of the regimen. The preferred components are zidovudine or tenofovir, and the alternatives are stavudine or abacavir.
4. The use of only two NRTI combinations is not recommended even in resource-limited areas since these regimens do not suppress viral replication adequately and are likely to produce resistance rapidly.
5. To enhance adherence, a combination of drugs in a single pill is recommended. The family and community members should be advised to encourage the patient to take pills regularly.
6. A triple-NRTI regimen should be considered as an alternative for first-line ART in situations where NNRTI options provide additional complications and to preserve the PI class for second-line treatment. Recommended triple NRTI combinations are zidovudine + lamivudine + abacavir or zidovudine + lamivudine + tenofovir.
7. It is recommended that PIs be reserved for second-line therapy because their use in an initial treatment regimen essentially rules out second-line options in a setting of limited formularies. With this important caveat, PIs as initial therapy with a standard dual-NRTI backbone are an option for the treatment of viral types with intrinsic resistance to NNRTIs (e.g. HIV-2), for women with CD4 counts of 250–350 cells/mm^3, or for individuals for whom NNRTI drugs are severely toxic and triple-NRTI therapy is deemed inappropriate.

Second-Line Antiretroviral Regimens

In a resource-limited setting where viral loads are difficult to assess, treatment failure is evaluated primarily on the basis of clinical response (if patient worsens to stage 4 or develops stage 4 again after initial improvement) or worsening CD4+ cell count (fall of CD4 count to pre-therapy baseline, or 50% fall from the on-treatment peak value or persistent CD4 levels below 100 cells/mm^3).

The second-line regimens generally include a ritonavir-enhanced PI combination. NFV can be considered as an alternative for PI component if RTV-enhanced PI is not available. The NRTI components in the regimen should also be changed, e.g., ddI + ABC or TDF + ABC or TDF + 3TC if patients were on ZDV + 3TC or d4T + 3TC.

It is recommended that countries that are planning to implement ART programmes should also implement an HIV drug resistance surveillance programme so as to detect potential drug resistance at the population level and modify recommendations as and when required.

Monitoring of Antiretroviral Treatment

A few baseline tests are mandatory before initiating ART. Haemoglobin level should be ascertained as zidovudine, one of the most frequently used NRTIs can produce anaemia as one of its side effects. Other tests include a white cell count and differential count (to permit the assessment of neutropenic side effects and to get baseline total lymphocyte count), serum transaminases (to assess the possibility of hepatitis), serum creatinine or blood urea (to assess baseline renal function), serum glucose and pregnancy test in women. If facilities are available, CD4+ cell counts and lipid profile should be done. Follow-up of patients on ART should include detailed clinical examination and total lymphocyte counts.

NACO guidelines for the initiation of antiretroviral treatment is given in Table 7.8.

Table 7.8 **Initiation of ART Based on CD4 count and WHO Clinical Staging**[25]

Classification of HIV-associated Clinical Diseases	*WHO Clinical Staging*	*CD4 Test Not Available or Result Pending*	*CD Test Available*
Asymptomatic	1	Do not treat	Treat if CD4 <200
Mild symptoms	2	Do not treat	
Advanced symptoms	3	Treat	Consider treatment if CD4 <350 and initiate ART before CD4 drops below 200
Severe/advanced symptoms	4	Treat	Treat irrespective of CD4 count

TLC is no longer used as global evidence has shown that it is a poor parameter for deciding the initiation of ART, especially in asymptomatic persons, and monitoring the response to ART.

Tuberculosis and Antiretroviral Treatment

Tuberculosis is common in patients from a resource-limited country, and this may complicate the use of ARV treatment. WHO recommends[24] that people with tuberculosis and HIV should complete their intensive phase of treatment for tuberculosis prior to beginning ARV treatment unless there is a high risk of HIV progression and death during that period (i.e., CD4+ cell count <50/mm^3). The recommendations for treating HIV infection in patients with tuberculosis are shown in Table 7.9.

Table 7.9 **Treatment of Tuberculosis in HIV Patients in a Resource-limited Country**

CD4 cell count	*ART recommendations*	*Timing of ART in relation to start of ATT*
$<200/mm^3$	Recommend ART	Between 2 and 8 weeks
$200\text{-}350/mm^3$	Recommend ART	After 8 weeks (after intensive phase)
$>350/mm^3$	Defer ART	Re-evaluate at 8 weeks and at the end of ATT
Not available	Recommend ART*	Between 2 and 8 weeks

*See text for indications to start ART when CD4 counts are not available.

CONCLUSION

Advances in the pathogenesis of HIV and development of new, potent drug regimens have resulted in more effective therapies for HIV infection. The use of newer modalities (alone or in combination) of treatment may lead to the ultimate goal of curing HIV infection.

REFERENCES

1. Powderly WJ. The pathogenesis of HIV infection. In: Powderly WJ, edr. Manual of HIV therapeutics. 2nd ed. Philadelphia: Lippincott William & Wilkins; 2001. p. 23-34.
2. Fischl MA, Richman DD, Hansen N, et al. The safety and efficacy of zidovudine (AZT) in the treatment of subjects with mildly symptomatic human immunodeficiency virus type 1 (HIV) infection. A double blind, placebo-controlled trial. AIDS Clinical Trial Group. Ann Intern Med 1990; 112: 727-37.
3. Hamilton JD, Hartigan PM, Simberkoff MS, et al. A controlled trial of early versus late treatment with zidovudine in symptomatic human immunodeficiency virus infection. Results of the Veterans Affairs Cooperative Study. N Engl J Med 1992; 326: 437-43.
4. Richman DD. Resistance of clinical isolates of human immunodeficiency virus to antiretroviral agents. Antimicrobial Agents Chemother 1993; 37: 1207-13.
5. Safrin S. Antiviral agents. In: Katzung BG, edr. Basic and Clinical Pharmacology. 8th ed. New York: Mc Graw Hill; 2001. p. 823-43.
6. Hammer SM. Nucleoside analogue reverse transcriptase inhibitor options: a re-examination of the class. Top HIV Med. 2006; 14: 140-3.
7. Piacenti FJ. An update and review of antiretroviral therapy. Pharmacotherapy. 2006; 26: 1111-1133.
8. Chearskul P, Rongkavilit C, Al-Tatari H, et al. New Antiretroviral Drugs in Clinical Use. Indian J Pediatr 2006; 73: 335-41.
9. Fortgang IS, Belitsos PC, Chaisson RE, et al. Hepatomegaly and steatosis in HIV-infected patients receiving nucleoside analog antiretroviral therapy. Am J Gastroenterol 1995; 90: 1433-6.
10. Harris M, Tesiorowski A, Chan K, et al. Lactic acidosis complicating antiretroviral therapy: Frequency and correlates. Antiviral Therapy 2000; 5 (Suppl 2): 31.
11. Sweet DE. Metabolic complications of antiretroviral therapy. Top HIV Med. 2005; 13: 70-4.
12. Campiani G, Ramunno A, Maga G, et al. Non-nucleoside HIV-1 reverse transcriptase (RT) inhibitors: Past, present, and future perspectives. Current Pharmaceutical Design, 2002; 8: 615-57.

13. Panel on Antiretroviral Guidelines for Adult and Adolescents. Guidelines for the use of antiretroviral agents in HIV-infected adults and adolescents. Department of Health and Human Services. October 10, 2006; 1-113. Available at http://www.aidsinfo.nih.gov/ContentFiles/AdultandAdolescentsGL.pdf.
14. Hicks CB, Cahn P, Cooper DA, et al. Durable efficacy of tipranavir-ritonavir in combination with an optimised background regimen of antiretroviral drugs for treatment-experienced HIV-1-infected patients at 48 weeks in the Randomized Evaluation of Strategic Intervention in multi-drug reSistant patients with Tipranavir (RESIST) studies: an analysis of combined data from two randomised open-label trials. Lancet 2006; 368: 466-75.
15. Carr A, Samaras K, Thorisdottir A, et al. Diagnosis, prediction and natural course of HIV-1 protease-inhibitor associated lipodystrophy, hyperlipidemia and diabetes mellitus: a cohort study. Lancet 1999; 353: 2093-9.
16. Winston A, Boffito M. The management of HIV-1 protease inhibitor pharmacokinetic interactions. J Antimicrob Chemother 2005; 56: 1–5.
17. Egger M, May M, Chene G, et al. Prognosis of HIV1-infected patients starting highly active antiretroviral therapy: a collaborative analysis of prospective studies. Lancet 2002. 360: 119-29.
18. Durant J, Clevenbergh, Halfon P, et al. Drug-resistance genotyping in HIV-1 therapy: The VIRADAPT rando-mized controlled trial. Lancet 1999; 353: 2195-9.
19. del Rio C. Current concepts in antiretroviral therapy failure. Top HIV Med. 2006; 14: 102-6.
20. Surjushe AU, Jindal SR, Kamath RR, et al. Immune reconstitution inflammatory syndrome. Indian J Dermatol Venereol Leprol 2006; 72: 410-4.
21. Navas E, Martin-Davila P, Moreno L, et al. Paradoxical reactions of tuberculosis in patients with the acquired immunodeficiency syndrome who are treated with highly active antiretroviral therapy. Arch Intern Med 2002; 162: 97-9.
22. Wendel KA, Alwood KS, Gachuhi R, et al. Paradoxical worsening of tuberculosis in HIV infected persons. Chest 2001; 120: 193-7.
23. BHIVA treatment guidelines for TB/HIV infection February 2005. Accessed at http://www.bhiva.org/guidelines/2005/tb/TB_HIV_FINAL2005.pdf.
24. Antiretroviral therapy For HIV infection in adults and adolescents: Recommendations for a public health approach. http://www.who.int/hiv/pub/guidelines/artadultguidelines.pdf
25. Antiretroviral therapy guidelines for HIV infected adult and adolescents and post exposure prophylaxis. NACO policies and guidelines. www.nacoonline.com

8 HIV IN PREGNANCY

Suneeta Mittal, Pakhee Aggarwal

In this chapter

- Magnitude of Problem
- Prevention of Parent to Child Transmission (PPTCT)
- Mother to Child Transmission (MTCT)
- Prevention of MTCT (PMTCT)

INTRODUCTION

The health and wellbeing of women is the key to the health and wellbeing of their families, communities and societies. The Safe Motherhood Initiative was started in 1987 to improve maternity services and to protect the health of mothers and their infants. HIV presents a formidable challenge to this end. The United Nations Millennium Development Goal No. 6 on combating HIV/AIDS aims to halt and reverse the spread of HIV/AIDS by 2015[1].

MAGNITUDE OF THE PROBLEM

As of July 2006, 38.6 million people were living with HIV/AIDS. In terms of the recent trend of the epidemic, 4.9 million people became newly infected with HIV in 2005, including 700,000 children (25% of which were in South East Asia), mostly infected by perinatal transmission[2]. Fifteen hundred children are infected daily as a result of mother-to-child transmission (MTCT)[3]. Of the 8.3 million HIV infected persons living in Asia, 5.7 million live in India alone[4]. The estimates for India are based on anonymous testing data from antenatal and STD clinics[5]. Prevalence rates of HIV sero-positivity have been taken as a good indicator of HIV infections in the community, although sentinel surveillance may underestimate the prevalence by a factor of 0.75, mostly due to sub-fertility and increased early pregnancy loss in HIV infected women[6,7]. The prevalence of HIV infection in India is 0.91% in general adult population and 0.3% in pregnant women, although it may be higher than this in some states[8].

Epidemiology

There are two main types of HIV virus - type 1 and type 2, with type 1 infection being the commonest one. HIV transmission among humans occurs in three ways: unprotected sexual intercourse, and homosexual or heterosexual behaviour; through blood or blood products, donated semen or organs; and from an infected mother to her child. In developing countries, 70% of infections are due to heterosexual spread, and 90% of infections in children are due to MTCT[9,10].

> **Declaration of Commitment to HIV/AIDS of the United Nations General Assembly Special Session on HIV/AIDS: preventing HIV among infants and young children:** "By 2005, reduce the proportion of infants infected with HIV by 20 per cent, and by 50 per cent by 2010, by ensuring that 80 per cent of pregnant women accessing antenatal care have information, counselling and other prevention services available to them, increasing the availability of and by providing access to HIV infected women and babies to effective treatment to reduce mother-to-child transmission of HIV, as well as through effective interventions in HIV infected women, including voluntary and confidential counselling and testing, access to treatment, especially anti-retroviral therapy, and where appropriate, breast milk substitutes and the provision of a continuum of care."

PREVENTION OF PARENT-TO-CHILD TRANSMISSION

The Prevention of Parent to Child Transmission of HIV/AIDS (PPTCT) programme was started in the country in 2002 following a feasibility study in 11 major hospitals in the 5 high HIV prevalence states. Currently there are more than 4000 Integrated Counselling and Testing Centres (ICTCs) in the country, most of them in government hospitals, offering PPTCT services to pregnant women. Of these, 502 are located in Obstetrics and Gynaecology Departments and Maternity Homes where the client load is predominantly comprised of pregnant women.

The Joint Technical Mission on PPTCT (2006) estimated that, out of 27 million annual pregnancies in India, 189,000 occur in HIV-positive women. In the absence of any intervention, an estimated cohort of 56,700 infected babies will be born annually. The PPTCT programme aims to prevent the perinatal transmission of HIV from an HIV infected pregnant mother to her newborn baby. The programme entails counselling and testing of pregnant women in ICTCs. Pregnant women who are found to be HIV-positive are given a single dose of Nevirapine at the time of labour; their newborn babies also get a single dose of Nevirapine immediately after birth.

The PPTCT services cover about 10% pregnancies in the country. In 2006, 2.1 million pregnant women accessed this service. Of these, more than 16,500 pregnant women were HIV-positive. In order to provide universal access to these services, a further scale-up has been planned up to the level of Community Health Centres, and Primary Health Centres, as well as forging public-private partnerships. Through these measures NACO hopes to achieve the UNGASS target of reducing the proportion of infants infected with HIV/AIDS by 50% by 2010.

The susceptibility to HIV infection is influenced by various biological and socio-cultural factors. In general, women in developing countries are more susceptible to HIV infection due to[11]:

1. Biological factors: vulval and vaginal inflammation, pelvic inflammatory diseasepartially treated/silent Chlamydia infections which act as cofactors for HIV, and other STDs like syphilis and herpes genitalis
2. Socio-cultural factors: poverty, gender-bias, unemployment, low education forcing women into prostitution, high-risk behaviour of male partners, poor condom usage, and desire and pressure for pregnancy precluding the use of barrier methods.

Effects of Pregnancy on HIV

Pregnancy is a state of suppressed immune function. However, this has not been shown to affect the natural history of HIV infection unless the patient has full-blown AIDS, where the risk of maternal mortality is increased[12,13].

Although earlier reports had suggested that preg-nancy has a suppressive effect on cell-mediated immunity, which may accelerate the course of HIV disease, recent studies have refuted this concept by showing that the markers of disease progression are not affected in women who have had pregnancy as compared to those who have not[14,15].

Pregnancy does not alter disease progression in asymptomatic women and those with early disease, although there may be a more rapid progres-sion in women with late-stage HIV infection[16]. CD4 and CD8 percentages are stable in seropositive women in late pregnancy and postpartum period[17].

Effects of HIV on Pregnancy

Adverse pregnancy outcomes including increased rates of spontaneous abortions, ectopic pregnancy, preterm labour, stillbirths and low birth weight babies have been reported more often in developing countries than in developed ones[18]. Pregnancy may be complicated by bacterial pneumonia, urinary tract infections, genital infections, and opportunistic infections like tuberculosis, Herpes zoster and Kaposi's sarcoma[19]. It was initially thought that babies born to HIV-positive women may have more neonatal complications, e.g. prematurity IUGR and HIV-syndrome. But recent data show no more fetal adverse effects or differences in birth weights than in HIV-negative pregnancy in developed nations[20].

Postpartum infectious complications are high in HIV-positive women, especially those with low CD4 counts[21].

MOTHER-TO-CHILD TRANSMISSION (MTCT)

Transmission of HIV from mother to child may occur in-utero, during labor and delivery, and/or through breastfeeding. The overall transmission risk is 15-25% in developed nations, and 20-45% in South-East Asian region[22] in the absence of any intervention to prevent it. The maximum transmission occurs late in pregnancy and during labour[23].

The factors which affect MTCT are briefly described as under:

1. Maternal factors: viral load, clinical, immunological and nutritional status, drug use and

sex practices, and availability of antiretroviral therapy. Of these, maternal viral load is the strongest predictor of vertical transmission. While there is no known level of viremia below which transmission does not occur, it is reported to be very low if HIV RNA <1000 copies/ml (<1%). With a viral load of >100,000 copies/ml, the transmission rate is 41%. Low levels of vitamin A in serum are associated with a risk of increased transmission[24].

2. Obstetric factors: duration of ruptured membranes, mode of delivery, intrapartum haemorrhage, obstetrical procedures and inva-sive fetal monitoring. With rupture beyond 4 hours, the risk rises from 14 to 25% and continues to rise by 2% every hour upto 24 hours. Elective caesarean reduces transmission rates[25], while obstetric procedures like external cephalic version, amniocentesis, operative vaginal delivery, fetal scalp electrode and invasive fetal testing increase the risk.
3. Fetal factors: prematurity, multiple pregnancy, breastfeeding, genetic susceptibility and immature gastrointestinal and immune system. Premature infants have a 3.7 times higher risk of intrapartum transmission due to increased fetal cell susceptibility to HIV infection, reduced functional immune response, incompetent mucosal barrier and reduced level of acquired maternal antibody. First-born twins have a twofold higher risk of transmission[26].

The total risk of transmission is 25-40% in the absence of any intervention. The distribution of risk is as follows:

- Antepartum: 10-15% mainly transplacental spread in-utero
- Intrapartum: 65-75% secondary to direct contact with infected blood/cervicovaginal secretions and passage through an infected birth canal. Transmission during labour may also be due to transplacental microtransfusion as placental integrity is disrupted.
- Postpartum: 10-15% through breast milk

The WHO strategy to prevent new infections among mothers and children involves a four-pronged approach[27]:

- Primary prevention among women and children
- Prevention of unwanted pregnancies
- Prevention of HIV transmission from infected women to their children (PTCT)
- Provision of treatment, care and support for women with HIV, their children and family (PPTCT Plus)

The antenatal care of HIV infected mothers require a multidisciplinary approach and should include:

- Regular antenatal checkup and assessment of fetal growth, detailed anomaly scan, especially after first trimester exposure to HAART
- Nutritional support - provide iron/folic acid/ calcium/multivitamins
- Screen for STI/Hepatitis B/C, tuberculosis
- Avoid procedures like external cephalic version/invasive fetal tests
- Prophylaxis for opportunistic infections like *Pneumocystis Carinii* pneumonia, toxoplasmosis, tuberculosis - *Mycobacterium avium complex*, varicella zoster, hepatitis A and B
- Plasma viral load and CD4 T-lymphocyte count three-monthly to advise regarding choice and timing of antiretroviral therapy
- Monitor for drug toxicity in women on antiretroviral therapy

PREVENTION OF MTCT

The interventions to prevent MTCT are:

1. Universal screening of antenatal women, offer therapeutic termination if positive
2. Behavioural interventions
3. ART in pregnancy
4. Elective caesarean section
5. Avoid breastfeeding
6. Neonatal ART
7. Contraception

1. **Universal screening of antenatal women** The discovery of HIV infection in early pregnancy is traumatic for a patient and leading her to emotional dilemma. However, the benefits of early detection far outweigh the cosequences. Universal screening in high seroprevalence areas and selective screening of high-risk cases in low prevalence areas has been suggested, although there are concerns that such a strategy would leave out a large number of infected women.
   HIV screening in pregnancy can be done in one of the two ways[28]:

   Opt-in strategy: The patient requests for HIV testing after informed consent and proper pre-test counselling followed by post-test counselling.

   Opt-out strategy: The screening is universal with informed consent, but the patient has the right to decline testing.

   The opt-out strategy encourages higher screening rates[29]. Screening is ideally carried out at the first prenatal visit, in the first trimester itself[30]. Pre and post-test counselling should be the norm. The diagnosis of HIV is made by either 3 rapid tests or 2 ELISA-based tests.

2. **Behavioural interventions** Behavioural interventions include reduction in the frequency of unprotected intercourse during pregnancy, reduction in the number of sexual partners, and avoidance of drug use and smoking during pregnancy.

3. **ART in pregnancy** The goals of ART in pregnancy are twofold:

   - To reduce MTCT (i.e., for the baby's health)
   - To prevent disease progression in the mother (i.e., for the mother's own health)

All HIV-positive women should receive ART during pregnancy and delivery.

ART to Prevent MTCT

Pregnant mothers require ART from 28 to 32 weeks onwards until delivery to prevent perinatal transmission. The first of these protocols to prevent MTCT was the Pediatric AIDS Clinical Trials Group Protocol (PACTG) 076, which recommended 100 mg Zidovudine (AZT) five times a day, initiated between 14 and 34 weeks gestation and continued throughout pregnancy. In the intrapartum period, intravenous AZT is given in a one-hour loading dose of 2 mg/kg, followed by continuous infusion of 1 mg/kg/hour until the infant is delivered. AZT levels in newborn are almost equivalent to those in mother as this regime as initial dose ensures rapid attainment of virucidal levels, while continuous infusion results in stable levels regardless of the duration of labour. The infant can receive AZT syrup 2 mg/kg four times a day for the first 6 weeks of life, started within 8-12 hours after birth. This will show a 70% reduction in the MTCT[31].

Subsequently, the National AIDS Control Organization (NACO) has recommended oral Nevirapine (NVP) single dose 200 mg stat at onset of labour to the mother, and syrup NVP single dose 2 mg/kg within 72 hours of delivery to the neonate. NVP is a non-nucleoside reverse transcriptase inhibitor with very long half-life and good efficacy but associated with rapid development of drug resistance. NVP reduces the risk of transmission by 50%.[32] However, there is no statistically significant difference in efficacy between short course AZT and SD-NVP[33].

The WHO has prepared guidelines for use of ART in developing countries[34,35].

For women in the antenatal period, the ART prophylaxis recommended is shown in Table 8.1.

Table 8.1 **ART Regimens for Prevention of HIV Transmission in Pregnancy**

	Pregnancy	*Labour*	*Postpartum*
For women detected during antenatal period			
Recommended	AZT 300 mg BD (>28 weeks gestation)	Sd – NVP + AZT 600 mg at onset of labour or 300 mg at onset of labour, 3-hourly until delivery + Lamivudine(3TC) 150 mg at onset of labour, 12 hourly until delivery	Mother: AZT/3TC × 7 days Infant: Sd – NVP 2 mg/kg oral + AZT × 7 days
Alternative	AZT 300 mg BD (>28 weeks gestation)	Sd – NVP 200 mg at onset of labour	Infant: Sd – NVP 2 mg/kg oral + AZT × 7 days
For women seen for the first time in labor			
Recommended		Sd – NVP + AZT/3TC	Mother: AZT 300 mg BD + 3TC 150 mg BD × 7 days Infant: Sd – NVP 2 mg/kg oral + AZT × 4 weeks
Alternative		AZT/3TC	Mother: AZT/3TC × 7 days Infant: AZT 4 mg/kg + 3TC 2 mg/kg × 7 days
For infants born to HIV-positive mothers who did not receive antepartum or postpartum prophylaxis			
Recommended	Sd – NVP immediately after birth + AZT × 4 weeks		
Alternative	Sd – NVP immediately after birth + AZT × 1 week		

Sd: Single dose

High levels of HIV-neutralizing antibodies in maternal plasma have been found to reduce the risk of transmission, independent of the viral load. The frequency and quantity of HIV in genital secretions is higher in pregnant HIV-positive women, than in non-pregnant HIV-positive women[36].

ART to Prevent Disease Progression

WHO recommends ART in pregnancy for mothers for their own health if they are in[35]:

- Clinical stage 3 or 4 disease
- Stage 1 or 2 disease with CD4 counts <350 cells/mm^3, particularly if closer to 200-250 cells/mm^3, or with absolute lymphocyte count <1200/mm^3 with symptomatic disease where CD4 testing is not available

These women should be prescribed a combination of three or more antiretroviral drugs, known as HAART, which usually includes AZT. Zidovudine (AZT) 300 mg BD + Lamivudine (3TC) 150 mg BD + Nevirapine (NVP) 200 mg BD (if CD4 <250) is given in antepartum, intrapartum and postpartum periods. Alternatively, AZT + 3TC + Efavirenz (EFV) can be given if CD4 is between 250 and 350 but initiation should be delayed to 2nd trimester as EFV is embryotoxic.

The infant should receive AZT 2 mg/kg × 7 days.

If the mother had received <4 weeks of AZT or HAART, then infant AZT should be continued for at least 4 weeks. If the mother had received at least 4 weeks of AZT before delivery, omission of maternal NVP may be considered.

In general, the side effects of ART are:

- Preterm labour
- Anaemia
- Hyperglycemia
- Hepatotoxicity

Rarely a woman becomes pregnant while on ART; in such cases, if she is on Efavirenz (EFV)-containing regimen in first trimester, it should be substituted with NVP, although exposure to EFV is not an indication for abortion. Women who are receiving EFV in the second or third trimester of pregnancy can continue the current regimen.

4. **Role of elective caesarean and intrapartum care** Elective caesarean at 38 weeks should be discussed and offered to all HIV infected women who are not on HAART and with HIV-RNA load >1000 copies/ml, as it has been shown to reduce MTCT. Doubtful benefit is observed with elective caesarean in women who are already on HAART and who have a viral load <1000 copies/ml. In such cases, decision regarding mode of delivery should be individualized[37].
   Universal precautions should be followed in labour and delivery. Avoid prolonged membrane rupture and invasive fetal monitoring like fetal blood sampling, scalp electrodes and operative vaginal delivery to minimize fetal contact with maternal blood and cervicovaginal secretions. The role of vaginal lavage with chlorhexidine is controversial. Prophylactic antibiotics are given as routine policy. Early cord clamping and immediate baby bath also minimize intrapartum transmission[38].
   Waste disposal after delivery should be appropriately done. Placenta should be soaked in 1% sodium hypochlorite for 30 min before discarding in a disposable plastic bag for incineration. Contaminated linen and delivery items should also be treated with 1% sodium hypochlorite before mixing with other items.

5. **Breastfeeding practices** Since HIV DNA is present in breast milk, HIV transmission can occur through breastfeeding, with maximum chances in the first few months. This exposure increases in the event of cracked nipples, mastitis, mixed feeding and oral candidiasis in the infant[39]. The exact mechanism of transmission through breast milk is still not well understood. It may involve:

   - Infection via cell-free HIV in breast milk or via HIV infected cells
   - Susceptibility of immature neonatal GI tract to virus
   - GI tract mucosal damage

   Transmission rates increase with increasing duration of breastfeeding[40]. Breast milk contains both cell-associated and cell-free virus, and where a safe and economically feasible alternative is not available, it forms a major route of transmission[41]. The efficacy of ART prophylaxis regimens is decreased by postpartum exposure through breastfeeding[35].
   UNAIDS issued a revised statement stating that women should be offered HIV counselling and testing, be informed of risks and benefits of breastfeeding if the mother is HIV-positive, and should make a decision that takes into account the individual and family situations. The ideal substitute is sterile artificial feeds which fulfil the AFASS criteria (Acceptable, Feasible, Affordable, Sustainable and Safe).
   In women of low socio-economic status, after counselling and discussing the risks, the patient should be advised exclusive breast milk (EBM) for 4 months followed by abrupt weaning. Mixed feeding is strongly condemned as it significantly increases MTCT due to immune factors and growth factors in breast milk and mucosal damage associated with mixed feeding[42].

6. **Neonatal ART** Blood sample of the neonate should be taken for assessment of ART

requirement. If the virus is detectable by PCR within 48 hours of birth, the fetus is assumed to be infected in utero, while intrapartum infection is suspected when viral studies are negative within the first week but become positive between 7 and 90 days. HIV status of the infant should be determined by a DNA-PCR at 6-8 weeks and ELISA at 18 months[43]. Neonatal ART is given as outlined earlier.

Contraception

In dual contraception, one barrier method which is moderately effective against pregnancy, but highly efficacious in preventing HIV transmission should be combined with another regular contraceptive like oral pills, intrauterine devices, implants or even voluntary sterilization which is highly effective but does not prevent HIV transmission to the partner[44].

REFERENCES

1. The Millennium Development Goals Report 2005, Report of the United Nations, published by the UN Department of Public Information DPI/2390-May 2005-35M.
2. UNAIDS. Report on the global HIV/AIDS epidemic. Geneva: Joint United Nations Programme on HIV/AIDS, July 2006.
3. Schwartlander B, Grubb I, Perriens J. The 10-year struggle to provide antiretroviral treatment to people with HIV in the developing world. Lancet 2006; 368: 589.
4. The Global HIV/AIDS pandemic, 2006. MMWR Morb Mortal Wkly Rep 2006; 55: 841.
5. Steinbrook R. HIV in India – a complex epidemic. N Eng J Med 2007; 356: 1089.
6. Borgdorff M, Barongo L, van Jaarsveld E, et al. Sentinel surveillance for HIV-1 infection: how representative are blood donors, outpatients with fever, anaemia, or sexually transmitted diseases, and antenatal clinic attenders in Mwanza Region, Tanzania. AIDS 1993; 7: 567-72.
7. Gray RH, Wawer MJ, Serwadda D, et al. Population-based study of fertility in women with HIV-1 infection in Uganda. Lancet 1998; 351: 98-103.
8. HIV/AIDS epidemiological surveillance & estimation report for the year 2005. Available from URL: www.nacoonline.org.
9. HIV/AIDS: the global epidemic. Geneva: Joint United Nations Programme on HIV/AIDS, 1996 (fact sheet).
10. Fowler MG, Melnick SL, Mathieson BJ. Women & HIV. Epidemiology & Global Overview. Obstet Gynecol Clin North Am 1997; 24: 705-29.
11. HIV in Pregnancy: A review. WHO Occasional Paper 2. Geneva. WHO/CHS/RHR/99.15. UNAIDS 99.35E, 1999.
12. Taha TE, Miotti P, Liomba G, et al. HIV, maternal death and child survival in Africa. AIDS 1996; 10: 111-2.
13. Ryder RW, Nsuami M, Nsa W, et al. Mortality in HIV-1-seropositive women, their spouses and their newly born children during 36 months of follow-up in Kinshasa, Zaïre. AIDS 1994; 8: 667-72.
14. French R, Brocklehurst P. The effect of pregnancy on survival in women infected with HIV: a systematic review of literature & meta-analysis. Br J Obset Gynaecol 1998; 105: 827-35.
15. Brettle RP. Pregnancy and its effects on HIV/AIDS. Balliere's Clin Obstet Gynecol 1992; 6: 125-36.
16. Temmerman M. Human immunodeficiency virus and women. J Obstet Gynecol 1994; 14: S70-5.
17. Miotti PG, Chiphangwi JD, Dalbetta G. The situation in Africa. Balliere's Clin Obstet Gynecol 1992; 6: 165-85.
18. Temmerman M, Plummer FA, Mirza NB, et al. Infection with HIV as a risk factor for adverse obstetrical outcome. AIDS 1990; 4: 1087-93.

19. Minkoff HL, Willoughby A, Mendez H, et al. Serious infections during pregnancy among women with advanced human immunodeficiency virus infection. Am J Obstet Gynecol 1990; 162: 30-4.

20. Markson LE, Turner BJ, Houchens R. Association of maternal HIV infection with low birth weight. J Acquir Immune Defic Syndr Hum Retrovirol. 1996; 13: 227-34.

21. Bulterys M, Chao A, Dushimimana A et al. Fatal complications after Cesarian section in HIV-infected women. AIDS. 1996; 10: 923-4.

22. Working group on mother-to-child transmission of HIV. Rates of mother to child transmission of HIV-1 in Africa, America & Europe: results from 13 perinatal studies. J Acquir Immune Defic Syndr Hum Retrovirol. 1995; 8: 506-10.

23. Mofenson LM. Mother-child HIV-1 transmission: timing & determinants. Obstet Gynecol Clin North Am 1997; 24: 759-84.

24. Semba RD, Miotti PG, Chiphangwi JD et al. Maternal vitamin A deficiency and mother-to-child transmission of HIV-1. Lancet 1994; 343: 1593-7.

25. The European Mode of Delivery Collaboration. Elective cesarean-section vs. vaginal delivery in prevention of vertical HIV-1 transmission: a randomized control trial. Lancet 1999; 353: 1035-9.

26. Duliège AM, Amos CI, Felton S et al. Birth order, delivery route, and concordance in the transmission of human immunodeficiency virus type 1 from mothers to twins. International Registry of HIV-Exposed Twins. J Pediatr 1995; 126: 625-32.

27. Mahendra S, Mudoi R, et al. Continuum of care for HIV-positive women accessing programs to prevent parent-to-child transmission: Findings from India. Horizons Final Report. Washington, DC: Population Council, 2007.

28. Walmsley S. Opt in or opt out: What is optimal for prenatal screening for HIV infection? CMAJ 2003; 168: 707-8.

29. Kiarie J, Nduati R, Koigi K. HIV-1 testing in pregnancy: acceptability and correlates of return for test results. AIDS 2000; 14: 1468-70.

30. Mofenson LM, McIntyre JA. Advances and research directions in the prevention of mother-to-child HIV-1 transmission. Lancet 2000; 355: 2237-44.

31. Connor EM, Sperling RS, Gelber R, et al. Reduction of matermal-infant transmission of human munodeficiency virus type 1 with zidovudine treatment. Pediatric AIDS Clinical Trials Group Protocol 076 Study Group. N Engl J Med 1994; 331: 1173-80.

32. Preventing Parent to Child Transmission. http://www.nacoonline.org/directory_ptct.htm

33. Comparing short AZT+SD NVP with other short course ARV regimens Comparative 6 week efficacy in breast feeding populations. The Ghent Group. AIDS 2005; 19: 1865-75.

34. Van Praag E, Fernyak S, Katz AM (eds.). The implications of antiretroviral treatments. Informal Consultation April 1997. Geneva: WHO (WHO/ASD/97.2)

35. Antiretroviral drugs for treating pregnant women and preventing parent to child transmission of HIV. Guidance & recommendations. WHO, UNICEF, UNFPA, UNAIDS, CDC, USAID, EGPAF Joint Technical Mission, India. January 2006.

36. Henine Y, Mandelbrot L, Henronin R, et al. Virus excretion in cervicovaginal secretions of pregnant & non pregnant HIV-infected women. J Acquir Immune Defic Syndr 1993; 6: 72-5.

37. American College of Obstetricians & Gynecologists Committee Opinion. Scheduled cesarean delivery and the prevention of vertical transmission of HIV infection. Number 134, May 2000. Int J Gynecol Obstet 2001; 73: 279.

38. European Collaborative Study. Cesarean section and the risk of vertical transmission of HIV infection. Lancet 1994; 343: 1464-7.

39. Kuhn L, Stein Z. Infant survival, HIV infection & feeding alternatives in less-developed countries. Am J Public Health, 1997; 87: 926-31.

40. Miotti PG, Taha TE, Kumwenda NI, et al. HIV transmission through breastfeeding: a study in Malawi. JAMA 1999; 282: 744-9.

41. Lewis P, Nduati R, Kreiss JK, et al. Cell-free human immunodeficiency virus type 1 in breast milk. J Infect Dis 1998; 177: 34-9.

42. HIV and infant feeding. Geneva: Joint United Nations Programme on HIV/AIDS 1997: 1-2.

43. Sivapalasingam S, Patel U, Itri V, et al. A Reverse transcriptase assay for early diagnosis of infant HIV infection in resource-limited settings. J Trop Pediatr. 2007 Jun 11; [Epub ahead of print].
44. World Health Organization (WHO). Improving access to quality care in family planning: medical eligibility criteria for contraceptive Use. Second Edition. Geneva, Switzerland: WHO, 2000; WHO. Improving Access to Quality Care in Family Planning: Medical Eligibility Criteria for Contraceptive Use. Third Edition. Geneva, Switzerland: WHO, 2004.

9 HIV/AIDS IN CHILDREN

K Neeladri Raju

In this chapter

- Transmission in children
- Clinical Manifestations
- WHO and NACO Paediatrics AIDS Case Definition
- Opportunistic Infections and Systemic Manifestations in Children
- Diagnosis
- Monitoring Paediatric HIV Infection
- Antiretroviral (ARV) Therapy
- WHO Treatment Guidelines
- Cotrimoxazole as Prophylaxis in HIV Exposed
- Immunization in HIV Infected Children
- Conclusion

INTRODUCTION

The first acquired immunodeficiency syndrome (AIDS) case in female was reported in 1981[1]. In 2004, UNAIDS estimated 4.2 crore people living with HIV and AIDS (PLWHA) in the world, and around 51 lakh PLWHA were in India. The National AIDS Control Organisation (NACO) revised the estimate to 2.5 million PLWHA in 2006. Perinatal transmission of HIV was first described in 1982[2], and transmission through breast milk has been proposed in 1985[3,40]. States in which antenatal prevalence is more than 1% are called high prevalence states. The high prevalence states in India were Andhra Pradesh, Maharashtra, Tamilnadu, Karnataka, Nagaland and Manipur with average prevalence in ANC mothers being 1.6%. Surveillance data in India showed that 36,750 female AIDS cases were reported from 1986 to August 2006. The total reported cases of AIDS in the age group of 0-14 years were 5,596 cases. Effective PMTCT regimens and awareness programmes will reduce the risk of mother-to-child transmission of HIV. HIV/AIDS epidemic has spread largely among pregnant women and children with serious economic and psychological consequences.

The number of infants infected with HIV through mother-to-child transmission decreased from an estimated peak of 1,750 infants born each year during early to mid-1990s to 280–370 infants in 2000. This decrease was largely due to the use of antiretroviral therapy during pregnancy and labour. HIV/AIDS in pregnancy is discussed in a separate chapter.

TRANSMISSION IN CHILDREN

Perinatal transmission is the predominant mode of transmission of HIV to children. The other less common routes of transmission are through blood transfusion and sexual abuse. Close child-to-child contact with extensive exposure to blood or body fluids may be a rare mode of transmission. Hence universal precautions need to be undertaken to prevent exposure of blood or body fluids. Isolation procedures are not recommended for HIV infected children in school or day care settings as no cases of HIV transmission has been reported.

Breastfeeding has accounted for 5-15% of perinatal transmission in population with infant feeding practices. Some observational studies have found that, when the mother was infected prenatally, the additional risk of transmission through breast milk would be 14% as compared to 29% increased risk of transmission in woman infected with HIV postnatally. The risk of HIV transmission to breastfed infant was reported to be 0.7% per month during the first 6 months of life and decreases with time due to immaturity of the immune system with high cellular content in early breast milk.

Colostrum intake may play a lesser role in the transmission of HIV through breast milk because of its contents like IgA, IgM and high levels of Vitamin A. These antibodies and Vitamin A have some neutralizing activity against HIV. It was demonstrated that epidermal growth factor in breast milk plays a protective role by enhancing maturation and integrity of gut epithelium and thus preventing the entry of HIV. Oral sores in newborns, neonatal hypochlorhydria, cracked nipple and mastitis may facilitate HIV transmission while breastfeeding. Prolonged breastfeeding may enhance the risk of HIV transmission to the infant. High HIV RNA viral load and lower CD4+ count in breast milk may be a risk factor in the transmission of HIV to the infant.

Glycosaminoglycans found in breast milk could be protective as it inhibits the binding of CD4+ to HIV envelope glycoproteins.

Replacement feeding (RF), especially bottle feeding, may be a choice in HIV infected mothers to prevent breast milk-induced HIV transmission. However, RF may be associated with infections like diarrhoea and acute respiratory infections in countries with high infant mortality (e.g., Brazil). WHO recommends RF by HIV infected mothers if affordable and safe to use. Undiluted cow's milk instead of formula feeds can be offered as it is easily available and cheap. Mixed feeding, i.e. infants given breast milk and any other liquid, has been associated with higher rates of HIV transmission. Thus the mother can choose between exclusive breastfeeding or exclusive RF. The highest rate of

HIV transmission from breastfeeding occurs in the first months of infant's life. Exclusive breastfeeding (no other foods or drink) is associated with less HIV transmission than mixed feeding. Early weaning could significantly reduce the risk of acquiring HIV infection from breastfeeding.

CLINICAL MANIFESTATIONS

Most HIV infected children are asymptomatic at birth. HIV infected children show different patterns of clinical manifestations. CDC case definition for paediatric HIV classification was based on two parameters: clinical status and immunological status.

Many children with HIV do not grow or gain weight normally. They usually suffer from childhood bacterial infections. These bacterial infections cause fever, diarrhoea, dehydration, pneumonia and seizures. Candidiasis that can cause oral thrush and diaper skin rash is frequently found in children with HIV. As the disease progresses, neurological manifestation such as difficulty in walking, seizures and other symptoms of HIV encephalopathy may be present. Motor skills and mental development such as speaking may be delayed.

CDC established a revised classification system of clinical manifestations in children in 1994, which is still in use. Among the clinical categories, category N includes children with no signs or symptoms of HIV. Category A includes children with two or more conditions listed in Table 9.1 and none of the conditions listed in Category B or C. Category B is moderately symptomatic and the conditions listed are other than those in Category A or C. Category C includes children with severely symptomatic AIDS-defining clinical conditions except lymphoid interstitial pneumonitis (LIP), which is included in Category B.

Table 9.1 **1994 Revised Human Immunodeficiency Virus Infection - Paediatric Classification System**

Clinical Categories
Category N: Not Symptomatic
Children who have no signs or symptoms considered to be the result of HIV infection or who have only one of the conditions listed in category A.
Category A: Mildly Symptomatic
Children with two or more of the following conditions but none of the conditions listed in categories B and C:
* Lymphadenopathy (0.5 cm at more than two sites; bilateral - one site) * Hepatomegaly, splenomegaly, dermatitis, parotitis * Recurrent or persistent upper respiratory infection, sinusitis or otitis media
Category B: Moderately Symptomatic
Children who have symptomatic conditions, other than those listed for category A or category C, that are attributable to HIV infection. Examples of conditions in clinical category B include but are not limited to the following:
Anaemia (8 gm/dL), neutropenia (1,000/mm) or thrombocytopenia (100,000/mm^3) persisting >30 days Bacterial meningitis, pneumonia or sepsis (single episode); Candidiasis, oropharyngeal (i.e. thrush) persisting for >2 months in children aged >6 months; Cardiomyopathy.
Cytomegalovirus infection with onset before one month of age

(Contd.)

Diarrhoea, recurrent or chronic; Hepatitis; Herpes simplex virus (HSV) stomatitis, recurrent (i.e. more than two episodes within one year); HSV bronchitis, pneumonitis or oesophagitis with onset before age of one month; Herpes zoster (i.e. shingles) involving at least two distinct episodes or more than one dermatome; Leiomyosarcoma; Lymphoid interstitial pneumonitis (LIP) or pulmonary lymphoid hyperplasia complex; Nephropathy; Nocardiosis; Fever lasting >1 month; Toxoplasmosis with onset before one month of age; Varicella, disseminated (i.e. complicated chickenpox).

Category C: Severely Symptomatic

Children who have any condition listed in the 1987 surveillance case definition for acquired immunodeficiency syndrome, with the exception of LIP (which is a category B condition).

Centres for Disease Control and Prevention. 1994 Revised classification system for human immunodeficiency virus infection in children less than 13 years of age [MMWR, 1994. 43 (No. RR-12): p. 1-10].

WHO AND NACO CASE DEFINITIONS FOR PAEDIATRIC AIDS

WHO Case Definition for Paediatric AIDS

WHO (2006) case definitions are defined in relation to clinical staging and immunological classifications to facilitate HIV-related surveillance and treatment of HIV infection where diagnostic facilities for HIV are limited.

When HIV infection has been confirmed, WHO clinical classification of established HIV infection has been taken into account. It has described four HIV-associated symptoms and four clinical stages as asymptomatic (clinical stage 1), mild symptoms (clinical stage 2), advanced symptoms (clinical stage 3) and severe symptoms (clinical stage 4). An additional clinical criterion for presumptive diagnosis of severe HIV disease among HIV-retro positive children aged under 18 months is suggested in situations where virological diagnosis is not readily available. WHO clinical classification and staging of established HIV infection is depicted in Tables 9.2 and 9.3.

Table 9.2 WHO Clinical Classification of Established HIV Infection

HIV Associated Symptoms	*WHO Clinical Stage*
Asymptomatic	1
Mild symptoms	2
Advanced symptoms	3
Severe symptoms	4

Table 9.3 WHO Clinical Staging of HIV/AIDS for Children with Confirmed HIV Infection

Clinical Stage 1
Asymptomatic Persistent generalized lymphadenopathy
Clinical Stage 2
Unexplained persistent hepatosplenomegaly Papular pruritic eruptions Extensive warts

(*Contd.*)

Extensive molluscum contagiosum
Fungal nail infections
Recurrent oral ulcerations
Unexplained persistent parotid enlargement
Linear gingivial erythema
Herpes zoster
Recurrent or chronic upper respiratory tract infections (otitis media, otorrhoea, sinusitis or tonsillitis)

Clinical Stage 3

Unexplained moderate malnutrition not adequately responding to standard therapy
Unexplained persistent diarrhoea (14 days or more)
Unexplained persistent fever (above 37.5°C intermittent or constant, for longer than one month)
Persistent oral candidiasis (after first 6-8 weeks of life)
Oral hairy leukoplakia
Acute necrotizing ulcerative gingivitis or peridontitis
Lymph node tuberculosis
Pulmonary tuberculosis
Severe recurrent bacterial pneumonia
Symptomatic lymphoid interstitial pneumonitis
Chronic HIV-associated lung disease including bronchiectasis
Unexplained anaemia (<8 g/dl), neutropaenia (<0.5×10^9 per litre)
Chronic thrombocytopaenia (<50×10^9 per litre)

Clinical Stage 4

Unexplained severe wasting, stunting or severe malnutrition not responding to standard therapy
Pneumocystis pneumonia
Recurrent severe bacterial infections (such as empyema, pyomyositis, bone or joint infection or meningitis but excluding pneumonia)
Chronic herpes simplex infection (orolabial or cutaneous of more than one month's duration or visceral at any site)
Extrapulmonary tuberculosis
Kaposi's sarcoma.
Oesophageal candidiasis (or candidiasis of trachea, bronchi or lungs)
Central nervous system toxoplasmosis (after one month of life)
HIV encephalopathy
Retinitis or cytomegalovirus infection affecting another organ, with onset at age older than one month
Extrapulmonary cryptococcosis (including meningitis)
Disseminated endemic mycosis (extrapulmonary histoplasmosis, coccidiomycosis)
Chronic cryptosporidiosis
Chronic isosporiasis
Disseminated non-tuberculous mycobacterial infection
Cerebral or B-cell non-Hodgkin lymphoma
Progressive multifocal leukoencephalopathy
Symptomatic HIV-associated nephropathy or HIV-associated cardiomyopathy.

Table 9.4 Clinical Criteria for Presumptive Diagnosis of Severe HIV Disease among Infants and Children Aged Under 18 Months in Situations where Virological Testing is Not Available

A presumptive diagnosis of severe HIV disease should be made if the infant
* is confirmed as being HIV antibody-positive
and diagnosis of any AIDS indicator conditions can be made;
Or
* is symptomatic with two or more of the following:
* oral thrush
* severe pneumonia
* severe sepsis

Other factors that support the diagnosis of severe HIV disease in HIV-seropositive infants include:

* recent HIV-related maternal death or advanced HIV disease in the mother :
* CD4 <20%

Confirmation of the diagnosis of HIV infection should be sought as soon as possible.

AIDS indicator conditions include some but not all HIV clinical stage-4 conditions in children such as pneumocystis pneumonia, oesophageal candidiasis, cryptococcal menin-gitis, cerebral toxoplasmosis, HIV wasting and Kaposi's sarcoma.

NACO Case Definition of AIDS for Children Upto 12 Years of Age[5]

1. Two positive tests for HIV infection (by ERS test) in children older than 18 months or confirmed maternal HIV infection for children <18 months.
   and
2. Presence of at least two major and two minor signs in the absence of known causes of immunesuppression.

Major Signs

(a) Loss of weight or failure to thrive, which is not known to be due to medical causes other than HIV infection.
(b) Chronic diarrhoea (intermittent or continuous) >1 month duration.
(c) Prolonged fever (intermittent or continuous) >1 month duration.

Minor Signs

(a) Repeated common infections (e.g. pneumonitis, otitis, pharyngitis, etc.)
(b) Generalized lymphadenopathy
(c) Oropharyngeal candidiasis
(d) Persistent cough for more than 1 month
(e) Disseminated maculopapular dermatitis

At birth, viral load is usually low (<10,000 copies/ml) and then slowly rises within the first 2 months of life to values above 100,000 copies/ml and only slowly decreases after the age of 4-5 years. These viral dynamics are significantly different from the rapid increase and decrease of viral load seen in untreated adults within a few months following acute HIV infection. In children, the higher viral load is associated with the somatic growth of lymphatic system and the inability of the immature immune system in children to mount an HIV-specific response.

Variations in Clinical Features and Opportunistic Infections

Clinical manifestations of HIV in children may greatly vary from that of adults. In adults, typical manifestations of acute HIV seroconversion illness include fever, sore throat, lymphadenopathy and a mononucleosis-like disease. HIV seroconversion illness has not been described in perinatally-infected children.[21] Thrush is the most common manifestation which occurs in more than 80% of HIV infected children. It frequently extends to the oesophagus and also disseminates. In children, recurrent bacterial infections, PCP and LIP are more commonly encountered opportunistic infections than in adults. Failure to grow and thrive may occur in children, while adults may have HIV-related wasting. CNS manifestations occur in the early stage of HIV infection in children, while AIDS dementia complex occurs late in adults. Malignancies are uncommon in children. Children may develop opportunistic infections at higher CD4 cell counts than in adults. Parotitis is a concern in paediatric HIV, and children are more likely to have enlarged liver, spleen and lymph nodes.

OPPORTUNISTIC INFECTIONS AND SYSTEMIC MANIFESTATIONS IN CHILDREN

Opportunistic infections in HIV infected children have been associated with immunodeficiency and may be caused by bacterial, fungal, viral and protozoal pathogens. The commonly encountered systemic and rare manifestations in paediatric HIV are discussed here.

Bacterial Infections

Bacterial infections in HIV infected children are caused by *Streptococcus pneumoniae*, *H. influenzae*, *Salmonella* spp., *Staphylococcus* and *Pseudomonas aeruginosa*. These bacterial infections may be related to immune disturbances with altered T and B lymphocyte functions. Abnormal B cell function results in disturbances in chemotactic and bactericidal function of neutrophils and macrophages. The common bacterial infections in children with HIV are sinusitis, pneumonia, skin and soft tissue infection, otitis media and bacteremia. Catheter-related infections are most commonly encountered due to staphylococcus. Antiretroviral therapy has been reported to lower the frequency of bacterial infections. Prophylaxis with TMP 150 mg/m^2/day given daily in two divided doses may prevent recurrent bacterial infections.

In HIV infected children with hypogammaglobulinemia, intravenous immunoglobulin (IVIG) (IgG 400 mg/kg/day) should be used to prevent serious bacterial infections.

Tuberculosis

It is one of the most common opportunistic infections in HIV infected children. *M. tuberculosis* spreads via respiratory droplets. Congenital TB can occur to the new borns of HIV infected women with active tuberculosis. Clinical features of congenital TB are non-specific and include fever, poor feeding, failure to gain weight, progressive pneumonia, hepatosplenomegaly and meningitis. Children with pulmonary TB may be asymptomatic, or non-specific symptoms such as fever and weight loss may occur. X-ray may be normal or show paratracheal lymphadenopathy obstructive emphysema and atelectasis. Clinical manifestations of older children and adults may show similar features seen in HIV infected adults.

Extrapulmonary tuberculosis may occur in various organs such as lymphnodes, central nervous system, haematogenous (miliary), bone, pericardium, pleura and peritoneum. Extrapulmonary and miliary TB are more common among children <4 years of age. Disseminated disease commonly occurs in patients with low CD4 count. Skin reaction with induration of >5 mm to a standard PPD is considered positive in HIV infected children. In patients with low CD4 counts, cutaneous anergy to Mantoux test may give negative results, and this cannot be used to rule out tuberculosis. The progression of HIV infection is more rapid in tuberculosis patients, and the level of plasma viremia declines with treatment of tuberculosis. Sputum for acid-fast bacilli (AFB) positivity is more common in HIV-positive children than in HIV-negative children. Diagnosis of tuberculosis in children is difficult as they are not able to give sputum for demonstration of AFB, tuberculin test may be negative, and X-ray of the chest may be non-specific. Diagnosis of tuberculosis in children needs a high index of suspicion. Clinical and radiological clues for tuberculosis include history of adult contact suffering from tuberculosis, child getting cough, fever that is not responding to appropriate antibiotics, and X-ray showing lymphadenopathy and parenchymal infiltrates unresponsive to antibiotics. For diagnostic purpose, a tuberculin test showing induration of >5 mm is suggestive of tubercular infection. An attempt should be made to obtain sputum for AFB; if that is not possible, then early morning gastric aspirate for 3 consecutive days may be obtained in young children. Radiometric culture technique demonstrates the presence of *M. tuberculosis* within 10-21 days. Drug susceptibility tests are available to detect drug resistance. Diagnosis of extrapulmonary tuberculosis is made by the examination of direct smears from tissues. PCR test can be used on sputum, pleural fluid and CSF to diagnose tuberculosis.

Treatment with anti-tuberculous drugs shows similar response in both HIV-positive and HIV-negative patients. The four-drug regimen consisting of isoniazid (5 mg/kg/day), rifampin (10-20 mg/kg/day), pyrazinamide (25-30 mg/kg/day) and ethambutol (15 mg/kg/day) or streptomycin (20-30 mg/kg/day) may prevent possible drug resistance in an individual patient. The duration of treatment for pulmonary tuberculosis is 6-12 months, and in extrapulmonary disease, the duration of treatment can be extended to further 12 months. Co-administration of rifampin with NNRTI and PI is contraindicated. As rifampin lowers the drug concentrations of PI and NNRTI, rifampin may be replaced by rifabutin. The administration of rifabutin with antiretrovirals such as nevirapine and ritonavir is not recommended. The drug regimen in such cases is modified and recommended as follows. Isoniazid, pyrazinamide and streptomycin daily for two months and then 2-3 times weekly for another 7 months. Direcly observed therapy is the preferred approach as it prevents multidrug- resistant tuberculosis. Treatment of TB should be initiated 4–8 weeks before initiating antiretroviral medications to improve adherence and to better differentiate potential side effects.[6]

Atypical Mycobacterial Infections

In immunocompetent children, *Mycobacterium avium complex* (MAC) may be confined to the respiratory tract. In HIV cases, MAC may disseminate and cause multisystem disease. This rarely occurs until CD4 count falls below 50 cells/mm^3. Clinical manifestations of disseminated MAC are characterized by recurrent fever, night sweats, weight loss, abdominal pain, diarrhoea, hepatomegaly, osteomyelitis, meningoencephalitis, intra-abdominal abscess and rarely intestinal perforation. MAC is the most common intrahepatic opportunistic infection and may present with jaundice. The laboratory abnormalities include abnormal liver function tests with elevated alkaline phosphatase. Diagnosis is made by the identification of MAC from blood, tissue biopsy of lymph node, bone marrow, liver or gastrointestinal tract. Positive culture results of sputum or stool may reflect colonization but do not confirm diagnosis. Treatment can suppress the infection. The recommended therapy includes two agents. These drugs are azithromycin (or clarithromycin) and ethambutol. The third drug is added in the form of either rifabutin, rifampin, ciprofloxacin or amikacin. In children receiving antiretroviral therapy, MAC infections are rarely reported. Drug interactions with antiretroviral drugs are to be considered. Drug prophylaxis can be offered to high-risk children according to CD4+ counts. Oral suspensions of clarithromycin or azithromycin may be offered as prophylactic agents in children. Rifabutin liquid formulation is not available for children. Lifelong prophylaxis is recommended in children with a history of disseminated MAC to prevent recurrences.

Pneumocystis jiroveci (formerly *P. carinii*) Pneumonia

It is one of the most commonly identified opportunistic infections in children with HIV and occurs frequently during infancy. PJP remains the most common AIDS-indicator disease among HIV infected children.[25] It can be prevented with antibiotic prophylaxis before 2 months of age.

Pneumocystis were originally classified as protozoa. Some suggested that it was a member of fungi based on its affinity for fungal stains, ultrastructural features and presumed airborne mode of transmission. The analysis of pneumocystis ribosomal RNA supports that *P. carinii* is a member of fungi. The infection can appear early in the first weeks of life. Its clinical course consists of cough, fever, tachypnoea, dyspnoea and severe hypoxia. Chest radiography findings demonstrate bilateral diffuse interstitial infiltrates. In a few cases, nodular lesions, lobar infiltrates and pleural effusion may be seen. Initial presentation in patients receiving aerosolized pentamidine may manifest as upper lobe cavitory disease.

Diagnosis is made by identification of the organism in either induced sputum or bronchoalveolar lavage fluid. Stains used for the identification of *P. jiroveci* include methenamine silver, Giemsa, toluidine blue and immunoflourescent technique. PCR technique is under evaluation for demonstration of the organism in induced sputum, bronchoalveolar fluid or peripheral blood. Open-lung biopsy is the most sensitive diagnostic technique, but because it requires thoracotomy and often chest tube drainage, it is not routinely recommended.[5]

The first choice for treatment of PJP is TMP-SMX. The recommended dosage is intravenous TMP 15-20 mg/kg/day and 75-100 g/kg/day of SMX in four divided doses. Adjunctive therapy with intravenous methylprednisolone (2 mg/kg/24 h in divided doses for every 6 or 12 h for 5-7 days) may decrease morbidity and benefit the infant. Indications for corticosteroid treatment include a PaO_2 value of <70 mm Hg or an alveolar-arterial gradient of >35 mm Hg.[25] Oral treatment with TMP/SMX is to be continued for a total of 21 days after clinical improvement with IV TMP/SMX. Alternative treatment for PCP includes intravenous pentamidine with a dosage of 4 mg/kg/24 h. For PCP/PJP prophylaxis, refer to Appendix IIC.

Lymphoid Interstitial Pneumonitis (LIP)

LIP is an AIDS-defining condition included in category B of revised paediatric classification. Its aetiology and pathogenesis are unknown. EBV may play a synergistic role with HIV or an exaggerated immunopathological response to inhaled or circulating antigen, which may contribute to LIP.[7] It generally presents as a chronic progressive interstitial lung disease in the second or third year of life. The clinical course in LIP includes insidious cough, digital clubbing , salivary gland enlargement, lymphadenopathy, hepatosplenomegaly, normal auscultatory findings and laboratory abnormalities with elevation of serum immunoglobulins.

At present, diagnosis can be confirmed by lung biopsy. Radiographic diagnosis of LIP is made by the demonstration of reticulonodular infiltrate with or without hilar adenopathy. Treatment with prednisolone 2 mg/kg/day may improve the clinical condition of the child. Gammaglobulins and supportive care with oxygen and bronchodilators are needed.

Toxoplasmosis

Toxoplasma gondii, a coccidian protozoan, is a causative organism for toxoplamosis. It begins as an asymptomatic infection and reactivates in HIV immunocompromised children. Majority of infants with congenital toxoplasmosis (70-90%) are asymptomatic at birth. The clinical manifestations are characterized by low birth weight, hepatosplenomegaly, icterus and CNS manifestations such as microcephaly, hydrocephaly, mental retardation, convulsions and intracranial calcification. The mechanism of transmission is by eating raw meat or undercooked meat. Transplacental transfer of *Toxoplasma gondii* causes congenital infection in the infant. Diagnosis of congenital toxoplasmosis is made by identification of toxoplasma-specific IgM, IgA or IgE in infants within the first six months of life or by finding specific IgG antibody beyond 12 months of age. IgA might be more sensitive for detection of congenital infection than IgM or IgE.[5] PCR can be used for the identification of DNA. CT or MRI may show multiple ring-enhancing lesions in the brain. Definitive diagnosis can be made by brain biopsy. The recommended treatment for congenital toxoplasmosis is as follows:

Sulphadiazine 100 mg/kg as a loading dose followed by 85-120 mg/kg/day in two or four divided doses. Pyrimethamine 1-2 mg/kg/day for 2 days followed by 1 mg/kg/day for 6 months and then 1 mg/kg/day thrice a week. Folinic acid is supplemented to this therapy to prevent anaemia. The duration of therapy for congenital toxoplasmosis is 12 months, and it should be followed by life-long prophylaxis. Alternate therapy with clindamycin, pyrimethamine and folinic acid may be recommended. In CNS toxoplasmosis, pyrimethamine 2 mg/kg /day (maximum 50 mg/day) for 2 days followed by 1 mg/kg/day (maximum 25 mg/day); sulfadiazine 75 mg/kg/day as a loading dose followed by 5 mg/kg/day, folinic acid 5-20 mg/day thrice a week is indicated. The duration of therapy is for 4-6 weeks beyond complete resolution of symptoms. The therapy should be followed by life-long prophylaxis.

Viral Infections

Herpes simplex viruses (HSV) present as a primary or reactivation disease in HIV infected children. HSV stomatitis with recurrence (i.e. more than two episodes within a year) is included in category B of revised HIV paediatric classification. HSV lesions present as vesicles or ulcers on lips, tongue, gums, palate and oropharynx. It causes oesophagitis with ulceration, chest pain, odynophagia and may be complicated by local and cutaneous dissemination. AIDS patients with systemic HSV infections may present with pneumonitis, hepatitis, meningoencephalitis, shock and sepsis-like syndrome.

Laboratory diagnosis is made by the examination of Tzanck smear to detect multinucleated giant cells.Other laboratory tests to diagnose HSV infection include fluorescent antibody (FA) and culture. Culturing takes 2-3 days and 95% of them are positive within 5 days. FA results are available within 24 h. The recommended treatment of HSV infection is oral acyclovir (ACV) 80 mg/kg/day in four divided doses for 10 days. ACV-resistant cases may be treated with IV foscarnet 120 mg/kg/day in 2-3 divided doses until the lesions are healed. Suppressive oral ACV 200 mg tid or 400 mg bid p.o. is recommended for HIV patients with relapses.

Varicella zoster virus (VZV), the aetiological agent of chicken pox, manifests as a primary infection, and it may be severe and prolonged and has rarely been documented to progress to visceral dissemination with involvement of lungs, liver, brain and pancreas. The course is fulminant in immunocompromised children. Diagnosis is made by clinical examination and laboratory tests that include demonstration of VZV antigens in skin lesions and cultures of the specimen. PCR is a sensitive and specific test for diagnosis. The following regimens can be used to treat VZV infection: (i) ACV 1500 mg/m^2/day in three divided doses for 7-10 days or until no new lesions appear, (ii) oral acyclovir 80-mg/kg/day in four divided doses, (iii) IV foscarnet 120-180 mg/kg/day in 2-3 divided doses in the treatment of ACV-resistant VZV strains. HIV infected children exposed to chicken pox should be given varicella zoster immunoglobulin (VZIG) within 96 h of exposure. Suppressive oral ACV is recommended in relapses.

In children, herpes zoster occurs in early HIV disease and it appears soon after varicella. In immunocompetent children, it is dermatomal. It may be multidermatomal, recurrent or disseminated in HIV infected children. Systemic dissemination of herpes zoster with constitutional symptoms, retinitis, hepatitis, pneumonitis and encephalitis may occur. Post-herpetic neuralgia is common. Diagnosis of herpes zoster can be made clinically with Tzanck test, FA and culture of the specimen. The disease can be treated with the following regimens: (1) oral ACV 80 mg/kg/day in four divided doses, (2) IV foscarnet 120-180 mg/kg/day in 2-3 divided doses in ACV-resistant cases.

Cytomegalovirus (CMV) infections are endemic and occur without any seasonal variation. The spread of infection is through close contact with infected secretions. It may present as an acute infection usually early in life after which it remains in a latent state. Disseminated CMV can occur when the CD4+ cell count falls below 50 cells/mm^3. Retinitis, oesophagitis, colitis, pneumonitis, hepatitis and encephalitis are manifestations in disseminated CMV infection. Diagnosis of CMV is made by upper endoscopy, biopsy and viral cultures of biopsy specimens. The recommended therapy for CMV disease is IV ganciclovir 10 mg/kg/day divided in two doses administered over 1-2 h for 21 days. Alternatively, IV foscarnet 180 mg/kg/day in three divided doses for 14-21 days can be used. Life-long prophylaxis with IV ganciclovir 5 mg/kg/day for 5 days/week is indicated to prevent recurrence of CMV infection. Annual screening for retinitis in CMV infected children is recommended. Other viral infections like measles may occur inspite of immunization and may present without typical rash.

Fungal Infections

Candidiasis is the most common fungal infection and manifests as oral candidiasis or oesophageal disease in HIV infected children. The clinical manifestation of oropharyngeal candidiasis includes white patches or plaques on an erythematous base on tongue and buccal mucosa. When it extends to oesophagus, children may present with vomiting, dysphagia, substernal pain and weight loss. Diagnosis is made by the demonstration of pseudohyphae on KOH preparation. Oesophageal candidiasis can be diagnosed by endoscopy and biopsy. Topical nystatin at a dose of 100,000 units/ml, 2-5 ml every six hours for 14 days, clotrimazole troches and amphotercin B solution may be effective for oral thrush. Oral fluconazole therapy at a dosage of 4-6 mg/kg/24 h for 14 days is recommended for oesophagitis. Itraconazole therapy can be given but there is limited experience with this drug. IV amphotercin B 0.5-1 mg/kg/day is recommended in refractory candidial oesophagitis or disseminated candidiasis. Primary prophylaxis is generally not indicated in HIV infected infants. In severe recurrent mucocutaneous candidiasis, particularly in infants with oesophageal candidiasis, suppressive therapy with systemic azoles should be considered. Deep fungal infections like disseminated histoplasmosis, cryptococcosis or coccidiodomycosis are not common in children.

Gastrointestinal Tract Disorders

Diarrhoea is a common gastrointestinal disorder in children with HIV infection. It may be due to various organisms such as protozoa, bacteria, viruses and fungi. Clinical features are characterized by abdominal pain, watery stool, dehydration, fever and weight loss.

Protozoal Infections

Cryptosporidium is a coccidian protozoan that inhabits the microvillus region of epithelial cells. This was first identified in humans in 1976. The most common site of infection is the small bowel, and the pathogenesis of this infection is uncertain. The organism lies on the surface of enterocyte and may be enveloped by the host cell membrane where it produces modest inflammatory response and cell injury. In AIDS patients, cryptosporidiosis is characterized by bloating, intermittent abdominal cramps, diarrhoea, nausea and weight loss. The illness may be related to the degree of immunity in the host. It may cause biliary tract disease, and the right upper quadrant pain suggests biliary tract involvement. Cryptosporidia have also been found in pulmonary specimens.

In intestinal cryptosporidiosis, diagnosis is often made by using acid-fast stain of the stool. The sucrose flotation or formalin-ethyl acetate method may be used to concentrate oocysts from stool samples. A sample is then stained by using a modified Kinyoun acid-fast stain and examined for small (4–6 μm in diameter) acid-fast positive oocysts.[5] The stain shows the organisms as bright red spherules similar in size to red blood cells. The stool examination is negative in cases where cryptosporidia may be identified in small bowel or rectal biopsies. The cryptosporidium infection is self-limited in immunocompetent hosts and usually does not require any treatment. Boiled water usage can prevent cryptosporidium infection. HAART is the most effective form of therapy for cryptosporidiosis. The treatment consists of paromomycin 25-35 mg/kg/day PO in 3-4 divided doses, antimotility agents and fluid support. The somatostatin analog octreotide is not consistently effective. Nitazoxanide has been tried in some cases.

Isospora belli is a coccidian protozoan endemic in Asia, Africa, South America and Haiti, and causes infection in the proximal small intestine with severe diarrhoeal manifestation. In AIDS patients, cryptosporidium and isospora produce similar clinical manifestations. Diagnosis of isospora is made by identification of the organism in stool specimen or duodenal secretions using acid-fast stain. Intestinal mucosal biopsy can be used to identify *Isospora belli* infections. Isosporiasis can be effectively treated with sulfonamides, pyrimethamine alone or with folinic acid, and ciprofloxacin oral therapy with TMP-SMX, 20 mg TMP/kg/day in four divided doses for 10 days and then bid for 21 days is recommended. Maintenance therapy is indicated to prevent relapse.

Microsporidia are obligate intracellular protozoa, and the disease presents with manifestations of chronic watery non-bloody diarrhoea, malabsorption and weight loss. Five genera have been identified as human pathogens in HIV (enterocytozoon, septata, nosema, pleistophora and encephalitozoon). Intestinal and hepatobiliary infections may be caused by *Enterocytozoon bienusi* and *Encephalitozoon intestinalis*. The organisms may be seen by electron microscopy at the luminal enterocyte surface, and the merozoite vacuole may be identified intracellularly near the enterocyte nucleus. There is little inflammation of tissues and rarely associated with atrophy of villi and cell degeneration. Microsporidia have been noted in a rarity of organs including eye, muscles and liver, and can be associated with conjunctivitis or hepatitis. Diagnosis is based on modified Trichrome staining of stool or small bowel biopsy specimen. The sensitivity of stool specimen with polymerase chain reaction is high, but it is now available as a research tool. There is no effective therapy for microsporidiosis. Albendazole 400 mg bd is used for *E. intestinalis* but not effective for *E. bienusi.* Treatment with metronidazole and atavoquone may show improvement. Like cryptosporidia, the initiation of HAART may result in loss of pathogen from stool and in small intestinal biopsy and show improvement in diarrhoea. Symptomatic treatment with antidiarrhoeal agents and nutritional support may be helpful in refractory cases.

Giardiasis is a water-borne disease that infects the small intestine and is often found in association with amoebiasis. The clinical features of giardiasis are characterized by abdominal cramps, diarrhoea, bloating and nausea. The organisms can be identified by multiple stool examinations. Trophozoites and cysts can be identified in stool and duodenal aspirates. The confirmation of diagnosis is made by small bowel biopsy. Giardia antigen in stool may be demonstrated by immunoassay. Treatment of giardiasis is with oral metronidazole 15 mg/kg/day in three divided doses for 5 days.

Bacterial Infections

Campylobacter jejuni infection presents with self-limiting watery or bloody diarrhoea with fever and abdominal pain. Mucous or frank blood may be present in stool. Campylobacterial infections may be more severe, persistent or recurrent and often associated with bacterial infections outside the bowel in HIV infected patients. Diagnosis is made by the isolation of the organism from stool by culture on selective media in a microaerophilic atmosphere. However, it is difficult to grow campylobacter and the patient may have negative stool cultures. The organisms can be identified only by culturing the tissue biopsy material. The recommended treatment for campylobacter infections is oral azithromycin 10 mg/kg on 1st day, followed by 5 mg/kg/day once a day for 4 days (or) oral erythromycin 30-50 mg/kg/day in 3-4 divided doses for 7 days or oral ciprofloxacin 20 mg/kg/day for 5 days.

Salmonella have been associated with four types of clinical presentation, namely enteric (typhoid) fever, acute gastroenteritis, septicaemia with or without focal or systemic lesions and asymptomatic carrier state. *Salmonella bacteremia* is transient in immunocompetent host. Recurrent *Salmonella bacteremia* in an HIV infected individual is diagnostic of AIDS. Their frequent recurrences may presumably be due to impaired reticuloendothelial clearance because of HIV infection of splenic or hepatic macrophages

(Kupffer cells). Diagnosis is made by the isolation of the organism from stool culture on selective media. The following antimicrobial therapy is recommended for 10-14 days to treat salmonella infections: (1) oral ciprofloxacin 15-30 mg/kg/day or IV in two divided doses, (2) IV cefotaxime 150-200 mg/kg/day in 3-4 divided doses, (3) IV ceftriaxone 100 mg/kg/day in 1-2 doses. Cotrimoxazole can be used to prevent recurrent salmonella and isospora infections.

Shigella species are the cause of dysentery. *S. sonnei* and *S. flexneri* are responsible for most of the infections in US. Shigella is highly infectious, and the transmission of the organism occurs rapidly and localized outbreaks are commonly attributed to contaminated food and water. The clinical features of shigellosis are characterized by an abrupt onset of diarrhoea, bloody or mucoid stool, abdominal cramps, tenesmus and fever. The infection may have complications such as toxic megacolon. These infections tend to be prolonged and recurrent in AIDS patients. Diagnosis is established by the culture of stool on selective media. Treatment is usually supportive. Antimotility drugs are not recommended. The following drugs may be recommended to treat shigella infections: (1) oral ampicillin 100 mg/kg/day for 10 days, (2) oral cefixime 8 mg/kg/day in two divided doses for 5 days, (3) ceftriaxone IV 50 mg/kg/day once daily for 5 days. Tab ciprofloxacin in bid dosage is usually effective.

Clostridium difficile was first demonstrated in 1935 from the faeces of infants, and it has been associated with antibiotic-associated colitis. Assays of stool for *C. difficile* enterotoxin may reveal diagnosis. Antibiotics such as ampicillin, tetracyclines and clindamycin have been found to be responsible for pseudomembranous colitis. Metronidazole or vancomycin may be recommended to treat *C. difficile* infection.

Viral Infections

Viral infections that cause diarrhoea in HIV patients include rotavirus and adenoviruses. The treatment is generally supportive. Nutritional support and treatment of dehydration are indicated.

Idiopathic AIDS Enteropathy

This is a chronic diarrhoeal illness in AIDS patients with no pathogens identified. Enteric HIV infection may lead to mucosal atrophy with impairment of small bowel absorption, which in turn may lead to diarrhoea and weight loss.[8] Altered intestinal permeability and malabsorption that suggests cellular dysfunction can be found even in patients with no detectable infection and minimal morphological changes.[9-10]

Decreased CD4/CD8 ratio of intestinal lymphocytes has been reported with HIV infection of the gut.[31-32] The intestinal infection may be due to reduced total CD4 cells in intestines. There were reports of decreased IgA plasma cells in intestinal mucosa of AIDS patients in association with increased IgM plasma cells, and the role of local HIV infection in producing these changes is not known.

The mechanism of AIDS enteropathy may be due to the effect of enteric HIV on autonomic nerves. Griffin et al. found degeneration of nerve axonal in HIV infected patients and then patients may have risk for motility disturbances.

Haematological Disorders

Eythrocytes, platelets, neutrophils and lymphocytes are affected by HIV infection. Most children may present with normocytic or microcytic anaemia. It may be due to iron deficiency, chronic infection, autoimmune phenomenon or side effects of drugs. Subcutaneous recombinant erythropoietin is recommended to treat children with low erythropoietin levels.

Neutropenia occurs in 10% of patients, which may be due to drugs used to treat HIV or opportunistic infections. It is benign and responds to bacterial infections when compared with neutropenia that develops after chemotherapy or radiation.

Treatment with intravenous immunoglobulin (IVIG) or subcutaneous granulocyte colony-stimulating factor offers some benefit in neutropenia or leucopenia. Lymphopenia is present in 30% of cases, and it is a marker for advanced disease.

Thromobocytopenia occurs in 10-15% of patients. Diminished platelet levels may be, present reportedly 20,000 to 45,000/mm^3. The cause may be drug-induced or immunological with platelet-associated antibodies. AZT therapy for HIV-associated thrombocytopenia improves platelet count. The counts rise from 100,000 to 400,000 platelets/mm^3 on therapy with AZT, but there is usually a fall if the drug is withdrawn. Treatment with IVIG, anti-D and corticosteroid shows improvement in some cases. In advanced HIV disease, deficiency of clotting factors (e.g. factors II, VII and IX) may be found, and it can be treated with Vitamin K.

Polyclonal hypergammaglobulinemia, thrombotic thrombocytopenic purpura and diffuse infiltrative CD8 lymphocytosis syndrome have been associated with HIV infection.

Central Nervous System Disorders

CNS involvement in HIV infected children may present as progressive encephalopathy and is characterized by cognitive deterioration, and motor and behavioural impairment with loss of developmental milestones. Older children may have learning disabilities or behavioural problems. CT scan shows cerebral atrophy, decreased attenuation of the white matter, and basal ganglia calcification. Seizures and focal neurological signs are not common, and they may represent tumour, opportunistic infections or other pathological processes. Differential diagnosis includes CNS lymphomas, toxoplasmosis, CMV, JC virus and HSV infections.

Cutaneous Manifestations

Cutaneous manifestations in children with HIV are more severe and more frequently recurrent than in immunocompetent children. Oral and oesophageal candidiasis, herpetic gingivo stomatitis, herpes zoster, molluscum contagio-sum, anogenital warts, and *Staphylococcus aureus* skin infections that include cellulitis, abscess, impetigo and staphylococcal folliculitis are common cutaneous manifestations in children with HIV infection. Seborrhoeic dermatitis, atopic dermatitis, drug eruption, and nutritional deficiencies (e.g., acrodermatitis enteropathica) because of malabsorption associated with chronic diarrohoea are other cutaneous disorders in paediatric population with HIV infection. Kaposi's sarcoma is less frequently reported in children than in adults. Non-specific findings in children with HIV include long eye lashes, patchy alopecia, pyoderma gangrenosum and erythema dyschromicum perstans (ashy dermatosis).

Growth Failure

Growth failure is common due to malnutrition, diarrhoea, HIV-associated anorexia and hypermetabolism. Congenital HIV dysmorphism with facial malformation may be a contributing factor for growth failure.

Renal Disease

A direct effect of HIV on renal epithelial cells was suggested as a cause for HIV-associated nephropathy, and it was not a common finding. Other possible causes for renal disease in HIV are nephrotoxic drugs and immune complexes. Histologically focal glomerulosclerosis, segmental necrotizing glomerulonephritis and mesangial hyperplasia have been reported. Nephrotic syndrome is the most common manifestation in HIV infected children. It may be present with oedema, proteinuria, and hypoalbuminemia, and blood pressure may be normal.

Cardiovascular System

Symptomatic HIV infected children may present with dilated cardiomyopathy and left ventricular hypertrophy. Sinus arrhythmia and resting sinus tachycardia have also been reported. Echocardiography and ECG testing should be done for cardiac evaluation.

DIAGNOSIS

The diagnosis of HIV infection is usually based on laboratory criteria. WHO provides case definitions for (a) HIV infection and (b) advanced HIV (including AIDS) reporting for adults and children.

WHO Case Definition for HIV Infection

- **Children younger than 18 months**

  Maternal antibodies can be detected in children up to the age of 18 months. Therefore, a direct method of detecting HIV is necessary. Identification by PCR is highly sensitive and specific.
  HIV infection is diagnosed based on a positive virological test for HIV or its components (HIV-RNA or HIV-DNA or ultrasensitive HIV p24 antigen) and confirmed by a second virological test obtained from a separate determination taken more than 4 weeks after birth. Cord blood is not useful for diagnosis because maternal cells may be present in it and may give a false positive test result.[21]
  Positive antibody testing is not recommended for definitive or confirmatory diagnosis of HIV infection in children upto 18 months of age.

- **Children 18 months or older and adults**

  HIV infection is diagnosed based on positive HIV antibody testing (rapid or laboratory-based enzyme immunoassay). This is usually confirmed by a second HIV antibody test (rapid or laboratory based enzyme immunoassay) relying on different antigens or of different operating characteristics.
  and/or
  A positive virological test for HIV or its' components (HIV-RNA or HIV-DNA or ultrasensitive HIV p24 antigen) and confirmed by a second virological test obtained from a separate determination.

Criteria for Diagnosis of Advanced HIV (including AIDS) for Children and Adults

- **Clinical criterion for diagnosis of advanced HIV in children and adults with confirmed HIV infection**

  Presumptive or definitive diagnosis of any stage-3 or stage-4 condition

- **Immunological criterion for diagnosing advanced HIV in children 5 years or older and adults with confirmed HIV infection**

  CD4 count less than 359 per mm^3 of blood in an HIV infected child or adult

- **Immunological criterion for diagnosing advanced HIV in a child younger than 5 years of age with confirmed HIV infection**

  % CD4+ <30 among those younger than 12 months
  %CD4 + <25 among those aged 12-35 months
  %CD4 + <20 among those aged 36-59 months

The WHO proposed immunological classification for established HIV infections is given in Table 9.5.

The detection of HIV infection in women before or during pregnancy allows the identification of HIV exposed infants and ensures care for the infected. The serological tests include ELISA and supplemental tests such as Western blot or immunofluorescence assay to confirm positive ELISA tests. Passive transfer of maternal HIV antibodies across placenta to the foetus may give rise to positive antibody tests in all newborn infants. As the HIV antibody may be present in uninfected infants upto the age of 18 months, a positive test for HIV antibody cannot be used for definitive diagnosis in infants younger than 18 months. HIV infection can be identified by the demonstration of IgA or IgM anti-HIV antibodies in infants because these maternal immunoglobulins do not cross the placenta. HIV-IgA antibody assay is insensitive for the detection of infection in the first 3 months (17% at first month, 67% at 3 months), but it is a very sensitive assay in infants 6 months of age (94% detected at 6 months, 100% detected at 9 months). Hence the use of IgA assay in the diagnosis of HIV infection in infants is limited.

Table 9.5 WHO Proposed Immunological Classification for Established HIV Infection

HIV Associated Immunodeficiency	*Age-related CD4 Values*			
	<11 months (% CD4+)	12-35 months (% CD4+)	36-59 months (% CD4+)	>5 years (absolute number per mm^3 or % CD4+)
None or not significant	>35	>30	>25	>500
Mild	30-35	25-30	20-25	350-499
Advanced	25-29	20-24	15-19	200-349
Severe	<25	<20	<15	<200 or < 15%

Viral diagnostic tests (PCR, viral culture) can be used to definitely diagnose HIV infection. Definitive diagnosis can be made in most cases by age 1 month and possibly in all cases by age 6 months. A positive virological test indicates possible HIV infection and should be confirmed by a second virological test. Virological tests in HIV exposed infants should be performed within the first 48 hours of age and at 14 days as test sensitivity is rapidly increased during the second week. Repeat testing is recommended at age one to two months and at age three to six months if the initial tests were negative. HIV infection in non-breastfed children may be reasonably excluded with two or more negative virological tests performed at age greater than 4 weeks, and one of those being performed at age greater than 16 weeks. Loss of HIV antibody in a child with previously negative virological tests definitely confirm the child is uninfected.

Perinatally exposed infants may be considered as "seroreverters" if they have become antibody-negative after 6 months of age, have no other laboratory evidence of infection, and have not met any AIDS-defining condition. The median age of seroreversion in uninfected children is 10 months, but in a few cases, the presence of HIV antibody can be demonstrated until 18 months of age. Hence definitive diagnosis cannot be established before 18 months of age with HIV antibody tests.

The acquisition of HIV infection occurs during intrauterine and intrapartum periods. Early (i.e. intrauterine) infection is considered in infants with a positive virological test at or before 48 h of life. Late (i.e. intrapartum) infection is considered in infants who have a negative virological test during the first week of life and subsequent positive tests in the later period.[11] Infants with early infection may tend to have more rapid disease progression and need more aggressive therapeutic approach than those with late infection.

HIV infection in infants and children can be detected by several laboratory methods, which include HIV culture, HIV DNA or RNA by PCR, HIV p24 antigen and immune complex dissociated p24 antigen (ICD-p24). HIV DNA PCR is the preferred virological method as it is sensitive to diagnosing HIV infection during the neonatal period. HIV RNA PCR method can be used in HIV exposed infants, but its sensitivity and specificity are more limited when compared to HIV DNA PCR for early diagnosis. By age of 28 days, HIV DNA PCR would have 96% sensitivity and 99% specificity to identify HIV proviral DNA.[12]

HIV culture has sensitivity similar to that of DNA PCR, but it is more expensive and results may not be available until 2-4 weeks. The sensitivity of ICD-p24 antigen is less and is not considered for routine use. The p24 antigen assay in infants less than a month of age is not recommended because of high frequency of false positive tests.

MONITORING OF PAEDIATRIC HIV

Laboratory tests and clinical evaluation should be done to monitor disease progression in HIV infected children. These include (1) immunological criteria, (2) plasma viral load and (3) clinical aspects.

Immunological Criteria

In HIV infected children, CD4+ T cell absolute count and percentage are markers of disease progression. In healthy infants, a higher CD4+ T cell absolute count and percentage have been observed when compared to healthy adults, and these counts reach adult values by age of 6 years. CD4+ T cell percentage in each immunological category does not change with age. CD4+ T cell absolute count has been found to change with age. Hence CD4+ percentage is taken into consideration in identifying disease progression in children.

The CD4+ T cell count declines as HIV infection progresses, and a patient with lower CD4+ T cell counts has poorer prognosis than a patient with higher counts. Transient decrease in CD4+ T cell count and percentage may occur in the presence of mild illness or vaccinations, and those values should be measured when the patients recover from illness. Due to higher CD4+ T cell counts in children, age-adjusted CD4+ T cell values are taken into account in identifying the disease progression. CD4+ T cell values should be measured immediately in a HIV infected child and every 3 months thereafter. Frequent monitoring is needed in children with immunological or clinical deterioration or to confirm an abnormal value. The risk of disease progression associated with a specific CD4 percentage or count varies with the age of the child. Infants in the first year of life experience proportionately higher risks than older children for any given CD4 stratum.[34] However, all age groups demonstrate rapid increases in risk as CD4 percentage decreases below 15–20%.[12]

Two CD4+ T cell measurements are needed with a minimum of one week gap between measurements when modification in therapy is recommended (Table 9.6).

Table 9.6 **Laboratory Parameters for Age-related CD4 Values**

Immunological Marker	*Age-specific Recommendation to Initiate ART*		
	<18 months	18 months – 5 years	>5 years
CD4%*	<25%	<15%	<10%
CD4 count**	<1500 cells/mm^3	<500 cells/mm^3	<200 cells/mm^3
Total *lymphocyte* count (where CD4 assays are not available)	<3400 cells/mm^3	<2300 cells/mm^3	<1200 cells/mm^3

* Immunological markers supplement clinical staging.

** CD4 cell percentage is preferred in children aged under 5 years; for all other children, CD4 count should be used.

Plasma Viral Load

Quantitative HIV RNA assays can determine viral load in peripheral blood. HIV RNA copy number and CD4 percentage or count are independent predictors of disease progression and mortality risk in both HIV infected children and adults, and the use of these two markers defines prognosis more accurately. HIV viral load should be assessed at once the child is tested positive for HIV by virological tests and every 3-4 months thereafter. The test may be repeated to confirm an abnormal value or when initiating or changing antiretroviral therapy. As untreated infants under 6-12 months of age show rapid disease progression, HIV RNA load is done more frequently, i.e. for every 1-2 months to identify those with rapid progression and start antiretroviral therapy.

Primary infection in adults show high HIV RNA levels. Humoral and cell-mediated immune response to HIV may lead to decline in HIV RNA levels to about 2-3 log^{10} copies and reaches a virological set point approximately within 6-12 months following primary infection. Several studies have indicated that infected adults with high HIV RNA set points have rapid progression than those with lower HIV RNA set points.

Perinatally infected infant's HIV RNA pattern takes a different course from that in infected adults. Some studies have shown that low HIV RNA levels were found at birth and reached peak values at about 2 months of age and then slowly declined. The mean HIV RNA levels within the first year of age was 185,000 copies/ml.[13] In contrast to the adult pattern, HIV RNA levels have shown decreased levels after one year of age, and these levels would continue to fall in the next few years of life.[35-38] This pattern may be due to an immature immune system in infants in controlling viral replication.

Interpretation of HIV RNA Assays

Plasma HIV RNA can be measured by three different assays. These include

(1) HIV-1 reverse transcriptase quantitative polymerase chain reaction assay (Amplicor HIV-1 Monitor Test, version 1.5, Roche Diagnostics; lower limit of detection differs between "ultrasensitive" assay (<50 copies/ml) and "regular sensitivity" assay (<400 copies/ml)
(2) HIV-1 nucleic acid sequence-based amplification test (nuclisens HIV-1 QT, bioMerieux)
(3) HIV-1 in vitro signal amplification, branched chain nucleic acid probe assay (bDANA) (VERSANT HIV-1 RNA 3.0 Assay)

The lower limit of detection for the assays differs (<50 copies/ml for the Amplicor assay, <80 copies/ml for the Nuclisens assay, and <75 copies/ml for the VERSANT assay). When a single specimen is subjected to two different assays for viral load, the absolute HIV RNA copy number can differ by twofold (0.3 log_{10}) or more.[14-17] Therefore, one method should be used consistently to estimate the viral load.

In young children, the choice of HIV RNA assay can be determined by the amount of blood required for the test. The least amount of blood (i.e. 100 μl of plasma) is required by the Nuclisens test followed by the Amplicor (i.e. 200 μl of plasma), and the VERSANT assays need 1 ml of plasma.

Biological variation in viral load tends to occur and is greater in infected infants and young children than in infected adults. This variation in a stable infected adult may vary as much as threefold (0.5 log_{10}) in either direction in a day or on different days.[18-20] Infected infants and young children may have grater biological variation in HIV RNA levels.

In perinatally infected children, there is a slow decline of viral load even without therapy in the early age. The HIV RNA load may be at higher levels than in most infected adults.[21-23]

The biological variation in HIV RNA levels should be taken into account while interpreting changes in HIV RNA load, since an average decline of approximately 0.6 log_{10} per year occurs during the first 12-24 months of age, and these values further decrease by about 0.3 log_{10} per year until 4-5 years of age. This biological variability must be taken into consideration when interpreting changes in viral load in children. Further viral load change greater than fivefold (0.7 log^{10}) in children aged <2 years of age and those greater than three fold (0.5 log_{10}) in children >2 years of age should be considered as a significant change. Two HIV RNA measurements should be taken before a change in therapy in considered.

The predominant subtype in the United States is B, whereas non-B subtypes are predominant in other parts of the world. Initial assays were used to can detect subtype B only. However, current kits detect and quantitate all viral subtypes except the uncommon O subtype.[20,24]

ANTIRETROVIRAL (ARV) THERAPY

WHO Guidelines for the Treatment of HIV Infection in Infants and Children in Resource-limited Settings (2005 Revision)

The ideal ART should provide a clinical, immunological and virological benefits in children. Treatment with HAART has a major impact on the health of HIV infected children, and substantial decrease in mortality rate has been reported. Adherence to therapy is important and lack of adherence to recommended regimen may lead to subtherapeutic levels of ARV drugs with subsequent development of drug resistance and virological failure. Antiretroviral drugs may be classified into four categories given below:

NRTI/NTRTI	NNRTI	PI	FUSION INHIBITORS
• Zidovudine (AZT)	• Nevirapine (NVP)	• Amprenavir (APV)	• Enfuvirtide (Fuzeon, T-20)
• Didanosine (DDI)	• Efavirenz (EFV)	• Atazanavir (ATV)	
• Zalcitabine (DDC)	• Delavirdine (DLV)	• Darunavir (DRV)	
• Stavudine (D4T)		• Fosamprenavir (F-APV)	
• Lamivudine (3TC)		• Indinavir (IDV)	
• Abacavir (ABC)		• Lopinavir/Ritonavir (LPV/RTV)	
• Emtricitabine (FTC)		• Nelfinavir (NFY)	
• Tenofovir Disoproxil Fumarate (TDF)		• Ritonavir (RTV)	
		• Saquinavir (SQV Hard Gel Capsules)	
		• Tipranavir (TPV)	

Initiation of ART in Children

ART should be initiated in HIV infected children to provide improvement in neurodevelopment, growth, immunological and virological parameters. A WHO working group has proposed the following guidelines for the treatment of HIV infected children.

(A) Clinical criteria: infants and children with confirmed HIV infection

- WHO paediatric clinical stage IV disease: treat all children irrespective of laboratory parameters
- WHO paediatric clinical stage III disease: treat all children irrespective of CD4; in children aged over 18 months, treatment is guided by CD4 where available, especially in children with lymphocytic interstitial pneumonia, oral hairy leukoplakia, or low platelet count
- WHO paediatric clinical stage II disease treat by CD4 guidance or, where CD4 is not available, guided by total lymphocyte count
- WHO paediatric clinical stage I disease: treatment only guidance by CD4; if CD4 is not available, children should not be initiated on ARV therapy

WHO recommends treatment for all children with ARV combination therapy under paediatric clinical stage IV irrespective of laboratory parameters, or WHO paediatric clinical stage III irrespective of the CD4 count; in children >18 months of age, treatment is guided by CD4 count if available, especially in children with oral hairy leukoplakia, lymphocytic interstitial pneumonia, or low platelet count.

For children with WHO clinical stage I or II disease, offer treatment as guided by CD4. If CD4 is not available, children should not be offered treatment in WHO clinical stage I, and treatment is guided by total lymphocyte count in WHO clinical stage II.

(B) Clinical criteria: symptomatic infants and children with unconfirmed HIV infection

For infants and children under 18 months of age where virological testing or p24 antigen is not available to confirm HIV infection status, WHO recommends the use of presumptive diagnosis of clinical stage IV HIV disease. This should be made if:

- The child's HIV exposure is confirmed by antibody testing.
- The child is symptomatic with two or more of the following:
  - Oral thrush
  - Severe pneumonia (as defined in IMCI)
  - Severe wasting/malnutrition (as defined in IMCI)
  - Severe sepsis (as defined in IMCI)
  - CD4 percentages, where available, below 25%

Other factors that support presumptive diagnosis of clinical stage IV HIV disease in an HIV seropositive infant include:

- ❖ Recent HIV-related maternal death
- ❖ Advanced HIV disease in the mother.

WHO GUIDELINES FOR TREATMENT

Recommended First-line Regimens

At present three different types of combination regimens are used in treatment-naïve children, namely NNRTI based (1NNRTI+ 2NRTI), PI based (1-2 PI + 2NRTI), and triple NRTI based regimens. In resource-limited settings, a limited number of first-line and second-line regimens are used. Selection of the ARV treatment regimen is individualized and takes a number of factors into consideration that include potency, side effect profile, adherence, comorbidity or conditions such as tuberculosis, Hepatitis B and/or C, drug interactions, resistant viral strains and potential for maintenance of future treatment options.

General Guidelines

Selection of dual NRTI is the backbone of initial combination therapy. Currently six NRTIs that include zidovudine, didanosine, lamivudine, stavudine, abacavir and emtricitabine are approved by FDA for use in children less than 13 years of age. Dual NRTI combinations are the backbone of HAART regimens in HIV infected children.

Extensive experience with well-known combination including Zidovudine + Lamivudine, Stavudine + Didano-sine, and Didanosine + Lamivudine has shown that they are preferred dual NRTI combinations for initiation of therapy in children. However, as DDI absorption is decreased after food, it is recommended that DDI can be given under fasting conditions when possible.

Another NRTI combination is Abacavir in combination with Zidovudine, Lamivudine or Stavudine. Abacavir-containing regimens are shown to be as or possibly more potent than Zidovudine + Lamivudine. But abacavir has been associated with possible life-threatening hypersensitivity reactions. Stavudine-containing regimens are used as dual NRTI backbone regimens, but it has shown higher risk of lipoatrophy and hyperlactemia than other NRTI drugs. As Zidovudine with Stavudine combination has antagonistic effect on HIV-1, this combination should not be used.

NNRTIs

Nevirapine and Efavirenz have been approved in children. Delaviridine was found to be having least potent antiretroviral activity in adults, and this drug has neither been studied in children nor recommended as initial regimen. Nevirapine is available as liquid formulation, while Efavirenz is available as a capsule or tablet. The advantages of NNRTI use are that there is a lower pill burden and they preserve PIs for future therapy. The major disadvantage of NNRTI drugs is cross-resistance of the entire class when a single NNRTI confers drug resistance. These drugs are associated with life threatening skin and hepatic toxicities the and reactions are most frequent with Nevirapine. Efavirenz in combination with two NRTIs is preferred in children >3 years of age based on clinical experience, in children and the results are comparable to those seen in adults. Nevirapine is the preferred NNRTI in children <3 years of age as initial therapy who require a liquid formulation.

PIs

Lopinavir/ritonavir regimens have very potent virological activity in treatment-naïve patients. Ritonavir in low doses when combined with other PIs acts as a "pharmacokinetic booster" by inhibiting the metabolism of other PIs, and increase drug exposure by prolonging the half-life of the second drug. Nelfinavir is well tolerated but virological potency has wide variability between studies, with virological suppression ranging from 26 to 69%.

The advantages of PI-based regimens include excellent virological potency and high barrier for development of drug resistance. However, the drugs have multiple drug interactions and metabolic complications such as fat maldistribution, dyslipidemia and insulin resistance.

Preferred Option

The combination of two NRTI and one NNRTI is the preferred ART regimen. It was proposed to add abacavir (ABC) as an additional NRTI option in regimen in view of treatment outcomes. HAART is recommended for initial treatment of infected children because it preserves immune function and delays disease progression.

Dual NRTI backbone	NNRTI
AZT + 3TC D4T + 3TC ABC + 3TC AZT + ABC D4T + ABC	NVP: Infants and children <3 years of age EFZ: Infants and children >3 years of age

Alternative Option

A triple nucleoside regimen (i.e. AZT + 3TC + ABC) remains an alternative option to treat HIV infected children when NNRTI-based or a PI-based regimen cannot be used because of concerns of toxicities, regimen complexity and drug interactions. The advantages of three NRTI regimens are lower pill burden, fewer drug-drug interactions and availability as a fixed dose combination (Zidovudine + Lamivudine + Abacavir combined as Trizivir). However, several clinical trials have shown that three NRTI-based regimens had inferior virological response when compared to Efavirenz-based and PI-based regimens. Rifampin in the treatment of tuberculosis infected children has drug interactions with NNRTI and PI regimens. As rifamycin lowers the drug concentrations of NNRTIs and PIs, a triple-nucleoside regimen is indicated for children who receive concurrent treatment for tuberculosis.

Second-line on Failure of First-line Regimens

The choice of second-line regimen depends on the success of the first-line regimen given earlier, and any second-line treatment requires the use of a protease inhibitor.

In the event of failure of initial first-line therapy, the following regimens may be chosen as a choice of second-line therapy (Table 9.7). The dose and side effects of drugs used in paediatric HIV infection are summarised in Table 9.8.

Table 9.7

For Failure on First-line Regimen	*Change to Second-line NRTI Component*		*Change to Second-line PI Component*
AZT *or* d4T + 3TC + NVP *or* EFV°	ddl + ABC		LPV/r *or*
ABC + 3TC + NVP *or* EFV°	ddl + AZT	+	SQV/r[1] *or*
AZT *or* d4T + 3TC + ABC	ddl + EFV°/[3] *or* NVP		NFV[2]

°EFV should not be used in children aged less than 3 years or weighing less than 10 kg.
[1]Saquinavir/ritonavir (SQV/r) should not be used in children weighing less than 25 kg.
[2]Nelfinavir (NFV) can be used instead of lopinavir/ritonavir LPV/r or SQV/r where no cold chain is in place.
[3]Tenofovir (TDF) is currently not approved for clinical use in infants and children.

Table 9.8 **Antiretroviral Drugs Used in Paediatric HIV**

Drug	*Dose*	*Side Effects*
NRTIs/NtRTIs Zidovudine (AZT, ZDV)	Neonatal/infant dose (age <6 weeks) oral: 2 mg/kg every 6 hrs . Paediatric dose (6 wks to 12 years) oral: 160 mg per m^2 of body surface area every 8 h	Headache, macrocytic anaemia, neutropenia, myopathy, liver toxicity and increased risk of hypospadias

(*Contd.*)

Drug	*Dose*	*Side Effects*
Didanosine (ddi)	90-150 mg/m^2 every 12 h.	Diarrhoea, abdominal pain, nausea, vomiting, peripheral neuropathy, electrolyte abnormalities, pancreatitis, increased liver enzymes and retinal depigmentation
Zalcitabine (ddc)	0.01 mg/kg every 8 h	Gastrointestinal disturbances, oral ulcers, oesophageal ulcers, skin rashes, peripheral neuropathy, pancreatitis, hepatic toxicity, lactic acidosis and severe hepatomegaly with steatosis
Lamivudine (3TC)	Neonatal dose: 2 mg/kg twice daily. Paediatric dose: 4 mg/kg (maximum dose: 150 mg) twice daily	Headache, nausea, diarrhoea, skin rash, anaemia, pancreatitis, peripheral neuropathy, fat redistribution, decreased neutrophil count. Lactic acidosis and severe hepatomegaly with steatosis. Rarely severe anaemia has been reported with use of 3 TC and ZDV combination
Stavudine (d4T)	Neonatal/infant dose (at birth to 13 days): 0.5 mg/kg every 12 h. Paediatric dose (age 14 days up to weight of 30 kg): 1 mg/kg every 12 h	Headache, GI disturbances, skin rashes, lipoatrophy, peripheral neuropathy, pancreatitis, lipodystrophy, hepatomegaly with steatosis, lactic acidosis and motor weakness
Abacavir (ABC)	Neonatal/infant dose: not approved in infant age less than 3 months. Paediatric dose (age > 3 months): 8 mg/kg BID (maximum dose 300 mg) twice daily	Diarrhoea, fever, nausea, vomiting, skin rashes. Fatal hypersensitivity reaction, and symptoms may include fever, diarrhoea, nausea, vomiting, and skin rashes. Lactic acidosis with hepatic steatosis and pancreatitis
NNRTIs **Nevirapine (NVP)**	Neonatal/infant dose (through age 2 months): 5 mg/kg or 120 mg/m^2 once daily for 14 days followed by 120 mg/m^2 every 12 h for 14 days, followed by 200 mg/m^2 every 12 h.	Skin rash, Stevens-Johnson syndrome, toxic epidermal necrolysis, fever, fatal hepatotoxicity and hypersensitivity reactions.
	Paediatric dose: 120–200 mg/m^2 twice daily Note: Initiate therapy with 120 mg/m^2 once daily for 14 days, later 120-200 mg/m^2 twice daily	

(*Contd.*)

Drug	*Dose*	*Side Effects*
Efavirenz (EFV)	Not approved in neonates/ infants. No data available for children <3 years of age. Children >3 years: 10 to 15 kg: 200 mg (270 mg = 9 ml) once daily 15 to <20 kg: 250 mg (300 mg = 10 ml) once daily 20 to <25 kg: 300 mg (360 mg = 12 ml) once daily	Skin rash, increased transaminase levels. Central nervous system abnormalities primarily reported in adults (e.g. somnolence, insomnia, abnormal dreams, abnormal thinking, hallucinations and depersonalization).
Protease inhibitors	25 to <33 kg: 350 mg (450 mg = 15 ml) once daily 33 to <40 kg: 400 mg (510 mg = 17 ml) once daily Maximum dose: 40 kg: 600 mg once daily	
Lopinavir/Ritonavir (LPV/RTV) for individuals receiving concomitant NVP or EFV or APV	Not approved in neonates / infants. Paediatric dose: 7 to <15 kg: LPV 13 mg/kg + 3.25 mg/kg RTV twice daily with food 15–50 kg: LPV 11 mg/kg + 2.75 mg/kg RTV twice daily with food >50 Kg: LPV 533 mg/ 133 mg RTV twice daily with food (same as adult dose) or 300 mg LPV/m^2 body surface area/ RTV 75 mg/m^2 body surface area twice daily with food (up to a maximum dose of 533 mg LPV/RTV 133 mg)	Headache, diarrhoea, nausea, vomiting, fat redistribution, elevations in triglycerides and cholesterol, hyperglycemia, new onset diabetes mellitus, exacerbation of preexisting diabetes mellitus, ketoacidosis, spontaneous bleeding in hemophilics, hemolytic anaemia, elevations in serum transaminases, hepatitis and pancreatitis
Nelfinavir (NFV)	Neonatal/infant dose not approved. Paediatric dose (2 to 13 years): 45-55 mg/kg BID	More common side effects are diarrhoea, flatulence, abdominal pain and rash. Lipodystrophy syndrome, new onset diabetes mellitus and exacerbation of previous hyperglycemia, ketoacidosis, spontaneous bleeding in hemophiliacs and elevated serum transaminases
Amprenavir (APV)	Not approved in neonates / infants. Paediatric dose: not approved in children <4 years of age. Children 4- 12 years or	GI disturbances, rash, Stevens-Johnson syndrome, perioral paresthesias, lipodystrophy, neutropenia, fat redistribution, new onset diabetes mellitus, hyperglycemia,

(*Contd.*)

Drug	*Dose*	*Side Effects*
	13-16 years of age weighing <50 kg, oral solution: 22.5 mg/kg twice daily (max daily dose: 2,800 mg) Caps: 20 mg/kg bid (max daily dose: 2,400 mg) Children 13-16 years wt >500 kg, oral solution: 1400 mg bid	diabetic ketoacidosis, spontaneous bleeding in hemophilics, hemolytic anaemia, elevated serum transaminases and creatine kinase levels and acanthosis nigricans
Ritonavir (RTV)	Not approved for use in neonates/infants. Paediatric dose: 400 mg/m^2 twice daily (not to exceed 600 mg per dose). Start with 250 mg/m^2 bid and increase at 2-3 day intervals by 50 mg/m^2 bid to full dose as tolerated	GI disturbances, circumoral paraesthesia, lipid abnormalities, hepatitis, fat redistribution, new onset diabetes mellitus, hyperglycemia, diabetic ketoacidosis, spontaneous bleeding in hemophiliacs and pancreatitis
Indinavir (IDV)	Not approved for use in neonates/infants. Paediatric dose: Not approved for use in children. Investigational dose: 500 mg/m^2 three times a day in children aged 4-15 years	Metallic taste, dizziness, asymptomatic hyperbilirubinemia (10%), nephrolithiasis (4%), lipid abnormalities, new onset diabetes mellitus, hyperglycemia, diabetic ketoacidosis, exacerbation of preexisting diabetes mellitus, spontaneous bleeding in hemophilics and hepatitis.

Insufficiency of Data in Drug Combinations

Data are preliminary or insufficient for the following drugs or drug combinations for use as initial therapy in children:

- Dual PIs with the exception of Lopinavir/ritonavir. PIs other than LPV/r can be used as secondary treatment regimens for children who have failed initial therapy
- NRTI plus NNRTI plus PI
- Tenofovir-containing regimens
- Enfuvirtide (T20)-containing regimens
- Atazanavir-containing regimens
- Darunavir-containing regimens
- Fosamprenavir-containing regimens
- Tipranavir-containing regimens

Evidence against use of ARV regimens in children includes:

1. Overlapping toxicities may occur and/or
2. Use may be virologically undersirable

An account of ARV regimens not recommended to children is given below.

Drugs	*Disadvantages*
Monotherapy	Inferior antiviral activity Rapid development of resistance
2 NRTIs alone	Inferior antiviral activity Rapid development of resistance
APV oral solution in children <4 years	Large amount of propylene glycol in oral liquid may be toxic to the child
APV oral solution + ritonavir oral solution	APV oral solution contains large amount of propylene glycol which may compete with ethanol in ritonavir oral solution for same metabolic pathway. It leads to the accumulation of ether with resulting toxicity
Amprenavir + fosamprenavir (APV + f-APV)	f-APV is a prodrug of Amprenavir. No additional benefit by combination of both drugs and may increase toxicity
Atazanavir + indinavir	Additive hypobilirubinemia
Dual NRTI combinations (Lamivudine + Emtricitabine)	3 TC should not be used with FTC because of similar resistance profile and no additional benefit
ZDV + d4T	Antagonism with this combination on HIV
Zalcitabine-containing combinations	Lack of paediatric formulation
Tenofovir + didanosine + (Lamivudine or Emtricitabine)	High rate of early virological nonresponse
Tenofovir + abacavir + (Lamivudine or Emtricitabine)	High rate of early virological nonresponse
Saquinavir	Appropriate dose of SQV alone and in combination with second PI has not been determined in children

COTRIMOXAZOLE AS PROPHYLAXIS IN HIV EXPOSED[34]

According to WHO recommendation, cotrimoxazole prophylaxis is recommended for

- All HIV exposed children (born to HIV infected mothers) from 4-6 weeks of age (whether or not part of a prevention of mother-to-child transmission programme)
- Any child identified as infected with any clinical signs or symptoms suggestive of HIV, regardless of age or CD4 count

The recommended dosage of 6-8 mg/kg once daily should be used. If the child is on ARV therapy, cotrimoxazole can be stopped only when evidence of immunerestoration has occurred. This can be assumed where the child is over 18 months of age and CD4% >15 at two measurements at least 3 to 6 months apart. If the CD4 count is not available, cotrimoxazole should not be stopped before full 6 months of successful adherence to ARV therapy, and then only when clinical evidence of immunerestoration is present. Continuing cotrimoxazole may provide benefit although the child has clinically improved. If ARV therapy is not available, cotrimoxazole should not be discontinued.

IMMUNIZATION IN HIV INFECTED CHILDREN

HIV infection has been associated with immunosuppression and progressive deterioration in children making them susceptible to various types of infections. Inactivated vaccines (e.g. DTP, polio, hepatitis B) in immuno-compromised children may give varied response and may be inadequate. All inactivated vaccines are found safe in HIV patients. As there is suboptimal or poor immunological response in HIV infected children, a double dose is recommended (e.g. hepatitis B vaccine) to induce maximum response. Use of live vaccines can result in severe vaccine-associated illness in children. In general, live vaccines are contraindicated in immunodeficient patients. However, some immunocompromised patients may have benefit from its use. Immunization recommendations for HIV infected children are shown in Table 9.9.

Table 9.9 **Immunization Recommendations in HIV Infected Children**

Vaccine	*WHO/UNICEF*	*Symptomatic HIV Infection*
BCG	Yes (at birth)	No
DTP	Yes (at 6, 10, 14 weeks)	Yes
OPV	Yes (at 6, 10, 14 weeks)	Yes
Measles	Yes (at 6 and 9 months)	Yes
Hepatitis B	Yes (as for uninfected children)	Yes
Hib	–	–
Pneumococcal	–	–
Influenza	–	–
Varicella	–	–
Meningococal	–	–

Prognosis

Two different patterns of disease progression have been observed in children. In the first group about 20% of children develop serious infections in the first year of life. This group is characterized by rapid progression of disease and most children die in the first 4 years of life. In the remaining 80% of cases, HIV-related symptoms develop at a slower rate and most of them may not develop serious symptoms until school age or even adolescence. Opportunistic infections are more often observed in HIV infected children with severe decline in CD4+ count. In children, opportunistic infections present as primary infections, whereas in adults they represent reactivation of a latent infection.

CONCLUSION

An effort to identify HIV in pregnant mothers ensures early recognition of HIV infection in the infant. HIV counselling to all pregnant women and educating about prevention of MTCT with antiretroviral prophylaxis regimens and risks in breastfeeding will drastically reduce the number of victims in the future. The management of HIV in children is to be carried out in close cooperation between paediatrician and physician dealing with the case.

REFERENCES

1. Centers for Disease Control: Follow up on Kaposi sarcoma and pneumocystis pneumonia. MM WR 1981; 30: 277.
2. Centers for Disease Control: Unexplained immunodeficiency and opportunistic infections in infants New York, New Jersey, California. MMWR 1982; 31: 665.
3. Zeigler JB, Cooper DA, Jhohnson RO, et al: Postnatal transmission of AIDS-associated retrovirus from mother to infant. Lancent 1985; 1: 896-8.
4. CDC HIV/AIDS FACT SHEET. Mother-to-Child (Perinatal) HIV Transmission and Prevention, http://www.cdc.gov/hiv/resources/factsheets/perinatl.htm.
5. NACO. Specialist's training and reference module, New Delhi: National AIDS Control Organization. http://www.nacoonline.org.
6. CDC. Treating Opportunistic Infections Among HIV-Exposed and Infected children, MMWR December 3, 2004/53(RR14); 1-63. http://www.cdc.gov/mmwr/preview/mmwrhtml/rr5314a1.htm.
7. Connor EM. Lymphocytic interstitial pneumonitis. Wilfert C, edr. Pediatric AIDS. 2nd edn. Baltimore: Williams & Wilkins; 1994. p. 467-481.
8. Zeitz M, Ullrich R, Schneider T, et al.: Cell differentiation and proliferation in the gastrointestinal tract with respect to the local immune system . Ann N Y Acad Sci 1994; 733: 75-86.
9. Keating J, Bjarnason I, Somasundaram S, et al: Intestinal absorptive capacity , intestinal permeability and jejunal histology in HIV and their relation to diarrhoea Gut 1995; 37: 623-9.
10. Batman PA, Kapembwa MS, Miller ARO et al : HIV enteropathy: comparative morphometry of the jejunal mucosa of HIV - infected patients resident in the United Kingdom and Uganda. Gut 1998; 43: 350.
11. Bryson YJ, Luzuriaga K, Sullivan JL, et al. Proposed definitions for in utero versus intrapartum transmission of HIV-1. N Engl J Med, 1992. 327: 1246-7.
12. UNAIDS. Joint WHO/UNAIDS/UNICEF statement on use of cotrimoxazole as prophylaxis in HIV exposed and HIV infected children. http://data.unaids.org/Media/Press-Statements01/ps_cotrimoxazole_22nov04_en.pdf
13. Shearer WT, Quinn TC, LaRussa P, et at. Viral load and disease progression in infants infected with human immunodeficiency virus type 1. Women and Infants Transmission Study Group. N Engl J Med, 1997; 336: 1337-42.
14. Goetz MB, Moatamed F, Howanitz JH. Measurement of plasma HIV viral load (VL) by bDNA versus RT PCR (PCR) assays. Clin Infect Dis 1997; 25: 394. (Abstract 207).
15. Brambilla D, Leung S, Lew J, et al. Absolute copy number and relative change in determinations of human immunodeficiency virus type 1 RNA in plasma: effect of an external standard on kit comparisons. J Clin Microbiol 1998; 36: 311-4.
16. Vandamme AM, Schmit JC, Van Dooren S, et al. Quantification of HIV -1 RNA in plasma: comparable results with the NASBA HIV-1 RNA QT and the AMPLICOR HIV monitor test. J Acquir Immune Defic Syndr Hum Retrovirol 1996; 13: 127-39.

17. Raboud JM, Montaner JSG, Conway B, et al. Variation in plasma RNA levels, CD4 cell counts, and p24 antigen levels in clinically stable men with human immunodeficiency virus infection. J Infect Dis 1996; 174: 191-4.
18. Centers for disease control and prevention guidelines for using antiretroviral agents in HIV infected adults and adolescents. MMWR. Last update. October 10, 2006: URL: http:// AIDSinfo.nih.gov- see this web site for most updated guidelines.
19. Hughes MD, Johnson V A, Hirsch MS, et al. Monitoring plasma HIV-1 RNA levels in addition to CD4+ lymphocyte count improves assessment of antiretroviral therapeutic response. ACTG 241 Protocol Virology Sub study Team. Ann Intern Med 1997; 126: 929-38.
20. Antunes R, Figueiredo S, Bartolo I, et al. Evaluation of the clinical sensitivities of three viral load assays with plasma samples from a pediatric population predominantly infected with human immunodeficiency virus type 1 subtype G and BG recombinant forms. J Clin Microbiol 2003; 41: 3361-7.
21. McIntosh K, Shevitz A, Zaknun D, et al. Age- and time-related changes in extracellular viral load in children vertically infected by human immunodeficiency virus. Pediatr Infect Dis J 1996; 15: 1087-91.
22. Mofenson LM, Korelitz J, Meyer WA, et at. The relationship between serum human immunodeficiency virus type 1 (HIV-l) RNA level, CD4 lymphocyte percent, and long-term mortality risk in HIV-l-infected children. National Institute of Child Health and Human Development Intravenous Immunoglobulin Clinical Trial Study Group. J Infect Dis 1997; 175: 1029-38.
23. Palumbo PE, Raskino C, Fiscus S, et at. Predictive value of quantitative plasma HIV RNA and CD4+ lymphocyte count in HIV-infected infants and children. JAMA 1998; 279: 756-61.
24. Plantier JC, Gueudin M, Damond F, et al. Plasma RNA quantification and HIV-1 divergent strains. J Acquir Immune Defic Syndr 2003; 33: 1-7.

10 | COUNSELLING IN HIV/AIDS

Dinesh Mathur, Veena Acharya

In this chapter

INTRODUCTION

HIV prevalence in India is lower than that previously estimated; however, its epidemic still continues to affect a large number of people. New and more accurate estimates of HIV indicate that approximately 2.5 million (2-3.1 million) people in India are living with HIV, with a national adult HIV prevalence of 0.36%.

WHAT COUNSELLING IS

It is a confidential dialogue between a client and a care provider aimed at enabling the client to cope with stress and take personal decisions related to HIV/AIDS. The counselling process includes an evaluation of personal risk of HIV transmission and facilitation of preventive measures. This includes information, education and psychosocial support, and allows individuals to make decisions that facilitate coping and preventive behaviours (WHO).

Counselling has become an integral part of prevention, diagnosis, management, care and support, of people living with HIV/AIDS. Even a doubt of the possibility of having an infection brings profound emotional, social, behavioural and medical consequences, and one has to deal with each one and its effects in different stages of life. Counselling enables a person's coping capacity to come out of difficult situations during the course of HIV disease. Since HIV infection is a dynamic, evolutionary and lifelong process, it makes new and changing demands on the patients, their relations and community. Counselling takes into account not only their immediate medical requirements but also their social relationships and attitudes about HIV/AIDS. It also provides information and education relevant to day-to-day life including the patient's sexual and occupational needs and general aspirations.

Both health education and counselling aim at changing risk behaviour. Although both use two-way interaction, they have a contrasting difference: education is emotionally neutral, whereas counselling has strong emotional overtones despite the detachment of the provider who augments the coping capacity of the client.

BASIC PURPOSES OF COUNSELLING

1. To motivate the person to prevent the spread of infection by helping in change of behaviour and lifestyle, improving quality of life and enabling to make future decisions with the acquisition of correct knowledge of reproductive and sexual health
2. To provide psychosocial support to the individual and family

THE PROCESS OF COUNSELLING

The process of counselling differs from place to place; however, risk assessment is the essential element. The counselor should not pre-judge the risk factors of any person, nor should be biased by the "appearance" of the patient, or the area where they come from should not be taken as an indicator of a risk factor.

In view of the many variables in defining risk, it is essential for the counselor to carry out a comprehensive sexual and lifestyle history of the patient. History-taking includes intravenous drug abuse, past history of blood transfusions, use of blood products for the treatment of haemophilia, sickle cell anemia or operations prior to the introduction of HIV screening of donors, intensive procedures carried out under non-sterile conditions such as circumcision, cosmetic procedures, and repeated infections.

In all counselling situations, there are some basic principles to be observed as follows:

- ❑ Welcoming the patient and using acceptable traditional greeting practices depending on local customs in that area.
- ❑ The room should be as comfortable as possible with diffuse light.
- ❑ The counselor should be seated facing the patient and not behind a table.
- ❑ The patient should be given a chance to pause or ask questions.
- ❑ The counselor should ask open-ended questions which would offer the patient a chance to answer or not to answer.

- Tell the patient directly, without evasion. Listen carefully.

Basic Micro-counselling Skills

Active attending and listening, reflection of feeling, effective questioning, paraphrasing and interpretation are essential skills in counselling.

Qualities of an Effective Counselor

- Positive regard or respect for people
- Open, non-judgmental and high level of acceptance
- Caring and empathetic
- Self-aware and self-disciplined
- Knowledgeable and informed about the subject
- Culturally sensitive
- Patient and good listener
- Ability to maintain confidentiality
- Objective and having clarity

Effective Feedback

In order to get effective feedback, questions should start with "I", as it reflects only subjective feelings and views. Some one else may feel differently about the same issue. So make statements beginning with "I feel", "I think" etc.

Give positive comments and offer alternatives or suggestions. Use simple words and short sentences. Do not interrupt or side-talk during interaction.

Essential Stages of Counselling

- Stage one: forming rapport and gaining the client's trust
- Stage two: defining and understanding roles, boundaries and needs
- Stage three: process of ongoing, supportive counselling.
- Stage four: closure or ending the counselling relationship

Elements of Counselling

The fundamental elements of any counselling programme can be summarized by a mnemonic "GATHER", which is used in counselling situations like family planning.

The GATHER approach could be understood as follows.

G – Greet the client politely
A – Ask about their needs, doubts, concerns
T – Tell the client about the facts, side effects and give options
H – Help the client to choose
E – Explain about the different issues
R – Return for follow-up

TYPES OF HIV/AIDS COUNSELLING

1. Pre-test counselling: counselling before the test for HIV
2. Post-test counselling: counselling after the HIV test is done, whether positive or negative
3. Risk reduction assessment
4. Counselling after a diagnosis of AIDS has been made
5. Family and relationship counselling
6. Bereavement counselling
7. Outreach counselling
8. Crisis counselling
9. Telephone and hotline counselling

Counselling in HIV-positive women regarding reproductive health issues includes the following:

1. Counselling for preventing pregnancy
2. Counselling for MTP (medical termination of pregnancy)
3. Counselling for the use of ARV during pregnancy, postpartum period and to the neonate
4. Counselling for breastfeeding
5. Counselling for family members to develop positive attitude and to support HIV infected women during pregnancy, delivery and nursing of mothers.

WHO CAN PROVIDE COUNSELLING

Any dedicated person who has got basic information and training in different issues of HIV/AIDS and counselling skills can provide counselling. These persons include primarily health care providers namely doctors, nurses, paramedical staff, psychologists, psychotherapists and social workers. Non-health care providers such as teachers, health educators, religious and community leaders, youth workers and traditional healers can also provide counselling after suitable training.

Where Counselling Can Be Provided

Counselling can be provided in any setting where discussion about HIV/AIDS can take place such as out-patient departments in hospitals, STD, ANC and family planning clinics, blood banks, drug deaddiction centers, prisons, community health centers and schools.

Indications for Counselling

People who are candidates for testing of STDs and HIV, identified patients of HIV disease, and people seeking help/assistance because of their current or past high risk behaviour should be given counselling (Table 10.1).

Table 10.1 Indication for HIV Counselling and Testing

- Clinical indications
- Acute HIV seroconversion symptoms
- Signs and symptoms of HIV (e.g. unexplained weight loss, fever, atypical pneumonia or oral thrush)
- Confirmation, if prior reported positive test is not documented
- Prior risk behaviour
- Multiple sex partners, sex partner at risk, prior or recent STD diagnosis, injection drug use and transfusion of blood and its products before screening for HIV, haemophilics who received factor VIII before screening for HIV, men who have sex with men (MSM)
- Pregnant women
- Exposure to HIV
- Occupational exposure
- Sexual or drug abuse
- Persons who request HIV testing

Pre-test counselling: Counselling is very much needed when a person is offered a test to know about his or her HIV status. Pre-test counselling (Table 10.2) should include accurate and updated information about transmission and prevention of HIV and other STDs. Inform about the window period of the HIV test, i.e. a period of 12 weeks since the last possible exposure to HIV should have elapsed by the time of testing. Explain clearly what a test can do, i.e. it looks only for the antibodies to HIV and it is not a test for AIDS, the difference between HIV-positive and AIDS, and how would the client cope personal resources, support network of friends, family members and community. Inform that the HIV-positive status has to be disclosed to the sex partner under the course of law. Inform from where the results of test are to be collected in person.

Table 10.2 Components of HIV Pre-test Counselling

- Ascertain risk
- Discuss likelihood and meaning of positive, negative and indeterminate test results
- Assess understanding of HIV transmission and natural history, psychological stability, social support, impact of a positive result
- Discuss confidentiality provisions and anonymous testing
- Ensure that follow-up is available (especially important when testing occurs in urgent care settings)
- Emphasize the importance of obtaining test results
- Discuss risk reduction plan and referral to other services if needed
- Obtain informed consent for HIV antibody testing

Post-test counselling: The results of a HIV test should always be given in person and under all precautions of keeping confidentiality. If a person is HIV-negative with a possibility of window period, he or she should be asked to come again and get the test done later. They should also be given all information regarding safer practices so that chances of they contracting HIV/AIDS in future also become less (Table 10.3).

Table 10.3 Components of HIV Post-test Counselling

- Ensure the client is ready to receive results
- Disclose test results and provide interpretation (positive, negative, indeterminate) in the context of person's risk of infection

If a person is HIV-positive, then break the bad news in an appropriate manner. Recommended manner of breaking a bad news is eliciting the person's understanding, exploring his or her knowledge and breaking the news in manageable chunks. Acknowledge immediate reactions and allow time to absorb initial shock. The counselor has to deal with emotional reactions and offer support as appropriate. The counselor has also to give correct information about future management and refer to an appropriate agency to manage his or her clinical or social problems. It has been frequently observed that the client invariably denies the bad news, and this denial is a valid mechanism of coping which may be total (rare) or ambivalent. Sometimes relatives may also encourage denial.

Other psychological events encountered are:

- ❑ Initial shock of diagnosis and hopelessness for the future
- ❑ Anxiety and fear of uncertain prognosis, incurability of the disease and reactions of family members
- ❑ Anger and frustration of becoming infected and development of sense of guilt
- ❑ Depression due to possible social, occupational and sexual rejection

COUNSELLING HIV-SERONEGATIVE PERSONS

Readdress and Reinforce Risk Reduction Plan

Discuss the need for repeat testing for those with recent (<6 months) exposure or ongoing risk behaviour.

COUNSELLING PERSONS WITH INDETERMINATE HIV-1 WESTERN BLOT

Discuss prevalence and risk factors for indeterminable cases; for persons with p24 bands and for those with risk behaviour, discuss the possibility of acute HIV infection and need for serological follow-up at 1, 3 and 6 months; discuss safe sexual and drug use behaviour until indeterminacy is resolved.

Consider performing supplemental assays (e.g. polymerase chain reaction) to more quickly identify seroconverters and reassure those with HIV infection.

COUNSELLING HIV-SEROPOSITIVE PERSONS

- ❑ Explain the meaning of a positive HIV test (HIV infected and thus potentially infectious)
- ❑ Differentiate between being HIV infected and having AIDS
- ❑ Emphasize the importance of clinical interventions (ability to alter disease progression through antiretroviral therapy and prophylaxis against opportunistic infections)
- ❑ Discuss ways to avoid transmitting HIV to others (abstinence, condoms, not sharing needles if IDU)
- ❑ Assess the need for psychological support
- ❑ Provide referrals for medical, psychological or social services, if necessary
- ❑ Confirm HIV antibody test if positive test is not consistent with risk history
- ❑ Schedule follow-up visit to assess psychological status and to address partner notification issues

COUNSELLING ON FUTURE MANAGEMENT

Significant developments have occurred in the area of therapeutics of HIV. Knowledge about opportunistic infections and drugs to prevent them should be imparted to the patient together with side effects of antiretroviral therapy. Importance of treatment adherence, signs and symptoms of possible drug resistance and failure should also be told.

CONFIDENTIALITY

Confidentiality has always been an ethical and legal requirement for health professionals, and one should always take all precautions to keep confidentiality in dealing with HIV/AIDS patients. However, health care providers need to share information with colleagues to ensure proper care of the client. Doctors may need to discuss relevant health care information with patients and their family. Nurses have an obligation to document observations and care given (charting/report writing) to the patient. "Private" information may be disclosed with the patient's consent only.

COUNSELLING FOR ADOLESENTS

Teen AIDER is a comprehensive risk assessment and counselling plan for testing and risk reduction for adolesents (AIDER is a pnemonic for Assess, Inquire, Discuss, Educate, Readi-ness).

1. Create a confidential atmosphere
    - ❑ Assure youth about confidentiality of visit and ability to consent for testing
    - ❑ Assure youth that testing is their choice
    - ❑ Acknowledge the fact that it may be embarrassing to discuss sexual behaviours
    - ❑ Help youth to identify a supportive adult who is aware that the youth is being tested
2. HIV/AIDS knowledge
    - ❑ Allow adolescents to verbalize the understanding of HIV, clarify misconceptions and fill in gaps in knowledge
    - ❑ Assess feelings about testing and previous HIV testing experiences
    - ❑ Inquire if youth knows anyone with HIV/AIDS (e.g. sex partner, family member)

3. Sexual risk assessment
   - ❑ Assess sexual behaviours without making assumptions about sexual orientation; not all youth are heterosexual and not all youth who engage in same-sex behaviour self-identify as lesbians or gays
   - ❑ Assess number of partners, age differential and partner's known risks
   - ❑ Assess frequency of substance use in the context of sexual behaviour
   - ❑ Assess consistency of condom use and obstacles such as unassertiveness, desire to become pregnant, fear of violence and religiosity
   - ❑ Assess for history of sexual abuse or rape
4. Substance use and other risk assessments
   - ❑ Assess level of drug and alcohol use and reasons and context in which use occurs
   - ❑ Review risk of impaired judgment that may lead to unsafe sex
   - ❑ Assess potential need for drug treatment
   - ❑ Assess violence and substance use in home and community
5. Discuss and educate
   - ❑ Discuss abstinence
   - ❑ Discuss sexual activities that do not involve exchange of body fluids
   - ❑ Demonstrate proper condom use on anatomical models and provide opportunity for practice
   - ❑ Rehearse effective ways to communicate risk reduction with sexual partner(s)
   - ❑ Discuss personalized sex for youth who are not sexually active
   - ❑ Determine referral needs (e.g. medical, psychosocial, school/vocational, substance abuse, reproductive health, legal, housing, psychiatric)
6. Reading for HIV testing and referral
   - ❑ Adolescents should be informed about both anonymous and confidential testing
   - ❑ Provide education about partner notification and other options for disclosure to partners
   - ❑ Assess understanding of meaning of positive and negative test results
   - ❑ Assess understanding of benefits of early intervention
   - ❑ Determine with youth if testing should occur at this time and obtain informed consent
   - ❑ Strategies for coping (how to relieve stress and anxiety during the testing process)
   - ❑ Arrange follow-up appointment and ways for confidentially contacting youth, if needed

REFERENCES

1. HIV/AIDS Counselling training Manual for Trainers-A Document of NACO, Ministry of Health and Family Welfare, Govt. of India.
2. Chippindale S, French L. HIV Counselling and the psychosocial management of patients with HIV or AIDS. BMJ 2001; 322: 1533-5.
3. Counselling about HIV/AIDS- Role of Dermatovenerologists- Dr. Dinesh Mathur-Abstract from Oration in the 27th National Conference of IADVL, 1999, Bhuvaneshwar.
4. A Guide to clinical care of women with HIV. Editor Anderson JR Rockvilli, Maryland 2001.
5. AIDS epidemic update: December 2007.Joint United Nations Programme on HIV/AIDS (UNAIDS) and World Health Organization (WHO).

11 INTERACTION OF HUMAN IMMUNODEFICIENCY VIRUS AND SEXUALLY TRANSMITTED DISEASES

H K Kar

In this chapter

- Relationship between STDs and HIV Infection
- STDs as a Cofactor for HIV Transmission
- Effect of STDs Management on HIV Transmission
- Impact of HIV Infection/AIDS on other STDs and their treatment
- Conclusion

INTRODUCTION

Globally the majority of HIV epidemics is through heterosexual transmission; HIV infection is thus, by definition, one among the sexually transmitted infections (STIs) or diseases (STDs). The complex interaction between STDs and HIV has been demonstrated in many epidemiological, in vitro and clinical studies over the last many years.

The explosive spread of HIV 1 in areas where classic STDs are epidemic (e.g., sub-Saharan Africa, Thailand) has encouraged a remarkable number of studies designed to examine the association between these STDs (urethritis, cervicitis, and genital ulcers) and HIV 1 infection.[1,2] Demonstrating that STDs were indeed a cofactor was initially difficult, because HIV 1 and STDs share the same mode of transmission, and so associations seen in epidemiological studies may well have resulted from the confounding effect of risky sexual behaviours. Longitudinal studies provide strong evidence and show substantial relative risks for HIV 1 infection associated with various STDs. Classic STDs could facilitate HIV 1 transmission by increasing the infectiousness of the index case, the susceptibility of the partner, or both.[1,2]

RELATIONSHIP BETWEEN STDs AND HIV INFECTION

The relationship between STDs and HIV infection is complex and manifold, and both are acquired through sexual transmission.

1. STDs are biological cofactors for acquisition and transmission of HIV infection.
2. Concurrent HIV infection alters the natural history of classic STDs.
3. STDs are markers for high-risk behaviour for HIV infection.
4. Many of the measures for prevention of HIV and STDs are the same as are the target audiences for these interventions.
5. STD clinical services are important access points not only for diagnosis and treatment but also for prevention and counselling for HIV infection.
6. The management of STDs may reduce HIV transmission, particularly in developing countries.
7. Trends in STD incidence and prevalence can be a useful indicator of changes in sexual behaviour and, therefore, valuable for determining the impact of HIV/AIDS control programmes.

STDs AS A COFACTOR FOR HIV TRANSMISSION

During the last decade, from different epidemiological, clinical, biological and in vitro studies, overwhelming evidence has accumulated that both ulcerative and non-ulcerative STDs promote HIV transmission by augmenting HIV infectiousness and HIV susceptibility via different biological mechanisms.[3]

There is increased risk of HIV infection associated with common STDs (Table 11.1). Six out of ten studies in Kenya and Zaire found that people with genital ulcers caused mainly by chancroid were 2–5 times more likely to be infected with HIV than people without ulcers. Nine out of 11 studies of syphilis and HIV have found an association. Syphilis increased the risk of HIV infection three-to ninefold for heterosexual men. In three out of six studies of genital herpes and HIV infection, herpes doubled the risk of HIV infection for women and heterosexual men. Besides the genital ulcer disease (GUD), other studies have found that many non-ulcerative STDs like chlamydia infection, gonorrhoea and trichomoniasis could increase the risk of HIV transmission to women by three- to fivefold. Many studies from different regions of India show gradual but increasing prevalence of HIV infection among STD clinic attendees.[4-7] The prevalence was found higher among GUD patients than in non-ulcerative STD patients. The relative importance of ulcerative and non-ulcerative STDs appears to be complex. Owing to the greater frequency of non-ulcerative STDs in many populations, these infections may be responsible for more HIV transmission than genital ulcers.[3]

The possible mechanisms of the cofactor effect of ulcerative and non-ulcerative STDs on HIV transmission are as follows:

1. Lack of mechanical skin/mucous membrane/endocervical epithelium barrier makes easy viral entry due to ulceration or microulceration.[8-10]
2. Among HIV-seronegative individuals, genital ulcers may increase the susceptibility to HIV not only by disrupting mucosal and skin integrity but also by increasing the presence and activation of HIV susceptible cells in the genital tract (the susceptibility cofactor effect). *Haemophilus ducreyi*, for example, evokes a cell-mediated immune response which attracts HIV susceptible cells to the ulcer surface.[11] In fact, *H. ducreyi* may contain specific T cell-stimulating antigens which further predispose T cells to infection by HIV. In addition, viral STDs such as herpes interact in the genital tract, which promotes the establishment of HIV infection. For example, in tissues coinfected with HSV-1, the virions are able to infect keratinocytes despite the lack of CD4 receptors. In gaining access to the cells, HIV may also take advantage of changes in cellular chemokine receptors that had resulted from infection with other viruses, as shown in recent studies of cytomegalovirus.
3. Genital ulcers bleed frequently during sexual intercourse, resulting in a potential increase in HIV infectiousness (the infectivity cofactor effect).
4. The presence of HIV in genital ulcer exudates in HIV infected individuals confirmed by culture and PCR[12] (the infectivity cofactor effect).
5. Increased number of HIV-containing white blood cells in both ulcerative and inflammatory genital secretions (the infectivity cofactor effect).
6. Increased shedding of HIV virus in the genital tract (the infectivity cofactor effect), particularly in non-ulcerative STDs, probably by recruiting HIV infected inflammatory cells as part of the normal host response. Investigators have noted a significant increase in the detection of HIV 1 DNA in cervicovaginal fluids of patients with gonorrhoea and chlamydial infection.[13]

Table 11.1 Association between STDs and HIV Infection

STDs	*Increased Risk for HIV Acquisition*		*Clinical Exacerbation*
N. gonorrhoeae infection	+\-	3 to 5 times	+\-
Chlamydial infection	+	3 to 5 times	+\-
Trichomonas vaginalis infection	+	3 to 5 times	–
Bacterial vaginosis	+	2 to 5 times	–
Chancroid	+	2 to 5 times	+
Syphilis	+	3 to 9 times	+
Genital herpes	+	2 times	+
Granuloma inguinale	+	+\-	
Human papillomavirus infection	+	+	
LGV	+	+\-	
Hepatitis B	—	+	

7. Increasing HIV replication by certain ulcerative STD pathogens (e.g. *Treponema pallidum* lipoproteins)[14] and increasing the number of receptors expressed per cell receptive to HIV 1 (e.g. *H. ducreyi* lipo-oligosaccharide may increase the number of CCR5 receptors on a macrophage cell line).[1]

9. For cervicitis specifically, three potential mechanisms have been suggested to explain the observed relationship of cervicitis and HIV infection.[15]

    (a) Recruitment of inflammatory cells to the cervical mucosa may result in increased concentration of HIV infected CD4 lymphocytes and monocytes-macrophages.
    (b) In the presence of an inflammatory milieu, HIV replication is enhanced, perhaps through the generation of reactive oxygen products secreted by granulocytes[16] and secondary to cell activation which is mediated by inflammatory cytokines (interleukin-1 or tumour necrosis factor-alpha).[15]
    (c) Cervicitis is associated with micro-ulceration and friable mucosal tissue that provides a portal of exit or entry for virus or infected cells.

10. Bacterial vaginosis (BV) may facilitate HIV transmission.[17,18] It requires a special mention since it is a common vaginal infection in women, and the relative risk of transmission of HIV is 2 to 5 times in the presence of BV. Schmid et al[19] have summarized all possible mechanisms from research studies of different workers:

    (a) Lactobacilli produce lactic acid that maintains vaginal pH and inhibits the growth of many organisms, including those associated with BV. Some lactobacilli particularly those posted against the development of BV produce hydrogen peroxide which is toxic to a number of organisms including HIV.
    (b) Low vaginal pH may inhibit CD4 lymphocyte activation and, therefore, decrease HIV target cells in the vagina. Therefore, a high vaginal pH due to the presence of BV may make the vagina more conducive to HIV survival and adherence.
    (c) BV has also been shown to increase the intravaginal levels of interleukin-10, which increases the susceptibility of macrophages to HIV.
    (d) A heat-stable protein elaborated by *Gardnerella vaginalis* increases the production of HIV by as much as 77-fold. *Mycoplasma hominis* is the most potent inducer of HIV 1 expression among several vaginal bacterial species studied.

EFFECTS OF STD MANAGEMENT ON HIV TRANSMISSION

If STD cofactor effects are strong and STDs are highly prevalent, STD control via improvement of STD management can be a strong strategy.[20]

In a study conducted in Malawi, the results showed that HIV 1 positive men with urethritis had eight times higher HIV 1 concentrations in seminal plasma than that in seropositive men without urethritis. After treatment, the concentration of HIV 1 RNA in semen decreased significantly.[21] Ghys and coworkers[14] found a significant increase of HIV 1 DNA in cervicovaginal lavage samples from patients with gonorrhoea chlamydia infection, cervicovaginal ulcer or cervical mucopus. A week after STD treatment, the detection of HIV 1 in these secretions decreased from 42 to 21%; however, changes in detection rate were not observed in women whose STDs were not cured.

A compelling body of evidence shows that prevention, early diagnosis and treatment of STDs can be important in a HIV prevention strategy. This is particularly true when treatment of symptomatic STDs is addressed. The syndromic approach is endorsed by WHO and National AIDS Control Organization (NACO), Government of India, Ministry of Health and Family Welfare, as an effective means to treat symptomatic STDs when rapid and sensitive laboratory tests are not available. A randomized control trial was done to evaluate the impact of improved STD case management as per the WHO recommended syndromic STD management guidelines at primary care level in rural Tanzania over a two-year period. The trial demonstrated a 42% reduction in new sexually transmitted HIV infection in intervention communities as compared with control communities.[22]

However, in another community-based randomized trial conducted in the Rakai district, Uganda between 1994 and 1998, no effect on HIV incidence was seen, either overall or in subgroups, including in initially discordant couples or pregnant women. Some reductions in curable STDs were seen in both studies. The unexpected result from Rakai studies might be due to several factors as mentioned below.[23]

(a) Differences in the stage of HIV 1 epidemic (16% in Rakai and 4% in Mwanza population)
(b) Potential difference in the frequency of incurable STDs like genital herpes (45% of all genital ulcers in Rakai, whereas it is less than 10% in Mwanza)
(c) Greater importance of symptomatic than asymptomatic STDs in HIV 1 transmission
(d) Greater effectiveness of continuously available services (Mwanza) than intermittent mass treatment to control rapid STD re-infection in Rakai.

Clearly the two trials tested different intervention and used different methods for evaluation in different epidemiological environments; therefore, the divergent results may be complementary rather than contradictory.[23]

Even if STD cofactor effects on HIV transmission would be weaker than previously thought, improving STD management remains an important component of HIV prevention programmes.[20] An association between STDs and HIV, whether casual or not, indicates that STD patients are at high risk of contracting and transmitting HIV. Education, counselling, condom promotion and provision, contact tracing and treatment as part of comprehensive STD management can be an effective means of targeting HIV prevention strategies to those in need.

IMPACT OF HIV INFECTION/AIDS ON OTHER STDs AND THEIR TREATMENT

The natural history, manifestations and treatment of classic STDs may be altered by concurrent HIV infection. The impact of HIV and its resulting immunosuppression on classic manifestations and management of STDs has been noted from the beginning of AIDS epidemic.

Syphilis

In most cases of HIV coinfection, syphilis presents as it does in non-HIV infected patients. However, from several reports, HIV appears to affect the epidemiology, clinical manifestations and treatment of syphilis (Table 11.2). Although the incidence of syphilis raised dramatically in the United States in late 1980s, especially among African-American communities, no such trend was reported from India.[6,24,25,26,27]

Unusual or severe manifestations of syphilis have been reported increasingly in HIV infected patients due to some degree of immunodeficiency, and there is reduced response to conventional therapeutic regimens in these individuals. In HIV infected patients with moderate to advanced immunodeficiency, who become infected with *T. pallidum*, the following variations from the expected course of syphilis (Table 11.2) have been noted.

Antibody Response

Limited or absent antibody response to infection with repeatedly negative reagin and treponemal antibody testing due to defective B and T cell functions leading to abnormal immune response makes serological diagnosis of syphilis unreliable. A delayed serological serum titre response was seen in HIV infected patients after treatment of diverse stages of syphilis in four studies, while three other studies showed a normal serological response.[28]

Increased rate of false negative nontreponemal serologies has been observed due to the prozone phenomenon caused either by blocking the

Table 11.2 Variations in Syphilis Incidence in Individuals with HIV Infection

Clinical finding	Primary syphilis	Painless ulcer becomes painful due to super infection, giant chancre, multiple ulcers (up to 25%)
	Secondary syphilis	Lues maligna - secondary syphilis with vasculitis manifested by fever, malaise, headache, nodules, indurated plaques with or without hyperkeratoses and/or ulceration, sclerosis, ocular diseases
	Latent and tertiary syphilis	Shorter latent period with rapid progression to tertiary disease within the first year of infection, i.e. meningovascular syphilis. Concomitant primary and symptoms of tertiary syphilis reported. Multiple cases of cerebral gummas published; however, cutaneous gummas continue to be rare. Maharajan and Kumar[32] reported higher prevalence and faster progression of cardiovascular involvement
	Serological response to syphilis	Numerous case reports of limited or absent antibody response to syphilis with repeatedly negative reagin and treponemal antibody testing in serum or CSF, increased rate of false negative nontreponemal serologies due to prozone phenomenon caused by either blocking antibody or high antibody titres. Failure to clear or sufficiently drop nontreponemal titers by 1 year despite adequate treatment (serofast phenomenon) has been reported (5% in non-HIV patients) at higher rates (18%)
Diagnosis		In the absence of negative serological tests, dark field microscopy, biopsy of the lesion and direct fluorescent antibody staining of material from lesion or PCR may be helpful
Treatment		Syphilis treatment is relatively unchanged in HIV coinfected patients, but regular follow-up is required because of increased rates of treatment failure

antibody or high antibody titers.[29] Failure to clear or sufficiently drop nontreponemal titres by 1 year despite adequate treatment (serofast phenomenon) has been reported (5% in non-HIV patients) at higher rates (18% in HIV-positive patients).[33]

Clinical Manifestations

(i) **Primary lesion:** The usually painless chancre becoming painful due to secondary infection, risk of multiple chancres in primary syphilis, and development of giant primary chancre have been reported.[29,30,35]

(ii) **Secondary lesion**: The finding, include lues maligna (malignant syphilis)[35,36] chracterized by nodulo-ulcerative lesions with systemic symptoms, florid cutaneous and mucocutaneous lesions, pustular, nodular necrotizing secondary lesions, hyperkeratotic verrucous plaque-type lesion[37]; rapid progression to secondary syphilis with persistence of primary chancre[38] enhances HIV transmission.

(iii) **Latent period:** Shorter latent period before development of meningovascular syphilis, increased incidence of early neurosyphilis along with primary and secondary lesions and concomitant primary and symptoms of tertiary syphilis were reported.[29,39] Multiple cases of cerebral gummas were published; however, cutaneous gummas continue to be rare.[31] Maharajan and Kumar reported higher prevalence and faster progression of cardiovascular involvement.[32]

Diagnosis

When clinical findings suggest syphilis but serological tests are negative or inconclusive, alternative tests such as dark field microscopy, biopsy of the lesion for histopathological examination, direct fluorescent antibody staining of materials obtained from the lesions or PCR may be needed. The diagnosis of neurosyphilis is especially difficult in HIV-seropositive patients, because both HIV and syphilis can cause mononuclear pleocytosis and elevated protein in CSF, and CSF VDRL can be negative in persons with neurosyphilis.[40] Some experts believe that CSF pleocytosis should be considered significant if the count is higher that 20 WBC/μL in patients who have a coinfection (>5 WBC/μL in neurosyphilis alone). RPR titre equal to or greater than 1:32 and CD4 cell count less than or equal to 350/μL are at significant risk of neurosyphilis in dual infection, and therefore requires lumbar pucture with CSF examination.[41] CSF examination of HIV infected patients with late latent syphilis, or latent syphilis of unknown duration is mandatory, preferably as part of initial diagnostic programme before treatment.

All patients with syphilis should be strongly encouraged to undergo testing for HIV because of the high frequency of dual infection and its implications in clinical assessment and management. Neurosyphilis should be considered in differential diagnosis of neurological diseases in HIV infected individuals. In cases of congenital syphilis, the mother should be encouraged to undergo testing for HIV infection. If her test is positive, the infant should be referred for follow-up.

Treatment

Syphilis treatment is relatively unchanged in HIV coinfected patients. However, there were reports of lack of response to penicillin therapy and relapse without re-exposure despite adequate treatment in many studies.[42-44] Immunodeficiency induced by HIV appears to render benzathine penicillin G treatment ineffective in a substantial proportion of cases.[25]

Jarisch-Herxheimer reaction in syphilis is more frequent among HIV infected early syphilis patients as compared to non-HIV infected controls.[34]

Early syphilis (primary, secondary and early latent): As per the CDC (2006)[45] and WHO (2005)[46] guidelines for management of STDs, recom-mended therapy for early syphilis in HIV infected patients is no different from that in non-HIV infected patients. Penicillin regimens should be used whenever possible for all stages of syphilis in HIV: single dose of benzathine penicillin G 2.4 million IU IM as for HIV-seronegative individuals for early syphilis. However, some authorities advise examination of the CSF and additional treatments (e.g., benzathine penicillin G administered at weekly intervals for 3 weeks as recommended for late syphilis) in addition to benzethine penicillin G 2.4 million units IM.

Follow-up: In all cases, careful follow-up is necessary to ensure adequacy of treatment and treatment failure with quantitative VDRL at 3, 6, 9, 12 and 24 months after treatment. Although of unproven benefit, some specialists recommend a CSF examination 6 months after therapy (CDC-2006)[45].

HIV infected persons who meet the criteria for treatment failure (i.e. signs and symptoms persisting and those who have fourfold increase in nontreponemal test titre) should be managed in the same manner as HIV-negative patients (i.e. a CSF examination and retreatment). CSF examination and retreatment should also be reconsidered for persons whose nontreponemal test titres do not decrease fourfold within 6-12 months of therapy. A majority of specialists prefer to re-treat patients with benzathine penicillin G administered as 3 doses of 2.4 million units IM each at weekly intervals even if CSF examination is normal (CDC-2006)[45]. If CSF shows abnormality, it could be due to HIV-related infection, neurosyphilis or both. *T. pallidum* may persist in the CNS of HIV infected patients in spite of adequate antibiotic therapy.

Patients who are allergic to penicillin can be prescribed doxycycline or ceftriaxone. However, in HIV infected patients, these alternative methods are not well studied. A single dose of oral azithromycin, an azole with longlife and good CSF penetration, has been reported as a possible alternative to penicillin. Recently, in a randomized control trial performed in Tanzania, Reider and colleagues reported 97.7% cure rates with oral azithromycin versus 95% cure rates with standard IM penicillin treatment. Around 70% of their patient poplaion comprised women consisting of bar workers and HIV coinfected individuals.[47] However, a mutation, in the 23S ribosomal RNA gene responsible for azithromycin-resistant *T. pallidum* was found in approximately one-third of patients among HIV infected MSM in Seattle, Dublin and San Francisco. These data raised concerns for treatment failure in future with azithromycin. Therefore, at present, its use is questionable in HIV-negative as well as coinfected patients.[48]

Late syphilis (late-latent syphilis, latent syphilis of unknown duration, gummatous and cardiovascular syphilis): Patients with late-latent syphilis or syphilis of unknown duration and a normal CSF examination can be treated with weekly doses of benzathine penicillin G 2.4 million IU IM for 3 weeks unless contraindicated by penicillin allergy (CDC-2006)[45]. Patients who have CSF findings consistent with neurosyphilis should be treated and mana-ged like a case of neurosyphilis. Patients with cardi-ovascular or aggressive gummatous disease may require individualized treatment.

Follow-up: Patients should be evaluated clinically and serologically at 6, 12, 18 and 24 months after therapy. If, at any time, clinical symptoms develop or nontreponemal titre does not decline fourfold, CSF examination should be repeated and treatment administered accordingly. (CDC-2006)[45]

Neurosyphilis

Adequate treatment relies on attaining sufficient CSF antibiotic levels. Therefore, aqueous crystalline penicillin G is recommended at 18 to 24 million units per day, 3 to 4 millions units administered intravenously every 4 hours, or by continuous infusion for a period of 10 to14 days. Additionally, HIV coinfected patients whose serologies fail to drop adequately or increase should be re-treated.

Since the efficacy of alternative nonpenicillin regimens in HIV infected patients has not been well studied, in case of penicillin allergy, the patient should be desensitized and treated with penicillin. Limited clinical studies, along with biological and pharmacological evidence, suggest that ceftriaxone might be effective. However, optimal dose and duration of ceftriaxone therapy have not been defined.[45]

Chancroid

Chancroid, caused by *H. ducreyi,* may be both a marker for increased risk of HIV infection and a cofactor for HIV transmission. Since the advent of HIV infection in Africa, several studies suggest a change in the natural history of chancroid.

The following variations are noticed in natural history and therapy of chancroid (Table 11.3):

(a) Genital ulcers tend to be larger and persist longer.[49]
(b) Chacroid with multiple inguinal buboes.
(c) Frequent occurrence of giant and phagedenic ulcer.
(d) Less responsive to standard antibiotic therapy. Single-dose therapies such as azithromycin and ceftriaxone also have been associated with a three- to fourfold higher failure rate in the treatment of chancroid among HIV-seropositive as compared to seronegative men.[50, 51]

A definite diagnosis of chancroid requires the identification of *H. ducreyi* on special culture media; however, the sensitivity is <80%. No FDA-cleared PCR test for *H. ducreyi* is available.

HIV infected patients who have chancroid should be monitored closely because, as a group, these patients are more likely to experience treatment failure and have ulcers that heal more slowly. HIV infected patients might require longer duration of therapy than that recommended for HIV-negative patients. Treatment failure can occur with any regimen. Because evidence is limited concerning the therapeutic efficacy of recommended regimens (azithromycin, 1 g orally in a single dose or ceftriaxone, 250 mg IM in a single dose) in HIV infected patients, these regimens should be used in such patients only if follow-up can be ensured. Some specialists prefer the erythromycin (500 mg orally 4 times a day for 7days) regimen in treating HIV infected persons.[45]

Herpes Genitalis

Herpes simplex virus (HSV) infections occur more frequently and is more severe in immunocompromised patients with HIV infection (Table 11.3).[52-54] There is a synergistic relationship between HSV and HIV leading to enhanced replication of viruses and potentiation of HIV transmission.[55]

Clinical Presentation

It ranges from those described in immunocompetent patients to life-threatening disseminated infections. The severity and frequency of recurrence increase over time as HIV-induced immunosuppression progresses. The lesions may persist or progress to produce erosions that enlarge into painful ulcers with raised margin involving larger areas of perianal, scrotal or penile skin. The ulcer may bleed. Non-healing perianal ulcerative herpes simplex was initially an opportunistic infection described in homosexual men with HIV infection. Chronicity parallels with immunosuppression. Antiretroviral therapy reduces the severity and frequency of symptomatic genital herpes; however, frequent subclinical shedding still occurs.[56]

Diagnosis of HSV Infection

Clinical diagnosis is insensitive and non-specific. The isolation of HSV in cell culture is the gold standard test for patients seeking medical treatment for genital ulcers or mucocutaneous lesions; however, sensitivity is low especially for recurrent lesions and declines rapidly as lesions begin to heal. PCR assays for HSV DNA are more sensitive and have been used instead of viral culture. The FDA-cleared glycoprotein G-based type-specific assays (ELISA G2 for HSV-2 and G1 for HSV-1) became commercially available since 1999. The sensitivity for HSV-2 antibody varies from 80-98%, and false negative results can occur at early stage of infection. The specificities of these assays are equal to or more than 96%. False positive results can occur especially in patients with a low likelihood of HSV infection. Repeat or confirmatory testing might be indicated in some settings, especially if a recent acquisition of genital herpes is suspected.

Some specialists believe that HSV serological testing should be included in a comprehensive evaluation for STDs among persons with HIV infection, multiple sex partners, and among MSM at increased risk for HIV infection.

Treatment

Acyclovir, famciclovir or valacyclovir is safe for use in immunocompromised patients in doses recommended for treatment of genital herpes.

Treatment might be extended if healing is incomplete after 7-10 days of therapy. For severe HSV disease, initiating therapy with acyclovir 5–10 mg/kg body weight IV every 8 hours might be necessary.

If lesions persist or recur in a patient receiving antiviral treatment, HSV resistance should be suspected, and a viral isolate should be obtained for sensitivity testing if facility is available. All acyclovir-resistant strains are resistant to valacyclovir, and the majority is resistant to famciclovir. Foscarnet, 40 mg/kg body weight IV every 8 hours until clinical resolution is attained, is often effective. Topical cidofovir gel 1% applied to lesions once daily for 5 consecutive days might be effective.

Suppressive or episodic therapy is effective in decreasing the clinical manifestations of HSV among HIV-positive persons.[45]

Recommened regimens for daily suppressive therapy

Acyclovir 400-800 mg orally twice to thrice a day
Or
Famciclovir 500 mg orally twice a day
Or
Valacyclovir 500 mg orally twice a day

Recommended regimens for episodic infection

Acyclovir 400 mg orally thrice a day for 5-10 days
Or
Famciclovir 500 mg orally twice a day for 5-10 days
Or
Valacyclovir 1.0 g orally twice a day for 5-10 days

Granuloma Inguinale

In the presence of HIV infection with moderate to severe immunodeficiency, the lesion of granuloma inguinale may clinically be larger, extensive and the pseudo bubo may burst producing ulceration, and there may be slow response to treatment (Table 11.3).

Persons with both granuloma inguinale and HIV infection should receive the same regimens as those who are HIV-negative. Recommended regimens are doxycycline 100 mg orally bid or erythromycin 500 mg orally qid for at least 3 weeks or until all lesions have completely healed.[45] Alternatively, azithromycin may be taken 1 g orally once per week for at least 3 weeks or until all lesions have completely healed. Adding gentamycin 1 mg/kg IV every 8 hours to the above regimen may be suggested if improvement is not evident within the first few days of therapy in HIV-positive patients.[45]

Lymphogranuloma Venereum

There may be an acute inflammation with bilateral inguinal bubo, which may burst into ulceration in cases with moderate to severe immunodeficiency due to HIV infection (Table 11.3).

Persons with both LGV and HIV infection should receive the same regimens as those who are HIV-negative. Prolonged therapy may be required, and delay in resolution of symptoms may occur (CDC-2006).[45] Recommended CDC 2006 and WHO 2005 regimen is doxycycline 100 mg orally bid for 21 days[45,46] or erythromycin base 500 mg orally four times a day for three weeks.[45]

Urethritis and Cervicitis

Gonococcal urethritis, chlamydial urethritis and nongonococcal, nonchlamydial urethritis may facilitate HIV transmission. Patients who have urethritis and also infected with HIV should receive the same treatment regimen as those who are HIV-negative.

Similarly, patients who have cervicitis and also infected with HIV should receive the same treatment regimen as those who are HIV-negative. Cervicitis increases cervical HIV shedding. Treatment of cervicitis in HIV infected women reduces HIV shedding from cervix and might reduce HIV transmission to susceptible sex partners.[45]

Bacterial Vaginosis and Trichomoniasis

Patients who have either of those infections and also infected with HIV should receive the same treatment regimen as those who are HIV-negative. BV appears to be more persistent in HIV-positive women.

Vulvovaginal Candidiasis

Vaginal candida colonization rates in HIV infected women are higher than among seronegative women with similar demographic characteristics and high risk behaviours. The colonization rates correlate with increasing severity of immunosuppression. Symptomatic vulvovaginal candidiasis (VVC) is more frequent in seropositive women and similarly correlates with the severity of immunodeficiency. In addition, among HIV infected women, systemic azole exposure is associated with the isolation of non-albicans Candida species from vagina.

Therapy for VVC should be same as that for seronegative women. Long-term secondary prophylactic therapy with fluconazole at a dose of 200 mg weekly is effective in reducing *C. albicans* colonization and symptomatic VVC particularly in recurrent infection. However, recurrent VVC should not be considered as an indication for HIV testing (CDC-2006).[45]

Table 11.3 Variations in Other STDs in Individuals with HIV Infection

Chancroid	Clinical findings	Genital ulcers tend to be larger and persist longer. Multiple inguinal buboes Frequent occurrence of giant and phagedenic ulcer
	Treatment	Treatment failure can occur with single-dose therapy with azithromycin and ceftriaxone. Some suggest erythromycin, 500 mg 6 hourly for 7 days[45]
Herpes genitalis	Clinical findings	As immunosuppression progresses, lesion may persist or progress to chronic enlarged painful ulcers with raised margin; ulcer may bleed
	Treatment	Acyclovir, famciclovir or valacyclovir are safe for use in immunocompromised patients in doses recommended for treatment of genital herpes. Treatment might be extended if healing is incomplete after 7-10 days of therapy. For severe HSV disease, initiating therapy with acyclovir 5–10 mg/kg body weight IV every 8 hours might be necessary. Suppressive therapy includes acyclovir 400-800 mg bid or tid[45]
Granuloma inguinale	Clinical findings	Lesion may be larger, extensive, pseudo bubo formation which may burst producing ulceration; slow response to treatment
	Treatment	Doxycycline 100 mg orally bid or erythromycin 500 mg orally qid for 2-3 weeks[45,46] If no improvement, addition of gentamycin 1 mg\kg IV suggested
LGV	Clinical findings	Acute inflammation with bilateral inguinal bubo which may burst into ulceration
	Treatment	Same regimen (doxycycline, 100 mg orally bid or erythromycin, 500 mg orally qid for 21 days[45,46], but prolonged therapy may be required

Epididymitis

Patients who have uncomplicated acute epididymitis, confirmed or suspected to be caused by *N. gonorrhoeoa* or *C. trachomatis* and also infected with HIV should receive the same treatment regimen as those who are HIV-negative. Fungi and mycobacteria, however, are more likely to cause acute epididymitis in immunosuppressed patients than in immunocompetent patients.

Human Papilloma Virus Infection

Human papillomavirus (HPV) infection, one of the very common STDs, presents as genital warts to carcinoma in HIV-positive patients. The incidence of venereal warts was 8.2% compared with 0.8% per 100 person-years of follow up for HIV 1 seronegative women. In a study examining HIV infected women in the United States, Europe, East Africa and West Africa, genital HPV DNA in 8% to >50% of HIV-seronegative women and 37% to 78% HIV-seropositive cases was reported. Among women in whom cervical HPV DNA was detected, HIV seropositive cases were more likely to harbour high-risk HPV types 16 and 18 than were HIV seronegative women. The causal link between invasive cervical squamous cell carcinoma and cervical intraepithelial neoplasia (CIN) in women is well demonstrated.[57] Women who are HIV-positive are at a higher risk of both HPV infection and CIN changes than HPV-negative women.[58,59] The immune status of women with HIV has been shown to influence the progression of CIN.[60] Cervical cancer is now considered as AIDS-defining illness in women.[61] The association between HPV and anal carcinoma in both men and women with HIV is almost certain.[62] The incidence of anal carcinoma in homosexual men with AIDS was 40 times that of general population and significantly higher than that of seronegative homosexual men.

In immunocompromised patients, genital warts may be more florid, disseminated and often refractory to treatment and might have more frequent recurrences after treatment. Squamous cell carcinomas arising in or resembling genital warts may occur more frequently among immunosuppressed persons, thus requiring biopsy for confirmation of diagnosis. Because of increased incidence of anal cancer in HIV infected homosexual men, screening for squamous intraepithelial lesion (SIL) by cytology is advocated by some specialists.[45]

After obtaining a complete history of previous cervical disease, HIV infected women should be provided a comprehensive gynaecological examination, including pelvic examination and Pap test, as part of their initial evaluation. A Pap test should be obtained twice in the first year after diagnosis of HIV infection and, if the results are normal, annually thereafter. Women who have a cytological diagnosis of high-grade SIL or squamous cell carcinoma should undergo colposcopy-directed biopsy. HIV infection is not an indication for colposcopy in women who have normal Pap smear.

Molluscum Contagiosum

Molluscum contagiosum (MC) began to receive more attention with the advent of AIDS.[63-65] Among AIDS patients, MC does not just occur in male homosexuals but throughout all races and in all groups when sufficiently immunocompromised. Despite recalcitrant MC in HIV patients, all are not sexually transmitted. The lesions are usually in clusters, pearly with an umbilicated centre. Hundreds of lesions may be found between the umbilicus and the genitals in sexually active young adults. On the pubis and external genitalia, they often coexist with genital warts and thus may represent a therapeutic challenge.

Hepatitis B

Hepatitis B and HIV coinfection has been reported among 2.85% of STD clinic attendees in a study from Chennai.[66] HBV infection in HIV infected persons is more likely to result in chronic HBV infection. HIV infection also can impair the response to hepatitis B vaccine. Therefore, HIV infected persons should be tested for HBsAg 1-2 months after the third vaccine dose. Revaccination with three more doses should be considered for persons who do not respond initially to vaccination. Those who do not respond to additional doses should be counselled on the use of methods to prevent HBV infection.

Hepatitis C

The role of sexual activity in the transmission of HCV has been controversial.[45] Case control studies have reported an association between acquiring HCV infection or exposure to multiple sex partners. Case reports of acute HCV infection among HIV-positive MSM who deny injecting drug use have indicated that this occurrence is frequently associated with other STDs.[67,68]

Because of the high prevalence of HIV/HCV coinfection and because of critical clinical management issues for coinfected persons, all HIV infected persons should be tested for HCV. A small percentage of coinfected persons fail to acquire HCV antibodies. Therefore, HCV RNA should be tested in HIV-positive patients with unexplained liver disease who are HCV antibody- negative. The course of liver disease is more rapid in HIV/HCV coinfected persons, and the risk of cirrhosis is nearly twice that in persons with HCV infection alone.

Treatment of HCV in coinfected persons might improve tolerance to highly active antiretroviral therapy (HAART) for HIV infection because of the increased risk for hepatotoxicity from HAART with HCV infection. However, anti-HCV treatment in coinfected persons is still investigational, and based on the ongoing clinical trials, more data are needed to determine the best regimens.[45]

Pelvic Inflammatory Disease

Differences in clinical manifestations of PID between HIV infected women and HIV-negative women have not been well delineated. In recent, more comprehensive observational and controlled studies, HIV infected women with PID had similar symptoms when compared with uninfected control.[69-71] They were more likely to have tuboovarian abscess, but responded equally well to standard parenteral and oral antibiotic regimens when compared with HIV-negative women.

Microbiological findings for HIV-positive and HIV-negative were similar, except for (a) higher rates of concomitant *M. hominis*, candida, streptococcal and HPV infection and (b) HPV-related cytological abnormalities among those with HIV infection.

Whether the management of immunodeficient HIV infected women with PID requires more aggressive intervention (e.g., hospitalization or parenteral antimicrobial regimen) has not been determined.[45]

Pediculosis Pubis

Pediculosis pubis patients who are also infected with HIV should receive the same treatment regimen as those who are HIV-negative (permethrin 1% cream applied to the affected areas and washed off after 10 minutes). Alternative regimens include malathion 0.5% lotion applied for 8-12 hours and washed off, or ivermectin 250 μg/kg repeated in 2 weeks.

Scabies

Crusted scabies is an aggressive infestation that usually occurs in HIV infected persons and other immunodeficient patients. It is associated with greater transmissibility than scabies. Substantial treatment failure might occur with single topical scabicide (permethrin cream 5% applied to all areas of the body from neck down and washed off after 8-14 hours or lindane 1% as alternative) or ivermectin treatment. Some specialists recommend combined treatment with a topical scabicide and oral ivermectin or repeated treatment with ivermectin 200 μg/kg on days 1, 15 and 29.[45] Lindane should be avoided because of risks of neurotoxicity with heavy applications and denuded skin. Patient's fingernail should be closely trimmed to reduce injury from excessive scratching.

Patients with uncomplicated scabies along with HIV infection should receive the same treatment regimen as those who are HIV-negative.

CONCLUSION

Effective treatment regimens are available for STIs at tertiary, middle and primary health care levels of the country. STI management is promptly applied along with other STI control measures such as provision of treatment to sex partner, constant condom use, health education and counselling. The NACO-2007guideline recommends that all persons who seek evaluation and treatment for STIs should be encouraged and recommended HIV testing after pre-test counselling and informed consent.[72] There should be a guarantee for confidentiality. HIV counselling and testing can either be performed in an STI clinic (if counsellor is available) or clients may be referred to the nearest integrated counselling testing centre (ICTC).[72] Detection and treatment of classic STIs must be undertaken in HIV-positive patients to reduce their infectiousness and in their partners to reduce susceptibility to infection.[1] In some cases of STIs, in the presence of HIV infection, larger doses and longer duration of drugs for different STIs may be required; these clients should be followed up regularly for longer duration.[72] Proper management of HIV infection involves a complex array of behavioural, psychological and medical services. Some of these services might not be available in all STI treatment facilities. Therefore, HIV-positive patients coinfected with other STIs must be advised to attend the nearest health care facilities where ART centers have been opened by the National AIDS Control Organization (NACO) and respective State AIDS Cell Society (SACS) for initiation of HAART and management of other HIV/AIDS-related complications, other support services and care.

REFERENCES

1. Cohen MS. Sexually transmitted diseases enhance HIV transmission: a hypothesis no longer. Lancet 1998; 351 (suppl III): 5-7.
2. Wasserheit JN. Epidemiological synergy: interrelationships between human immunodeficiency virus infection and other sexually transmitted diseases. Sex Transm Dis 1992; 19: 61-77.
3. Fleming DT, Wasserheit JN. From epidemiological synergy to public health policy and practice: the contribution of other sexually transmitted diseases to sexual transmission of HIV infection. Sex Transm Inf 1999; 75: 3-17.
4. Kar HK, Jain RK, Sharma PK, et al. Increasing HIV prevalence in STDs clinic attendees in Delhi, India: 6 year (1995-2000) hospital based study results. Sex Transm Inf 2001; 77: 393.
5. Kumar B, Gupta S. Rising HIV prevalence in STDs clinic attendees at Chandigarh (North India)- A relatively low prevalence area. Sex Transm Inf 2000; 76: 59.
6. Ray K, Bala M, Gupta SM, et al. Changing trends in sexually transmitted infections at a Regional STDs Centre in north India. Indian J Med Res, 2006; 124: 559-68.
7. Subramanian, Gupte MD, Mathai AK, et al. Factors associated with HIV seroprevalence among STDs patients attending a Govt. STDs clinic in Chennai, South India. Indian J Sex Transm Dis 2006; 27: 50-3.
8. Laga M, Nzila N, Goeman J. The interrelationship of sexually transmitted diseases and HIV infection: implications for the control of both epidemics in Africa (Review). AIDS 1991; 5: S55-63.
9. Wasserheit JN. Epidemiological synergy: interrelationships between human immunodeficiency virus infection and other sexually transmitted diseases (Review). Sex Transm Dis 1992; 19: 61-77.
10. Vernazza PL, Eron JJ, Fiscus SA, et al. Sexual transmission of HIV: infectiousness and prevention. AIDS 1999; 13: 155-66.
11. Magro CM, Crowson AN, Alfa M, et al. A morphological study of penile chancroid lesions in human immunodeficiency virus (HIV)- positive

and –negative African men with a hypothesis concerning the role of chancroid in HIV transmission. Human Pathol 1996; 27: 1066-70.

12. Plummer FA, Wainberg MA, Plourde P, et al. Detection of human immunodeficiency virus type 1 (HIV 1) in genital ulcer exudates of HIV 1-infected men by culture and gene amplification (letter). J Infect Dis 1990; 161: 810-1.
13. Ghys PD, Fransen K, Diallo MO, et al. The associations between cervicovaginal HIV shedding, sexually transmitted diseases and immunosuppression in female sex workers in Abidjan, Cote d' Ivoire. AIDS 1997; 11: 85-93.
14. Theus SA, Harrich DA, Gaynor R, et al. Treponema pallidum lipoproteins and synthetic lipoprotein analogues induce human immunodeficiency virus type 1 gene expression in monocytes via NF-Kb Activation. J Infect Dis 1998; 177: 941-50.
15. Kreiss J, Willerford DM, Hensel M, et al. Association between cervical inflammation and cervical shedding of human immunodeficiency virus DNA. J Infect Dis 1994; 170: 1597-1601.
16. Ho JL, He S, Hu A, et al. Neutrophils from human immunodeficiency virus (HIV) seronegative donors induce HIV replication from HIV-infected patient's mononuclear cells and cell lines: an in vitro model of HIV transmission facilitated by *Chlamydia trachomatis*. J Exp Med 1997; 181: 1403-1505.
17. Klebanoff SJ, Coomb RW. Virucidal effects of lactobacillus acidophilus on human immunodeficiency virus type-1: possible role in heterosexual transmission. J Exp Med 1991; 174: 289-92.
18. Cohen CR, Duer RA, Pruithithada N, et al. Bacterial vaginosis and HIV seroprevalence among female commercial sex workers in Chaing Mai, Thailand. AIDS 1995; 9: 1093-7.
19. Schmid G, Markowitz L, Joesoef R, et al. Bacterial vaginosis and HIV infection. Sex Transm Inf 2000; 76: 3-4.
20. Korenromp EL, Sake J, Vlas DE, et al. Estimating the magnitude of STDs cofactor effects on HIV transmission, how well can it be done? Sex Transm Dis 2001; 28: 613-21.
21. Cohen MS, Hoffman IF, Royce RA, et al. Reduction of concentration of HIV 1 in semen after treatment of urethritis: implications for prevention of sexual transmission of HIV 1. Lancet 1997; 349: 1868-73.
22. Grosskurth H, Mosha F, Todd J, et al. Impact of improved treatment of sexually transmitted diseases on HIV infection in rural Tanzania: randomized controlled trial. Lancet 1995; 346: 530-6.
23. Grosskurth H, Gray R, Hayes R, et al. Control of sexually transmitted diseases for HIV 1 prevention: understanding the implications of the Mwanza and Rakai trials. Lancet 2000; 355: 1981-7.
24. Wald A, Corey L, Handsfield HH, et al. Influence of HIV infection on manifestations and natural history of other sexually transmitted diseases. Ann Rev Publ Health 1993; 14: 19-42.
25. Chopra A, Dhaliwal RS,Chopra D. Pattern and changing trend of STDs at Patiala. Indian J Sex Transm Dis 1999; 20: 22-5.
26. Raj Narayan, Kar HK, Gautam RK, et al. Pattern of sexually transmitted diseases in a major hospital of Delhi. Indian J Sex Transm Dis 1996; 17: 76-8.
27. Kar HK. Incidence of secondary syphilis on rise and need for a separate flow chart for its syndromic management. Indian J Sex Transm Dis 2004; 25: 70-3.
28. Pieter C, Vader VV. Syphilis management and treatment. Dermatol Clin 1998; 16: 699-711.
29. Nnoruka EN, Ezepke AC. Evaluation of syphilis in patients with HIV infection in Nigeria. Trop Med Int Health 2005; 10: 58-64.
30. Rompalo AM, Lawlor J, Seaman P, et al. Modification of syphilis genital ulcer manifestations by coexistent HIV infection. Sex Transm Dis 2001; 28: 448-54.
31. Regal L, Demaerel P, Dubois B. Cerebral syphilic gumma in a human immunodeficiency virus-posititive patient. Arch Neurol 2005; 62: 1310-1.
32. Maharajan M, Kumar GS. Cardiovascular syphilis in HIV infection: a case-control study at the Institute of Sexually Transmitted Diseases, Chennai, India. Sex Transm Infect 2005; 81: 361.
33. Malone JL, Wallace MR, Hendrick BB, et al. Syphilis and neurosyphilis in a human

efficiency virus type-1 seropositive population: evidence for frequent serologic relapse after therapy. Am J Med 1995; 99: 55-63.
34. Rolfs RT, Joesoef MR, Hendershot EF, et al. Randomized trial of enhanced therapy for early syphilis in patients with and without HIV infection. N Engl J Med 1997; 337: 307.
35. Schofer H, Imhof M, Thoma-Greber E, et al. Active syphilis in HIV infection: A multicentre retrospective survey. Genitourin Med 1996; 72: 176.
36. Mohan KK, Rao GRR, Lakshmi P, et al. Changing patterns of secondary syphilis (a clinical study). Indian J Sex Transm Dis 2000; 2: 75-8.
37. happa DM, Hemanth RH, Karthikeyan, et al. Unusual manifestations of secondary syphilis in a patient with human immunodeficiency virus infection. Indian J Sex Transm Dis 1999; 20: 29-32.
38. Hutchinson C, Hook EW, Shepard M, et al. Altered clinical presentation of early syphilis in patients with HIV infection. Ann Intern Med 1994; 121: 94.
39. Pavithran K, Beena S. Primary chancre – associated syphilitic meningitis during HIV infection. Indian J Sex Trans Dis 1999; 20: 55-6.
40. Feraru ER, Aronow HA, Lipton RB. Neurosyphilis in AIDS patients: initial CSF VDRL may be negative. Neurology 1990; 40: 541-3.
41. Mara CM, Maxwell CL, Smith SL, et al. Cerebrospinal fluid abnormalities in patients with syphilis: association with clinical and laboratory features. Neurology 2004; 63: 85-8.
42. Dover JS, Johnson RA. Cutaneous manifestations of Human immunodeficiency virus infection. Arch Dermatol 1991; 127: 1549-58.
43. Fowler VG Jr, Maxwell GL, Myers SA, et al. Failure of benzathine penicillin in a case of seronegative secondary syphilis in a patient with acquired immunodeficiency syndrome: case report and review of the literature. Arch Dermatol 2001; 137: 1374-6.
44. Pavithran K. Chancre redux and tinea incognito in an HIV-infected person. Indian J Sex Transm Dis 1997; 18: 22-3.
45. Centers for Disease Control and Prevention (CDC), Sexually Transmitted Diseases Treatment Guidelines 2006 (http://www.cdc.gov/STDs/treatment/2006/toc.htm)
46. WHO Guidelines for management of Sexually transmitted and other reproductive tract infections 2005.
47. Reidner G, Rusizoka M, Todd J, et al. Single-dose azithromycin versus penicillin G benzathine for the treatment of early syphilis. N Engl J Med 2005; 353: 1236-44.
48. Lukehart SA, Godornes C, Molini BJ,, et al. Macrolide resistance in Trepanoma pallidum in the United States and Ireland. N Engl J Med 2004; 35; 154-8.
49. Latif AS. Epidemiology control of chancroid, 8th Int Soc STDs Res 1989 Copenhagen (Abstr. 66).
50. Tyndall M, Agoki E, Ombetti J, et al. A randomized, single blinded study of azithromycin in male patients with culture proven chancroid. 9th Int Soc STDs Res 1991 Banff. (Abstr. A-041)
51. Tyndall M, Malisa M, Plummer FA, et al. Ceftriaxone in the treatment of chancroid. 9th Int Soc STDs Res 1991 Banff. (Abstr. A-42)
52. Johnson R, Leef, Hadgu A, et al. Genital herpes trends during the first decade of AIDS: Prevalence increased in young whites and elevated in blacks. 10th International Meeting of the Int Soc for STDs Res 1993 Helsinki (Abstract).
53. Norris SA, Kessler HA, Fife KH. Severe progressive herpetic whitlow caused by an acyclovir resistant virus in a patient with AIDS. J Infect Dis 1987; 157: 209-10.
54. Safrin S, Asseykeen T, Follansby, et al. Foscarnet therapy for acyclovir resistant mucocutaneous herpes simlex virus in 26 AIDS patients. J Infect Dis 1990; 161: 1078-84.
55. Heng M, Heng S, Allen S. Coinfection and synergy of human immunodeficiency virus-1 and herpes simplex virus-1. Lancet 1994; 343: 255-8.
56. Posavad CM, Wald A, Kuntz S et al. Frequent reactivation og herpes simplex virus among HIV-1 infected patients treated with highly active antiretroviral therapy. J Infect Dis 2004; 190: 693-6.
57. Nash JD, Burkar TW, Hoskin WJ. Biological course of cervical human papilloma virus infection. Obstet Gynaecol 1987; 69: 160-2.

58. Byrne MA, Taylor-Robinson D, Munday PE, et al. The common occurrence of human papillomavirus infection and intraepithelial neoplasm in immunosuppressed women infected by HIV. AIDS 1989; 3: 379-82.
59. Vermund SH, Kelley KF, Klein RS, et al. High risk of human papillomavirus and cervical squamous intraepithelial lesions among women with symptomatic human immunodeficiency virus infection. Am J Obstet Gynecol 1991; 165: 392-400.
60. Silman J, Stanek A, Sedlis A, et al. The relationship between human papillomvirus and lower genital intraepithelial neoplasia in immunosuppressed women. Am J Obstet Gynaecol 1984; 150: 300-8.
61. Melbye M, Cote T, Biggar R, et al. High incidence of anal cancer among AIDS patients X International Conference on AIDS, 1993 Berlin. (Abstract po-b14-1636).
62. Kiviat MB, Human pappiloma virus and hepatitis viral infections in human immuno deficiency virus infected persons. In: Devita Jr VT, Hellman S, Rosenberg SA, Curran J, Essex M, Fauci AS, Eds. AIDS Aetiology, Diagnosis, Treatment and prevention, New York: Lippincott- Raven: 1997. p. 281-91.
63. Gottlieb SL, Myskowski PL. Molluscum contagiosum. Int J Dermatol 1994; 33: 453-61.
64. Myskowski PL. Molluscum contagiosum: New insights, new directions. Arch Dermatol 1997; 133: 1039-41.
65. Meadows KP, Tyring SK, Pavia AT, et al. Resolution of recalcitrant molluscum contagiosum lesion in human virus infected patients treated with cidofovir, Arch Dermatol 1997; 133: 987-90.
66. Rajesh R, Subramaniam K, Padmavathy BK, et al. Sero prevalence of HBV/HCV among STDs clinic attedees in the era of HIV/AIDS. Indian J Sex Transm Dis 2006; 27: 56-61.
67. Ghosen J, Pierre-Francois S, Thibault V, et al. Acute hepatitis C in HIV-infected men who have sex with men. HIV Medicine 2004; 5: 303-6.
68. Brown R, Asboe D, Gilleece Y, et al. Increased numbers of acute hepatitis C infection in HIV positive homosexual men; is sexual transmission feeding the increase? Sex Transmit Infect 2004; 80: 326-7.
69. Cohen CR, Sinei S, Reilly M, et al. Effects of human immunodeficiency virus 1 infection upon acute salpingitis: a laparoscopic study. J Infect Dis 1998; 18: 1352-8.
70. Bukesi EA, Cohen CR, Stevens CE, et al. Effects of human immunodeficiency virus 1 infection on microbial origins of pelvic inflammatory disease and on efficacy of ambulatory oral therapy. Am J Obstet Gynecol 1999; 18: 1374-81.
71. Irwin KL, Moorman AC, O'Sullivan MJ, et al. Influence of human Immunodeficiency virus infection on pelvic inflammatory disease. Obstet Gynecol 2000; 95: 525-34.
72. National guidelines on prevention, management and control of reproductive tract infections including sexually transmitted infections by Maternal Health Division and NACO, Ministry of Health and Family Welfare, Government of India, August 2007.

PART 3

Basics of Anatomy and Clinical and Laboratory Methods

12 APPLIED ANATOMY OF MALE AND FEMALE REPRODUCTIVE TRACT

Gurvinder P Thami

In this chapter

- Male Genitalia
- Female Genitalia
- Lymphatic Drainage of Genitalia
- Consequences of Lymphatic Blockade
- Anorectal Mucosa and Sexually Transmitted Diseases
- Oral Mucosa and Sexually Transmitted Diseases
- Normal Anatomical Variations In the Genital Region

INTRODUCTION

Sexually transmitted diseases (STDs) particularly affect the genitalia, anorectal area and oral mucosa. Majority of the symptoms and signs of STDs are dependant on anatomy and lymphatic drainage. A sound knowledge of anatomy of male and female genitalia is essential for accurate diagnosis and prompt treatment of STDs.

MALE GENITALIA

Male Urethra (Fig. 12.1)

The male urethra is a membranous canal for external discharge of urine and seminal fluid. It extends from the neck of urinary bladder to external urethral meatus and is 18-20 cm long. It has three parts, including proximally prostatic, membranous

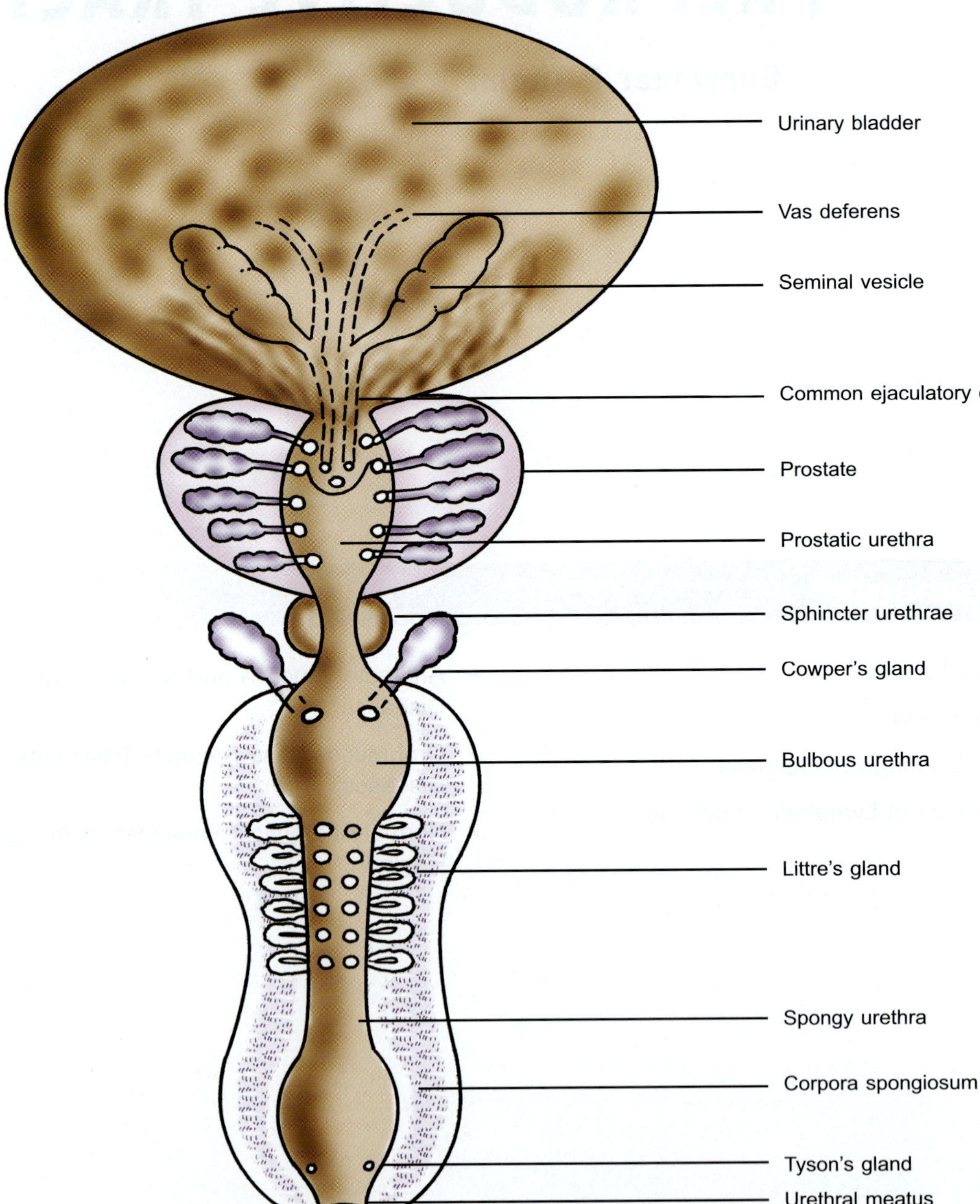

Fig. 12.1 Diagrammatic Representation of Coronal Section of Male Urethra

and spongy or penile urethra. The spongy or penile part is commonly referred to as anterior urethra, while the membranous and prostatic parts together constitute posterior urethra. The prostatic part is 3 cm, membranous part is 1.5-2 cm, and penile part is 15 cm in length. The spongy part of urethral mucosa is lined by pseudostratified columnar epithelium except in its distal (fossa navicularis) 10-12 mm, where it is lined by stratified squamous epithelium. The membranous and prostatic urethra are lined by transitional epithelium. Spongy or penile urethra can be felt running deep within corpora spongiosum along the median raphe of penis and scrotum ventrally. Palpation of urethra in this location can detect urethral strictures, and milking of urethra proximal to distal direction helps to bring out the urethral discharge for laboratory diagnosis.

Sphincter of the Urethra

1. The internal urethral sphincter or sphincter vesicae is involuntary in nature. It controls the neck of the bladder and the prostatic urethra above the opening of the ejaculatory ducts.
2. The external urethral sphincter or sphincter urethrae is voluntary in nature. It is made up of striated muscle fibres and is supplied by the perineal branch of pudendeal nerve (S2 to 4). It controls the membranous urethra and is responsible for voluntary holding of urine.

Vessels

The urethra is supplied by vessels of the prostate and the penis.

Lymphatics

The lymphatics from the prostatic and membranous parts of urethra pass mostly to the internal iliac nodes and partly to the external iliac nodes. Those from the spongy part pass mostly to the deep inguinal nodes; some may end in superficial inguinal and external iliac nodes.

Penis (Fig. 12.2)

(i) **Shaft or body of the penis** consists of erectile tissue constituted by corpora spongiosum penetrated by urethra throughout its length ending up in a bulb-like projection known as glans penis and two corpora cavernosa lying side by side.

(ii) **Glans penis** is the distal end of corpora spongiosum ending up in a bulb-like projection. It has a rim-like raised surface at its proximal end, which is termed as corona glandis. A circular groove, coronal sulcus runs along corona glandis and separates it from the shaft of penis. Small, pin head-sized projections studded over corona glandis in one or two rows are known as pearly penile papules, which may be confused with condyloma acuminata.

(iii) **Prepuce** is a specialized fold of skin which marks the junction between cutaneous and mucocutaneous areas of the penis. This fold of skin covers glans penis to form a potential space known as preputial sac. The mobility of prepuce makes it a vulnerable tissue for trauma during coitus and serves as a portal of entry for sexually transmitted agents. Preputial sac itself, due to its occlusive effect over glans and the undersurface of prepuce, makes this sac and glans penis vulnerable for inflammation, which is termed as balanoposthitis. Prepuce is attached to glans penis at its ventral surface near external urinary meatus with a fold of skin known as frenulum, which is prone to trauma and infection during sexual intercourse

Scrotum

Scrotum is a loose sac of skin which contains testes, epididymis, vas deferens and loose areolar tissue. Scrotal skin is vulnerable to genital ulcer disease due to its close proximity with penis.

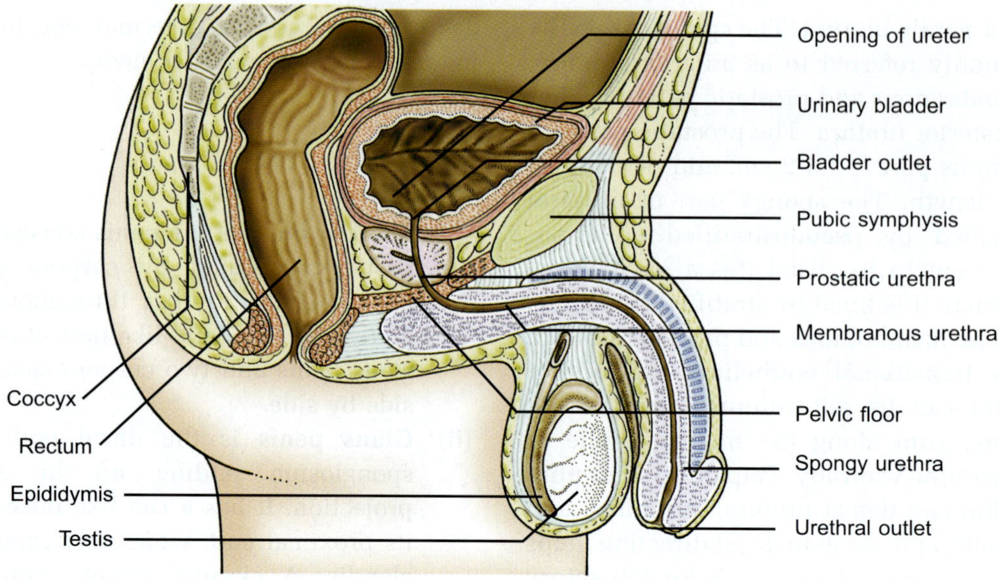

Fig. 12.2 Diagrammatic Representation of Saggital Section of Male Genital Organs.

Glands (Figs. 12.1 and 12.2)

(i) **Prostate** is a racemose type of branched glandular tissue with one middle and two lateral lobes which encircles the prostatic urethra throughout its length starting from the neck of bladder. The glandular tissue is lined by columnar epithelium and opens with multiple ducts into prostatic urethra. The common ejaculatory ducts formed by joining vas deferens and seminal vesicles opens up in prostatic urethra over veru montanum. The branching character of prostatic glandular tissue along with columnar epithelium makes it especially vulnerable for gonococcal and non-gonococcal infections, often leading to chronicity with consequent difficulty to eradicate the infection. Prostate can be felt through per rectal examination (feel like tip of the nose), and prostatic massage is useful to bring about prostatic secretions.

(ii) **Cowper's glands** or bulbourethral glands of Cowper are two in number, lying one on either side of membranous urethra, which is surrounded by the sphincter urethrae muscle. The gland and its duct are lined by columnar epithelium. Enlarged Cowper's gland can be felt one each on the side just below the prostate on per rectal examination.

(iii) **Littre's glands** are a group of mucous glands present in the roof and sides of penile urethra. These glands are also lined by columnar epithelium, hence a site of predilection for infection with gonococcus.

(iv) **Tyson's glands** are sebaceous glands present on each side of frenulum in parafrenal distribution and on the superior surface of corona of glans penis.

FEMALE GENITALIA

Vulva

Vulva constitutes the external female genitalia consisting of labia majora and minora, mons pubis, clitoris, vestibule, Skene's glands and greater vestibular (Bartholin's) glands.

(i) **Labia majora** are two folds of skin and subcutaneous tissue which cover the vaginal opening and other structures of external genitalia. These folds join anteriorly to form mons pubis, a rounded bulge of pad of subcutaneous fat covered with hair. Posteriorly these join to form a small transverse fold called posterior commissure. Labia majora are the female counterparts of scrotum.

(ii) **Labia minora** are smaller folds interior to labia majora with inner mucosal and outer cutaneous surface. Labia minora fuse anteriorly to form a fold of skin known as clitoral prepuce, and posteriorly they join at posterior commissure or fourchette. The fourchette is quite predisposed to trauma during sexual intercourse, hence a common site for genital ulcer diseases.

(iii) **Clitoris** is an erectile tissue analogous to penis in the male. It has a small rudimentary glans and a prepuce.

(iv) **Vestibule** is the space between two labia minora that is penetrated by the openings of urethral meatus, vaginal introitus, paraurethral glands of Skene and ducts of Bartholin's gland. A thin translucent membrane called hymen covers vaginal introitus during childhood and adolescence, and is usually ruptured due to trauma, physical exercise or sexual intercourse.

(v) **Bartholin's glands**, also known as greater vestibular glands homologous to Cowper's glands in male, lie in the lower third of labia majora on either side and their duct opens at the side of the hymen, between hymen and labia minora. These are compound racemose type of glands lined with columnar epithelium. Bartholin's glands get acutely inflammed with gonococcal infection (bartholinitis) and may rarely lead to bartholin abscess, which manifests as unilateral swelling of the lower end of labia majora with consequent difficulty in walking.

(vi) **Skene's glands** or paraurethral glands are analogous to prostate in the male, and lie adjacent to urethral meatus and open either directly in vestibule or just inside urinary meatus. Rarely these glands are involved in various STDs.

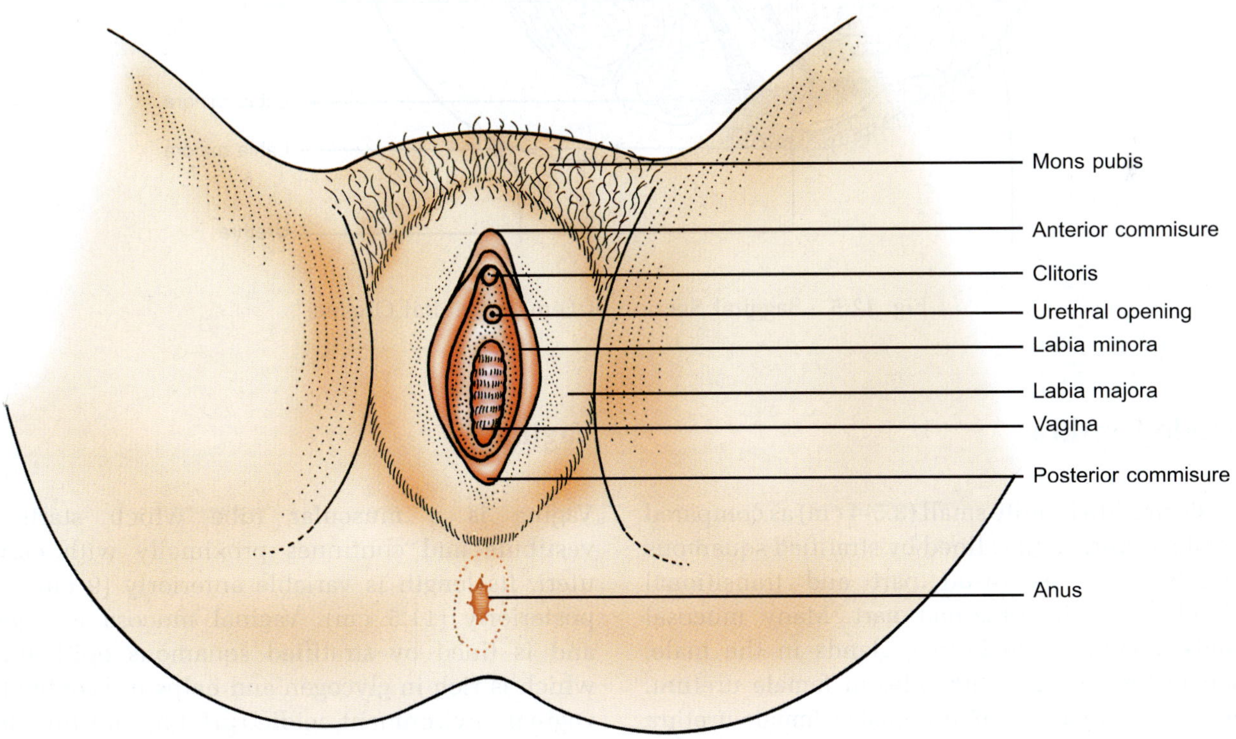

Fig. 12.3 Anatomical Structure of Female External Genitalia (Vulva).

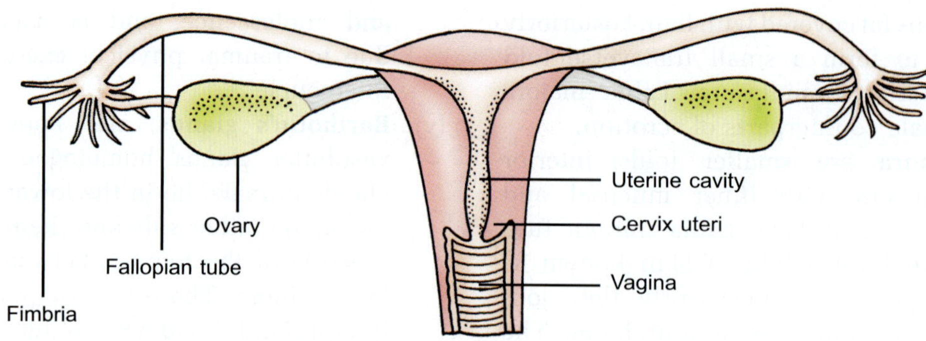

Fig. 12.4 Coronal Section of Female Genital Organs.

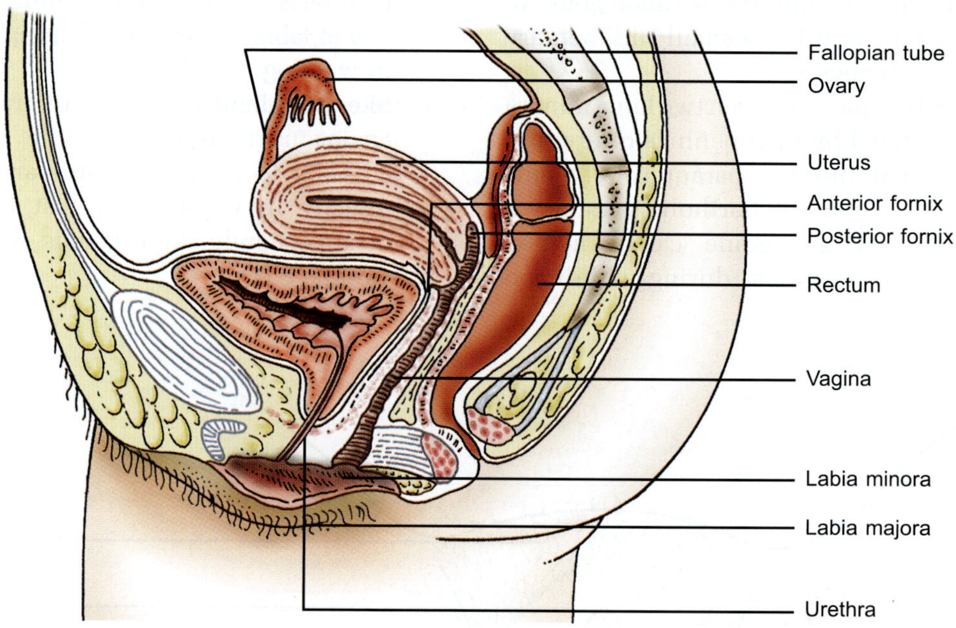

Fig. 12.5 Saggital Section of Female Genital Organs.

Female Urethra

Female urethra is quite small (3.5-4 cm) as compared to male urethra, and is lined by stratified squamous epithelium in its distal part and transitional epithelium in its proximal part. Many mucosal glands, analogous to Littre's glands in the male, open in the roof and the sides of female urethra. Lack of columnar epithelium makes female urethra relatively resistant to gonococcal infection.

Vagina

Vagina is a muscular tube which starts at vestibule and continues proximally with cervix uteri. Its length is variable anteriorly (9 cm) and posteriorly (11.5 cm). Vaginal mucosa is rugose and is lined by stratified squamous epithelium, which is rich in glycogen and helps in keeping the vaginal environment acidic (pH-4.5) and thus less susceptible to penetration by sexually acquired pathogens.

Uterus

(i) **Cervix uteri** or the neck of uterus is for its involvement in as cervicitis. Cervical canal is lined by columnar epithelium quite susceptible to gonococcal and non-gonococcal infections. Its projection into vagina divides the upper vaginal space into vaginal fornices where pooled secretions serve as an important sample for isolation of sexually transmitted pathogens. It serves as a good site for collecting diagnostic samples, as it is invariably involved in gonococcal and non-gonococcal infections.

(ii) **Body of uterus** is lined by thick endometrium and may get affected by ascending infections from the lower genital tract leading to endometritis and parametritis, which are common manifestations of pelvic inflammatory disease (PID) along with features of salpingitis.

(iii) **Fallopian tubes** arise from the side of uterus as tortuous structures which end up laterally as fimbriae, opening into the peritoneal cavity in the vicinity of ovaries. The tubes have different diameters at isthmus, ampulla and infundibulum. The ciliated columnar epithelium of fallopian tubes arranged in longitudinal folds is quite susceptible to infections with gonococcal and non-gonococcal pathogens resulting in acute salpingitis or acute pelvic inflammatory disease. The communication of fallopian tubes through fimbriae to the peritoneal cavity can lead to periappendicitis or perihepatitis due to either direct spread of sexual pathogens or as a sequel of PID.

LYMPHATIC DRAINAGE OF GENITALIA

Superficial structures of the genitalia drain chiefly into the inguinal group of lymph nodes constituting superficial and deep inguinal lymph nodes (Fig. 12.6).

Superficial Inguinal Lymph Nodes

This group of lymph nodes lies superficial to deep fascia of the thigh and have two subgroups: horizontal and vertical. The horizontal subgroup lies along the inguinal ligament and is further divided into medial and lateral chains. Medial chains are 2-3 nodes in number. They drain the external genitalia except glans penis or clitoris, lower parts of the vagina below hymen, and anal canal below the pectinate line. Some lymphatics from the superolateral angle of uterus also pass through the inguinal canal to drain into medial chain. The lateral chain of horizontal group of superficial inguinal lymph nodes drains lymphatics from the abdominal wall below umbilicus. The vertical group of superficial inguinal lymph nodes (4-5 nodes) lies along great saphenous vein and drain lymphatics from thigh and leg. All efferents from superficial inguinal lymph nodes ultimately drain into deep inguinal lymph nodes and external iliac lymph nodes.

Deep Inguinal Lymph Nodes

These are usually 1 to 3 in number with one of them usually lying within the femoral canal (node of Cloquet) into the deep fascia medial to femoral vein. Glans penis and clitoris directly drain into deep inguinal lymph nodes. Deep lymphatics of the lower limb and efferents from superficial inguinal lymph nodes drain into deep inguinal lymph nodes. Ultimately all lymphatics from inguinal lymph nodes drain through external and internal iliac lymph nodes to common iliac and para-aortic lymph nodes.

Different parts of genitalia drain their lymphatics into different lymph nodes:

(i) **Penis:** Lymphatics from the skin of the penis drain into the medial chain of horizontal group of superficial inguinal lymph nodes, while deep structures including anterior urethra drain into deep inguinal lymph nodes and posterior urethra drain into deep iliac nodes. Lymphatics from glans penis drain directly into deep inguinal lymph nodes.

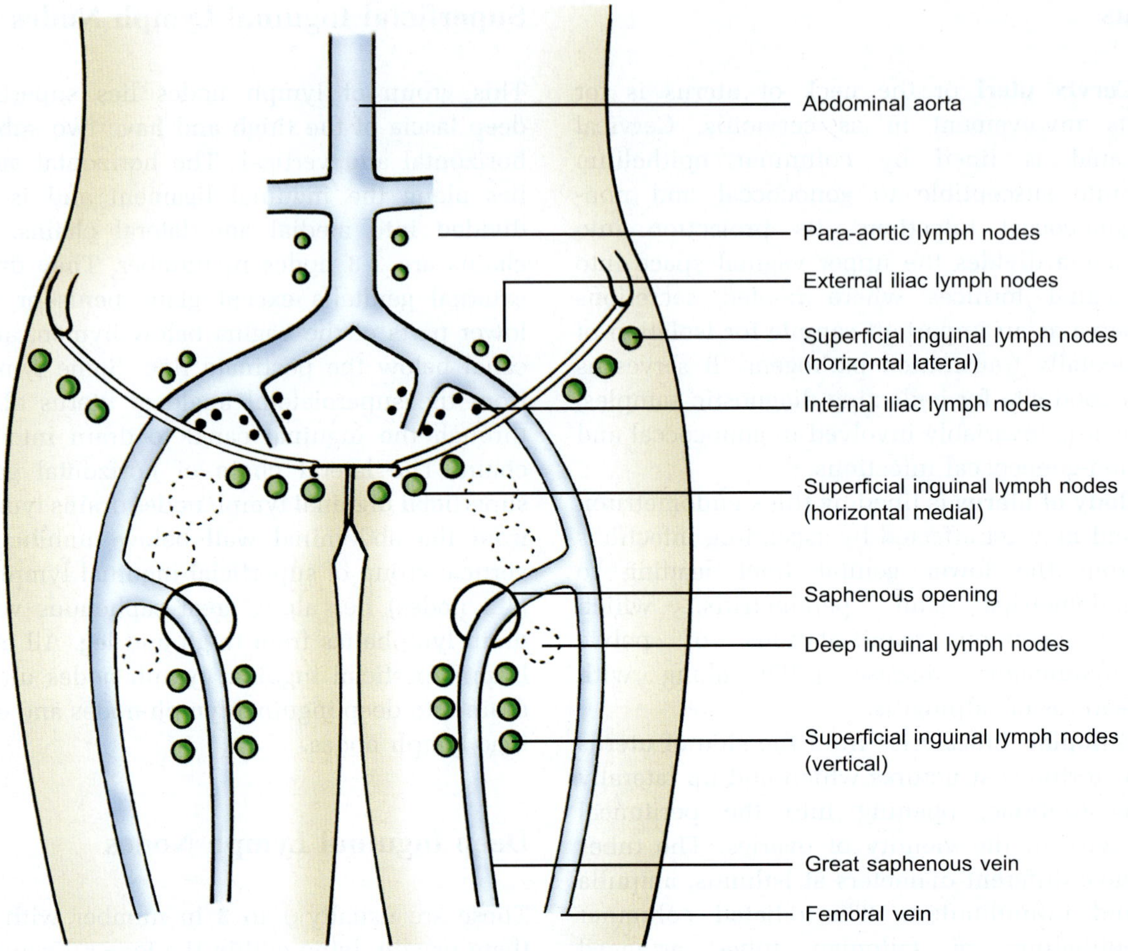

Fig. 12.6 Lymphatic Drainage of Genital Organs.

(ii) **Scrotum:** Lymphatics from the skin of scrotum drain into the medial chain of horizontal group of superficial inguinal lymph nodes, while testes and epididymis drain into the pre- and para-aortic group of lymph nodes.

(iii) **Prostate:** Lymphatics from prostate drain into the internal iliac and sacral lymph nodes and partly into the external iliac lymph nodes.

(iv) **Vulva:** Lymphatics from vulval structures drain into the medial chain of horizontal group of superficial inguinal lymph nodes and also femoral nodes. Some of the lymphatic vessels from vestibule also drain into the common iliac and sacral lymph nodes.

(v) **Vagina:** Lymphatics from the upper third of vagina drain into external iliac, middle third into internal iliac, and lower third into medial chain of horizontal group of superficial inguinal lymph nodes.

(vi) **Cervix:** Lymphatics from cervix drain into external and internal iliac and sacral lymph nodes. Some of the lymphatics pass directly to the common iliac and lower para-aortic nodes.

(vii) **Uterus:** Lymphatics from uterus are divided into upper lymphatics which drain into the para-aortic group of nodes, middle group to external iliac lymph nodes, and lower lymphatics running along the round ligament pass through inguinal canal to drain into the medial chain of horizontal group of superficial inguinal lymph nodes.

(viii) **Fallopian tubes:** Lymphatics from fallopian tubes drain predominantly into para-aortic lymph nodes. The lymphatics from isthmus drain into superficial inguinal lymph nodes

(ix) **Ovaries:** Lymphatics from ovaries drain into para- and pre-aortic lymph nodes.

Enlargement of the regional lymph nodes is invariably observed in all STDs, and is of considerable clinical significance in the diagnosis of genital ulcer disease. Variable morphology of inguinal lymphadenopathy in genital ulcer disease forms the basis of various inguinal syndromes or buboes. The separation of enlarged superficial inguinal lymph nodes from deep-seated femoral lymph nodes by inguinal ligament or fascia is the basis of genesis of 'groove sign of Greenblat' initially regarded to be characteristic of lymphogranuloma venereum. Similar groove sign has, however, been observed in the manifestation of other infections and malignancy affecting inguinal lymph nodes.

CONSEQUENCES OF LYMPHATIC BLOCKADE

Inguinal lymph nodes are by far the most important lymph nodes from the viewpoint of STDs. The destruction of these lymph nodes through any process like infection, carcinoma, irradiation, etc. leads to the blockage of lymphatic drainage of external genitalia and lower limb. Long-term sequelae of genital lymphoedema and subsequent elephantiasis are not uncommon in infections like lymphogranuloma venereum, donovanosis, filariasis, carcinoma, tuberculosis and irradiation. Pseudoelephantiasis is a condition where lymphatics rather than lymph nodes are destroyed due to local infiltration of the tissues with the offending pathogen.

Perineum is the diamond-shaped space at the lower end of the trunk and situated between two thighs. The boundaries are outlined by scrotum in males and mons pubis in females anteriorly, posteriorly by the buttocks and laterally by medial side of the thighs. This site is commonly overlooked and lesions like condylomata lata, genital warts or ulcers can occur in this region. Lymphatics of perineum drain into the superficial medial group of inguinal lymph nodes.

ANORECTAL MUCOSA AND SEXUALLY TRANSMITTED DISEASES

Anorectal mucosa has a complex lining of epithelium. The perianal area up to anal verge is lined by keratinized stratified squamous epithelium similar to other mucocutaneous junctions. This is followed by the conversion of squamous epithelium to stratified cuboidal epithelium of anal canal and true columnar epithelium of rectum. Almost all pathogens capable of producing STDs over the genitalia can affect anorectal mucosa and perianal skin. Lesions of STDs within the anal canal and perianal area are extremely painful and produce tenesmus and painful spasm of anal sphincter due to rich nerve supply in this area. Similar lesions in rectum are usually painless but may produce bleeding per rectum and mucopurulent discharge.

Anorectal mucosa is quite vulnerable to infection with sexually transmitted pathogens in females due to close proximity of vulva and anal orifice. Rectal mucosa is predisposed to infection with gonococcus in females, and rectal involvement has been observed in 50-60% of cases of genital infection. Lymphatics from perianal skin and anal canal below the pectinate line drain into the medial chain of horizontal group of superficial inguinal lymph nodes, while those from rectal mucosa drain into internal iliac lymph nodes.

ORAL MUCOSA AND SEXUALLY TRANSMITTED DISEASES

Oral mucosa lined with stratified squamous epithelium is equally vulnerable to sexually transmitted agents as anorectal mucosa. Pharynx and tonsils are common sites affected by sexual pathogens, and most infections in these areas are asymptomatic. The presence of lymphoid tissue in oral mucosa in the form of tonsils makes these infections less amenable to treatment with the same regimen as used for a similar infection in the genital area. Lymphatics from the oral mucosa drain into submandibular, submental, jugulodiagastric, jugulo omohyoid and other groups of superficial and deep cervical lymph nodes.

NORMAL ANATOMICAL VARIATIONS IN THE GENITAL REGION

Some anatomical variations within normal limits can mimic STDs. These include the following:

(i) Pearly penile papules are small monomorphous fibromas present in a row or two over the corona glandis. They are most common in uncircumcised men. These are asymptomatic but may cause apprehension in a patient and mimic genital warts.

(ii) Vestibular papillomatosis is characterized by small raised papillae over mucous membranes of introitus. These are normal variants and may be an incidental finding with any other symptoms over the genitalia. Like pearly penile papules, these may also be mistaken for genital warts.

(iii) Fordyce spots are ectopic sebaceous glands present over prepuce or inner aspect of labia minora. These lesions are often mistaken for genital warts.

(iv) Physiological hyperpigmentation is observed primarily in dark-skinned individuals. Hyperpigmentation is around the edges of labia minora in females, scrotum and penile skin in males, and perianal skin in both sexes. Therapy may be unnecessary.

REFERENCES

1. Hollinshead WH. Anatomy for surgeons. (The thorax, abdomen and pelvis). New York: Harper and Row and John Weatherhill; 1966. p. 749-909.
2. McMinn RMH. Last's Anatomy: Regional and applied. Edinburgh: Churchill Livingstone; 1991. p. 385-412.
3. Williams PL. Gray's Anatomy. The anatomical basis of medicine & surgery. London: Churchill Livingstone; 1995. p. 1813-76.
4. Agur AMR. Grant's Atlas of Anatomy. Philadelphia: Williams & Wilkins; 1991. p. 147-98.
5. Moore KL. Clinically oriented anatomy. Philadelphia: Williams & Wilkins; 1992. p. 295-322.
6. Snell RS. Clinical anatomy for medical students. London: Little, Brown and Company; 1995. p. 347-79.
7. Graney DO, Vontver LA. Anatomy and physical examination of the female genital tract. In: Holmes KK, Sparling PF, Mardh PA, et al, eds. Sexually Transmitted Diseases. New York: McGraw Hill; 1999. p. 685-98.
8. Krieger JN, Graney DO. Clinical anatomy, histology and physical examination of male genital tract. In: Holmes KK, Sparling PF, Mardh PA, et al, eds. Sexually Transmitted Diseases. New York: Mc GrawHill; 1999. p. 699-710.
9. Orient JM. Sapira's Art and Science of Bedside Diagnosis. Philadelphia: Lippincott Williams & Wilkins; 2002. p. 157-162.
10. Tindall VR. Jeffcoate's Principles of Gynaecology, Oxford: Butterworth-Heinmann; 1997. p. 16-52.

13 SIDE LABORATORY PROCEDURES IN SEXUALLY TRANSMITTED DISEASES

Vinod K Sharma, G Sethuraman

In this chapter

- Dark Field Microscopy
- Gram Staining
- Tzanck Smear or Giemsa Stain
- Wet mount (direct microscopy without staining)
- KOH Wet Mount
- Acetic Acid Test
- Whiff Test or Sniff Test
- Two and Three Glass Test
- Aspiration of Bubo

INTRODUCTION

Sexually transmitted diseases are a group of communicable diseases, which are acquired primarily through heterosexual or homosexual intercourse. STDs still remain an important major public health problem not only because of their complications, sequelae and social stigma but also because they increase the risk for transmission of HIV. Hence a good clinical assessment and appropriate laboratory tests are mandatory for the diagnosis and management of different STDs. A number of bacteria, spirochaetes, viruses, fungi, chlamydiae and protozoa are known to cause STDs. The identification of these diverse organisms requires skilled laboratory personnel and good laboratory infrastructure. In this chapter, the common laboratory diagnostic procedures performed in an outpatient department are described (Table 13.1).

Table 13.1 Side Lab Procedures in STDs

1. Dark field microscopy
2. Gram stain
3. Giemsa stain
4. Wet mount
5. KOH wet mount
6. Whiff or sniff test
7. Bubo aspiration
8. Acetic acid test
9. Two- and three-glass test

DARK FIELD MICROSCOPY[1]

Dark field microscopy, commonly referred to as dark ground illumination (DGI), is the only method for demonstrating *Treponema pallidum*, the causative agent for syphilis. The organism is imposible to be stained by ordinary reagents, and is so thin that it cannot be visualized under a normal light microscope.[2] In dark field microscopy, only light rays hitting the organism at an oblique angle enter the microscope objective to give a luminous appearance against a black background, making the visualization of *T. pallidum* much easy.

Requirements

- Dark field microscope
- Thin glass slides (1 mm)

Collection of Specimen for Dark Field Microscopy

T. pallidum can be identified in serous fluid from the lesions of primary and secondary syphilis and early congenital syphilis. Rarely it may be identified in lymph node aspirate.

- Clean the lesion carefully with sterile gauze soaked in saline.
- Gently abrade the lesion with dry gauze, wipe off any blood stained serum and squeeze the lesion to produce clear serous exudate.
- The serous exudate is transferred on to the glass slide either by pressing the cover slip directly on to the serous exudate or by Pasteur pipette.
- If serous exudate is sufficient, cover with cover slip and examine.
- If the material is not sufficient it, then mix it with a drop of saline to give a homogenous suspension.
- Seal the edges of the cover slip with petroleum jelly.
- Examine immediately.

Setting the Microscope for Examination

- Bring down the condenser of the dark field microscope.
- Put a drop of liquid paraffin on the condenser of dark field microscope.
- Place the slide on the microscope stage.
- Raise the condenser until there is good contact between oil and bottom of the slide.
- Avoid trapping of air bubbles in oil.

Focussing

Bring the specimen into focus with a low power objective (10x). Centre the light onto the field by adjusting the centering screws located on the condenser and focus the condenser by raising and lowering it until the smallest possible diameter of light is obtained. Recentre the light if necessary. Put a drop of liquid paraffin on coverslip and examine under 100x oil immersion lens. Bring the specimen into focus and examine the slide carefully. The contrast will be better when microscopy is carried out in the dark. Avoid bright daylight. If Brownian movements can be seen clearly, the slide is focussed.

WHO[1] claims that *T. pallidum* can be seen through a dry 40x lens, but it is not a common practice in India.

Reading

T. pallidum appears white, illuminated on a dark background. The organism is identified by its typical morphology, size and movements. It is a thin spiral organism 6-14 μm long. It has 8-14 spirals which are regular and pronounced. It rotates relatively slowly about the longitudinal axis (like a corkscrew). The rotation is accompanied by sudden bending at acute angle which is most typical, or twisting in the middle of the organism. Other movements which may be observed are lengthening, shortening and distortion in tortuous convolutions. Obstruction of the treponemes by heavier objects might distort the coil. The pathogenic *T. pallidum* can be differentiated from other non-pathogenic spirochaetes in whom the movements take the form of a writhing motion with marked flexion and frequent relaxation of the coils.

The presence of *T. pallidum* confirms the diagnosis of syphilis. Ideally the test should be done on three consecutive days since single dark field microscopy has a sensitivity of no more than 50%. Dark field microscopy is less useful for lesions in the oral cavity which is usually colonized by other spirochaetes.[1,3]

Reasons for Testing Negative

- Non-syphilitic ulcer
- Natural resolution of the lesion
- Treated patients
- Prior topical application of antiseptics or antibiotics
- Number of organisms present in the specimen is insufficient

GRAM STAINING[4,5]

Gram staining is useful in the diagnosis of gonococcal and non-gonococcal urethritis, muco-purulent cervicitis, chancroid, bacterial vaginosis and candidal infections.

Requirements

- Crystal violet:
  Dissolve 2 gm of crystal violet (methylrosanilinium chloride) in 20 ml of 96% ethanol and then add 80 ml of 0.08 mol/l (1%) ammonium oxalate.
- Iodine solution:
  2 gm of iodine crystals are dissolved in 10 ml of 1 mol/l NaOH solution; make up to 100 ml with distilled water.
- Decolourizing solution:
  10 ml of analytical grade acetone is mixed with 50 ml of 96% ethanol.
- Counter stain solution (either fuschsin or safranin):
  Fuschsin 0.3 gm of basic fuschsin is dissolved in 10 ml of 96% ethanol. 5 gm of phenol is dissolved in 95 ml of distilled water. Mix the solutions slowly with vigorous stirring. Add 950 ml of distilled water. Allow the mixture to stand for 2-3 days. Filter through a 0.22 μm filter before use.
  Safranin 1 gm of safranin O is dissolved in 20 ml of 96% ethanol and 10 ml of this solution is diluted with 90 ml of distilled water.

Collection of Specimen for Gram Staining

Sterile cotton, calcium alginate or polyethylene terephthalate (PET) swabs can be used for collecting the specimen. In India, sterile cotton wool swab is routinely used.

Gonorrhoea

Neisseria gonorrhoeae produces lower urogenital tract infection and pelvic inflammatory disease (PID) in women, urethritis and epididymitis in men, and proctitis, pharyngitis, conjunctivitis and disseminated infections in both sexes. The appropriate site for specimen collection will depend on age, sex, sex practices and clinical symptoms.

Site for collection of specimen

The primary collection site in heterosexual men is the urethra, and in homosexual men the urethra, rectum and oropharynx. In women, the material is collected from the endocervical canal. The secondary sites of specimen collection in women include urethra, vagina, rectum and oropharynx. Direct microscopic examination is generally not recommended for the diagnosis of rectal and pharyngeal infection.

Methods of collection of specimen

Urethra: Urethral specimen is collected at least 1 hour after the patient has urinated. Retract the prepuce, clean the tip of the meatus with normal saline and collect the pus directly onto the swab. If no discharge is seen, milk the urethra from root of penis towards glans to express the pus. If no pus is obtained, insert a thin sterile swab 2-3 cm into the urethra and gently scrape the mucosa by rotating the swabs for 5-10 seconds. The organisms can also be demonstrated in the sediments of early morning urine sample. In women, massage the urethra against pubic symphysis and use the same technique as for men.

Endocervical specimen: The routine use of antiseptics, analgesics or lubricants should be avoided. The vaginal speculum is inserted after moistening with warm water. Clean the exocervix using forceps with sterile cotton swab. Insert another sterile swab 2 cm into the cervical canal, rotate and move from side to side for 5-10 seconds and withdraw.

Vagina: Vaginal specimens are collected from prepubertal girls and from women who have had a hysterectomy. The material is taken from the posterior fornix with a swab either with or without a speculum.

Non-gonococcal Urethritis and Mucopurulent Cervicitis

The specimen is collected in the same manner as in gonorrhoea, but as the discharge in NGU may be scanty, the samples are collected after holding the urine for 3-4 hours.

Chancroid

The specimen is usually collected from the edge of the ulcer. First clean the ulcer with a saline-soaked gauze and then with dry gauze; take a sterile swab and roll it in one direction on the edge of undermined ulcer. After doing so, reroll the swab in the reverse direction on a glass slide and stain it. The organisms may be demonstrated from the material aspirated from an intact bubo.[3]

Bacterial Vaginosis

It is caused by the replacement of lactobacilli of the vagina by the characteristic group of bacteria. Here the specimen is collected from the posterior or lateral wall of vagina with a sterile swab soaked in saline.

Procedure

A. Preparation of smear

- ⥣ Take a clean glass slide, wipe it with gauze piece and pass it through the flame twice or thrice and wipe it again.
- ⥣ Draw two vertical lines 2.5 cm apart with a glass marking pencil on the central part of the slide.
- ⥣ Roll the swab with the specimen over the marked area and spread it to make a smear of 2 × 1 cm size.
- ⥣ Label the smear on the right or left corner of the slide.

B. Fixing the smear

- ⥣ Fixing kills the organism, sticks it to the slide, prevents autolytic changes and makes the organisms permeable to dye and harmless to the person handling the smear.
- ⥣ Hold the slide with the smear facing upwards.
- ⥣ Pass the slide over the flame of a Bunsen's burner or spirit lamp twice or thrice.
- ⥣ Allow the fixed smear to cool.
- ⥣ Heating should be appropriate and tolerable to the back of the hand.

C. Staining

- ⥣ Cover the fixed smear with crystal violet for 1 minute and then rinse it with tap water.
- ⥣ Flood the slide with Gram's iodine solution for 1 minute. Drain off the solution and gently rinse with running water.
- ⥣ Decolourize with acetone-ethanol until the drops falling off the slide are no longer blue. This usually takes 10 to 20 seconds depending on the thickness of the smear. Excessive decolourization must be avoided. Rinse quickly under running water to stop decolourization and drain off excess water.
- ⥣ Counterstain with safranin or fuschsin for 1 minute. Gently wash in running water and blot the slide with absorbent paper.

Smear reading

Examine the slide under a light microscope. Scan the smear first and focus on a good field. Put a drop of liquid paraffin without air trapping and examine under 100x oil immersion objective. Push the condenser up and open the iris diaphragm so that maximum light passes through the slide.

The presence of onococcus which appear as intracellular Gram negative kidney or coffee bean-shaped diplococci, 0.6-0.8 μm in size, confirms the diagnosis of gonorrhoea **(Fig. 13.1)**. Sometimes the organism may be extracellular. In addition, clumps of pus cells are also seen. Non-pathogenic Neisseria other than *N. meningitidis*, which are morphologically indistinguishable from *N. gonorrhoeae*, are generally not cell-associated. Acinetobacter species are bipolar-taining Gram negative bacilli.[6]

The presence of five or more polymorphonuclear leucocytes (PMN) in the absence of intracellular Gram negative diplococci is suggestive of non-gonococcal urethritis.[7] Cervical Gram stain with more than 30 PMN/high power field in women of menstruating age is suggestive of mucopurulent cervicitis[8].

Haemophilus ducreyi, the causative agent of chancroid, appears as small Gram negative bacilli grouped in chains or "school of fish" or "railroad track" appearance. The sensitivity of Gram staining in chancroid is less than 50% as the typical arrangement is seen only infrequently on smears. Often the ulcers harbour polymicrobial flora due to contamination resulting in false positive diagnosis.

The presence of "clue cells" is highly diagnostic of bacterial vaginosis (BV). Clue cells are squamous epithelial cells coated with many small coccobacillary organisms giving a stippled or granular appearance **(Fig. 13.2)**. The edge of the cells is usually indistinct. In BV, a mixture of normal exfoliated vaginal epithelial cells and 20% or more clue cells are seen. The organisms are usually *Gardenerella vaginalis*, which are Gram variable to Gram negative small rods (1.5-2.5 μm × 0.5 μm) showing pleomorphism. Sometimes other anaerobes like *Prevotella* spp and *Mobiluncus* spp are seen as slender (0.3-0.4 μm), slightly curved rods either singly or in pairs with the appearance of gull wings.[9]

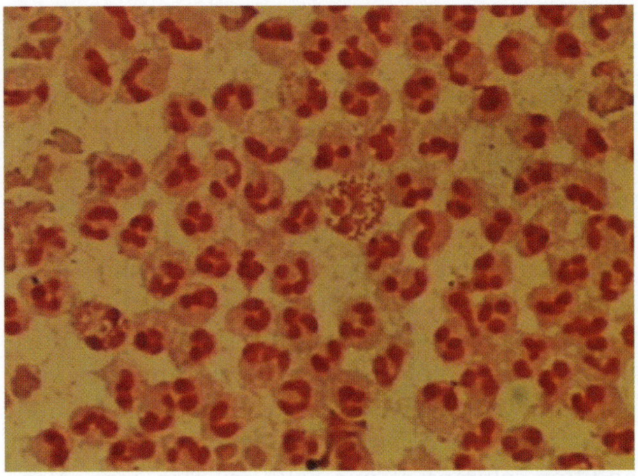

Fig 13.1 Gonorrhoea – Gram Negative Intracellular Diplococci (Gram Stain, 100x)

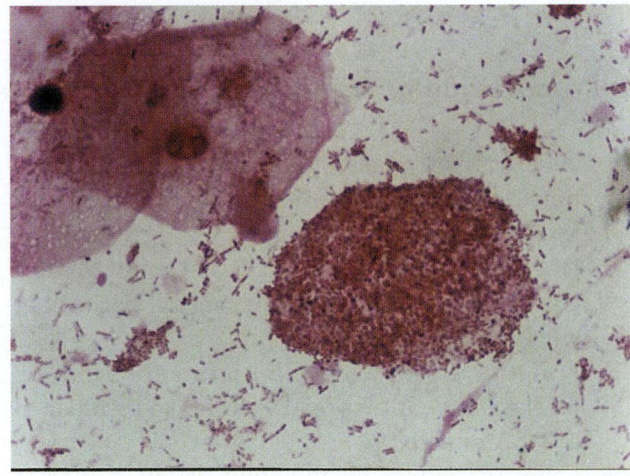

Fig 13.2 Bacterial Vaginosis – Clue Cell, Gram Stain (100x).

Gram staining may also be used in the diagnosis of vulvovaginal candidiasis and balanoposthitis which show Gram positive budding yeast cells looking like "figure of 8" and yeast hyphae. However, KOH wet mount examination may improve diagnostic sensitivity.[9]

TZANCK SMEAR OR GIEMSA STAIN[10,11]

Tzank smear or Giemsa stain is a simple bed-side test used in the diagnosis of various STDs like genital herpes, molluscum contagiosum, donovanosis and chancroid.

Requirements

- Giemsa stock: It is prepared by dissolving 4 gm Giemsa powder in 250 ml glycerol at 60°C and then adding 250 ml methanol.
- 4 ml of stock solution is added to 96 ml of distilled water or buffered water at pH 7.0-7.2.

Collection of Specimen in Various STDs

Herpes Progenitalis

The intact roof of the vesicle or blister is opened along one side and folded back. Scrape the under-surface of the roof of vesicle and the floor of ulcer with a curette or scalpel and smear the obtained material on a clean glass slide.[12,13]

Donovanosis

Clean the granulomatous ulcer at the edge with gauze soaked in saline and then with dry gauze. A small piece of tissue is removed with forceps or a curette. Local anaesthesia may be required. Alternatively, the ulcer may be scraped with a scalpel. Place the tissue specimen over a clean glass slide. Keep another slide over the specimen and press it firmly so that the tissue is crushed between the two slides. Spread the crushed tissue and allow the smear to dry. Direct impressions on the glass slide are not usually adequate because surface debris and other bacteria are liable to obscure the picture.[14]

Molluscum Contagiosum

The central semisolid core is removed and stained.

Procedure

- ⥣ Initial preparation of the slide is same as in Gram's stain.
- ⥣ The smear is fixed in methanol. Dip the slide for 5 minutes in Coplin jar containing methanol.
- ⥣ Allow the smear to dry.
- ⥣ Dilute the Giemsa stain 10 times, or 1 ml of Giemsa stain is added to 9 ml of distilled water.
- ⥣ Cover the slide with diluted Giemsa stain and leave it to stand for 20-30 minutes.
- ⥣ Wash the slide with distilled water or buffer.
- ⥣ Allow the smear to dry.

Smear Reading

The smear is first examined under a low power objective and then under oil immersion objective. Herpes progenitalis will show the characteristic multinucleated giant keratinocytes **(Fig. 13.3)**. The cells show ballooning degeneration sometimes reaching a diameter of 60-80 μm. The nuclei show blurring of the chromatin pattern and loss of staining. Intranuclear inclusion bodies surrounded by a subtle halo are highly diagnostic of herpetic infection but difficult to find in the smear.[12]

The demonstration of intracellular donovan bodies is the gold standard for the diagnosis of donovanosis. They appear as coccobacilli within the large vacuoles (80-90 μm in diameter) in the cytoplasm of large histiocytes and rarely in plasma cells and PMN. They are bluish purple in colour and resemble "safety pins" **(Fig. 13.4)**. A wide variety of stains may be used for demonstrating the donovan bodies, viz. Leishman or Wright's stain and Delafield's haematoxylin with a small amount of eosin.[14]

Molluscum contagiosum will show the characteristic molluscum or Henderson–Patterson's bodies. They are the largest inclusion bodies (30-35 μm). They are basically virus-transformed keratinocytes that appear as ovoid, deeply basophilic bodies with the hyaline homogenous structure surrounded by, membrane.[12] Although molluscum bodies can be identified in the smear, the diagnosis is generally made on clinical grounds.[15]

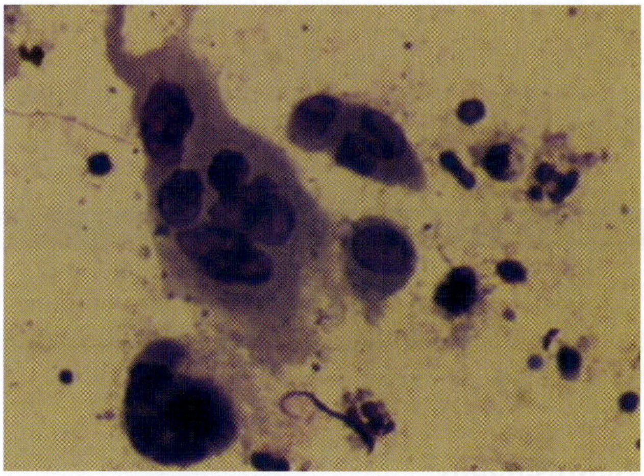

Fig 13.3 Genital herpes – Multinucleated Giant Cells, Giemsa Stain (100x).

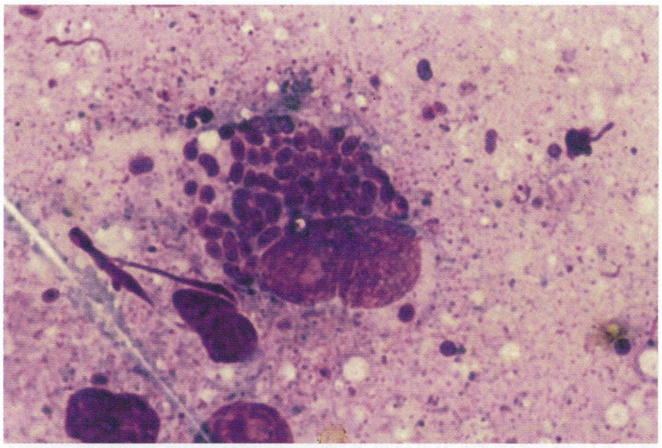

Fig 13.4 Donovan Bodies, Haematoxylin and Eosin 100x.

WET MOUNT (DIRECT MICROSCOPY WITHOUT STAINING)[5]

This method is mainly used for the diagnosis of trichomoniasis, BV and candidiasis in women and occasionally in men with urethral discharge in whom trichomoniasis is suspected.

Collection of Specimen

Vaginal discharge is obtained with cotton tipped swab from the posterior fornix. In men, the sample is collected by inserting a sterile swab into the urethra for 1-2 cm.

Procedure

The sample is placed on a clean glass slide, diluted with a drop of saline, and then a coverslip is placed. It is examined under a light microscope immediately under 40x with reduced illumination.

Reading

In trichomoniasis, *Trichomonas vaginalis* is identified by its typical jerky movements. They are clear pear-shaped organisms about the size of a pus cell with four anterior flagellae and an axostyle that traverses the body to end in a spine. They have a lateral undulating membrane. In addition, large numbers of leucocytes are seen in most of the patients.

Although clue cells of bacterial vaginosis can be seen in wet mount, they are better visualized with Gram stain. Yeast cells of candidiasis can also be seen in wet mount, but 10% KOH mount is better.

KOH WET MOUNT[16]

KOH wet mount is used for the diagnosis of candidal infection of the genital tract.

Requirement

10 or 20% KOH

Collection of specimen

In females, the discharge is collected from the posterior fornix. In men with balanitis, a swab moistened in saline is rubbed against the glans penis.[9]

Procedure

- Take a clean microscopic slide.
- Place the specimen on the slide.
- Add 2 drops of 10% KOH to the specimen.
- Put a clean coverslip over the specimen. Ensure that no air bubble is trapped under the coverslip.
- The prepared smear is examined under a light microscope first scanning the material under low power (10x) and then using 40x magnification.

Reading

The identification of yeast usually confirms the diagnosis of candidiasis. Yeasts are round to ovoid cells, 4 µm in diameter showing typical budding (blastoconidia) and the pseudohyphae.

ACETIC ACID TEST[17]

The acetic acid test is used to detect subclinical genital human papilloma virus (HPV)-associated infections.

Requirements

- Acetic acid 3 to 5%
- Swab sticks

Procedure

- ⇑ Clean the area to be tested with gauze soaked in saline and then with dry gauze.
- ⇑ Apply acetic acid with the swab.
- ⇑ Wait for 2 to 3 minutes for lesions of vulva and penis. In uterine cervix, the reaction appears within 1 minute.

Reading

The affected area becomes whitish, distinctly demarcated and thickened, sometimes with elevated borders and centrally located epithelial fissures. In men, the surface of affected areas may look red because of hypervascularization. The whitish appearance of the epithelium is due to over-expression of cytokeratin 10 in HPV infected suprabasal cells. The epithelial cells of HPV infected areas are undifferentiated and contain large nuclei and their protein content is very high. Acetic acid application causes denaturation of these proteins, which results in whitish appearance of the epithelium.

Limitation

The test is not specific for HPV infection as acetic acid-induced whitish reaction of the genital epithelium can occur in other non-specific inflammation. But in HPV infection, the reaction occurs much slower.

WHIFF TEST OR SNIFF TEST[5]

Whiff test is diagnostic of bacterial vaginosis. The addition of 1 or 2 drops of 10% KOH solution to the specimen of vaginal discharge on a glass slide causes enhancement of typical fishy odour.

TWO- AND THREE-GLASS TEST[18]

This test is mainly used to differentiate anterior urethritis from posterior urethritis or infection of the bladder. The patient is asked to pass urine into two separate glasses. In case of anterior urethritis, the first specimen is cloudy or hazy with pus or mucous threads and the specimen in the second glass is clear. Haziness in the second specimen suggests the involvement of posterior urethra. If both the specimens are hazy, then bacterial cystitis should be suspected. For greater accuracy, it is necessary to apply the three-glass test, in which the anterior urethra is irrigated with a colourless antiseptic solution (such as 1:8000 oxycyanide of mercury) until the washings contained in the first glass seem to be clear. The patient then passes urine into two other separate glasses. If the first sample of urine contains pus, the posterior urethra is infected. If there is pus in the second glass, then infection has extended into the bladder. But at present, it is used infrequently.

ASPIRATION OF THE BUBO

Aspiration of the bubo is carried out for fluctuant bubo associated with chancroid and LGV. Once the bubo becomes fluctuant, it may continue to progress despite antimicrobial therapy.

Procedure

The patient is made to lie on a couch in supine position. Skin is sterilized with iodine and bubo is aspirated using a 16-18 G needle with 10 or 20 ml syringe. Aspiration is done from the non-dependent fluctuant part of the bubo and continued till all parts of the swelling are reduced. The material is collected and culture sent for *H. ducreyi*, chlamydia and anaerobes, and smear for Gram stain and direct immunofluorescene for chlamydia.

REFERENCES

1. Dyck EV, Meheus AZ, Piot P, eds. Syphilis. In: Laboratory diagnosis of sexually transmitted diseases. Geneva: World Health Organization; 1999. p. 36-49.
2. Young H. Syphilis-serology. Dermatol Clin 1998; 16: 691–8.
3. Arndt KA, Bowers KE, eds. Sexually transmitted diseases. In: Manual of dermatologic therapeutics. Philadelphia: Lippincott Williams and Wilkins; 2002. p. 196-208.
4. Dyck EV, Meheus AZ, Piot P, eds. Gonnorrhoea. In: Laboratory diagnosis of sexually transmitted diseases. Geneva: World Health Organization: 1999; 1-21.
5. Management of patients with sexually transmitted diseases. Geneva: World Health Organization, 1991.
6. Hook EW, Handsfield HH. Gonococcal infections in the adult. In: Holmes KK, Mardh P, Sparlin FP, et al, eds. Sexually transmitted diseases. New York: McGraw Hill; 1999. p. 407-22.
7. Stary A. Urethritis: Diagnosis of nongonococcal urethritis. Dermatol Clin 1998; 16: 723-6.
8. Stamm WE. *Chlamydia trachomatis* infection of the adult. In: Holmes KK, Mardh P, Sparling PF, et al, eds. Sexually transmitted diseases. New York: McGraw Hill; 1999. p. 407-22.
9. Dyck EV, Meheus AZ, Piot P, eds. Vaginitis in adults. In: Laboratory diagnosis of sexually transmitted diseases. Geneva: World Health Organization; 1999. p. 70-80.
10. Dyck EV, Meheus AZ, Piot P, eds. Media, reagents, stains (Annex 2). In: Laboratory diagnosis of sexually transmitted diseases. Geneva: World Health Organization; 1999. p. 102-12.
11. Dyck EV, Meheus AZ, Piot P, eds. *Chlamydia trachomatis* infection. In: Laboratory diagnosis of sexually transmitted diseases. Geneva: World Health Organization; 1999. p. 22-35.
12. Ruocco V, Ruocco E. Tzanck smear, an old test for the new millennium: when and how. Int J Dermatol 1999; 38: 830-4.
13. Yeung-Yue KA, Brentjens MH, Lee PC, et al. Herpes simplex viruses 1 and 2. Dermatol clin 2002; 20: 249-66.
14. Richens J. The diagnosis and treatment of donovanosis (granuloma inguinale). Genitourin Med 1991; 67: 441-52.
15. Perna AG, Tyring ST. A review of the dermatological manifestations of pox virus infection. Dermatol Clin 2002; 20: 343-6.
16. Warren NG. Taxonomy and introduction. Dermatol Clin 1996; 14: 1-7.
17. Strand A, Rylander E. Human papilloma virus. Subclinical and atypical manifestations. Dermatol Clin 1998; 16: 817-22.
18. King A, Nicol, Rodin P, eds. 'Non specific' urogenital infections; Non gonococcal genital infections in children; Non gonococcal ophthalmia. In: Venereal diseases. 4th edn. London: ELBS; 1980. p. 274-93.

PART 4

Sexually Transmitted Diseases

14 SYPHILIS: CLINICAL FEATURES AND NATURAL COURSE

R S Misra, Joginder Kumar

In this chapter

Syphilis simulates every other disease. It is the only disease necessary to know. One then becomes an expert dermatologist, an expert laryngologist, an expert alienist, an expert oculist, an expert internist and an expert diagnostician,

Sir William Osler

INTRODUCTION

Syphilis is a sexually transmitted infection caused by a spirochaete bacterium, *Treponema pallidum* subspecies *pallidum*. The untreated syphilis runs through several decades manifesting in various stages involving various organs of the body.

With its protean manifestations due to multiorgan involvement syphilis is not an exclusive domain of the venereologists. The disease is systemic right from its inception. In fact occasionally it has been transmitted by blood transfusion even during its incubation period in the donor. Early world literature talks of genital ulcers or chancres, skin rashes and bone pains as its clinical manifestations. The disease was known to occur during coitus or through surgical instrumentation. The redoubtable experiment of John Hunter[1] (1728-1793) gave rise to the misconception of common aetiology of syphilis and gonorrhoea. He had inoculated a patient's urethra with genital discharge from a prostitute. The development of a chancre as well as gonorrhoeal discharge made him propagate this concept. Later, Philip Ricord[2] in 1838 proved the concept to be erroneous and established syphilis and gonorrhoea as two distinct disease entities. John Hunter's patient had probably been suffering from both the diseases. John Hunter, however, had observed that the genital chancres could be classified into two distinct types—hard ones and soft ones. He reported the latter as non-specific. Another worker Bassereau in 1852 detected that patients with hard or soft chancre transmitted similar lesions to their contacts and separated both as two different venereal diseases.[3] The hard chancre was said to be of syphilis and the soft chancre was called chancroid. But it had been diffcult to link some of symptoms and signs to syphilis. Syphilitic origin of aortic aneurysm had been suspected in early eighteenth century, but consensus could only be reached on this aspect in 1903, when the histopathological picture had become clear.[4] Clustering of tabes dorsalis patients and patients with general paresis of insane among past sufferers of syphilis led to the suggestion of their relationship with syphilis.

CLASSIFICATION OF SYPHILIS

The disease presents in a congenital or an acquired form. The acquired form may be early or late depending upon whether the infection was acquired within the last two years or earlier than that. The most accepted classification of syphilis is as shown below:

Acquired Syphilis

Early Syphilis (infectious phase)

- Primary syphilis
- Secondary syphilis
- Early latent syphilis

Late Syphilis (non-infectious phase)

- Late latent syphilis
- Tertiary syphilis
  - Benign tertiary
  - Cardiovascular syphilis
  - Neurosyphilis

Syphilis derives its name from a poem, *Syphilis sive morbus gallicus* written by a physician, Girolamo Fracastoro. In the poem syphilus happens to be the name of a shepherd who suffered this disease as a curse for insulting the god Apollo. The disease had also been known as *morbus gallicus* and *Lues venereum* in the past. It was brought to India by the Europeans and had been referred to as English disease, French disease, Portuguese disease or Firang disease in the various parts of the country.

The term tertiary syphilis is used to include benign tertiary, cardiovascular and neurosyphilis.

Congenital Syphilis

- Early congenital syphilis
- Late congenital syphilis
- Stigmata of congenital syphilis

BIOLOGY OF *TREPONEMA PALLIDUM*

The causative bacterium of venereal syphilis was first demonstrated by Fritz Schaudin and Erich Hoffman in 1905 from the syphilitic lesion. It was identified as *Treponema pallidum* subspecies *pallidum* and classified under the order spirochaetales and family spirochaetaceae (spiro: coiled + chaete: hair). The important genera in this order are *Treponema*, *Borrelia* and *Leptospira*. The genus *Treponema* (trepo: turn + nema: a thread = turning thread) includes:

T. pallidum subspecies *pallidum* — causative agent of venereal syphilis

T. pallidum subspecies *pertenue* — causative agent of yaws

T. pallidum subspecies *endemicum* — causative agent of endemic syphilis

T. carateum — causative agent of pinta

T. pallidum subspecies *pallidum* (= pale, pallid) cannot be differentiated from other subspecies either by morphology or by antigenic character. However genetic studies have revealed some nucleotide sequence differences between *T. pallidum* subspecies *pallidum* and other subspecies of *T. pallidum*[5]. One other treponeme, called Reiter strain having antigenic relationship to *T. pallidum* is a nonvirulent, cultivable treponeme and now has been named as *T. phagedenis*.

For T.Pallidum,man is the only natural host.

Treponema pallidum subspecies *pallidum* is a slender, thread-like, motile, flexible, unencapsulated, coiled structure with tapering ends. There are about 8-24 coils placed at regular intervals. The organism is Gram negative but stains pale pink with prolonged Giemsa staining. The Unstained organism can only be visualized by the dark field microscope because of its thinness and appears as a white wave. Silver impregnation technique makes the organism easy to be visualized under the microscope. It measures about 6-20 μm in length, 0.10 to 0.18 μm in diameter and has regular tight spirals with a coil length of about 1.1 μm and an amplitude of 0.2 to 0.3 μm[6]. The distinct features as revealed by electron microscopy include a central protoplasmic cylinder, 6 – 8 periplasmic flagella and a multilayered cell envelope. The protoplasmic cylinder runs through the entire length of the organism and has nucleoid, ribosomal structures and other cytoplasmic material. It is bounded by the cytoplasmic membrane. Running along the inside of the cytoplasmic membrane is a cluster of 6-8 cytoplasmic fibrils (intracytoplasmic tubules) while just outside the cytoplasmic membrane, in the periplasmic space, are the periplasmic flagella (also called endoflagella). These endoflagella, usually 6 in number, originate as a group of 3 from both ends of the organism, run towards the centre and wind around the protoplasmic cylinder in a spiral manner. The flagella from both the sides overlap considerably in the central part of the organism and terminate after crossing into the opposite half of the organism. The multilayer cell envelope is composed of an outer membrane, a thin peptidoglycan layer and an inner cytoplasmic membrane. The peptidoglycan layer is closely adhered to the cytoplasmic membrane and provides some rigidity to the organism. As compared to other bacteria,very few protein molecules have been observed on its outer surface thereby limiting the antigenicity of the organism[7].

The various movements of *T. pallidum* are attributed to the presence of the above endoflagella. These movements are helpful in identifying the organism under dark field microscope and include slow forward-backward motion, compression– expansion, bending or angling on its long axis and burrowing or cork-screw like movement. Less common movements include looping, buckling and undulation. The spiral shape and the internal location of the flagella help the organism to move even in viscous fluids of synovia, eyes and extracellular matrices of the skin.[8]

The organism is very fragile and is readily destroyed on drying or heating. At 41-42°C,it is destroyed within one hour while it can survive for 2-4 days at 0-4°C. The susceptibility to high temperature has served as the basis of artificially induced fever therapy in the past. Common antiseptics and antimicrobials may also inactivate it. Even centrifugation and incubation may be sufficient to inactivate the treponeme.[9]

T. pallidum is a microaerophilic organism and multiplies by transverse binary fission with 'in vivo' generation time of about 30 hrs. *T. pallidum* has been found to have a small genome[10] that lacks many biosynthetic pathways,making it dependent upon the host molecules for its survival. This possibly explains the failure to cultivate it on artificial culture media. However, some success has been made in cultivating *T. pallidum* in monolayer tissue culture of cottontail rabbit epithelial cells.[11,12] The animal models used for experimental study include rabbit (intradermal or intratesticular inoculation), hamsters and guinea pig. Most often the organism is grown in rabbit testicles and can be maintained and propagated further by serial passage. The invitro intradermal infection of rabbit's skin results in a lesion that broadly resembles the primary chancre in humans[13].

INCUBATION PERIOD

The primary syphilitic lesions appear within 9 to 90 days as an ulcer (chancre) at the site of inoculation. Mostly, the chancre appears at 2-6 weeks with a average incubation period of about 3 weeks. The incubation period is inversely proportional to the number of treponemes inoculated. The three-week incubation period corresponds to an inoculum containing 500 to 1000 organisms. Trauma during sexual intercourse is as other factor that can decrease the incubation period. The disease manifests when the organisms multiply to a density of 10^7 per gram of tissue.[14]

TRANSMISSION OF THE DISEASE: MODE OF INFECTION

T. pallidum does not survive in environment and man is the only natural host and reservoir. The organism is very sensitive to temperature and drying. It is the moist skin or mucosal lesion that transmits the disease. The prime route of acquiring infection is through sexual contact. Majority of the patients are heterosexual, acquiring infection through peno-vaginal intercourse. The probability of getting infected throughthis route is around 30%. With the changing sex practices, oral sexual contact also is emerging to be as important mode of disease especially among homosexuals[15,16]. In one such outbreak, as many as one third of the patients transmission,reported to have had oral sex as the only risk factor.[16]

The primary chancre and secondary syphilitic mucosal or moist cutaneous lesions are the sources of treponemes to transmit the disease onto the contacts. The 50% infectious dose has been worked out to be 57 organisms using Nichol's strain of the treponeme.[17]

Apart from sexual route, other modes of transmission include vertical transmission from infected mother to the foetus (congenital syphilis). Kissing, fondling an infant having early congenital syphilis, accidental inoculations among medical personnel by needle pricks on the digits or spilling of syphilitic material in eyes have also caused the disease. Improved modern blood storage techniques have almost eliminated the possibility of transmission by blood transfusion.

Handling of inanimate objects can transmit the disease only if it contained moist infected body fluids. An outbreak of syphilis in the cities of medieval Europe could be traced to a ritual of cupping (a procedure to bleed out 'bad fluids') in the social bathhouses. The primary lesions have been restricted to the sites of cupping. No fresh cases were seen after the restiction of these bathhouses.[18]

PROGRESSION OF THE DISEASE: COURSE OF UNTREATED SYPHILIS

Philip Ricord in 1838 had classified syphilis into primary, secondary and tertiary stages. But the exact progression of the disease could be known only when the report of Oslo study (Boeck-Bruusgaard study) became available. Professor Caesar Boeck had withheld the treatment of 1978 patients with primary and secondary syphilis between the period 1891 and 1910, as the treatment available at that time was inadequate. This study was carried on further by Bruusgaard[19] in 1929 and later by Gjestland[20] in 1955. The limitation of the study was that the basis of diagnosis was based only upon clinical criteria. Clark and Danbolt[21] reinvestigated the available clinical material and concluded that a history of great majority of these patients had early syphilis. The other works dealing with the natural course, Tuskegee study[22] and Rosahn study[23] are said to be biased for some or the other reason. These studies have shown spontaneous cure in some patients.

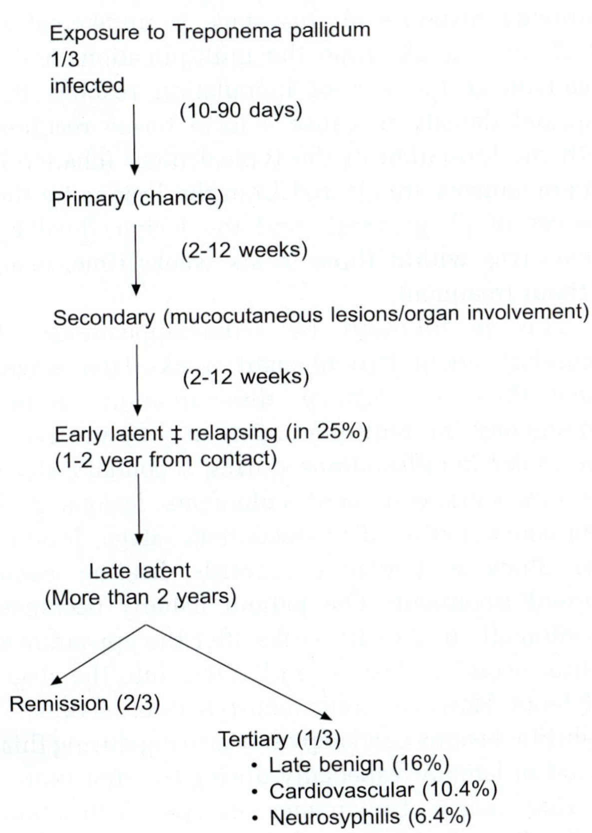

Fig. 14.1 Natural Course of Untreated Syphilis.

After an incubation period of about 3 weeks, about 30% of people having unprotected sex with infected partners developed chancre of primary syphilis. These lesions heal in about 3 to 8 weeks.

After 2 to 12 weeks of appearance of primary chancre, lesions of secondary syphilis appear. About 25% of the patients in secondary syphilitic stage had not reported the history of primary lesion. Almost all patients undergo secondary phase[24] though the manifestations may be mild and subtle to be noticeable. The lesions of secondary syphilis heal in about 3 months but may show waxing and waning up to 9 months before complete disappearance.

The patient thereafter enters into the phase of latency. There are no active lesions at this stage. About 25% of the patients in latent phase experience one or more self-remitting relapses conforming to lesions of secondary syphilis. In the Oslo study, mouth, throat and anogenital lesions predominated in these relapses. Over 75% patients had relapsed within 6 months and 93% within one year. No relapses were seen after 5 years.

Still further along the time scale, about two thirds of the latent syphilitics either remit spontaneously or persist in latent phase without any symptom throughout their life. The remaining one-third progress to the next stage of the disease, tertiary syphilis (late benign, cardiovascular and neurosyphilis).

Late benign syphilis develops in about 16% of the total syphilitic patients. In the Oslo study, the majority had developed this form within first 15 years (one to 46 years). The lesions of benign tertiary syphilis remitted and relapsed at one or the other place. About 25% of males and 34.7% females had 2 to 7 such episodes. Solitary, single structure lesions were seen in 90%. About 70% lesions were on the skin.

Cardiovascular syphilis manifests about 10-40 years after the initial infection, and neurosyphilis is seen after about 3-35 years.

In the Oslo study, cardiovascular syphilis developed in 10.4% and neurosyphilis in 6.4%. The patients infected before the age of 15 years did not develop cardiovascular syphilis and patients infected after 40 years of age did not acquire neurosyphilis. The risk of cardiovascular complications was twice in males as compared to females. Untreated syphilis was the cause of death in about 11% of the total syphilitics. It is significant that 60%-70% of the patients lived without any major problem *attributable* to syphilis.

In the present era of antibiotics, the course of syphilis is likely to be changed. Late syphilis has almost disappeared from the scene possibly due to effective treatment of early syphilitic stage. Use of penicillin or other antibiotics for treating some other disease also could be a probable cause of this reduced morbidity of late syphilis. However, on the other hand, these antimicrobials may only suppress the growth but fail to completely eliminate treponemes because of inadequate dosage or duration. In these cases, the disease may run a subclinical course and manifest later on or is detected only after serology. Scientists are already seeing an increase in patients of secondary syphilis without any history of primary lesion. Latent syphilis is also being detected with increased frequency. These findings have been corroborated by other workers.[25] By the same analogy one can expect resurgence of late syphilis in the near future though expression of the disease may change. Some subtle and atypical forms of neurosyphilis have already been reported,[26] thereby justifying its title 'the greatest imitator of all diseases'. The whole picture may be further confused by the emergence of HIV infection.

EARLY SYPHILIS

Pathogenesis

Early syphilis is said to be infectious, while late syphilis is non-infectious, but there is no strict dividing line. The exact pathogenetic mechanisms in the evolution of the disease are still being elucidated. Some orthologs for production of virulent factors similar to bacterial hemolysin have been identified in *T. pallidum* genome, but its pathogenetic significance could not be ascertained so far.[10] The reasons for the appearance and disappearance of the lesions and inactivity of the organisms after primary stage or during the phase of latency are yet to be answered. Observations over the last few decades have revealed some cyclic trends with periodic exacerbations in incidence every 8-11-year period.[27] This periodicity has been attributed to the endogenous natural dynamics of the disease rather than to the social or behaviour al trends.

After inoculation, the treponemal proteins help the organism to adhere to the host cell receptors, especially the surface fibronectin.[28] Subsequent multiplication and migration of *T. pallidum* across the anatomical barrier is still an unsettled issue. The cork-screw motility of the treponemes is useful but is not the only factor for its penetration into the host tissues.[29] Once inside the tissues, the organisms not only multiply but also disseminate rapidly. The experiments have shown the presence of treponemes in the blood as well as in the lymphatics within few hours of inoculation.[30] *T. pallidum* enters the circulation by its capacity to penetrate through intercellular junctions of the endothelial cells of blood vessels[31] and soon disseminates throughout the body. Antibody response at this stage is undetectable. At about 3 weeks time the multiplication of the organism at the site of inoculation reaches the required density to cause a local tissue reaction with the formation of the typical ulcer (chancre). The organisms are cleared from the lesions by the process of phagocytosis and the lesions heal by themselves within three to six weeks time, even without treatment.

This is followed by the appearance of secondary about two to eight weeks later stage. Since there is vascular dissemination of the treponemes, the multiple organs may be involved. The major manifestations during secondary stage are mucocutaneous and cutaneous lesions and lymphadenopathy. The secondary stage lesions also show a tendency towards healing even without treatment. The patient usually becomes asymtomatic in 2 to 12 weeks after the appearance of the secondary lesions and enters into the stage of latency. However, some recurrences of secondary syphilitic lesions can keep on occurring during this period of latency, especially during the first year.

How some treponemes escape destruction by the immune system of the body to cause the secondary stage is not known. That the immune system is active against *T. pallidum* is evidenced by (1) spontaneous healing of the lesions without any of treatment, (2) the patients harbouring *T. pallidum*, in active or latent phase, are immune to reinfection (however this immunity is lost after treatment) and (3) presence of high levels of the treponemicidal antibodies in the host.Possible mechanisms of their survival include rapid dissemination before immune system incapacitates them at inoculation site. After dissemination, they escape from immune system by lodging in some anatomic sites, which are rather not amenable to the immune mechanisms. These sites may be central nervous system, eyes, bones, lymph nodes and perilymph of the middle ear. Moreover the paucity of exposed antigenic molecules on the outer surface may also diminish the host immune response[7]. As other hypothesis for escaping the host deferce is antigenic variation through gene conversion[32]. This is evidenced by the observation that Th1 response seen in primary syphilis shifts to a Th2 response in the secondary stage, which probably occurs somewhat prematurely, allowing incomplete clearance of the treponemes.[33]

Primary Syphilis

(Primary sore or chancre, hard sore or chancre, Hunterian chancre)

As expected the disease occurs in reproductive age group, most commonly involving people of 20-30 years of age but occurs in older people too, because of Freudian lust. Children are unfortunate victims due to child abuse or the prevailing misconception that sex with a child may cure the sexually transmitted diseases. It is more commonly seen among males because they have more opportunities to venture out.

The primary syphilis is presented as an ulcer or chancre usually situated on genitalia. The lesion starts as a dusky red, painless, non-itchy macule of about 0.5–1 cm in size. The patient usually fails to notice this. It soon becomes elevated to form a papule that increases in size and ulcerates. The resulting chancre or ulcer is variable in size but rarely exceeds 2 cms. It is painless, causing only little discomfort to the patient, and often the patient postpones his visit to the clinician. The chancre is rounded with well-defined regular edges that may be raised, rolled out or may imperceptibly merge with the surrounding tissue. The floor is clean-looking with dull, red granulated tissue. The chancre is non-tender **(Fig. 14.2, 14.3, 14.4)**.

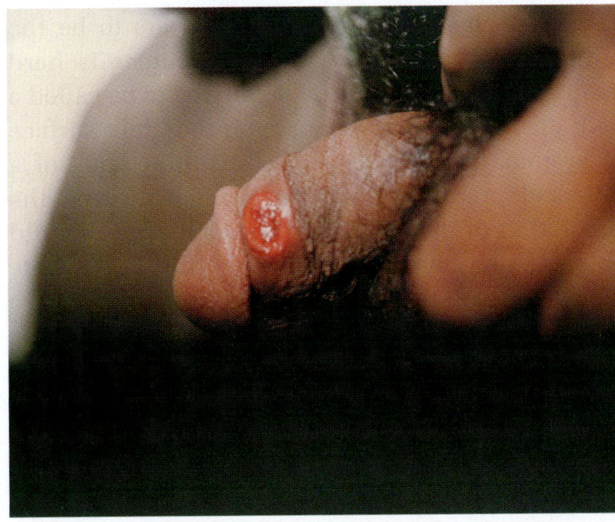

Fig 14.2 Primary chancre-Single, well defined, clean ulcer.

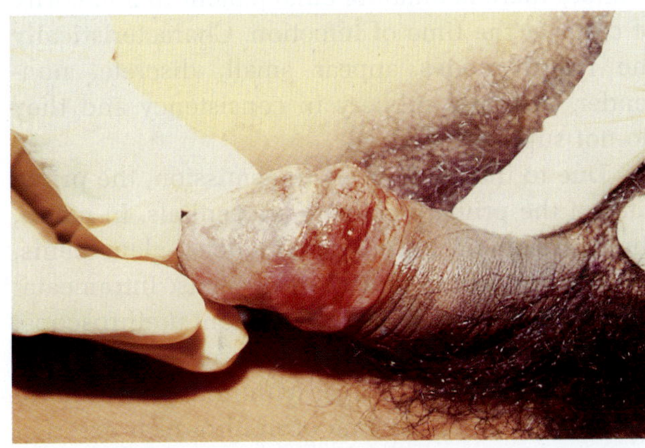

Fig. 14.3 Atypical primary chancre in HIV positive patient.

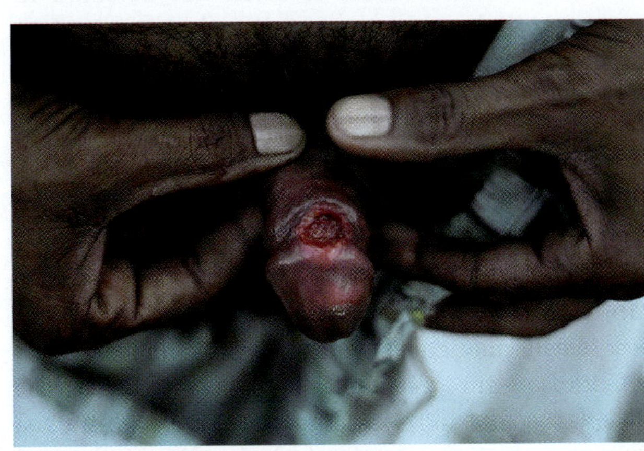

Fig. 14.4 Primary chancre.

The most characteristic feature appears to be the induration of its base, which sometimes is hard enough to feel like a button, justifying to be called a hard chancre. A hard chancre on the inner surface of prepuce may result in the snapping back of a retracted prepuce (Dory flap sign). However, the induration of the lesions on coronal sulcus should be cautiously interpreted as any other lesion here may also feel indurated. Non-indurated chancre can also occur. In the majority, the chancre tends to be single, but multiple lesions can occur simultaneously or soon after the appearance of initial chancre. The manipulation of the chancre leads to exudation of serous fluid, which is highly contagious.

The regional lymph nodes become enlarged within 7-10 days, initially unilateral, but soon other side also becomes involved. In case of ano-genital chancre there is bilateral enlargement in a majority of cases at the time of infection. Characteristically the lymph nodes appear small, discrete, non-tender, firm and rubbery in consistency and they do not suppurate.

Due to the mode of its transmission, the prime sites of the primary chancre are genitals. In males, the common sites are coronal sulcus, glans penis, prepuce, frenulum and shaft of penis. Intrameatal chancre cannot be visualized without urethroscope, and suspicion rests on the presence of scanty, serous urethral discharge with the palpation of indurated area in the line of urethra near external urinary meatus. In females the common sites of primary chancre are labia, fourchette, around urethra, clitoris, cervix, perineum and vaginal wall. A cervical chancre is often not detected in woman and she may present directly to secondary stage. Nearly 5% of chancres may be at extragenital sites.

Morphology of the chancre could be modified due to drying of exudates or formation of scab. The tissue around the chancre may become oedematous. The chancre may become tender due to secondary infection and so do the regional lymph nodes. The application of certain indigenous products, not necessarily medicated ones, may also interfere with detection picture. At times the prepuce may not be retractable due to associated oedema or phimosis. On deep palpation, one may feel a localized indurated area underneath the prepuce, which represents the chancre. The chancre in pregnant women is often larger and more indurated due to increased vascularity.

Non-chancre synptoms include multiple erosive lesions especially on glans penis and balanoposthitis. Primary lesions are observed in the form of about 1-2 cm, localized, non-ulcerated, indurated plaques on the genitalia from which treponemes can be recovered. Rarely, development of a firm, rubbery unilateral labial swelling in females may be due to deep-seated chancre.[34] Proctitis has been reported among homosexuals.[35]

Extragenital Sites of Primary Chancre

Virtually any part of the body can be involved , especially the erogenous zones. Many of these may be painful. Lymphadenopathy is usually unilateral in these cases, except in anorectal lesions. Oral, anorectal, breast, digital lesions rank next to genital sites. Lip**(Fig. 14.5, 14.6)**,tongue and other oral

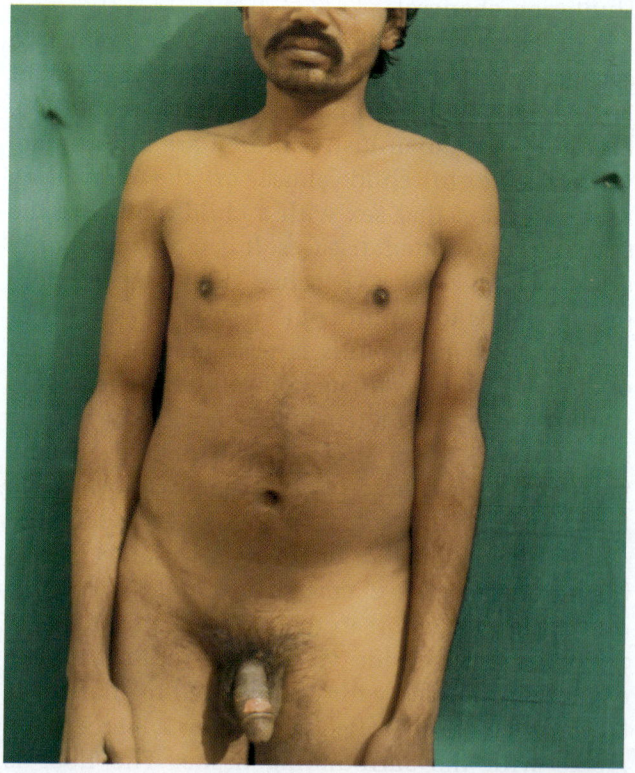

Fig. 14.5 Primary Chancre, Genital and Lip Lesions.

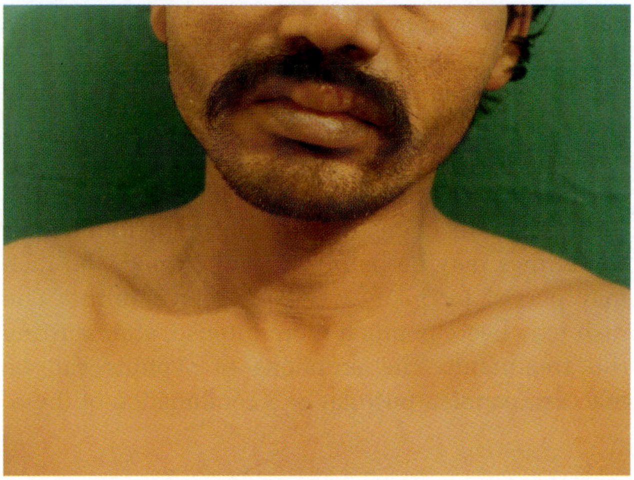

Fig. 14.6 Primary Chancre, Lip Lesion.

sites can be involved by kissing or oral sex. Oral lesions have also been reported to have occurred by drinking vessels, pipes, toothpicks,etc. when used after a syphilitic having oral lesions. Anal chancres are being seen among homosexuals with increasing frequency. They may be painful and may have an atypical appearance. Chancres on fingers can occur due to accidental exposure among the medical personnel, especially the dentists, and present as classical chancre or a chronic whitlow. Fingers can also become infected due to sexual foreplay practices.

Healing of Primary Chancre

The spontaneous healing of the chancre is rather slow without treatment. It takes about 3-8 weeks leaving behind a thin, atrophic scar in some patients. With adequate treatment the ulcer heals in one to two weeks time. Enlargement of the lymph nodes may persist for an indefinite time.

Histopathology of Primary Syphilis[36]

Vascular changes comprising of endarteritis and periartetitis are the fundamental changes observed in early syphilis.

In the primary stage, the initial change is seen in the form of epidermal hyperplasia with intense lymphohistiocytic and neutrophilic infiltrate with a few plasma cells in the dermis. The clinical induration of the primary chancre appears to be due to large amount of mucoid content.[37] After the development of chancre, the epidermis under the ulcer is edematous and may become thin or even absent. The surface of the ulcer is covered with fibrin exudates, necrotic tissue fragments, and polymorphonuclear leukocytes. The adjacent epidermis is acanthotic and shows spongiosis with some degrees of exocytosis of lymphocytes and neutrophils. The dermis is edematous and dense with mixed inflammatory infiltrate, consisting of lymphocytes, histiocytes, plasma cells, and sometimes neutrophils. The infiltrate is concentrated more in the perivascular areas, and the changes are more marked in the papillary dermis. The blood vessels show endarteritis obliterans in the form of swelling and proliferation of endothelial cells with edema of vessel wall. Using silver stains, the *T. pallidum* can be demonstrated in most of the specimens.[38] These are seen at the dermoepidermal junction and within and around the blood vessels.

Diagnosis of Primary Syphilis

Diagnosis is based on demonstration of the trepo-nemes from the chancre and serological tests for syphilis. The organisms in the lesions are demonstrated by performing a dark-field microscope examination of the exudate. The ulcer is cleaned by normal saline and it is pressed to exude fluid, which is collected on a cover slip. The cover slip is then inverted on a thin glass slide, and the preparation is examined under dark-field microscope. In case of likely delay in the examination, the preparation is sealed by vaseline. However, in hot weather, the vaseline may seep under the cover slip and interfere with the examination *may cause confusion*. The organisms can be demonstrated in the chancre in about 80% of the cases. In case of dry lesions or inaccessibility of the chancre, one can demonstrate the organism by aspiration of enlarged lymph node. For this, a lymph node is fixed, and overlying skin is made taut with one hand, and 0.05–0.1 ml normal saline is injected into the lymph node. The Lymphis their drawn out using syrings out. The fluid is spread on a thin glass slide, covered with a cover slip and subjected to dark-ground microscopy.

Serological tests become positive 5-6 weeks after infection or 2-3 weeks after appearance of primary chancre. Reagin tests are positive in about 80% of the patients with primary syphilis. Positivity is seen generally in dilution of less than 1:32.

Differential Diagnosis

Major ulcers of venereal origin include chancroid, donovanosis, lymphogranuloma venereum (LGV) and herpes genitalis. Other ulcers include traumatic ulcers, Behcet's disease and malignant ulcer. The details are discussed in Chapter 42.

Secondary Syphilis

The secondary stage begins 2-12 weeks after the appearance of primary chancre. About 25-35% of the patients who are probably still recovering from the primary chancre begin to show symptoms of secondary syphilis *becomes manifest*[39]. The term 'syphilis d'emblee' denotes those cases where primary syphilitic stage is absent, and the patient directly presents with the features of secondary syphilis. It can happen when treponemes have been deeply inoculated as in the case of a puncture wound or during transmission by blood transfusion.

Secondary stage represents the dissemination of the disease involving many organs of the body. Commonly involved tissues are skin, mucous membranes and lymph nodes. A few involves bones, eyes, nervous system and abdominal organs. Many patients develop constitutional symptoms in the form of low-grade fever, malaise, headache and anorexia. Persistent severe headache may signify nervous system involvement. More often ,the patient with secondary syphilis lands up in a dermatology clinic with skin rash.

Mucocutaneous Involvement

Cutaneous involvement takes the form of different types of eruptions. Characteristically ,these eruptions are (1) non-vesicular ,(2) non-pruritic ,(3) widespread and bilaterally, symmetrically distributed, but few patients do complain of pruritus, and at times the rash may be confined to only one anatomical area as palms and soles or genitalia. The rash may show polymorphism in the same patient. A good daylight is essential to visualize the rash, which at times may be faint enough to be noticed. Tilting the patient to change the angle of incident light sometimes may be helpful. If not treated, the rash may persist for many weeks or even months. The rash may become much more intense, after starting the treatment. The eruptions of syphilis can be macular, papular, pustular or a combination of these.

Macular Syphilide

Appearing at about 8 weeks macular syphilicide is the earliest eruption to become noticeable and may be evanescent. The eruption may be pinkish or coppery red, but more frequently, it is grayish among Indians. The macules are discrete, non-scaly, round or oval in shape, usually less than one Centimeter in size. They are concentrated on trunk, shoulders and flexor aspects of upper arms. Palms and soles are more frequently involved sites **(Fig. 14.7)**, and rash here appears more dramatic in dark skinned individuals, as skin in these areas is lighter. Rash may be sparse and often overlooked by the patient. It may disappear in a few days or evolves into papular rash. Occasionally it may persist as such.

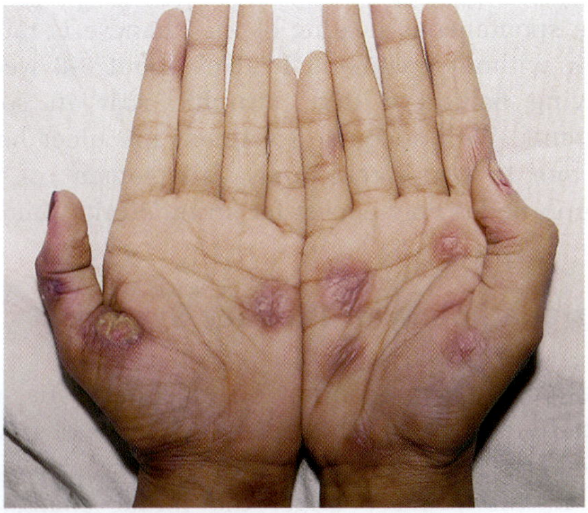

Fig. 14.7 Secondary Syphilis – Lesions on the Palms.

Papular Syphilide

Papular syphilide is the most characteristic rash of syphilis. It evolves from macular rash through a maculo-papular phase or manifests as such. In fact the maculopapular rash is the commonest rash of secondary stage but frequently goes unnoticed. The papular syphilide appears around 3 months post-infection. The papules are dull red and measure less than 1 cm. In dark-skinned patients, they are skin coloured or grayish. The eruption is non-scaly initially, but lesions can be scaly afterwards. The papules are firm to feel. Lichenoid, acneiform and nodular lesions can occur. Lichenoid lesions may itch **(Fig. 14.8, 14.9)**. The rash is wide spread with a distribution on trunk, extremities, face, and genitals. The papules are usually discrete but may be arranged in circinate, annular or a corymbose pattern **(Fig. 14.10)**. Their linear arrangement along the forehead hairline has been referred to as 'corona veneris'. Annular syphilides are mostly seen on the face. The corymbose syphilide resembles a spatter of a liquid with a large papule in the centre and a few small ones around it. A deep tenderness can be elicited over the rash in many patients by pressing the papule directly with a small blunt object such as the head of a common pin (Buschke Ollendorf sign).

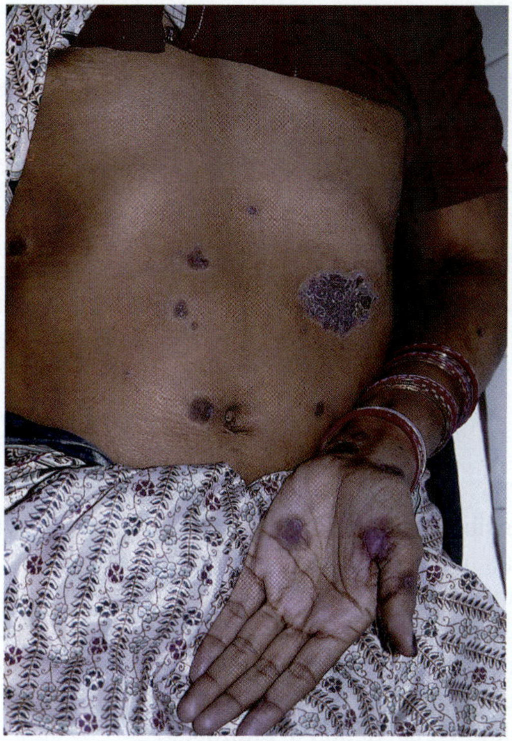

Fig. 14.8 Secondary Syphilis – Lichenoid Variety.

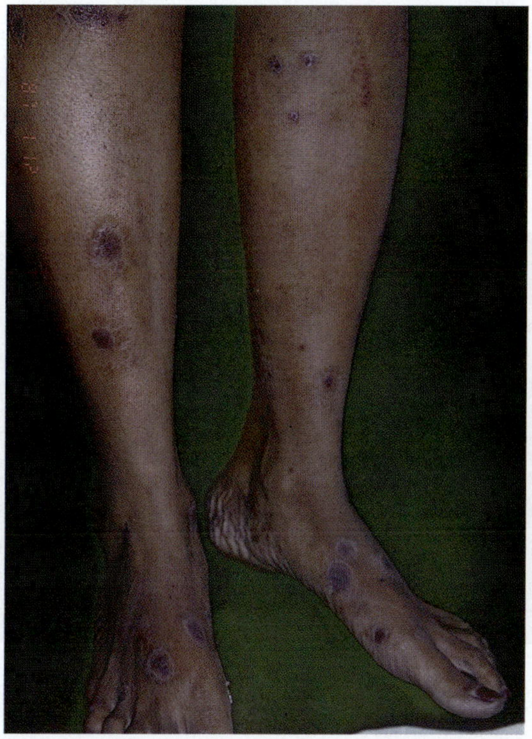

Fig. 14.9 Secondary Syphilis – Lichenoid Variety.

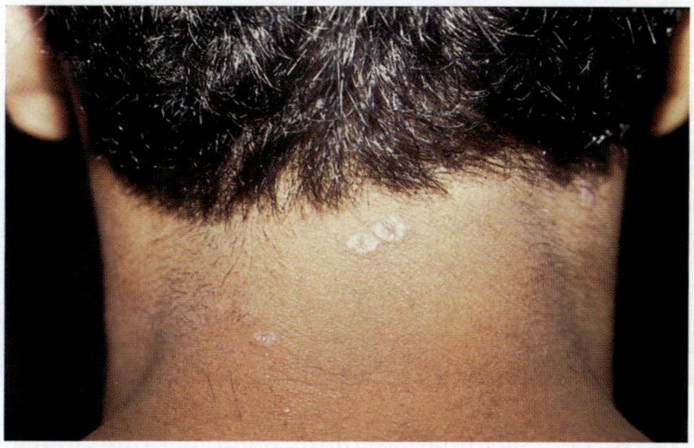

Fig. 14.10 Secondary Syphilis – Annular Variety.

The papules on the moist intertriginous areas tend to become large and coalescent to form large fleshy masses with flat tops and broad bases. Due to maceration they appear grayish white and may be eroded. These are 'condyloma lata' or flat lesions of syphilis, which are highly infectious because of the fluid they continue to exude. Many believe that they evolve their evolution from direct spread of treponemes from the primary chancre, as at times they are seen independent of appearance of skin rash.[40] The common sites of condyloma lata are perianal, between thigh and scrotum, vulva and perineal regions **(Fig. 14.11, 14.12)**. These have also been seen at the areas of mouth, axillae and other moist part of the body. The fissured condyloma lata may sometimes appear as split papules especially at commissures of the mouth **(Fig. 14.13)**. Rarely, condyloma lata in between the toes and on the upper eyelid have been described.[41,42]

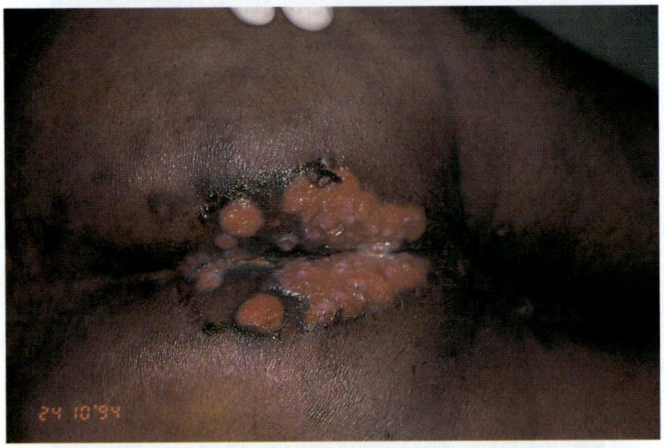

Fig. 14.11 Secondary Syphilis–Perianal Condylomata Lata.

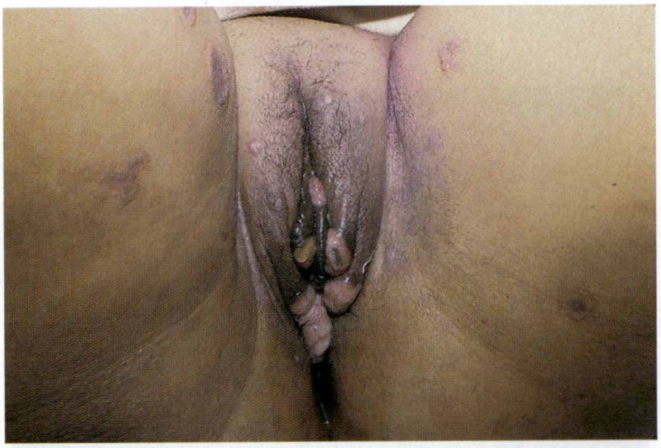

Fig. 14.12 Secondary Syphilis – Vulval Condylomata Lata.

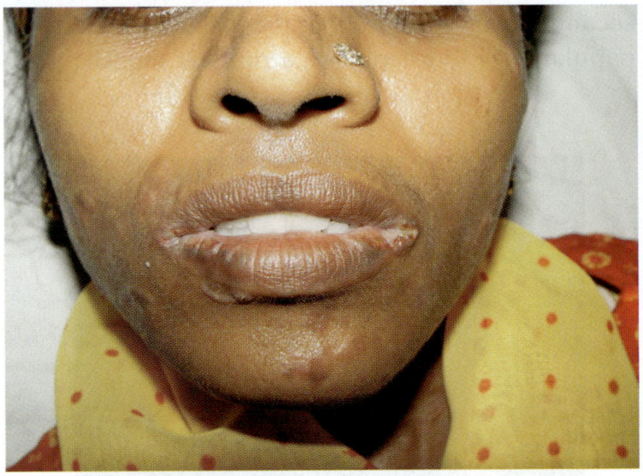

Fig. 14.13 Secondary Syphilis – Split Papules on Angles of the Mouth.

The acuminate follicular papular lesions are responsible for the 'moth eaten' alopecia, which appears as irregular patches of non-scarring hair loss on the occipital and parietal regions of the scalp. The alopecia can also involve other hairy parts of the body. The appearance of small clusters of miliary follicular eruption on the trunk and extremities has been known as 'lichen syphiliticus'.

Nail involvement can occur in late secondary stage. Nail bed or nail matrix can be involved in by papular syphilide. The nails loose luster and become brittle. Pitting, splitting, onycholysis, shedding and distortion of the nail can occur in secondary syphilis. Nailfold involvement can result in paronychia.

Papulosquamous syphilide is essentially a papular eruption in which scaling is prominent, and lesions may form plaques. Presence of scaly plaques may resemble the clinical picture of psoriasis.

Pustular Syphilide

Pustular syphilide evolves from papular lesions, which have undergone central necrosis due to endarteritis obliterans. Rarely seen these days, pustular syphilitic lesions tend to develop in patients who are debilitated **(Fig. 14.14, 14.15)**. The lesions may be rupioid with heaped-up crusts. 'Malignant syphilis' is a rare form of pustular syphilide with deep cutaneous ulcerations, visceral involvement and severe toxemia, which can prove fatal.

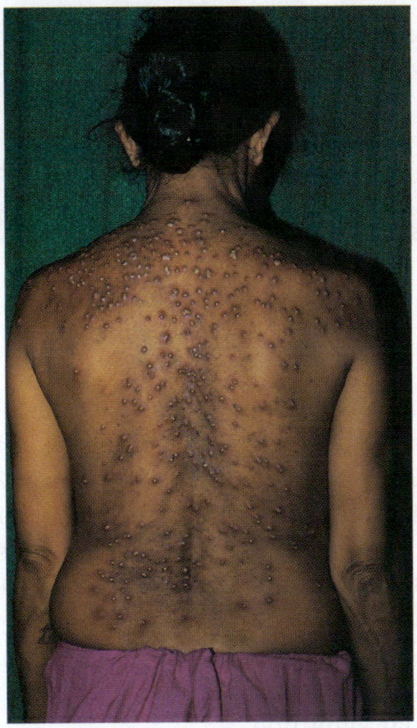

Fig. 14.14 Secondary Syphilis–Pustular Variety.

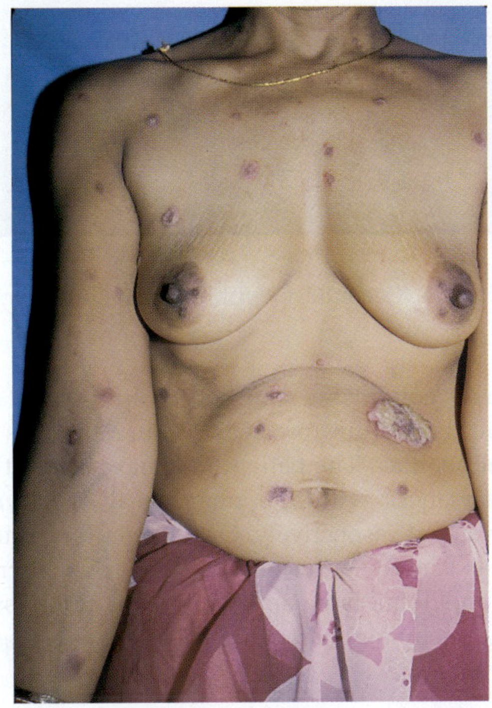

Fig. 14.15 Secondary Syphilis-Pustular Variety.

Healing of Cutaneous Lesions: Pigmentary Changes

Cutaneous rashes may be a part of early relapsing syphilis in which the rash appears and disappears. Macular lesions heal without any trace. Papular lesions may leave behind hyperpigmented or hypopigmented areas. Hyperpigmentation usually fades up with time. The term 'leukoderma colli' or 'collar of venus' denotes a residual depigmentation of the neck area. Depigmentation may be confused with vitiligo. Sometimes atrophic macules may persist at the place of papular rash. The pustular lesions, especially of malignant syphilis, develop due to tissue necrosis, and they heal by scarring. Secondary anetoderma can occur.

Mucous Membrane Lesions

These are painless lesions and take the form of dull red erythematous macules, mucous patches and condyloma lata. Sometimes papules and plaques can also occur. So called mucous patches are erosive lesions of the mucosa that appear at the same time as papular syphilide. A mucous patch starts as grayish-white plaque, its surface gets eroded, forming a sharply defined superficial erosion **(Fig. 14.16, 14.17)**. It is surrounded by a dull red areola. These are highly infectious lesions. Confluence of these lesions form irregular, serpiginous erosions or ulcers that have been called 'snail track ulcers'. Mucous patches are seen in oral as well as genital mucosa. Lips, buccal mucosa, palate, tongue,and fauces are the common oral sites, and glans penis, prepucial and vulvar mucosa, vaginal orifice,

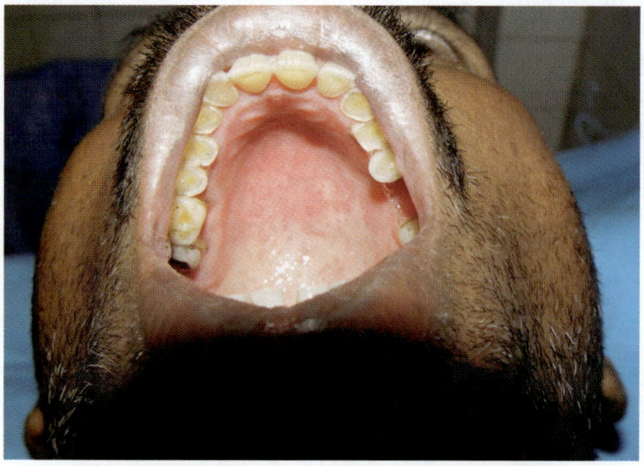

Fig. 14.16 Secondary Syphilis – Mucous Patches.

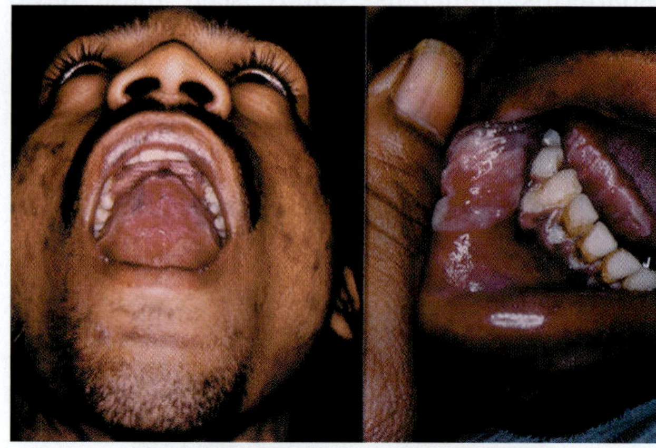

Fig. 14.17 Secondary Syphilis – Mucous Patches.

posterior commisure and cervix are genital sites. On the tongue they are seen as smooth areas with loss of papillae. The patient may have a sore throat or hoarseness with the pharyngeal or laryngeal involvement respectively. On the genitals, mucous patches can be confused with primary chancre.

Condyloma lata can involve oral commissures and have similar characteristics as the same lesions elsewhere.

Malignant Syphilis or Lues Maligna[43,44]

Malignant syphilis, also known as Lues maligna, is an explosive form of syphilis that was first described before the turn of the 20th century. This rare form of syphilis is characterized by a prodrome of fever, headache, and muscle pains followed by a papulopustular eruption that soon becomes necrotic, resulting in sharply marginated ulcers with a thick, rupioid crust. Mucous membranes are involved in more than one third of patients and hepatitis may be associated. Histologic study shows an intense plasma cell and histiocytic infiltrate obscuring blood vessels, and there is obliterative vasculitis of medium sized vessels at the dermal subcutaneous junction with associated necrosis of the overlying skin. It has become more prevalent after the advent of HIV infection.

Most of the clinical description of early syphilis is based on old studies.[19–20] In a recent study spanning over 10 years, Kumar et al[45] from India in an analysis of 53 cases of early syphilis (34 males, 19 females) reported that skin rash was found in 38 (71.7%), lymphadenopathy in 26 (49%), persistent chancre in 4 (7.5%), nodular syphilide in 2 (3.8%), lues maligna in 2 (3.8%), mucous patches in 6 (11.3%), condylomata lata in 14 (26.4%), split papules in 2 (3.8%) and healed scar of primary chancre in 5 (9.5%) patients. Three patients were HIV-positive and each had lues maligna, lichenoid and nodular syphilide.

Histopathology of Syphilitic Skin Rash

The histological changes vary with the clinical pattern of the skin rash. The changes are very much similar to those seen in the primary syphilis and include epidermal hyperplasia, spongiosis and exocytosis of lymphocytes. There is dermal edema with inflammatory infiltrate, especially of perivascular areas consisting of varying proportions of lymphocytes and histiocytes. The vascular changes include endothelial swelling and vessel wall edema. In the older lesions, granulomatous inflammation may be seen. With silver staining, *T. pallidum* can be demonstrated in large majority of the cases.[38] The condyloma lata lesions show marked epithelial hyperplasia with intraepithelial micorabscesses.

Pandhi et al[46] studied 40 biopsies of mucocutaneous lesions and observed a spectrum of changes, ranging from minimal infiltrate to granulomatous inflammation throughout the dermis. The pattern of inflammation correlated well with the type of skin lesions, with macules showing the least and nodules the most prominent changes. The predominant cell type in infiltrate was lymphocytes. Plasma cells were seen infrequently except in condylomata lata. Endothelial proliferation, the classical feature of histopathology of syphilis, was noted infrequently.

Systemic Manifestations of Secondary Syphilis

The systemic involvement is represented by nonspecific constitutional symptoms like fever, malaise, myalgia, arthralgia and headache,or the manifestations may be due to specific organ involvement.

Lymphadenitis: The lymhadenopathy is one of the common findings of secondary syphilis, It is said to be generalized, though one or the other groups of the lymph nodes are involved more frequently. Bilateral inguinal lymphnode involvement is commonly seen, followed by axillary, cervical, epitrochlear and femoral in order of frequency.[47] Other groups can rarely be involved. Characteristically the involved lymph nodes are non-tender, discrete, mobile, nonsuppurative and bilaterally symmetrical. Their consistency is firm and rubbery with a size usually less than 1 cm, often appearing as 'lead shot' like.

Ophthalmologic involvement is rare. It is seen during late phase of secondary syphilis, and patient complains of pain in the eye, photophobia, excessive lacrimation and redness of one or both eyes. There is unilateral or bilateral anterior uveitis or iritis. Rarely choroidoretinitis and occlusion of retinal vessels may occur. In a study, syphilitic uveitis accounted for about 4% of total uveitis cases.[48]

Musculoskeletal system involvement is rarely seen clinically. The involvement includes periostitis, joint effusion, bursitis, osteomyelitis and myopathy. Tendon sheaths may be involved. Patient presents with local aching *pains* over bones, especially over tibia with signs of inflammation. Joint effusion may limit the movements. Radiologically the bones show destructive or productive lesions. The lesions may take one year to resolve completely. Muscle involvement causes generalized muscle weakness, pain, and tenderness.

Gastrointestinal system involvement includes hepatitis and stomach lesions. Hepatitis can be observed among 10% of cases, and in a small number the treponemes can be recovered.[49] It is usually subclinical though jaundice may manifest in some patients, and liver enzymes may be raised. Stomach lesions are even rarer and endoscopy reveals erosions, ulcers or nodular lesions.[50] The patient complains of abdominal pain, vomiting and loss of weight. Hepatitis as well as stomach lesions responds to anti-syphilitic therapy.

Renal involvement is rare and may result in nephrotic syndrome due to acute membranous glomerulonephritis. Its pathogenesis appears to be due to immune complex deposition.[51]

Cardiac involvement is rare and causes conduction defects.

Neurological involvement may be asymptomatic with abnormalities of cerebrospinal fluid (CSF) or is symptomatic with signs and symptoms pertaining to meningitis, raised intracranial pressure and cranial nerve palsies. The patient presents with headache, vomiting and papilloedema. Signs of acute meningeal involvement are usually absent. Damage to eighth cranial nerve can cause deafness. The CSF abnormalities include high cell count, raised proteins and positive reagin and specific tests for syphilis.

Haematological abnormalities include mild to moderate anaemia, raised erythrocyte sedimentation rate and leukocytosis.

Diagnosis

The diagnosis is established by demonstration of *T. pallidum* from moist lesions, mucous membrane lesions or in the lymph node aspirate and by serological tests. Dark-field microscopy from oral lesion is not reliable because of the presence of *T. microdentium*, a commensal of mouth. However, fluorescent staining can be used. Reagin and specific tests are invariably positive in secondary syphilis.

Differential Diagnosis

- Macular syphilide – viral exanthemata, drug rash, pityriasis rosea, glandular fever.
- Papular syphilide – pityriasis rosea, lichen planus, papular urticaria, pityriasis lichenoides, drug rash.
- Papulosquamous syphilide – psoriasis, seborrhoeic dermatitis, drug rash.
- Follicular lesions – lichen scrofulosorum, lic-hen spinulosus, lichen planus, pityriasis rubra pilaris,
- Condylomata lata – condyloma acuminata, pro-lapsed hemorrhoids.
- Oral mucosal lesions – aphthous ulcers, pemphigus, Behcet's disease, Stevens-Johnson syndrome, lichen planus, Vincent's angina, tonsillitis.
- Genital mucosal lesions – herpes genitalis, primary chancre, Behcet's disease, fixed drug eruptions.

Viral exanthem usually starts with fever and a flu-like illness. It is self limiting and rarely persists beyond 15–20 days. Drug rashes are characterized by itchy eruptions preceded by a variable interval after drug intake. Lymph node involvement is uncommon. Pityriasis rosea can be most confusing. There is a larger herald patch and rashes are is aligned along the skin creases on the back. Generalized lymphadenopathy can occur. The rash usually resolves within 6 weeks.

EARLY LATENT SYPHILIS

After healing of secondary syphilitic lesions and occasionally immediately after primary stage, the patient enters into the long phase of latency. Detection of latent syphilis within two years of infection is referred to as early latent syphilis. The dividing line of two years between early and late latent syphilis indicates substantially diminished infectivity potential after 2 years of infection. However, the dividing line is not a strict one (CDC - the Centres for Disease Control, USA, has put the limit about one year). There are no clinical symptoms and signs, and diagnosis is based on finding positive reaginic and specific tests of syphilis. A common problem with regards to latent syphilis is the exact categorization of early or late syphilis due to lack of information regarding the incriminating sexual intercourse. It is better to treat these 'difficult-to-categorize' patients as late latent syphilis.

Sometimes the term 'syphilis incognito' is used to denote a form of latent syphilis where seropositivity has been detected (i.e. incidentally) without any past or present manifestation of syphilis. It is likely to assume more significance in future[52] because of a rise in asymptomatic infections.[25,53]

EARLY RELAPSING SYPHILIS

Relapses occur in about 25% of the patients during latent phase among untreated syphilitics. About 75% relapses are observed during the first six months, 90% within the first year and none after five years. In the Oslo study on natural course, 18.5% had experienced two and 22.5% patients had experienced four relapses. Some of the cases relapse after inadequate treatment. The relapse may be clinical or only serological. Clinical relapses conform to a picture of secondary syphilis though the disease is less extensive. Predominantly there are oral and anogenital mucocutaneous lesions, which at times may be the only manifestations. Skeletal, visceral, ophthalmic and nervous system lesions can also be seen.

Occasional occurrence of a relapsing lesion resembling a primary chancre at the site of initial primary chancre has been referred as 'monorecidive' or 'chancre redux'. It is the result of proliferation of the residual treponemes at the initial site.

The serological relapse without clinical manifestations may precede clinical relapse. It is defined as rising titres of antibodies or a negative serological test turning into a positive one.

INFECTIVITY OF EARLY SYPHILIS

Infection has been known to be transmissible by the process of blood transfusion even during incubation period but such cases might be only few. The primary chancre, moist and ulcerated lesions of secondary syphilis are contagious, while dry, healing non-ulcerated lesions are not. Condylomata and mucous patches are highly infectious. Contact tracing studies[54,55] spanning over a three-month period have shown an almost similar infectivity of primary and secondary syphilis that ranged from 46 to 58%. How the remaining contacts escaped the disease is not clear. The body fluids such as saliva, blood and semen may contain enough treponemes during secondary stage to be infective.[56] The disease could be transmitted by CSF in animal models.[57] Lesions of relapsing secondary syphilis are infectious in a similar way. Even after the lesions of secondary syphilis have disappeared in their natural course, the body fluids remain infective during the latent phase, usually upto two years. However the patient's infectivity potential declines with the passage of time, even in untreated disease, especially after two years. No infectivity has been observed after 10 years. Treatment can abort infectivity.

LATE SYPHILIS

After 2 years, the disease enters the non-infective stage. For the majority of untreated patients, it remains latent without any clinical manifestations and can be suspected only during blood testing during blood donation, antenatal check up or check ups for immigration purposes. Since in all these cases the VDRL serology is positive in low dilutions, it needs to be confirmed by specific tests for syphilis, and in all such cases more serious asymptomatic neurosyphilis needs to be excluded by CSF examination. The tell-tale signs of early syphilis like a penile scar of healed primary sore or leukoderma of neck or macular atrophy of earlier secondary syphilis may be evident.

Lesions of tertiary syphilis start appearing 3-10 years after primary infection. The tissues most commonly involved during this stage are:

- Covering structures: skin, mucous membranes, subcutaneous tissue.
- Supporting structures: bones, joints, muscles, ligaments.
- Visceral regions: gastrointestinal tract, liver, spleen and other abdominal organs.

Incidence

The incidence of late benign syphilis had considerably decreased to the point of becoming non-existent except for occasional case-reports. The increased incidence of HIV with concomitant immunosuppresion has, however, enhanced the fear of rise in incidence of late syphilis. A critical review of 1147 untreated patients of Boeck-Brussgaard study in 1955 reported that 15.8% of patients sooner or later developed late benign lesions of the skin, mucous membranes, bones or joints. These were more frequent in women (17.3%). Of these, about a quarter or more had 2-7 episodes of these manifestations with more than one tissue involvement in some.

Pathogenesis

The characteristic lesion in late syphilis is gumma, which may be single or multiple and varying in size from pin-head to a few centimeters in diameter. It has a central area of tissue necrosis resembling caseous material surrounded by a zone of granulation tissue with a narrow zone of tough fibrous tissue at the outer and peripheral margin. The intima of the blood vessels shows cellular hypertrophy due to endarteritis. *T. pallidum is* rarely demonstrated due to supervening local tissue allergy in the host. The gummatous lesion heals with central scarring but spreads peripherally. In contrast to localized gummatous lesions, the diffuse gummatous reaction is seen in tongue and testis with diffused interstitial fibrosis.

Gummatous Lesions of Covering Structures

1. **Nodular lesions:** Nodular lesions **(Fig. 14.18)** are seen as deep indurated nodules varying in size from pin-head to pea-size. The multiple nodules adapt an arciform pattern with predilection for face, scapular, interscapular area and extremities. Nodular lesions break down to become nodulo-ulcerative form, which lead to atrophic noncontractile scarring. Lesions heal with prompt treatment.

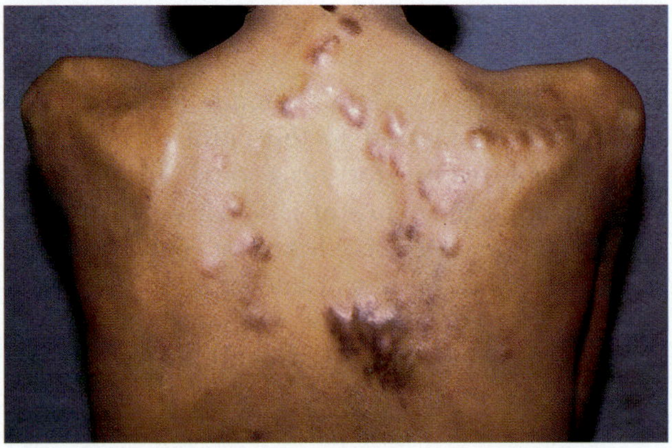

Fig. 14.18 Tertiary Syphilis – Nodulo-plaques in Annular Arrangement.

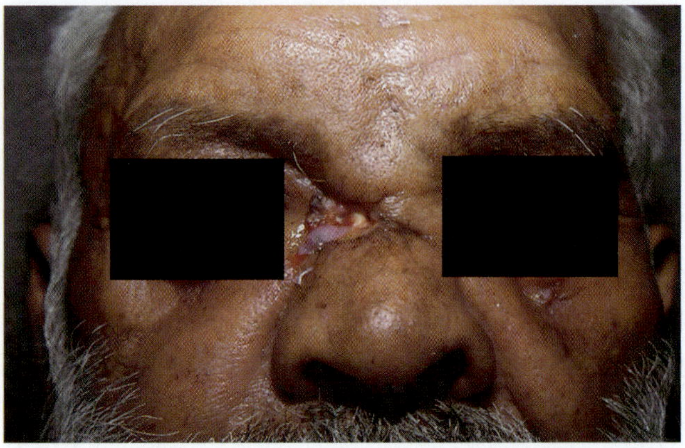

Fig. 14.19 Tertiary Syphilis – Gummatous Ulcer on the Nose.

2. **Psoriasiform or scaly lesions:** Here the tissue reaction is more intense leading to waxy scaling. Such lesions are seen on palms and soles. On scraping, in contrast to psoriasis, the Auspitz sign is negative, i.e., no capillary pinpoint bleeding is seen after removing scales.

3. **Subcutaneous gumma:** Single or multiple painless subcutaneous lesions over which the overlying skin gradually gets attached taking a dull-red hue. They break down to form punched out ulcers with rounded or polycyclic margin **(Fig. 14.19, 14.20)**. The walls of the ulcer are vertical giving the appearance of a well-punched-out ulcer with wash leather slough on the walls and floor. Such subcutaneous gummata are seen on legs, scalp and face along with involvement of sternum and sterno-clavicular joints. These subcutaneous nodules may originate from or extend to periosteum of the underlying bone which may form the floor. These gummatous ulcers heal by tissue paper scarring.

4. **Mucosal surface involvement:** The involvement of the mucosal surface may be localized, or diffused. The localized gumma are seen in mouth, throat, palate, pharynx, larynx or nasal septum. On breaking down, they leave behind a characteristic punched out ulcer **(Fig. 14.21)**. The destructive lesions may cause dysfunction in the area involved and over long period of

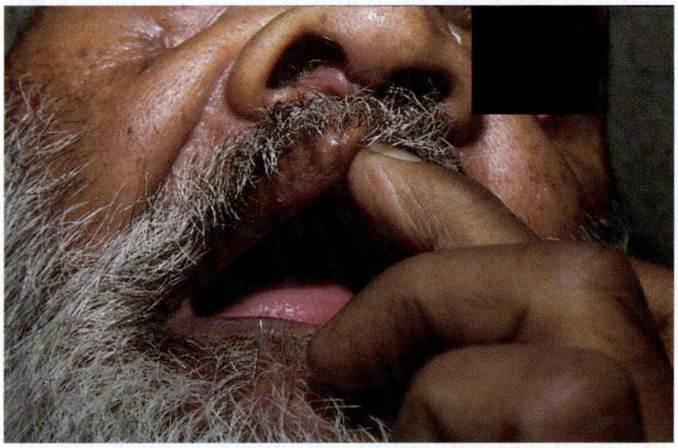

Fig. 14.20 Tertiary Syphilis – Gummatous Ulcer on the Upper Lip

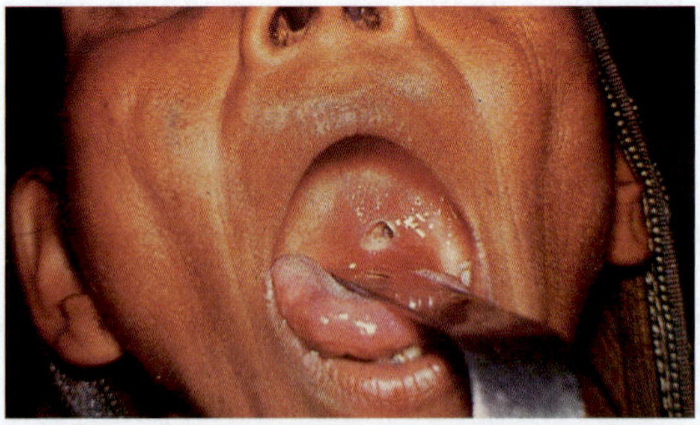

Fig. 14.21 Tertiary Syphilis – Gumma on the Palate with Perforation.

time, are prone to malignant changes. The tongue has diffuse gummatous involvement, and as a result the tongue becomes swollen leading finally to chronic superficial glossitis. Such patients may complain of discomfort on taking hot, spicy food with swoller tongue. Due to interstitial fibrosis, there may be deep, irregular furrowing of tongue and patches of necrotic epithelium may lead to leukoplakia. Also due to loss of filiform papillae, the sides and tip of the tongue may look smooth and glazed.

The gummatous lesions of skin and mucous membranes need to be differentiated from other granulomatous conditions, like tuberculosis, leprosy, deep fungal infections and non-granulomatous conditions, like psoriasis, seborrheic dermatitis, superficial dermatophytes, squamous cell epithelioma as per involvement of area and surface. The leg ulcers need to be differentiated from stasis ulcers, sporotrichosis and erythema induratum.

Gummatous Lesions of Supporting Structures

1. **Bones:** The bones are affected in tertiary syphilis 5-25 years after the original infection. It is more commonly seen in men. The bones commonly involved are long bones, bones of skull and shoulder girdle. There is deep-seated boring pain at the site of involvement in 50% cases, which becomes worse at night. The involvement of the skull bones at times gives rise to continuous severe headache. In case the subcutaneous bone is involved, there may be a tender swelling at that site. Disability due to bone involvement is rare. The overlying subcutaneous tissue and skin may get involved, giving rise to gummatous ulceration and necrotic bone. The hard palate and nasal septum involvement may lead to perforation at site, which is obvious on examination.

   Etiopathogenesis: There is involvement of fibrous layer of periosteum with infiltration of lymphocytes, plasma cells and a few epitheloid cells and occasional giant cells with large number of fibroblasts. The inflammation in turn stimulates osteoblastic activity, leading to new bone formation; but the new bone is laid in irregular fashion and lacks usual cortical pattern and is sclerotic in nature. The bone involvement is patchy, and the transition from healthy to diseased bone is abrupt. Due to new bone formation, there is no tendency to bending or pathological fractures.The gummatous involvement of medullary cavity leads to syphilitic osteomyelitis. In contrast to long bones, in membranous bones of skull, nasal septum, hard palate, destruction outpaces the new bone formation and periosteal reaction is slight, leading to rounded areas of destruction starting from outer table and extending on to inner table. This destructive process falls short of duramater and thus cerebral cortex is spared. The gummatous osteoperiostitis of skull bones is local and is termed as worm-eaten skull.

   A radiological study of 115 bones of 67 patients showed the following patterns of bone involvement[58]:

   - Periosteitis, periosteal thickening with increased density in laminated layers: 27 bones.
   - Gummatous osteitis, destructive or osteomyelitic lesions, usually with periosteal or endosteal changes and sclerosis of the surrounding bones: 72 bones.
   - Sclerosing osteitis, in which the increased density and periosteal changes hide the gummatous lesion: 16 bones.

2. **Muscles:** Primary muscle involvement is rare, but they may get involved due to gumma in subcutaneous tissue or underlying bone.

3. **Joints, bursae and tendonsheath:** They are rarely involved in tertiary syphilitic lesions. Hard fibrous nodules found along tendon-sheaths or subcutaneously near joints, called juxta-articular nodes of late syphilis, disappear after anti-syphilitic treatment.

Gummatous Lesions of Viscera

1. Gastrointestinal involvement

In an analysis of 200 patients of syphilis, 87% patients gave 'stomach trouble' as their chief complaint. Of them only 8 (4%) had true symptoms of the stomach. Neurosyphilis is primarily the cause of gastric complaints.

2. Liver, spleen and other organ involvement

Liver is used to be the most common abdominal organ involved in syphilis. This is either in the form of diffuse interstitial cirrhosis or in the form of focal gumma of the liver, progressing to irregular fibrosis (hepar lobatum).

The portal cirrhosis was found in equal frequency in syphilitics as well as non-syphilitics.

The patient with syphilitic liver involvement presents with complaints of loss of weight, jaundice, pain or tenderness in right hypochondrium. In some cases, symptoms like vomiting, haematemesis due to varicosity of oesophageal venous plexus are observed; and abdominal mass may be palpated. On clinical examination, besides hepatic enlargement, ascites may be found with portal hypertension. Abnormal LFT and positive serological test for syphilis confirms the diagnosis. The condition needs to be differentiated from other causes of acute abdomen.

Other organ involvement, e.g., lung, urinary tract, reproductive organs, is rarely reported in syphilitic gumma.

CARDIOVASCULAR SYPHILIS

Manifestations of cardiovascular syphilis, like other forms of tertiary syphilis, are likely to be due to immunological response and manifest quite late, ranging from 10 to 40 years from the onset of infection. Its incidence in untreated patients ranged from 10% in caucasians to 25 to 50% in Negroes. The cardiovascular system is not affected in early syphilis, but evidence of infection is present in upto 80% of patients with tertiary syphilis though most of them do not have clinical disease. In the post-antibiotic era, cardiovascular syphilis is considered rare, even in patients with AIDS[59,60], yet it has been considered to be the cause of death in 1492 patients between 1976 and 1985.[34] It has been suggested that a late stage of syphilis should be considered in the differential diagnosis of cerebrovascular lesions in young patients. Men have a more frequent and earlier age of onset than women. History of primary or secondary stage may not be available in all cases and about 40% cases may have associated involvement of the nervous system. Depending on the site of involvement, it can be broadly categorized as syphilis of the heart, syphilis of the great vessels, and syphilis of the medium-sized vessels.

Syphilis of the Heart

Myocardial disease is rare and accounts for 2.4% cases of cardiovascular syphilis. It may take the form of diffuse myocarditis or gumma. Gumma commonly involves left ventricle and septum and presents as ventricular arrythmias and valve dysfunction.

Syphilis of the Great Vessels

Lesions may occur in the aorta, in the pulmonary artery or in the great vessels emerging from the aorta. Spirochaetes reach the aorta in the early stage of the disease, lodge there in a dormant state for many years, and cause gradual changes of endarteritis, commencing from the vasovasorum to the proximal part of the aorta. Subsequently , all three layers of aortic wall are affected by the same process. Media destruction causes dilatation of the aortic wall with different sequelae; minimal dilatation causes uncomplicated aortitis, extension of the dilatation to the aortic ring causes aortic regurgitation and gross dilatation at any point causes aortic aneurysm. The damaged intima becomes the site for atherosclerotic patches and calcification and presence of such changes coupled with fibrotic changes near the openings of the coronary ostia leads to coronary ostial stenosis.[59]

Uncomplicated Aortitis

It accounts for 27 to 36% cases of cardio-vascular syphilis. The ascending part of the aorta is involved in most cases, less than 10% cases show involvement of the abdominal aorta; only 2% cases involve the portion below the renal artery.[34] Clinical suspicion can be made when a loud and *tambour* like second sound (bruit de Tabourka) is heard in a patient who has neither hypertension nor atherosclerosis. Radiological suspicion can be made when linear calcifications can be seen on the anterolateral wall of the ascending aorta.[59]

Aortic Aneurysms

They comprise 20% cases of cardiovascular syphilis. Saccular and fusiform aneurysms are characteristic; dissecting aneurysm does not occur. Over 60% of aneurysms involves the ascending portion of the thoracic aorta and 25% involve the transverse arch. They remain asymptomatic for many years and commonly present as a palpable pulsating mass on the anterior chest wall **(Fig. 14.22)**. They may manifest with host of other features like chest discomfort, dyspnoea, cough, haemoptysis, hoarseness, backache, drowsiness, seizures, flush-ing and features of superior vena caval syndrome. If neglected, one-third of patients may die due to spontaneous rupture.

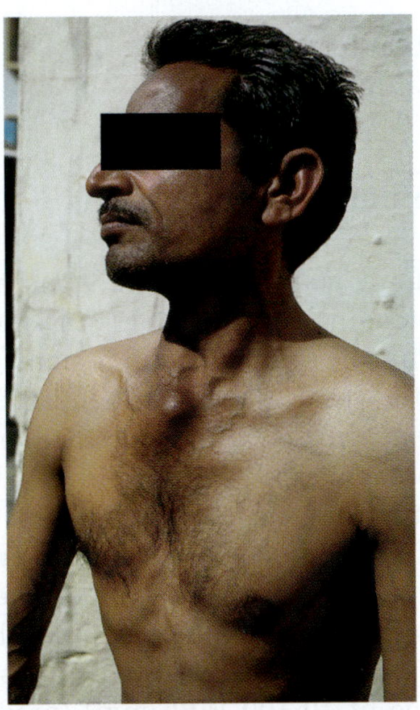

Fig. 14.22 Cardiovascular Syphilis –Aortic Aneurysum.

- On auscultation, heart beats are found to be tambouric.
- Chest X-ray may show characterstic egg shell calcification.

Coronary Artery Disease

Coronary ostia or the most proximal part of coronary arteries are preferentially involved in cardiovascular syphilis; coronary artery stenosis accounts for 25 to 30% cases of cardiovascular syphilis. Patients commonly present with congestive cardiac failure and angina pectoris; acute myocardial infarction almost never occurs. When a patient with either a history of syphilis or other presenting feature of cardiovascular syphilis shows evidence of isolated right or left main coronary ostial narrowing on angiography without atherosclerotic changes, the diagnosis of a syphilitic pathology should be considered.

Aortic Valve Disease

Aortic valvular incompetence is a relatively late manifestation, occurring mostly in patients who are 50 years or older. If there is associated aortic stenosis, the possibility of a syphilitic cause is almost excluded. On auscultation, soft diastolic blowing murmur is heard along the lower left sternal border. A ventricular diastolic gallop with tambour-like quality or a 'Austin flint' murmur may be heard at the apex.

Syphilis of the Medium Sized Vessels

The cerebral and spinal arteries are affected in cardiovascular syphilis, but as the clinical manifestations are neurological, they are categorized under neurosyphilis. Rarely, the hepatic, carotid, mesenteric, renal, iliac or femoral arteries may be involved by the syphilitic process. But except for occasional cases of gangrene of the extremities, diagnosis is mostly performed on at autopsy.

NEUROSYPHILIS

In the pre-penicillin era, physicians were well conversant with the manifestation of neurosyphilis, accounting for about 29% of cases in some hospitals. The common forms were asymptomatic neurosyphilis and tabes dorsalis. In the antibiotic era, prior to and during the early years of HIV epidemic, penicillin and incidental antibiotic therapy brought down these cases considerably. Number of admissions with symptomatic syphilis came down from 4.3 cases in 100,000 population in 1946 to 0.4 cases per 100,000 population in 1960. However, with the upsurge of HIV infection, the incidence of an early form of neurosyphilis, 'acute syphilitic meningitis' has increased up and also the presence of later forms of the disease like paresis, gumma, ophthalmic disease and otologic complications has become more familiar.[60] Development of meningovascular syphilis even after therapy for primary syphilis necessitates the need for appropriate serologic follow-up.[61] A relatively high incidence of neurosyphilis (17.5%) was observed in men involving multiple sex partner with neurological symptoms and in a study from India, in the absence of any associated HIV infection.[62]

Despite the re-emergence of neurosyphilis in the AIDS era, a consideration of neurosyphilis is often neglected in patients with aseptic meningitis and mental changes who are negative for HIV, culminating in high mortality rates. Hence, a high index of suspicion and early inclusion of young patients with cognitive decline in the differential diagnosis of neurosyphilis are mandatory.[63] Haematogenous invasion of the meninges by *T. pallidum* occurs early. There may be spontaneous resolution, some may develop acute symptomatic meningitis, while a few others remain asymptomatic to manifest 5 to 35 years later with meningovascular, parenchymatous and gummatous disease in brain and spinal cord. Classification is difficult because of the various anatomical sites involved with variable histological reactions; manifesting in the form of various clinical syndromes and significant overlap. The following classification for neurosyphilis is commonly followed:

Classification of Neurosyphilis

Asymptomatic

- Early
- Late

Meningeal

- Acute syphilitic meningitis
- Meningovascular
- Cerebral
- Spinal form

Parenchymatous

- General paresis
- Tabes dorsalis
- Taboparesis (mixed)
- Optic atrophy

Gummatous

- Cerebral form
- Spinal form

Asymptomatic Neurosyphilis

It refers to a state of finding abnormalities in the cerebrospinal fluid (CSF) in the absence of any clinical symptoms and signs. The CSF abnormalities peak at 12-18 months from onset of infection and is also a predictive indicator of development of neurosyphilis; absence of abnormalities beyond 2 years almost rules out chances of developing neurosyphilis. Persistence of CSF abnormalities beyond 5 years of infection (late asymptomatic neurosyphilis) increases the chances of neurosyphilis upto 87%. CSF picture shows cells in the range of 10-100 WBC/mm^3 (predominantly lymphocytes), or protein content of 50-100 mg/dl, a reactive non treponemal antibody test and positive blood serology in most cases. Treated or untreated, this stage may progress to neurosyphilis.[60]

Meningeal Neurosyphilis

This may occur early or late. Meningitis may be the first clinical manifestation in one fourth of patients with neurosyphilis. Acute syphilitic meningitis occurs at a time when secondary rash may still be present, in less than 1 year from infection. The symptoms are like any other aseptic meningitis and may manifest as headache, fever, photophobia, nausea, vomiting, stiff neck (Kernig's sign) and confusion. Acute syphilitic hydrocephalus may occur, between 3 months to 6 years of primary infection in one third of cases. Papilloedema is a principal finding of hydrocephalus.

Syphilitic meningitis with cerebral changes account for one fourth of the cases of early neurosyphilis. Forty percent cases present with cranial nerve palsies, unilateral or bilateral due to basal meningitis. Frequently involved cranial nerves are 3rd, 6th, 7th and 8th. Reversible sensorineural deafness is a common accompaniment (20%) of cranial nerve involvement, and may develop abruptly within 1 or 2 weeks or may develop gradually.[60] Involvement of the meninges of the vertex and underlying cortex present in the form of convulsions, aphasias, mental confusion, papilloedema with normal pupillary reaction, and mono or hemiplegia. Subependymal gliosis may disrupt the fibres of the light reflex, *pupillary* resulting in loss of pupillary light reflex, but accommodation reflex is preserved.

Involvement of the meninges of the spinal cord may lead to involvement of the pyramidal tract and other motor tracts, producing lower motor neuron lesions. Meningitis in the dorso lumbar and cervical regions may manifest as:

- Erb's syphilitic spastic paraplegia
- Hypertrophic cervical pachymeningitis
- Syphilitic amyotrophy

The current serum RPR is positive in most cases of acute syphilitic meningitis. CSF examination shows elevated intracranial pressure, mononuclear pleocytosis of 10-200 cells/mm^3 (may be as high as 1000-2000 cells/mm^3), protein content as high as 200 mg/dl, elevated globulin level and/or reduction in the glucose content. The CSF VDRL is positive in most cases.

Histopathology shows inflammatory changes not only in the meninges, but also in the ependyma (granular ependymitis), cells predominantly being lymphocytes and plasma cells. Progressive inflammation produces endarteritis, with subsequent vascular thrombosis, occlusion, and cerebral infarction.[60]

Meningovascular Neurosyphilis

It constitutes 10% of all cases of neurosyphilis and may involve both the cerebrum (cerebrovascular) and the spinal cord (spinal meningovascular).

Cerebrovascular Syphilis

It is caused by endarteritis of the medium and large arteries (Heubner's arteritis) or small arteries and arterioles (Nissl's arteritis).[34] More than 12% of patients have involvement of more than one cerebral artery, commonest being middle cerebral artery. Symptoms may begin as early as 2 years but onset after 4 to 7 years is more common. Manifestations may be sudden or there may be prodromal signs like headache, dementia, dizziness and sleep disturbances. Various neurological features may be seen, depending on the vessel involved. Commoner presentations are hemiparesis or hemiplegia, aphasia and seizures. Other presentations like homonymous hemianopia, cerebellar ataxia, and various syndromes like Horner's syndrome, Walkenberg's syndrome, Weber's syndrome and Dejerine-Roussy syndrome may be encountered. Such features are more prevalent in untreated patients; the present era is more conversant with atypical manifestations like 'drop attacks', suggestive of vertebrobasilar artery disease. Blood and CSF tests for syphilis are positive.[60,64]

Angiography shows diffuse irregularity and 'beading' of anterior and middle cerebral arteries, and segmental dilatation of the pericallosal artery. Computer tomography shows low density areas with variable degrees of contrast, suggestive of multifocal infarction. Magnetic Resonance Imaging shows focal regions of high signal density, suggestive of foci of ischaemia. Histology shows inflammatory changes and occlusive pathology to the vasovasorum, medium and small sized arteries.[60]

Spinal Meningovascular Syphilis

Spinal Meningovascular syphilis comprises of two forms, syphilitic meningomyelitis and spinal vascular syphilis (acute syphilitic transverse myelitis). The basic pathology is chronic spinal meningitis, which leads to parenchymatous degeneration of the cord directly or due to a vascular thrombosis. Syphilitic meningomyelitis is more common and manifests insidiously after a latency of 20-25 years with paraesthesia and weakness of the legs, sensory loss, sphincter disturbances, pain and muscular atrophy. Abdominal reflexes are absent, deep reflexes are hyperactive and extensor plantar response can be elicited. Acute transverse myelitis or spinal vascular syphilis produces sudden paraplegia, sensory loss and urinary retention, simulating the Brown-Sequard syndrome[34,60]. Blood and CSF tests are positive for syphilis.

Parenchymatous Neurosyphilis

It can be categorized under three types: general paresis of the insane,tabes dorsalis and optic atrophy.

General Paresis of the Insane (GPI)

Paretic neurosyphilis or dementia paralytica is a meningoencephalitis associated with direct cerebral invasion by *T. pallidum* and accounts for 10% cases of neurosyphilis.[60,64] Cerebrocortical function is severely affected due to degenerative changes, gross atrophy of the frontal and temporal lobes occur. The symptoms are either psychiatric, neurologic or both. Early complaints are of a psychiatric nature and manifest as memory loss, delusion (mostly of grandeur), megalomania, disinhibition, emotional lability, erratic behaviour, deterioration of personal habits and hygiene and disintegration of symbolic thoughts resulting in professional disaster and social catastrophy. Paresis may manifest with adult onset seizures in 15 to 20 % of patients, without any accompanying mental aberrations.[65] Most common neurologic signs are pupillary abnormalities (Argyll Robertson pupil), flattening of facial lines, impaired writing and speech, tremors of lips, tongue, facial muscles and fingers. More extensive involvement may lead to apathy, hypotonia, dementia, cranial nerve palsies, long tract signs, clumsiness, incoordination and sphincter incontinence.[64] Blood and CSF tests are positive for syphilis. Computer tomography shows decreased attenuation in the cerebral white matter of the frontal and parietal lobes, with enlarged cortical sulci and ventricular dilatation. Histopathology shows granular ependymitis, form-ed by whorls of subependymal astrocytes.

Tabes Dorsalis

Locomotor ataxia is a late manifestation of syphilis due to parenchymatous involvement of the spinal cord. It is commoner in men and occurs later than GPI, approximately 20-25 years after the primary infection. The early features are those of posterior root and posterior column dysfunction, manifesting as lightening pain, paraesthesia, diminished deep tendon reflexes, and poor pupillary responses to light. Lancinating or stabbing types of repeated, clustered pain develops for several days or longer, primarily affecting the legs and less frequently, the trunk and arms. Visceral crisis occur concurrent with lightening pain, manifesting as severe abdominal pain, vomiting, paralytic ileus, and bladder and bowel crisis. Hypotonia follows loss of deep tendon reflexes and hypermobility of joints sets in; this combined with sensory impairment leads to grossly swollen and disorganized joints, known as Charcot's joints. Postural ataxia, unsteady gait and painless, penetrating trophic ulcer on the base of the toe (mal perforans) are some other features. Optic atrophy occurs commonly as also occulomotor palsies resulting in a characteristic 'tabetic' facies. Other forms of neurosyphilis frequently co-exist. CSF and blood show positive changes of syphilis, except in advanced 'burnt out' cases.[60]

Syphilitic Optic Atrophy may occur as an isolated manifestation of neurosyphilis or as an accompaniment of tabes dorsalis. It occurs due to damage to the optic nerve fibers from chronic inflammatory changes and manifests as progressive visual loss, involving first one and then both eyes.[34]

Gumma of the Brain and Spinal Cord

Gumma of the brain is a rare lesion and may involve the meninges by virtue of extension from skull bones. They are rubbery nodules, single or multiple and usually produce space-occupying signs and symptoms.

Gumma of the spinal cord is essentially a granuloma with features of spinal cord compression, manifesting as root pain, spastic paraplegia, urinary and faecal incontinence and sensory loss below the lesion.

Syphilitic Osteitis

Syphilitic osteitis of the skull and vertebra is more of a historical entity now, and signs are secondary to pressure changes on the spinal cord and brain.[64]

Congenital Neurosyphilis

Asymptomatic neurosyphilis is encountered in upto one-fourth of the patients with congenital syphilis, over the age of 2 years. Symptomatic neurosyphilis is much rarer, and once it develops, it manifests after adolescence with juvenile paresis and other adult onset features like tabes dorsalis, syphilitic encephalitis (general paresis) and local gummata.[66]

Neurosyphilis and HIV

HIV infection has had a significant impact on the manifestation of neurosyphilis. Some researchers are of the opinion that HIV infected patients have a greater chance of developing secondary syphilis, atypical manifestations of neurosyphilis and atypical serological tests including false positive tests for syphilis.[64] Both the processes affect the neurological system and can hence produce confounding clinical manifestations. Others believe that the disease is not 'atypical' but in fact, present with manifestations that are typical of early neurosyphilis. Amongst the manifestations, acute syphilitic meningitis was found to be the commonest.

Cardiovascular syphilis is exceedingly rare and has not been reported except for occasional case reports[67,68] Neurosyphilis is also becoming progressively uncommon, however, cases are still occurring especially in HIV positive cases. Neurosyphilis has also been described in HIV carriers.[69] In a recent study from Madurai, a cohort of 40 patients (34 males, 6 females) presenting with neurologic symptoms and history of multiple sexual exposures was evaluated.[62] Seven (17.5%) males were found to have neurosyphilis. None of them were HIV positive. It suggests that there are still pockets of infection where late syphilis is still present. Similarly, benign tertiary syphilis has become uncommon, but cases are still occurring but are not being reported.

The interaction of syphilis and HIV is discussed in a separate chapter.

IMMUNOLOGICAL HYPOTHESIS OF SYPHILIS[70,71]

Syphilis immunology is an enigmam, and despite 400 years of its occurrence we are unable to decipher it completely. The part of difficulty is inability to culture the organism and cumbersome procedures of animal inoculation and their maintenance. Both cell mediated immunity (CMI) and humoral immunity play a role in development of different stages of syphilis. After the inoculation of *T. pallidum* the tissues are initially infiltrated by polymorphonuclear cells which are later replaced by lymphocytes, macrophages and plasma cells. The ratio of CD4+ to CD8+ T-lymphocytes is high in skin and serum at this time and Th1 cytokines can be detected. It results in the development of indurated chancre due to massive infiltrate by the lymphocytes and plasma cells. In due course of time the *T. pallidum* reaches the draining lymph nodes which initiates an antibody response. The combined cell mediated and humoral immunity is unable to clear the infection and even though the primary sore subsides, the treponemas continue to proliferate and produce secondary syphilis. It has been demonstarated that serum of syphilis patients has immunosuppressive factor that can be removed by treatment with hyaluronidase. It was proposed that it is the capsular mucopolysacchride that may be immunosuppressive. Similar findings have been documented in experimental syphilis.[72] The secondary syphilis has a rash, lymphadenopathy, hepatosplenomegaly and can have arthritis and nephritis, a clinical picture of immune complex disease. It is associated with high level of antibodies to cardiolipin and treponemal antigens and CMI is suppressed temporarily though there is resistance to newer infection. There is waxing and waning of immunological response as secondary rash slowly disappears, but there may be relapse. Gradually, most organisms are eliminated and a state of balance is reached. In this stage antibodies are still demonstrable and person is infectious, especially in first two years. During secondary stage, *T. pallidum* is widely distributed, reaches almost all the organs and continues to persist in protected sites like central nervous system, eyes, aorta, bones, lymph nodes and perilymph of middle ear. In late syphilis, this equilibrium is disturbed and organisms again elicit CMI and cellular infiltrate and granulomas develop resulting in tertiary syphilis. *T. pallidum* has been demonstrated in gummas by polymerase chain reaction.

REFERENCES

1. Power DA. Hunterian oration 1925. John Hunter: a martyr to science. In: selected writings. 1877-1930. Oxford: Clarendon pres, p. 1-28.
2. Ricord P. In: letters sur la syphilis. 2nd edition. Paris: 1856. p. 348.
3. Bloomfield AL. A Bibliography of internal medicine. Chicago: University of Chicago Press; 1958. p. 309-10.
4. Bloomfield AL. A Bibliography of internal medicine. Communicable diseases. Chicago University of Chicago press. 1958. p. 318.
5. Centurian-Lara A, Castro C, Castillo R et al. The flanking region sequences of the 15-k Da lipoprotein gene differentiate pathogenic treponemes. J Infect Dis 1998; 177: 1036-40.
6. Smibert RM: Treponema Schaudinn 1905, 1728. In Holt JG (ed): Bergey's Manual of Systemic Bacteriology. Vol 1, 2nd ed. Baltimore: Williams and Wilkins; 1984. p. 49-57.
7. Radolf JD, Norgard MV, Schulz WW. Outer membrane ultrastructure explains the limited antigenicity of virulent *Treponema pallidum*. Proc Natl Acad Sci USA 1989; 86: 2051.
8. Charon NW, Greenberg EP, Koopman MB, et al. Spirochete chemotaxis, motility and the structure of the spirochetal periplasmic flagella. Res Microbiol 1992; 143: 597–603.
9. Stamm LV, Hodinka RL, Wyrick PB, et al. Changes in cell surface properties of *Treponema pallidum* that occurs during in vitro incubation of freshly extracted organism. Infect Immun 1987; 55: 2255–61.
10. Fraser CM, Norris SJ, Weinstock GM et al. Complete genome sequence of *Treponema pallidum*, the syphilis spirochaete. Science 1998; 281: 375-88.
11. Fieldsteel AH, Cox DL, Moeckli RA. Cultivation of virulent *Treponema pallidum* in tissue culture. Infect Immun 1981; 32: 908.
12. Cox DL. Culture of *Treponema pallidum*. Methods Enzymol 1994; 236: 390.
13. Sell, Norris SJ. The biology, pathology and immunology of syphilis. Int Rev Exp Pathol. 1983; 24: 204-76.
14. Lukehart SA, Holmes KK. Spirochaetal diseases: syphilis. In: Isselbacher KJ, Braunwald E, Wilson JD, et al eds: Harrison's principles of medicine. 13th Ed. New York: McGraw-Hill; 1994. p. 720-6.

15. Transmission of Primary and Secondary syphilis by oral sex – Chicago, Illinois, 1998 – 2002. MMWR 2004; 53(41): 966-8.
16. Poulton M, Dean GL, Williams DI, et al. Surfing with spirochaetes; on ongoing syphilis outbreak in Brighton. Sex Transm Dis 2001; 77: 319-21.
17. Magnuson HJ. Inoculation syphilis in human volunteers. Medicine 1956; 35: 33-82.
18. Oriel JD. The French disease. In: The scars of Venus: a history of venereology. London: Springer-Verlog Ltd; 1994. p. 11-23.
19. Bruusgaard E. Ober das schicksal der nicht specifisch behandelten leuktiker. Arch Dermatol Syph (Berlin) 1929; 157: 309.
20. Gjestland T. The Oslo study of untreated syphilis. Acta Dermato- Venereologica (Stockh). 1955; 35 (suppl 34): 11-368.
21. Clark EG, Danbolt N. The Oslo study of natural course of untreated syphilis: An epidemiologic investigation based on a restudy of Boeck-Bruusgard material. Med Clin North Am 1964; 48: 613-23.
22. Talbot MD, Morton RS. The Tuskegee study of untreated syphilis. Eur J Sex Transm Dis 1984; 125-32.
23. Rosahn PD. Autopsy studies in syphilis. U.S. Public Health Service, venereal disease division. J Vener Dis Inf 1947; 21(suppl).
24. Sanchez MR. Infectious syphilis. Seminars Dermatol 1994; 13: 234-42.
25. Gurvinder PT, Sukhjot K, Amrinder JK. The changing face of syphilis: from mimic to disguise. Arch Dermatol 2001; 137: 1373-4.
26. Hooshmand H. Neurosyphilis: A study of 241 patients. JAMA. 1972; 219: 726.
27. Grassly NC, Fraser C, Garnett GP. Host immunity and synchronized epidemic of syphilis across the United States. Nature 2005; 433(7024): 417-21.
28. Baseman, Hayes EC. Molecular characterization of receptor binding proteins and immunogens of Virulent *Treponema Pallidum*. J Exp Med 1980; 151: 573-86.
29. Fitzgerald JJ, Repesh LA. Toxic Activities of *Treponema pallidum*. In: Schell RF, Musher DM, eds: Pathogenesis and immunology of treponemal infection. New York: Marcel Dekker And Basel Inc; 1983. p. 173-93
30. Willcox RR. Early acquired venereal syphilis. In: Textbook of venereal diseases and treponemtoses. 2nd Ed. London: Willium Heinmann Medical Books Ltd; 1964. p. 166-87.
31. Thomas DD, Navab M, Haake DA, et al. *Treponema pallidum* invades intercellular junction of endothelial cell monolayers. Proc Natl Acad Sci. USA 85: 3608-12.
32. Peeling RW, Hook EW. The pathogenesis of syphilis: the Great Mimicker, revisited. J Pathol. 2006; 208: 224-32.
33. Fitzgerald TJ. The Th1/Th2-like switch in syphilitic infections: Is it detrimental? Infect Immun 1992; 60: 3475-9.
34. Sanchez MR. Syphilis. In: Freeberg IM, Eisen AZ, Wolff K, et al eds: Fitzpatrick's Dermatology in General Medicine. 5th ed. New York: McGraw-Hill; 1999. p. 2551-81.
35. Klausner JD, Kohn R, Kent C. Etiology of clinical proctitis among men who have sex with men. Clinical Infectious Diseases 2004; 38: 300-2.
36. Crowson AN, Magro C, Mihm M Jr: Treponemal Diseases. In Elder DE (ed): Lever's histopathology of the skin. 9th ed (Indian). Philadelphia: Lippincot Williams & Wilkins. 2005. p. 591-602.
37. Mckee Ph: Syphilis. In Pathology of the skin with clinical correlations. 2nd ed Barcelona: Mosby-Wolfe. 1996. p. 4.26-4.30.
38. Engelkens HJ, ten Kate FJ, Vuzevski VD, et al. Primary and secondary syphilis: a histopathological study. Int J STDs AIDS. 1991; 2: 280-4.
39. Mindel A, Tovey SJ, Timmins DJ, et al. Primary and secondary syphilis, 20 years experience . 2. Clinical fearures. Genitour Med. 1989; 65: 1-3.
40. Mushel DM. Early syphilis. In: Homes KK, Marth PA, Sparling, PF et al. eds: Sexually Transmitted Diseases. 3rd edn. New York: McGraw-Hill, 1999. p. 479-85.
41. Sharma VK, Chander R, Kumar B, et al. Condylomata lata of eyelids. Genitour Med 1989; 65: 124-5.
42. Rosen T, Hwong H. Pedal interdigital condylomata lata: a rare sign of secondary syphilis. Sex Trans Dis 2001; 28: 184-6.
43. Sharma VK, Kumar B. Malignant syphilis or syphilis simulating malignancy. Int J Dermatol 1991; 30: 676–7.
44. Kumar B, Muralidhar S. Malignant syphilis: a review AIDS patient care. Sex Tran Dis 1998; 12: 921-5.

45. Kumar B, Gupta S, Muralidhar S. Mucocutaneous manifestations of secondary syphilis in north Indian patients: a changing scenario? J Dermatol 2001; 28: 137-44.
46. Pandhi RK, Singh N, Ramam M. Secondary syphilis: clinicopathologic study. Int J Dermatol 1995; 34: 240-3.
47. Chapel T. The Signs and symptoms of secondary syphilis. Sex Trans Dis 1980; 7: 161-4.
48. Barile GR, Flynn TE. Syphilis exposure in patients with uveitis. Ophthalmology 1997; 104: 1605-9.
49. Fehr J Feher J, Somogyi T, Timmer M et al. Early syphilitic hepatitis. Lancet 1975; 2: 896-8.
50. Winters HA, Notar-Francescov, Bromberg K, et al. Gastric Syphilis: Five recent cases and a review of literature. Ann Intern Med 1992; 116: 314-9.
51. Gamble CN, Reardan JB. Immunopathogenesis of syphilitic glomerulonephritis. N Eng J Med 1975; 292: 449–54.
52. Stratigos JD, Katoulis AC, Hasapi V, et al. An epidemiological study of syphilis incognito, an emerging public health problem in Greece. Arch Dermatol. 2001; 137: 157-60.
53. Nessa K, Waris SA, Huq M, et al. Sexually transmitted infections among brothel-based sex workers in Bangladesh: high prevalence of asymptomatic infection. Sex Transm Dis 2005; 32: 13-9
54. Schober PC, Gabriel G, White P, et al. How infectious is syphilis? Br J Ven Dis 1983; 59: 217-9.
55. Von Werssowetz AJ. The incidence of infection in contacts of early syphilis. J Vener Dis Inform 1948; 29: 132-7.
56. Willcox RR. Syphilis: history and experimental infection. In: Textbook of venereal diseases and treponematoses. 2nd ed. London: William Heinemann Medical Books Ltd; 1964. p. 127-47.
57. Tuner TB. Infectivity Tests in Syphilis. Br J Vener Dis 1969; 45: 183-96.
58. Grin EI. Epidemiology and Control of Endemic Syphilis: Report on a Mass Treatment Campaign in Bosnia. WHO Monography Series. Geneva, WHO, 1953.
59. Cardiovascular syphilis. In: King A, Claude Nicol C, Rodin P, eds. Venereal disease. 4th edn. London: ELBS; 1980. p. 67-80.
60. Swartz MN, Healy BP, Musher DM. Late syphilis. In: eds. Holmes KK, Mardh PA Sparling PF, et al. Sexually Transmitted Diseases. 3rd edn. New York: McGrawHill 1999. p. 487-509.
61. Moskovitz BL, Klimek JJ, Goldman RL. Meningovascular syphilis after 'appropriate' treatment of primary syphilis. Arch Intern Med 1982; 142: 139-40.
62. Ganesh R, Stanley A, Ganesh N. Prevalence of neurosyphilis at Government Rajaji Hospital, Madurai, India. Int J STDs AIDS. 1994; 5: 290-2.
63. Schiff E, Lindberg M. Neurosyphilis. South Med J 2002; 95: 1083-7.
64. Milne A. Encephalitis and other brain infections. In: Donaghy M eds Michael Donaghy Brain's Diseases of the Nervous System 11th edition. London: Oxford University Press; 2001. 1118-80.
65. Dawson-Butterworth K, Heathkote PR. Review of hospitali-zed cases of general paralysis of the insane. Br J Vener Dis 1970; 46: 295-302.
66. Wile U, Mundt LK. Congenital syphilis. A statistical study with special regard to sex incidence. Am J Syph Gon Vener Dis 1942; 26: 70-83.
67. Hemdevarajan, Williams J, Gopikishanan. Syphilitic abdominal aortic aneurysm in middle aged married villager. Int J STDs AIDS 2000; 11: 485-6.
68. Rathore AS, Ray K, Ramesh V, et al. Periodic syphilis profile in a New Delhi hospital. J Commun Dis 1998; 30: 153-7.
69. Tien RD, Gean Marton AD, Mark AS. Neurosyphilis in HIV carriers. MR findings in six patients. Am J Roentgenol 1992; 158: 1325.
70. Turk JL. Contribution of modern immunlogical concepts to an understanding of diaeases of skin. BMJ 1970; 3: 363-8.
71. Fitzgerald JT. Pathogenesis and immunology of *Treponema pallidum*. Ann Rev Microbiol 1981; 35: 29-54.
72. Centurion-Lara A, Castro C, Shaffer JM, et al. Detection of *Treponema pallidum* by sensitive reverse transcriptase PCR. J Clin Microbiol 1997; 35: 1348-52.

15 CONGENITAL SYPHILIS

Sanjeev Handa

In this chapter

- Incidence
- Pathology
- Classification
- Early Congenital Syphilis
- Late Congenital Syphilis
- Diagnosis
- Evaluation and Treatment of Infants During the First Month of Life
- Evaluation and Treatment of Older Infants and Children
- Follow-Up
- Prevention and Control of Congenital Syphilis
- Conclusion

INTRODUCTION

Congenital syphilis is the result of syphilitic infection of the mother and is the oldest recognized congenital infection. It is the infection of fetus in utero and refers to all outcomes of pregnancy; whether spontaneous abortion (during 2nd and early 3rd trimester), stillbirth (in up to 30% cases) or a live syphilitic child. Several observations were made with regard to congenital syphilis during the 19th century and were accorded the status of laws. **Colles's law** (1837) states that syphilitic infants could transmit the disease to previously healthy wet nurses but never to their own mothers. Profeta's law (1865) states that a healthy infant born to a syphilitic mother is immune to the disease. **Kassowitz's law** (1876) states that the untreated syphilitic mother tends to improve on her past performances. Diday and Hutchinson had made the same observation.[1-3]

The cornerstone of congenital syphilis control is antenatal screening and treatment of mothers with penicillin. A syphilitic mother treated adequately before the fourth month of pregnancy gives birth to a normal child. Treatment after 18 weeks generally brings about an in utero cure, though it may not prevent neural deafness, keratitis or bone disease.[1,3,4]

INCIDENCE

The occurrence of congenital syphilis is an indication of STDs in a given population. While it is rare in affluent countries, in many poor countries, including Eastern Europe and the former Soviet Union, the numbers are high and still increasing. In sub-Saharan Africa, approximately 10% of pregnant women are affected by syphilis. The incidence of congenital syphilis varies from place to place. It depends upon the prevalence of infectious syphilis in the population at a given point of time and reflects upon the availability of treatment to the infected pregnant woman. There was a dramatic decline in the incidence in USA from 1943 to 1958 following the introduction of penicillin in 1943. But the incidence began to rise again by 1959 despite penicillin treatment. It was only by 1978 that it reached the lower earlier figure of 3.8 cases per 100,000 live births. The incidence of congenital syphilis is rising once more since then. Thus besides the availability of treatment, there are a host of socioeconomic factors that influence its incidence.[1,5,6] Most reports from India are case reports. The incidence of congenital syphilis in childhood STDs is less than 1/1000 in Indian patients.[7-11]

PATHOLOGY

The pathology of fetal syphilis depends on the gestational age at which the abortus is examined. Early congenital syphilis is due to direct bacterial infection which interferes with organogenesis. It may prove fatal, or it may interfere with normal development at various stages of intrauterine and extra uterine life. Late congenital syphilis is possibly not the direct effects of treponemal activity, but believed to be phenomenon of hypersensitivity.[1]

The commonly held belief that infection of the fetus does not occur before 18 weeks is now proved wrong. It was thought that the prominent Langhans' cell layer of the cytotrophoblast prior to midgestation provides a barrier against the infection of the fetus and its regression thereafter leeaves the fetus vulnerable to spirochetal infection. Now it is evident that early gestational syphilis is not appreciated because of the incapability of the fetus to mount an inflammatory response before 18-20 weeks. Even in the latter part of gestation, the major fetal pathology is small perivascular inflammatory foci and a lymphocytic infiltrate, resulting in reduced growth of parenchymal cells and fibrosis. When the pregnancy ends in stillbirth, gross placental changes are found. The placenta is bulky, heavy, pale and greasy. Syphilitic endarteritis produces alterations in the chorionic villi with a subsequent decrease in the blood vessels, with an increase of connective tissue and infarcts. Placental histopathology may reveal necrotizing funisitis, villous enlargement and acute villitis. Demonstration of *T. pallidum* in the placenta clinches the diagnosis. Once the treponemes enter the fetal circulation, dissemination to all the tissues occurs at once, inciting the cellular inflammatory response of small lymphocytes and plasma cells. The fetus may be overwhelmed by the infection and may die. The stillborn fetus may have a macerated appearance with collapse of the skull and a protuberant abdomen with enlarged liver and spleen. The skin may have hemorrhagic bullae. Erythroblastosis is also seen in stillborn infants with congenital syphilis. The addition of histological evaluation to conventional diagnostic evaluations improved the detection rate for congenital syphilis from 67 to 89% in live-born infants, and 91 to 97% in stillborn infants.[1,12,13]

CLASSIFICATION

The clinical course of congenital syphilis can arbitrarily be divided into early congenital syphilis –features typically appearing within the first two years of life and late congenital syphilis with features that occur later than two years.

EARLY CONGENITAL SYPHILIS[1,4,13,16-20]

The child may be born with manifestations of the disease or apparently normal. A period of 2-6 weeks may elapse after birth before the signs of congenital syphilis appear in nearly all cases within three months. By this time the serology for syphilis also becomes positive. The primary stage is absent in congenital syphilis as the disease is already blood borne.

The baby may be premature or born full term. Where the neonates lack manifestations at birth, they may present with nonspecific complaints several weeks later such as rhinitis, pneumonia or failure to thrive. Those born with the disease carry a worse prognosis and are most likely to show the classical presentation of "marasmic syphilis" –the wizened, pot-bellied, hoarse baby looking like old man with withered brown skin and runny fissured nose. These neonates are also prone to intercurrent infections.

Skin Lesions

There is no primary stage and signs are similar to those of secondary stage of acquired syphilis. The lesions of early congenital syphilis are contagious. Vesiculobullous rash distributed symmetrically over the palms and soles is the earliest and most specific sign. It is also known as pemphigus syphiliticus, which is actually a misnomer. The bullae may also be seen around the oral cavity, the trunk, buttocks and the genitalia. They are mostly multiple, discrete and tense blisters over a normal looking skin, containing a serous or seropurulent fluid which is teemed with spirochetes. The floor of a ruptured bulla is dull red, elevated and indurated.

Some weeks later, a papulosquamous rash similar to that described in secondary syphilis may appear. It may involve the face, mouth, anterior nares, buttocks, palms and soles.

Condylomata lata characterized by flat topped, hypertrophic, moist papules which are greyish white and distributed over the angle of the mouth, nose, perianal and vulvar area may be seen. Movement of the lips tends to produce radiating fissures at the angles of the mouth, which upon healing may leave linear scars (rhagades). Syphilitic paronychia occurs due to involvement of the nail folds. It leads to an atrophic nail and a claw nail deformity. Patchy alopecia may be noticed on the scalp. Hair are brittle and sparse. Infantile alopecia affecting the eyebrows may be observed.

Mucous Membrane Lesions

These are typically smooth grayish white mucous patches occurring on the palate, tongue, buccal and genital mucosa, pharynx and the larynx. They may lead to erosions and snail track ulcers. Similar lesions in the nasal mucosa cause syphilitic rhinitis, presenting as a watery nasal discharge (snuffles). It becomes thicker, purulent and bloody later. Nasal blockage due to the discharge may cause breathing and suckling difficulties. It may lead to ulceration and perforation of the nasal septum with flattening of the nasal bridge, forming the characteristic saddle nose. Throat lesions may cause pharyngitis and obstruction of the larynx, leading to a characteristic hoarse cry (syphilitic aphonia) and cough.

Lymph Nodes

Generalized lymphadenopathy may be seen in up to 50% of the cases. The nodes are multiple, discrete, firm and non-tender. Epitrochlear lymph nodes are considered pathognomonic in 20% cases of lymphadenopathy.

Bone Lesions

Earliest characteristic involvement during the first six months of life is osteochondritis of the long bones namely the upper end of tibia, distal end of radius and the ulna. It may be asymptomatic and detected only on radiological examination, or the child may have severe pain and tenderness while handling with consequent loss of movement of the affected limbs, the syphilitic pseudo paralysis. There is a periosteal reaction with deposition of new bone under the periosteum, appearing as a thin line on the surface of the cortex. There may be saw tooth appearance of the epiphyses. Epiphyseal separation may be occasionally seen. Loss of density on the medial side of the upper end of the tibia, characteristic of congenital syphilis and known as Wimberger's sign may be seen **(Fig. 15.1)**.

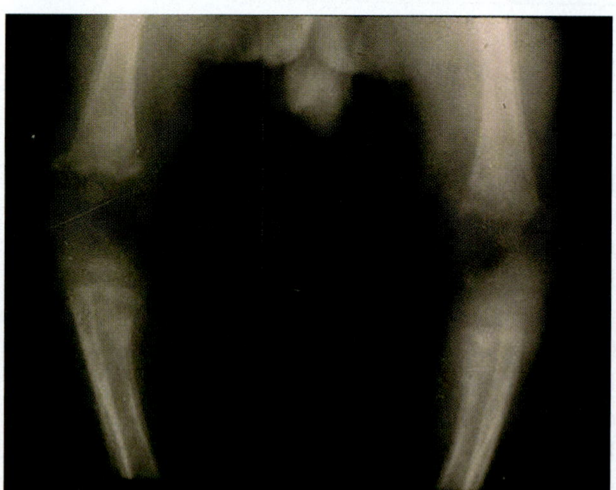

Fig. 15.1 Congenital Syphilis – X-ray of Lower Limbs Showing Wimberger Sign.

Osteochondritis tends to disappear by the second six months of life, but periostitis persists. Successive layers of bone are laid down on the surface of the cortex in a 'onion-peel' appearance. Painless, fusiform swellings of the digits, osteochondritis of phalanges, *'syphilitic dactylitis'* occur in the second year of life'. Proximal phalanges of one or several digits are affected and the fingers are involved more frequently than the toes.

Eyes

Choroidoretinitis, glaucoma and uveitis may be seen in early congenital syphilis. Choroidoretinitis may be detected only as stigmata in later life as pepper-and-salt fundus showing black pigment and white atrophic patches.

Central Nervous System

Neurological involvement is rare and similar to that seen in acquired secondary syphilis. It may be asymptomatic, presenting as abnormal CSF findings only without any clinical disease or it may be symptomatic syphilis due to meningeal or meningoencephalitic involvement. It may then present as convulsions, bulging fontanelles, stiffness of the neck and hydrocephalus along with CSF findings. Most infants with CNS involvement can be diagnosed by physical examination, laboratory tests and radiographic studies. The use of additional tests including IgM immunoblotting and PCR assay may be required. Spirochetes in the CSF may be seen in 22% patients.

Other Organ Systems

Liver and Spleen

Mild to severe hepatosplenomegaly and ascites may cause a protuberant abdomen. It may be associated with jaundice and hypoproteinaemia.

Kidneys

Involvement of the kidneys is evident by the presence of albumin and hyaline and granular casts in the urine. Proliferative or membranous glomerulonephritis may be found.

Lungs

In the absence of clinical signs wide spread infiltration of the lungs known as 'white pneumonia or pneumonia alba' may be found at autopsy in infants who die of congenital syphilis.

Other Systems

Involvement of pancreas and intestines may lead to syphilitic diarrhea. Myocarditis has also been reported.

Coomb's test negative anaemia, probably due to autoimmune hemolysis, leucocytosis or leucopenia, monocytosis, thrombocytopenia and raised ESR may occur. The anemia is also often associated with reticulocytosis and erythroblastosis. There may be associated cryoglobulinemia.

LATE CONGENITAL SYPHILIS[1,4,13,17,18,21,22]

Late stage of congenital syphilis is seen beyond the 2nd year of life. Eighty percent of children with congenital syphilis go through the early stage unnoticed. The late manifestations correspond to the tertiary phase of acquired syphilis. Management of other intercurrent infections with broad spectrum antibiotics has modified the expression of the disease to such an extent that classic syndromes of late congenital syphilis are now rare. The clinical manifestations are either stigmata, or hypersensitivity or inflammatory reactions.

Stigmata

Stigmata are the scars or deformities resulting from congenital syphilis. Some of them are characteristic and remain as permanent evidence of infection. Frontal and parietal bossing due to chondritis and focal osteitis is seen in 30-87% of symptomatic cases. It produces a 'hot cross bun' look of the cranium. Other stigmata include Olympian brow, saddle nose **(Fig. 15.2)**, short maxillae, a high arched palate and prominent mandible 'bull dog jaw'. Sequelae, of periostitis include anterior bowing of tibia 'sabre tibia', scaphoid shape of the scapulae, and thickening of medial third of clavicle called Higoumenakis' sign.

Hutchinson's teeth: Seen at 6 years of age or later the permanent upper central incisors are shorter than the lateral incisors, widely spaced, have a notch in the biting edge as a result of defective enamel formation and assume a peg or screw driver shape **(Fig. 15.3)**. X-ray findings permit the diagnosis even when unaffected deciduous teeth are in place. Other incisors may also be affected.

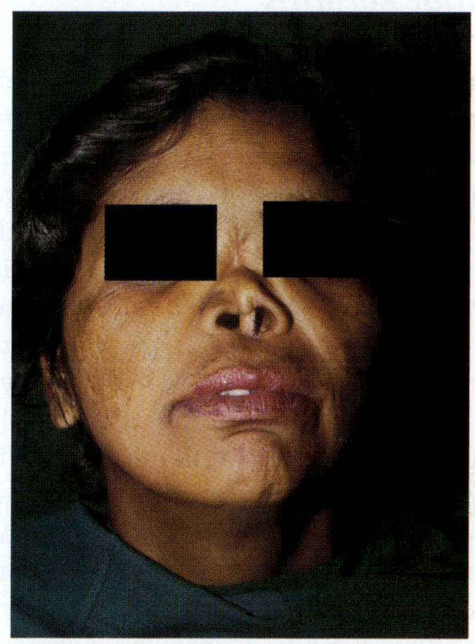

Fig. 15.2 Congenital Syphilis – Saddle Nose Deformity.

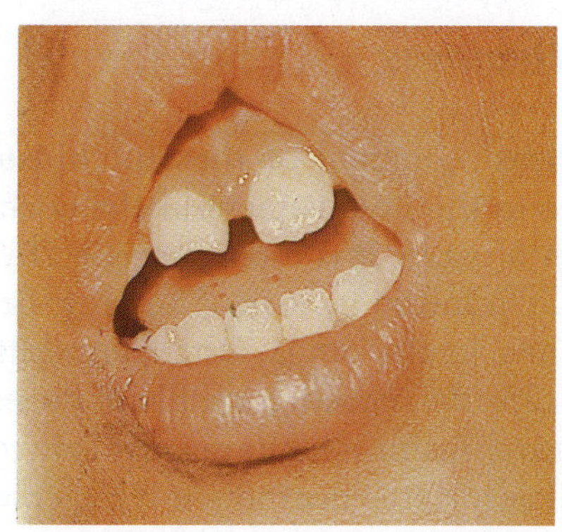

Fig. 15.3 Congenital Syphilis – Hutchinson's Teeth.

Mulberry or Moon's molars: The first lower molars are most often affected with cusps that are under developed and poorly enameled. The biting surface looks dome-shaped, with small projections of the ill-developed cusps. The affected molars are very prone to caries and are usually lost early in life.

Corneal opacities, salt and pepper fundus, optic atrophy and rhagades are the other stigmata. The stigmata are diagnostic, if they present with positive serological tests for syphilis.

Hutchinson's triad is considered as a pathognomonic sign of late congenital syphilis. It includes Hutchinson's teeth, interstitial keratitis, and eighth nerve deafness.

Interstitial Keratitis

It is the most common late manifestation of congenital syphilis (in up to 50%) and is a component of Hutchinson's triad. Onset is between 5-15 years of age and the symptoms are unilateral photophobia, pain, excessive watering of the eyes and blurred vision. It appears first as circumcorneal vascularization, clinically obvious as a dull pink patch at the periphery of the cornea, the so-called "Salmon patch". This is followed by vascular infiltration extending from the sclera into the deep layers of the cornea and cellular exudation into the deep corneal structures. It usually starts in one eye but the other eye is likely to be involved within a matter of weeks. It has a self limited course that ends in corneal ground glass appearance (syphilitic nebulae). The condition may be aggravated by associated iridocyclitis.

Neural Deafness

It is the least common of the Hutchinson's triad and is due to the involvement of the cochlear part of the eighth nerve. It is often preceded by tinnitus and vertigo followed by loss of hearing, first in one ear and then in the other. Osteochondritis affects the otic capsule, causing cochlear degeneration. Sensorineural deafness may arise due to involvement of the ossicles. Nerve deafness is a hypersensitivity reaction to the treponemes because it takes its course irrespective of antisyphilitic treatment but may be modified by steroid therapy.

Nervous System

The clinical manifestations may be asymptomatic or symptomatic. The clinical features and CSF findings are similar to acquired syphilis. Juvenile paresis has been observed more frequently than juvenile tabes. It may precede a varying degree of dementia. Optic atrophy may be associated.

Skin and Mucous Membrane Lesions

Gummas are the usual presenting features. They may manifest as nodules, noduloulcerative and subcutaneous lesions. They lead to nasal septal and palatal perforation **(Fig. 15.4)**, which may cause a nasal twang and regurgitation of food. Leucomelanoderma of the palms has been described from India.

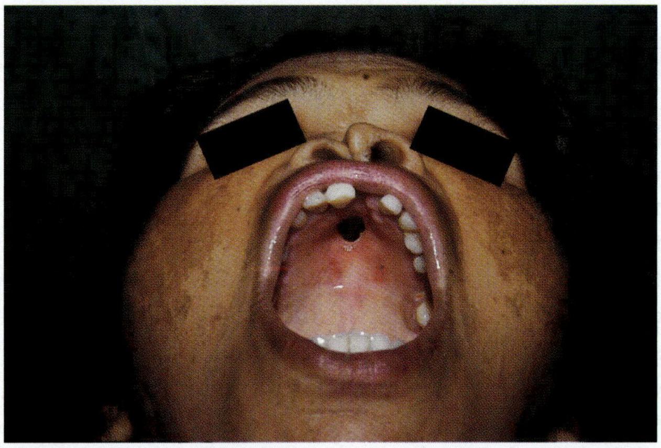

Fig. 15.4 Congenital Syphilis – Palatal Perforation.

Bone Lesions

Gummas may involve the long or flat bones and manifest as diffuse or localized gummatous osteoperiostitis. The bones are not only thickened but also tender. The tibia is most frequently involved, and thickening of its middle third causes anterior bowing called "sabre tibia". Localized osteoperiostitis of the bones of the skull cause the formation of rounded, bony swelling, called

Parrot's nodes. Thickening of the inner end of the clavicle (Higoumenaki's sign) and dactylitis are occasionally found in cases of late congenital syphilis.

Clutton's Joint

Perisynovitis of the knee joint occurs in up to 3% children between the ages of 8-15 years. It was initially described by Clutton and leads to hydroarthrosis. There is a painless swelling insidious in onset and chronic in course. Usually both knee joints are involved, often simultaneously, but occasionally months or years may lapse before the second joint gets affected. Mobility is preserved and there is no impairment of function. X-ray of the knee joint shows enlargement of the joint space with no bony change. Occasionally the elbow joints are involved. Since it is due to hypersensitivity, it does not respond to antisyphilitic treatment. *T. pallidum* has not been detected in the joint fluid in these cases. There is gradual improvement in these cases.

Other Organs

Visceral involvement is rare. Liver is occasionally involved and similarly cardiovascular syphilis is quite rare in late prenatal syphilis.

Paroxysmal Cold Haemoglobinuria

It is seen in both congenital and acquired syphilis and is due to the presence of a thermolabile haemolysin in the blood of patients with syphilis. This antibody first sensitizes the red cells during the period of chilling, then hemolyses them in the presence of complement when the body temperature returns to normal. This is known as the Donath-Landsteiner reaction and can be performed in vitro as a diagnostic test. The patients manifest with malaise, headache, pain in the back, fever and urticaria. They pass "coca-cola" coloured urine which clears in 1-2 days. Antisyphilitic treatment usually cures the condition and prevents further attacks.

DIAGNOSIS[1,4,13,17,18,23-25]

Demonstration of *T. pallidum* by direct examination from the nasal discharge or from early lesions of congenital syphilis confirms the diagnosis.

A positive non-treponemal test in a titre higher than the mother or a rising titre in serial monthly tests suggests a prenatal infection, and the infant should be treated. In any doubtful situation it is better to offer treatment. Blood taken from the umbilical vein (cord blood) or from the infant may give positive results, but these results do not necessarily indicate infection of the infant and may be due to the presence of reagin and specific antibodies, which have passed from the maternal to the foetal circulation.

An active infection can be ruled out in these cases from an FTA-ABS test using fluorescent-labeled IgM conjugate in place of an ordinary fluorescent labeled anti-human globulin. Also a negative blood test at birth does not exclude infection, as it may become positive later in a few weeks or months. This also applies to the FTA-IgM test so that follow-up of an infant for at least 3 months is essential before the infection can be excluded.

In infants of mothers who have been inadequately treated in pregnancy, the use of new diagnostic techniques,e.g., Western blot supplementing fluorescent treponemal antibody-absorption [FTA-ABS] IgM tests on serum, and polymerase chain reaction [PCR] tests on cerebrospinal fluid may yield better results.

EVALUATION AND TREATMENT OF INFANTS DURING THE FIRST MONTH OF LIFE[26]

The diagnosis of congenital syphilis is complicated by the transplacental transfer of maternal antibodies to the fetus (both nontreponemal and treponemal). Thus the interpretation of reactive serologic tests for syphilis in infants is difficult. Treatment decisions are made on the basis of (1) identification of syphilis in the mother; (2) adequacy of maternal treatment; (3) presence of clinical, laboratory, or radiographic evidence of syphilis in the infant; and (4) comparison of maternal (at delivery) and infant nontreponemal serologic titers by using the same test and the same laboratory,procedures

All infants born to mothers who have reactive nontreponemal and treponemal test results should be evaluated with a quantitative non-treponemal serologic test (RPR or VDRL) performed on infant serum, because umbilical cord blood can become contaminated with maternal blood and could yield a false-positive result. Conducting a treponemal test (i.e., TPPA or FTA-ABS) on a newborn's serum is not necessary. No currently available immunoglobulin (IgM) test is recommended.

All infants born to women who have reactive serologic tests for syphilis should be examined thoroughly for evidence of congenital syphilis (e.g., nonimmune hydrops, jaundice, hepatosplenomegaly, rhinitis, skin rash, and/or pseudoparalysis of extremity). Pathologic examination of the placenta or umbilical cord, using specific fluorescent antitreponemal antibody staining is suggested. Darkfield microscopic examination or direct fluorescent antibody staining of suspicious lesions or body fluids (e.g., nasal discharge) should be performed.

The following scenarios describe the evaluation and treatment of infants for congenital syphilis:

Scenario 1. Infants with proven or highly probable disease and

1. An abnormal physical examination that is consistent with congenital syphilis,
2. A serum quantitative nontreponemal serologic titer that is fourfold higher than the mother's titer, or
3. A positive darkfield or fluorescent antibody test of body fluid(s).

Recommended Evaluation

- CSF analysis for VDRL, cell count, and protein
- Complete blood count (CBC) and differential and platelet count
- Other tests as clinically indicated (e.g., long-bone radiographs, chest radiograph, liver-function tests, cranial ultrasound, ophthalmologic examination, and auditory brainstem response)

Recommended Regimens

Aqueous crystalline penicillin G 100,000–150,000 units/kg/day, administered as 50,000 units/kg/dose IV every 12 hours during the first 7 days of life and every 8 hours thereafter for a total of 10 days

OR

Procaine penicillin G 50,000 units/kg/dose IM in a single daily dose for 10 days

If more than 1 day of therapy is missed, the entire course should be restarted. Data are insufficient regarding the use of other antimicrobial agents (e.g., ampicillin). When possible, a full 10-day course of penicillin is preferred, even if ampicillin was initially provided for possible sepsis. The use of agents other than penicillin requires close serologic follow-up to assess adequacy of therapy. In all other situations, the maternal history of infection with *T. pallidum* and treatment for syphilis must be considered when evaluating and treating the infant. The absence of a fourfold or greater titer for an infant does not exclude congenital syphilis.

CSF test results obtained during the neonatal period can be difficult to interpret; normal values differ by gestational age and are higher in preterm infants. Values as high as 25 white blood cells (WBCs)/mm^3 and/or protein of 150 mg/dL might occur among normal neonates; some specialists, however, recommend that lower values (i.e., 5 WBCs/mm^3 and protein of 40 mg/dL) be considered the upper limits of normal. Other causes of elevated values should be considered when an infant is being evaluated for congenital syphilis.

Scenario 2. Infants who have a normal physical examination and a serum quantitative nontreponemal serologic titer with same or less than fourfold the maternal titer and the

1. Mother was not treated, inadequately treated, or has no documentation of having received treatment;
2. Mother was treated with erythromycin or other non penicillin regimen see Notel or
3. Mother received treatment <4 weeks before delivery.

Recommended Evaluation

- CSF analysis for VDRL, cell count, and protein
- CBC and differential and platelet count
- Long-bone radiographs

A complete evaluation is not necessary if 10 days of parenteral therapy is administered. However, such evaluations might be useful; a lumbar puncture might document CSF abnormalities that would prompt close follow-up. Other tests (e.g., CBC, platelet count, and bone radiographs) may be performed to further support a diagnosis of congenital syphilis. If a single dose of benzathine penicillin G is used, then the infant must be fully evaluated (i.e., through CSF examination, long-bone radiographs, and CBC with platelets), the full evaluation must be normal, and follow-up must be certain. If any part of the infant's evaluation is abnormal or not performed, or if the CSF analysis is rendered uninterpretable because of contamination with blood, then a 10-day course of penicillin is required see Notel.

Recommended Regimens

As Scenario 1
OR
Benzathine penicillin G 50,000 units/kg/dose IM in a single dose

Some specialists prefer the 10 days of parenteral therapy if the mother has untreated early syphilis at delivery.

Notel : woman treated with a regimen other than those recommended in these guidelines for treatment should be considered untreated.

Notel : If the infant's nontreponemal test is nonreactive and the likelihood of the infant being infected is low, certain specialists recommend no evaluation but treatment of the infant with a single IM dose of benzathine penicillin G 50,000 units/kg for possible incubating syphilis, after which the infant should receive close serologic follow-up.

Scenario 3. Infants who have a normal physical examination and a serum quantitative nontreponemal serologic titer the same or less than fourfold the maternal titer and the

1. Mother was treated during pregnancy, treatment was appropriate for the stage of infection, and treatment was administered >4 weeks before delivery; and
2. Mother has no evidence of reinfection or relapse.

Recommended Evaluation

No evaluation is required.

Recommended Regimen

Benzathine penicillin G 50,000 units/kg/dose IM in a single dose·

Some specialists may not treat the infant but would provide close serologic follow-up in those whose mother's nontreponemal titers decreased fourfold after appropriate therapy for early syphilis or remained stable or low for late syphilis.

Scenario 4. Infants who have a normal physical examination and a serum quantitative nontreponemal serologic titer the same or less than fourfold the maternal titer and the

1. Mother's treatment was adequate before pregnancy, and
2. Mother's nontreponemal serologic titer remained low and stable before and during pregnancy and at delivery (VDRL <1:2; RPR <1:4).

Recommended Evaluation

No evaluation is required.

Recommended Regimen

No treatment is required; however, some specialists would treat with benzathine penicillin G 50,000 units/kg as a single IM injection, particularly if follow-up is uncertain.

EVALUATION AND TREATMENT OF OLDER INFANTS AND CHILDREN

Children who are identified as having reactive serologic tests for syphilis after the neonatal period (i.e., aged >1 month) should have maternal serology and records reviewed to assess whether the child has congenital or acquired syphilis. Any child at risk for congenital syphilis should receive a full evaluation and testing for HIV infection.

Recommended Evaluation

- CSF analysis for VDRL, cell count, and protein
- CBC, differential, and platelet count
- Other tests as clinically indicated (e.g., long-bone radiographs, chest radiograph, liver function tests, abdominal ultrasound, ophthalmologic examination, and auditory brain stem response)

Recommended Regimen

Aqueous crystalline penicillin G 200,000–300,000 units/kg/day IV, administered as 50,000 units/kg every 4–6 hours for 10 days.

If the child has no clinical manifestations of disease, the CSF examination is normal, and the CSF VDRL test result is negative, some specialists would treat with up to 3 weekly doses of benzathine penicillin G, 50,000 units/kg IM.

Any child who is suspected of having congenital syphilis or who has neurologic involvement should be treated with aqueous penicillin G. Some specialists also suggest giving these patients a single dose of benzathine penicillin G, 50,000 units/kg IM after the 10-day course of IV aqueous penicillin. This treatment also would be adequate for children who might have other treponemal infections.

FOLLOW-UP

All seroreactive infants (or infants whose mothers were seroreactive at delivery) should receive careful follow-up examinations and serologic testing (i.e., a nontreponemal test) every 2–3 months until the test becomes nonreactive or the titer has decreased fourfold. Nontreponemal antibody titers should decline by 3 months of age and should be nonreactive by 6 months of age, if the infant was not infected (i.e., if the reactive test result was caused by passive transfer of maternal IgG antibody) or was infected but adequately treated. The serologic response after therapy might be slower for infants treated after the neonatal period. If these titers are stable or increase after age 6–12 months, the child should be evaluated (e.g., given a CSF examination) and treated with a 10-day course of parenteral penicillin G.

Treponemal tests should not be used to evaluate treatment response because the results for an infected child can remain positive despite effective therapy. Passively transferred maternal treponemal antibodies can be present in an infant until. A reactive treponemal test after is diagnostic of congenital syphilis. If the nontreponemal test is nonreactive at this time, no further evaluation or treatment is necessary. If the nontreponemal test is reactive at age 18 months, the infant should be fully (re)evaluated and treated for congenital syphilis.

Infants whose initial CSF evaluations are abnormal should undergo a repeat lumbar puncture approximately every 6 months until the results are normal. A reactive CSF VDRL test or abnormal CSF indices that cannot be attributed to other ongoing illness requires retreatment for possible neurosyphilis.

Follow-up of children treated for congenital syphilis after the newborn period should be conducted as is recommended for neonates.

Special Considerations

1. Penicillin Allergy

Infants and children who require treatment for syphilis but who have a history of penicillin allergy or develop an allergic reaction presumed secondary to penicillin should be desensitized, if necessary, and then treated with penicillin. If a nonpenicillin agent is used, close serologic and CSF follow-up are indicated.

2. HIV Infection

Evidence is insufficient to determine whether infants who have congenital syphilis and whose mothers are coinfected with HIV require different evaluation, therapy, or follow-up for syphilis than is recommended for all infants.

3. Infants

For infants at risk for congenital syphilis without any clinical evidence of infection (Scenarios 2 and 3), use

Procaine penicillin G, 50,000 U/kg/dose IM a day in a single dose for 10 days;

OR

Benzathine penicillin G, 50,000 U/kg IM as a single dose.

If any part of the evaluation for congenital syphilis is abnormal, CSF examination is not interpretable, CSF examination was not performed, or follow-up is uncertain, Procaine penicillin G is recommended. A single dose of ceftriaxone is inadequate therapy.

4.Premature Infants

For premature infants at risk for congenital syphilis but who have no other clinical evidence of infection (Scenarios 2 and 3), and who might not tolerate IM injections because of decreased muscle mass, use ofIV ceftriaxone may be considered with careful clinical and serologic follow-up. Ceftriaxone dosing must be adjusted to age and birth weight.

PREVENTION AND CONTROL OF CONGENITAL SYPHILIS[27-31]

Congenital syphilis is a preventable disease. The prevention of congenital syphilis depends on adequate follow-up during pregnancy. An ideal routine for antenatal clinics would be to examine the pregnant woman and take blood for VDRL checkup as early and as late in pregnancy as possible. The control of congenital syphilis depends on adequate treatment being given to the infected pregnant woman at the earliest. High VDRL titers at treatment and delivery, earlier maternal stage of syphilis, the interval from treatment to delivery, and delivery of an infant at < or=36 weeks' gestation may be associated with the delivery of a congenitally infected neonate even after adequate treatment for maternal syphilis.

Other considerations of public health importance are -

Raising awareness of the need for antenatal care in affected communities

Effective campaigns that raise public awareness of problems associated with lack of adequate antenatal care should be a priority.

Provision of culturally appropriate services and involvement of the community

Public antenatal care programmes should truly meet the needs of those most at risk, and the services should be continually evaluated. Doubts in the mind of young women that prevents them seeking antenatal care must be addressed and a rapport established with communities where there is a high prevalence of syphilis.

Improved notification and surveillance systems

Healthcare professionals involved in antenatal care must be educated about the importance of notification and proper treatment and follow-up protocols.

Screening of unbooked pregnant women for syphilis

Pregnant women presenting to an obstetric unit without prior booking must be screened for syphilis, so that the result can be made available while they are still in the unit, and treatment provided if a positive diagnosis is made; similarly, their newborn infants should never be discharged from care until the mother's syphilis status is known.

Risk Factors for Transmission[1,32,33]

1. Transmission occurs when the infected woman becomes pregnant or when a pregnant woman becomes infected.
2. Time of acquiring infection-in the first 4 months of pregnancy it is thought that the Langhans cell layer provides a barrier against the infection of the fetus.
3. Delay in approach and treatment
4. Maternal cocaine use
5. Past history of sexually transmitted disease
6. Failure to repeat a serological test for syphilis in the third trimester when it tested negative at first booking
7. Multiple sexual partners
8. Displaced or marginalized population group (indigenous people, and people marginalized by chemical dependency, poverty, prostitution)

CONCLUSION

The minimum standard of care for the management of a pregnant woman with syphilis must include:

- Appropriate antibiotic therapy
- Careful screening for other STDs
- Referral of partner(s) to a sexual health clinic
- Instructions to refrain from sexual activity during treatment
- Regular follow-up of RPR or VDRL to ensure that titers steadily decline.

Despite apparently satisfactory treatment protocols treatment failures do occur. Hence careful review and follow-up of the newborn is mandatory.

REFERENCES

1. Radolf JD, Sanchez PJ, Schulz KF, et al. Congenital syphilis, In:Holmes KK, Sparling PF, Mardh P, Lemon SM, Stamm WE, Piot P, Wasserheit JN, eds. Sexually Transmitted Diseases. 3rd ed. New York: Mc Graw-Hill; 1999. p. 1165-90.
2. Wicher V,Wicher K. Pathogenesis of maternal – foetal syphilis revisited. Clin Infect Dis 2001; 33: 354-63.
3. Mavrov GI, Goubenko TV. Clinical and epidemiological features of syphilis in pregnant women: the course and outcome of pregnancy. Gynecol Obstet Int 2001; 52: 114-8.
4. Sanchez M. Syphilis, In: Fitzpatric TB, Eisen AZ, Wolf K, Freedberg IM, Austen FK, eds. Dermatology in general medicine. 4th ed. New York: Mc Graw-Hill; 1999. p. 2551-81.
5. Walker GJ, Walker DG. Congenital syphilis: a continuing but neglected problem. Semin Fetal Neonatal Med 2007; 12: 198-206.
6. Walker DG, Walker GJ. Forgotten but not gone: the continuing scourge of congenital syphilis. Lancet Infect Dis 2002; 2: 432-6.
7. Garg BR, Sardarilal. Changing pattern of sexually transmitted diseases. Indian J Sex Transm Dis 1982; 3: 41-2.

8. Rangiah PN. Syphilis and Infancy. Indian J Dermatol Venereol Leprol 1961; 27: 165-87.
9. Kumar GA, Lakshmi N, Babu SV. The incidence of congenital syphilis and hepatitis-B virus surface antigen carrier state among deaf mute children. Indian J Dermatol Venereol Leprol 1990; 56: 25-6.
10. Nair TV, Asha LK, Leelakumari PV. An epidemiological study of sexually transmitted diseases. Indian J Dermatol Venereol Leprol 2000; 66: 69-72.
11. Bhogal CS, Chauhan S, Baruah MC. Pattern of childhood STDs in a major hospital of East Delhi. Indian J Dermatol Venereol Leprol 2002; 68: 210-2.
12. Sheffield JS, Sanchez PJ, Wendel GD Jr, et al. Placental histopathology of congenital syphilis. Obstet gynecol 2002; 100: 126-33.
13. Willcox RR. Textbook of venereal diseases and treponematoses. 2nd ed. London: William Heinemann Medical Books Ltd; 1964. p. 231.
14. Peihong J, Zhiyong L, Rengui C, Jian W. Early congenital syphilis. Int J Dermatol 2001; 40: 198-202.
15. Thappa DM, Karthikeyan K. Late diagnosis of early congenital syphilis. Indian J Sex Transm Dis 2002; 23: 43-5.
16. Wendel GD Jr. Early and congenital syphilis. Obstet Gynecol Clin North Am 1989; 16: 479-94.
17. Arya OP, Osab AD, Benatt FJ. Syphilis. In: Tropical Venereology. 2nd ed. Edinburgh: Churchill Livingstone, 1988. p. 39-132.
18. Siddappa K, Ravindra K. Syphilis and nonvenereal treponematoses. In: Valia RG, Valia AR, eds. IADVL Textbook and Atlas of Dermatology. Mumbai: Bhalani Publishing House; 2001. p. 1390-1422.
19. Bennett ML, Lynn AW, Klein LE, et al. Congenital syphilis: subtle presentation of fulminant disease. J Am Acad Dermatol 1997; 36: 351-4.
20. Lim CT, Koh MT, Sivanesaratnam V. Early congenital syphilis - a continuing problem in Malaysia. Med J Malaysia 1995; 50: 131-5.
21. Sood VK, Dogra A, Minocha YC. Congenital syphilis - stigmata. Indian J Dermatol Venereol Leprol 1995; 61: 358-9.
22. Lal Sardari, Lamba PA. Leucomelanoderma in late congenital syphilis. Indian J Dermatol Venereol Leprol 1972; 38: 19-20.
23. Dorfman DH, Glaser JH. Congenital syphilis presenting in infants after the newborn period. N Eng J Med 1990; 323: 1299-1302.
24. Johnston NA. Neonatal congenital syphilis. Diagnosis by the absorbed fluorescent treponemal antibody (IgM) test. Br J Vener Dis 1972; 48: 464-9.
25. Michelow IC, Wendel GD Jr, Norgard MV, et al. Central nervous system infection in congenital syphilis. N Engl J Med 2002; 346: 1792-8.
26. Centers for Disease Control and Prevention, Workowski KA, Berman SM. Sexually transmitted diseases treatment guidelines, 2006. MMWR Recomm Rep. 2006; 55(RR-11): 1-94.
27. Connor N, Roberts J, Nicoll A. Strategic options for antenatal screening for syphilis in the United Kingdom: a cost effective analysis. J Med Screen 2000; 7-13.
28. Alexander JM, Sheffield JS, Sanchez PJ, et al. Efficacy of treatment for syphilis in pregnancy. Obstet Gynecol 1999; 93: 5-8.
29. Sheffield JS, Sánchez PJ, Morris G, et al. Congenital syphilis after maternal treatment for syphilis during pregnancy. Am J Obstet Gynecol 2002; 186: 569-73.
30. Walker GJ. Antibiotics for syphilis diagnosed during pregnancy. Cochrane Database Syst Rev 2001; (3): CD001143.
31. Humphrey MD, Bradford DL. Congenital syphilis: still a reality in 1996. Med J Aust 1996; 165: 382- 5.
32. Webber MP, Lambert G, Bateman DA, et al. Maternal risk factors for congenital syphilis: a case-control study. Am J Epidemiol 1993; 137: 415-22.
33. McFarlin BL, Bottoms SF, Dock BS, et al. Epidemic syphilis: maternal factors associated with congenital infection. Am J Obstet Gynecol 1994; 170: 535-40.

16 | LABORATORY DIAGNOSIS OF SYPHILIS

Madhu Vajpayee, Purva Mathur

In this chapter

- Direct Detection Methods
- Serological Diagnosis of Syphilis
- Polymerase Chain Reaction
- Laboratory Diagnosis of Different Stages of Syphilis

INTRODUCTION

Syphilis, caused by the spirochaete *Treponema pallidum* (subsp. *pallidum*) is a chronic infection with diverse clinical manifestations that occur in distinct stages. As *T. pallidum* cannot be readily cultured[1] or stained with simple laboratory tests, other laboratory methods to identify the infection in various stages of syphilis have been developed. The growing population of patients co-infected with syphilis and HIV has renewed interest in this disease, even in regions where it was showing a steady decline.[2,3] Tests for syphilis fall into four categories: (i) direct microscopic examination, used when lesions are present; (ii) nontreponemal tests, used for screening; (iii) treponemal tests that are confirmatory; and (iv) direct antigen detection tests currently used in research settings and as gold standards for test evaluation.

DIRECT DETECTION METHODS

Dark Field Microscopy

The most specific and easiest means of diagnosing syphilis is by direct detection of the organism if lesions are present. A positive result on microscopy is definitive evidence of syphilis, if infection with other pathogenic treponemes can be excluded. Dark field examination must be accomplished immediately after the specimen is obtained, because viability of the treponemes is necessary to distinguish *T. pallidum* from morphologically similar saprophytic spirochaetes within and near the genitalia. Dark field examination is most productive during primary, secondary, infectious relapsing and early congenital syphilis when lesions containing large number of treponemes are present. Dark field examination can also be carried out on lymph node aspirate when no moist skin lesions are present.

The lesions should be cleaned only if encrusted or obviously contaminated, and only tap water or physiological saline (without antibacterial additives) should be used. A minimum amount of liquid should be used for cleaning because large amounts may dilute organism and hinder the ability to recover treponemes. Antiseptics or soaps should not be used because they may kill the treponemes and invalidate interpretation of the dark field examination. After cleaning the lesion, abrasion should be done with gentle pressure and clear serum exudate should be collected. The material can be collected directly on the cover slip, which is then placed on glass slide and examined while organism is still motile. The specificity of dark field examination is dependent on the skill of the microscopist in distinguishing *T. pallidum* from other commensal spirochaetes (Table 16.1). Positive findings on dark field examination permit a specific and immediate diagnosis of syphilis. However, a negative dark field finding does not exclude the diagnosis of syphilis. The sensitivity of dark field examination is upto 80%.[4]

Refer to Chapter 13 for more details.

Direct Fluorescent Antibody (DFA) Test for *Treponema Pallidum*

Lesion samples for the DFA for *T. pallidum* (DFA-TP) examination are collected in the manner described for dark field examination. The test detects and differentiates pathogenic treponemes from non-pathogenic treponemes by an antigen antibody reaction; thus the organism is not required to be motile in the DFA-TP. It is applicable to samples collected from oral, rectal or intestinal lesions, because the conjugates used are specific for pathogenic strains of *Treponema species*. However, the test cannot distinguish between the pathogenic strains of *Treponema* spp. Smears are stained with FITC labeled anti *T.pallidum* globulins prepared from the sera of humans or rabbit with syphilis and that have been absorbed with Reiter's treponemes. More recently, mouse monoclonal antibody to *T. pallidum* has been used in the DFA-TP.[5]

Animal Inoculation

The oldest method for detecting infection with *T. pallidum* is animal infectivity testing. This technique probably is the most sensitive method for detecting infectious treponemes and is used as a gold standard for measuring the sensitivity of methods such as PCR.[6]

Table 16.1 Morphology and Motility of *T. pallidum* subsp. *pallidum* and Related Non-pathogenic Species

Organism	*Location*	*Coils*	*Length (μm)*	*Width (μm)*	*Wave length (μm)*	*Wave depth (μm)*	*Translation*	*Rotation*	*Flexion*
T. pallidum Subsp. *Pallidum**	Skin and mucosal lesions	Spiral shape 10-13 coils	Medium, 10	Very thin 0.13-0.15	Tight, 1.1 (1.0-1.5)	Deep, 0.5-0.7	Slow, deliberate	Slow to rapid like a cork-screw	Soft bending in middle; pops back into place with spring
T. refringens	Normal genital flora	Spiral shape 2-3 coils	Short, 5-8	Thick, 0.20-0.50	Loose, 1.8 (1.5-2.5)	Shallow 0.4-0.6	Rapid	Very rapid; serpentine-like	Marked bending, relaxed coils
T. phagedenis	Normal genital flora	Spiral shape 10-12 coils	Medium long, 10-12	Thick, 0.20-0.25	Loose, 1.4-1.6 (1.5-2.0)	Shallow, 0.4-0.6	Slow, jerky; deliberate	Slow to rapid; rotates without changing place	Jerky; twists or undulates from side to side
T. denticola	Normal oral flora	Spiral shape 6-8 coils	Medium, 8	Very thin 0.15-0.20	Tight 0.9 (0.8-1.2)	Deep, 0.4-0.6	Slow, deliberate	Slow to rapid, jerky	Soft bending; bends, twists, or undulates

*Reiter's treponeme

SEROLOGICAL DIAGNOSIS OF SYPHILIS

Except during the very early stage of infection, serology remains the mainstay of laboratory testing for syphilis, and certain characteristics of syphilis make it amenable to serological screening. There have been several developments in serological tests for syphilis in recent years, particularly the advent of enzyme immunoassays (EIA), and lately the commercial availability of recombinant antigen-based tests.

Natural History of Infection and Immune Response

Most of the information on the pathogenesis of syphilis is derived from animal models because of limited information from human studies. The natural history of syphilis is very variable; the course of the infection spans many years and may lead to a variety of clinical presentations including primary, secondary, latent and late syphilis, and may be further divided into early (infectious) and late (non-infectious) stages. The immune response to syphilis is complex and involves production of antibodies to a broad range of antigens, including non-specific antibodies (cardiolipin or lipoidal antibodies), and specific treponemal antibodies. The first demonstrable response to infection is the production of specific anti-treponemal IgM, which may be detected towards the end of the second week of infection, whilst anti-treponemal IgG appears later, at about 4 weeks.[7] By the time the symptoms are present, most patients have both detectable IgG and IgM antibodies.[8] The immune response can be affected by treatment and by HIV infection. The titres of non-specific antibody and specific IgM decline rapidly after adequate therapy of early syphilis but specific IgG antibody generally persists. HIV infection may lead to a reduced or delayed antibody response in primary syphilis but in most cases the response is normal or exaggerated.[9]

Serological Tests for Syphilis and Their Application

Serological tests for syphilis may be classified into two groups: non-treponemal tests, which detect non-specific treponemal antibody, eg. the Venereal Diseases Research Laboratory (VDRL) or rapid plasma reagin (RPR) tests, and treponemal tests, which detect specific treponemal antibody, e.g. *T. pallidum* haemagglutination assay (TPHA), fluorescent treponemal antibody-absorbtion (FTA-ABS) and enzyme immunoassay (EIA) **(Tables 16.2, 16.3).**

Table 16.2 **Basis of Non-treponemal Tests**

Capture System	*Test*	*Comments*
Liposomes in suspension producing visible flocculation with lipoidal antibodies	VDRL	
Liposomes in suspension + unattached charcoal particles producing dark coloured flocculation due to trapping of charcoal particles in lattice formed by antigen-antibody complex	RPR	USR (Unheated Serum Reagin), TRUST (Toluidine Red Unheated Serum Test)
VDRL antigen coated onto wells of microtitre plates and attached antibody detected by enzyme immunoassay	EIA (Reagin)	

Table 16.3 Basis of Treponemal Tests

Antigen	*Capture System*	*Test*
Intact Treponemes	Treponemes fixed onto microscope slides	FTA-ABS
Purified and sonicated treponemes	Attached to red blood cells	TPHA
	Attached to gelatin particles	TPPA
	Attached to microtitre plates	EIA
	Proteins separated by PAGE and transferred to filter paper by Western blotting	Immunoblots
Recombinant antigens	Attached to microtitre plates	EIA
	Attached to latex particles	Latex agglutination

PAGE – Polyacrylamide gel electrophoresis

Non-treponemal Tests

In 1906, Wassermann et al. adapted the complement fixation test, previously introduced by Bordet and Gengou in 1901, for serologic testing of syphilis.[5] The antigen previously used in the Wassermann test for syphilis was an extract of liver from newborns, who had died of congenital syphilis and later beef heart extracted in alcohol served equally well as an antigen.[10] Although the complement fixation tests contributed immensely to the diagnosis of syphilis, they were too complicated to perform and required many reagents and as long as 24 hours to complete. Kahn in 1922 introduced a flocculation test without complement that could be read macroscopically in a few hours, but the antigen, a crude extract of tissue, varied in quality.[11] Pangborn in 1941 successfully isolated from beef heart the active antigenic component, a phospholipid, cardiolipin.[12] Cardiolipin, when combined with lecithin and cholesterol, forms a serologically active antigen for the detection of syphilitic antibody. In contrast to the crude tissue extract antigens, the pure cardiolipin-cholesterol-lecithin antigens could be standardized chemically as well as serologically, thus ensuring greater reproducibility of test results both within and between laboratories.[13]

The non treponemal tests used are the VDRL, Toluidine Red Unheated serum test (TRUST), RPR card test, Reagin Screen Test (RST) and Unheated Serum Reagin Test (UST). Non-treponemal tests can be used as qualitative tests for initial screening or as quantitative tests to follow treatment. All four tests are based on an antigen composed of alcoholic solution, containing measured amount of cardiolipin, cholesterol and sufficient purified lecithin to produce standard reactivity. The nontreponemal (reagin) tests measure IgM and IgG antibodies to lipoidal material released from damaged host cell as well as to lipoprotein like material and possibly to cardiolipin released from treponemes. The antilipoidal antibodies are produced not only as a consequence of syphilis and other treponemal diseases but also in response to non-treponemal disease of an acute and chronic nature in which tissue damage occurs. Without some other evidence for the diagnosis of syphilis, a reactive nontreponemal test does not confirm *T. pallidum* infection. Serum is the specimen of choice for both treponemal and non treponemal tests. However plasma samples may also be used in the RPR card test and TRUST. Plasma cannot be used in the VDRL test, since the samples must be heated before testing, and it cannot be used in the treponemal test for syphilis. The VDRL is the only test that can be used for testing CSF. The CSF is not heated before the test is performed.[5]

False Positive Reaction

Antibodies against cardiolipin may also occur in the absence of treponemal infection and give what has been referred to as biological false positive

(BFP) reactions. BFP reactions are defined as those present in patients whose serum gives positive cardiolipin antigen test but negative specific treponemal antigen test in the absence of past or present treponemal infection. False positive reaction can be divided into two groups: (1)those that are acute false positive reactions of less than 6 months in duration, and (2)those that are chronic false positive reactions that persist for more than 6 months. Acute false positive nontreponemal reactions have been associated with hepatitis, infectious mononucleosis, viral pneumonia, chicken pox, measles, other viral infections, malaria, pregnancy and laboratory accident or technical error. Chronic false positive reactions have been associated with connective tissue diseases such as SLE or diseases associated with immunoglobulin abnormalities, which are more common in women. Other conditions associated with chronic false positive reactions are narcotic addiction, aging, leprosy and malignancy.[5]

Treponemal Tests

In 1949, Nelson and Mayer developed the first treponemal antibody test, the *T. pallidum* immobilization (TPI) test.[14] The TPI test uses *T. pallidum* (Nichol's strain) grown in rabbit's testes as the antigen and is based on the ability of patient's antibody and complement to immobilize living treponemes, as observed by dark-field microscopy. The TPI test was rapidly accepted as a specific test for syphilis. However, because the TPI test is complicated, technically difficult, time-consuming and expensive to perform, a simpler procedure was sought after In addition, studies[15] in the 1970's found that the TPI test was less sensitive and specific than the treponemal test that appeared in the 1960s.

In 1957, a major breakthrough in treponemal antigen tests occurred with the development of the fluorescent treponemal antibody (FTA) test.[16] The original FTA procedure used a 1:5 dilution of the patient's serum in saline solution, reacting with a suspension of killed treponemes. A flourescein-labeled anti-human immunoglobulin was used as the conjugate, and the test was read under a microscope with a UV light source. When an improved flourescein compound, flourescein isothiocynate (FITC) was used to prepare the labeled anti-human globulin conjugate, nonspecific reactions were encountered in approximately 25% of normal serum specimens. To eliminate these false-positive reactions, the test was modified by diluting the patients serum 1:200, the FTA-200.[17] However, the FTA-200 test, although highly specific, is not very sensitive. The nonspecific reactions of the original FTA test are found to arise because of shared antigens common to *T. pallidum* and the nonpathogenic treponemes that occur as part of the normal bacterial flora of humans.[18] Deacon and Hunter, by preparing a sonicate from cultures of the Reiter's spirochaete, removed the common antigens by absorption: their work led to the development of the more specific and sensitive FTA-ABS test.[19] The FTA-ABS and its counterpart, the FTA-ABS double-staining test, used with incident light microscopes, remain the standard treponemal tests for syphilis today.

In 1965, Rathlev reported the first reliable application of haemagglutination techniques (TPHA) to the serologic diagnosis of syphilis.[20] The antigen used in her procedure was formalinized, tanned sheep erythrocytes sensitized with ultrasonicated material from *T. pallidum* (Nichol's strain). The presence of treponemal antibody in the patient's serum was detected by indirect agglutination of the sensitized erythrocytes and the subsequent formation of a mat of erythrocytes upon their settling.

Testing Strategy

An important principle of syphilis serology is the detection of treponemal antibody by a screening test, followed by confirmation of a reactive screening test result by additional testing. The confirmatory test, or tests, should have equivalent sensitivity and ideally greater specificity compared to the screening test and should be methodologically independent, where possible, so as to reduce the chance of coincident false-positive reactions. A quantitative non-treponemal test and/or detection of specific treponemal IgM may be useful for assessment of the stage of infection and to monitor the effect of therapy. Serology cannot distinguish between the different treponematoses (syphilis, yaws, pinta and bejel or non-venereal 'endemic syphilis'). The cost effectiveness of screening tests for syphilis will depend on the prevalence of the disease in the population and the risk groups. While VDRL or RPR test alone is useful for screening infectious syphilis, it will fail to diagnose many primary and late syphilis cases.[21]

The testing strategy employed varies by using either a non-treponemal, or a treponemal test, or both in combination, depending on a number of factors including whether it is intended to detect all stages of syphilis or only infectious syphilis. In the United States, India and certain countries in Europe, e.g., France and Belgium, non-treponemal tests are used for screening.[22]

One advantage of this approach is that it does not detect most adequately treated cases, thus simplifying patient assessment. The disadvantages with this approach is screening undiluted specimens with a non-treponemal test alone can give rise to false-negative reactions in the presence of high titres of antibody, the prozone phenomenon. This phenomenon may occur in early infection and with concomitant HIV infection. In addition, non-treponemal tests lack sensitivity in late stage infection and screening with a non-treponemal test alone may also give rise to false-positive reactions (BFP) in a variety of acute and chronic conditions in the absence of syphilis. In some countries of Europe, eg. Germany and Netherlands, the TPHA is used for screening.[22] This provides a good screen for all stages of syphilis beyond the early primary stage but because more primary infections are detected by a combination of VDRL and TPHA tests, the use of TPHA test alone has found limited favour in diagnostic laboratories in UK, where screening with both VDRL and TPHA tests in combination has been common practice for many years.[23] The combination of VDRL and TPHA tests provides sensitive and specific screening for all stages of syphilis except very early primary infection. However, it is more labour intensive than a single screening test and requires subjective interpretation and cannot be easily automated.[23] With these practical disadvantages, and with the recent commercial availability of EIA, the VDRL and TPHA combination for screening is increasingly being replaced in various diagnostic microbiology laboratories by the use of EIA tests detecting treponemal IgG, IgM or both. The advantages of the EIA format include the production of objective results, the ability to link EIA plate readers directly to laboratory computer systems, hence reducing the potential for errors white transcribing results, and the facility for automation. These factors make EIA attractive for laboratories with large workloads.

The development of commercial EIA tests has occurred since the WHO recommended the use of a combination of a non-treponemal test and a treponemal test for screening and diagnostic purposes.[24] Although the treponemal IgG EIA is still regarded as an investigational test in the United States[5], there are published data showing that screening with a treponemal IgG EIA gives comparable results to the VDRL and TPHA combination[25] and that it may be a useful method for detecting treponemal antibody in patients who are infected with HIV.[26]

Confirmatory Tests

The FTA-ABS is still generally regarded as the 'gold standard', but in fact it has a number of limitations. It is a subjective test and difficult to standardize. The TPHA is more sensitive, than FTA-ABS except in the 3rd to 4th week of infection; and is also more specific.[7] In addition, false negative FTA-ABS results have been described in HIV infection and in association with autoimmune disorders.[27] Thus TPHA is the most appropriate test for confirming reactive EIA results at present; equally, if TPHA is used for screening, an EIA can be used as the confirmatory test.[23] Although immunoblotting has been suggested as a possible confirmatory test,[28] further evaluation is required in order to define its precise role.

Assessment of the Stage of Infection and Monitoring the Effect of Therapy

In treponemal infection, a quantitative non-treponemal test and/or a test for specific anti-treponemal IgM helps with the assessment of the stage of infection, and provides a baseline for monitoring the effect of therapy. In general, IgM becomes undetectable within 3 to 9 months after adequate treatment of early syphilis, although it may persist for 1 to 1.5 years after treatment of late disease. Detection of specific anti-treponemal IgM in patients without a history of recent treatment suggests active disease and the need for therapy. Quantitative non-treponemal tests such as the VDRL/RPR remain the method of choice for follow-up testing, the object being to demonstrate a decline in titre, depending on a range of factors including the initial titre, stage of infection when treated, treatment regimen and HIV status.[23]

To monitor the efficacy of treatment, quantitative nontreponemal test should be performed on the patient's serum samples, which are drawn at 3-month intervals for at least 1 year. Following adequate therapy for primary and secondary syphilis, there should be at least fourfold decline in titre by third or fourth month and an eightfold decline in titre by the six to eight months. Patients treated in the latent or late stages, or who have had multiple episodes of syphilis, may show a more gradual decline in titre.[29] As far as can be determined, this persistent seropositivity does not signify treatment failure or reinfection, and these patients are likely to remain serofast even if they are retreated.

The failure of nontreponemal test titres to decline after treatment with standard therapy has been documented for HIV-seronegative persons treated during latent stage or late-stage syphilis and in persons treated for reinfection. Therefore, the failure of titres to decline with treatment for syphilis in HIV-infected person is probably related to the stage of syphilis rather than to HIV status.

Summary

1. Follow-up of seronegative patients at recent risk of acquiring a sexually transmitted infection is essential because of the seronegative window in early primary syphilis.
2. Screening with a non-treponemal test alone is not recommended because of the potential for false-negative results.
3. A treponemal EIA alone (IgG or IgG/IgM), or a combination of a non- treponemal test (VDRL/RPR) and a treponemal test (TPHA), is most appropriate for screening.
4. Specimens that are reactive on screening require confirmatory testing with a different treponemal test of equal sensitivity and greater specificity.
5. Specimens giving discrepant treponemal test results on confirmatory testing need additional testing.
6. Following confirmation of a reactive specimen, a second specimen should be tested to confirm the results and the correct identification of the patient.
7. In treponemal infection, a quantitative non-treponemal test, and/or a test for specific treponemal IgM, should be performed as part of the assessment of the stage of infection and to monitor the efficacy of therapy.

POLYMERASE CHAIN REACTION (PCR)

PCR based tests have been developed by several laboratories either as potential diagnostic tests or to identify *T. pallidum*-infected animals in experimental animal systems.[30,31] Most of the tests have been based on membrane lipoproteins, of which a large number have been cloned and sequenced. Two PCR-based techniques were described almost simultaneously in 1991.[30,31] Since sensitive and inexpensive serologic tests are available for most stages of syphilis in adults, the investigators in these two articles concentrated on problem areas in which definitive diagnosis is beyond the abilities of most clinical laboratories. The first of these is based on the amplification of a 658-bp segment of the gene for the 47-kDa surface antigen: this is a lipoprotein that is antigenically dominant in the human immune response to *T. pallidum*.[5]

Several studies have indicated that *T. pallidum* can persist for long periods in the central nervous system, even apparently in patients who have received what was considered adequate antibiotic treatment.[32] Thus, a method that could detect the presence of *T. pallidum* in small samples of CSF could prove extremely valuable, especially in determining whether treatment was sufficient in cases where neurosyphilis is suspected or known to have occurred. Noordhoek et al.[31] used as their target the gene coding for a 39-kDa basic membrane protein.

PCR could be extremely valuable in diagnosing infection in congenital syphilis, neurosyphilis (the serologic test available presently is only 50% sensitive), early primary syphilis (the only tests available currently are microscopic), and in distinguishing new from old infections (presently only a rise in titre can be used).[5] PCR is also proving valuable in the diagnosis of syphilis in HIV positive patients.[2,3,33]

Real Time Polymerase Chain Reaction

A real time PCR assay has been developed that targeted the polA gene of *T. pallidum*. The assay is found to be fast and has a high sensitivity (94%) and specificity (100%).[34]

LABORATORY DIAGNOSIS OF DIFFERENT STAGES OF SYPHILIS

Early Syphilis

The finding of treponemes with characteristic appearance by dark field microscopic examination of fluid obtained from the surface of chancre is the most specific and sensitive method for verifying the diagnosis of primary syphilis. The dark field examination is actually the only test that specifically establishes the diagnosis of primary syphilis. Antibody to cardiolipin, as measured by the non treponemal test is present, often at a relatively low level in about 80% of patients at the time they come to medical attention for primary syphilis **(Table 16.4)**. In early syphilis, non treponemal test reactivity reflects activity of disease. This reactivity is expected to disappear with treatment. The non treponemal test is generally recommended even when the dark field examination is positive, in order to provide a baseline for follow-up after therapy.

Tests that measure antibody to surface proteins of *T. pallidum* by treponemal tests are positive in about 90% of patients at the time they seek medical attention for a chancre **(Table 16.5)**. Thus a negative result does not exclude the diagnosis.

Once *T. pallidum* infection has resulted in treponemal tests to be positive, these tests remain positive for life. Thus a positive result does not establish a diagnosis of primary syphilis in someone who has a lesion that might be syphilitic, since antibody may be present as a result of some earlier infection.[35] For these reasons, the search for treponemes by dark field examinations should be undertaken, even though it is time consuming and requires trained personnel.

Table 16.4 Sensitivity and Specificity of Nontreponemal Tests

Test	*% Sensitivity and Stage of Infection*				*% Specificity*
	Primary	*Secondary*	*Latent*	*Late*	*(onsyphilis)*
VDRL	78(74-87)	100	95 (88-100)	71 (37-94)	98 (96-99)
RPR	86 (77-100)	100	98 (95-100)	73	98 (93-99)
USR	80 (72-88)	100	95 (88-100)	99	
RST*	82 (77-86)	100	95 (88-100)	97	
TRUST	85 (77-86)	100	98 (95-100)	99 (98-99)	

*Reagin Screen Test

Table 16.5 **Sensitivity and Specificity of Treponemal Tests**

	% Sensitivity and Stage of infection				*% Specificity*
TEST	*Primary*	*Secondary*	*Latent*	*Late*	*(nonsyphilis)*
FTA-ABS	84 (70-100)	100	100	96	97 (94-99)
MHA-TP	76 (69-90)	100	97 (97-100)	94	99 (98-100)
FTA-ABS Double Staining	80 (69-90)	100	100	–	99 (97-100)

Secondary Syphilis

Treponemes can be easily found by dark field examination of material obtained from moist wet lesions in secondary syphilis. This test is usually not done on dry skin lesions. Serological tests give far more distinctive results in secondary than in primary syphilis. Antibody to cardiolipin is always present, usually at a high dilution (VDRL more than 1:32). Rarely, a prozone phenomenon occurs, in which a blocking antibody obscures a positive reading in undiluted serum, but the positive reaction is readily apparent with dilutions. In doing the non-treponemal test, most laboratories do not perform serum dilutions if the undiluted serum gives a negative result unless the physicians specifically indicates that the diagnosis of syphilis is suspected clinically; therefore in ordering a non treponemal test in a case of suspected secondary syphilis, a specification for dilutions should be made. In secondary syphilis, the treponemal tests are always positive.[36]

Latent Syphilis

At the present time, patients are diagnosed as having latent syphilis if they have a reactive non treponemal test in the absence of any apparent signs of the disease and the treponemal test is positive. If a patient admits to having had a chancre or a skin rash for which he did not seek treatment and he now has a reactive non treponemal with a positive treponemal test, the diagnosis of latent syphilis is apparent. However this would not always be the case. More often, the serological findings are present without any useful information on the medical history. Such patients are regarded as if they have latent syphilis from the public health point of view. It is worth mentioning however, that such a diagnosis is difficult. On the one hand, these serological abnormalities may have persisted after adequate treatment (serofast state) so that it may be difficult, to be certain whether the patient has partially treated syphilis, latent syphilis, or an adequately treated syphilis in which the serological abnormalities persist. On the other hand, the positive serological test may indicate unrecognized active disease after unrecognized chancre or lesion has healed and manifest late syphilis is not present. In this scenario, the patient may have asymptomatic neuro-syphilis which can only be excluded by documenting a normal cerebrospinal fluid. This leads to recommendations that a spinal tap be done and the CSF be negative in order to establish the diagnosis of latency.[36]

Syphilis and HIV infection

There is a steep rise in co-infection of syphilis and HIV across the globe.[2,3] The problems in the diagnosis of syphilis with HIV are (i) confusing clinical signs and symptoms[37]; (ii) lack of serologic response in a patient with a clinically confirmed case of active syphilis[38]; (iii) failure of nontreponemal test titres to decline after treatment with standard regimens; (iv) unusually high titres in nontreponemal test[39], perhaps as the result of B-cell activation; (v) rapid progression to late stages of syphilis and neurologic involvement even after treatment of primary or secondary syphilis[39]; and (vi) the disappearance of treponemal test reactivity over time. Biological false positive reactions for cardiolipin tests (VDRL and RPR) and prozone phenomenon can also occur.[21]

Aberrant results in the serological tests for syphilis appear to be related to abnormally low absolute CD4 cell counts and are relatively rare.[40] The diagnosis of syphilis in these cases was supported either by the observation of *T. pallidum* in material from typical lesions or by the appearance of serologic reactivity after treatment. The delay in development of a response to syphilis theoretically should be expected in persons with abnormal lymphocyte counts; however, the frequency of this occurrence is unknown.

Late Syphilis

The serum non treponemal test is positive in most cases of acute syphilitic meningitis. The CSF changes include elevated pressure, mononuclear pleocytosis of 10 to 200 cells per cubic millimeter, elevated protein concentration (200 mg/dl), elevated globulin level and a modest reduction in glucose in 45 percent of cases. The presence of a positive VDRL/RPR and a raised TPHA index in CSF indicates neurological involvement.[21] The VDRL test on CSF is reactive in most, but not all cases. It has been noted that patients who present with isolated involvement of the eighth cranial nerve are likely to have a normal CSF with a nonreactive VDRL test. Serum non treponemal test is positive in meningovascular syphilis. The CSF changes are those usually seen in neurosyphilis, in keeping with a smouldering low grade meningitis owing largely to vascular occlusive disease. The CSF VDRL test is positive in most but not all cases. Nontreponemal serological tests of blood and CSF are nearly uniformly positive in cases of paresis. Other CSF findings are typical of those in neurosyphilis. The CSF may be normal in a patient, whose neurosyphilis has been arrested by treatment, leaving persistent mental changes. A positive serum VDRL often is a clue to the presence of neurosyphilis. Specific anti treponemal antibody tests of CSF, such as FTA-ABS or MHA-TP have been studied as a tool to diagnose neurosyphilis in the occasional case in which the CSF VDRL is non reactive.[41] These tests may be reactive as a result of diffusion of serum immunoglobulin into the CSF or as a result of contamination of CSF by small amount of blood rather than because of local antibody synthesis in the CNS. Hence a careful collection of CSF sample, free of contamination by blood, is essential.[37] Another approach is to examine intrathecal antibody synthesis using the CSF–IgG index,[42] obtained by dividing the CSF to serum IgG ratio by the CSF to serum albumin ratio. A result of more than 0.7 is indicative of IgG synthesis within the CNS, but this finding is consistent with a variety of infectious or inflammatory processes.[43] Specificity is provided by demonstrating that the antibody is produced intrathecally, as determined by an intrathecal *T. pallidum* antibody index >100,[44] defined as

$$\text{CSF-TPHA titre} \Big/ \frac{\text{CSF albumin (mg/dl)} \times 10^3}{\text{Serum albumin (mg/dl)}}$$

Better evidence for intrachecal antitreponemal antibody synthesis may be obtained if the serum CSF ratio of TPHA is at least four times lower than the corresponding ratio for some other unrelated but ubiquitous antibody, such as adenovirus haemagglutination antibody.[45]

The potential usefulness of the MHA-TP index has been confirmed, but tests for antitreponemal IgM antibodies in CSF are rarely performed. There is much research going on for use of polymerase chain reaction (PCR) test for *T. pallidum* as a means of diagnosing neurosyphilis, but the sensitivity and specificity are still under investigation.[46]

Neurosyphilis in HIV Infected Persons

Neurosyphilis can usually develop rapildly when there is concomitant infection with HIV. CSF examination is necessary when there is evidence of clinical relapse or a four fold rise is noted in the titre of follow up serological tests on serum. It is generally agreed that the CSF should be examined in all patients with clinical neurosyphilis and in all syphilitic infections of more than 2 years, in order to exclude asymptomatic neurosyphilis. It is unnecessary to perform routine tests for syphilis on the CSF of patients with central nervous system symptoms in whom there is no suspicion of syphilis. A negative *T. pallidum* antigen such as the TPHA, on serum will virtually exclude active neurosyphilis and is a better screen for the detection of all forms of late syphilis than examination of the CSF. The latter should be reserved for cases selected on clinical grounds and backed by positive TPHA test on serum. A negative TPHA test on CSF excludes neurosyphilis. A negative VDRL test on CSF does not exclude neurosyphilis as a third to half of patients with clinically active neurosyphilis will give a negative VDRL result on the CSF.

Cardiovascular Syphilis

Screening serological tests are helpful because they are usually reactive, especially where there is extensive involvement of soft tissue. The serological test result may be of high titre. The prozone phenomenon has been a problem in some case, with serological test shown to be positive upon retesting in appropriate dilutions of serum. On the other hand, a negative reaction may accompany a localized lesion, as of bone.

REFERENCES

1. Fieldsteel AH, Cox DL, Moeckli. RA. Cultivation of virulent *Treponema pallidum* in tissue culture. Infect Immunol 1981; 32: 908-15.
2. Stevenson J, Heath M. Syphilis and HIV infection: an update. Clin Infect Dis 2007; 44: 1222-8.
3. Zetola NM. Syphilis and HIV infection: an update. Dermatol Clin 2006; 24: 497-507.
4. Romanowski B, Forsey E, Prasad E, et al. Detection of *Treponema pallidum* by a fluorescent monoclonal antibody test. Sex Transm Dis 1987; 22: 156-9.
5. Larsen SA, Steiner BM, Rudodph AH. Laboratory diagnosis and interpretation of tests for syphilis. Clin Microbiol Rev 1995; 8: 1-21.
6. Grimprel E, Sanchez PJ, Wendel GD, et al. Use of polymerase chain reaction and rabbit infectivity testing to detect *Treponema pallidum* in amniotic fluid. J Clin Microbiol 1991; 29: 1711-8.
7. Luger AFH. Serological diagnosis of syphilis: Current methods. In: Young H, McMillan A, eds. Immunological diagnosis of sexually transmitted diseases. New York: Marcel Decker; 1988: p. 249-74.
8. Baker-Zander SA, Hook EW, Bonin P, et al. Antigens of *Treponema pallidum* recognized by IgG and IgM antibodies during syphilis in humans. J Infect Dis 1985; 151: 264–72.
9. Rufli T. Syphilis and HIV infection. Dermatologica 1989; 179: 113-7.
10. Eagle H. The laboratory diagnosis of syphilis, St. Louis.The C.V. Mosby Co. 1937: 21-8.
11. Kahn RL. A simple quantitative precipitation reaction for syphilis. Arch Dermatol Syphilol 1922; 5: 570-8, 734-43; 6: 332-41.
12. Pangborn MC. A new serologically active phospholipid from beef heart. Proc Soc Exp Biol Med 1941; 48: 484-6.
13. Rudolph A H, Larsen SA. Laboratory diagnosis of syphilis, In: Demis DJ eds Clinical Dermatology, Lippincott Co: Philadephia. 1993: p. 1-16.
14. Nelson RA Jr, Mayer MM. Immobilization of *Treponema pallidum* in vitro by antibody produced in syphilitic infection. J Exp Med 1949; 89: 369-93.
15. Rein MF, Banks GW Logan LC, et al. Failure of the *Treponema pallidum* immobilization test to provide additional diagnostic information about contemporary problem sera. Sex Transm Dis 1980; 7: 191-205.
16. Deacon WE, Falcone VH, Harris A. A fluorescent test for treponemal antibodies. Proc Soc Exp Biol Med Biol Med 1957; 96: 477-80.
17. Deacon WE, Freeman EM, Harris A. Fluorescent treponemal antibody test. Modification based on quantitation (FTA-200). Proc Soc Ex Biol Med 1960; 103: 827-9.

18. Deacon WE, Hunter EF. Treponemal antigens as related to identification and syphilis serology. Proc Soc Exp Biol Med 1962; 110: 352-6.
19. Hunter EF, Deacon WE, Meyer PE. An improved FTA test for syphilis: the absorption procedure(FTA-ABS). Public Health Rep 1964; 79: 410-2.
20. Rathlev V. Haemagglutination tests utilizing antigens from pathogenic and apathogenic *Treponema pallidum*. WHO/VDT Res 1965; 77: 65.
21. Goh BT. Syphilis in adults. Sex Transm Infect 2005; 81: 448-52.
22. Young H. Syphilis: new diagnostic directions. Int J STDs AIDS 1992; 3: 391-413.
23. Young H. Syphilis serology. Dermatol Clin 1998; 16: 691-8.
24. World Health Organization. Treponemal infections. Technical reports series 674. Geneva: World Health Organization, 1982.
25. Young H, Moyes A, McMillan A, et al. Enzyme immunoassay for anti-treponemal IgG: screening or confirmatory test? J Clin Pathol 1992; 45: 37-41.
26. Young H, Moyes A, Ross JCD. Markers of past syphilis in HIV infection comparing with captia Syphilis G anti-treponemal IgG enzyme immunoassay with other treponemal antigen tests. Int J STDs AIDS 1995; 6: 101-4.
27. Erbelding EJ, Vlahov D, Nelson TC, et al. Syphilis serology in human immunodeficiency virus infection: evidence for false-negative fluorescent treponemal testing. J Infect Dis 1997; 176: 1397-400.
28. Byrne RE, Laska S, Bell M, et al. Evaluation of a *Treponema pallidum* western immunoblot assay as a confirmatory test for syphilis. J Clin Microbiol 1992; 30: 115-22.
29. Fiumara NJ. Reinfection primary, secondary and late latent syphilis. The serologic response after treatment. Sex Transm Dis 1980; 7: 111-5.
30. Grimprel E, Sanchez PJ, Wendel GD, et al. Use of polymerase chain reaction and rabbit infectivity testing to detect *Treponema pallidum* in amniotic fluid. J Clin Microbiol 1991; 28: 1711-8.
31. Noordhoek, GT, Wolters EC, De Jonge MEJ, et al. Detection by polymerase chain reaction of *Treponema pallidum* DNA in cerebrospinal fluid from neurosyphilis patients before and after antibiotic treatment. J Clin Microbiol 1991; 29: 197-8.
32. Hay PE, Clarke JR, Scrugnell RA, et al. Use of the polymerase chain reaction to detect DNA sequences specific to pathogenic treponemes in cerebrospinal fluid. FEMS Microbiol Lett 1990; 56: 233-8.
33. Kandelaki G, Kapila R, Fernandes H. Destructive osteomyelitis associated with early secondary syphilis in an HIV-positive patient diagnosed by *Treponema pallidum* DNA polymerase chain reaction. AIDS Patient Care STDs. 2007; 21: 229-33.
34. Koek AG, Bruisten SM, Dierdorp M, et al. Specific and sensitive diagnosis of syphilis using a real time PCR for *Treponema pallidum*. Clin Microbiol Infect 2006; 12: 1233-6.
35. Musher DM. Early syphilis. In: Holmes KK, Sparling PF, Mardh P, et al. eds. Sexually Transmitted Diseases. 3rd ed., New York: McGraw-Hill. 1999: p. 479-85.
36. Swartz MN, Healy BP, Musher DM, Late Syphilis. In: Holmes KK, Sparling PF, Mardh P et al, eds. Sexually Transmitted Diseases. 3rd ed, NewYork: McGraw-Hill. 1999: p. 487-509.
37. Dawson SB, Evans A, Lawrence AG. Benign tertiary syphilis and HIV infection. AIDS 1988; 2: 315-6.
38. Gregory N, Sanchez M, Buchness MR.. The spectrum of syphilis in patients with human immunodeficiency virus infection. J Am Acad Dermatol 1990; 22: 1061-7.
39. Musher DM. Syphilis, neurosyphilis, penicillin and AIDS. J Infect Dis 1991; 163: 1201-6.
40. Hicks CD, Benson PM, Lupton GP, et al. Seronegative secondary syphilis in a patient infected with the human immunodeficiency virus (HIV) Kaposi sarcoma. Ann Intern Med 1987; 107: 492-5.
41. Jaffe HW, Larsen SA, Peters M, et al. Tests for treponemal antibody in CSF. Arch Intern Med 1978; 138: 252-5.

42. Madiedo G, Ho KC, Walsh P. False positive VDRL and FTA in cerebrospinal fluid. JAMA 1980; 244: 688-91.
43. Pedersen NS, Kam-Hansen S, Link H, et al. Specificity of immunoglobulins synthesized within the central nervous system in neurosyphilis. Acta Pathol Microbiol Immunol 1982; 90: 97-104.
44. Prange HW, Moskophidis M, Schipper HI, et al. Relationship between neurological features and intrathecal synthesis of IgG antibodies to *Treponema pallidum* in untreated and treated human neurosyphilis. J Neurol 1983; 230: 241-52.
45. Gschnait F, Schmidt BL, Luger A. Cerebrospinal fluid immunoglobulins in neurosyphilis. Br J Vener Dis 1981; 57: 238-40.
46. Tomberlin MG, Holton PD, Owens JL, et al. Evaluation of neurosyphilis in human immunodeficiency virus-infected individuals. Clin Inf Dis 1994; 18: 288-92.

17 TREATMENT OF SYPHILIS

G Sethuraman, Vinod K Sharma

In this chapter

- Historical Perspectives
- Treatment Guidelines
- Treatment of Primary, Secondary and Early Latent Syphilis
- Treatment of Late Latent Syphilis
- Treament of Tertiary Syphilis (Gumma and Cardiovascular Syphilis)
- Treatment of Neurosyphilis
- Management of Sex Partners
- Treatment of Syphilis Among HIV Infected Patients
- Treatment of Syphilis During Pregnancy
- Penicillin Allergy
- Evaluation of patients with penicillin allergy

HISTORICAL PERSPECTIVES[1]

Syphilis ravaged the mankind for almost 350 years after it spreaded in the Europe in 16th century. The prevalence rates in early twentieth century were 5-10% at autopsy and in poor socioeconomic status it reached up to 25%. It was referred to as Great Pox compared to Small Pox because of its devastating nature. The all above remind us of current AIDS scenario. The development and use of penicillin was one of the landmark breakthroughs that made the treatment of Great Pox possible with one magic injection.

Until the introduction of penicillin in the year 1943, mercury and arsenic were used for the treatment of syphilis. In the beginning of twentieth century mercury was the only drug available for the treatment of syphilis. But its highly toxic nature limited its therapeutic use.

Later different forms of arsenic, Ehrlich's solution, and intravenous neoarsphenamine along with bismuth for a variable period of 9-15 months, depending upon the stage of the disease, was used. Subsequently, sulpharsphenamine, a trivalent arsenical compound, oxophenarsine or arsphenoxide, and tryparsamide have been used. Because of the serious side effects and longer duration of treatment, nowadays these drugs are no longer recommended.

Bismuth has been used as a therepeutic agent in patients with lesions suggestive of late syphilis and also to prevent Jarisch-Herxheimer reaction. Potassium iodide was used for many years as an adjuvant therapy, especially in the gummatous lesions and also as a therepeutic test along with bismuth.

Fever, induced by mechanical means or by inoculation of infective agents such as malaria had been used in the treatment of syphilis either alone or as an adjuvant.

Penicillin was first used in the treatment of syphilis in experimental animals and in man by Mahoney, Arnold and Harris in 1943. The impure amorphous penicillin consisted of a mixture of four different penicillins called G, F, X, and K, was given at a dose of 2.4 million units every 3 hours for a period of seven-and-half days (60 injections). Later in 1946, this treatment was proved to be ineffective due to the fact that the preparation consisted of a greater portion of penicillin K, which was not effective in syphilis. It was also found that penicillin G was the most effective component against treponemes and was used at a dose of 2.4 or 4.8 million units given every two or four hours day and night for a period of a week or more. Because of the usable too many injections necessitating admission and other discomfort, attempts were made to prepare long acting repository penicillins. One such preparation was calcium penicillin in arachis oil containing 4.8% of beewax and was used at a dose of 2 ml (each ml consisted of 3,00,000 units) intramuscularly daily for a period of 8 days. A single daily injection maintained an effective level for about 24 hours. But the drug was difficult to administer and had severe reactions. The next repository preparation was the procaine penicillin, a combination of procaine and penicillin. It is used as a watery suspension in daily doses of 6,00,000 units for a period of 8-10 days. Further modification in the preparation is the suspension of procaine penicillin in arachis oil along with 2% water repellent aluminium monostearate (PAM). The advantage of this preparation is that the dose of 3,00,000 to 6,00,000 units maintained the therapeutic level of penicillin for 72 hours, which allows the patients to take the injection on alternate days.

Later, modifications and developments came with the discovery of benzathine penicillin G (dibenzyl ethylene diamine dipenicillin G), the only antibiotic formulation, which provides serum drug concentration for several weeks following a single IM injection.[2]

TREATMENT GUIDELINES

Parenteral penicillin is the treatment of choice for the treatment of all stages of syphilis. The preparations used are benzathine, aqueous procaine and aqueous crystalline penicillin.[3] Oral penicillin can also be used in the treatment but is not recommended because of reduced efficiency and lack of compliance.[1]

Mechanism of Action[1]

Penicillin at the concentration of 0.0025 units/ml kills 50% *T. pallidum* within 16 hours. The recommended concentration of penicillin in syphilis is 0.03 units/ml for a period of 7 to 10 days in early syphilis and longer time in late syphilis. Penicillin binds irreversibly to the transpeptidase enzymes of the treponemes, which are required for the biosynthesis of outer envelopes and thereby prevents closing of the gaps in the envelope lattice. This results in high osmotic pressure within the protoplasmic cylinder, causing bulging of the inner membrane and bursting of the treponemes.

TREATMENT OF PRIMARY, SECONDARY AND EARLY LATENT SYPHILIS[3]

Recommended Regimen

- Benzathine penicillin G 2.4 million units intramuscular (IM) single dose (1.2 million units deep IM in each buttock).
- For children: Benzathine penicillin G 50,000 units/kg IM up to the adult dose of 2.4 million units in a single dose.

The treatment should be given after testing intradermal sensitivity for penicillin.

All the patients who have syphilis should be tested for HIV infection. If it is negative, a repeat test should be done after 3 months, especially in areas where the HIV prevalence is high. Patients with early syphilis who have features suggestive of meningitis or uveitis should be evaluated for neurosyphilis.

WHO[4] and NACO[5] recommend the following alternative regimen:

Procaine benzyl penicillin G 1.2 million IU daily IM for 10 days. (3 vials, each having combination of 1 lakh units of benzyl penicillin G sodium and 3 lakh units of procaine benzyl penicillin G.)

Alternative Regimen for Penicillin Allergic Patients

- Doxycycline 100 mg bid orally for 2 weeks or
- Tetracycline 500 mg qid orally for 2 weeks

The efficiency of these regimens is not well documented. Hence frequent follow up of the patients receiving these therapies is essential. The effectiveness of these therapies in HIV infected patients has not been studied. Although limited clinical studies suggest that azithromycin and ceftriaxone are effective in the treatment of syphilis, their use in the clinical practice is yet to be established.[6,7]

Follow-Up

Patients should be examined clinically and serologically at 6 and 12 months. There should be a fourfold decrease in the non-treponemal (VDRL) titre within 6 months. Patients who have persistent symptoms or recurrence, or who have four fold increase in the VDRL titre or failure of titre to decline four fold within 6 months should be re-evaluated for reinfection, treatment failure, HIV infection, or unrecognized CNS infection. All such patients should undergo a thorough neurological evaluation including CSF analysis and HIV testing. When they are retreated, they should preferably be given 3 weekly doses of benzathine penicillin G 2.4 million units, unless CSF examination indicates that neurosyphilis is present.

TREATMENT OF LATE LATENT SYPHILIS

All the patients who have latent syphilis should be evaluated for tertiary syphilis. CSF analysis is clearly indicated if any one of the following criteria is present.

- CNS or eye changes
- Evidence of active tertiary syphilis

- HIV infection
- Treatment failure
- Non treponemal titre ≥ 1:32

If the CSF analysis shows features of neurosyphilis then the patient should be treated for the same.

Late latent syphilis or latent syphilis of unknown duration should be treated with 3 weekly doses of benzathine penicillin G 2.4 million units IM.

Doses in Children

Three weekly injection of benzathine penicillin G at a dose of 50,000 units/kg up to an adult dose of 2.4 million units IM.

Alternate Regimen

Procaine benzylpenicillin G 1.2 million units IM daily for 20 days.

Follow-Up

Quantitiative non treponemal serologic test (VDRL) should be repeated at 6, 12 and 24 months. After treatment, the patient should be reevaluated for neurosyphilis if any of the following criteria is present.

- Fourfold increase in the titre of VDRL
- An initially high VDRL titre (≥1:32) failing to decline a least fourfold within 12-24 months of therapy
- The patient developing signs and symptoms of tertiary syphilis.

Alternative Regimen for Penicillin Allergic Patients

- Doxycycline 100 mg orally bid for 30 days or
- Tetracycline 500 mg orally qid for 30 days

TREAMENT OF TERTIARY SYPHILIS (GUMMA AND CARDIOVASCULAR SYPHILIS)

Three weekly doses of benzathine penicillin G 2.4 million units IM.

TREATMENT OF NEUROSYPHILIS

Patients with neurosyphilis, or syphilitic eye disease in the form of neuroretinitis, optic neuritis, uveitis or any other cranial nerve palsies should have CSF examination and be treated with aqueous crystalline penicillin G 18-24 millions units per day administered as 3-4 million units IV every 4 hours or continuous infusion for 10-14 days.

Alternative Regimen

Procaine penicillin G 2.4 million units IM daily for 14 days along with probenecid 500 mg orally qid for 14 days.

Benzathine penicillin G has no role in the treatment of neurosyphilis as it does not cross the blood barrier in sufficient quantity.

Follow-Up

CSF should be re-examined every 6 months until it becomes normal. CSF cell count should decrease by 6 months and CSF VDRL and protein levels by 2 years. If not, patient should be retreated.

MANAGEMENT OF SEX PARTNERS

The sex partners should be evaluated clinically and serologically and treated according to the following recommendations.

- Persons who are exposed within the 90 days preceding the diagnosis of primary, secondary or early latent syphilis in a sex partner might be infected even if seronegative; therefore such persons should be treated presumptively.

- Persons who were exposed >90 days before the diagnosis of primary, secondary, or early latent syphilis in a sex partner should be treated presumptively if serologic test results are not available immediately and the opportunity for follow up is uncertain.
- For purposes of partner notification and presumptive treatment of exposed sex partners, patients with syphilis of unknown duration who have high nontreponemal serologic test titres (i.e., >1:32) can be assumed to have early syphilis. However, serologic titres should not be used to differentiate early from late latent syphilis for the purpose of determining treatment
- Long term sex partners of patients who have latent syphilis should be evaluated clinically and serologically for syphilis and treated on the basis of the evaluation findings.

TREATMENT OF SYPHILIS AMONG HIV INFECTED PATIENTS[3]

Primary, Secondary, Early Latent Syphilis

Injection benzathine penicillin G 2.4 million units single dose IM. Some authors recommend 3 weekly doses.

Other Treatment Consideration

HIV infected persons with early syphilis are at increased risk of developing neurological complication. Hence some specialists recommend CSF examination before treatment and then it is treated accordingly.

Follow-Up

Clinical and serological follow-up are done at 3, 6, 9, 12 and 24 months. CSF examination and retreatment with 3 weekly doses of benzathine penicillin G are recommended in patients whose non-treponemal titres do not fall fourfold within 6-12 months of therapy.

Late Latent Syphilis

Patients with late latent syphilis or syphilis of unknown duration should undergo CSF examination. If it is normal, then 3 weekly doses of benzathine penicillin G 2.4 million units is given. If there are CSF abnormalities, then they are treated as neurosyphilis.

Follow-Up

Clinical and serological examination are repeated at 6, 12, 18 and 24 months after therapy. During the follow up, if clinical symptoms develop or non-treponemal titres rise fourfold, a repeat CSF examination is performed. If in 12-24 months the non-treponemal titres do not decline four fold, CSF examination is repeated and treated accordingly.

Treatment of Neurosyphilis[8]

Treatment of choice for neurosyphilis in HIV infected patients is intravenous administration of aqueous crystalline penicillin G at a dose of 18-24 million units daily for 14 days. (Same as in non HIV infected patients). If the intravenous injections cannot be given, then an alternative regimen of procaine penicillin G is given at a dose of 2.4 million units IM daily for 14 days along with probenecid 500 mg orally qid for 14 days. But, as far as possible, intravenous regimen is preferred to the IM penicillin. Some specialists recommended injection benzathine penicillin 2.4 million units IM to ensure prolonged antispirochetal activity.

Penicillin allergic patients should preferably be desensitized and given penicillin only.

Follow-Up

Patients after treatment for neurosyphilis may have a high index of suspicion for relapse. CSF examination should be done at 6-month interval until CSF is normal and reassessment of CSF should be undertaken when neurosyphilis is suspected.

TREATMENT OF SYPHILIS DURING PREGNANCY

Appropriate penicillin regimen should be given during pregnancy, depending upon the stage. Pregnant women who are allergic to penicillin should be desensitized and treated with penicillin. No alternatives to penicillin have been proved effective for the treatment of syphilis during pregnancy. However, WHO[4] and NACO[5] recommend erythromycin as an alternative regimen in pregnant woman who are allergic to penicillin as desensitization is a very cumbersome procedure and is not feasible in most of the primary health care settings. Patients receiving erythromycin regimen should be monitored frequently and closely. Azithromycin and ceftriaxone are other potential options for penicillin allergic pregnant women, but insufficient data on efficacy limit their use.[9]

The treatment of congenital syphilis is discussed in a separate chapter.

PENICILLIN ALLERGY

Allergic reactions to penicillin may occur in 10% of patients receiving therapy. Three types of reactions can occur:

1. Penicillin Reaction

It can be either toxic or allergic.

Toxic reaction is dose related, occurring in penicillin overdose or patients with renal impairment.

Allergic reaction is immune mediated and occurs in 10% of the patients. They are divided into four types.

Type I	:	IgE mediated - urticaria, angiodema, anaphylaxis
Type II	:	Characterized by haemolytic anaemia and leucopenia
Type III	:	Serum sickness
Type IV	:	Delayed type reaction manifesting as maculopapular rash, toxic epidermal necrolysis, etc.

2. Procaine Reaction (Hoigne Syndrome)

Acute psychotic episode, severe anxiety, agitation, vertigo, seizures, visual and auditory hallucinations. It is thought to be due to brain microembolism secondary to inadvertent injection of crystals of procaine penicillin intravenously.

3. Jarisch-Herxheimer Reaction[1,10]

Jarisch in 1895 first described this reaction in syphilitic patients, and subsequently Herxheimer in 1902 observed similar features. Since then it is known as Jarisch-Herxheimer (JH) reaction. It is also observed in other bacterial infections. The reaction occurs as "all or none phenomenon", with full potential if it occurs at all. Hence starting treatment with low dose of penicillin does not give any protection. It occurs most frequently (50%) with greater severity in early syphilis more so with secondary syphilis. The patients will manifest symptoms 2 to 12 hours after injection but within the first 24 hours after giving penicillin. The features in early syphilis are more like "flu like" syndrome with fever, headache, malaise, flushing and sweating, lasting for about 24 hours. The symptoms are often accompanied by local tissue reactions with temporary aggravation or flaring of primary and secondary lesions. The existing chancre may become swollen and oedematous or the patient may develop transient secondary rash. In pregnancy with early syphilis, the reactions may precipitate early labour and foetal distress.

In late syphilis, the reactions are milder and occur in no more than 25% of the patients except in general paralysis of insane in which it can occur in over 50% patients. Rarely serious side effects may occur in the form of oedema of the glottis in gummatous lesions, coronary artery occlusion, cerebral thrombosis and rupture of the aneurysmal sac in cardiovascular syphilis, intensification of psychosis, epilepsy, and severe attacks of lightning pain in neurosyphilis.

The exact pathogenesis of JH reaction is not known. But it has been attributed to the sudden destruction of the treponemes with the subsequent release of large amounts of antigens. The reactions are associated with an increase in circulating levels of TNF $\propto$ and interleukins.[6,8]

Treatment is supportive with fluids and NSAID.

Prevention: Prednisolone at a dose of 30-40 mg given 2 days prior to the injection and continued 2-3 days afterwards may prove to be beneficial.

Treatment of Penicillin Allergic Reactions[1]

Acute reactions: The treatment room should be well equipped with all the resuscitation measures. The patient should be given Inj. adrenaline 0.6 ml of 1:1000 solution IM along with Inj. aminophylline 250 mg in 10 ml of sterile distilled water to relieve the bronchospasm. After giving adrenaline patient may be given Inj.hydrocortisone at a dose of 250 mg followed by 1000 mg during the succeeding 24 hours.

Delayed reactions are treated with antihistamine and or steroids.

EVALUATION OF PATIENTS WITH PENICILLIN ALLERGY

Penicillins are low molecular weight compounds that covalenently bind to tissue carrier proteins and form drug-protein complexes or haptens which makes them immunogenic. Ninety five percent of tissue-bound penicillin is haptenated as benzyl penicilloyl and are termed as major antigenic determinants. The remaining 5% of the molecules are termed as minor antigenic determinants, which are benzylpenicillin, benzylpenicilloate and benzylpenilloate, and these are not immunologically cross reactive.[3]

Skin testing with both major and minor determinants is the gold standard for detecting penicillin allergy. It demonstrates the presence or absence of IgE antibodies against these determinants.[11] In the USA the major determinants are commercially available as benzylpenicilloyl –polylysine (PPL) [Prepen, Kremers Urban, Wisconsin]. Many researches use penicillin G at a concentration of 10,000 U/ml as a partial source of minor determinants.[12] Testing with major determinant and penicillin G identifies approximately 90 – 97% of the allergic patients. This increases to nearly 100% if it is tested with major and all the minor determinants.[11] A commercial kit containing both these determinants was available in Europe (Allergopen) but was withdrawn from the market in 2005. A new kit with both major and minor determinants has recently been commercialized in Spain for skin testing (Diater laboratories, Madrid, Spain). It has been shown that it is an equally effective and safe alternative for the diagnosis of penicillin allergy.[12-15]

Indication for Penicillin Testing

Penicillin skin testing is always indicated in all patients with suspected IgE mediated reactions (urticaria, angioedema and anaphylaxis). It is usually not indicated in patients with history suggestive of non IgE mediated reactions. Solensky et al,[16] in a large series of 1063 patients, demonstrated that 33% of patients with a history of penicillin allergy and positive penicillin testing had "vague" non IgE mediated reactions. They recommended that patients with such "vague" reactions should also be tested; otherwise many patients with IgE antibodies would be missed. In conclusion, penicillin skin testing may be useful in all patients with a history of penicillin allergy (both IgE and non IgE mediated reactions).[17]

Penicillin Skin Testing[3]

Patient should be tested in a tertiary care centre where an intensive care setting is available, in which treatment for anaphylaxis can be undertaken. Ideally the patients should not have taken antihistamines in the recent past. The major and minor antigenic compounds of penicillin are given in Table 17.1. Dilute the antigens to 100 fold for preliminary testing, if the patient has had a life threatening reaction to penicillin or 10 fold if the patient has had another type of immediate, generalized reaction to penicillin within the preceding year.

Table 17.1 **Skin Test Reagents for Identifying Persons at Risk for Adverse Reactions to Pencillin[3,12]**

- **Major Determinant**
  Benzylpenicilloyl poly-L-lysine (0.04mg/mL)
- **Minor Determinant**
  sodium benzylpenicillin (0.5 mg/mL)
  disodium benzylpenicilloate (0.5mg/mL)
  benzyl penicilloic acid (0.5 mg/mL)
- **Positive Control**
  Commercial histamine (1 mg/mL).
- **Negative Control**
  Diluent used to dissolve other reagents, usually phenol saline.

Epicutaneous (prick) Test

Duplicate drops of reagents for skin testing are placed on the volar surface of the forearm, and the underlying epidermis is pierced with a 26-gauze needle without drawing blood. Reading is taken after 15 minutes. The test is considered positive if the diameter of the wheal is 4 mm larger than that of negative control, otherwise the test is negative. A histamine control should be positive to ensure that results are not false negative because of the effect of antihistamines.

Intradermal Test

If the prick test is negative, then an intradermal test is done. A 0.02 ml antigenic solution is injected intradermally with a 26 or 27 G needle on a syringe, on the volar surface of the forearm. Reading is taken after 15 minutes. The test is said to be positive if the average wheal diameter is >2 mm larger than the initial wheal size and also is >2 mm larger than the negative control. Otherwise the test is negative.

Recommendations

If the skin test is negative, patients who report a history of penicillin reactions can receive the conventional penicillin therapy. Generally it is safe to administer penicillin in these patients; however a small percentage of patients can develop non-life threatening reactions. In a multicenter study,[18] 566 patients with history of penicillin allergy and negative skin test (to major determinant, penicillin G and minor determinants) were treated with penicillin, 1.2% of the patients developed non-life threatening reactions in the form of pruritus or urticaria. In another series,[19] 346 patients with negative skin tests to the major determinants and penicillin G received penicillin and 12% had adverse drug reactions. Of those 1% had IgE mediated reactions. Hence, it is concluded that 97%-99% of the patients with negative skin tests can tolerate the penicillin with no risk of an immediate severe reaction.

Skin test positive patients should be desensitized and it should be done orally, because it is safer than parenteral. The schedule begins by administering extremely small doses of penicillin with a doubling of the dose every 15 minutes. Full dose therapy should be completed and the overall time to complete the process of desensitization is approximately 4 hours. If a dose is missed, then desensitization is repeated. The oral desensitization protocol is given in Table 17.2. After desensitization, the patient can be given parenteral penicillin.

The process of desensitization induces immunotolerance by administartion of very small doses of antigen. Hypersensitivity to penicillin still persists, but antibodies of the IgE class bind to scanty amounts of antigen, hence the reaction is faint and remains subclinical.[20] If repeat administration of penicillin in the same patient is required in future, skin testing should be done again and if positive desensitization should be repeated.[21]

Table 17.2 Oral Desensitization Protocol for Patients with a Positive Skin Test

Pencillin V Suspension Dose	*Amount (units/mL)*	*mL*	*Units*	*Cumulative Dose (units)*
1	1,000	0.1	100	100
2	1,000	0.2	200	300
3	1,000	0.4	400	700
4	1,000	0.8	800	1500
5	1,000	1.6	1600	3100
6	1,000	3.2	3200	6300
7	1,000	6.4	6400	12700
8	10,000	1.2	12000	24700
9	10,000	2.4	24000	48700
10	10,000	4.8	48000	96700
11	80,000	1.0	80000	176700
12	80,000	2.0	160000	336700
13	80,000	4.0	320000	656700
14	80,000	8.0	640000	1296700

Note: Observation period: 30 minutes before parenteral administration of penicillin.
Adapted from CDC Treatment of Sexually Transmitted Diseases. 2006

REFERENCES

1. King A, Nicol C, Rodin P, eds: Treatment of syphilis in "Venereal diseases". 4th edn. London: ELBS; 1980. p. 144-64.
2. Markowitz M. Long-acting penicillins: historical perspectives. Pediatr Infect Dis 1985; 4: 570-3.
3. Centre for Disease Control. Sexually transmitted diseases. Treatment guidelines. MMWR, 2006; 55/RR-11.
4. WHO/RHR/01.10. Guidelines for the management of sexually transmitted infection. 2001
5. Sexually transmitted infection treatment recommendations. NACO 2004.
6. Links Zhou P, Gu Z, Xu J, et al. Study evaluating ceftriaxone as a treatment agent for primary and secondary syphilis in pregnancy. Sex Transm Dis 2005; 32: 495-8.
7. French P. Syphilis. BMJ 2007; 20; 334: 143-7.
8. Treponemal infection is HIV disease. In: Powderly WG edr. Manual of HIV therapeutics. 2nd edn. Philedelphia: Lippincott Williams & Wilkins; 2002. p. 229-38.
9. Wendel Jr GD, Sheffield JS, Hollier LM, et al. Treatment of syphilis in pregnancy and prevention of congenital syphilis. Clin Infect Dis 2002; 35: S200-209.
10. Van Voorst, Vader PC. Syphilis management and treatment. Dermatol Clin 1998; 16: 697-711.
11. Schafer JA, Mateo N, Parlier GL, et al. Penicillin allergy skin testing: what do we do now? Pharmacotherapy 2007; 27: 542-5.
12. Matheu V, Pérez E, González R, et al. Assessment of a new brand of determinants for skin testing in a large group of patients with suspected beta-lactam allergy.J Investig Allergol Clin Immunol. 2007; 17: 257-60.
13. Romano A, Viola M, Bousquet PJ, et al. comparison of the performance of two penicillin reagent kits in the diagnosis of beta-lactam hypersensitivity.Allergy 2007; 62: 53-8.
14. Rodríguez-Bada JL, Montañez MI, Torres MJ, et al. Skin testing for immediate hypersensitivity to betalactams: comparison between two commercial kits. Allergy 2006; 61: 947-51.

15. Treudler R, Simon JC. PPL and MDM skin test: new test kit is helpful in detecting immediate-type allergy to beta-lactams. J Dtsch Dermatol Ges 2007; 5: 286-92.
16. Solensky R, Earl HS, Gruchalla RS.Penicillin allergy: prevalence of vague history in skin test-positive patients. Ann Allergy Asthma Immunol 2000; 85: 195-9.
17. Park MA, Li JT. Diagnosis and management of penicillin allergy. Mayo Clin Proc 2005; 80: 405-10.
18. Sogn DD, Evans R, Shepherd GM, et al. Results of the National Institute of Allergy and Infectious Diseases Collaborative Clinical Trial to test the predictive value of skin testing with major and minor penicillin derivatives in hospitalized adults.Arch Intern Med 1992; 152: 1025-32.
19. Green GR, Rosenblum AH, Sweet LC.Evaluation of penicillin hypersensitivity: value of clinical history and skin testing with penicilloyl-polylysine and penicillin G. A cooperative prospective study of the penicillin study group of the American Academy of Allergy. J Allergy Clin Immunol 1977; 60: 339-45.
20. Sanchez MR. Syphilis. In: Freedberg IM, Eisen AZ, Wolff K, et al, eds. Dermatology in general medicine. 5th edn. New York: McGraw-Hill; 1999. p. 2551-2581.
21. Macy E, Mellan MH, Schatz M, et al. Drug allergy. In Adelman DC, Casale TB, Correu J, eds. Manual of allergy and immunology. 4th edn. Philedelphia: Lippincott Williams & Wilkins; 2002. p. 219-241.

18 ENDEMIC TREPONEMATOSES

Yogesh S Marfatia, Archana Sharma

In this chapter

- History
- Global Epidemiology
- Yaws
- Endemic Syphilis
- Pinta
- HIV and Endemic Treponematoses
- Diagnosis of Endemic Treponematoses
- Histopathology of Endemic Treponematoses
- Treatment
- Control

INTRODUCTION

Endemic treponematoses includes non-venereally transmitted treponemal infections namely yaws, endemic syphilis and pinta. These diseases are of great public health significance because of their easy communicability and crippling, invalidating and disfiguring sequelae. It is said that syphilis goes with civilization, while endemic treponematoses start where highway ends and overcrowding as well as poor socio-economic conditions prevail. It is postulated that all treponematoses are merely variants of a single disease, the expression of which has been modified by environmental factors, especially temperature.[1]

All these conditions are caused by subspecies of *Treponema pallidum* and hence show remarkable similarities in morphology and antigenic make up of causative organisms, as well as in immune response pattern in terms of serology by non-specific and specific tests. Differences have been demonstrated in the *tp*15, *gpd* and *tp*92 genes. A difference in the flanking region of a lipoprotein gene has been reported, and this 'genetic signature' can differentiate several subspecies.[2] The general pattern of clinical stages of various treponemal diseases is remarkably similar and characterized by initial primary lesions followed by more extensive secondary manifestations, and they all exhibit the phenomenon of latency.[3,4] The epidemiology and clinical features of various treponematoses are summarised in Table 18.1 and 18.2.

HISTORY

It has been postulated that *T. pallidum* originally arose from free-living treponemes in mud; *T. zulezerae* still remains as a representative of this form. These organisms ultimately evolved into human saprophytes. Diseases then developed as natural selection ensured the optimal survival of more virulent organisms.[5]

Treponematoses are the diseases of antiquity, and bones discovered in a cemetery of an ancient Greek colony in Southern Italy contain unequivocal evidence of the presence of syphilis or yaws in an era well before Columbus. Bone lesions with probable yaws have been traced down to AD 854 on the Mariana Islands in the West Pacific.[6]

GLOBAL EPIDEMIOLOGY

In early 1950s, there were estimated 50-150 million of cases, and hence WHO in collaboration with UNICEF launched Global Endemic Treponematoses Control Programme in the period 1952-1964. More than 50 million cases were treated with long-acting penicillin in 46 countries, reducing the overall disease prevalence by more than 95%. The control strategy subsequently was changed from a vertical programme to one that was integrated into basic health services. By the end of 1970s, resurgence of endemic treponematoses had occurred in many areas.[3]

According to an estimation in 1996, the population at risk is estimated at 34 millions i.e. 5% of the total world population (mainly infants, children and to a lesser extent, adolescents and young adults). They all live in the developing countries, with 21 million living in the so-called least developed countries. The regions most affected are Africa and South East Asia, with some foci in Central and South America, the Middle East and the Pacific Islands. The total number of cases estimated globally is 2.5 million and infectious cases 460,000, of which there are 400,000 cases in Africa. The number of disabled persons due to endemic treponematoses is estimated at 260,000 globally.[3]

Problem in India

A survey (1985) suggests that yaws continues to occur in India, although at a low level, in at least 3 states, viz. Andhra Pradesh, Chhattisgarh and Orissa; a total of 1349 yaws cases were diagnosed in these three states between 1983 and mid 1985. Whereas, in Andhra Pradesh yaws occurred exclusively among tribal population, in Orissa and Chhattisgarh both tribal and non-tribal populations were affected. The problem of yaws now is one of either "residual yaws" or "recrudescence" of yaws due to continued low levels of transmission in some areas.[7]

Table 18.1 Comparison of Epidemiologic Features of Treponematoses

Features	Yaws	Endemic Syphilis	Pinta	Venereal Syphilis
Organism	*T. pallidum* ssp. *pertenue*	*T. pallidum* ssp. *endemicum*	*T. pallidum* ssp. *carateum*	*T. pallidum* ssp. *pallidum*
Geographical distribution	Africa, Asia, South and Central America, Pacific Islands	North Africa, South East Asia, Arabian Peninsula	South and Central America, Mexico	Worldwide, more in developing countries
Climate	Humid, warm	Arid, warm	Semi-arid, warm	–
Age group	< 15 years (Early childhood)	< 15 years (Early childhood)	Late childhood	Adulthood
Mode of transmission	Skin to skin	Household contacts, mouth to mouth or via shared drinking/ eating utensils, insect vector?	Skin to skin	Sexual, transplacental

Table 18.2 Comparison of Clinical Features of Various Treponematoses

Features	Yaws	Endemic Syphilis	Pinta	Venereal Syphilis
Primary lesions	Ulcerating and vegetating papular lesions with satellites	Eroded papules (Rarely seen)	Non-ulcerating papules with psoriasiform plaques	Cutaneous ulcer (chancre)
Location	Extremities	Oral	Extremities, face	Genital, oral, anal
Secondary lesions	Papulosquamous lesions, warty nodules and palmoplantar 'crab yaws'	Florid mucocutaneous lesions (mucous patch, split papule, Condylomata lata)	Pintides (erythematous, psoriasiform scaly plaques), pigmentary changes	Mucocutaneous lesions, Condylomata lata
Tertiary lesions	Gummas, pintoid dyschromia, juxta-articular nodes, gangosa, goundou, keratoderma	Serpiginous gummas, juxta-articular nodes and on elbows only	Dyschormic hypochromic, achromic polychromatic patches	Granulomatous nodules, psoriasiform granulomatous plaques, gumma
Osseous	Yes	Yes	No	Yes
Cardiovascular	No	No	No	Yes
CNS manifestations	No	No	No	Yes
Congenital	No	No	No	Yes

(*Contd.*)

Infectious relapses	Common	Unknown	None	~ 25%
Positive serum tests for syphilis	Yes	Yes	Yes	Yes
Response to penicillin	Excellent	Excellent	Excellent	Excellent

YAWS

Nomenclature: *framboesia* (German and Dutch), *pian* (French), *parangi* (Sinhalese), *buba* (Spanish), *bouba* (Portugese)

Distribution: Exclusively found in the humid regions between the tropics of cancer and capricon, central and northern part of South America, the Caribbean, Africa, and South East Asia.

Epidemiology

The causative organism is *'Treponema pallidum* ssp. *pertenue'* discovered by Castellani in 1905. It is commonly found in early childhood, 2-10 years of age, incidence being more in males than females. It is a disease particularly of warm climates and rural environments. Transmission is among children or family members from moist early lesions by skin-to-skin contact. The entry is facilitated by excoriations, abrasions and bites. Thus, most primary lesions occur over exposed parts on legs, arms, buttocks or face.[5]

Indirect transmission by flies, *Hippelates pallipes,* has been suggested.

Clinical Features

The incubation period varies from 3 to 6 weeks.

Primary Stage

The initial lesion is known by a variety of names such as primary or 'mother yaw', *framboesia, pianoma, bubamadre,* and *mannanpian.* The 'mother yaw' begins as an erythematous infiltrated papule, which enlarges by extension at the periphery or by confluence with satellite nodules. Progressive growth gives rise to a large, raised, rounded or oval ulcer, papillomatous or vegetative, bearing some resemblance to a raspberry. The lesions then ulcerate and are covered by yellowish crust formed by exudates. The lesions are symptomless, highly infectious and vary in size from 1 to 5 cm. It may be accompanied by fever, joint pain or regional lymphadenopathy. It heals spontaneously after 3-6 months leaving atrophic and depressed scar with hypopigmented center sometimes surrounded by dark halo. 'Decapitated yaws' i.e. mother yaws is absent and the disease passes directly to its secondary stage in 10% of cases.[6]

Secondary Stage

The secondary stage starts few weeks after the appearance of mother yaw and is characterized by:

Cutaneous lesions: It resembles the mother yaws or tends to be smaller and widespread and is called 'daughter yaws' or "pianomas". The lesions are frequently located adjacent to body orifices and tend to expand, ulcerate and exudate fluid rich in treponema. The xudates attract flies. Occasionally peripheral extensions or coalescence of several lesions result in circinate and annular lesions, resembling tinea. These are referred to as 'tinea yaw' or 'circinate yaws'.[4] Condylomatous lesions in the axillae and groins are also seen.

Palmoplantar lesions: On palmoplantar surfaces, the lesions form thick hyperkeratotic plaques which crack and fissure (worm eaten sole), producing painful crab like gait (*Crab yaws*). Palmoplantar hyperkeratotic papules or macules mimicking secondary syphilis are not uncommon.

Papillomas arising in the nail fold cause a paronychia called 'pianic onychia'.

Bone and Joint lesions: Early bone lesions consist of painful periosteitis, polydactylitis and fusiform swelling of metatarsals and metacarpals.

Infectious secondary lesions reoccur during ensuing 5 years and lesions tend to be localized to axillae, perianal and circumoral areas. The disease then enters a non-infectious latent period.

Tertiary Stage (Late yaws)

Approximately 10% of the cases develop late yaws several years after the primary infection. This stage is characterized by destructive and ulcerated cutaneous lesions, palmoplantar keratoderma, lesions of the joint, bone, gangosa and gondou.

Cutaneous lesions: Keratoderma and hyperkeratosis of palms and soles are frequently seen in late yaws. There is formation of subcutaneous nodules, which undergoes abscess formation, central necrosis and ulceration. Ulcers may become secondarily infected, resulting in destruction of underlying deep structures. On healing, it may result into significant scarring, keloid formations, and contractures. There is a potential risk of development of squamous cell carcinoma in the ulcerative lesions of late yaws.

Painless minute craters surrounded by hyperkeratotic papules similar to keratoderma punctatum may be observed in late yaws known as "hormiguillo".

Bone and Joint lesions: Osseous lesions consist of hypertrophic periosteitis (pianic osteoperiosteitis), gummatous periosteitis, osteitis and osteomyelitis. Chronic osteitis of long bones, such as tibia can lead to curvature of the bone, producing sabre shins. '*Gondou*' is the exostoses of the nasal bones and neighbouring osseous structures, producing oval thickened bony masses on either side of the nasal bridge. '*Gangosa*' (deforming rhinopharyngitis) is mutilation of the central part of face. It includes destruction of the mucosa, cartilagenous and osseous structures of nasal septum, palate and posterior aspect of pharynx.

Neurologic and Ophthalmic manifestations: Although it is believed that yaws spares the nervous system and eyes, isolated cases of idiopathic optic atrophy and myeloneuropathies have been reported.

Attenuated Yaws

This is the mild form of the disease found in areas with low disease prevalence. It is characterized by a solitary or few lesions generally confined to skin folds. The lesions are dry and patients are less contagious. There is great potential for missing these cases during surveillance.[4]

Differential Diagnosis

Yaws must be differentiated from venereal syphilis clinically as no serological test can distinguish between the two. The skin lesions of yaws can be confused with eczema, psoriasis, keratoderma, calluses, verruca, bites and vitamin deficiencies. Leprosy, leishmaniasis, tropical ulcer, ecthyma, and deep mycoses can also resemble yaws. Bone lesions can be identical to those of venereal syphilis, endemic syphilis, tuberculosis and osteomyelitis. Nasopharyngeal lesions mimic mucocutaneous leishmaniasis, rhinosporidiosis, rhinosclerosis, leprosy and tuberculosis.

ENDEMIC SYPHILIS

Nomenclature: *Syphilis insontium*, *bejel* (Middle East), *njovera* (Zimbabwe), *siti*, *dichuchwa* (Botswana), *skeljevo*, *bishel or belesh* (Saudi Arabia), *firjal*, *loath*.

Distribution: Endemic syphilis is prevalent in dry, arid climates. It occurs among primitive population, in the areas bordering deserts like in Middle East, Northern Nigeria, Southern Morocco, Botswana, Zimbabwe and Nothern Australia.

Epidemiology

The causative organism is '*Treponema pallidum* ssp. *endemicum*'. The infection is prevalent in children between 2 and 15 years of age and has no sex predilection. The infection is transmitted from child to child by close skin contact, kissing, and fomites such as communal drinking vessels. Direct lesion-to-skin contact among children and contact with saliva are additional modes of transmission. Occasionally, a previously uninfected nursing mother will have a primary lesion on or near the nipple from her infected infant. Unlike venereal syphilis, congenital transmission is rare and mother does not have immunity against treponema. This represents reverse of Colle's law.[8]

Very few cases of venereal syphilis are seen in hyperendemic areas of endemic syphilis due to immunity in young adults with latent infection of *Treponema pallidum* endemicum. The venereal syphilis slowly emerges as the endemic disease overcomes and in this period of transition, mixed (endemic and venereal) disease will be found with considerable number of endemic syphilis cases in older group.[8]

Clinical Features

Primary Stage

Incubation period is 3 weeks. This stage is characterized by rare occurrence of small papules, ulcers on oropharyngeal mucosa and skin.

Secondary Stage

After 3 months, disease enters the secondary stage. The initial lesions occur as mucous patches, which are shallow, painless ulcers over the lips, tongue, tonsils, fauces and buccal mucosa. These are accompanied by regional lymphadenopathy. Split papules and condylomata lata over axillary and anogenital regions are other important secondary lesions. Non-pruritic papular eruptions and papulosquamous eruptions are also reported. Osteoperiosteitis of long bones occurs and causes nocturnal leg pain. Untreated secondary lesions last for 6-9 months.

Tertiary Stage

Gummata of nasopharynx, larynx, skin and bone develop 6 months to several years after inoculation and may progress to destructive chronic ulcers. In time they resolve, leaving characteristic atrophic, depigmented scars, surrounded by hyperpigmentation. Gross mutilation with loss of skin, mucous membrane, muscle, cartilage and bone with destructive lesions of palate and nasal septum are disfiguring features (saddle nose deformity, palate perforation, or gangosa) of untreated disease. There is no reported evidence of neurological or cardiac involvement, however, ophthalmologic manifestations like uveitis, choroiditis, chorioretinitis and optic atrophy are encountered.

Attenuated Endemic Syphilis

In attenuated endemic syphilis, the number, severity and duration of both early and late lesions are reduced and majority of seropositive persons have latent disease. Improvement in the hygiene and wide availability of antibiotics are the most accepted reasons for attenuated disease.[9] The most frequent finding in it is paining legs caused by osteoperiosteitis.

Differential Diagnosis

The most important and difficult disease to differentiate from endemic syphilis is venereal syphilis. Oral lesions must be differentiated from venereal syphilis, aphthosis, vitamin deficiencies and herpes. Mutilating nasopharyngeal endemic syphilis can be confused with tuberculosis, leprosy, rhinoscleroma, and rhinosporidiosis.

PINTA

Pinta (Mexico) which means spot or mark in Spanish, comes from the verb pintar 'to paint'.

Nomenclature: *Carate, cute* (Venezuela and Columbia), *mal del pinto, puru-pur, morados* and *azul* meaning 'the bluish ones'.

Distribution: It is found in remote areas of Mexico, Central and Northern South Americas and certain Islands of Caribbean.

Epidemiology

Pinta, caused by *Treponema pallidum* ssp. *carateum*, is unique in having only skin manifestations and affects persons of all ages. Majority of the cases occur in children younger than 15 years, and young adults are the main reservoir of infections. Mode of transmission is by repeated lesion to skin contact. Patients with late pinta are resistant to syphilis, but those with yaws and syphilis at any stage are susceptible to pinta.

Clinical Features

As in syphilis, there are three distinct clinical stages, but in contrast to syphilis, lesions from different stages may be present in a single patient.

Primary Stage

After an incubation period of 6 days to 4 months, with a mean of 8-10 days, minute papules or erythematous macules appear over the lower extremities and other exposed areas. The lesions grow by extending to periphery or fusioning with satellite lesions, forming ill-defined erythematous infiltrated plaque. Infection is confined to skin with the exception of occasional juxta-articular nodes.

Secondary Stage

The secondary lesions, '*pintides*' (three varieties-hypochromic, pigmentary and erythematosquamous) appear as small, scaly papules that gradually enlarge and coalesce, forming psoriasiform plaques. Initially they are red to violaceous and later become slate blue, brown gray or black. Several colours may exist within the same lesion. Primary and secondary stage lesions are highly infectious.

Tertiary Stage

Symmetric achromic lesions develop over body prominences, wrists, elbows, and ankles from 3 months to 10 years after the appearance of pintides, creating a mottled appearance. This spotted appearance is highly characteristic. Cutaneous atrophy, hyperkeratosis and pigmentation may also be present. Generalized lymphadenopathy is also seen. Cardiovascular and central nervous systems are not involved, and attenuated form of pinta has not been described.

Course and Prognosis

The disease runs a progressive course, with increasingly widespread involvement of the skin. Visceral complications of any type are not recorded. This disease is confined exclusively to the skin and even lesions of the nail apparatus are infrequent.

Differential Diagnosis

Early pinta may be difficult to distinguish from the other treponematoses, venereal syphilis, yaws and endemic syphilis. Eczema, pityriasis alba, psoriasis, leprosy, lupus erythematosus, pellagra, tinea corporis, and tinea versicolor can also mimic early pinta. The leukoderma of late pinta closely resembles vitiligo.

HIV AND ENDEMIC TREPONEMATOSES

The immunodeficiency due to HIV infection might lead to reactivation of latent treponemal infections. HIV infected persons are more likely to carry large number of treponemes and might disseminate pathogenic treponemes more effectively than HIV-negative persons.[4]

DIAGNOSIS OF ENDEMIC TREPONEMATOSES

In the past, clinical diagnosis was accepted in areas of high endemicity. After mass treatment campaigns, the clinical manifestations have changed and atypical attenuated disease is more commonly seen. Serologic tests for yaws, endemic syphilis and pinta are similar to those of venereal syphilis. The RPR, VDRL, FTA-ABS, TPI and TPHA have all been used. No serologic test can distinguish yaws, endemic syphilis, pinta and venereal syphilis. Dark field microscopic examination of lymph from primary, secondary or tertiary lesions of pinta as well as histopathological and radiological studies can aid in diagnosis and evaluation but are neither economical nor convenient. Eosinophilia has been described as a frequent feature of pinta.

HISTOPATHOLOGY OF ENDEMIC TREPONEMATOSES

Endemic syphilis does not show significant differences from that found in venereal syphilis.

In yaws, early lesion shows acanthosis and papillomatosis. There is neutrophilic exocytosis, giving rise to intraepidermal microabscesses. The dermis is infiltrated mainly by plasma cells, but other cells like neutrophils, eosinophils, lymphocytes and histiocytes may also be present. Blood vessels are affected usually only mildly in yaws, in contrast to syphilis.[10]

The early lesion in pinta is characterized by acanthosis, exocytosis of lymphocytes, loss of melanin and liquefaction degeneration in the basal layer. The dermis shows a mixed infiltrate of plasma cells, lymphocytes, histiocytes and neutrophils. Melanophages are seen in the upper dermis.[10]

TREATMENT

Penicillin was established as an effective treatment of treponematoses in the 1940s. The mass treatment campaigns of the 1950s and 1960s used procaine penicillin in 2% aluminium monostearate. Active infections in adults as well as non-infectious cases should be given Benzathine penicillin 2.4 MU intramuscularly in a single injection. The WHO recommends treating all cases and contacts over 10 years of age with 1.2 million units of benzathine penicillin in single intramuscular injection and 0.6 million units in children younger than 10 years old. Once injected, penicillin begins to destroy the treponemes within minutes and the lesions become non-infectious within 18-24 hours. Alternative drugs used in patients allergic to penicillin include tetracyclines or erythromycin 500 mg PO four times daily or chloramphenicol for a minimum of 5 days. In children, oral erythromycin in a dose of 8 to 10 mg/kg four times a day for 15 days is the alternative regimen.

When the prevalence of cases with active lesions is above 10% of the population examined, penicillin should be given to whole community, if between 5-10% it should be administered to patients, contacts and children of less than 5 years of age and if prevalence is less than 5% only active cases and their contacts should be treated.[6]

CONTROL

In contrast to smallpox, it is highly unlikely that endemic treponematoses will ever be eradicated, and that a treponemal vaccine may be developed in foreseeable future. In the former disorder, those afflicted develop life long immunity, remain contagious for brief periods and are usually symptomatic. However, victims of endemic treponematoses do not develop life long immunity, remain contagious for protracted periods of time and may harbour subclinical or mild disease. In mass treatment campaigns of 1950s and 1960s, though the diseases were controlled, subsequently, many countries failed to integrate continued active control measures into local health services. This led to gradual rebuilding and extension of treponemal reservoirs. For halting the transmission of the diseases, the mass treatment approach must be followed by periodic screening surveys of children and others at risk and by long-term sero-surveillance.[4]

The future may bring the emergence of plasmid-mediated antibiotic resistance among the non-venereal treponematoses. These diseases are not perceived as high priority because they are not fatal and are largely restricted to remote, poor and rural populations.

The enigma whether these organisms are truly different organisms or demonstrating various clinical expressions caused by divergent environmental conditions may be settled by newer molecular techniques.

REFERENCES

1. Sheila A. Lukehart. Endemic Treponematoses, In: Fauci AS, Braunwald E, Kasper DL, et al, Ed. Harrison's Principles of Internal Medicine, 15th edition, New York: McGraw Hill; 2001: 1053-5.
2. Antal GM, Lukehart SA, Meheus AZ. The endemic treponematoses. Microbes Infect 2002; 4: 83-94.
3. Meheus A, Tikhomirov E. Endemic Treponematoses. In: Holmes KK, Mardh PA, Sparling SF, et al. eds. Sexually Transmitted Diseases. 3rd edition. New York: McGraw Hill; 1999: 511-13.
4. Koff AB, Rosen T. Non-venereal treponematoses: Yaws, endemic syphilis and pinta. J Am Acad Dermatol 1993; 29: 519-35.
5. King A, Nicol C, Rodin P, eds. Yaws; Endemic syphilis; Bejel; Pinta. In: Venereal Diseases, 4th edition, London: Balliere Tindall; 1980: 333-45.
6. Morton RS, Kinghorn GR, Kerdel-Vegas F. The treponematoses. In: Tony Burns, Stephen Breathnach, Neil Cox, Christopher Griffiths, eds. Rook's Textbook of Dermatology. 7th edition. London: Blackwell; 2004: 30.1-30.36.
7. Park K, eds. Epidemiology of communicable diseases- Endemic Treponematosis. In: Park's textbook of preventive and social medicine. 18th edition. India: Banarsidas Bhanot; 2005: 269-71.
8. Willcox RR, Willcox JR. Venereological Medicine. Oxford: Oxford University Press; 1992: 151-60.
9. Castro LG. Nonvenereal treponematoses. J Am Acad Dermatol 1994; 31: 1075-6.
10. Balachandran C, Pai S. Endemic Treponematoses. In: Kumar B, Gupta S eds. Sexually Transmitted Infections. 1st edition. New Delhi: Elsevier; 2005: 312-7.

19 | CHANCROID

C Balachandran, Sathish Pai B

In this chapter

INTRODUCTION

Ulceration of the genitalia is a common presentation of sexually transmitted diseases (STDs). In developing countries, especially India and Africa, genital ulcers due to chancroid and granuloma inguinale are more common, whereas in developed countries most of the cases are due to genital herpes, or syphilis.[1]

Chancroid is also called as soft sore, soft chancre and ulcus molle. It is an acute infectious disease caused by a gram negative bacillus, *Haemophilus ducreyi* and is clinically characterized by one or more genital ulcers with inguinal lymphadenitis. It is referred to as a soft sore, because the lesions are usually not indurated. In contrast, a syphilitic chancre is non-tender and indurated.

HISTORY

Chancroid was first described as a separate disease from syphilis in 1838 by Ricord. In 1889, Ducreyi isolated the organism and described it as a short, compact streptobacillus[2]. The intradermal test for *H. ducreyi* was reported by Ito in 1913[3] and the work was confirmed by Reenstierna in 1923.[4]

INCIDENCE

Although chancroid is not a problem in industrialized nations[5], it is endemic in many developing countries.[6] In Kenya, Zambia and Zimbabwe chancroid is considered to be the most common cause of genital ulceration.[7] The disease is more prevalent in communities with low hygienic standards. Uncircumcised men are more susceptible to infection with *H. ducreyi*[8]. The male to female ratio ranges from 3:1 to 53:1.[7] The disease is transmitted from person to person mainly through heterosexual contact, and is usually acquired from prostitutes. Patients from lower socioeconomic groups, commercial sex workers, uncircumcised men are at higher risk for acquiring disease.[9] Over and Piot[10] estimated that the probability of transmitting chancroid from an infected male to an uninfected female during a single sexual exposure was 0.35, whereas the probability of transmitting chancroid from an infected female to an uninfected male during a single sexual exposure was 0.30. The duration of infectivity was estimated to be 45 days.[10]

Incidence of chancroid seems to be higher in males, which may be attributed to the facts like easy visibility on male external genitalia, asymptomatic vaginal or cervical ulcers in females, less common occurrence of lymphadenitis and bubo formation in females, and common spontaneous healing of lesions in females.[11]

CAUSATIVE ORGANISM

The causative organism of chancroid is the gram negative, facultative anaerobic bacillus *H. ducreyi*. It was originally classified as a Haemophilus species because of its growth requirements, biochemical properties, and antigenic relatedness to other species in the group[12]. However, by rRNA analysis and also by the fact that it differs from other true haemophili by the lack of requirement for nicotinamide adenine dinucleotide (NAD, V factor); its failure to produce H_2S, catalase or indole; and its production of alkaline phosphatase, it is now considered that[13] *H. ducreyi* is only remotely related to true *haemophili* such as *Haemophilus influenzae* and is now classified in the Actinobacillus cluster of the Pasteurellaceae.[14,15] Gram stain shows groups of organisms, which are often arranged in chains of two's or four's, giving the typical appearance of a "school of fish" or "rail road track". *H. ducreyi* is a strict human pathogen and naturally infects genital and nongenital skin, mucosal surfaces, and regional lymph nodes.[16] The organism can be easily demonstrated in the pus aspirated from an inguinal abscess, whereas open lesions on the genitalia may not reveal any *H. ducreyi* because of secondary bacterial infection.

Although several potential virulence factors have been identified in *H. ducreyi*, at present their roles in pathogenesis are poorly understood. All strains appear to have fine, tangled, surface fimbriae, 40 KDa and 18 KDa outer membrane proteins, lipooligosaccharide and a cytotoxin/haemolysin.[16] It is a fastidious organism and hence culturing is difficult. *H. ducreyi* also has a specific growth requirement for hemin (X factor). Both cell and humoral immunities occur in response to infection with *H. ducreyi*.

PATHOGENESIS

The organism is inoculated into the tissues, possibly through a minor abrasion or trauma, which occurs during the sexual intercourse. Once in the tissue, it induces secretion of interleukin 6 (IL-6) and interleukin 8 (IL-8). IL-8 induces polymorphonuclear neutrophils (PMNs) and macrophages to form intradermal pustules. IL-6 stimulates T cell IL-2 receptor expression, which in turn stimulates CD4 in the region.[17] The immune response to *H. ducreyi* has many features of a type 1 response, which usually facilitates phagocytosis, antibody responses, and bacterial clearance for extracellular bacterial pathogens. The antigen-specific $CD4^+$ cells recruited to the skin may eventually provide help for the development of antibody responses that usually occur late in the ulcerative stage of disease.[18] *H. ducreyi* preferentially infects mucosal epithelium and also infects keratinized sratified squamous epithelium. In the tissue, the organism is usually present within macrophages, neutrophils, and also as clumps in the interstitium. The tripartite cytolethal distending toxin (CDT) produced by the organism is an important virulence factor, which causes cell damage and may be responsible in the formation of an ulcer.

Both virulent and avirulent strains of *H. duceryi* have been demonstrated in animal and human studies. Virulent strain shows greater capacity than the avirulent strain to attach to the epithelial cells. Avirulent organisms are more susceptible to antimicrobial agents. Recently, the genome of *H. ducreyi* strain that is virulent in humans, 3500 HP (HP refers to human passaged), has been sequenced.[18] The genome is composed of a single 1.7-Mb chromosome.

Human immunodeficiency virus transmission is increased in the presence of chancroid. The two main chemokine receptors that are essential for entry of HIV are CCR5 and CXCR4, which are increasingly expressed on the macrophages present in the lesions of chancroid. Upregulation of these receptors and disruption of mucosal and skin barriers provide an ideal environment for the acquisition of HIV infection.

CLINICAL FEATURES

Chancroid presents as a painful ulcerative disease of the genitalia. The incubation period is usually short and ranges from 1 to 14 days[19], with a median of 7 days between inoculation and appearance of the first skin lesion.[5]

Initially, a small inflammatory papule surrounded by erythema develops on the genitalia, which rapidly progresses to a pustule. Multiple often foul smelling ulcerations develop quickly. Vesicles are not seen at any stage of the disease[13] Classically, the ulcers are painful, sharply circumscribed with ragged undermined edges **(Fig. 19.1, 19.2, 19.3)**. Multiple ulcers are seen in 50% of cases.[11] The floor of the ulcer may be covered by a yellow necrotic purulent exudate and removal of the exudate may reveal unevenly distributed highly vascular granulated tissue, which may bleed on scraping or gentle manipulation. Characteristically, the base of the ulcer is non-indurated. Autoinoculation results in multiple sites of infection in various stages of evolution. Thus, a typical chancroid lesion is characterized by the triad of undermined ulcer edge, purulent dirty gray base, and moderate to severe pain.[11] All the three features are present in less than 50% of the sufferers.

The common sites of infection are the external or internal surface of the prepuce, the frenulum, the coronal sulcus and occasionally external urinary meatus and the shaft of the penis may be involved. Extragenital chancroids are rare.

In women, chancroid may have a more variable course than in men. Most females with ulcers are unaware of their infection and the presenting symptoms may include pain on urination or defaecation, vaginal discharge and dyspareunia. The common sites of involvement are the fourchette, vestibule, labia, clitoris, vagina and the perianal area **(Fig. 19.4)**. *H. ducreyi* has not been shown to cause systemic infection. However, extra genital lesions can occur and are thought to be the result of autoinoculation.[10] Extragenital lesions on the breasts, fingers, thighs and in the oral cavity have been described. Female genital ulcers have been reported to heal faster than their male counterparts.[20]

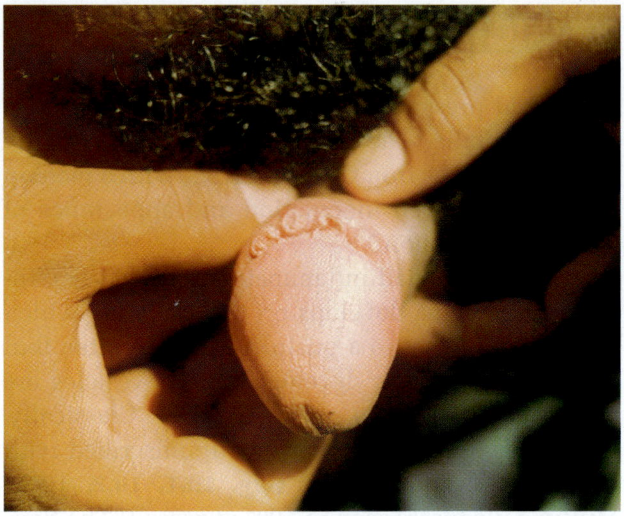

Fig. 19.1 Chancroid – Multiple Ulcers with Ragged Edge on the Coronal Sulcus.

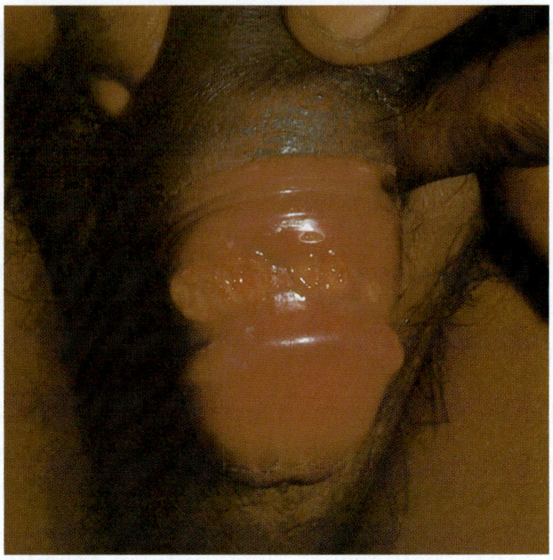

Fig. 19.2 Chancroid – Multiple necrotic Ulcers on the Undersurface of Prepuce.

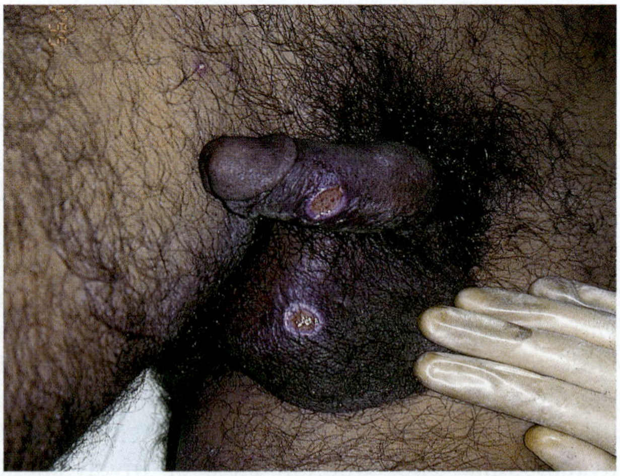

Fig. 19.3 Chancroid – Kissing Ulcers.

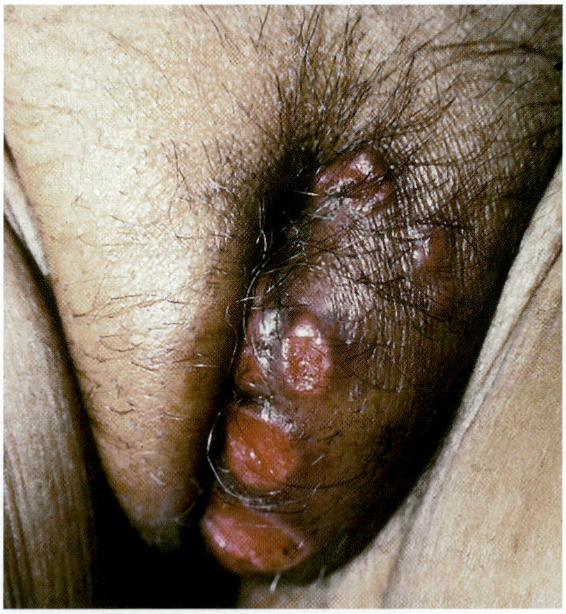

Fig. 19.4 Chancroid – Multiple Ulcers with Ragged Edge on the Labia Majora.

Clinical Variants[21]

1. Giant chancroid: a single lesion extends peripherally and shows extensive ulceration.
2. Large serpeginous ulcer: a lesion that becomes confluent, spreading by extension and autoinoculation.
3. Phagedenic chancroid: a variant caused by superinfection with fusospirochetes.
4. Transient chancroid: small ulcer that resolves spontaneously in a few days. It may be followed 2 to 3 weeks by regional lymphadenitis.
5. Follicular chancroid: multiple small ulcers in a follicular distribution.
6. Papular chancroid: a granulomatous ulcerated papule that might resemble donovanosis or condylomata lata.
7. Dwarf chancroid: lesions remain pustular and resemble pyogenic infection.
8. Pseudogranuloma inguinale is a variety of chancroid that closely resembles granuloma inguinale. **(Fig. 19.5)**[22,23] Clinically, the ulcers have the features of granuloma inguinale but on culturing *H. ducreyi* is grown.

Painful inguinal lymphadenitis develops in 30 to 60% of the patients within 1 to 2 weeks of the development of genital ulcers. This adenopathy is unilateral in most patients. The nodes become enlarged, tender and then matted together. If untreated, about 25% of patient's suppuration occurs with the formation of a unilocular abscess **(Fig. 19.6)** called as bubo.[24] The overlying skin is erythematous and shiny. The bubo if untreated, ruptures through the skin with the formation of a single sinus. The opening of the sinus may break down to form a chancroidal ulcer, which may then enlarge to form a giant ulcer. Most of the patients have genital ulcers along with the inguinal bubo. This clinical finding along with other features may help us to differentiate it from LGV bubo. Some patients may develop buboes during antibiotic therapy while the ulcers are healing.[25] Bubo pus is usually thick, creamy and viscous. In female patients, both lymphadenitis and bubo formation are less common. Scar formation, fibrosis and lymphedema may occur in affected patients.[25]

Other complications of chancroid include phimosis, paraphimosis, urethral fistula and phagedenic ulcerations. The phagedenic ulcers are due to superadded infection with Vincent's organisms, which causes widespread necrosis of the tissue, leading to the formation of large destructive ulcers.

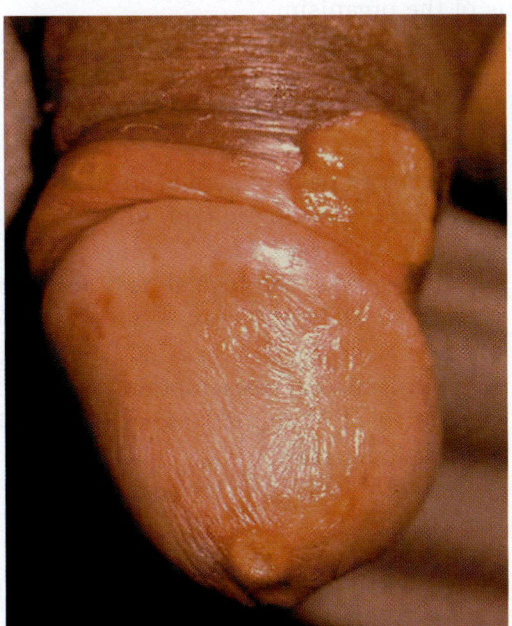

Fig. 19.5 Donovanosis-like Chancroid.

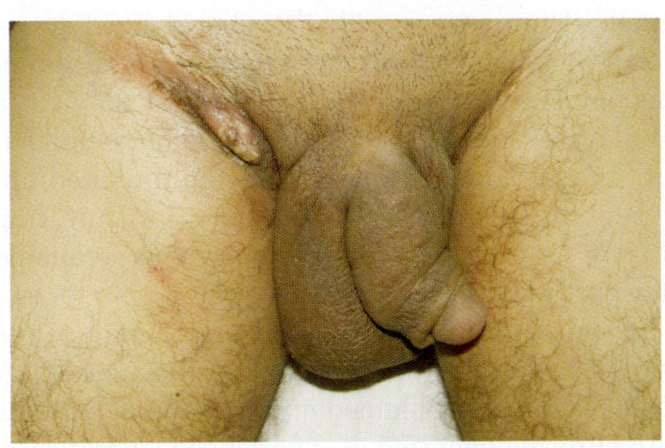

Fig. 19.6 Chancroid – Penile Oedema with Bubo.

DIAGNOSIS

Diagnosis of chancroid is basically made on clinical grounds, which has an accuracy rate of 30 to 50%.[26,27] Isolation of *H. ducreyi* from the genital ulcer or bubo is important in the diagnosis of chancroid.

Smears are taken with cotton swabs from beneath the undermined edges of ulcers and stained with Gram's or Wright's stain. Pleomorphic gram negative coccobacilli arranged in parallel chains of two's or four's described as "school of fish" may be demonstrated. The organisms are visualized extracellularly more often than intracellularly and tend to occur in close proximity to polymorphonuclear leukocytes. This finding may be suggestive of chancroid but lacks sensitivity and specificity for a definitive diagnosis.[28]

Ito-Reenstierna test is an intradermal test,wherein a cutaneous reaction is produced by intradermal injection of a vaccine containing killed *H. ducreyi* in a suspension. The test is said to be positive if an inflammatory papule of 0.5 to 1 cm diameter develops at the site after 48 hrs. This diagnostic test is now considered obsolete.

A definitive diagnosis of *H. ducreyi* infection requires growing of the organism in culture. *H ducreyi* is a fastidious organism. A special culture medium is required and the recovery rates have ranged from 0 to 80%. Selective artificial media used are gonococcal agar base with 2% bovine haemoglobin and 5% foetal calf serum and Mueller-Hinton agar with 5% chocolatized horse blood. Media are made selective by the addition of vancomycin. Cultures are incubated at 35°C in a candle jar. Patient's specimen must either be plated out directly on an appropriate culture medium or sent to microbiology laboratory for culturing as soon as possible. There is no widely available transport medium.

Small, non-mucoid, yellow-gray, semiopaque colonies appear 2 to 4 days after inoculation. A positive culture is obtained in about 80% of patients with clinical chancroid in experienced laboratories. Anaerobes like *B. melaninogenicus*, *B. fragilis* and anaerobic cocci were isolated more frequently from ulcers of chancroid associated with fluctuant bubo, suggesting that they may play a role in the development of a bubo.[29] Recent developments in the diagnosis are polymerase chain reaction (PCR)[30] and indirect immunofluorescence using monoclonal antibodies.[31] Recently, monoclonal antibody against haemoglobin receptor (HgbA) of outer membrane protein of *H.ducreyi* has shown a sensitivity of 100% and ability to detect 2×10^6 CFU, 8.5 ng of purified HgbA and holds promise of serodiagnosis of chancroid.[32] PCR is the most sensitive technique but is not commercially available. Multiplex test which combines PCR for *H. ducreyi*, *T pallidum* and HSV has been developed by Roche.[33] Indirect immunofluorescence (IF), using monoclonal antibodies (MAb) against lipo-oligosaccharide (LOS) of *H. ducreyi* was assessed by Ahmed et al. and is found to be superior to bacterial culture. It is a good method to be used in population with high chancroid prevalence.[11] DNA- DNA hybridisation techniques using labelled *H. ducreyi* derived probes have been developed but the usefulness of this method in clinical specimens has not been assessed widely.

Serological methods include enzyme immuno assays (EIA) using ultrasonicated whole cell antigen, purified LOS or OMP of *H. ducreyi* as antigen, DOT immunoblot, agglutination, and complement fixation test. A mass spectrometric method identifies *H. ducreyi* in short time (10 minutes). It is also helpful to detect the differed strains of the organism.

The Centres for Disease Control (CDC) proposes that a probable diagnosis of chancroid can be made if following are present:[32]

1. One or more painful genital ulcers.
2. Dark field examination of ulcer exudate is negative for *T. pallidum*.
3. A non-reactive serological test for syphilis performed at least 7 days after the onset of ulcers.
4. A typical clinical presentation with findings suggestive of chancroid along with regional lymphadenopathy.
5. A negative test for herpes simplex virus (HSV).

To summarise, till date, culture using specialized media is the most practiced method for diagnosis of infection with *H. ducreyi*. It has the added advantage that antimicrobial sensitivity of the organism can be tested at the same time. PCR is a superior method than other available means of diagnosis. Serology has limited usefulness in routine diagnosis of *H. ducreyi* infection, but it is helpful in epidemiological studies as a screening method for past infection.[34]

DIFFERENTIAL DIAGNOSIS

The differential diagnosis includes genital herpes especially in immunocompromised patients, primary chancre, granuloma inguinale, chancroidal ulcers and traumatic lesions with secondary bacterial infection. In about 10% of patients with chancroid there can be associated primary chancre or genital herpes. In chancroid, the ulcers are undermined, invariably tender and are deeper than herpetic ulcers. The ulcer is indurated and non tender in primary chancre. Co-infection with *T. pallidum* or HSV has been demonstrated in approximately 10% of patients with chancroid, which requires careful evaluation.

HISTOPATHOLOGY OF CHANCROID

Tissue biopsy is not a recommended diagnostic method for chancroid but may be useful as a means to exclude malignancy in nonhealing or atypical ulcers. Histopathology of the ulcer shows three distinctive zones, which is helpful in a presumptive diagnosis of chancroid in many instances. The zone at the top is narrow and consists of neutrophils, fibrin, erythrocytes and necrotic tissue. The middle zone is wide and is made up of newly formed blood vessels with marked endothelial cell proliferation. The lower zone contains a dense infiltrate of plasma cells and lymphoid cells. Biopsy samples seldom show *H ducreyi*.

MANAGEMENT

A painful ulceration associated with tender inguinal lymphadenopathy is suggestive of chancroid, whereas the development of associated suppurative adenopathy is almost pathognomonic.[35] Successful treatment cures infection, resolves clinical symptoms, and prevents further transmission of the disease to others.

General Advice

1. Patients should be advised to avoid unprotected sexual intercourse until they and their partners have completed treatment and follow-up.
2. Condoms, when correctly used, will prevent transmission in most cases.
3. Local hygiene with saline cleaning.

The CDC (2006) recommends the following regimens

a. Azithromycin 1 gm orally in a single dose

or

b. Ceftriaxone 250 mg intramuscularly in a single dose

or

c. Ciprofloxacin 500 mg orally two times a day for 3 days.

or

d. Erythromycin base 500 mg orally three times a day for 7 days.

Earlier a combination of trimethoprim-sulfamethoxazole (TMP-SMZ) was used widely in the treatment of chancroid. But because of the development of resistance to this drug, it is no longer recommended.[36,37]

β lactam antibiotics are effective against *H.ducreyi*[7]; however plasmid mediated β lactam resistance to *H ducreyi* has been described.[38] Many studies have demonstrated that *H. ducreyi* are capable of producing β lactamase.[7,39] So β lactamase resistant or inhibiting antibiotics are recommended in the treatment of chancroid e.g., ceftriaxone.

Quinolones have shown significant activity against *H. ducreyi* in vitro.[40] A cure rate of 95-100% has been demonstrated with ciprofloxacin.[40,41] Cordero in 1961 first used the macrolide antibiotic, erythromycin in the treatment of chancroid.[42]

Erythromycin and rosaramicin (another macrolide antibiotic) have been found to be effective in the treatment of culture proved *H. ducreyi* infections.[43,44] Macrolide antibiotics are inexpensive, well tolerated and widely available. Compliance can be a problem with erythromycin as it requires multiple daily doses for 1 to 2 weeks. Recently, thiamphenicol 5.0 g orally as a single dose was evaluated in a study of 1128 cases in Brazil, the treatment was successful in 99% cases.[45]

In centers where diagnostic facilities are not available the world health organization and NACO advocates the use of a syndromic approach for the therapy of genital ulcer disease (Appendix V). Men and women who present with genital ulcers are treated for syphilis and chancroid or genital herpes.

Management of Buboes

Fluctuant buboes should be aspirated using a wide bore needle from the non dependent part and adjacent healthy skin. Multiple aspirations were required prior to the advent of antimicrobial agents. With adequate antimicrobial treatment, a single aspiration is usually sufficient even in patients with large buboes.[13]

The antimicrobial agents have effect on genital ulcer as well as the inguinal bubo. In the presence of a bubo, the antimicrobial agents may have to be continued for a longer period till the bubo heals. Patients with inguinal lymphadenitis without suppuration usually respond without developing a bubo. Buboes less than 5 cm in diameter tend[20] to resolve along with the healing of genital ulcer whereas buboes more than 5 cm resolve slowly and healing does not correspond to the resolution of genital ulcers.[20]

A randomised study has shown that careful incision and drainage is an effective and safe method for treating fluctuant buboes and avoids frequent needle re-aspiration.[46]

Treatment for Pregnant or Lactating Mothers and Children

Antimicrobial agents like erythromycin and ceftriaxone can be used during this period. Ciprofloxacin is contraindicated during pregnancy, lactation, children and in adolescents less than 18 years of age. The safety of azithromycin during pregnancy and lactation has not been established.

HIV Infection and Chancroid

There is a complex interaction between STDs and the human immunodeficiency virus (HIV). On one hand, the natural history of STDs is altered by concurrent HIV infection and on the other, the transmission and course of HIV is modified. During the last decade enough evidence has been gathered to say that there is an increased risk of transmission of HIV in patients co-infected with an STDs.

Ulcerative STDs such as chancroid, primary syphilis and herpes simplex are all associated with an increased relative risk of infection. HIV sero conversion occurred more frequently in heterosexual men with genital ulcer disease (GUD) than in men without GUD.

Effect of HIV on Chancroid

- Healing of the ulcer is delayed in HIV infected persons.
- HIV infected men tend to have a greater number of ulcers than those who are not infected with HIV.
- Treatment failures are more common.
- Alteration of clinical picture. Extensive necrotising ulcers and multiple or multilocular buboes have been reported.

FOLLOW-UP

After initiating the treatment, patients should be reviewed at day 3 and day 7. Genital ulcers are likely to improve symptomatically within 3 days and significant re-epithelialisation occurs within 7 days. If there is no response to treatment suspect coinfections with *T pallidum* or HSV resistance.

REFERENCES

1. Rosen T, Brown TJ. Genital ulcers evaluation and treatment. Dermatol Clin 1998; 16:673-85.
2. Ducreyi A. Experimentelle Untersuchunger uber den Ansteckungstoff des weichen Schankers und uber die Bubonen. Monatshr Prakt Dermatol 1989; 9: 387.
3. Ito T. Kliniche und bacteriologische studies uber Ulcus Molle und Ducreysche streptobazillen. Arch Dermatol Syph 1913; 116: 341.
4. Reenstierna J. Chancre mou experimental chez le singe et le lapin. Acta Dermatol Venereol 1921; 2: 1.
5. Ronald AR, Plummer FA. Chancroid and *Haemophilus ducreyi*. Ann Intern Med 1985; 102: 705-7.
6. Bilgeri YR, Ballard RC, Duncan MO, et al. Antimicrobial susceptibility of 103 strains of *Haemophilus ducreyi* isolated in Johannesburg. Antimicrob Agents Chemother 1982; 22: 686-8.
7. Boyd AS. Clinical efficacy of antimicrobial therapy in *Haemophilus ducreyi* infections. Arch Dermatol 1989; 125: 1399-1405.
8. Hart G. Venereal disease in a war environment: Incidence and management. Med J Aust 1975; 1: 808-10.
9. Charles L.H. Chancroid. National Network of STDs/HIV Prevention Training Centers. 2004: 1-8.
10. David L.T, Stephen A.M. Chancroid and *Haemophilus ducreyi*: an Update. Clinical Microbiology Reviews 1995; 8: 357-75.
11. Inamadar A.C, Aparna P. Chancroid: An update. Indian J Dermatol Venereol Leprol 2002; 68: 5-9.
12. Morse SA. Chancroid and *Haemophilus ducreyi*. Clin. Microbiol. Rev 1989; 2: 137-57.
13. Ronald AR, Albritton W. Chancroid and *Haemophilus ducreyi* In: Holmes KK, Mardh P, Sparling PF, et al. 2nd edn. Sexually Transmitted Diseases. New York: McGraw Hill; 1990. p. 268.
14. De Ley J, Mannheim W, Mutters R, et al. Inter- and intrafamilial similarities of the rRNA cistrons of the Pasteurellaceae. Int J Syst Bacteriol 1990; 40: 126-37.
15. Dewhirst F E, Paster BI, Olsen I, and Fraser GJ. Phylogeny of 54 representative strains of species in the family Pasteurellaceae as determined by comparison of 16S rRNA sequences. J Bacteriol 1992; 174: 2002-13.
16. Winn WC, Allen SD, Janda WM, et al. Koneman's Colour Atlas and Textbook of Diagnostic Microbiology. 6th edn. Philadelphia: Lippincott Williams & Wilkins; 2006. p. 444.
17. Plummer FA, Nsanze H, Karasira P, et al. Epidemiology of chancroid and *Haemophilus ducreyi* in Nairobi, Kenya. Lancet 1983; 1293-5.
18. Spinola SM, Bauer ME, Munson RS. Immunopathogenesis of *Haemophilus ducreyi* infection (Chancroid). Infection and Immunity 2002; 70: 1667-76.
19. Felman YM, Nikitas JA. Sexually transmitted diseases: update on chancroid. Cutis 1983; 602: 607-8.
20. Fast MV, Nsanze H, Plummer FA, et al. Treatment of chancroid: a comparison of sulphamethoxazole and trimethoprim - sulphamethoxazole. Br J Vener Dis 1983; 59: 320-4.
21. Lautenschlager S, Eichmann A.R. Chancroid. *In:* Freedberg IM, Eisen AZ, Wolff K, Austen KF, Goldsmith LA, Katz SI, *eds.* Fitzpatrick's Dermatology in General Medicine, 6th edn., New York: McGraw-Hill 2003; 2193-8.
22. Rosen T, Dhir A. Chancroid, granuloma inguinale and lymphogranuloma venereum, In: Arndt KA, editor. Cutaneous medicine and surgery an integrated programme in dermatology. Philadelphia: WB Saunders; 1996. p. 973-82.
23. Werman BS, Herskowitz LJ, Olansky S, et al. A clinical variant of chancroid resembling granuloma inguinale. Arch Dermatol 1983; 119: 890-4.
24. Jones CC, Rosen T. Cultural diagnosis of chancroid. Arch Dermatol 1991; 127: 1823-7.
25. Kraus SJ, Kaufman HW, Albritton WL, et al. Chancroid therapy: a review of cases confirmed by culture. Rev Infect Dis 1982; 4: S-848-56.

26. Chapel TA, Brown WJ, Jeffries C, et al. How reliable is the morphological diagnosis of penile ulcerations? Sex Transm Dis 1977; 4: 150-2.
27. Sturm AW, Stolting GJ, Cormane RH, Zanen HC. Clinical and microbiological evaluation of 46 episodes of genital ulceration. Genitourin Med 1987; 63: 98-101.
28. Strakosch EA, Kendall HW, Craig KM, et al. Clinical and laboratory investigation of 370 cases of chancroid. J Invest Dermatol 1945; 6: 95-107.
29. Kumar B, Sharma VK, Bakaya V, et al. Isolation of anaerobes from clinical chancroid associated with fluctuant bubo in men. Indian J Med Res 1991; 93: 236-9.
30. Joseph AK, Rosen T. Laboratory techniques used in the diagnosis of chancroid, granuloma inguinale and lymphogranuloma venereum. Dermatol Clin 1994; 12: 1-8.
31. Karim QW, Finn GY, Easmon CSF, et al. Rapid detection of *Haemophilus ducreyi* in clinical and experimental infections using monoclonal antibody. Genitourin Med 1989; 65: 361-5.
32. Patternson K, Olsen B, Thomas C, et al. Development of a rapid immunodiagnostic test for *Haemophilus ducreyi*. J Clin Microbiol 2002; 40: 3694-702.
33. Radchiffe K, Jushuf IA, Cowan F, et al. National guideline for the management of chancroid. Sex Transm Inf 1999; 75: S43-5.
34. David A.L. Diagnostic tests for chancroid. Sexually Transmitted Infections 2000: 76; 137-41.
35. Brown TJ, Yen-Moore A, Tyring SK. An overview of sexually transmitted diseases. Part I. J Am Acad Dermatol 1999; 41: 511-32.
36. Van Dyck E, Bogaerts J, Smet H, et al. Emergence of *Haemophilus ducreyi* resistance to trimethoprim - sulfamethoxazole in Rwanda. Antimicrob Agents Chemother 1994; 38: 1647-8.
37. Kumar B, Sharma VK, Bakaya V. Sulphaphenazole, streptomycin and sulphaphenazole combination trimethoprim, and erythromycin in the treatment of chancroid. Genitourin Med 1990; 66: 105-7.
38. Brunton JL, Maclean IW, Ronald AR, et al. Plasmid mediated ampicillin resistance in *H. ducreyi*. Antimicrob Agents Chemother 1979; 15: 294-9.
39. Fast MV, Nsanze H, D'costa LJ, et al. Treatment of chancroid by clavulanic acid with amoxicillin in patients with beta-lactamase positive *Haemophilus ducreyi* infection Lancet 1982; 2: 509-11.
40. Reeves DS, Bywater MJ, Holt HA, et al. In vitro studies with ciprofloxacin: a new 4-quinolone compound. J Antimicrob chemother 1984; 13: 333-46.
41. Naamara W, Plummer FA, Greenblatt RM, et al. Treatment of chancroid with ciprofloxacin: a prospective randomised clinical trial. Am J Med 1987; 82: 317-20.
42. Cordero FA. Propionyl erythromycin ester lauryl sulphate in the treatment of treponematosis and chancroid. Antibiot Chemother 1961; 11: 764-71.
43. Carpenter JL, Back A, Gehle D, et al. Treatment of chancroid with erythromycin. Sex Transm Dis 1981; 8: 192-7.
44. Sng EH, Lim AL, Rajan VS, et al. Characteristics of *Haemophilus ducreyi*: a study. Br J Vener Dis 1982; 58: 239-42.
45. Belda Junior W, Siqueira LF, Fagundes LJ. Thiamphenicol in the treatment of chancroid. A study of 1128 cases. Rev Inst Med Trop Sao Paulo 2000; 42: 133-5.
46. Ernst AA, Marvez - Vells E, Martin DH. Incision and drainage versus aspiration of fluctuant buboes in the emergency department during an epidemic of chancroid. Sex Transm Dis 1995; 22: 217-20.

20 DONOVANOSIS

R Ganesh

In this chapter

- Synonyms
- History
- Epidemiology
- Etiology
- Pathology
- Clinical Features
- Morphological Variants
- Diagnosis
- Course and Prognosis
- Differential Diagnosis
- Treatment
- Follow Up

SYNONYMS

Granuloma venereum, Granuloma inguinale, Granuloma inguinale tropicum, Granuloma venereum genito-inguinale, Ulcerating granuloma of the pudenda, Ulcerating sclerosing granuloma, Infective granuloma and Serpiginous ulceration of the groin.

Donovanosis is a chronic destructive and slowly progressive, mildly contagious disease caused by *Calymmatobacterium granulomatis* and is characterized by granulomatous ulceration affecting primarily the genitalia.

HISTORY

McLeod first described the clinical aspect of donovanosis in 1882 who called it as serpiginous ulcer of the groin. Donovan discovered the causative organism, *Calymmatobacterium granulomatis* in 1905. It was Greenblatt and his associates who described the intracellular bodies in 1937. Anderson obtained the culture of the donovanosis microorganism, in 1943.[1-3] A monograph on donovanosis written by Rajam and Rangiah has been published by WHO in 1954.[2]

EPIDEMIOLOGY

The disease is endemic in southern China, the Far East, northern Australia, Africa (west and central), and West Indies. In India, donovanosis is endemic along the East Coast i.e., Orissa, Andhra Pradesh and Tamil Nadu. In USA sporadic occurrence of the disease has been reported. The disease is more prevalent among the blacks. The prevalence of the disease only in certain parts of the world may be related to the humidity and constant high temperature. Low socioeconomic conditions, overcrowding and poor hygiene have also been implicated as probable predisposing factors. It is far less common than syphilis, chancroid and herpes. The male to female ratio is 4:1.[1,2,4,5]

ETIOLOGY

Calymmatobacterium granulomatis, otherwise known as *Klebsiella granulomatis,* is a gram negative intracellular bacterium, measuring 1 to 1.5 × 0.5 to 0.7 μm, usually seen within the vacuoles of large mononuclear cells (histiocytes) or occasionally inside polymorphonuclear cells.[6] They reproduce in multiple foci resulting in 20 to 30 organisms occurring in a vacuole inside the host cell. The organism has a surrounding cell membrane and an overlying cell wall with a capsule in mature forms. Fimbriae (pili) like projections are seen on the cell wall.[1]

Two characteristic appearances of the organism have been described:

(i) A larger capsulated form with ovoid or bean shaped body, having well defined pinkish material surrounding a blue bacillary body with dark blue or black chromatin inclusions. These inclusions may be rounded, rod shaped and positioned centrally, peripherally or in a bipolar fashion.
(ii) The noncapsulated forms were described as minute deeply stained bodies of varying morphology-coccoid, bacillary, diplococcoid, often with a closed safety pin or telephone handle shape surrounded by a halo of unstained area. These forms are smaller, measuring 0.6 to 1 μm and both may coexist in the same host cell.

Apart from the organisms, certain inclusion bodies have been reported inside infected mononuclear cells. They may be sharply defined globular mass homogeneously staining deep pink or blue and lying away from the intact nucleus of the cell. Deeply staining spherical bodies almost filling the cell and obscuring the nucleus have also been documented. Such inclusions seem to be non-nuclear in origin, as the nucleus is intact.[2]

PATHOLOGY

The organism enters through a breach in the epithelium and causes granulomatous changes in the dermis. The marginal epithelium often shows pronounced proliferation with irregular acanthosis and elongation of rete pegs that may simulate early epithelioma (hence called peudoepitheliomatous change). Clusters of polymorphonuclear leucocytes (PMN) forming microabscess may be seen in the epidermis.

Large mononuclear cells, 25 to 90 μm in diameter, containing intracytoplasmic vacuoles filled with clusters of donovan bodies are the diagnostic hallmark of the disease **(Fig. 20.1)**. These cells are scattered diffusely throughout the dermis. Dense infiltrate of plasma cells along with scanty PMN and variable number of eosinophils is also seen. Fibrosis and oedema are seen in some of the patients. Capillaries with hypertrophy of the endothelium giving the appearance of solid cords of large pale staining cells is seen.[1,2]

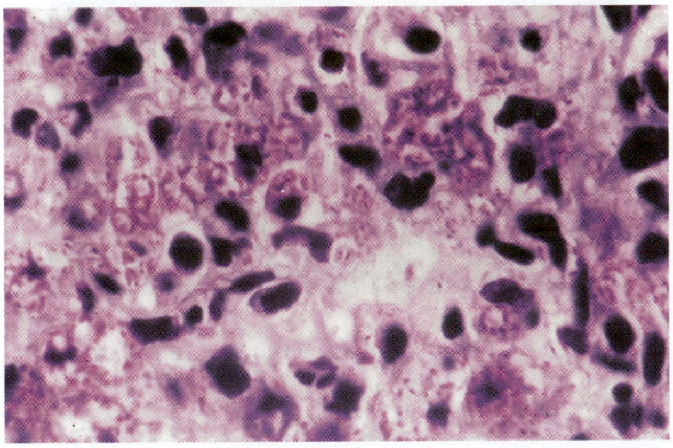

Fig. 20.1 Donovan Bodies in H & E Section.

CLINICAL FEATURES

The incubation period is variable and it may range from 3 days to 3 months. The average incubation period is 40 to 50 days. Rajam and Rangiah have experimentally produced the lesion in a volunteer in 17 days.[2]

The disease begins as single or multiple firm papules, which erode to form well defined granulomatous ulcer. The ulcer is usually painless, beefy red in colour and bleeds easily on touch. Phimosis or lymphoedema of distal tissues is common in active phase of the disease.

The genitalia are the most common sites involved in 90% of the cases. Other sites of involvement are inguinal region in 10%, anal region in 5-10% and other sites in 1-5%. Verrucous type of disease is usually seen in perianal area. Infection of oral cavity and face has also been reported.

Lymph nodes are not usually involved in donovanosis; however, in cases of secondary infections or coexisting syphilis or chancroid or rarely in malignant transformation, they can be involved. Infection spreads by direct continuity along the dermis of the skin or by autoinoculation of apposing surfaces or through fingernails. Lesions appearing in the groin may present like lymphadenopathy prior to rupture and have been referred to as pseudo bubo **(Fig. 20.2)**.

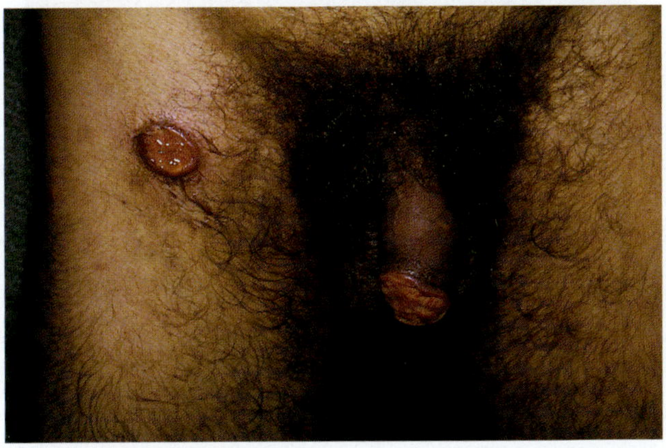

Fig. 20.2 Donovanosis - Ulcerogranulomatous Variety, Lesion on the Glans Penis and Inguinal Region.

Involvement of deeper parts of the vagina and cervix is usually associated with vulval lesions and occasionally it may be the primary lesion. The disease readily involves the perianal margins in the female as well as in homosexual men, but rectum is usually spared. It is hypothesized that while stratified squamous epithelium is susceptible, the columnar epithelium lining the urethra and rectum could be resistant to the disease. Rare cases of involvement of uterus and tubes, lips, gum, cheek, palate, pharynx, larynx, and neck have been reported.[5]

Rajam and Rangiah have reported liver and bone involvement besides extension of genital lesion to the trigone of the bladder in a female. Metastatic haemotogenous spread to bones, joints, lung and liver have been reported[2].

Based on the clinical and pathological features four morphological patterns are described:

- Classical granulomatous type **(Fig. 20.3)**
- Hypertrophic type: shows predominantly fibrous tissue reaction throughout the dermis **(Fig. 20.4, 20.5, 20.6)**.
- Sclerotic or cicatricial type **(Fig. 20.7)** hyalinised collagenous fibrous tissue dominates the histological picture.
- Destructive necrotic (phagedenic) variety shows extensive tissue destruction due to secondary fusobacillary infection.[2]

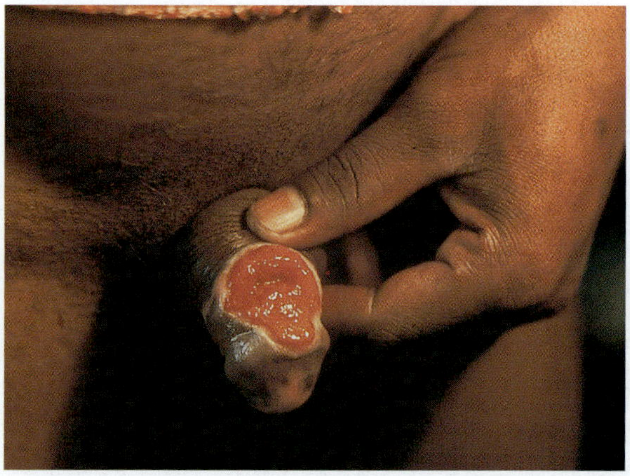

Fig. 20.3 Donovanosis – Ulcerogranulomatous variety.

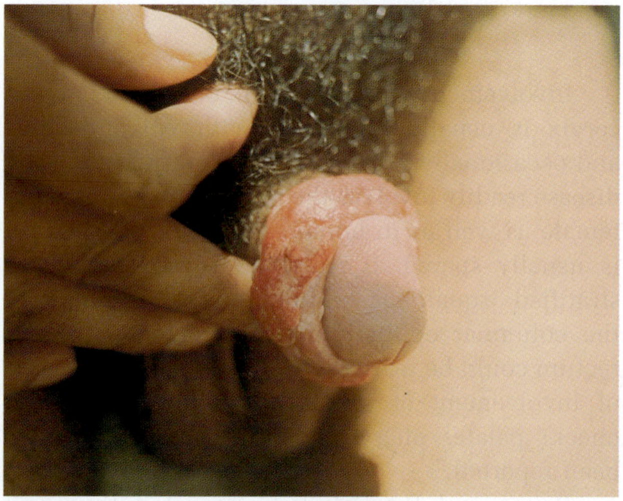

Fig. 20.4 Donovanosis – Hypertrophic Variety.

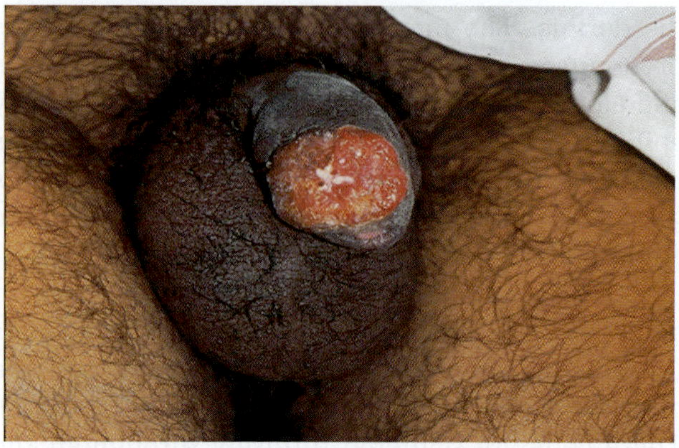

Fig. 20.5 Donovanosis – Hypertrophic Variety.

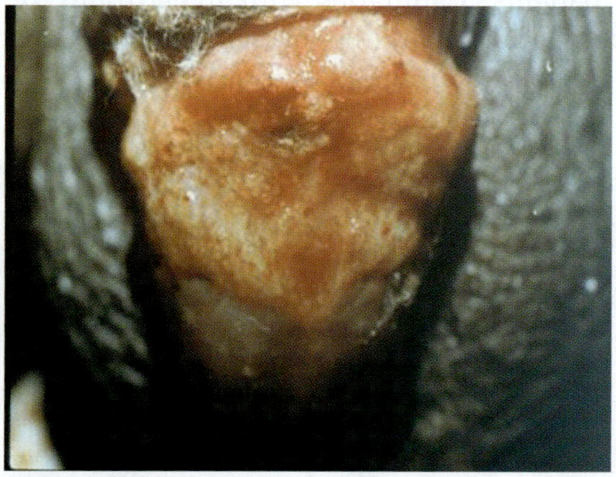

Fig. 20.6 Donovanosis – Hypertrophic Variety healing.

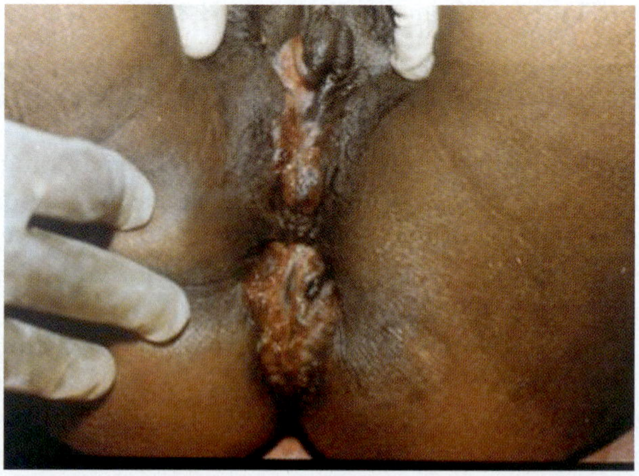

Fig. 20.7 Donovanosis involving Vulva and Perianal Area.

MORPHOLOGICAL VARIANTS

Classical or fleshy exuberant type is the most common presentation involving the inguinal region in both the sexes. The granulation tissue overflows the edges of the lesions, suggesting herniation of fleshy mass through the skin. The edge is thin and often undermined. Skin around the ulcer is slightly oedematous and infiltrated **(Fig. 20.3)**. Offensive serosanguinous discharge may be noticed. The young non-capsulated forms of the organism are found both inside and outside the mononuclear cells.

Hypertrophic type is also seen in both the sexes. The ulcer is raised above the surrounding skin and consists of pale red coarse, warty granulation tissue resulting in a buckled appearance. The edge is thickened **(Fig. 20.4, 20.5 and 20.6)**. There is no exudates and lesion is painless. Lesions may remain stationary for months. Capsulated intracellular organisms are seen only in the deeper parts of the lesion.

The sclerotic or cicatricial type is more common in women and is recognized by early and extensive formation of fibrous tissue. Breaking down of the scar by islands of active ulceration is a frequent occurrence. The hard fibrous tissue may result in deformities of the genitalia and demonstration of the organism is difficult.

The destructive, necrotic (phagedenic) type is often due to the superadded anaerobic infection, (fusospirillary) and is seen in chronic cases. It results in rapidly spreading necrotic inflammation with abundant foul smelling exudates. The ulcers are painful and the inflammation rapidly spreads both superficially and deeply with extensive tissue destruction. In female, rectovaginal fistula resulting in a cloaca has been reported.

In men, partial or complete amputation of the penis has been reported **(Fig. 20.8, 20.9, 20.10)**. Occasionally the condition can be fatal.[1,2,5] Extragenital donovanosis is a controversial subject but several cases have been reported.[8-9]

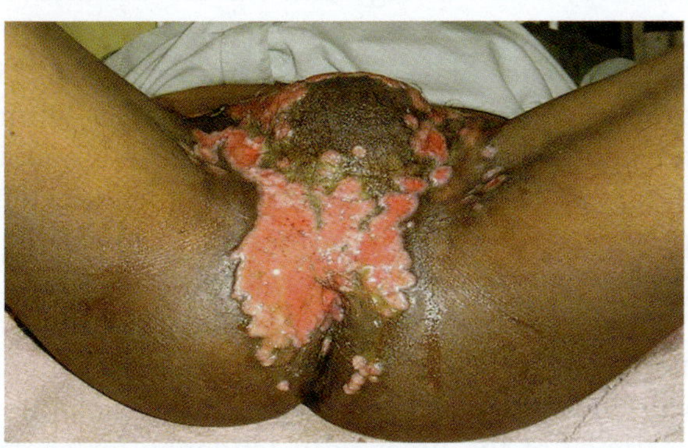

Fig. 20.8 Donovanosis – Amputation of Penis in a HIV 2 Positive Patient.

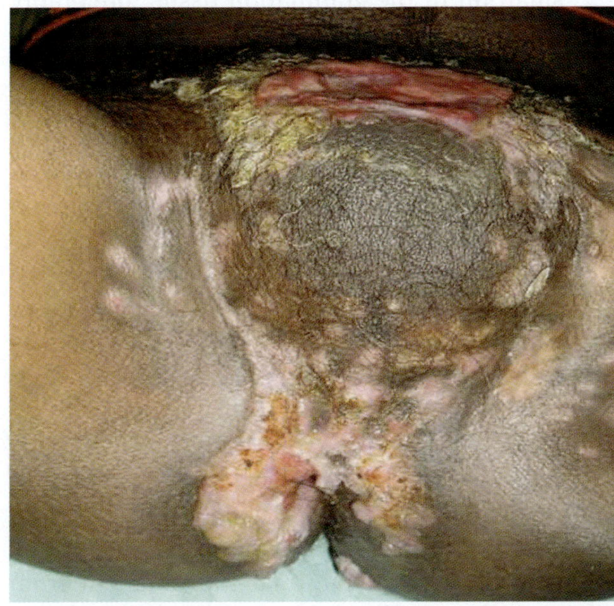

Fig. 20.9 Donovanosis – Healing after Treatment in HIV 2 Positive Patient.

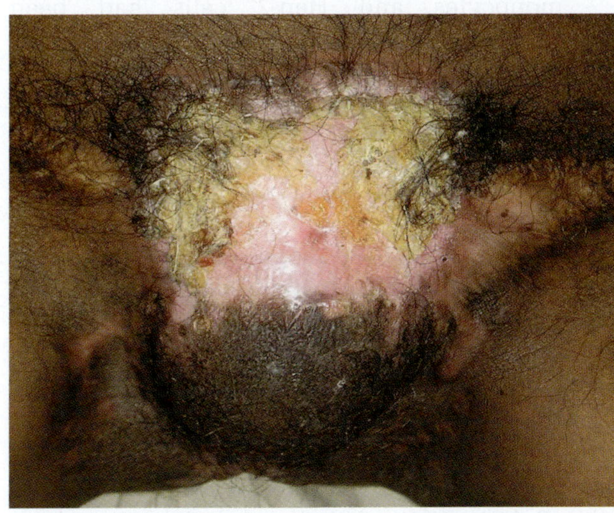

Fig. 20.10 Donovanosis – Healed with Amputation of Penis in HIV 2 Positive Patient.

DIAGNOSIS

1. Direct microscopy: The identification of intracellular donovan bodies is the gold standard for the diagnosis. It can be demonstrated by direct microscopy of crushed tissue smear stained with Giemsa or Leishman, obtained from the active lesion **(Fig. 13.4)**. Smear is prepared by taking a small bit of the granulation tissue, preferably from the edge of the ulcer, drying it with blotting paper, crushing it between two slides so as to make a clean well spreadout smear and then staining the dried smear with Giemsa or Lieshman. The slide is visualized under oil immersion microscope. Donovan bodies appear as pinkish organisms (due to bipolar condensation of the stain) within the cytoplasm of the large mononuclear cells. Papanicolaou smears may be used to identify Donovan bodies. Klebsiella granulomatis does not stain with eosin or hematoxylin.
2. Biopsy: It is less frequently used and is indicated in chronic ulcers with suspicion of malignancy.
3. Serological tests: Complement fixing technique and skin tests using material obtained from proved cases have not been found to be of reliable practical use.
4. Culture: Yolk sac of chick embryo,[3] and recently using human peripheral blood monocytes and Hep-2 cells had been successful but is not useful for routine use.[9] PCR technique has also been described.[10]
5. Recently, a colorimetric detection system for Calymmatobacterium granulomatis has been developed.[11]

COURSE AND PROGNOSIS

The disease progresses very slowly and the tendency for spontaneous healing is low and recurrence in already healed areas is not uncommon. Persistent edema of the distal tissues may result in pseudoelephantiasis, particularly in females (15 to 20%). Subsequent excoriation and ulceration result in deformities resulting in difficulty in micturition, defaecation, sexual intercourse and delivery. Even walking may be difficult for the patient with advanced disease.[5]

Females may suffer from stenosis of urethra, vulva or anal orifice, particularly in the sclerotic type. Healing may result in extensive scarring, leading to infibulation of the vaginal introitus. Rectovaginal fistula has also been reported. Epidermoid carcinoma has been documented in chronic cases (0.25%). Haematogenous spread to bones and joints, particularly during pregnancy has been reported.[1,2] Adhesion of penis to scrotum, partial or total amputation or lateral or backward deformity of penis has been reported in males.

Psoas and perinephric abscess and spinal cord compression has been documented as rare complications.[12] Secondary anaemia and tuberculosis may be seen in some patients.

In oral lesions, adhesion of lip and cheek to the gum may result in microstomia (difficulty in opening the mouth), difficulty in swallowing food and nasal regurgitation. Vertical transmission is rare, though lesions on the ears of infants borne to mothers with donovanosis have been documented.[13] Associated HIV infection may result in aggressive ulceration and poor tendency for healing.[14]

DIFFERENTIAL DIAGNOSIS

Syphilis

Primary chancre is differentiated by its classical button-like indurated non-bleeding ulcer and the associated rubbery lymphadenopathy. Dark field microscopy and serology can further confirm the diagnosis.

Condyloma lata of secondary syphilis, particularly in perianal margins may mimic donovanosis, but in the latter, the lesions are moist with broad base and flat top and teeming with treponemes, which can further be confirmed by dark field microscopy and serology.

Nodulo-ulcerative benign tertiary syphilis may sometimes confuse the clinician, especially due to the absence of lymphadenopathy. The punched-out appearance of the ulcer with tendency for central healing and peripheral spread besides positive serology help in making the diagnosis.

Chancroid

Chancroid is recognized by the short incubation period. The ulcers are multiple, painful with necrotic slough, and an undermined edge. It is often associated with painful suppurative lymphadenopathy and demonstration of Gram negative *H. ducreyi* bacilli in their classical "school of fish" appearance in microscopy.

Bubo of LGV

Bubo of LGV can be confused with pseudobubo of donovanosis. Late cases of LGV with elephantiasis may show secondary ulcerations and deformities, but the involvement of lymphnodes helps in clinical diagnosis. Serology using microimmunofluorescence assay for chlamydia is confirmatory.

Herpes Genitalis

When associated with advanced HIV infection, herpes genitalis may present with granuloma-like appearance (pseudogranuloma herpeticum). Absence of donovan bodies, presence of epithelial giant cells and response to acyclovir therapy help in diagnosis.

Amoebiasis

Amoebiasis of the genitalia in homosexuals may resemble donovanosis, and is differentiated by microscopy or therapeutic trial.

Malignancy

Particularly epidermoid carcinoma may mimic donovanosis in the early stages. Classical stony induration and lymphadenopathy differentiates the disease. Biopsy is confirmatory.

Donovanosis may coexist with other sexually transmitted infections, hence routine screening for them, particularly syphilis and HIV is mandatory.

Like other genito-ulcerative diseases, donovanosis can predispose to both acquiring and spread of HIV infection. Delayed response to therapy and relapse may be noticed in the presence of immune deficiency. The advent of syndromic approach to STDs and increased use of condoms in HIV era may be responsible for decreasing incidence of donovanosis in recent times.

TREATMENT

The following antimicrobials have been used successfully in various centres:

- Streptomycin 1 g IM bid for 10 to 14 days
- Gentamycin 1 mg/kg body wt IM 8 hourly for 2 weeks
- Chloramphenicol 0.5 g orally tid
- Tetracycline 0.5 g orally qid for 2 to 3 weeks
- Erythromycin 0.5 g orally qid
- Ampicillin 0.5 g orally qid for 12 weeks
- Cotrimoxazole 2 tablets bid for 3 weeks[15]
- Azithromycin 1 g once per week for 3 weeks[16]
- Erythromycin is the drug of choice in pregnancy and during lactation. Children borne to infected and untreated mothers must be closely monitored and a course of prophylactic antibiotics may be considered.
- Recently trovofloxacin and ceftriaxone have been successfully used in the treatment of chronic donovanosis.[17-18]

Recommended Regimen by CDC (2006)[19]

Recommended regimen

Doxycycline 100 mg orally twice daily for atleast 3 weeks and until all lesions have healed completely.

Alternative Regimens

Azithromycin 1g orally once per week for atleast 3 weeks or until all lesions have healed completely

or

Ciprofloxacin 750 mg twice daily for atleast 3 weeks or until all lesions have healed completely or

Erythromycin 500 mg orally four times a day for atleast 3 weeks or until all lesions have healed completely

or

Cotrimoxazole DS one tablet twice daily for atleast 3 weeks or until all lesions have healed completely.

Associated HIV infection may necessitate prolonged antimicrobial therapy and more frequent review. Addition of aminoglycoside (gentamycin) to one of the oral regimens may be considered if there is no response to the above treatment.

Recommended Regimen by NACO (2004)

Doxycycline 100 mg orally bid for 14 days

or

Tetracycline 500 mg orally qid for 14 days

or

Erythromycin base/stearate 500 mg orally qid for 14 days

or

Cotrimoxazole double strength 2 tablets twice a day for 14 days or until lesions have completely healed.

All sex partners (within 60 days of onset of patient's symptoms) should be examined and offered therapy. Empirical treatment is not recommended routinely. Local hygiene is generally enough. Surgical repair of scar tissues may not be rewarding.

FOLLOW UP

Patients must complete the recommended course. Review is preferable monthly for first 3 months when concomitant syphilis and HIV can also be ruled out. Subsequent follow up depends on level of healing and possible relapse. Partner notification and safe sex education with condom promotion must be emphasized.

REFERENCES

1. Hart G. Donovanosis. In: Holmes K, Mardh PA, Sparling FP, et al. eds. Sexually Transmitted Diseases. 3rd edn. New York: McGraw-Hill; 1999. p. 393-7.
2. Rajam RV, Rangiah PN. "Donovanosis" (granuloma inguinale, granuloma venereum) WHO Monograph 1954; 24: 1-72.
3. Anderson K, De Monbreun WA, Goodpasture EW. An etiological consideration of Donovania granulomatis cultivated from granuloma inguinale (three cases) in embryonic yolk. J Exp Med 1943; 8: 25-40.
4. Goldberg J. Studies on granuloma inguinale: Some epidemiological considerations of the disease. Br J Vener Dis 1964; 40; 140-5.
5. Sehgal VN ed. Donovanosis. New Delhi: Jaypee Brothers; 1-49.
6. Carter JS, Bowden FJ, Bostain I, et al. Phylogenetic evidence of reclassification of *Calymatobacterium granulomatis as Klebsiella granulomatis comb. nov.* Int J Systematic Bacteriol 1999; 49: 1695-700.
7. Rao MV, Thappa DM, Jaishankar TJ, et al. Extragenital donovanosis of the foot. Sex Trans Infect 1998; 74: 298-9.
8. Sanders CJ. Extragenital donovanosis in patients with AIDS. Sex Trans Infect 1998; 74: 142-3.
9. Carter J, Hutton S, Sriprakash KS, et al. Culture of the causative organism of donovanosis in HEp-2 cells. J Clin Microbiol 1997; 35: 2915-7.
10. Carter J, Bowden FJ, Sriprakash KS, et al. Diagnotic polymerase chain reaction for donovanosis. Clin Infect Dis 1999; 28: 1168-9.

11. Carter J, Kemp BJ. A colorimetric detection system for *Calymmatobacterium granulomatis*. Sex Transm Infect 2000; 76: 134-6.
12. Paterson DL. Disseminated donovanosis (granuloma inguinale) causing spinal cord compression; Case report and review of donovanosis involving bone. Clin Infect Dis 1998; 26: 379-83.
13. Govender D, Naidoo K, Chetty R. Granuloma Inguinale; an unusual case of otitis media and mastoiditis in children. Am J Clin Pathol 1997; 108: 510-4.
14. Jamkhedkar PP, Hira SK, Shroff HJ, et al. Clinico epidemiologic features of granuloma inguinale in era of acquired immunodeficiency syndrome. Sex Transm Infect 1998; 25: 196-200.
15. Lal S, Garg BR. Further evidence of the efficacy of co-trimoxazole in donovanosis. Br J Vener Dis 1980; 56: 412-3.
16. Bowden FJ, Mein J, Plunkett C, et al. Pilot study of azithromycin in the treatment of genital donovanosis. Genitourin Med 1996; 72: 17-9.
17. Hsu SL, Chia JK. Trovofloxacin for the treatment of chronic granuloma inguinale. Sex Transm Infect 2001; 77: 137.
18. Merianos A, Gilles M, Chuah J. Ceftriaxone in the treatment of donovanosis in central Australia. Genitourin Med 1994; 70: 84-9.
19. Centers for Disease Control and Prevention (CDC). Sexually transmitted diseases treatment guidelines, 2006. MMWR Recomm Rep 2006; 55: 1-94.

21 GONORRHOEA

VS Dorairaj, K Venkateswaran

In this chapter

INTRODUCTION

The word *gonorrhoea* is derived from combination of gonos, '*seed*' and rhoea, '*flow*'. It was considered that gonorrhoea and syphilis are caused by the same organism until Albert Neisser identified the organism to be *Neisseria gonorrhoeae* in 1879.

Gonorrhoea is one of the commonest sexually transmitted diseases. The infection affects the urethra in both the sexes, but it may spread to paraurethral glands, cervix, endometrium, fallopian tubes and peritoneum in females. The risk of acquiring urethral infection for a man following single episode of vaginal intercourse with an infected women is estimated to be 20%, rising to an estimated 60-86% following four exposures. The prevalence of infection in women who had sexual contact with men having gonococcal urethritis has been reported to be 50-90%. Anorectal and oropharyngeal infections are common with persons who practice anal or oral sex. In children, gonorrhoea is mostly sexually transmitted[1] and rarely through accidental inoculation. Occasionally, the gonococcal infection can present as disseminated form in immunocompromised patients, and it accounts for less than 3% of the cases.[2] The commercial sex workers are the main source of infection in a developing country like India. However, the incidence seems to be higher in homosexual men.[3]

AETIOLOGY

Neisseria gonorrhoeae is a gram-negative, non-motile, non-spore forming diplococci. The organism is present intracellularly in the polymorphonuclear leucocytes(PMN). Of the Neisseria species *N. gonorrhoeae* and *N. meningitidis* are pathogenic, and *N. cartarrhalis*, *N. pharyngis sicca*, *N. lactamica* and *N. subflava* are usually non-pathogenic.

MOLECULAR BIOLOGY

The structure of *N. gonorrhoeae* consists of a capsule, trilaminar membrane and pili[(1)].

The capsule possesses polyphosphate, and the trilaminar membrane has outer membrane, peptidoglycan and cytoplasmic membrane. The piliserve as the attachment units of gonococci.

The outer membrane is gram negative, and consists of proteins, phospholipid and lipo oligo saccharides (LOS). Outer membrane proteins are Type 1 protein (Por), which are of two types, PorA & PorB, that mediate invasion and penetration of host cell, and the monoclonal antibody serotyping is based on Por protein only. Type 2 Protein (Opa Protein) mediates adhesion to epithelial cells via CD66 Opa receptors. All pathogenic Neisserria, including all gonococci, contain RMP protein. This protein is of importance in pathogenesis, because many blocking antibodies that prevent serum bactericidal activity are directed against this antigen.

Peptidoglycan: Gonococcal petidoglycan is similar to that of other gram-negative bacteria, which contain muramic acid and N-acetyl glucosamine producing tissue toxin. Penicillin and cephalosporins inhibit its synthesis

Cytoplasmic membrane contains penicillin-binding proteins.

Pili: Pili are filaments, composed of protein pilin, emanating from the bacterial cell surface. The attachment of gonococci to mucosal surfaces is of primary importance in their interactions with the genito-urinary tract of the human host. This process may be, in part, mediated by pili. Long pili are pathogenic whereas short pili are non pathogenic.

There are 70 different strains of *N. gonorrhoeae* and can be differentiated by auxotyping, serotyping and genotyping. Auxotype AHU (arginine, hypoxanthine, uracil) requiring gonococci are of epidemiologic importance as they have resistance to killing by normal human serum, propensity for asymptomatic male urethral infection and increased likelihood of causing bacteremia.

PATHOGENESIS

Primary infection commonly occurs in the columnar epithelium of the urethra, para-urethral ducts and glands, cervix, conjunctiva, Bartholin's ducts, and rectum. Primary infection may also occur in the stratified squamous epithelium of the vagina in prepubertal girls (gonococcal vulvovaginatis). The female urethra often escapes infection, owing to its lining with stratified squamous epithelium. The male urethra is lined with columnar epithelium and favours penetration of gonococcus.

Penetration of the organisms takes place through the intercellular spaces and they reach the sub epithelial connective tissue on the third and fourth day of infection. Total process of tissue infection occurs in the stages **(Fig. 21.1)**:

1. Adherence
2. Invasion
3. Tissue damage

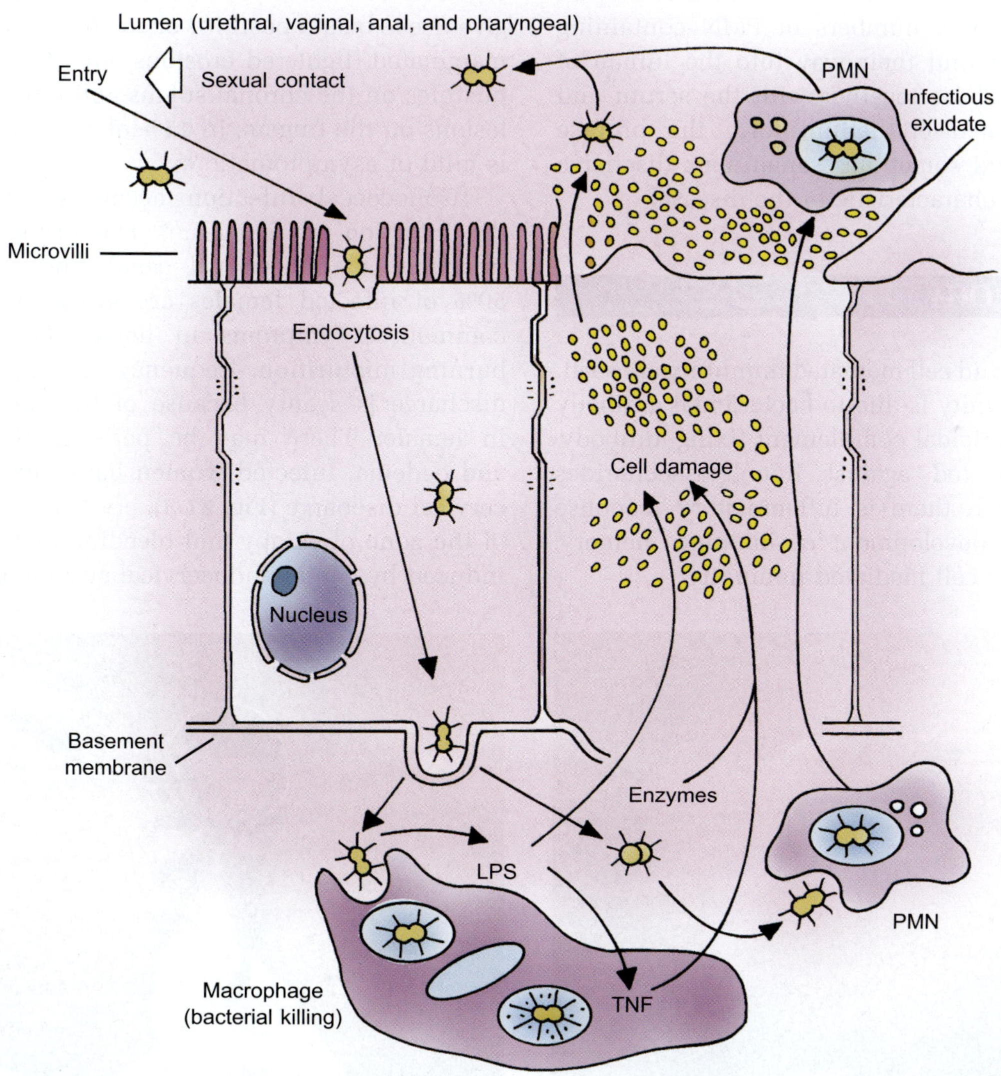

Fig. 21.1 Mechanism of N. gonorrhoeae Infection.

1. **Adherence:** Gonococci are able to invade and persist in the blood stream by evading host defense[2]. Pili E and Opa are adherence ligands. Antigenic variants of pili and Opa help to escape gonococci from immune response.

2. **Invasion:** Endocytosis and pseudopod formation occur after invasion and then transported to the base of the cell called exocytosis, followed by multiplication intracellularly.

3. **Tissue damage:** Occurs due to lipo oligo saccharide (LOS) and peptidoglycan, which stimulates production of tissue necrosis factor (TNF). Neutrophils are attracted to the site and large numbers of PMN containing gonococci find their way into the lumen of urethra. These together with the serum and desquamated epithelium form the profuse yellow and sometimes sanguinous discharge which is characteristic of the disease.

IMMUNOLOGY

Both humoral and cell mediated immunity are seen. Humoral immunity is due to bactericidal antibody IgM, and bactericidal complement fixing antibody, which is directed against lipooligosaccharides (LOS). Although there is inflammatory response there is little development of immune memory, leading to poor cell mediated immunity.

CLINICAL FEATURES

Incidence of asymptomatic gonococcal infection in general population has been estimated at approximately 1-3%. The incubation period ranges from 1 to 14 days, but majority of men develop symptoms within 2 to 5 days.[4] Anterior urethritis is the most common manifestation of gonococcal infection in men. It starts with mild irritation, scanty mucopurulent or mucoid discharge per urethra in men. As it progresses, within 24 hours the dischrage becomes thick, purulent and profuse **(Fig. 21.2)** with intense burning and pain during micturition[5]. It is associated with increased frequency and urgency. The direct contact of the discharge may give rise to balanoposthitis characterized by sharply marginated, light red erosions along with discrete pustules on the coronal sulcus and rarely pustular lesions on the fingers. In 15% of males the disease is mild or asymptomatic.[6]

Gonococcal infection accounts for 90% of the infection in females.[7,8] The primary site of infection is endocervical canal, and only about 50% of infected females are symptomatic.[9] The commonest symptoms in female are moderate burning micturition, frequency and urgency. The discharge is scanty because of the short urethra in female. There may be peri-meatal erythema and oedema. Infected women have mucopurulent cervical discharge **(Fig. 21.3)**, erythema and edema of the zone of ectopy and bleeding that is usually induced by gentle endocervical swabbing.

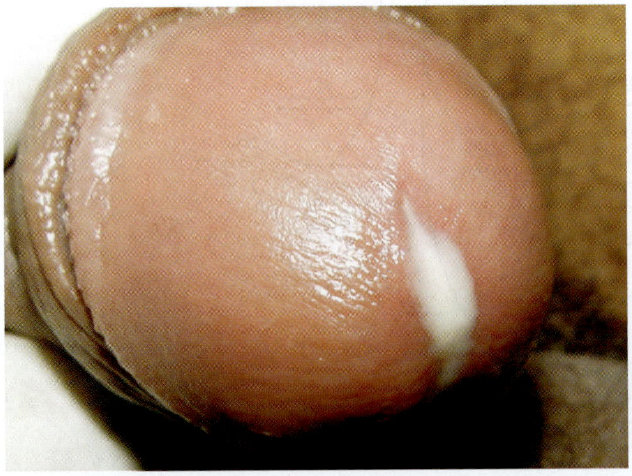

Fig. 21.2 Gonorrhoea in Male - Mucopurulent Urethral Discharge.

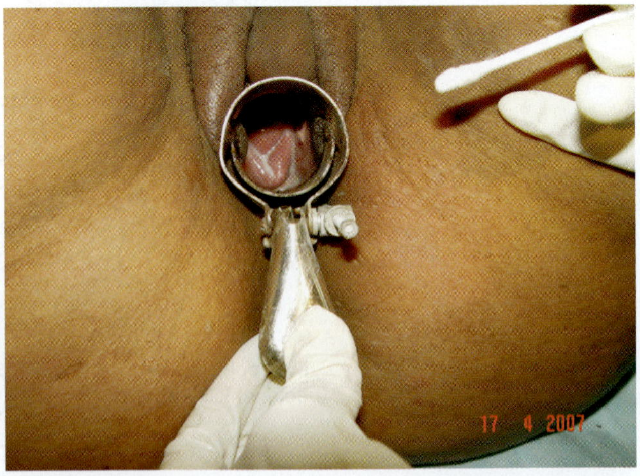

Fig. 21.3 Gonorrhoea in Female - Mucopurulent Discharge from the Cervix.

Ano-rectal Gonorrhoea

The rectal mucosa is infected in 35% to 50% of women with gonococcal cervical infection and is the only site of infection in 5% of women with gonorrhoea. Ano-rectal gonorrhoea may be primary or secondary. Secondary infection occurs chiefly in women and prepubertal girls with a primary genito-urinary infection and occasionally due to bursting of gonorrhoeal abscesses into the rectum. Primary infection usually results from anal intercourse but may be accidental, and in many cases it has followed the insertion of contaminated thermometers or enema nozzles.

In MSM, rectal infection is due to direct inoculation through receptive anal intercourse.

Symptoms of rectal infection are anal pruritus, painless mucopurulent discharge, proctitis, including severe rectal pain, tenesmus and constipation. Inspection of anus shows erythema and abnormal discharge, but anoscopy often reveals mucoid or purlent exudate, erythema, edema, friability or other inflammatory mucosal changes.

Pharyngeal Infection

The pharynx is the sole site of infection in less than 5% of patients irrespective of gender or sexual orientation[7]. Infection is sexually transmitted to the pharynx by urogenital sexual contact and is more efficiently acquired by fellatio than by cunnilingus. Transmission of gonorrhoea from patients with pharyngeal infection to their sex partner is inefficient and is relatively rare.

Although pharyngeal gonococcal infection may cause acute pharyngitis or tonsillitis and occasionally associated with fever or cervical lymphadenopathy, over 90% of the infections are asymptomatic. Pharyngeal infection may now be an important source of urethral gonorrhoea in MSM.

COMPLICATIONS IN MEN

These include posterior urethritis, infection of Cowper's and Tyson's glands, epididymitis, acute or chronic prostatitis, seminal vesiculitis and periurethral abscess. The disease may reach both diaphragmatic and bulbar portions of the glands of Cowper, either by way of the columnar lined duct, which opens on the floor of the bulb or by lymphatic route. Inflammation, often subacute throughout, may progress to abscess formation. A diaphragmatic abscess rarely remains localized between the two layers of the urogenital diaphragm, the pus tracking either downwards presenting as perianal, ischiorectal or perianal abscess, or upwards to form a perirectal or peri-prostatic abscess. Chronically inflamed Cowper's glands are hard and brick-like consistency, size varying from that of a pea to hazelnut. Untreated gonorrhoea may rarely lead to periurethral abscess and watercan perineum **(Fig. 21.4, 21.5)**.

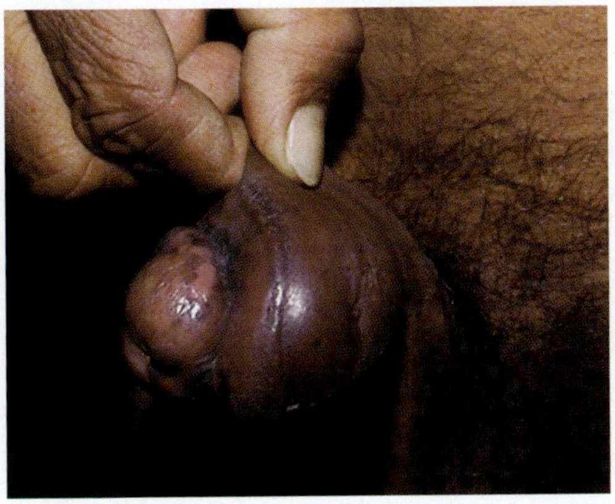

Fig. 21.4 Gonorrhoea - Periurethral Abscess.

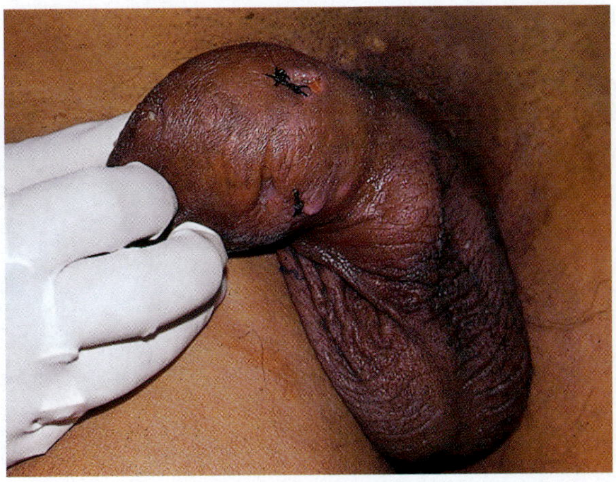

Fig. 21.5 Gonorrhoea in Male - Watercan Perineum.

Epididymitis

Involvement of the epididymis is the most frequent complication before the introduction of the sulphonamides and penicillin that usually follows trauma to the posterior urethra. Gonococci penetrate the columnar epithelium of the tubules of the epididymis. The only distinctive feature is the formation of multiple miliary abscesses in the subepithelial connective tissue, which rarely coalesce to form extensive abscesses. There is often an associated inflammation of the rete testis and an inflammatory hydrocele.

Acute Prostatitis

Acute inflammation of the prostatic ducts and gland with peri-glandular inflammation may cause swelling of one or both lateral lobes, which may progress to form prostatic abscess.

Infection may also spread by continuity in the columnar epithelium of the short ejaculatory ducts or by the lymphatic vessels to one or both of the seminal vesicles.

COMPLICATIONS IN WOMEN

Salpingitis

It is usually bilateral, may present as acute, subacute and mild form. There is tendency for the tubes to get closed to form hydrosalpinx or pyosalpinx. Acute salpingitis or pelvic inflammatory disease (PID) is the most common complication of gonorrhoea in women. They present with lower abdominal pain, dysparuenia, abnormal periods, etc. The details are discussed in chapter on PID.

Bartholin's Gland Abscess

Inflammation is commonly unilateral and remain confined to the ducts and the periglandular tissues. The orifice often has a red halo, exudes pus on pressure **(Fig. 21.6)**. It may develop a small indurated swelling, or a large abscess, often preceded by cystic swelling of the duct or gland.

COMPLICATIONS IN INFANTS

Ophthalmia Neonatorum

Primary gonococcal infection of the conjunctiva occurs rarely in adults but is common in babies, starting within 21 days of birth. It accounts for 5-15% of conjuctivitis in the new born. It produces an acute purulent conjunctivitis, which appears 2-5 days after birth. It is characterized by intense redness and swelling of the conjunctiva, associated with a profuse purulent and often blood stained discharge. The ocular conjunctiva, swollen with an inflammatory oedema, bulges over the cornea and for the same reason the upper lid may overlap the lower **(Fig. 21.7)**. An intense inflammatory reaction develops in the subepithelial connective

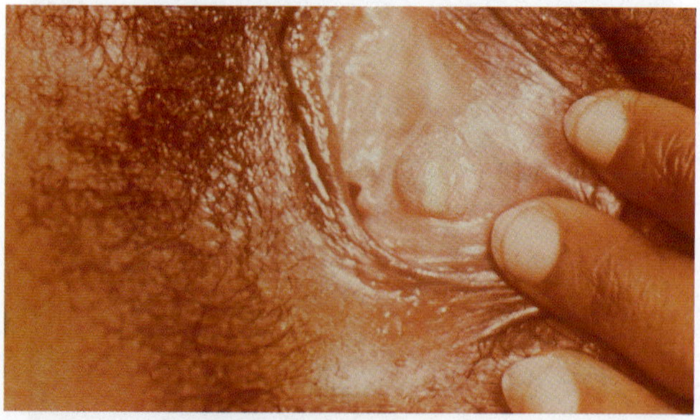

Fig. 21.6 Gonorrhoea in Female – Pus at the Opening of Bartholin's Duct.

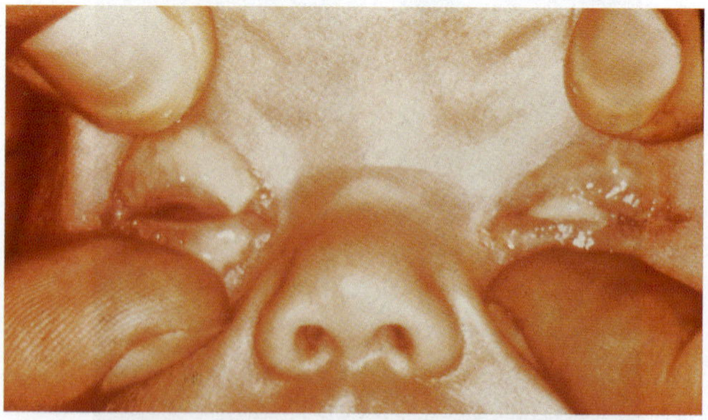

Fig. 21.7 Gonorrhoea - Ophthalmia Neonatorum.

tissue of the conjunctiva during the first 24 hours and gonococci can be demonstrated on the second day of the disease. If treatment is delayed, *N. gonorrhoeae* penetrates through intact corneal epithelium, producing perforation, scarring, blindness and sometimes infection with two or more microorganisms.

METASTATIC COMPLICATIONS

Disseminated Gonococcal Infection

Disseminated gonococcal infection (DGI) is the most common systemic complication of acute gonorrhoea.[2] It manifests as acute arthritis-dermatitis syndrome. The syndrome has been estimated to occur in 0.5 to 3 percent of patients with untreated gonorrhoea. DGI results from gonococcal bacteremia and is most often manifestated by acute arthritis, tenosynovitis, dermatitis or combination of these findings. The most common clinical manifestation of DGI is joint pain and skin lesions, the arthritis-dermatitis syndrome. Skin lesions present as macules, papules, pustules, petechiae, bullae, or ecchymoses. The skin lesions tend to be located on distal portions of the extremities. Approximately 30 to 40 percent of patients with DGI have overt arthritis. Any joint may be involved, although DGI most often involves wrist, metacarpophalangeal, ankle and knee joints. Iris, conjunctiva, endorcardium, pericardium, meninges and nerves are also involved. In more than 80% of the DGI patients, *Neisserria gonorrhoeae* may be cultured from the primary mucosal site of infection Disseminated gonococcal infection is more common in women than in men.

Gonococcal Arthritis

Gonococcal inflammation of the joints is commonly polyathritic. The joints most often involved are the knees, ankles, and small joints of the feet. It may occur at any stage of the disease and has usually an acute onset; a subacute onset is rare. There are three main types of acute joint infection in gonorrhoea: arthralgia, acute synovitis, and acute arthritis which includes serofibrinous arthritis and the purulent form. The details are discussed in a separate chapter.

Meningitis

The complication may be blood borne from primary foci. Autopsy showed patches of purulent exudates containing gonococci in the subarachnoid space, the exudates being most obvious in the frontal and parietal regions, as seen in other type of purulent meningitis. *N. gonorrhoeae* cannot be distinguished from N. meningitidis on gram stain of cerebrospinal fluid.

Endocarditis

Gonococcal endocarditis is an uncommon complication of gonococcal bacteremia. The aortic valve appears to be infected most often in patients with gonococcal endocarditis.

LAB DIAGNOSIS

The diagnosis of gonorrhoea includes microscopy and culture. VDRL and HIV serology testing should be done after getting the informed consent.

Microscopy

Specimen is collected with help of sterile cotton wool swabs. If no discharge is present, urethral or prostatic massage is performed and specimen is collected from the distal urethral meatus. In female specimen is collected from the endocervix, urethra, rectum or oropharynx. The urethral discharge is homogenously spread over the slide by rolling the swab onto a clean slide. Allow the smear to dry before it is stained. Fix the dried smear by passing the slide rapidly three to four times over a flame. The slide is stained with Gram stain and examined under oil immersion 100 x objective. The gonococci are seen as gram-negative diploccocci within PMN cells **(Fig. 13.1)**. The specificity of gram stain is 95-97% from the culture of positive male urethral discharge, 40-60% from endocervical secretion and in asymptomatic patients, the smear is mostly negative.[10]

Culture

The culture is the most specific investigation and the commonly used selective media for *N. gonorrhoeae*, are modified Thayer Martin (MTM), Chacko Nayar Medium (Trypsin digested beef extract), Martin Lewis (ML) media, and New York City (NYC) medium. The direct plating of organism has better success in growing organism. If direct plating is not available, the swabs are transported to the laboratory in Stuart's medium or Amie's medium. The inoculated plates are placed in an atmosphere containing 5% CO_2 at 37°C and examined every 18-24 hours until 48-72 hours.[10] Small pinpoint colonies of 0.5 to 1mm diameter of *N. gonorrhoeae* can be seen.

Gonococci are fastidious organisms, requiring an enriched culture media for their growth, which also selectively supress the normal flora. Vancomycin, colistin, trimethoprim and nystatin are added to inhibit the growth of bacterial and fungal organisms

The isolation rate decreases with increase in time difference between the specimen collection and inoculation, 90% within 12 hours and 100% within 6 hours of obtaining specimen and the acceptable result can be expected if the transport time is <2 days.[10] The oxidase reaction aids the search for gonococcal colonies in mixed cultures. A drop of tetra methyl-*p*-phenylene diamine hydrochloride is poured over suspected gonococcal colonies, which quickly turn pink and then dark blue.

The sugar fermentation reaction is done to differentiate *N. gonorrhoeae* from the other group of Neisseria organisms. Gonococcus produces acid only with glucose while meningococcus with both glucose and maltose.

Monoclonal antibodies for fluorescence, co-agglutination or enzyme are highly sensitive and specific to *N. gonorrhoeae* and they have the advantage of identifying *N. gonorrhoeae* 24 hours before the conventional culture technique.[10]

Recently, polymerase chain reaction (PCR), ligase chain reaction (LCR) and other nucleic acid amplification techniques are also being developed to diagnose gonorrhoea.

The specificity of DNA hybridization is superior to the ELISA.

Serology

The complement fixation, latex agglutination immunofluorescence and anti-surface pili assays, haemagglutination, radioimmunoassay, ELISA and immunoblotting can be used to detect serum antibody against *N. gonorrhoeae,* but it is not useful as it cannot differentiate between the present and past infection.

The acidometric method, iodometric test and chromogenic cephalosporin test are used to detect the resistance of *N. gonorrhoeae* to penicillin.[10] β lactamase, an extra cellular enzyme produced by many strains of bacteria, specifically hydrolyze amide bond inβ lactam ring of penicillin analogues, rendering the antibiotic inactive. Penicillinoic acid is formed with a resulting colour change. A rapid carbohydrate utilization test (RCUT) is used for β lactamase production by Neisseria species. The production of β lactamase from *N. gonorrhoeae* can be detected by the change in colour of the phenol red pH indicator from red to yellow. The test can thus be used both for identification and testing for β lactamase production.

TREATMENT[11]

Uncomplicated Gonococcal Infections of the Cervix, Urethra and Rectum

Cefixime 400 mg orally in a single dose

or

Ceftriaxone 125 mg IM in a single dose

or

Ciprofloxacin 500 mg orally in a single dose

or

Ofloxacin 400 mg orally in a single dose

or

Levofloxacin 250 mg orally in a single dose
plus
If Chlamydial infection is not ruled out
Azithromycin 1 g orally in a single dose
or
Doxycycline 100 mg orally bid a day for 7 days

Uncomplicated Gonococcal Infections of the Pharynx

Ceftriaxone 125 mg IM in a single dose
or
Ciprofloxacin 500 mg orally in a single dose
plus
If Chlamydial infection is not ruled out
Azithromycin 1 g orally in a single dose
or
Doxycycline 100 mg orally bid for 7 days

Gonococcal Conjunctivitis

Ceftriaxone 1 g IM in a single dose
Note: Consider lavage of the infected eye with saline solution once.

Disseminated Gonococcal Infection (DGI)

Ceftriaxone 1 g IM or IV every 24 hours.
Alternative regimens
Cefotaxime 1 g IV every 8 hours
or
Ceftizoxime 1 g IV every 8 hours
or
Ciprofloxacin 400 gm IV every 12 hours
or
Ofloxacin 400 mg IV every 12 hours
or
Levofloxacin 250 mg IV daily
or
Spectinomycin 2 g IM every 12 hours
All of the preceding regimens should be continued for 24-48 hours after improvement begins, at which time therapy may be switched to one of the following regimens to complete at least 1 week of antimicrobial therapy.

Cefixime 400 mg orally bid daily
or
Ciprofloxacin 500 mg orally bid daily
or
Ofloxacin 400 mg orally bid daily
or
Levofloxacin 500 mg orally od daily

Gonococcal Meningitis and Endocarditis

Ceftriaxone 1-2 g IV every 12 hours
Therapy for meningitis should be continued for 10-14 days; therapy for endocarditis should be continued for at atleast 4 weeks. Treatment of complicated DGI should be undertaken in consultation with a specialist.

Ophthalmia Neonatorum Caused by *N. gonorrhoeae*

Ceftriaxone 25-50 mg/kg IV or IM in a single dose, not to exceed 125 mg
Note: Topical antibiotic therapy alone is inadequate and is unnecessary if systemic treatment is administered.

Management of Sex Partners

All sex partners of patients who have *N. gonorrhoeae* infection should be evaluated and treated for both *N. gonorrhoeae* and *C. trachomatis* infections if their last sexual contact with the patient was within 60 days before onset of symptoms or diagnosis of infection in the patient.

FOLLOW UP

Treated patients with CDC regimen need not follow up to confirm their cure but the patient with persistent symptoms may be tested for antimicrobial susceptibility and other cause and treated accordingly.

REFERENCES

1. Neinstein LS, Goldenring J, Carpender S. Nonsexual transmission of sexually transmitted diseases: an infrequent occurrence. Paediatrics 1984; 74: 67-76.
2. Disseminated gonococcal infection. Lancet 1984; I: 832-833.
3. Hook EW, Holmes KK. Gonococcal infection. Ann Intern Med 1985; 102: 229-243.
4. Hay RJ, Adriaans BM. Bacterial infection. In: Champion RH, Burton JL, Burns DA, Breathnach SM, eds. Rook Textbook of Dermatology. Oxford: Black well Science; 1998. p. 1140-1.
5. Gonorrhoea in males. In: King A, Nicol C, Rodin P eds.Venereal diseases. 4th edn. London: ELBS; 1980. p. 200-213.
6. Feingold DS, Peacocke M. Gonorrhoea. In. Freedberg IM, Elisen AZ, Wolff K, et al. eds. Dermatology in general medicine. 5th edn. McGraw Hill: New York ,1999: 2598-2603.
7. Thin RN, Shav EJ. Diagnosis of gonorrhoea in women. Br J Vener Dis 1979; 55: 10-13.
8. Barlow D, Phillips. Gonorrhoea in women: Diagnosis clinical and laboratory aspects. Lancet 1978; 1: 761-4.
9. Tiwari VD, Talwar S, Grewal RS. Urethritis, pelvic inflammatory disease and Reiter's disease. In: Valia RG, Valia AR, eds. IADVL Textbook and atlas of Dermatology. 2nd ed. Mumbai: Bhalani publishing house; 2001. p. 1423-42.
10. Gonorrhoea . In: Dyck EV, Meheus AZ, Piot P, eds.. Laboratory diagnosis of sexually transmitted diseases. Geneva: WHO; 1999. p. 1-21.
11. Centers for Disease Control and Prevention (CDC). Sexually transmitted diseases treatment guidelines, 2006. MMWR Recomm Rep 2006; 55: 1-94.

22 NON-GONOCOCCAL URETHRITIS AND CHLAMYDIA INFECTIONS

Usha Gupta, D K Gupta

In this chapter

- Non Gonococcal Urethritis
- Clinical features
- Management
- HIV Infection
- Recurrent and Persistent NGU
- Post-Gonococcal Urethritis
- Chlamydial Infections
- Chlamydial Life Cycle
- Persistence
- Lab Studies
- Treatment

NON GONOCOCCAL URETHRITIS

Urethritis, or inflammation of the urethra, is a multifactorial condition which can be sexually acquired. It is characterised by discharge and/or dysuria or may be asymptomatic. Urethritis is described as either gonococcal, when *Neisseria gonorrhoeae* is detected, or non-gonococcal (NGU) when it is not. The term non-specific urethritis (NSU) was used for non-gonococcal non-chlamydial urethritis and should be avoided. Men with NGU may have symptoms of urethritis or may be asymptomatic. Microscopy of Gram stained specimens of their urethral discharge reveals pus cells but no Gram-negative intracellular diplococci. Urethral inflammation with >5 pus cells/HPF on urethral smear can occur without a known pathogen being isolated from the large number of patients even using more sensitive detection methods.[2-5]

Mucopurulent cervicitis is the female equivalent of urethritis with approximately 40% of cases being due to *Chlamydia trachomatis*.[1]

The distinction between gonococcal and non-gonococcal urethritis became possible with the identification and culturing of *N. gonorrhoeae* from 1880 onwards, although cell culture for isolation of *C. trachomatis* was not available until 1965. Approximately 10% of men attending genitourinary medicine clinics in the UK are diagnosed with nongonococcal urethritis (NGU).

The aetiology of NGU[6-16] is summarized in Table 22.1.

Table 22.1 Aetiology of NGU

Organism	*Isolated in (% of Cases)*	*Estimated Cause in (% of cases)*
Chlamydia trachomatis	20–50%	20–50%
Ureaplasma urealyticum	20–80%	10–20%
Mycoplasma genitalium	10–30%	10–20%
Trichomonas vaginalis	1–17%	1
Other organisms: Herpes simplex, Adenovirus, Candida spp., Coliforms associated with UTI, Staphylococcus saprophyticus, Haemophilus species, Neisseria meningitidis, Streptococcus pneumoniae	Rare	Rare
Non-infective Other causes*	–	Rare
No cause found: 'true' non-specific urethritis	20–50%	20–50%

* Other causes including trauma, chemical, neoplasm, foreign body e.g. catheterisation, pre-existing urethral stricture, alcohol, allergy, abstinence, excess sexual activity, dehydration and masturbation etc.

The commonest organisms implicated are *C. trachomatis* and *M. genitalium* with the latter perhaps causing more symptoms.[4,6] Chlamydia is more likely to be isolated in younger patients than *M. genitalium* and the two organisms rarely coexist in the same individual.[3] However in large number of patients either of them is not isolated and this can be as high as 30-80%.[2-5,16-22]

The isolation of *Trichomonas vaginalis* is dependent on the prevalence of the organism in the community, being more common in non-white ethnic groups. *T. vaginalis* isolation is greater in men >30 years.[24] The exact role of ureaplasmas in NGU has been controversial due to the conflicting observations in clinical studies. *U. urealyticum* biovar 2 may account for 5-10% of cases of acute NGU.[25] UTI may account for 6.4% of cases, although there is only one study evaluating this.[26] Adenoviruses may be responsible for 2-4% of symptomatic patients and is often associated with conjunctivitis.[22,27] HSV 1 and 2 are less commonly associated with NGU (2-3%).[22,28] *N. meningitidis*, Haemophilus sp., Candida sp., urethral stricture and foreign bodies have been reported in a few cases and probably account for a small proportion of NGU.[29]

Asymptomatic urethritis, without an observable discharge, may have a different aetiology from symptomatic urethritis, with *C. trachomatis*[30,31,32] and *M. genitalium* being detected less frequently[20,33] and at lower quantities. There is also a possible association of asymptomatic NGU with bacterial vaginosis.[34,35]

It is assumed that the aetiological agents of sexually acquired male NGU could potentially cause genital tract inflammation in women, in particular pelvic inflammatory disease (PID). This is undoubted with chlamydial and gonococcal infection and possible with *M. genitalium*[3,36,37,38] but remains to be substantiated for pathogen-negative NGU. Asymptomatic chlamydia-negative NGU was reported in male partners of women with PID, but *M. genitalium* was not tested.[39]

CLINICAL FEATURES

NGU may be asymptomatic or may present with clear, creamy white, yellow or green urethral discharge with or without dysuria. The discharge may not have been noticed by the patient or may only be present on urethral massage. There may be associated variable dysuria. Sometimes, urethral itch or discomfort may be the only symptom.

The incubation period of NGU is often longer, and the discharge is less purulent than that of gonococcal urethritis, but these differences do not permit diagnosis on clinical grounds.Occasionally, men presenting with NGU gives no history of sexual contact. Occasionally, conjunctival infection, reactive arthritis or epididymo-orchitis may be present in men with NGU.

Herpes Simplex Virus (HSV) Urethritis

When urethral discharge is accompanied by flu-like systemic symptoms or groin, buttock or leg pain, the possibility of HSV urethritis should be considered. Severe dysuria with scant discharge can also point to this diagnosis. Other features with which HSV urethritis can present, include severe dysuria, blood stained discharge (sometimes with haematuria), inguinal lymphadenopathy and intrameatal ulceration.

Urethritis Associated With Urinary Tract Infection

When discharge is accompanied by frequency, haematuria, abdominal pain, severe dysuria and/or systemic symptoms and urethritis associated with UTI should be considered. Microscopy of a Gram-stained, mid-stream clean-catch urine with more than one bacterium per high-power field supports the diagnosis. Other points that could help in diagnosis are:

- Gram-stained slide of urethral smear containing pus cells but no Gram-negative diplococci (GNDC)
- Positive Dipstick test for haematuria, proteinuria and presence of nitrites and leukocyte esterase in a midstream urine sample.
- Sterile midstream sample of urine positive for bacterial culture

Potential Complications

- Epididymo-orchitis
- Sexually acquired reactive arthritis/Reiter's syndrome

These are infrequent, occurring in fewer than 1% of cases, though incomplete forms may be more common.

Diagnosis

The diagnosis of urethritis must be confirmed by demonstrating PMNLs in the anterior urethra. This can be done by means of:

(i) A Gram stained urethral smear containing >5 PMNL per high power (x1000) microscopic field (averaged over five fields with greatest concentration of PMNLs)[30]

and/or

(ii) Positive leukocyte esterase test on first-voided urine or a gram stained preparation from a centrifuged sample of a first passed urine (FPU) specimen, containing ≥10 PMNL per high-power (x1000) microscopic field (averaged over five fields with greatest concentration of PMNLs).

Either test can be used: both tests will identify cases missed by the other test.[32] Either a 5 mm plastic loop or cotton-tipped swab can be used and should be introduced about 1 cm into the urethra. There are no published data comparing the two but the former is probably less traumatic to the patient.

Positive leucocyte esterase activity on dipstick on FPU specimen correlates with NGU and the detection of chlamydia[8] and is considered diagnostic by some authorities.[40] However, it does not have adequate sensitivity to be considered a reliable rapid diagnostic test for acute NGU.[41,42] Moreover its positive predictive value for *C. trachomatis* in asymptomatic patients is poor.[8]

There is controversy as to the need to perform microscopy in asymptomatic patients.[43,44] Treatment will be delayed in up to 30% of those infected with *C. trachomatis* who are asymptomatic.[43,45,46,47] Also, a single nucleic acid amplification test (NAAT) may miss up to 3% of men with urethral chlamydia[48] and will miss 5-6% of asymptomatic men infected with *M. genitalium*.[43,49,50] It is however, unclear if microscopy would identify a substantial proportion of these patients. On the other hand, omitting microscopy in asymptomatic men will prevent diagnosing 77-87% of men as having a sexually transmitted infection in whom neither of the above organisms will be isolated.[7,50] Indeed, relying on microscopy alone will miss up to 37% of *C. trachomatis* and up to 23% of *M. genitalium* urethral infections[5,7,9,51] There is, therefore, little justification in performing urethral microscopy in asymptomatic men. It does of course remain an important test in symptomatic men for the diagnosis of gonococcal urethritis.

The traditional two-glass test adds little to the diagnosis and should be abandoned.[52] The 'two-glass' urine test, consisting of first-passed urine (FPU) and midstream urine has been used for diagnosing urethritis. Threads (casts of mucus or mucopus washed from the urethral glands) in the first sample but none in the midstream is supportive of urethritis. The test's main use in modern practice is to obtain threads for Gram staining and microscopy.

MANAGEMENT

General advice

The following should be discussed and clear written information provided:

- An explanation of the causes of NGU, including non-infective causes, and possible short term and long term implications for the health of the patient and his partner.
- The side-effects of treatment and the importance of complying fully with it.
- The importance of their sex partner(s) being evaluated and treated.
- Advice to abstain from sexual intercourse, or if that is not acceptable, the consistent use of condoms, until he has completed therapy and his partner(s) have been treated.
- The importance of complying with follow-up.

Treatment

Treatment should be initiated as soon as the diagnosis is made and without waiting for the results of tests for chlamydia and cultures for *N. gonorrhoeae*.

Ideally, treatment should be effective (microbiological cure rate for *C. trachomatis* >95%), easy to take (not more than twice daily), with a low side-effect profile, and cause minimal interference with daily lifestyle.

However assessing treatment efficacy is problematic, as no pathogen is identifiable in over 60% of cases, and the inflammatory process may not reflect persistent infection.[29] It is important to note that the inflammatory exudate may persist for an unknown length of time even when the putative organism has been eliminated.[40]

Tetracyclines are generally effective against *C. trachomatis* though sporadic reports of treatment failure have been reported.[41] While the general treatments that are effective against *C. trachomatis* appear to be also effective in NGU. Tetracyclines in the doses used do not consistently eradicate *M. genitalium*[53,54,55] and this may also be the case with stat dose of azithromycin.[54,55] Single-dose regimens though have the advantage of improved compliance and directly observed treatment.

Recommended regimens for NGU(CDC 2006)

Doxycycline 100 mg twice a day for 7 days
Or
Azithromycin 1g orally in a single dose

Alternative Regimens

Erythromycin base 500 mg orally four times a day for 7 days
or
Erythromycin ethylsuccinate 800 mg orally four times a day for 7 days
or
Ofloxacin 300 mg orally twice a day for 7 days
or
Levofloxacin 500 mg orally once daily for 7 days

Partner notification

Where available, all men with NGU should be referred to a trained health adviser on diagnosis. They should be offered a choice of self-notification, provider notification or conditional notification.

Treatment of Contacts of Men with NGU

According to CDC 2006, all sex partners in last 60 days should be evaluated and treated.

Greater priority should be given to tracing female contacts of men with Chlamydia-positive NGU.) Female partners of men with NGU should be treated whether or not Chlamydia is isolated.

Follow-Up

- Men with NGU should be reviewed 2–3 weeks after treatment to confirm resolution of symptoms and treatment of sexual contacts
- Results of tests for other infections will be available at this time
- Routine repeat microscopy of the urethral smear is not indicated in men whose symptoms have resolved.

HIV INFECTION

Gonococcal, chlamydial, and nongonococcal, nonchlamydial urethritis might facilitate HIV transmission. Patients who have NGU and also are infected with HIV should receive the same treatment regimen as those who are HIV negative.

RECURRENT AND PERSISTENT NGU

This is empirically defined as persistent or recurrent symptomatic urethritis occurring 30-90 days following treatment of acute NGU[45] and occurs in 10-20% of patients.[56-59]

According to CDC 2006, persistent symptoms alone, without documentation of signs or laboratory evidence of urethral inflammation, are not a sufficient basis for retreatment. Objective signs of urethritis should be present before initiation of antimicrobial therapy.

Patients with recurrent and persistent urethritis should be retreated if they did not comply with treatment or if there is rexposure to an untreated partner. Otherwise, *T. vaginalis* culture should be performed using an intraurethral swab or a first void urine specimen and should be treated as given below.

Metronidazole 2 g orally in a single dose
or
Tinidazole 2 g orally single dose
plus
Azithromycin 1 g orally in a single dose (if not used in initial episode)

Pathogenesis and Clinical Practice

Chemotactic markers of inflammation persist for weeks after treatment of acute NGU and are less marked in chlamydial than in non-chlamydial NGU.

The type of antibiotic used and the duration of treatment in the management of acute NGU does not affect the probability of development of recurrent or persistent NGU.

Reinfection with and persistence of *C. trachomatis* appears to be rare, but both *M. genitalium* and *U. urealyticum* have been implicated as causing persistent or recurrent NGU. A persistent immune response to chlamydial heat-shock protein (HSP)[60] has also been suggested as a cause.

Persistent NGU, whether symptomatic or asymptomatic, does not cause structural damage to the urethra or affect fertility.

Retreatment

1st line: Erythromycin 500 mg twice daily for two weeks plus Metronidazole 400 mg twice a day for five days.
2nd line: Erythromycin 500 mg four times daily for three weeks.

POST-GONOCOCCAL URETHRITIS

Men treated for gonorrhoea with penicillin, ciprofloxacin or aminoglycosides may have a recurrence of discharge containing polymorphonuclear leukocytes (PMNLs) but no *N. gonorrhoeae* on microscopy or culture. This may reflect the longer incubation period of infection with *C. trachomatis* compared to that of *N. gonorrhoeae*. The aetiology of this condition appears to be similar to that of NGU, although the role of *U. urealyticum* and other Mycoplasma spp. is even less clear.

Approximately 25% of heterosexual men with urethral *N. gonorrhoeae* infection are co-infected with *C. trachomatis,* and it is common practice to give treatment for both organisms when *N. gonorrhoeae* is identified. Co-infection is less common in homosexual men in most settings.

CHLAMYDIAL INFECTIONS

Chlamydia (from the Greek word meaning "cloak") is a common sexually transmitted disease (STD) caused by the bacterium, *Chlamydia trachomatis.* Chlamydia is a major infectious cause of human eye and genital disease.

They are small gram-negative obligate intracellular microorganisms that preferentially infect squamo-columnar epithelial cells.[60]

Chlamydia trachomatis is one of the 4 species (also including *Chlamydia puerorum*, *Chlamydia psittaci,* and *Chlamydia pneumoniae*) in the genus Chlamydia. *C. trachomatis* can be differentiated into 18 serovars (serologically variant strains) based on monoclonal antibody–based typing assays. Serovars A, B, Ba, and C are associated with trachoma (a serious eye disease that can lead to blindness), serovars D-K are associated with genital tract infections, and L1-L3 are associated with lymphogranuloma venereum ([LGV]).[60]

C. trachomatis is naturally found living inside human cells and is one of the most common sexually transmitted infections in people worldwide about 2.8 million cases of chlamydia infection occur in the United States each year.[61] Chlamydia can be transmitted during vaginal, anal, or oral sex, and can be passed from an infected mother to her baby during vaginal childbirth. Many people with Chlamydia exhibit no symptoms of infection. Between half and three-quarters of all women who have chlamydia have no symptoms and do not know that they are infected. If untreated, chlamydial infections can cause serious reproductive and other health problems with both short-term and long-term consequences. Chlamydia is easily treated with antibiotics.

Table 22.2 Human Diseases Caused by Chlamydia

Species	*Serovar*	*Disease*
C. psittaci	Many identified serotypes	Psittacosis
C. pneumoniae	TWAR	Respiratory disease
C. trachomatis	L1, L2 ,L3	Lymphogranuloma venerum (LGV)
C. trachomatis	A, B,Ba, C	Hyperendemic blinding trachoma
C.trachomatis	B, D, E, F, G,H, I,J,K	Inclusion conjunctivitis (adult and newborn), NGU and others

CHLAMYDIAL LIFE CYCLE

Chlamydiae are obligate intracellular bacterial pathogens, which mean they are unable to replicate outside the host cell. However, to disseminate effectively, these pathogens have evolved a unique biphasic life cycle wherein they alternate between two functionally and morphologically distinct forms.[62]

The pathophysiologic mechanisms of chlamydiae are poorly understood at best. The initial response to infected epithelial cells is a neutrophilic infiltration followed by lymphocytes, macrophages, plasma cells, and eosinophilic invasion. The release of cytokines and interferons by the infected epithelial cell initializes this inflammatory cascade.[60]

Infection with chlamydial organisms invokes a humoral cell response, resulting in secretory immunoglobulin A (IgA) and circulatory immunoglobulin M (IgM) and immunoglobulin G (IgG) antibodies and a cellular immune response. Recent studies have implicated a 40-kd major outer membrane protein (MOMP) and a 60-kd heat-shock protein (hsp60) in the immunopathologic response, but further studies are needed to better understand these cell-mediated immune responses.[60]

The elementary body (EB) is infectious, but metabolically inert (much like a spore), and can survive for limited amount of time in the extracellular milieu. Once the EB attaches to a susceptible host cell, it mediates its own internalization through pathogen-specified mechanisms (via type III secretion system) that allows for the recruitment of actin with subsequent engulfment of the bacterium.

The internalized EB, within a membrane-bound compartment, immediately begins differentiation into the reticulate body (RB). RBs are metabolically active but non-infectious, and in many regards, resemble normal replicating bacteria. The intracellular bacteria rapidly modify their membrane-bound compartment into the so-called chlamydial inclusion so as to prevent phagosome-lysosome fusion **(Fig. 22.1)**. According to published data, the inclusion has no interactions with the endocytic pathway and apparently inserts itself into the exocytic pathway as it retains the ability to intercept sphingomyelin-containing vesicles.

PERSISTENCE

Chlamydia have the ability to establish long-term associations with host cells. When an infected host cell is starved for various nutrients such as amino acids (e.g. tryptophan),[2] iron, or vitamins, this has a negative consequence for Chlamydia since the organism is dependent on the host cell for these nutrients.

The starved chlamydiae enter a persistent growth state wherein they stop cell division and become morphologically aberrant by increasing in size.[2] Persistent organisms remain viable as they are capable of returning to a normal growth state once conditions in the host cell improve.

There is much debate as to whether persistence has in vivo relevance. Many believe that persistent chlamydiae are the cause of chronic chlamydial diseases. Some antibiotics such as β-lactams can also induce a persistent-like growth state, which can contribute to the chronicity of chlamydial diseases.

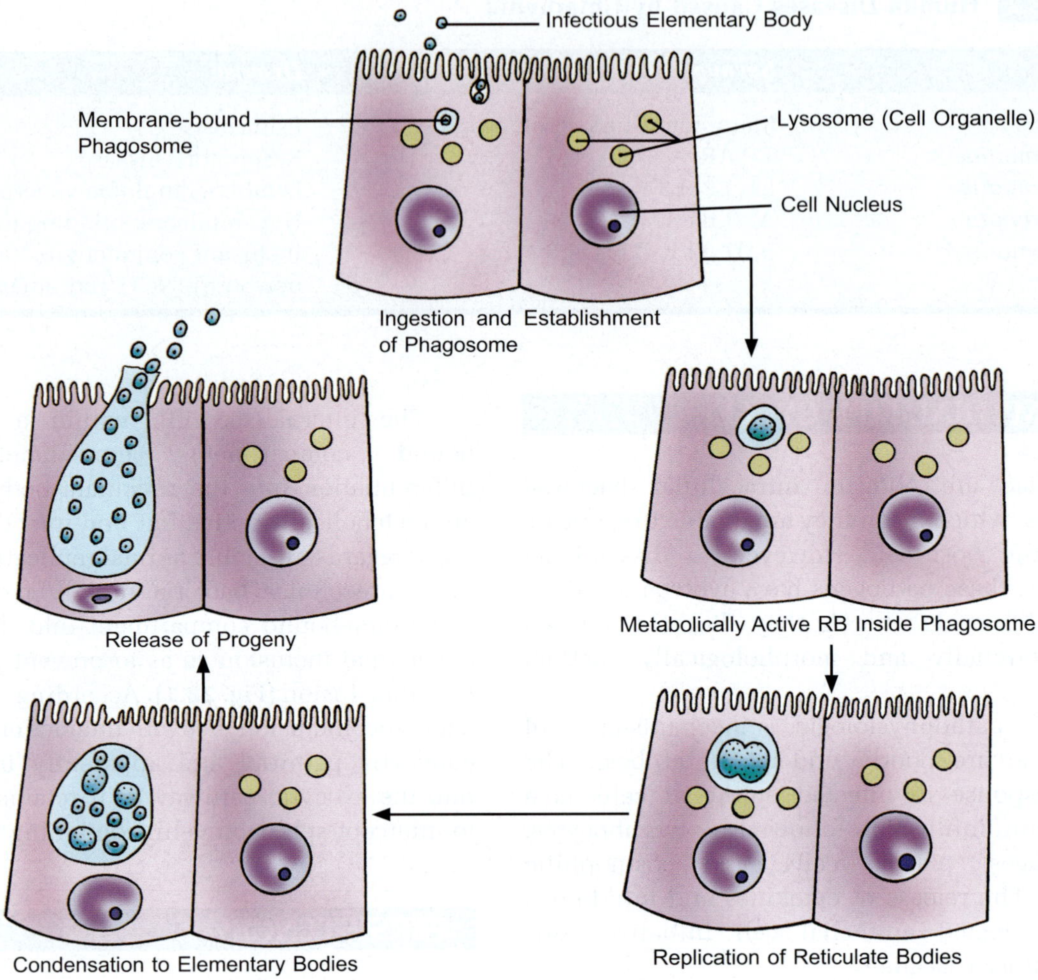

Fig. 22.1 Life Cycle of Chlamydia

Epidemiology

In 1995, the World Health Organization (WHO) estimated[89] a million cases of *C trachomatis* infection worldwide.[60] The incidence of chlamydial infection is not related to race per se but rather to the sexual histories of the individuals, including age of first sexual exposure and the frequency of exposure and use (or nonuse) of barrier protection.[60] Although the presence of asymptomatic infection with genitourinary chlamydiae can differ, acquisition of the infection is similar for both sexes.[60]

Chlamydia has been isolated in approximately 40-60% of males presenting with nongonococcal urethritis. Recent epidemiological studies indicate a high prevalence rate of asymptomatic men who act as a reservoir for chlamydial infections. A study by Quinn et al. (1996) demonstrated that transmission probability in both men and women is estimated at 68%.[65]

The risk factors identified for the disease are nonwhite race, multiple sex partners, age younger than 19 years, poor socioeconomic conditions, single marital status and nonbarrier contraceptive use.

Clinical Course

The incubation period is highly variable. Although it is considerd as 1-3 weeks, shorter and considerably longer incubation periods are also described.

The usual presentation is with low-grade urethritis with scanty or moderate mucoid or mucopurulent urethral discharge and variable dysuria, but in a majority of cases the appearance of the discharge and the severity of the condition make it clinically indistinguishable from gonococcal urethritis. In a small number of cases the discharge is accompanied by haematuria and symptoms of cystitis, when it is usually called 'acute abacterial haemorrhagic cystitis'. On the other hand, subclinical urethritis tends to be common. The patient does not notice the condition but it may be found in course of routine examination or when the patient presents with complications.

Table 22.3 **Clinical Syndromes Caused by *C. trachomatis***

	Site of Infection	*Clinical Syndrome*
Men	Urethra	NGU, PGU
	Epididymis	Epididymitis (Infertility)
	Systemic	Reiter's Syndrome
Women	Urethra	Urethritis (NGU/NSU)
	Bartholin's glands	Bartholinitis
	Cervix	Cervicitis
	Fallopian tubes	Salpingitis
		Ectopic pregnancy (spontaneous abortion)
	Uterus	Endometritis
	Liver	Perihepatitis
	Systemic	Arthritis
		Dermatitis
Both	Conjunctiva	Conjunctivitis
	Heart	Endocarditis
	Pharynx	Pharyngitis
	Inguinal lymph nodes	LGV
	Rectum	Proctitis
	Large intestine	Crohn's disease
	Systemic	Sexually acquired reactive arthritis (SARA)
Infants & Children	Conjunctiva	Conjunctivitis, Trachoma
	Lung	Pneumonia
		Chronic lung disease
	GIT	Gastroenteritis

Infections in Men

The prevalence of chlamydial urethral infection ranges from 3-5% of asymptomatic men seen in the general medical settings to 15-20% of all men seen in STDs clinics.[66,67] Of 1221 patients screened for urethral infection in a STDs clinic, 5% and 14% of homosexual and heterosexual men respectively had positive urethral cultures for *C. trachomatis*.[68] Serologic studies showed that chlamydial infection increased with age in homosexuals, but appeared relatively constant with increasing age in heterosexual and bisexual men. The incidence of chlamydial infections in men has not been well defined since in most countries, these infections, either not reported or microbiologically diagnosed or being asymptomatic, escape attention.

Urethritis

Clinically it is very difficult to differentiate between chlamydia positive and chlamydia negative NGU on the basis of signs and symptoms. Both usually present after a 7 to 21 day incubation period with dysuria and mild to moderate whitish or clear urethral discharge. Examination reveals no abnormalities other than discharge in most cases, associated adenopathy, focal urethral tenderness and meatal or penile lesions should suggest herpetic urethritis. Neither abnormal prostatic examination nor prostatic inflammation has been convincingly linked with chlamydial urethritis.[69]

Post-gonococcal urethritis (PGU) occurring in heterosexual men, like NGU, frequently results from *C. trachomatis*. These patients probably acquire gonorrhoea and chlamydial infection simultaneously but because of the longer incubation period of the latter, develop a biphasic illness if the gonorrhoea is treated with an agent that does not eradicate chlamydia. This has given rise to the development of the concept of syndromic approach.

Littritis

This is inflammation of Littre's glands, which are present in the wall of the urethra. It is probably inevitable in the course of any urethral infection.

Epididymitis

It has been proposed that *C. trachomatis* causes most cases of what was previously termed idiopathic epididymitis in young, heterosexually active males. Clinically, chlamydial epididymitis presents as unilateral scrotal pain, swelling, tenderness and fever in a young male who often has associated chlamydial urethritis. The urethritis, however, may often be asymptomatic and evident only as urethral inflammation on Gram stain. Men with chlamydial epididymitis improve rapidly with tetracycline treatment, supporting the causal role of *C. trachomatis*. However, one must exclude epididymo-orchitis, testicular torsion and malignancy before treatment.

Prostatitis

It should be more accurately called prostatovesiculitis due to simultaneous involvement of seminal vesicles. Despite several studies, the role of *C. trachomatis* in causing non-bacterial prostatitis (NBP) remains unclear[69], with NBP being the most common form of prostatic inflammation (40-60% of all prostatitis).[70] Some authors[71] point to an autoimmune aetiology and the role of urine reflux into the canaliculi of the gland causing chemical inflammation. The patient is generally asymptomatic, or may present with discomfort on passing urine and vague pain in the perineum, groins, thighs, penis, suprapubic region or back. There may also be painful ejaculation.

Proctitis

The clinical manifestations of rectal infection in infants and adult women have not been studied extensively. The clinical syndrome in homosexual men usually presents with subacute manifestations like proctocolitis and hyperplasia of intestinal and perirectal lymphoid tissue (lymphorrhoids) or late/chronic manifestations such as perirectal abscesses, ischiorectal fistula and rectal stricture or stenosis.

In men, the rectal mucosa can be infected directly with chlamydia during receptive anal intercourse or by lymphatic spread from the male posterior urethra. Most *C. trachomatis* infected patients have abnormal numbers of PMNL in their rectal mucous a on Gram stain and on sigmoidoscopy, those with symptoms exhibiting friable rectal mucosa and mucopus. In the pre-AIDS era, *C. trachomatis* appeared to be responsible for up to 15% of proctitis seen in homosexual males.[60] Proctitis is diagnosed by presence of >1 PMNL/hpf in rectal smear.

Reiter's Syndrome

Both Reiter's syndrome (urethritis, conjunctivitis, arthritis and characteristic mucocutaneous lesions) and reactive tenosynovitis or sexually acquired reactive arthritis (SARA) without the other components of Reiter's syndrome has been related to genital infection with *C. trachomatis*. Studies of untreated men with characteristic Reiter's syndrome using serology indicate that preceding or concurrent infection with *C. trochomatis* is present in 69% of the men who had signs of urogenital inflammation at the time of examination. The class 1 HLA –B27 haplotype appears to confer a ten fold increased risk of developing Reiter's syndrome, and 60-70% of persons with the syndrome are HLA-B27 positive.

Infections in Women

Cervicitis

The prevalence of chlamydial infections has ranged from 3-5% in asymptomatic women to over 20% of those attending STD clinics. The incidence of *C. trachomatis* infection in women is even less well-defined[68] than in men because the former produces no specific symptom, is rarely confirmed microbiologically and is not reported. Virtually no data on incidence is available. *C. trachomatis* causes cervicitis and is responsible for 60% of pelvic inflammatory disease (PID)[73] in Northern European countries. Genital tract infection in women is usually asymptomatic as compared to 5-10% of men attending genitourinary medicine (GUM) clinics.[74]

Although women with chlamydia isolated from the cervix are usually asymptomatic, at least one third of them generally have signs of infection on gynaecological examination. The most common presentation is a mucopurulent discharge **(Fig. 22.3)** (37%) and hypertrophic ectopy (19%).[58] The latter refers to an area of ectopy, which is oedematous, congested, and bleeds easily. The number of PMNL in cervical mucous is correlated with chlamydial infection of the cervix.[69] There appears to be a wide range of normal leukocyte values in women without cervical infection, possibly due to the influence of the menstrual cycle, contraceptive practices, sexual activity and other infections. One study[75] showed that on univariate analysis age, combined oral contraceptives and ectropian were risk factors for the laboratory detection of *C. trachomatis*. There was a reported association between the week of the menstrual cycle and the detection of *C. trachomatis*.[75] *C. trachomatis* was detected more often in the later part of the cycle, but others have found no such association.[76,77,78] The variation in the detection of *C. trachomatis* with the menstrual cycle could be either due to a direct hormonal effect on chlamydial replication or alternatively, due to an indirect effect acting through local immune factors, or a combination of both.[75]

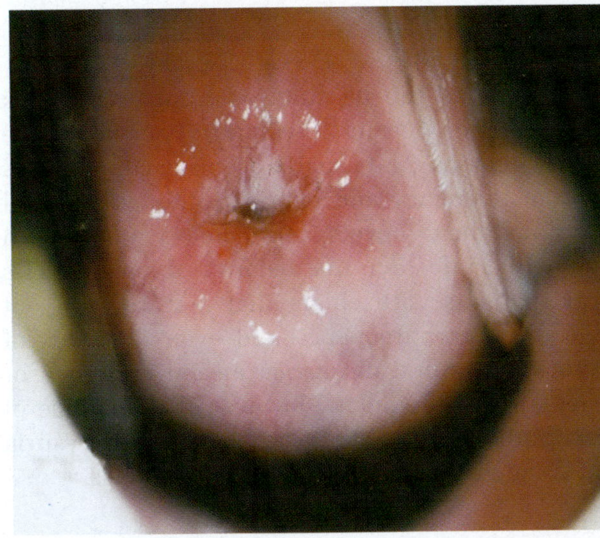

Fig. 22.2 Chlamydial Cervicitis in a Female Patient Mucopurulent Discharge, Erythema and Inflammation.

Clinical recognition of chlamydial cervicitis depends on a high index of suspicion and a careful cervical examination. There are hardly any genital symptoms which can specifically be correlated with chlamydial cervical infection. The clinical findings on examination suggestive of chlamydial infection include easily induced endocervical bleeding, mucopurulent endocervical discharge and oedema within an area of ectopy. The differential diagnosis of mucopurulent discharge from the endocervical canal in young, sexually active women includes gonococcal endocervicitis, salpingitis, endometritis and IUCD induced inflammation. Gram stain of appropriately collected mucopurulent endocervical discharge from patients having chlamydial endocervicitis usually shows more than 30 PMNL per 1000 field, absence of gonococci and occasional other bacteria.[69] Nearly all women with endocervical chlamydial infection have or develop antibodies to *C. trachomatis* in serum (20-30% have IgM antibody) assessed by micro-IF assay.

Urethritis

C. trachomatis can be cultured from both cervix and urethra in 50% of cases and either site alone in 25% of cases. The usual presenting complaint is dysuria, frequency and pyuria. Although urethral symptoms may develop in some women with chlamydial infection, the majority of female STDs clinic patients with chlamydial urethritis do not have dysuria or frequency and even the signs of urethritis (urethral discharge, meatal erythema or oedema) are infrequent. However, the presence of mucopurulent cervicitis in a woman with dysuria and frequency should suggest the diagnosis.

Bartholinitis

C. trachomatis may produce an exudative infection of Bartholin's ducts in a way similar to gonococci. Purulent Bartholinitis may be owing to chlamydial infection, either alone or with simultaneous gonococcal infection or some anaerobic organisms viz. *Bacteroides* spp.

Endometritis

Histological evidence of endometritis, often with immunohistological and or cultural evidence of *C. trachomatis* is present in about 50% of patients suffering from chlamydial mucopurulent cervicitis and in almost all patients having chlamydial salpingitis. There may also be associated abnormal vaginal bleeding, menorrhagia and metrorrhagia. Chlamydial endometritis is characterized by infiltration of the endometrial stroma by plasma cells and infiltration of the endometrial superficial epithelium by PMNL. Besides nonpuerperal endometritis, association of intrapartum fever and late post-partum endometritis with untreated antenatal *C. trachomatis* infection has been suggested.

Salpingitis

The proportion of acute salpingitis due to *C. trachomatis* varies geographically and with the population studied. Cases of chlamydial salpingitis are usually associated with mild or absent symptoms and signs. Despite progressive tubal scarring, they result in ectopic pregnancy and infertility, thus giving rise to the term "silent salpingitis".

Perihepatitis (Fitz-Hugh-Curtis Syndrome)

Previously, perihepatitis occuring after or with salpingitis was considered a complication of gonococcal infection. But studies in the last 15 years suggest that chlamydial infection is in fact more commonly associated with perihepatitis than with *N. gonorrhoeae*.[69] Perihepatitis should be suspected in young, sexually active women who develop right upper quadrant pain, fever, nausea or vomiting. It may present as an acute abdomen, and may also mimic acute cholecystitis. A recent study has demonstrated that perihepatitis is strongly associated with extensive tubal scarring, adhesions, and inflammation observed at laparoscopy as well as with high titres of antibody to the 57-kDa chlamydial heat shock protein.

Infection in Pregnancy

Chlamydial infection in pregnancy can cause (1) spontaneous abortion, (2) neonatal conjunctivitis, (3) low birth weight (LBW) (4) prematurity and (5) preterm delivery. Postnatal infection can cause (1) neonatal conjunctivitis, (2) ophthalmia neonatorum, (3) pneumonia and (4) chronic lung or eye diseases.

C. trachomatis infection of neonates results from perinatal exposure to the mother's infected cervix. Neonatal ocular prophylaxis with silver nitrate solution or antibiotic ointments does not prevent perinatal transmission of *C. trachomatis* from mother to infant in contrast to gonococcal opthalmia neonatorum. Initial *C. trachomatis* perinatal infection involves the mucus membrane of the eye , oropharanyx, urogenital tract and rectum and might be asymptomatic in these locations. It is most frequently recognized as conjunctivitis that develops at 5-12 days after birth. *C. trachomatis* can also cause a subacute, afebrile pneumonia with onset at ages 1-3 months.

LAB STUDIES[60]

- Cytologic diagnosis
  Cytologic diagnosis has been used to evaluate endocervical scrapings, but interpretation is difficult and sensitivity and specificity have been low.

- Isolation in cell culture
  - *C. trachomatis* grows well in a variety of cell lines (e.g, McCoy, HeLa cells) that can be maintained in tissue culture.
  - A carefully collected sample of columnar epithelial cells from the cervix or urethra is necessary and specimens composed purely of PMNL or mucopurulent discharge are inadequate.
  - For culture, specimens may be collected with a cotton tipped swab (wooden sticks are not recommended as they are inhibitory to chlamydial growth). For endocervical specimens, a cytobrush may increase the culture sensitivity due to collection of more cells. Specimens must be placed in specific transport media and kept refrigerated until they are inoculated within 24 hours onto cell culture plates.
  - Incubation in tissue culture takes 40-72 hours, depending on the cell type and specific biovar.
  - Intracytoplasmic inclusions can be detected either by Giemsa stains or by immunofluorescent staining with monoclonal antibodies.
  - Because of its high specificity (100%) and sensitivity, cell culture is the only test that should be used to establish the presence or absence of infections in cases with legal implications such as rape or sexual abuse.

- Antigen detection
  - By direct fluorescent antibody (DFA) and enzyme-linked immunosorbent assay
  - Antigen detection tests use monoclonal or polyclonal antibody against chlamydial lipopolysaccharide (LPS) or MOMP
  - Advantage: This is simpler, rapid and less expensive. Most studies report sensitivities greater than 70% and specificities of 97-99% in populations of men and women with a prevalence of infection of 5% or more.
  - Disadvantage: It is less sensitive when compared to tissue culture. In low-prevalence populations (i.e, <5% infected), a highly significant proportion of positive test results are false-positive. Therefore, verification of a positive test result is desirable in certain cases. Such verification can be by culture (i.e, a second nonculture test that identifies a different chlamydial antigen or nucleic acid sequence than the first test), a blocking antibody, or competitive probe.

- Nucleic acid hybridization
  - Detection of chlamydial ribosomal RNA (rRNA) by hybridization with a DNA probe
  - Commercially available as PAGE 2 assay by Genprobe.
  - It detects but does not amplify chlamydial nucleic acid and results on endocervical and urethral specimens are comparable to that of DFA and the best EIAs.

- Detection of chlamydial genes by DNA amplification tests
  - Polymerase chain reaction (PCR) and Ligase chain reaction (LCR)
  - Both of these tests can be used for cervical, urethral and urine specimens from both males and females. Although the PCR uses primers, nucleotides and the enzyme taq-polymerase, the LCR is based on the ligation of oligonucleotide probes that serve as a copy of the original target sequence and are immediately adjacent to each other.
  - The specificity of these tests has consistently been above 99%, with sensitivity comparable to that with urogenital swab specimens.
  - Another methodology, transcription-mediated amplification assay, amplifies specific chlamydial rRNA sequences

- Serology
  - o Using complement fixation test or micro-immunofluorescence test
  - o All patients with LGV or psittacosis have complement-fixing antibody titers of greater than 1:16, but among superficial genital tract infection, only 15% of men with urethritis and 45% of women with endocervical infection have titers 1:16 or greater. Women with salpingitis and perihepatitis have higher titres, over 1:256 and 1:1024 respectively
  - o Microimmunofluorescence test is, however, more sensitive than complement fixation test. Results are positive in 99% or more of women with cervicitis and in 80-90% of men with urethritis.

- Problems with serological tests
  - o Due to lack of an abrupt onset of symptoms in a lot of chlamydia infected patients, they are seen during periods when IgM antibody could not be demonstrated. So, antichlamydia IgM is uncommon in adults with genital tract infection
  - o The prevalence of antichlamydia IgG is high in sexually active adults, even in those who do not have an active infection, and is likely to be due to past infection.
  - o Cross reacting antibody developing to *Chlamydia pneumoniae* may obscure serodiagnosis.
  - o The sensitivity, specificity, and predictive values are not high enough to make any serology clinically useful in the diagnosis of active disease. Therefore, chlamydial serologies are not recommended for diagnosis of genital tract disease.

A summary of the diagnostic criteria in different clinical syndromes in men and women are given in Tables 22.4 and 22.5

Table 22.4 Diagnosis of *C. trachomatis* in Men

Clinical Syndrome	*Clinical Criteria*	*Laboratory Criteria*	
		Presumptive	*Diagnostic*
NGU	Dysuria, urethral discharge	Urethral GS* with >5 PMNL/HPF (× 1000) Pyuria on FVU	Positive culture or nonculture tests (urethra or FVU)
Acute epididymitis	Fever, epididymal or testicular pain, evidence of NGU, epididymal tenderness or mass	As for NGU	As for NGU; Positive test on epididymal aspirate
Acute proctitis (Non-LGV stain)	Rectal pain, discharge, bleeding, abnormal anoscopy (mucopurulent discharge, pain, spontaneous or induced bleeding)	Rectal GS with >1 PMNL/HPF (× 1000)	Positive culture or direct FA (rectal)
Acute proctocolitis (LGV strain)	Severe rectal pain, discharge, hematochezia, markedly abnormal anoscopy (as above) with lesions extending to colon; fever, lymphadenopathy	Rectal GS with > 1 PMNL/HPF (× 1000)	Positive culture or direct FA (rectal), complement fixation antibody litre

*GS = Gram Stain; PMNL = Polymorphonuclear leukocytes; NGU = Non-gonococcal urethritis, HPF = High-power Field; FA = Fluorescent antibody; FVU = First void urine; LGV = Lymphogranuloma venereum.

Table 22.5 Diagnosis of C. trachomatis Infections in Women[69]

Clinical Syndrome	*Clinical Criteria*	*Laboratory Criteria*	
		Presumptive	*Diagnostic*
Mucopurulent cervicitis	Mucopurulent cervical discharge, cervical ectopy and oedema, spontaneous or easily induced cervical bleeding	Cervical GS* with > 30 PMNL/HPF (× 1000) in NMW.	Positive culture or non-culture test (cervix, FVU).
Acute urethral syndrome	Dysuria–frequency syndrome in young, sexually active women, recent new sex partner, often > 7 days of symptoms.	Pyuria, no bacteria.	As above
PID	Lower abdominal pain; adnexal tenderness on pelvic exam; evidence of MPC often present.	As for MPC; cervical GS positive for gonococcus. Endometritis on endometrial biopsy.	Positive culture or non-culture test (cervix, FVU, endometrium, tubal).
Perihepatitis	Right upper quadrant pain, nausea, vomiting, fever, young sexually active women; evidence of PID.	As for MPC and PID.	High titre IgM or IgG antibody to *C. trachomatis*

*GS = Gram stain; PMNL = Polymorphonuclear leukocytes; HPF = High power field; NMW = Non-menstruating women; PID = Pelvic inflammatory disease; MPC = Mucopurulent cervicitis

TREATMENT

Treatment of *Chlamydia trachomatis* infections is tabulated below:

	WHO (2003)[79]	CDC (2006)[80]
Uncomplicated Anogenital Infection		
Recommended regimens	Doxycycline, 100 mg orally, twice daily for 7 days or Azithromycin, 1 g orally, in a single dose	Azithromycin, 1 g orally, in a single dose or Doxycycline, 100 mg orally, twice daily for 7 days
Alternative regimens	Amoxycilin, 500 mg orally, 3 times a day for 7 days or Erythromycin, 500 mg orally, 4 times a day for 7 days or Ofloxacin, 300 mg orally, twice a day for 7 days or Tetracycline, 500 mg orally, 4 times a day for 7 days	Erythromycin, 500 mg orally, 4 times a day for 7 days or Erythromycin ethylsuccinate 800 mg orally four times a day for 7 days or Oflaxcin 300 mg orally twice a day for 7 days or Levofloxacin 500 mg orally once daily for 7 days

(*Contd.*)

	WHO (2003)[79]	CDC (2006)[80]
Chlamydial infection during pregnancy		
Recommended regimens	Erythromycin, 500 mg orally, 4 times a day for 7 days or Amoxycillin, 500mg orally, 3 times a day for 7 days	Azithromycin, 1 g orally, in a single dose or Amoxycillin, 500mg orally, 3 times a day for 7 days
Alternative regimens		Erythromycin base 500 mg orally four times daily for 7 days or Erythromycin base 250 mg orally four times a day for 14 days or Erythromycin ethylsuccinate 800 mg orally four times daily for 7 days or Erythromycin ethylsuccinate 400 mg orally four times daily for 14 days
Neonatal chlamydial conjunctivitis		
Recommended regimens	Erythromycin syrup, 50 mg/kg per day orally, in 4 divided doses for 14 days	Erythromycin base or ethyl succinate syrup, 50 mg/kg per day orally, in 4 divided doses for 14 days
Alternative regimens	Trimethoprim 40 mg with sulfamethoxazole 200 mg orally, twice daily for 14 days	
Infantile pneumonia		
Recommended regimens	Erythromycin syrup, 50 mg/kg per day orally, in 4 divided doses for 14 days	Erythromycin base or ethyl succinate syrup, 50 mg/kg per day orally, in 4 divided doses for 14 days

Follow up: Patients should be instructed to return for evaluation if symptoms persist or recur after completion of therapy. Symptoms alone, without documentation of signs or laboratory evidence of urethral inflammation, are not a sufficient basis for retreatment. Patients should be instructed to abstain from sexual intercourse until 7 days after therapy is initiated, provided their symptoms have resolved and their sex partners have been adequately treated. Persistence of pain, discomfort, and irritative voiding symptoms beyond 3 months should alert the clinician to the possibility of chronic prostatitis/chronic pelvic syndrome in men.

Management of Partner: According to CDC 2006, persons with NGU should refer evaluation and treatment for all sex partners within proceeding 60 days.

Prognosis

The natural history of NGU suggests that it is a self limiting disease even without treatment. Nowadays, the local complications are relatively uncommon as compared to the premicrobial era. Complications are similar to those seen in gonorrhoea but milder. Dissemination, however, to other sites is known. 1-2% of both *C. trachomatis* positive and negative individuals develop epididymitis and another 1-2% develop conjunctivitis. The frequency of NGU patients developing Reiter's disease and SARA is also very low; however, its rate can be decreased by initiating therapy in both chlamydial NGU and NCNGU patients, even in HLA-B27-positive individuals. In certain individuals, NGU creates significant psychologic turmoil and counselling from a psychologist is needed.

Acknowledgement

The authors acknowledge the contribution of Dr S Mazumdar and Dr GC Saha who were authors of this chapter in first edition of this book.

REFERENCES

1. Marrazzo JM. Mucopurulent cervicitis: no longer ignored, but still misunderstood. Infectious Disease Clinics of North America 2005; 19: 333-49.
2. Deguchi T, Maeda S. Mycoplasma genitalium: another important pathogen of nongonococcal urethritis. Urology 2002; 167: 1210-7.
3. Jensen JS. Mycoplasma genitalium: the aetiological agent of urethritis and other sexually transmitted diseases. Journal of the Europ Acad Dermatol Venereol 2004; 18: 1-11.
4. Falk L, Fredlund H, Jensen JS. Symptomatic urethritis is more prevalent in men infected with Mycoplasma genitalium than with *Chlamydia trachomatis*. Sex Transm Infect 2004; 80: 289-93.
5. Haddow LJ, Bunn A, Copas AJ, et al. Polymorph count for predicting non-gonococcal urethral infection: a model using *Chlamydia trachomatis* diagnosed by ligase chain reaction. Sex Transm Infect 2004; 80: 198-200.
6. Centers for Disease Control and Prevention. Sexually transmitted diseases treatment guidelines 2002. MMWR 2002; 51 (no. RR-6): 30–2. www.cdc.gov/stds/treatment/rr5106.pdf.
7. *Chlamydia trachomatis*: summary and conclusions of CMO's Expert Advisory Group. London; Department of Health: 1998.
8. Duncan B, Hart G, Scoular A et al. Qualitative analysis of the psychosocial impact of diagnosis of *Chlamydia trachomatis*: implications for screening. BMJ 2001; 322: 195-8.
9. Guaschino S, De Seta F. Update on *Chlamydia trachomatis*. Ann N Y Acad Sci 2000; 900: 293-300.
10. Horner P, Owen C E. Clinical effectiveness guideline for the management of *Chlamydia trachomatis* genital tract infection 2002. www.bashh.org/guidelines/C4A%2009%2001c.pdf.
11. Management of genital *Chlamydia trachomatis* infection. SIGN Publication number 42. Edinburgh; SIGN Secretariat: 2000.
12. McMillan S, McKenzie H, Flett G, et al. Which women should be tested for *Chlamydia trachomatis*? Br J Obstet Gynaecol 2000; 107: 1088-93.
13. Paavonen J, Eggert-Kruse W. *Chlamydia trachomatis*: impact on human reproduction. Hum Reprod Update 1999; 5: 433-47.
14. Ross JD. Outpatient antibiotics for pelvic inflammatory disease. BMJ 2001; 322: 251-2.
15. Sellors J, Mahony J, Goldsmith C et al. The accuracy of clinical findings and laparoscopy in pelvic inflammatory disease. Am J Obstet Gynecol 1991; 164: 113-20.

16. Sweet RL. Role of bacterial vaginosis in pelvic inflammatory disease. CID 1995; 20 (Suppl 2): S271–S275.
17. Leung A, Eastick K, Haddon L et al. Mycolpasma genatalium is associated with symptomatic urethritis. Int J of STDs AIDS 2006; 17: 285-8.
18. Geisler WM, Yu S, Hook EW III. Chlamydial and gonococcal infection in men without polymorphonuclear leukocytes on gram stain: implications for diagnostic approach and management. Sex Trans Dis 2005; 32: 630-4.
19. Marrazzo JM, Whittington WL, Celum CL, et al. Urine-based screening for *Chlamydia trachomatis* in men attending sexually transmitted disease clinics. [erratum appears in Sex Transm Dis 2001; 28: 429]. Sexually Transmitted Diseases 2001; 28: 219-25.
20. Mena L, Wang X, Mroczkowski TF, et al. Mycoplasma genitalium infections in asymptomatic men and men with urethritis attending a sexually transmitted diseases clinic in New Orleans. Clin Infect Dis 2002; 35: 1167-73.
21. Horner PJ, Thomas B, Gilroy CB, et al. Do all men attending departments of genitourinary medicine need to be screened for non-gonococcal urethritis. Int J of STDs AIDS 2002; 13: 667-73.
22. Bradshaw CS, Tabrizi SN, Read TR et al. Etiologies of nongonococcal urethritis: bacteria, viruses, and the association with orogenital exposure. [see comment]. J of Infect Dis 2006; 193: 336-45.
23. Schwebke JR, Lawing LF. Improved detection by DNA amplification of *Trichomonas vaginalis* in males. Journal of Clin Microbiol 2002; 40: 3681-3.
24. Joyner JL, Douglas JM Jr, Ragsdale S. Comparative prevalence of infection with *Trichomonas vaginalis* among men attending a sexually transmitted diseases clinic.[see comment]. Sex Transm Dis 2000; 27: 236-40.
25. Povlsen K, Bjornelius E, Lidbrink P, et al. Relationship of Ureaplasma urealyticum biovar 2 to nongonococcal urethritis. Europ J Clin Microbiol Infect Dis 2002; 21: 97-101.
26. Leung A, Horner P. Urinary tract infection in patients with acute non-gonococcal urethritis. Int J STDs & AIDS 2003; 13: 801-4.
27. Tabrizi SN, Ling AE, Bradshaw CS, et al. Human adenoviruses types associated with non-gonococcal urethritis. Sex Health 2007; 4: 41-4.
28. Srugo I, Steinberg J, Madeb R, et al. Agents of non-gonococcal urethritis in males attending an Israeli clinic for sexually transmitted diseases. [see comment]. Israel Medical Association Journal: Imaj 2003; 5: 24-7.
29. Shahmanesh M. Problems with non-gonococcal urethritis. Int J STDs AIDS 1994; 5: 390-9.
30. Swartz SL, Kraus SJ, Herrmann KL et al. Diagnosis and etiology of nongonococcal urethritis. J Infect Dis 1978; 138: 445-54.
31. Rietmeijer CA, Judson FN, Van Hensbroek MB et al. Unsuspected *Chlamydia trachomatis* infection in heterosexual men attending a sexually transmitted diseases clinic: evaluation of risk factors and screening methods. Sex Transm Dis 1991; 18: 28-35.
32. Janier M, Lassau F, Casin I,et al. Male urethritis with and without discharge: a clinical and microbiological study. Sex Trans Dis 1995; 22: 244-52.
33. Iser P, Read TH, Tabrizi S, et al. Symptoms of non-gonococcal urethritis in heterosexual men: a case control study. Sex Transm Infect 2005; 81: 163-5.
34. Dupin N, Bijaoui G, Schwarzinger M, et al. Detection and quantification of Mycoplasma genitalium in male patients with urethritis. Clin Infect Dis 2003; 37: 602-5.
35. Jensen JS, Bjornelius E, Dohn B, et al. Use of TaqMan 5' nuclease real-time PCR for quantitative detection of Mycoplasma genitalium DNA in males with and without urethritis who were attendees at a sexually transmitted disease clinic. J Clini Microbiol 2004; 42: 683-92.
36. Simms I, Eastick K, Mallinson H, et al. Associations between Mycoplasma genitalium, *Chlamydia trachomatis* and pelvic inflammatory disease. J Clin Pathol 2003; 56: 616-8.
37. Ross JD. Pelvic Inflammatory Disease: how should it be managed. Curr Opin Infect Dis 2003; 16: 37-41.
38. Ross JD, Jensen JS. Mycoplasma genitalium as a sexually transmitted infection: implications for

screening, testing, and treatment. Sex Transm Infect 2006; 82: 269-71.
39. Kamwendo F, Johansson E, Moi H, et al. Gonorrhea, genital chlamydial infection, and nonspecific urethritis in male partners of women hospitalized and treated for acute pelvic inflammatory disease. Sex Transm Dis 1993; 20: 143-6.
40. Centers for Disease Control and Prevention. 1998 guidelines for the treatment of sexually transmitted diseases. MMWR 1998; 47: 11.
41. Patrick DM, Rekart ML, Knowles L. Unsatisfactory performance of the leukocyte esterase test of first voided urine for rapid diagnosis of urethritis. Genitourin Med 1994; 70: 187-90.
42. Fraser PA, Teasdale J, Gan KS, et al. Neutrophil enzymes in urine for the detection of urethral infection in men. Genitourin Med 1995; 71: 176-9.
43. Horner PJ. Should we still be testing for asymptomatic non-specific urethritis in departments of genitourinary medicine? Int J STDs AIDS 2005; 16: 273-7.
44. O'Mahony C. View from the frontline. Int J STDs AIDS 2004; 15: 498.
45. Manavi K, McMillan A, Young H, et al. Genital infection in male partners of women with chlamydial infection. Interna J STDs AIDS 2006; 17: 34-6.
46. Tait IA, Hart CA. *Chlamydia trachomatis* in non-gonococcal urethritis patients and their heterosexual partners: routine testing by polymerase chain reaction. Sex Transm Infect 2002; 78: 286-8.
47. Marcos AR. The incidence of sexually related conditions in asymptomatic vesus symptomatic patients. Intern J STDs AIDS 2007; 18: 610-2.
48. Chernesky MA, Martin DH, Hook EW, et al. Ability of new APTIMA CT and APTIMA GC assays to detect *Chlamydia trachomatis* and *Neisseria gonorrhoeae* in male urine and urethral swabs. J Clin Microbiol 2005; 43: 127-31.
49. Foo C, Browne R, Boag F. Retrospective review of the correlation of symptoms, signs and microscopy with the diagnosis of *Chlamydia trachomatis* in men. Int J STDs AIDS 2004; 15: 319-21.
50. Anagrius C, Lore B, Jensen JS. Mycoplasma genitalium: prevalence, clinical significance, and transmission. Sex Transm Infect 2005; 81: 458-62.
51. Jensen JS, Bjornelius E, Dohn B, et al. Comparison of first void urine and urogenital swab specimens for detection of Mycoplasma genitalium and *Chlamydia trachomatis* by polymerase chain reaction in patients attending a sexually transmitted disease clinic. Sexu Transm Dis 2004; 31: 499-507.
52. National Guidelines (2007) on the management of Non-gonococcal urethritis. Clinical effectiveness group (British Association for Sexual Health and HIV- BASHH). www.bashh.org/guidelines 2007/2007_NGU_national_guideline.pdf
53. Falk L, Fredlund H, Jensen JS. Tetracycline treatment does not eradicate Mycoplasma genitalium. Sex Transm Infect 2003; 79: 318-9.
54. Mroczkowsky TF, Mena L, Nsuami M. A randomized comparison of azithromycin and doxycycline for the treatment of Mycoplasma genitalium (MG) positive urethritis. 16th Biennial Meeting of the International Society of Sexually Transmitted Disease (ISSTDR), Amsterdam, The Netherlands 2005; 304-5.
55. Wikstrom A, Jensen JS. Mycoplasma genitalium: a common cause of persistent urethritis among men treated with doxycycline. Sex Transm Infect 2006; 82: 276-9.
56. Horner P, Thomas B, Gilroy C, et al. The role of Mycoplasma genitalium and Ureaplasma urealyticum in acute and chronic non-gonococcal urethritis. Clin Infec Dis 2001; 32: 995-1003.
57. Horner PJ, Cain D, McClure M, et al. Association of antibodies to *Chlamydia trachomatis* heat-shock protein 60 kD with chronic nongonococcal urethritis. Clin Infect Diseases 1997; 24: 653-60.
58. Munday PE. Persistent and recurrent non-gonococcal urethritis. In: Taylor-Robinson D, editor. Clinical problems in sexually transmited diseses. Dordrecht: Martinun Nijhoff; 1985. 15-34.
59. Hay PE, Thomas B, Gilchrist C, et al. A reappraisal of chlamydial and non-chlamydial

urethritis. International Journal of STDs AIDS 1992; 3, 191-5.

60. Lutwick LI. Chlamydial genitourinary infections: Article Last Updated: Nov 26, 2007. www.emedicine.com/med/topic340.htm
61. www.chlamydiae.com (professional) - Taxonomy diagram. Chlamydia fact sheet from the Centers for Disease Control and Prevention. Retrieved on 2007; 10-27.
62. www.chlamydiae.com (professional) Retrieved on 2007; 10-27.
63. Leonhardt RM, Lee SJ, Kavathas PB, et al. Severe Tryptophan Starvation Blocks Onset of Conventional Persistence and Reduces Reactivation of *Chlamydia trachomatis*. Infect. Immun 2007; 75: 5105-17.
64. Mpiga P, Ravaoarinoro M. Chlamydia trachomatis persistence: an update. Microbiol. Res 2006; 161: 9-19.
65. Quinn TC, Gaydos C, Shepherd M. Epidemiologic and microbiologic correlates of *Chlamydia trachomatis* infection in sexual partnerships. JAMA 1996; 276: 1737-42.
66. Thelvin I, Wennstrom AM, March PA. Contact tracing in patients with genital chlamydial infections. Br J Vener Dis 1980; 56: 259-64.
67. McMillan A, Sommer Ville RG, Mckie PMK. Chlamydial infection in homosexual men. Frequency of isolation of *Chlamydia trachomatis* from urethra, anorectum and pharynx. Br J Vener Dis 1981; 57: 47-9.
68. Tiwari VD, Talwar S, Grewal RS. Urethritis Pelvic inflam-matory disease and Reiter's Disease Valia RG, Valia AR, eds In. IADVL Textbook of Dermatology. 2nd Ed. Bhalani Publishing House; 2001. Mumbai: p. 1423-52.
69. Stamm WE. *Chlamydia trachomatis* infections eds. adult. In: Holmes KK, Mardh PA, Sparling SF, et al. eds. Sexually Transmitted Diseases, 3rd ed. New York: McGraw–Hill; 1999. p. 407-22.
70. Ostaszewska I, Zdrodowska-Stefanow B, Badyda J. et al. *Chlamydia trachomatis*: probable cause of prostatitis. Int J STDs AIDS 1998; 9: 350-3.
71. Keetch DW, Humphrey P, Ratliff TL. Development at mouse modal for nonbacterial prostatitis. J Urol 1994; 10: 274-80.
72. Shahmanesh M, Pandit PG, Round R. Urethral lymphocyte isolation in non-gonococcal urethritis. Genitourin Med 1996; 72: 362-4.
73. Westrom L, Wolmer–Hanssen P. Pathogenesis of pelvic inflammatory disease. Genitourin Med 1993; 69: 9-17.
74. Taylor–Robinson D. *Chlamydia trachomatis* and sexually transmitted disease. BMJ 1993; 308: 150-1.
75. Crowley T, Horner P, Hughes A, et al. Hormonal factors and the laboratory detection of *Chlamydia trachomatis* in women: implications for screening? Int J STDs AIDS 1997; 8: 25-31.
76. Arya OP, Mallinson H, Goddard AD. Epidemiological and clinical correlates of chlamydia infection of the cervix. Br J Ven Dis 1981; 57: 118-24.
77. Tait A, Rees E, Hobson D et al. Chlamydia infection of the cervix in contacts of men with non-gonococcal urethritis. Br J Ven Dis 1979; 8: 37-45.
78. Orien JD, Johnson AL, Nayyar U et al. Infection of the uterine cervix with *Chlamydia trachomatis*. J Infect Dis 1978; 137: 443-51.
79. WHO guidelines for the management of sexually transmitted infections 2003; 36-8.
80. Centers for Disease Control and Prevention. Sexually transmitted diseases treatment guidelines 2006. MMWR 2006; 55 : 35-7.

23 LYMPHOGRANULOMA VENEREUM

A K Bajaj, Rajeev Sharma

In this chapter

- Synonyms
- Definition
- Prevalence
- Aetiological Agent
- Transmission
- Clinical Stages
- Inguinal Syndrome (Bubo)
- Genito-Ano-Rectal Syndrome
- Rare Manifestations
- Diagnosis
- Treatment

SYNONYMS

Climatic bubo, Tropical bubo, Lymphopathia venereum, Lymphogranuloma inguinale, Durand-Nicholas-Favre disease

Description of lymphogranuloma venereum (LGV) dates back to 1833 when Walkee first identified the condition. It was extensively studied and described in detail by Durand, Nicolas and Favre. It was Frei, in 1925 who for the first time developed a intradermal test. *Chlamydia trachomatis* was first identified as the causative agent of LGV in 1927. The causal relationship was established by inoculating monkeys (intracerebral) by Favre and Hellerstom. The first successful drug for treating LGV was a sulphonamide. LGV was first described from India in 1902 by Caddy.[1]

DEFINITION

Lymphogranuloma venereum (LGV) is a sexually transmitted infection affecting primarily the lymphatic system, caused by *Chlamydia trachomatis* serovars L1, L2 and L3. It is characterized by regional suppurative lymphadenopathy, which is preceded by a small transient, inconspicuous lesion at the site of inoculation, usually the genitalia.

PREVALENCE

LGV has a worldwide distribution and no predilection for any race, colour or religion. However, it occurs more commonly in the tropical and the subtropical regions. It is endemic in India and South-East Asia, East and West Africa, South America and the Caribbean islands.[2] Cases have been reported from Europe, North America and Australia mostly in people travelling to or living in the endemic area.[3]

Actual prevalence in India is not known. The data from STDs clinics in different parts of India indicates a prevalence rate of 6%, ranging from 0.27% to 11.5%.[4-20] A higher incidence (8%) was reported from Madagascar.[21] It is a relatively uncommon sexually transmitted disease (STD). Recently there was an epidemic of LGV with HIV infection with crack cocaine use in Bahamas,[22] later in Europe, United Kingdom and Australia, especially in men having sex with men (MSM) presenting with symptomatic proctitis and high prevalence of HIV coinfection.[23,24]

AETIOLOGICAL AGENT

Chlamydia are gram-negative, intracellular, obligate parasites. They measure from 0.3 to 1.0μ. In their infective state they have a cell wall, contain both DNA and RNA and divide by binary fission. *Chlamydia* are divided into four species, *Chlamydia trachomatis, Chlamydia psittcai, C. pneumoniae and C. pecorum.*[23] *C. trachomatis* has two major biovars, Trachoma (TRIC) and LGV. There are 15 serotypes and types L1, L2 and L3 cause LGV.[22] Infection occurs by a metabolically inactive form of *Chlamydia* called 'elementary bodies'. These undergo changes to form a metabolically active 'reticular body' in 6-8 hours of infection. The organisms lack the ability to synthesize high-energy compounds such as ATP. They multiply in the host cells by binary fission. After a few such fissions, the reticular body cells condense and form an elementary body. The newly formed elementary bodies burst out of the host cells. The complete cycle takes about 48-72 hours. Human beings are the sole natural hosts for *C. trachomatis*. It can be experimentally transmitted to monkeys, mice and guinea pigs. It can be readily grown in the yolk sac of developing chick embryo, HeLa 229 cell line culture, and McCoy tissue culture.[25,26] It is inactivated by low concentrations of formalin, phenol or ether and by heat (56°C).[1]

TRANSMISSION

LGV is a sexually transmitted infection. Rarely it can be transmitted by non-sexual contact.[25] There is no vertical transmission of the infection but infection may occur while passing through an infected birth canal.[2]

CLINICAL STAGES

The incubation period is usually around a week (3-12 days) or longer. LGV has early as well as late manifestations.[2] The clinical features can be divided into a primary stage, secondary (inguinal stage) and a tertiary stage (complications).[26,27]

The primary lesion is almost never noticed. The primary lesion, if present, usually last for 2-3 days. About one fourth of the patients, present with a papule, a vesicle, erosion or an ulcerated area at the site of inoculation. The site usually is the coronal sulcus of glans in men, and posterior vaginal wall in the women. The lesions may also occur on fraenum, prepuce, shaft of penis, urethra and scrotum in men and fourchette, vulva and posterior lip of cervix in women. In both sexes, the lesions may have anal, rectal or oral localization according to their sexual practice. Non-specific urethritis may be a manifestation in a rare case.[28] Very rarely primary lesions of LGV may occur in the tonsils, nasolabial folds, and submammary and umbilical regions.

Lymphangitis occurs on the dorsal aspect of the penis and soon a chord like swelling called bubonulus makes its appearance in men. Very often lymphangitis leads to phimosis in men and genital swelling in women. The disease then localizes in the regional lymph nodes.[1,2]

INGUINAL SYNDROME (BUBO)

A characteristic unilateral inflammatory swelling of the inguinal lymph nodes and their corresponding draining lymph nodes, is the most common presentation of LGV in men **(Fig. 23.1)**. The involvement may be bilateral in about one third cases **(Fig. 23.2)**. The interval between appearance of bubo and the time of exposure varies from 10 days to 6 months, but on an average, it takes about 10-30 days.[1,2]

Initially the superio-medial group of inguinal lymph nodes is involved in most cases but in some cases, the lateral group may also get involved. Pain accompanies a firm elastic swelling. The pain gradually increases in severity and forces the patient to walk with a limp, bending forward to control pain. The bubo then becomes fluctuant within 1 to 2 weeks The whole chain of lymph nodes in the inguino-cruro-iliac group may get involved. The lymphnodes soon become matted, the overlying skin becomes thick and dusky, and soon the bubo becomes ready to rupture.[1,2]

In about 20% of patients femoral group of lymph nodes are also involved and may be separated by the Poupart's ligament from the enlarged inguinal lymphnodes, producing the **groove sign of Greenblat (Fig. 23.3)**.[2]

Constitutional symptoms often precede or follow the development of the bubo. Symptoms accompanying bubo are fever, chills, sweating, loss of appetite, joint pains and myalgia. Pain and fever are relieved once the bubo ruptures.[1,2] Suppuration **(Fig. 23.4)** occurs in majority (60-70%) of the cases while spontaneous resolution in 25-30 percent cases, while in another 5 percent cases the adenitis may persist for months. The sites of suppuration are the inguinal lymph nodes at multiple foci, giving rise to multiple sinuses.

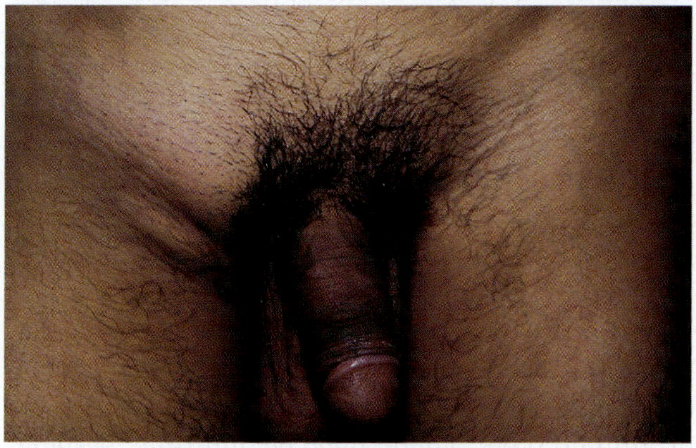

Fig. 23.1 Lymphogranuloma Venereum–Unilateral Bubo.

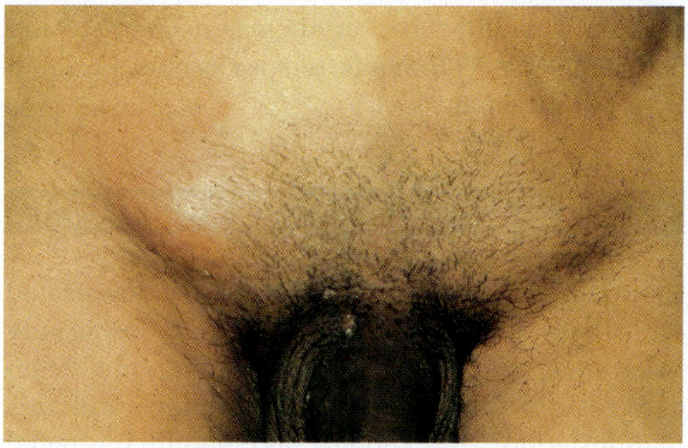

Fig. 23.2 Lymphogranuloma Venereum – Bilateral Bubo.

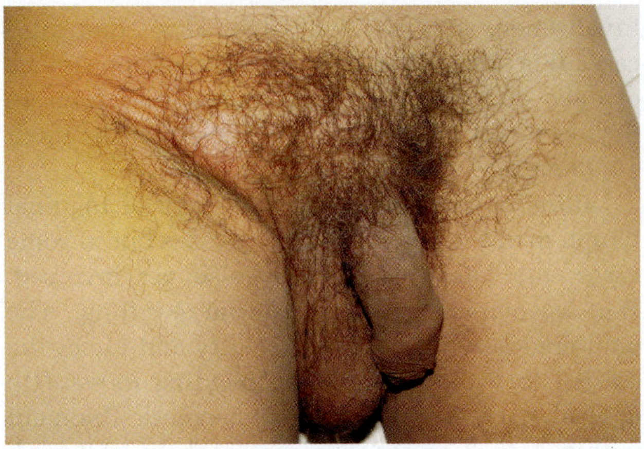

Fig. 23.3 Lymphogranuloma Venereum – Groove Sign.

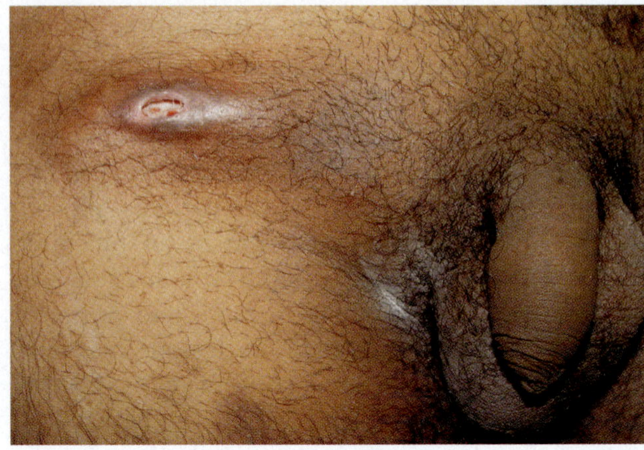

Fig. 23.4 Lymphogranuloma Venereum – Bubo with Discharging Sinus.

These sinuses may persist for few weeks to many months. Secondary infection is common. Healing is very slow and leaves behind contracted scars in the inguinal region. The iliac lymph nodes may rarely suppurate, but they usually undergo spontaneous resolution.[1,2]

Bilateral inguinal lymph node involvement leads to elephantiasis of the genitalia. Less than one third of the female patients with LGV develop inguinal lymphadenopathy. About one third complain of lower abdominal and back pain despite having no anorectal involvement, indicating the involvement of the deep pelvic and lumbar lymph nodes.[2]

Rarely, dissemination of the organism may occur via blood stream and produce systemic disease, which may present clinically as hepatitis, pneumonitis, spondyloarthritis, endocarditis, erythema multiforme, erythema nodosum, and ocular disease.[1,2] Bubonic relapse occurs in about 20% of untreated cases.[2]

GENITO-ANO-RECTAL SYNDROME

Genital involvement in LGV may be associated with hyperplastic ulcerative lesions, especially in women with LGV. Such lesions are often associated with ano-rectal involvement and this manifestation is known as genito-ano-rectal syndrome.[1] The characteristic features being proctocolitis, hyperplasia of the lymphatic tissue (lymphorrhoids), abscess formation, fistulae, stricture formation, chronic ulceration and scarring. The commonly affected sites are rectum and vagina.[2,26]

Anorectal involvement occurs mostly in women and homosexual men. It follows inoculation of the rectal mucosa by *Chlamydia* during peno-anal intercourse. It may also occur secondary to involvement of the posterior urethra in men, and by direct spread from vaginal secretions or by lymphatic dissemination from the cervix or posterior vaginal wall in women.[2] Perianal oedema associated with diffuse oedema of the anorectal mucosa is the only early change noticed. It may present as pruritus ani in the first few weeks. This is followed by development of multiple fissures around the anal margin. The examining finger encounters a pebbled anorectal mucosa but the elasticity of the mucosa is retained.[1]

Submucosal swellings develop as the anorectal and pararectal lymphnodes are enlarged. The rectal mucosa may have an ulcerated or granulomatous appearance on proctoscopy. The patient may have tenesmus and blood stained rectal discharge. After 3-6 months, the anorectal mucosa becomes rigid and rugose with narrowing of the lumen secondary to involvement of all layers of the bowel. Later on, fully developed stricture can be felt on every rectal examination. The stricture may be annular, tubular or funnel type. There may be multiple perianal swellings and tags associated with strictures.[1]

Complications

Lymphatic obstruction leads to elephantiasis of the genitalia. The manifestation in men can be in form of (i) ram-horn penis, and (ii) saxophone penis; both being result of chronic, massive oedema of the penis.

In women, chronic oedema leads to enlargement of the vulva (elephantiasis) often referred to as 'esthiomene' **(Fig. 23.5)**.[2,29] The appearance clinically may vary from swelling of one lip to giant lobulated masses hanging and obstructing the vaginal cleft. Fistulae involving the rectum and vagina, urethra and vagina, cervix and vagina or vulva may occur in women.[1] Stricture of the urethra, prostatitis, seminal vesiculitis and epididymo-orchitis may occur rarely in men.[1] Carcinoma of the rectum is known to develop in 2-5% cases of rectal stricture due to LGV.

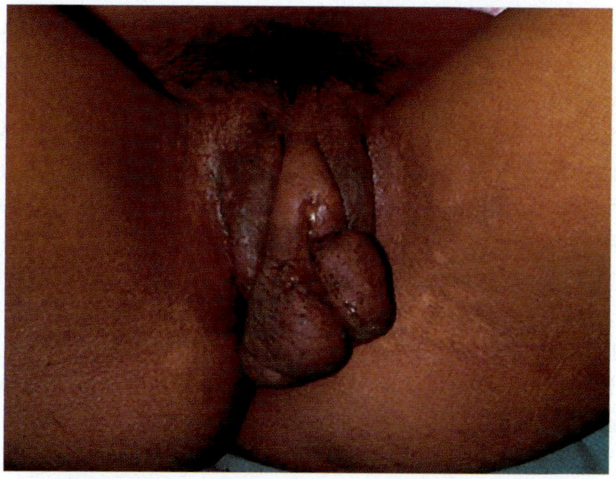

Fig. 23.5 Lymphogranuloma Venereum - Esthiomene.

RARE MANIFESTATIONS

Papillary growths on the urinary meatus in women may lead to various urinary symptoms.[2] Uretro-genito-perineal syndrome may manifest as multiple penile, scrotal or perineal sinuses with or without urethral stenosis.[30] Generalized exanthem-papular, papulopustular, nodular, erythema nodosum and erythema multiforme have been reported.

Unilateral follicular conjunctivitis with regional lymphadenopathy may be a presenting feature after autoinoculation.[30] Rarely bilateral conjunctivitis, episcleritis, keratitis or iritis may develop during the course of LGV.[31] Extragenital LGV may lead to enlargement of the axillary or cervical lymph nodes[2,32] and psoas abscess.[33]

Table 23.1 **LGV versus Chancroid Bubo**

LGV Bubo	*Chancroid Bubo*
Genital ulcer not present	Genital ulcer present
Bubo is less painful	Bubo is painful
Constitutional symptoms present	Constitutional symptoms present
Seen in 66.7% cases	Seen in 40% cases
Bilateral in 1/3 cases	Mostly unilateral but can also be bilateral
Groove sign is positive	Groove sign may be positive
Matting of lymph nodes is present	Absent
Multilocular suppurative swelling	Unilocular suppurative swelling
Ruptures to form multiple sinuses	Ruptures to form an ulcer
Heals slowly with scarring	Heals with treatment with less scarring

DIAGNOSIS

The main differential diagnosis is chancroid and clinical differences of LGV and chancroid bubo are given in Table 23.1.

The diagnosis is established after taking careful history and proper clinical examination, looking specially, for painful adenopathy.

Laboratory tests often help in establishing the clinical suspicion. Mild leukocytosis with an increase in monocytes and eosinophils is often seen in early bubo and anogenital stage of LGV. Presence of polymorphonuclear leukocytosis would indicate secondary infection in LGV buboes and abscesses.[2]

Laboratory diagnosis of LGV can be made by (i) a positive serology for *C. trachomatis*, (ii) isolation of *C. trachomatis* from infected tissue, and (iii) identification of *C. trachomatis* from infected tissue or bubo pus.

Serological Tests

Complement fixation test: It is more sensitive than Frei's test because it is the first test to become positive. It has low specificity as it cross reacts with psittacosis and other *Chlamydia*. Low titres may persist for years. Titres greater than 1:64 are supportive of clinical diagnosis of LGV.[2]

Immunofluorescence Tests

The single L-type immunofluorescence test is more sensitive than complement fixation test but it also cross-reacts with other chlamydial antigens. Newer tests using type specific antigens can be more useful in detecting active infection.[31,32]

ELISA based tests using monoclonal antibodies are also available for LGV.[36]

Identification of *C. trachomatis* in Tissues

Presence of elementary and inclusion bodies can be demonstrated in the infected tissue or bubo pus by using special stains such as Giemsa-Romanowsky, Iodine or Macchiavello stains.[2] Immunofluorescent methods using polyclonal or monoclonal antibodies may also be used for demonstrating *C. trachomatis*.

Electron microscopy, though helpful in identifying the organism, is not used widely in making or confirming the diagnosis.[37]

Polymerase chain reaction (PCR) method using primers of 16S ribosomal DNA can also be used to identify the organism in infected tissue or bubo pus.[37]

Histology

Histology of an infected lymph node shows multiple stellate abscesses, representing areas of tissue necrosis with surrounding granulomatous infiltrate.[37]

Isolation of *C. trachomatis*

C. trachomatis can be isolated from infected tissue or bubo pus using mouse brain, yolk sac or tissue culture. Various cell lines such as McCoy, HeLa 229, L929 treated with agents to prevent replication are used. The yield is usually poor (24-30%).[31]

Frei's Test

It was originally performed using the pus from an unruptured bubo, diluted with saline and sterilized by heating. The antigen was available commercially in the past. The test now remains one of historic interest in the absence of a readily available antigen. The procedure consists of injecting 0.1 ml of the antigen into the skin on the volar aspect of a forearm and a similar amount of yolk sac or dilutent is injected on the other forearm as control. Reading is taken at 48 hours. A papule at least 6 mm in diameter, indicates a positive result provided the control arm showed a papule measuring 5mm or less.[2]

The test becomes positive after the appearance of buboes. It may indicate infection with non-LGV serovars of *C. trachomatis*. The test remains positive for many years after clinical cure.[2]

Others

Barium enema is done to locate the level of stricture and to know the level of stricture and the resultant deformity. It is also used to differentiate it from carcinoma of the rectum.[2]

Lymphography, CT scan or MRI scan may be used to know the extent of lymph node involvement.[2]

TREATMENT

The treatment is aimed at eliminating the organism to render the patient non-infectious and prevent complications.

Centre for disease control, Atlanta, USA[38] recommends, either

(i) Doxycycline 100 mg orally bid for 3 weeks or

(ii) Erythromycin base 500 mg orally qid for 3 weeks (specially for pregnant and nursing mothers, children under 8 years of age and patients sensitive to doxycycline)

Azithromycin 1 gm orally once a week for 3 weeks is also a recommended mode of therapy though adequate trials are lacking. It is also recommended to either aspirate with a wide bore needle through normal skin or incise and drain the buboes as and when required.[38]

Other drugs used for treating LGV are:

(i) Sulphadiazine 500 mg orally qid for 2-3 weeks[39]

(ii) Cotrimoxazole 2 tablets orally bid for 2 weeks.[39]

(iii) Tetracycline hydrochloride 500 mg orally qid for 2-3 weeks.

(iv) Minocycline 300 mg initially then 200 mg orally bid for 10 days.[40]

(v) Rifampicin 450 mg orally on empty stomach od for 10 days.

(vi) Azithromycin 1gm orally one dose with doxycycline 100 mg bid for 7 days.[41]

The recommendations are same for HIV positive cases but they may require longer duration of treatment.[38] Sexual contacts must be treated simultaneously. Follow up must be done at every 3 months for 1 year. A surgeon or a gynecologist, depending on the merit of the case, best deals with rectal strictures and fistulae surgically.

REFERENCES

1. Siddappa K, Rangaiah PN. Lymphogranuloma venereum. In: Valia RG, Valia AR, eds. IADVL Textbook and colour atlas of Dermatology. 2nd edn. Mumbai: Bhalani Publishing House; 2001: p. 1466-75.
2. Perine PL, Stamm WE. Lymphogranuloma venereum. In: Holmes KK, Sparling PF, Mardh PA, et al, eds. Sexually transmitted diseases. 3rd ed. New York: McGraw Hill; 1999. p. 423-32.
3. Abrams AJ. Lymphogranuloma venereum. JAMA 1968; 205: 199-202.
4. Chopra A, Mittal RR, et al. Pattern of sexually transmitted diseases at Patiala. Indian J Sex Transm Dis 1990; 11: 43-5.
5. Bansal NK, Khare AK, Upadhay OP. Pattern of sexually transmitted diseases in and around Udaipur. Indian J Dermatol Venereol Leprol 1988; 54: 90-2.
6. Nigam P, Mukhija RD. Pattern of sexually transmitted diseases at Gorakhpur. Indian J Sex Transm Dis 1986; 7: 70-3.
7. Singh KG, Joshi MK, Bajaj AK. Pattern of sexually transmitted diseases in Allahabad. Indian J Sex Transm Dis 1990; 11: 6-8.
8. Chaudhary SO, Bhatia KK, Bansal RK, et al. Pattern of sexually transmitted diseases in Rohtak. Indian J Sex Transm Dis 1988; 9: 4-7.
9. Sahib KPM, Pai GS, Pinto J, et al. Pattern of genital ulcers in and around Mangalore. Indian J Sex Transm Dis 1990; 11: 52-3.
10. Arora SK, Sharma RC, Sardari Lal. Pattern of sexually transmitted diseases at Smt. Sucheta Kripalani Hospital, New Delhi. Indian J Sex Transm Dis 1984; 5: 5-7.

11. Siddappa K, Jagannath Kumar V, Ravindra K. Pattern of STD's at Davangere. Indian J Sex Transm Dis 1990; 11: 39-42.
12. Garg BR, Baruah MC, Sait MA. Pattern of sexually transmitted diseases at JIPMER, Pondicherry. Indian J Sex Transm Dis 1985; 6: 41-3.
13. Kapur TR. Pattern of sexually transmitted diseases in India. Indian J Dermatol Venereol Leprol 1982; 48: 23-4.
14. Vora NS, Dave IN, Mukhopadyay AK, et al. A profile of sexually transmitted diseases at Apex ESIS Hospital, Ahmedabad. Indian J Sex Transm Dis 1994; 15: 36-8.
15. Rajanarayan, Kar HK, Gautam RK, et al. Pattern of sexually transmitted diseases in a major hospital of Delhi. Indian J Sex Transm Dis 1996; 17: 76-8.
16. Khanna N, Pandhi RK, Lakhanpal S. Changing trends in sexually transmitted diseases: A hospital based study from Delhi. Indian J Sex Transm Dis 1996; 17: 79-81.
17. Jaiswal AK, Bhushan B. Pattern of sexually transmitted diseases in North Eastern India. Indian J Sex Transm Dis 1994; 15: 19-20.
18. Arora PN, Romasastry CV, Chatterjee RG. Changing pattern of sexually transmitted diseases in Indian armed forces: Retrospective study from 1961 to 1990. Indian J Sex Transm Dis 1993; 14: 34-7.
19. Reddy BSN, Garg BR, Rao MV. An appraisal of trends in sexually transmitted diseases. Indian J Sex Transm Dis 1993; 14: 1-4.
20. Rege VL, Shukla P. Profile of genital sores in Goa. Indian J Sex Transm Dis 1993; 14: 10-4.
21. Behets FM, Andriamadana J, Randrianasolo D, et al. Chancroid, primary syphilis, genital herpes and lymphogranuloma venereum in Antananarivo, Madagascar. J Infect Dis 1999; 180: 1382-5.
22. Bauwens JE, Orlander H, Gomez MP, et al. Epidemic lymphogranuloma venerum during epidemics of crack cocaine use and HIV infection in Bahamas. Sex Transm Dis 2002; 29: 253-9.
23. Hering A, Richens J. Lymphogranuloma venerum. Sex Trans Infect 2006; 82 (suppl IV): 23-5.
24. Simms I, Ward H, Martin I, et al. Lymphogranuloma venerum in Australia. Sex health 2006; 3: 131-3.
25. Schachter I, Caldwel[1] KD. Chlamydiae. Ann Rev Microbiol 1980; 34: 285-309.
26. Schachter J, Osoba AO. Lymphogranuloma venereum. Br Med Bull 1983; 39: 151-4.
27. Gupta S, Ajith C, Kanwar AJ, Sehgal VN et al. Genital elephantiasis and sexually transmitted infection revisited. Int J STDs AIDS 2006: 17: 157-65.
28. Watson DJ, Parker AI, Macleod TI. Lymphogranuloma venereum of the tonsil. J Laryngols, Otol 1990; 104: 331-2.
29. Gupta S, Gupta U, Gupta DK. A gigantic esthiomene. Indian J Sex Transm Dis 1997; 18: 75-6.
30. Coutts WE. Lymphogranuloma venereum: a general review. Bull WHO 1950; 2: 545-62.
31. Kamprneir RH, Smith OW, Larsen RM. Human chlamydial infection. Am J Med Sci 1939; 198: 516.
32. Heaton ND, Yates-Bell A. Thirty-year follow-up of Iymphogranuloma venereum. Br J Urol 1992; 70: 693-4.
33. Speers D. Lymphogranuloma venereum presenting with psoas abscess. Aust NZ J Med 1999; 29: 563-4.
34. Van Dyck E, Piot P. Laboratory techniques in the investigation of chancroid, lymphogranuloma venereum and donovanosis, Genitourin Med 1992; 68: 130-3.
35. Joseph AK, Rosen T. Laboratory techniques used in the diagnosis of chancroid, granuloma inguinale and lymphogranuloma venereum. Dermatol Clin 1994; 12: 1-7.
36. Mittal A, Sachdeva KG. Monoclonal antibody for the diagnosis of lymphogranuloma venereum: a preliminary report. Br J Biomed Sci 1993; 50: 3-7.
37. Hadfield TL, Lamy Y, Wear DI. Demonstration of *Chlamydia trachomatis* in inguinal lymphadenitis of lymphogranuloma venereum: a light microscopy, electron microscopy and polymerase chain reaction study. Modern Pathology 1995; 8: 924-9.

38. Sexualy transmitted diseases. Treatment guidelines, 2006. www.cdc.gov
39. Expert Group Recommendations on National Sexually Transmitted Diseases Control Programme. New Delhi: DGHS, Govt. of India, Sept. 26-28, 1991; 23.
40. Sowmini CN, et al. Minocycline in the treatment of lymphogranuloma venereum. J Am Vener Dis Assoc 1976; 2: 19-22.
41. Levine WC, Berg AO, Johnson RE, et al. Development of sexually transmitted diseases treatment guidelines 1993. Sex Transm Dis 1994; 21(Suppl.2): S96-S101.

24 | BACTERIAL VAGINOSIS

Devinder M Thappa, Balaji Adityan

In this chapter

- Synonyms
- Historical Aspects
- Epidemiology
- Aetiopathogenesis
- Risk Factors
- Clinical Features
- Diagnosis
- Differential Diagnosis
- HIV and Bacterial Vaginosis
- Complications
- Bacterial Vaginosis and Other Genital Tract Infections
- Bacterial Vaginosis and Pregnant Women
- Treatment
- HIV Infections
- Prevention

SYNONYMS

Haemophilus vaginalis vaginitis; Gardnerella vaginalis vaginitis; Anaerobic vaginosis; Vaginal bacteriosis

INTRODUCTION

Bacterial vaginosis (BV) is a common cause of abnormal vaginal discharge in women of reproductive age.[1] It is a polymicrobial syndrome involving the replacement of the normal vaginal lactobacilli by a variety of anaerobic bacteria and mycoplasmas.[2] Little is known about the incubation period of BV, but recurrences are common.[1] The importance of BV with respect to women's health is emphasized by the association between BV and pelvic inflammatory diseases (PID), adverse outcome of pregnancy, postpartum endometritis, and cuff cellulitis.[3]

HISTORICAL ASPECTS

Gardner and Dukes first described the syndrome as "Haemophilus vaginalis vaginitis" in 1955. They concluded that it was a sexually transmitted disease (STD) as the isolated aetiological agent, *H. vaginalis* (now renamed *Gardnerella vaginalis*), was found in the male contacts of the female cases.[4] However, Leopold had previously described a Gram negative non-motile rod isolated from men and women with symptoms characteristic of BV and it is now known that *G. vaginalis* occurs in up to 50% of women without BV.[5] Further research has implicated a wide range of other microorganisms, including *Prevotella spp, Mycoplasma hominis, Mobiluncus spp, peptostreptococcus*, and *fusobacterium* in the syndrome.[2]

EPIDEMIOLOGY

The incidence of BV varies according to the population studied and the geographic location, with recorded prevalence ranging from 4% in university students to 33% in GUM clinics.[1] BV was the most common infection (26%) among the 319 women with vaginal discharge attending a reproductive health clinic in New Delhi, India. At least one STD was detected in 21.9% of women. The prevalence of *Chlamydia trachomatis* infection was 12.2%, trichomoniasis 10% and syphilis 2.2%.[6] In another study from New Delhi, BV was seen in 50% of symptomatic cases with vaginitis (out of 544 cases) and 21.8% of asymptomatic women (out of 258 cases) based on the clinical criteria and Gram's stain.[7] Bacterial vaginosis significantly correlated with increasing years since marriage, lower socio-economic status and a parity of more than two, but not with age, stage of menstrual cycle and hours since last intercourse. In a report from Chennai[8], 150 symptomatic and 50 asymptomatic women in second trimester of pregnancy in the age group of 20-30 years were screened for bacterial vaginosis by Gram stained smear of vaginal discharge utilizing the scoring system of Nugent et al. They found that 38.5% of symptomatic and 16% of asymptomatic women had BV. In JIPMER at Pondicherry, in a group of 100 women with abnormal vaginal discharge, 16% of them were found to have BV by Amsel's criteria and it was the commonest cause of abnormal vaginal discharge (unpublished data). The prevalence of bacterial vaginosis was 37.5% among the 80 randomly selected married women from Mumbai, based on Gram's stain and Amsel's criteria.[9] In a study of hundred women with vaginal discharge at Patiala, BV was seen in 48%, candidiasis in 26% and trichomoniasis in 13% of the cases.[10] In a study conducted in South Indian rural population, the prevalence of bacterial vaginosis was found to be 20% by smear examination and 17% by culture in married women of sexually active age group. The most common organisms identified were *Gardnerella* followed by *Prevotella* and *Peptostreptococcus*.[11] Among patients consulting STI clinics, the incidence of BV may be as high as 40%.[12] The consistently highest figures for BV cases are reported for sex workers: in Africa 40%[13] and in Asia 33%.[14] As many as 47% of HIV seropositive patients also have BV.[15]

AETIOPATHOGENESIS

The vagina is a dynamic ecosystem that is sterile at birth.[16] Under the influence of mother's estrogen, the glycogen content of vaginal epithelial cells get elevated and the infant vagina is colonized by lactobacilli. In most instances, this flora continues to dominate throughout the individual's lifetime, and this is also the case with the vaginal flora though it is influenced by hormone-instigated changes in the vagina's physiological environment during the life cycle. As the level of oestrogen diminishes, the glycogen also disappears and – with it – preconditions for survival of lactobacilli.

The vaginal flora of the infant girl is interspersed with contributions of coagulase-negative staphylococci, streptococci, *E. coli,* and other intestinal bacteria.[16] Small quantities of lactobacilli are there, which under the influence of the oestrogen get propagated and become the dominant vaginal flora of the adult female. This microflora composition continues until menopause, when it is replaced by a mixed flora unlike that of the infant female, but with a considerable portion of mycoplasma species and small quantities of anaerobic bacteria (including *Gardnerella vaginalis*). Hormone replacement therapy, when used, will cause lactobacilli to continue as the dominant flora.[16]

The vaginal pH in premenarchal females is near neutral (pH 7.0).[17] At the time of puberty, under the influence of estrogen, the vaginal epithelium increases to about 25 cells thick with increased glycogen levels, the predominant flora changes to lactobacilli and vaginal pH decreases to less than 4.5 due to production of lactic acid. This low pH is maintained until menopause, when vaginal pH rises above 6.0. In BV, this symbiotic relationship is broken in one or more places and leads to overgrowth of bacteria associated with BV (the bacterial shift from the normally occurring lactobacilli species: *L. crispatus*, *L. gasseri*, *L. jensenii*, and *L. iners* to a mixed flora dominated by anaerobic bacteria).[16,17]

In BV, the normal vaginal ecosystem is lost, instead a profuse mixed flora is established.[16] This consists of *G. vaginalis*, *Mobiluncus*, *Prevotella*, *Mycoplasma hominis*, *Bacteroides ureolyticus*, *Porphyromonas*, *Peptostreptococcus*, *Corynebacterium spp.*, *Streptococcus viridans*, *coagulase-negative staphylococci,* and *Enterococcus faecalis*. One can also find a quantitative change in the flora, the total concentration of bacteria being 100-1000 times the normal. The anaerobic bacteria produce amines by decarboxylation of aminoacids and fatty acids. This elevates the vaginal pH and further promotes the growth of anaerobic species.[16,18,19]

There are several hypotheses in the pathogenesis of BV, one hypothesis states that women who risk BV lack an adequate IgA response against Gvh (a hemolytic toxin produced by *G. vaginalis*).[16] Another hypothesis is that hydrolytic enzymes like sialidase and protein dipeptidase produced by *Prevotella*, *Mobiluncus*, and *G. vaginalis*, lyse mucin and help in the adherence of bacteria.[16]

The pathogenetic mechanisms that lead to BV among a subpopulation of women is still unknown.[16] The consequences of any interaction between different species of bacteria are not clear. All in all, however, it seems that an increased level of proinflammatory cytokines in conjunction with a disruption of the vaginal flora does not evoke an inflammatory effect in the usual clinical sense, but that it nonetheless is a host response to a growing potential threat.

Synergistic relations between different BV associated organisms have now been demonstrated. The prevalence of *M. hominis* and *G. vaginalis* are known to increase following an increased prevalence of various anaerobes.[20] The stimulation of *G. vaginalis* growth has been observed with the production of amino acids by anaerobes and ammonia by *Prevotella bivia*.

RISK FACTORS

BV is related to sexual activity, though it is hard to confirm that its development is entirely determined by those variables. It could be a marker of specific sexual practices or may be related to changing biological mechanisms, with means a woman's susceptibility increases with age.[1] The risk of BV is greatest among black Caribbean women. Those with a history of a bacterial STDs (gonorrhoea or *Chlamydia trachomatis*) are at a greater risk of BV.[1] Previous studies have reported that the prevalence of BV also increases with the number of lifetime sexual partners and is more common in those with a lower age of first intercourse.[21]

BV is more prevalent in lesbians. In a report from London, 33% of lesbians were infected compared with 13% of heterosexuals.[22] Lesbians usually have lower rates of STDs and this fact together with studies that have found BV in virgins indicate that specific practices and not sexual intercourse with an infected partner predisposes to BV.

In an Australian study, bacterial vaginosis was associated with indicators of high-risk sexual behaviour such as a new sexual partner and greater number of male partners in the last year, increased number of lifetime sexual partners, less than 13 years of education, a past history of pregnancy, and smoking ($P < .05$).[23]

CLINICAL FEATURES

BV is the commonest cause of vaginal discharge occurring in women attending the gynaecological clinics in our country.[9] Patients often present with a malodorous vaginal discharge although many are asymptomatic. BV and "other non-sexually transmitted conditions" exhibit an age profile in direct contrast with the known STDs. Both showed prevalence peaking in the over 30's, when one would expect lower rates of sexual partner change than in younger adults.[1] Non-viscous homogenous, white non-inflammatory discharge that smoothly coats the vaginal walls, often visible on the labia and fourchette with characteristic odour are the features of BV.[19] The vaginal mucosa and vulva appear normal and because of this lack of inflammation, it has been called as vaginosis instead of vaginitis. The majority of women with BV note a foul odor in the genital area immediately following intercourse when alkalinization of the vaginal secretions by semen occurs, leading to volatilization of polyamines. In addition to vaginal discharge, BV patients may have other symptoms like pruritus, pain during coitus, and lower abdominal pain.[16]

DIAGNOSIS

Most types of infectious diseases are diagnosed by culture, by isolating an antigen or RNA/DNA from the microbe, or by serodiagnosis to determine the presence of antibodies to the microbe.[24] This is not the case for BV, since the ultimate cause of the disease is not yet known. Therefore the patient must satisfy clinical or laboratory criteria which do not include the presence of a specific bacterium in a specified quantity. Therefore PCR and similar nucleic acid amplification methods have not gained ground in diagnostics. Also since BV implies a disrupted vaginal flora with a superfluity of anaerobic bacteria, anaerobic cultures cannot be employed economically to diagnose BV as they require a great deal of time and resources. For this reason, quantitative anaerobic cultures have not gained a footing in BV diagnostics.[24]

The method of choice for diagnosing BV is Amsel's clinical criteria and in a laboratory setting Nugent scoring/Gram staining.[4,25] Amsel et al[26] proposed a set of practical diagnostic criteria for the clinical diagnosis of BV that is now often accepted as the "gold standard." Diagnosis requires three or more of the following clinical/diagnostic features:

1. Excessive homogeneous uniformly adherent vaginal discharge
2. Elevated vaginal pH > 4.5
3. Positive amine test (Whiff test)
4. Clue cells (20%)

1. **Vaginal discharge:** The discharge should be thin, homogenous and uniformly adherent to the vaginal walls. It must not have any granular material.[24]

2. **Elevated vaginal pH >4.5:** The pH of vaginal secretions should be determined by using a strip of narrow range pH paper (about 4.0 to 5.5), which may be applied to the withdrawn speculum or directly inserted into the vagina.[1] It is unusual for BV to have a pH more than 5.5, if it happens it will in most cases be caused by cervical secretion.[24]

3. **Whiff test:** The odour of vaginal secretions should be tested by smelling the withdrawn speculum.[18,19,24] Normal vaginal secretions do not have an unpleasant odour. If this test is negative, a more sensitive procedure for detecting the amines is performed by adding a few drops of 10% KOH to a few drops of

vaginal secretions and immediate smelling ("whiffing") of the specimen for the transient "dead fish" odour that is characteristic of BV. Menses, semen or douching may affect the pH and a weakly positive whiff test may be produced by menstrual blood or semen. It is thought that amines produced by the microbial flora, perhaps by microbial decarboxylases, account for the characteristic abnormal fishy odor produced. The aromatic amines include putrescine, cadaverine, and trimethylamine. *Mobiluncus* is known to produce trimethylamine but other microbial sources of amines are still unknown.

4. **Clue cells:** Wet mount and Gram's stain of vaginal secretions should be done to look for 'clue cells', epithelial cells covered with G. vaginalis that Gardner and Dukes called "clues" to the diagnosis of BV. Detection of clue cells is the most useful single procedure for diagnosis of BV.[19] Gram's staining of vaginal secretions is even more reliable than wet mount, with a sensitivity of 93 percent and specificity of 70 percent, but it is underused.[18] Some older literature states that there must be atleast 20% clue cells to fulfill the clue cell criterion; however this is not seen in conventional Amsel criterion.[24]

BV is diagnosed conventionally when at least three of four composite criteria are fulfilled. Vaginal pH has the greatest sensitivity of the four clinical signs, but the lowest specificity. Amsel criteria is however laborious. Alternatively, Gram's staining of the smear has been shown to be a simple, inexpensive, sensitive, specific, and reproducible way to diagnose BV.[27] Spiegel et al[28] defined criteria that made it easy to diagnose BV by scoring Gram-stained vaginal secretion smears, and this procedure was refined by Nugent et al. **(Table 24.1)**.[29] Nugent's criteria for diagnosis of BV on Gram stained smear, has the sensitivity of 86 to 89% and specificity of 94 to 96% compared to the Amsel's criteria.[19]

Table 24.1 Nugent Scoring System

Bacterial Morphological Type	*Score*				
	None	*1+*	*2+*	*3+*	*4+*
Lactobacilli type (large, elongated, Gram positive bacteria)	4	3	2	1	0
Gardnerella type (small Gram variable coccobacteria)	0	1	2	3	4
Mobiluncus type (Curved Gram negative bacilli)	0	1	2	3	4

Interpretation:
<1/oil immersion field – 1+
1-5/oil immersion field – 2+
6-30/oil immersion field – 3+
>30/oil immersion field – 4+

Score: 0-3 Normal; 4-6 intermediate (test to be repeated later); 7-10 Bacterial vaginosis

The Hays/Ison system is another scoring system based on the observation of gram stains to estimate the ratios of the observed morphotypes rather than the exact number of bacteria.[30,31] Originally, the observations were divided into three categories- normal, intermediate or BV. But in order to obtain a more precise classification, two additional categories have been introduced in this scoring system as compared to Nugent scoring. The new groups define those preparations that contain no bacteria at all (group 0) and those that contain large amounts of gram-positive cocci, such as *Streptococcus* or *Staphylococcus* morphotypes. These morphotypes have previously been included in the intermediate flora classification but will now make up a class of their own (class 4).

Schmidt's scoring system of wet smears of vaginal fluid (wet smear criteria) resembles Nugent scoring in that it ranks the quantities of lactobacilli and cocci in the same way, although the demarcations of the intervals differ.[32] Moreover, the Schmidt system does not recognize *Mobiluncus*. The Schmidt method has been validated for diagnosis of BV in primary care populations.

For STI populations, a combination of whiff test, pH testing, observation of clue cells and absence of lactobacilli can be applied.[24]

Several other alternative methods have also been used to develop easy, inexpensive and reproducible diagnostic methods such as the rapid nucleic acid hybridization test, proline aminopeptidase activity and the amine test.[3] Laboratory diagnosis by gas liquid chromatographic identification of fatty acids is useful as a research tool.[17] A ratio of the succinate to lactate peaks of more than 0.4 is highly predictive of BV.

Some recent methods to diagnose BV include self-test pH glove (In this screening procedure one finger of a medical examination glove has an attached pH indicator paper, which the patient can introduce into her vagina and then read the measured result), electronic sensor array 'electronic nose' (the idea of using sensor arrays coupled with software interpretation of the resulting signals "electronic nose" for the diagnosis of BV is based on the assumption that the signal pattern thus detected might be an electronic counterpart to the human sensation of smell and has attracted some attention. The results so far are generally disappointing), determination of sialidase activity and DNA probe for G.vaginalis rRNA in vaginal discharge.[24]

DIFFERENTIAL DIAGNOSIS

The three major causes of vaginitis (bacterial vaginosis, trichomoniasis and candida vaginitis) and their differentiating features are discussed in chapter 46 on vaginal discharge[18,33] Other possible differential diagnosis includes ulcerative vaginitis due to *Staphylococcus aureus*, vaginal ulceration associated with the use of vaginal tampons or cervical caps or spermicide, infections associated with other intravaginal foreign bodies, postmenstrual atrophic vaginitis, allergic or chemical reactions and contact dermatitis.

HIV AND BACTERIAL VAGINOSIS

An understanding is emerging of how BV might enhance the susceptibility to HIV infection.[34] Lactobacilli produce hydrogen peroxide, which is toxic to a number of microorganisms, including HIV. BV is characterized by the absence of lactobacilli and thus an elevated pH. A low vaginal pH may inhibit CD4 lymphocyte activation and therefore decrease HIV target cells in the vagina; conversely, an elevated pH may make the vagina more conducive to HIV survival and adherence. BV has also been shown to increase intravaginal levels of interleukin-10, which increases susceptibility of macrophages to HIV. In addition, the mucin degrading enzymes in BV will make it easier for HIV to infect by breaking down the cervicovaginal mucosa. It has also been hypothesized that the level of acidity within the vagina may affect CD4 lymphocyte activation. The more alkaline the environment, the more likely it is that CD4 lymphocytes will be activated and thus act as suitable target cells for HIV.[35]

COMPLICATIONS

Women with BV have fivefold increased risk of late miscarriage or preterm delivery.[27] Studies are underway to determine whether intervention can prevent a woman with BV having a late miscarriage and preterm delivery. Other reported complications in pregnancy are low birth weight, premature rupture of membranes (PROM), chorioamnionitis and amniotic fluid infection. Causal relations have also been established between BV and postpartum endometritis, vaginal cuff cellulitis (occurs when vaginal bacteria contaminate the operative field during a hysterectomy), post abortion and spontaneous PID.[19]

BACTERIAL VAGINOSIS AND OTHER GENITAL TRACT INFECTIONS

BV is present most frequently as a co infection with other STIs.[35] Those presenting with BV are more likely to have a concurrent infection with gonorrhoea, but less likely to be diagnosed with a protozoal, viral, or fungal infection.[36] An inhibitory effect of the bacterial amines, putrescine and cadaverine on the cell division and germ tube formation of Candida albicans has recently been reported.[36] The leading hypothesis to explain the coexistence of BV with other STIs is that the absence of protective lactobacilli in BV facilitates the acquisition of other STIs.[35]

BACTERIAL VAGINOSIS AND PREGNANT WOMEN

BV during pregnancy is associated with adverse pregnancy outcomes, including PROM, preterm labour, preterm birth, postpartum endometritis, and intraamniotic infections.[25] The results of several investigations indicate that treatment of pregnant women who have BV and who are at high risk for preterm delivery (i.e., those who previously delivered a premature infant) may reduce the risk for prematurity. All symptomatic pregnant women should be tested and treated. Metronidazole 250 mg orally three times a day for 7 days or Metronidazole 500 mg orally twice a day for 7 days or Clindamycin 300 mg orally twice a day for 7 days is the recommended treatment.[25] Metronidazole is not recommended for use in the first trimester of pregnancy, but it may be used during the second and third trimesters.[37]

Currently, pregnant women with asymptomatic bacterial vaginosis are not routinely screened or treated for this syndrome.[38] As the treatment of BV in asymptomatic pregnant women at high risk for preterm delivery with a recommended regimen has reduced preterm delivery in three of four randomized controlled trials, some specialists recommend the screening and treatment of these women during the first prenatal visit.[25]

TREATMENT

The treatment of bacterial vaginosis as recommended by CDC, WHO and NACO is summarised in Table 24.2.

Table 24.2 **Treatment of Bacterial Vaginosis**

WHO (2003)[37]	*CDC (2006)*[25]	*NACO (2004)*[39]
Recommended regimen Metronidazole, 400 mg or 500 mg orally, twice daily for 7 days. **Alternative regimen:** • Metronidazole, 2 g orally, as a single dose (or) • Clindamycin 2% vaginal cream, 5 g intravaginally, at bedtime for 7 days. (or) • Metronidazole 0.75% gel, 5 g intravaginally, twice daily for 5 days. (or) • Clindamycin, 300 mg orally, twice daily for 7 days.	**Recommended Regimens** Metronidazole 500 mg orally twice a day for 7 days. Or Metronidazole gel, 0.75%, one full applicator (5 g) intravaginally, once a day for 5 days. Or Clindamycin cream, 2%, one full applicator (5 g) intravaginally at bedtime for 7 days. **Alternative Regimens** Clindamycin 300 mg orally twice a day for 7 days. Or Clindamycin ovules 100 mg intravaginally once at bedtime for 3 days.	**Recommended regimens** Metronidazole 400 mg orally twice daily for 7 days Or Metronidazole 2 g orally as a single dose. Or Tinidazole 2 gm orally as a single dose However in symptomatic women in the first trimester and those intolerant to Metronidazole or Tinidazole, Imidazole pessaries cream may be given for 7 days

Recurrence

Recurrent BV is defined as 4 or more appearances of infection in one year.[33,40] When BV recurs, it is most likely to be a reactivation rather than a reinfection. Optimal treatment for recurrent BV is unknown. Options include re-treatment with metronidazole or clindamycin and local therapy with clotrimazole. Other treatment modalities include supplement of H_2O_2, vaccination with lyophilized *Lactobacillus acidophilus* and intravaginal Lactobacillus capsules. If an intrauterine device is present, its removal should be considered.

Partner Treatment

Treatment of the male sex partner has not been beneficial in preventing the recurrence of BV.[25]

HIV INFECTION

Patients who are co-infected with HIV and BV may receive the same treatment regimen as those who are HIV-negative.[25]

PREVENTION

It is difficult to define useful approaches for the prevention of this condition in the scenario of poorly understood host factors and agents involved. Since BV is associated with sexual activity, abstinence may represent the most effective means to prevent its occurrence.[19]

REFERENCES

1. Morris MC, Rogers PA, Kinghorn GR. Is bacterial vaginosis a sexually transmitted infection? Sex Transm Infect 2001; 77: 63-8.
2. Krohn M, Hillier S, Eschenbach D. Comparison of methods for diagnosing bacterial vaginosis among pregnant women. J Clin Microbiol 1989; 27: 1266-71.
3. Wolrath H, Forsum U, Larsson PG, et al. Analysis of bacterial vaginosis-related amines in vaginal fluid by gas chromatography and mass spectrometry. J Clin Microbiol 2001; 39: 4026-31.
4. Gardner H, Dukes *C. Haemophilus vaginalis* vaginitis: a newly defined specific infection previously classified "non-specific vaginitis". Am J Obstet Gynecol 1955; 69: 962-76.
5. Leopold S. Heretofore undescribed organism isolated from the genitourinary system. US Armed Forces Med J 1953; 4: 263-6.
6. Vishwanath S, Talwar V, Prasad R, et al. Syndromic management of vaginal discharge among women in a reproductive health clinic in India. Sex Transm Inf 2000; 76: 303-6.
7. Bhalla P, Kaushika A. Epidemiological and microbiological correlates of bacterial vaginosis. Indian J Dermatol Venereol Leprol 1994; 60: 8-14.
8. Mathew R, Kalyani J, Bibi R, et al. Prevalence of bacterial vaginosis in antenatal women. Indian J Pathol Microbiol 2001; 44: 113-6.
9. Saharan SP, Surve C, Raut V, et al. Diagnosis and prevalence of bacterial vaginosis. J Postgrad Med 1993; 39: 72-3.
10. Chopra A, Mittal RR, Kanta S, et al. Vaginitis and vaginal flora – Study of 100 cases. Indian J Sex Transm Dis 1993; 14: 52-4.
11. PS Rao, S Devi, A Shriyan, et al. Diagnosis of bacterial vaginosis in a rural setup: Comparison of clinical algorithm, smear scoring and culture (smauc) by semiquantitative technique. Indian J Med Microbiol 2004; 22: 47-50.
12. Tchoudomirova K, Stanilova M, Garov V. Clinical manifestations and diagnosis of bacterial vaginosis in a clinic of sexually transmitted diseases. Folia Med (Plovdiv) 1998; 40: 34-40.

13. Riedner G, Rusizoka M, Hoffman O, et al. Baseline survey of sexually transmitted infections in a cohort of female bar workers in Mbeya region, Tanzania. Sex Transm Infect 2003; 79: 328-7.
14. Cohen CR, Duerr A, Pruithithada N, et al. Bacterial vaginosis and HIV seroprevalence among female commercial sex workers in Chang Mai, Thailand. AIDS 1995; 9: 1093-7.
15. Warren D, Klein RS, Sobel J, et al. A multicenter study of bacterial vaginosis in women with or at risk for human immunodeficiency virus infection. Infect Dis Obstet Gynecol 2001; 9: 133-41.
16. Forsum U, Holst E, Larsson PG et al. Bacterial vaginosis-a microbiological and immunological enigma. APMIS. 2005; 113: 81-90.
17. Schmid GP, Arko RJ. Vaginitis. In: Morse SA, Moreland AA, Thompson SE, eds. Slide Atlas of Sexually Transmitted Diseases. New York: Gower Medical Publishing; 1992. p. 1-8.
18. Sobel JD. Vaginitis. New Engl J Med 1997; 337: 1896-902.
19. Hilliers S, Holmes KK. Bacterial vaginosis. In: Holmes KK, Mardh PA, Sparling PF, et al. eds. Sexually Transmitted Diseases. 3rd edn. New York: McGraw-Hill; 1999: p. 563-86.
20. Pybus V, Onderdonk AB. Microbial interactions in the vaginal ecosystem, with emphasis on the pathogenesis of bacterial vaginosis. Microbes Infect 1999; 1: 285-92.
21. Larsson P, Platz-Christensen J, Sundstrom E. Is bacterial vaginosis a sexually transmited disease? Int J STDs AIDS 1991; 2: 362-4.
22. Bump R, Buesching W. Bacterial vaginosis in virginal and sexually active adolescent females: evidence against exclusive sexual transmission. Am J Obstet Gynecol 1988; 158: 935-9.
23. Bradshaw CS, Morton AN, Garland SM, et al. Higher-risk behavioural practices associated with bacterial vaginosis compared with vaginal candidiasis. Obstet Gynecol 2005; 106: 105-14.
24. Forsum U, Hallen A, Larsson PG. Bacterial vaginosis -a laboratory and clinical diagnostics enigma. APMIS 2005; 113: 153-61.
25. Centre For Disease Control. Sexually transmitted diseases: Treatment guidelines 2006. MMWR 2006; 55 (No.RR-11): 50-2.
26. Amsel R, Totten P, Spiegel CA, at el. Non-specific vaginitis: diagnostic techniques and microbial and epidemiologic associations. Am J Med 1983; 74: 14-22.
27. Hay PE, Lamont R, Taylor-Robinson D, et al. Abnormal bacterial colonization of the genital tract and subsequent preterm delivery and late miscarriage. BMJ 1994; 308: 295-8.
28. Spiegel CA, Amsel R, Holmes KK. Diagnosis of bacterial vaginosis by direct Gram stain of vaginal fluid. J Clin Microbiol 1983; 18: 170-7.
29. Nugent RP, Krohn MA, Hillier SL. Reliability of diagnosing bacterial vaginosis is improved by a standardized method of Gram stain interpretation. J Clin Microbiol 1991; 29: 297-301.
30. Hay PE, Lamont RF, Taylor-Robinson D, et al. Abnormal bacterial colonisation of the lower genital tract as a marker for subsequent preterm delivery and late miscarriage. BMJ 1994; 308: 295-8.
31. Ison CA, Hay PE. Validation of a simplified grading of Gram stained vaginal smears for use in genitourinary medicine clinics. Sex Transm Infect 2002; 78: 413-5.
32. Schmidt H, Hansen JG. Diagnosis of bacterial vaginosis by wet mount identification of bacterial morphotypes in vaginal fluid. Int J STDs AIDS 2000; 11: 150-5.
33. Celum CL, Wilch E, Fennell Cet, et al. The Practitioner's Handbook for the Management of Sexually Transmitted Diseases, revised second edition, Seattle, WA: Health Sciences Centre for Educational Resources, University of Washington: 1998; p. 31-34, p. 76-7.
34. Schmid GP, Markowitz LE, Joesoef R, et al. Bacterial vaginosis and HIV infection. Sex Transm Inf 2000; 76: 3-4.
35. Schwebke JR. Abnormal vaginal flora as a biological risk factor for acquisition of HIV infection and sexually transmitted diseases. J Infect Dis 2005; 192: 1315-7.
36. Rodrigues AG, Mardh PA, Pina-Vaz C, et al. Is the lack of concurrence of bacterial vaginosis and vaginal candidosis explained by the presence of bacterial amines? Am J Obstet Gynecol 1999; 181: 367-70.

37. Guidelines for the management of sexually transmitted infections. WHO/HIV/AIDS 2003: 1-89.
38. Hillier SL, Nugent R, Eschenbach D, et al. Association between bacterial vaginosis and preterm delivery of a low birth weight infant. N Engl J Med 1995; 333: 1737-42.
39. Guidelines for treatment of sexually transmitted diseases NACO (2004).
40. Larsson PG, Forsum U. Bacterial vaginosis –a disturbed bacterial flora and treatment enigma. APMIS 2005; 113: 305-16.

25 HERPES GENITALIS

Joseph A Sundharam

In this chapter

- Aetiology
- Structure
- Epidemiology
- Transmission and Viral Shedding
- Pathology
- Clinical Manifestations
- Differential Diagnosis
- Laboratory Tests
- Management
- Prevention of Transmission of Genital Herpes

INTRODUCTION

Genital herpes simplex virus infections are now one of the commonest sexually transmitted diseases (STD), afflicting both men and women. The incidence has increased manifold in the last two decades and has assumed major public health significance, especially because of its association with HIV infection. The reasons for this increase in genital herpes infections include a decreasing incidence of treatable bacterial STDs, high rates of both clinical and asymptomatic recurrences, and transmission of the disease in the absence of symptoms. The morbidity of the illness is due to the severity of the primary infections as well as to the high recurrence rates. The high mortality and morbidity in neonates is also of great concern to both patients and health care workers.

AETIOLOGY[1]

Herpes genitalis is caused by a DNA virus, Herpesvirus hominis. There are two types—type 1 and type 2. The predominant type isolated from the genital area is type 2, although in a third of the cases, type 1 may be isolated. There is evidence that genital HSV-1 infections are becoming increasingly common, particularly among adolescents and young women.[2]

Herpes simplex virus (HSV) infections are characterized by persistence in the sensory nerve ganglia after primary infection (i.e., latency). During this period of latency, the virus cannot be detected by the host defence mechanisms. Following various triggers, the virus may be reactivated, travel peripherally to the skin and mucous membranes, and replicate to cause recurrent disease. Virus shedding may occur even without lesions (asymptomatic shedding); however, the number of virus particles shed is considerably less than from active lesions (up to a 1000 times less).

Thus, herpes genitalis may be defined as a chronic persistent infection of the sensory ganglia with varying unpredictable degrees of epithelial expression (i.e., asymptomatic or symptomatic recurrences).

STRUCTURE

The herpes simplex virus has four basic components

- The core—which consists of a linear double stranded DNA, coding for over 70 different polypeptides.
- The capsid—a 20 sided (icosahedral) protein shell which protects the DNA core. The capsid is composed of 162 structural units known as capsomeres.
- The tegument—an amorphous proteinaceous material which covers the capsid
- The envelope—a lipid membrane derived from the host-cell nuclear membrane. The envelope contains 11 glycoproteins which are the major targets of the humoral and cellular immune response.

EPIDEMIOLOGY

Spreading occurs through direct contact with infected secretions. The incubation period varies from 5 to 14 days. All patients with HSV infections are potentially contagious, whether or not lesions are visible. Transmission often occurs in the absence of lesions because of asymptomatic shedding.

The epidemiology of type 1 and type 2 infections differ. In developing countries, the majority of the adult population is infected in childhood by the type 1 virus; in the developed countries the proportion is lower.[3] Type 2 virus infection is typically post pubertal. There is a paucity of community-based Indian studies on the prevalence of herpes genitalis. Most statistics are based on the incidence in STD patients at various clinics and these may vary according to the criteria used (clinical, or based on tests such as Tzanck smears or viral cultures). In a recent review of the scenario of STDs in India, Sharma & Khandpur concluded that the incidence and prevalence of genital herpes has been increasing.[4] They compiled statistics reported from various STD clinics across the country and noted that the rate of herpes genitalis among attendees to these clinics ranged from 4% to 27.9% in different regions.

The prevalence of genital herpes has increased markedly between the 1960's and 1990's. These increases have been seen not only in STD clinics in India but also all over the world, and 6 to 10 fold increases have been reported from centres in the UK and USA.[5]

In the US, approximately 25% of the population is seropositive to HSV type 2. Orogenital contact may lead to transmission of type 1 virus to the genitalia[6] and up to a third of genital HSV infections are caused by the type 1 virus.

A study published from Sweden challenges the traditional view that HSV 2 infections remain confined below the waist, while HSV 1 tends to cause infections on the upper half of the body.[7] In this study, cultures from lesions at all sites were taken over a four-year period. While among 631 orofacial isolates, 96% were HSV 1, of 3085 anogenital isolates, 29% were HSV 1 and the rest (71%) were HSV 2. On the fingers and hands, 46% of 69 isolates were HSV 2, while at other sites (such as the foot and abdomen), 40% of 95 isolates were HSV 2. It seems, therefore, that except for the orofacial region, both viral types are capable of and well adapted to infecting other body regions.

Both humoral and cell mediated immune responses follow primary infection. These, however, do not fully prevent either recurrences or reinfection. Infection with HSV of a different type produces a first episode nonprimary infection. This is usually milder. The importance of the immune system is demonstrated by the prolonged and atypical course of herpes in immunodeficient individuals such as patients on immunosuppressive or cytotoxic drugs following organ transplantation or malignancy, and in patients with AIDS.

The importance of the immune system is also demonstrated by neonatal transmission of the disease. In maternal primary infection at the time of delivery, transmission occurs in 50% of neonates and is often severe and fatal. However, transmission to the neonate is less frequent and serious morbidity is rare in nonprimary, first episode or recurrent genital infection during pregnancy or at delivery, since maternal antibodies protect the foetus.

TRANSMISSION AND VIRAL SHEDDING[1,8]

Infection with the herpes simplex virus follows contact with infected secretions through oral to oral, oral to genital or genital to genital contact. Some factors influencing the transmission of HSV are listed in Table 25.1.

Table 25.1 Factors Influencing HSV Transmission

- Gender
- Previous infection with HSV
- Frequency of recurrence
- Presence of active lesions at intercourse
- Use of barrier contraceptives
- Use of HSV suppressive therapy in the partner with herpes

In couples where one partner has a history of herpes, serologic tests show that in 25% of these couples, both partners are seropositive, suggesting that infection had already been transmitted. In the couples who were serologically discordant for HSV antibodies, the mean rate of transmission was 12% per year.[9]

PATHOLOGY

The herpes simplex virus infects the epidermal cell. Oedema of the cytoplasm produces the characteristic "ballooning degeneration". Giant cells formed from epidermal keratinocytes containing 2 to 15 nuclei, and intranuclear inclusions can also be seen.

Vesicles in the epidermis are formed by coalescence of intercellular oedema as well as degeneration of epidermal cells. Polymorphonuclear leukocytes infiltrate the dermis and subsequently the epidermis.

CLINICAL MANIFESTATIONS[1]

The severity and frequency of clinical manifestations (Table 25.2) may be influenced by a number of viral and host factors. Viral factors include the viral type (type 1 or type 2), while host factors include the immune status of the host and prior exposure to autologous or heterologous virus type.

Table 25.2 Classification of Herpes Virus Infections

- First episode

  True primary—in a seronegative individual

  Nonprimary—first episode in a previously infected individual
- Recurrent

The first time that a nonimmune (i.e., seronegative) person develops herpes is known as a primary infection. The first episode of herpes in an immune person (i.e., infected by another virus type) is termed a nonprimary first episode. Recurrences may follow first episode infections in a proportion of individuals. The first episode of infection is usually more severe and more frequently associated with systemic symptoms. However, the acquisition of infection in many individuals may go unnoticed and without any associated signs or symptoms, and in one study almost half of seroconversions of HSV 2 infections were asymptomatic.[10]

Only fifty percent of patients who present with their first episode of genital herpes have a true primary infection with either HSV 1 or 2. In the remainder, there is serological evidence of earlier infection, usually with HSV 1. About a fourth of patients presenting with their first episode of clinical HSV 2 infection have serological evidence of previous HSV 2 infection, in these cases, this is not a primary infection, but probably a recurrence in an individual with an asymptomatic first episode.

Prior nongenital HSV 1 infection protects against acquisition of genital HSV 1 infection, but protection against genital HSV 2 infection is incomplete. However, prior HSV 1 infection reduces the severity of first episode genital herpes.

Primary Genital Herpes

In primary genital herpes, systemic symptoms (fever, headache, myalgias and malaise) are prominent and prolonged. The disease is more severe in women and systemic symptoms are experienced by more than three fourth of women, but less than half the men. Symptoms are maximal in the first few days after onset of lesions. Painful ulcers are present in almost all patients and may last up to 2 weeks. The severity of local symptoms is similar with both types of HSV infection. Urethral and vaginal discharge and local lymphadenopathy are common but suppurative lymphadenopathy does not occur.

The lesions start as grouped vesicles **(Fig. 25.1, 25.2)** but rapidly become pustular and ulcerate . During presentation, large coalescent areas of

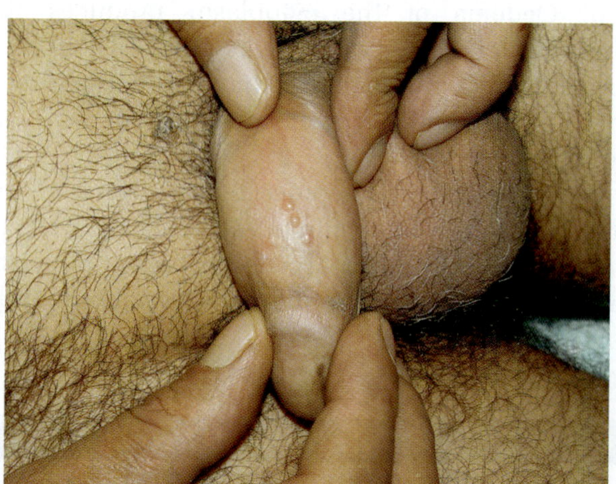

Fig. 25.1 Genital Herpes – Vesicular Stage.

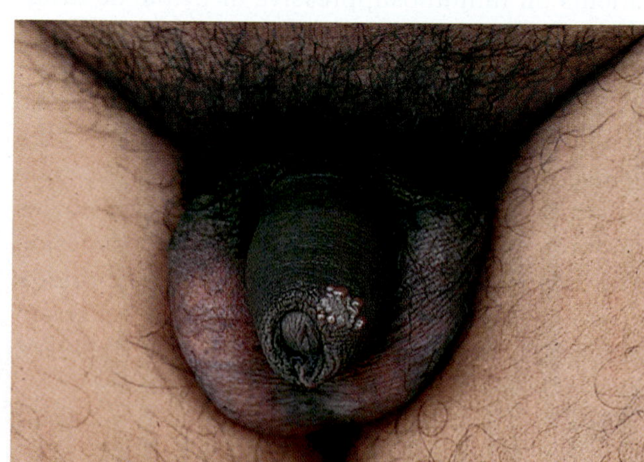

Fig. 25.2 Genital Herpes – Vesicular Stage.

ulceration, often with polycyclic margins are usually present **(Fig. 25.3)**. New lesions continue to form in the first 8 to 10 days and complete re-epithelization may take as long as three weeks or more. Viral shedding usually continues for the first two weeks. Scarring is uncommon.

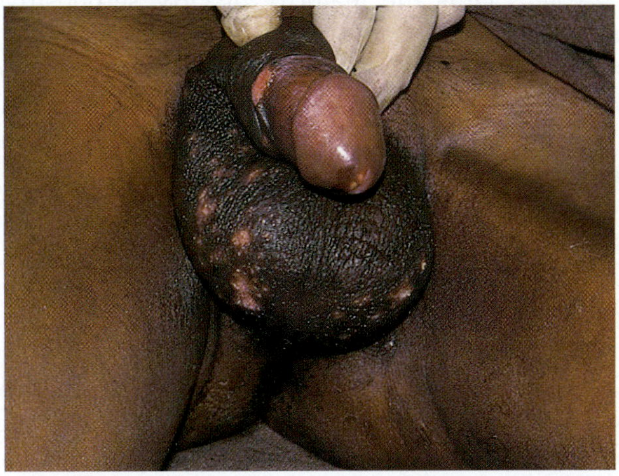

Fig. 25.3 Genital Herpes – Multiple Polycyclic, Superficial Ulcers.

Systemic signs and symptoms are uncommon in patients with first episode nonprimary genital HSV 2 infections.

Cervicitis is commonly (upto 90%) associated in first episode HSV 2 infections in women and it is often ulcerative or necrotic. However, an examination of the cervix is usually not performed in the presence of painful vulval lesions. Proctitis caused by the herpes simplex virus is more commonly seen in homosexual men, and is the most common cause of nongonococcal proctitis. It is frequently severe and associated with severe systemic symptoms. It is usually limited to the lower third of the rectum. Anorectal infections may be occasionally seen in women and may be related to recurrences in the sacral ganglion rather than anal intercourse. Pharyngeal infection is often associated. In 20% of patients it may be the presenting complaint and may be associated with orogenital exposure. Autoinoculation during the course of primary gingivo-stomatitis to the genitalia sometimes occurs in children.

Complications of First Episode Genital Herpes

CNS involvement: Aseptic meningitis, transverse myelitis and sacral radiculopathy have been reported. HSV may be isolated from the CSF. Pleocytosis in the CSF may occur. Autonomic dysfunction (urinary retention, constipation, perineal hyperaesthesia or anaesthesia) may also be seen in the more severe cases.

Extragenital lesions: Extragenital lesions are frequent on the thigh, buttock or groin, but occasionally on the hand or eye. They are more common in women and with primary HSV 1 infection (25%) as compared to primary HSV 2 infection (9%) and usually appear in the second week. Autoinoculation, rather than viremic spread is probably the mode of spread.

Disseminated infection: This is rare, viremic spread occurs early, and it is associated with more severe disease. Disseminated infection is often associated with aseptic meningitis, hepatitis or pneumonitis. Pregnancy, immunosuppression, atopic eczema may predispose to disseminated infection.

Secondary infection: Bacterial superinfection, manifesting as cellulitis and secondary pyoderma, is not uncommon. Fungal vaginitis may be associated and usually emerges in the second week.

Recurrent Genital Herpes

Recurrences generally follow first episodes of infection, but in many cases the first episode may be asymptomatic or so mild as to remain unrecognized. Recurrent episodes are milder, lasting only 5 to 7 days. Over 90% of patients with recurrent disease have prodromal symptoms, varying from a mild tingling sensation to shooting pains from an hour to up to 5 days prior to the appearance of the lesions. In a fifth of episodes, there may be only prodromal symptoms without appearance of lesions.

Recurrent genital herpes is milder in men as compared to women, and is usually confined to one side. The duration of viral shedding is usually about 3 to 4 days and healing is usually complete by 7 to 10 days. However, even in the same patient there may be considerable variation in severity between episodes. The same strain of virus may have markedly different patterns of reactivation between persons and even in the same individual. The intervals between recurrence and duration of consecutive episodes are unpredictable.

Recurrences may not always be "typical" with grouped vesicles leading to crusting in a few days. In one study, a third of the women in whom HSV was isolated, only linear superficial fissures or erosions were seen which were initially thought to be traumatic or monilial in origin.[11]

Rate of Recurrences

After the primary episode, patients with HSV 2 infections have more frequent recurrences and earlier recurrences than those with HSV 1. The time to first recurrence after primary infection was about 10 months for HSV 1 infection but only about 6 weeks for HSV 2 infection.[12] Patients with more severe and prolonged first episode disease (> 5 weeks) have more frequent recurrences than those without. Genital herpes caused by HSV 2 may recur up to six times more frequently than that caused by HSV 1. During the first year, after a symptomatic episode of primary genital herpes caused by HSV type 2, almost 90% have at least 1 recurrence, 38% have more than six and 20% may have more than 10 recurrences. Recurrences are more common in men. The number of recurrences varies from 4 to 5 per year.

The frequency of recurrences shows a declining trend over the initial years of infection at the rate of about 1 recurrence per year. However, this is variable and up to a fourth of these patients may actually show an increase in the number of recurrences in the fifth year.[13]

In contrast to HSV 2, only 60% of patients with HSV 1 will have a recurrence in the first year of follow up. Rates of recurrence are also low at about 1 recurrence per year and less than 5% of patients with HSV 1 average more than 4 recurrences, that too mostly in the first year.

Asymptomatic Shedding

Although HSV infections are frequent, less than 20% of patients are aware that they are infected. Among HIV negative homosexual men, asymptomatic shedding from anogenital sites occurs on an average 2.2% of days sampled (range 1-24%).[14] Thus the majority of HSV seropositive individuals are unaware of their infection and yet are capable of shedding the virus and hence of transmitting the infection. Asymptomatic viral shedding is responsible for at least 70% of viral transmission.[15]

Genital Herpes Complicating Pregnancy[16]

There are no studies addressing the seroprevalence of HSV type 2 infections in Indian women and hence the extent of the problem is unknown. In the US, approximately 25% of women in the reproductive age group are infected with the HSV 2 virus, more blacks (55%) being seropositive as compared to whites (19%). In studies from antenatal clinics, HSV 2 seroprevalence rates vary from less than 10% (UK, Japan, Italy and Spain) to intermediate (11 to 30%) reported from Australia, Finland, France and Sweden to high (more than 30%) in USA and Brazil.[17] Most of these patients are unaware of the fact and only a fourth of infected women report signs and symptoms suggestive of recurrent herpes.

It is important to classify genital herpes in pregnancy accurately based on typing of the genital isolate and serotyping the patient with type-specific serologic assays as the incidence and severity of neonatal infection depend on the HSV subtype.

First Episode Genital Herpes in Pregnancy

Genital herpes is acquired for the first time during pregnancy in 2-3% of the pregnant women. Among seronegative pregnant women who have seronegative partners, the rate of transmission (acquisition) of herpes is 13% by the end of pregnancy. Most of these cases of herpes acquired during pregnancy are asymptomatic, and since in most cases seroconversion has occurred by the time of labour, the foetus is not in any danger. However, in patients acquiring infection late in pregnancy in which HSV seroconversion has not been completed by the time of labour, there is a 40% risk of transmission of herpes to the newborns.

Recurrent Genital Herpes in Pregnancy

The progressive decline in the immune competence that occurs during pregnancy results in an increase in the frequency, duration and severity of symptomatic recurrences as pregnancy progresses. During and around the time of labour, approximately 2% of seropositive women suffer a symptomatic recurrence, with another 2% having a culture positive asymptomatic shedding, and about 20% showing PCR positive tests.

Symptomatic recurrences during advancing gestation may be atypical and more severe, sometimes even resembling first episode disease. To complicate matters, some seropositive women who have been earlier asymptomatic, may experience a first-ever recurrence in advanced pregnancy. In one study of 29 women who presented with what appeared clinically to be primary genital herpes in the latter half of pregnancy, it was determined serologically that only 4 (14%) of these were actually true first episode disease and all the remaining were HSV seropositive and experiencing a first ever recurrence.[18] It is important, in view of both implications to the socity and as implications to the newborn that type specific serology should be determined as well as culture and typing of the viral strain isolated from the genitalia – antibodies to the same viral type isolated from the genitalia would indicate that the infection most likely antedated the pregnancy.

Transmission During Pregnancy and Delivery

Despite the frequency of genital herpes infection in women, the transmission of genital herpes to neonates is relatively rare, and is estimated to be less than 3%. The risk increases more than ten fold if a woman acquires genital HSV in the third trimester and delivers prior to the development of antibodies. Currently available data suggest that the risk of transmission to the infant from a mother with primary HSV infection of either type is 50%, while in a first episode (nonprimary) HSV 2 infection in a woman with a past HSV 1 infection is 20%. In recurrent HSV 2 the risk of neonatal transmission is less than 1%.[1]

Neonatal Herpes

Transmission of HSV 2 infection to a neonate during delivery is one of the most disastrous consequences of maternal herpes virus infection. The problem is compounded by the fact that less than 10% of HSV-2 seropositive individuals are aware of their serological status[19-22] and many cases of neonatal herpes transmission have occurred in asymptomatic HSV-2–infected mother.[23]

Neonatal herpes is a serious and frequently fatal disease and is of major concern to patient with genital herpes. This is the most serious complication of genital herpes occurring during pregnancy. The prevalence varies with the prevalence rate of maternal infection and reported rates range from up to 50 per 100,000 live births in the US to 6/100,000 in Sweden, 8/100,000 in Australia and 3/100,000 in the UK.[17] A large study from the US published in 2003, reported an incidence of 1 in 3200 live births.[24]

Eighty percent of the infants in whom neonatal herpes develops have mothers who report no history of exposure to HSV and are asymptomatic at delivery. Some 25% of infants who contract herpes at delivery will develop disseminated herpetic infection, which has a high mortality (>40%) despite antiviral therapy. Congenital infection is rare and can occur through transplacental transmission of the virus. It may lead to spontaneous abortion, prematurity and a host of other abnormalities.

Only 5% of infants with neonatal HSV are born with the disease (suggesting in utero transmission), with most infections being acquired during labour or delivery. It is estimated that about two-thirds of these infections are caused by asymptomatic first episode genital herpes.

HSV type 1 is more easily transmitted to the newborn as compared to HSV 2. However, neonatal HSV 2 infections are more serious, with frequent dissemination to the CNS and fatal outcome, as compared to HSV 1 infections which are usually limited to the skin, eyes and mucous membranes.

The diagnosis of neonatal herpes is often overlooked early on and made late in the course of the disease. This may happen because lesions in the mother may be absent (asymptomatic) or not recognized or hidden (e.g., on the cervix), or the fact that the long incubation period (5 to 21 days) allows the mother to take home a healthy looking newborn that sickens at home. Further, the initial manifestations are non-specific (irritability, lethargy, poor feeding) and skin lesions are present only in a minority of infants.

Most cases of neonatal herpes cannot be anticipated and hence are not preventable even with the best of antenatal and obstetric care. It has been estimated that even if every patient entering pregnancy with symptomatic recurrent genital herpes was delivered by a caesarean section, only a minority of cases of neonatal herpes would be prevented.

Unrecognized HSV 2 Infection

In a large survey in the US, only 9% of HSV 2 infected persons reported a history of genital herpes. Of individuals with genital HSV infection, approximately 20% have symptomatic disease that they recognize as genital herpes, another 60% have symptoms that they attribute to genital herpes only after being taught about the manifestation of infection, and the remaining 20% lack any sign or symptom of genital herpes.

In a more recent study, of 328 men enrolled, 148 (46%) had HSV-2 antibodies.[25] However only 14 (4.3%) reported a history of GH when queried as part of a list of other STD; on more detailed questioning 75 (21.1%) participants admitted to having a history of a recurring genital sore, ulcer, or zipper cut.

Herpes Genitalis in Patients with Concomitant HIV Infection[26]

A study from Trivandrum noted an incidence of herpes genitalis of 7.3% among patients with HIV,[27] while Syal et al. reported that 17.6% of patients with herpes genitalis had concomitant HIV infection.[28]

Current seroprevalence studies suggest that HSV is the most common opportunistic infection occurring among HIV infected adults. In developed countries, up to 90% of men who have sex with men, and 40–60% of injection-drug users have antibodies to HSV-1, HSV-2 or both, while studies from Africa suggest that most (up to 90%) persons infected with HIV are co-infected with HSV-2.[29] It is probable that the persistent genital ulcers of HSV **(Fig. 25.4, 25.5)** facilitate the transmission of HIV.

Atypical presentations are common in patients with AIDS. These include deep progressive infection, disseminated infections and prolonged viral shedding (Table 25.3).

Table 25.3 Atypical Presentations of Herpes Genitalis in Patients with AIDS

- Deep progressive ulceration
- Haemorrhagic and ecthyma-like lesions
- Hyperkeratotic verrucous lesions resembling condylomata
- Pseudotumour of the tongue
- Esophagitis, hepatitis, pneumonitis or life threatening disseminated infections associated with viremia
- Continuous and prolonged viral shedding

DIFFERENTIAL DIAGNOSIS

Many clinicians are under the impression that genital herpes has a characteristic appearance, comprising of easy-to-recognize blisters or ulcers. However, these so-called 'typical' signs and symptoms of herpes in clinical practice are not the commonest signs of herpes genitalis, and recurrent episodes of viral shedding may be associated with

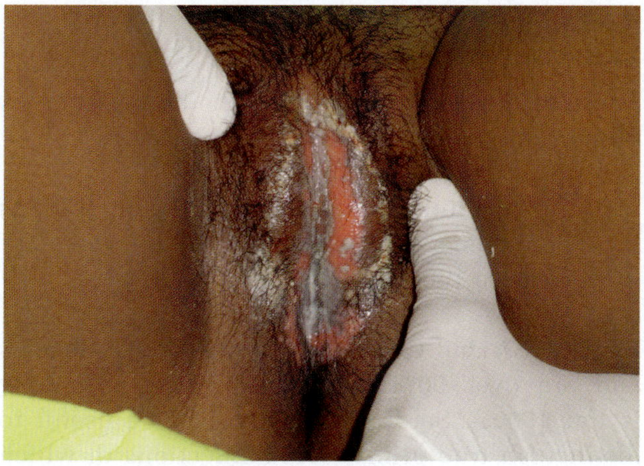

Fig. 25.4 Genital Herpes–Multiple erosions over the Vulva in a HIV Positive Patient.

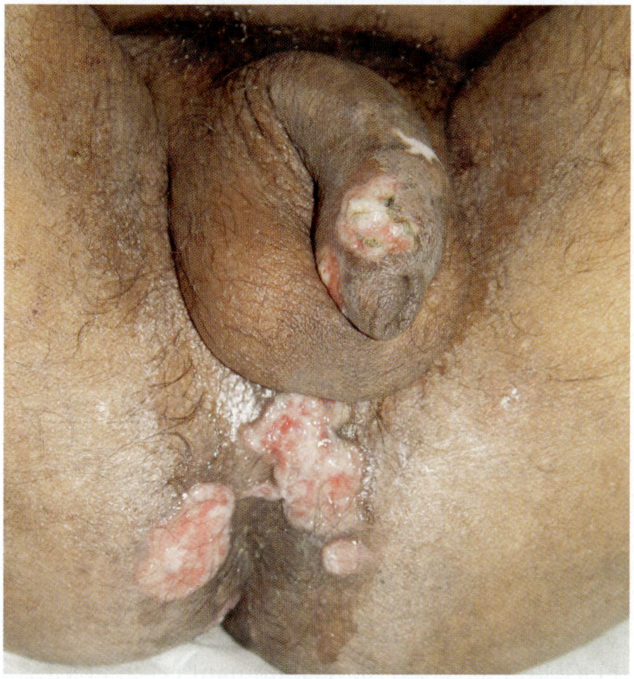

Fig. 25.5 Ano-genital Herpes – Extensive Ulceration in a HIV Positive Patient.

a wide variety of non-specific signs and symptoms such as erythema, small fissures, excoriated skin and burning or itching which frequently fail to be recognized as herpes. It should be emphasized also, that owing to the distribution of sacral sensory nerves, recurrences may occur anywhere below the waist; particularly common sites are on the buttocks, lower back, thighs and around the anus.

LABORATORY TESTS

The diagnosis of herpes genitalis is usually made clinically in typical cases. The sensitivity of clinical diagnosis is low—in one study, while the specificity was 96%, the sensitivity was only 39%.[10] However, in view of the fact that herpes may masquerade as a number of genital diseases with ulceration such as syphilis or chancroid, or even as non-specific lesions such as erosions or fissures, and in a proportion of cases may be asymptomatic, laboratory tests are frequently necessary to resolve the issue. As a thumb rule, all genital lesions regardless of appearance must be evaluated for herpes.

Laboratory tests available for the diagnosis of herpes virus infection include

- Tzanck smear
- Histopathology
- Viral culture
- Serology
- PCR

Tzanck Smear

A smear taken from the base of a vesicle or erosion and stained with Giemsa stain may show multinucleate giant cells **(Fig. 25.6)**. This test is not sensitive and may be negative in later lesions.

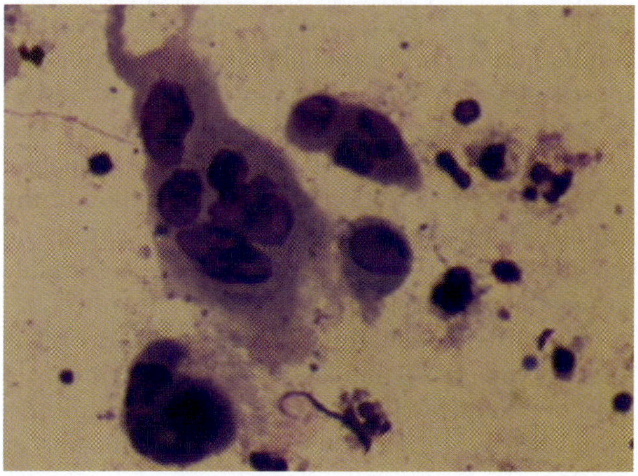

Fig. 25.6 Genital Herpes – Multinucleated Giant Cells-Giemsa stain (100X).

Specimens cannot be taken from dry lesions or crusts. Varicella-zoster virus infections may show a similar picture, although the clinical picture usually is distinctive enough to avoid confusion. Also, the Tzanck smear does not distinguish between HSV 1 and 2 infections.

Immunofluorescence staining of a Tzanck smear increases the sensitivity and specificity of the Tzanck test, but is not available in most laboratories.

Histopathology

Genital lesions are rarely biopsied. The presence of balloon cells and multinucleate giant cells will confirm the diagnosis of herpes. Histopathology is occasionally necessary in chronic herpes virus infections in HIV infected individuals wherein the morphology and clinical course are atypical. As in the case of the Tzanck smear, the presence of giant cells does not distinguish between type 1 and 2 herpes simplex virus infections, nor does it exclude varicella zoster virus infections.

Viral Culture

This is the definitive means for diagnosis of herpes. The technique is demanding. The material for culture is collected with special (Dacron) swabs, placed in a viral transport medium which is then refrigerated and transported to the laboratory. Refrigeration is necessary, as otherwise negative results may occur. In the laboratory, the swabs are inoculated into either human diploid fibroblast cultures or green monkey kidney (GMK) cell cultures. The virus grows rapidly, and cytopathic effects are visible within a few days, although the cultures are observed for two weeks if there is no growth. Virus cultures are generally not available in most laboratories.

Cultures are usually positive in primary or first episode infections, but may be negative in up to 50% of patients with recurrent infections. Cultures are also frequently negative from dry erosions or crusts.

Serology[30,31]

These tests detect antibodies to the herpes simplex virus in the blood and include

- Enzyme linked immunosorbent assay (ELISA)
- Complement fixation test (CFT)
- Western Blot

Both ELISA and CFT detect circulating antibodies and are over 90% sensitive but the specificity is low (50%). Serologic testing may be useful to distinguish true primary HSV infections in which there is only increased IgM from first episode nonprimary infections (increased IgG with or without increased IgM). The Western Blot is another serologic technique which distinguishes between HSV 1 and HSV 2 with high sensitivity and specificity (>99%).

Earlier tests based on envelope proteins of HSV-1 and HSV-2 which induce cross-reactive antibody responses were misleading, inaccurate and had low sensitivity and specificity. The current generation of tests based on enzyme immunoassays is highly sensitive and specific and uses type-specific glycoproteins gG1 and gG2 from HSV 1 and HSV 2 respectively. Kits have been developed for office use with results within hours. The Pockit tests can detect HSV 2, antibodies within 15 days on an average, although response times vary from 3 to 102 days (within 4 weeks in over 80% of episodes) Because of the wide variation in seroconversion, negative results should be repeated after 3 months for confirmation.

The FDA-approved commercially available type-specific ELISA, the HerpeSelect 2 ELISA (FOCUS2), is based on recombinant gG-2. FOCUS2 and other commercial gG-2-based assays showing high performance for sera from individuals resident in the United States and Europe 32 show significantly lower specificity in sub-Saharan Africa populations owing to the lower prevalence of HSV2.

The gG2 protein can be cleaved into a secreted portion (sgG-2) and a highly O-glycosylated mature portion (mgG-2). The performances of sgG-2 and mgG-2antigens as an ELISA test were compared with a commercially available assay (FOCUS2) in a recent study conducted in Tanzania 32 and concluded that native purified mgG-2 showed the highest accuracy for detection of HSV-2 in patient sera and was suitable for seroprevalence studies as well as in clinical settings.

Unfortunately, the serological tests being performed at most commercial laboratories in India still utilize the older generation ELISA tests.

PCR

A large number of studies[33-37] comparing virus culture with PCR in mucocutaneous swabs have uniformly demonstrated that the superiority of PCR for HSV detection. Despite the widespread use of HSV PCR for testing of CSF, only a minority of laboratories have adopted PCR for the processing of genital swabs. With the use of herpes cultures one third of symptomatic patients receive a false negative result, preventing appropriate counselling and often triggering additional clinic visits and investigations. It has been recommended that PCR should replace virus culture as the diagnostic method of choice for genital herpes[38].

In a survey of laboratories in the UK providing diagnostic services for genital herpes, virus culture was the preferentially used diagnostic method in most laboratories.[38] Although HSV-PCR for DNA detection in cerebrospinal fluid (CSF) was available in many laboratories, it was generally not used in the diagnosis of genital herpes, despite evidence indicating that its sensitivity is much higher than viral culture. Only 2/25 (8%) laboratories offered HSV type specific serology. In the Indian scenario, viral cultures are unavailable except in institutional settings, and although HSV-PCR is available, its high cost prevents its use in the clinical setting.

MANAGEMENT[39]

When a patient presents with suspected genital herpes, the clinician should establish a working diagnosis and a swab should be taken for confirmation if possible. Coexisting STDs should be looked for, and appropriate screening tests should be performed. The importance of evaluating the sexual partners should be discussed with the patient.

The patient with herpes should be counseled and should receive a comprehensive diagnostic evaluation, information and ongoing support. Patients confronted with a diagnosis of herpes genitalis frequently report feelings of depression, isolation, loss of self esteem, and a fear of rejection and discovery; although these tend to subside over time, many patients report that these feelings never totally disappear even after many years. Although effective antiviral drugs are now available, cure of the infection is not possible, and therefore strategies to avoid contracting and transmitting infection are important and should be discussed. A professional, but non-judgemental and non-patronizing approach is essential to maintain a rapport with the patient.

Drugs available for use in herpes simplex virus infections are given in Table 25.4. Immunomodulators and vaccines are still in their infancy, while many drugs and modalities of treatment used in the past have now been shown to be ineffective (a few of the more popular ones are listed).

Table 25.4 Drugs Used for the Treatment of HSV Infections

Current Drugs	*Vaccines and Immunomodulators*	*Ineffective Drugs (Used in the Past)*
Acyclovir	To reduce recurrences	Vidarabine
Valacyclovir	Imiquimod	Idoxuridine
Famcyclovir	Resiquimod	Ether
Cidofovir	Vaccines	Chloroform
Trifluridine		Povidone iodine
Foscarnet	For prevention of acquisition	Photodynamic dyes
	Vaccines	BCG vaccine
		Nonoxynol-9

There are currently three drugs approved for the treatment of herpes genitalis – acyclovir, famcyclovir and valacyclovir. They are nucleoside analogues and prevent replication of herpes simplex virus by interfering with the formation of viral DNA. They are active only in herpes virus infected cells, making them extremely safe and well tolerated. Acyclovir's only drawback is poor bio-availability and less than a fifth of each dose is absorbed. Famcyclovir is the oral prodrug of penciclovir, which has a similar, but not identical mechanism of action to acyclovir. Famcyclovir is well absorbed orally, making twice daily oral therapy possible. Valacyclovir is metabolized to acyclovir in vivo, and has the same mechanism of action as acyclovir. Valacyclovir is almost completely absorbed orally so, lower doses and less frequent dosage is possible. Drugs less commonly used, usually only in special circumstances such as acyclovir resistance, include foscarnet, cidofovir and trifluridine. Foscarnet is a viral DNA polymerase inhibitor; it has potent antiviral activity, but its insolubility precludes oral formulations. Intravenously, it is used in doses of 40 mg/kg every eight hours, but is toxic to the kidney and may produce hyperphosphatemia. It has been shown to be efficacious in acyclovir resistant recurrent HSV infections as a 0.3% and 0.1% cream.

Cidofovir is an acyclic nucleoside phosphonate which is phosphorylated only by cellular enzymes and hence is active against thymidine kinase deficient acyclovir resistant HSV strains. Intravenous cidofovir is effective, but is toxic to the kidney. Topical cidofovir, as a 0.3 and 1% gel formulation has been shown to help healing of non healing skin lesions of HSV in AIDS patients, however, almost one fourth of the treated patients had mild to moderate local side effects. Trifluridine is a topical antiviral (since it is toxic when given internally). Interferon alpha sign may poten-tiate its antiviral effect. It could become a useful alternative in acyclovir resistant HSV infections.

Drug Regimens

Available antivirals may be used in different ways including:

- Symptomatic management using only applications designed to reduce symptoms and improve healing
- Episodic (intermittent) therapy: to abort or reduce the duration of the episodes
- Continuous antiviral therapy-suppressive therapy to prevent recurrences

In 'episodic' treatment, oral antiviral therapy is used intermittently by the patient whenever a recurrence is experienced. In 'suppressive' (preventive) treatment the patient takes antiviral therapy continuously to prevent recurrences. While episodic therapy may only decrease the duration of lesions by one to one-and-a-half days. Some patients may find this effect clinically significant. Suppressive therapy generally reduces the number of recurrences and virus shedding by 85-90 percent.

Dosage schedules used to treat initial and recurrent episodes of herpes genitalis are given in Table 25.5. The probability of recurrences should be discussed with the patient after an initial episode and the decision to use episodic or suppressive treatment should be evolved in consultation with the patient. The potential benefits of antiviral therapy should be discussed with all patients. As many patients are unaware of the options available to them, the responsibility lies with the clinician to provide patients with sufficient information to enable them to participate fully in management decisions. Once the patient is fully informed about the options available, the patient and clinician together should agree upon a management strategy.

Patients who have four or less recurrences per year are best managed with episodic therapy. Patients managed by episodic antiviral therapy can start therapy themselves each time they detect the first signs of a recurrence. Self initiation allows each recurrence to be treated more expeditiously than if a physician had to be consulted. Education directed at recognition of early signs and symptoms, including the prodrome, is very important. Allowing patients to self initiate treatment without having to go back to the physician also returns control of the infection to the patient.

Table 25.5 Treatment of Herpes Genitalis

Initial episodes	Acyclovir	400 mg thrice daily for 7-10 days
	Valacyclovir	1 g twice daily for 7-10 days
	Famcyclovir	250 mg twice daily for 7-10 days
Recurrent episodes	Acyclovir	400 mg orally three times a day for 5 days
	Acyclovir	800 mg orally twice a day for 5 days
	Acyclovir	800 mg orally three times a day for 2 days
	Famcyclovir	125 mg orally twice daily for 5 days
	Famcyclovir	1000 mg orally twice daily for 1 day
	Valacyclovir	500 mg orally twice a day for 3 days
	Valacyclovir	1.0 g orally once a day for 5 days

Adapted from CDC 2006 Guidelines for treatment of sexually transmitted diseases.[39]

Short Course Therapy for Herpes Genitalis

Short-course therapy is based on the fact that viral replication occurs within the first 24 hours, and that the subsequent events such as erythema, swelling, vesiculation, and ulceration are caused by the immune response to epidermal damage by the virus and the ensuing wound healing process. Although patients usually have well developed lesions by the time of presentation to the physician, many patients can predict the appearance of lesions during the prodrome. Prodromal symptoms include itching, burning or pain. Self-administered therapy (patient initiated therapy) generally involved treatment periods of 5 days in the past.

A number of studies have compared shorter courses of antivirals with the traditional longer courses and have found them uniformly equally effective. A study by Leone et al. in 800 men with herpes genitalis, concluded that 3 days of 500 mg valacyclovir given twice daily was as effective as 5 days when they were required to self administer therapy no later than 24 hours after the onset of symptoms.[40] Another placebo-controlled trial of 2-day acyclovir therapy (800 mg TDS) by Wald and coworkers[41] in eighty-four immunocompetent HSV-2–infected patients with a history of ≥3 recurrences in the previous 12 months showed a decreased time to healing and episode duration by 2 days compared with placebo. Aoki et al. performed a randomized, double-blind, patient-initiated, placebo-controlled trial to assess the efficacy and safety of patient initiated, single-day famcyclovir 1000 mg twice daily in 329 immunocompetent adults with recurrent genital herpes.[42] Not only did single-day treatment with famcyclovir shorten the time to healing of nonaborted genital herpes lesions by approximately 2 days, and the time to healing of all lesions by 1.5 days, it aborted the lesions (i.e., no lesions developed after the prodrome) in 23% of the patients.

Famcyclovir is the only drug that has been proven to be effective in preventing a full herpes outbreak with a single-day treatment regimen.[43] Patient initiated episodic therapy with this single-day regimen may help to increase compliance, which in turn could help to decrease the severity of a recurrence, or prevent a full outbreak from occurring altogether.

Not only are these shorter course regimens as effective and more convenient as the recommended 5-day course (thus likely leading to increased patient compliance) there are also added gains in the form of a reduction in dose, and thus the cost.

Suppressive Therapy

Suppressive therapy should be considered for patients with severe, frequent or distressing recurrences (Table 25.6)

In the original benchmark study of suppressive therapy with acyclovir (400 mg twice daily), 20% of patients remained recurrence free for the entire period of 5 years.[44] In the multicentre trial of 1100 patients with over 12 episodes of herpes genitalis per year, in the first year of treatment the recurrence rate was only 1.7 during the first year and 0.8 in the fifth year. There were no serious side effects, nor was there any cumulative toxicity. Some patients required higher doses up to 800 mg twice daily. A study comparing 250 mg famcyclovir twice daily with 500 mg valacyclovir once daily found the latter to be marginally superior for suppression of genital herpes and associated shedding.[45]

Table 25.6 Suppressive Therapy

Immunocompetent patients	Acyclovir	400 mg twice daily
	Famcyclovir	250 mg twice daily
	Valacyclovir	500 mg once daily (<10 recurrences per year)
		1000 mg once daily(> 10 recurrences per year)
Immunocompromised patients	Acyclovir	400 - 800 mg twice or thrice daily
	Famcyclovir	500 mg twice daily
	Valacyclovir	500 mg twice daily

Immunomodulation

Resiquimod, an immune response modifier, is a potential treatment option for genital herpes. Unlike nucleoside analogues, immune response modifiers have no direct antiviral activity. Resiquimod stimulates the innate immune response to produce cytokines such as tumour necrosis factor α, interleukin 12 and interferon γ as well as the antigen-presenting cells (APC) present in the skin. Once HSV in neurons has reactivated and translocated to cells in the skin, it can be recognized by skin-based APC stimulated by resiquimod. Thus resiquimod stimulates the development of Th1 acquired, cell mediated immune response against HSV infected cells, thereby preventing HSV recurrences. Results from a Phase II clinical trial of resiquimod (0.01 or 0.05% gel for 4 to 9 doses) as a treatment for genital herpes in patients have been promising, with a tripling of time to recurrences from 57 to 169 days in the resiquimod treated patients.[46] Another recent study has shown that topical resiquimod 0.01% gel decreases herpes simplex virus type 2 genital shedding.[47]

Management of Herpes Genitalis in Pregnancy[48]

The American College of Obstetricians and Gynecologists (ACOG) have published guidelines for the management of herpes in pregnancy in June 2007.[48] Herpes virus infections prior to labour have no effect on pregnancy outcome. Antiviral chemotherapy is indicated only for the treatment of maternal disease and should be restricted only to treat the more severe infections – whether recurrent or first episode.

All the three antiviral agents that are commonly used to treat HSV infections - acyclovir, famcyclovir, and valacyclovir are all FDA pregnancy category B medications. Acyclovir has been extensively used during pregnancy and is considered safe while there are insufficient data on valacyclovir and famcyclovir exposure in the pregnancy registry for analyses.[48] Acyclovir is readily transferred to the amniotic fluid with an amniotic fluid to serum concentration of 5:1. At term, the maternal serum to cord blood ratio is approximately 1.15:1.

Management of HSV Infections at Labour

It has been suggested by some workers in the past that all women with symptomatic genital herpes should be delivered by caesarean section. As discussed earlier, however:

1. Most neonates who develop herpes have mothers who either have no past history of

herpes and have no active lesions at the time of delivery
2. Most of symptomatic lesions at term are recurrent HSV 2 which usually does not lead to infection of neonates.
3. Most neonatal herpes is a consequence of asymptomatic first episodes and caesarean section for all symptomatic lesions at term will prove ineffective in preventing neonatal HSV infection
4. HSV 1 infections during pregnancy and at term are rare but more easily transmissible to the neonate.

Since acyclovir is safe, two studies have been conducted using suppressive acyclovir treatment at term in pregnant women, and it was shown to be effective in suppressing symptomatic recurrences at term. However, this strategy is not advocated for routine use for prevention of HSV neonatal infections.

Recommendations for the Management of HSV Infections in Pregnancy

The ACOG in its guidelines[48] concludes that:

- Women with active recurrent genital herpes should be offered suppressive viral therapy at or beyond 36 weeks of gestation.
- Cesarean delivery is indicated in women with active genital lesions or prodromal symptoms, such as vulvar pain or burning at delivery, because these symptoms may indicate an impending outbreak.
- In women with premature rupture of membranes, there is no consensus on the gestational age at which the risk of prematurity outweigh the risk of HSV.
- Cesarean delivery is not recommended for women with a history of HSV infection but no active genital disease during labor.
- Routine antepartum genital HSV cultures in asymptomatic patients with recurrent disease are not recommended. Routine HSV screening of pregnant women is not recommended.

A simple strategy could involve asking all women at their first antenatal visit if they or their partner have ever had genital herpes. Female partners of men with genital herpes, but without a history of genital herpes, should be strongly advised not to have sex at the time of lesional recurrence. The regular use of condoms throughout pregnancy may diminish the risk of acquisition. Pregnant women should be advised of the risk of acquiring HSV 1 as a result of oro-genital contact.

All women, not just those with a history of genital herpes should undergo careful vulval inspection at the onset of labour to look for clinical signs of herpes infection. Mothers, staff, and other relatives/friends with active oral lesions should be advised about the risk of postnatal transmission.[23]

Management of Genital Herpes in HIV-Infected Patients[26]

The management of genital herpes in human immunodeficiency virus (HIV)-infected (HIV positive) patients differs from that in individuals not infected with HIV (HIV negative) for three reasons. Firstly, recurrent herpes simplex virus (HSV) genital infection in HIV positive patients tends to be persistent rather than self-limiting as in HIV negative individuals. This is particularly true in cases where the CD4 positive cell count falls below 100×10^6 cells/l. Secondly, HSV infection increases the replication and possibly the transmission of HIV infection. Finally, HIV immunosuppression increases the likelihood that antiviral therapy will lead to the emergence of drug-resistant mutants and with it, the associated failure of therapy.

Management of Primary and Initial Genital Herpes HIV-infected Patients

Initial genital herpes infection in HIV negative patients may be severe and prolonged but resolves spontaneously. In HIV infected patients, primary genital herpes may not resolve spontaneously but rather cause progressive, severe, multifocal and coalescing mucocutaneous anogenital lesions.

Conventionally used doses of acyclovir, valacyclovir or famcyclovir frequently effective in primary and initial genital herpes but higher doses of acyclovir (400 mg three to five times daily) have been recommended for HIV infected patients with severe genital infection and continuation of treatment until all lesions have crusted or re-epithelized This will generally exceed the 5–10-day duration of treatment that is recommended for HIV-negative patients.[26]

Management of Recurrent Genital Herpes in HIV Infected Patients

Genital herpes disease in HIV-infected patients may recur more frequently than in HIV-negative patients, especially those with a CD4 positive cell count of $<50 \times 10^6$ cells/l, and cause extensive, severe anogenital ulceration that does not resolve spontaneously.

Managing recurrent genital herpes in HIV-infected patients requires close attention both to the treatment of the HIV infection itself and to the recurring HSV infection. Highly active antiretroviral therapy (HAART) has been shown to reduce the risk of retinitis due to reactivation of another herpes virus, cytomegalovirus (CMV) by 83%, and extrapolating these results, optimizing the control of HIV disease is of fundamental importance for the management of genital herpes in these individuals.[26]

Episodic Therapy for Recurrent Genital Herpes in HIV Infected Individuals

Collectively, the available data support the choice of acyclovir 200–400 mg five times daily, famcyclovir 500 mg twice daily or valacyclovir 1 g twice daily for 5–7 days for episodic treatment of recurrent genital herpes in HIV positive individuals.[26] Although short courses of treatment of recurrent genital herpes are effective in HIV-negative adults, the appropriate duration of therapy in HIV infected adults appears to be at least 5–10 days (Table 25.7).

Table 25.7 CDC Recommended Regimens for Episodic Infection in Persons Infected with HIV[39]

Acyclovir	400 mg orally three times a day for 5–10 days 200 mg five times a day for 5–10 days,
Famcyclovir	500 mg orally twice a day for 5–10 days
Valacyclovir	1.0 g orally twice a day for 5–10 days

Suppressive Therapy of Recurrent Genital Herpes in HIV Infected Individuals

In addition to the indications for suppressive antiviral therapy of recurrent genital herpes discussed in non-HIV infected individuals earlier, recurrent disease that is either slow to respond to treatment or has a marked adverse psychological impact may be added. HIV infected patients with recurrent genital herpes lesions should initially be treated with one of the regimens for episodic therapy to achieve lesion resolution, after which a suppressive regimen as for HIV-negative individuals can be initiated. Until optimal drug regimens are defined, available data indicate that valacyclovir 500 mg twice daily should be the preferred regimen for suppressive therapy of recurrent genital herpes in HIV infected individuals. Breakthrough recurrences may occur, but if frequent may necessitate an upward revision of the dose or assessment for resistance to the drug.

Special Situations in Herpes Genitalis in Patients with HIV Infection

Holmes et al. reported the successful use of thalidomide in dose of 100 mg twice daily for 8 weeks in a single patient with disfiguring hypertrophic genital herpes associated with human immunodeficiency virus.[49] This patient was receiving antiretroviral therapy and had failed treatment with valacyclovir, cidofovir, and foscarnet.

Management of Acyclovir-resistant Infection

Acyclovir-resistant strains of HSV were first reported over 20 years back but are only now assuming significance with the epidemic of AIDS. Drug resistance appears to be uncommon in the immunocompetent population but more common in HIV-infected patients with prevalence rates of 4 to 7%. Acyclovir-resistance is most commonly due to a mutation in the gene encoding HSV thymidine kinase (TK), resulting in TK that either possesses reduced affinity for acyclovir or is not synthesized (TK–). Moreover, as famcyclovir and ganciclovir are also subject to the same initial phosphorylation activation step mediated by TK, acyclovir resistance also extends to famcyclovir and ganciclovir. Acyclovir-resistance may also be due to a mutation in the HSV DNA polymerase that results in a reduced affinity for acyclovir-triphosphate. Infection caused by isolates with altered TK or reduced affinity of HSV DNA polymerase should theoretically respond to higher doses of acyclovir and indeed, successful treatment of a patient with acyclovir-resistant HSV that had a TK with altered affinity, using intravenous acyclovir 1.5–2.0 mg/kg per hour for 6 weeks has been reported.

Long-term management of genital herpes in patients with resistant disease is unsatisfactory. Although both foscarnet and adenine arabinoside show in vitro activity against acyclovir-resistant HSV, a controlled clinical trial demonstrated healing of mucocutaneous lesions due to acyclovir-resistant HSV only in recipients of foscarnet 120 mg/kg per day for an average of 14 days but not in those treated with adenine arabinoside 15 mg/kg per day intravenously; the latter was also associated with significant toxicity (neurotoxicity). Unfortunately, recurrences, mostly with acyclovir resistant virus occurred a median of 14 days after foscarnet was stopped in most of the treated patients.

Topical trifluridine alone or in combination with interferon-alpha, cidofovir gel and foscarnet 1% cream have been reported to have clinical utility for the treatment of acyclovir-resistant HSV genital ulcers.

The Role of Antiherpes Drugs in the Management of HIV and HSV Co-infection[29]

HSV infection increases HIV replication, and possibly the transmission of HIV infection, raising the possibility of a role for antiherpes drug therapy in controlling HIV disease and reducing HIV transmission. Epidemiological observations suggest that HSV-2 infection facilitates HIV transmission. HSV is a potent stimulator of HIV replication in co-infected CD4-positive cells in vitro. A survival benefit of treatment with acyclovir, 3200–4800 mg per day, has been demonstrated by a meta-analysis of eight randomized trials in patients with HIV and herpes virus infections.[29] The advantage was seen specifically in studies in which the incidence of HSV and varicella zoster virus (VZV) clinical disease was high, with >25 cases per 100 patient years. Acyclovir decreased HSV and VZV but not CMV infections as well as reducing mortality. These data suggest an important pathogenetic interaction between HIV and the herpes viruses, HSV and VZV.

A recent randomized, double-blind, placebo-controlled trial of HSV suppressive therapy with valacyclovir (at a dose of 500 mg twice daily) in Burkina Faso among women who were seropositive for HIV-1 and HSV-2 but were ineligible for highly active antiretroviral therapy showed that the HSV suppressive therapy significantly reduced genital and plasma HIV-1 RNA levels in dually infected women.[50] The same group of workers had earlier reported[51] that valacyclovir reduced the proportion of visits with detectable genital HSV-2 DNA but had no significant impact on the frequency or quantity of genital HIV-1 RNA in women on HAART.

Complementary And Alternative Medicine

The fact that herpes genitalis is not curable and the fear of side effects drive many patients to use a variety of complementary and alternative medicine (CAM) treatments. Perfect and his colleagues superscript 52 reviewed available scientific data on six commonly used treatments (echinacea, eleuthero, L-lysine, zinc, bee products and aloe) besides listing a number of other products and concluded that there was insufficient clinical data to be confident of the efficacy and safety of any of these products for the treatment of genital herpes.

PREVENTION OF TRANSMISSION OF GENITAL HERPES

The only methods currently available for preventing transmission of genital herpes infections are male and female condoms. There have been no studies evaluating the efficacy of female condoms in preventing the transmission of herpes simplex virus infections. In one recent large study of over 500 serodiscordant couples enrolled in a candidate HSV 2 vaccine trial, where participants were followed for 18 months,participants using condoms are less likely to acquire HSV 2.[53] The efficacy of condoms was especially marked among women.

In a analysis of data collected as part of a recent clinical trial of an ineffective candidate vaccine for HSV-2, Wald and her coworkers found that consistent use of condoms was associated with lower rates of infection with HSV-2 and should be routinely recommended.[54] In a recent multicentric study of sex practices in patients who were aware that they had herpes genitalis, Rana et al.[55] found that although the majority of people with GH either abstained from intercourse or "always" used condoms during symptomatic periods of GH, condom use was relatively low during asymptomatic periods. These results highlight that further education on GH prevention is warranted, particularly for symptomatic periods. Data presented here indicate that a large proportion abstain from sex during symptomatic periods. However, condoms were used irregularly. A focus of prevention must continue to highlight the importance of regular and consistent condom use during both symptomatic and asymptomatic periods.

Altering sexual behaviours represents a cost-effective and safe measure that may significantly reduce new infections. Consistent and correct use of latex condoms appears to protect women from HSV 2 infection, and should be emphasized in pregnant women at risk of HSV 2 to prevent neonatal herpes.[56] Unfortunately, condoms are not acceptable to all users and the male condom does not provide coverage of all susceptible surfaces.

HSV vaccines are still in development. There are currently over nine types of live attenuated as well as inactive vaccines under evaluation. Although vaccines may not offer absolute protection, it is possible that they might ameliorate the disease or reduce recurrences. However, recent trials of some of the vaccines have not been very encouraging showing only minimal protection.[57]

Table 25.8 **Potential Methods of Preventing Transmission of Genital Herpes**

Condoms
Vaccines
Microbicides
Monoclonal antibodies
Antivirals eg. valacyclovir

Another approach is the use of topical microbicides. These have been investigated in the prevention of other STDs and have been found to be useful. Among the first such topical agents to be used was nonoxylenol-9. A variety of novel microbicides are in various stages of development[58] and these include sulphated polymer based inhibitors, acid buffers and surfactants. Sulphated polymer-based inhibitors interfere with transmission by binding to pathogens and/or target cells and preventing the pathogen from attaching to its target. Acid buffers are designed to maintain the natural vaginal acidity in the presence of the alkalinizing effects of semen, thereby inactivating acid sensitive pathogens. Surfactants solubilize membranes and viral envelopes.

In contrast to the topical microbicides which are non-specific, monoclonal antibodies are highly specific. Monoclonal antibodies have been shown in experimental studies to protect against other sexually transmitted infections such as *Candida albicans, Chlamydia trachomatis and Human papilloma virus* among others.

Monoclonal antibodies can also be used for preventing vertical transmission (neonatal herpes).[58] Microbicidal agents such as vaginally applied chlorhexidine have been used in the past to prevent neonatal transmission of HSV, HIV and other sexually transmitted infections. Based on the fact that antibodies prevent vertical transmission of hepatitis B and varicella zoster and also that maternal antibodies to HSV are associated with low transmission to infants by infected women systemically delivered anti-HSV monoclonals given to women at risk for neonatal transmission have been suggested as an alternative to or in conjunction with suppressive acyclovir therapy. Systemically delivered HSV specific antibodies have been shown to protect neonatal mice and guinea pigs from mucosal challenge, even when administered 2 days after viral challenge, and prevent oral transmission of infection in a neonatal macaque model.

Fife and his coworkers[59] have recently shown that patients administered 1 g/d of suppressive valacyclovir therapy had a 71% reduction in days with total shedding and a 58% reduction in subclinical days with shedding as compared to patients on placebo. Seventy percent of the valacyclovir patients had no days of shedding. There was also a significant reduction in the average log HSV-2 DNA copy number per day for all shedding days for valacyclovir compared with placebo.

An earlier large randomized, controlled clinical trial of 500 mg of valacyclovir used once a day by the infected source partner, in combination with safer sex counselling of heterosexual couples discordant for HSV-2 infection demonstrated reduced transmission of clinical HSV-2 infection to the susceptible partner by 75% and overall HSV-2 infection by 48%. In this study, there was a 73% reduction in total (clinical and subclinical) days of viral shedding and a 64% reduction in days of subclinical viral shedding in infected source partners receiving valacyclovir compared with those receiving placebo.[60] Fifty-one percent of the valacyclovir patients in that substudy had no days of shedding.

A recent comparison of efficacy of valacyclovir and famcyclovir shows that the former was more effective in suppressing herpes simplex virus-2 (HSV-2) shedding. However, the clinical implications of this finding are unclear, as the time to disease recurrence with both drugs is about the same.[61]

REFERENCES

1. Corey L and Wald A. Genital herpes. In: Holmes KK, Mardh PA, Sparling PF, et al. eds. Sexually Transmitted Diseases. 3rd Edition. New York: McGraw-Hill; 1999. p. 285-312.
2. Roberts CM, Pfister JR, Spear SJ. Increasing proportion of herpes simplex virus type 1 as a cause of genital herpes infection in college students. Sex Transm Dis 2003; 30: 797-800.
3. Xu F, Schillinger JA, Sternberg MR, et al. Seroprevalence and coinfection with herpes simplex virus type 1 and type 2 in the United States, 1988-1994. J Infect Dis 2002; 185: 1019-24.
4. Sharma VK, Khandpur S. Changing patterns of sexually transmitted infections in India. Natl Med J India 2004; 17: 310-9.
5. Kumar B, Sahoo B, Gupta S, et al. Rising incidence of genital herpes over two decades in a sexually transmitted disease clinic in North India. J Dermatol 2002; 29: 74-8.
6. Cherpes TL, Meyn LA, and Hillier SL. Cunnilingus and vaginal intercourse are risk factors for herpes simplex virus type 1 acquisition in women. Sex Transm Dis 2005; 32: 84-9.
7. Lowhagen GB, Tunback P, Bergstrom T. Proportion of herpes simplex virus (HSV) Type 1 and Type 2 among genital and extragenital isolates. Acta Derm Venereol 2002; 82: 118-20.
8. Wald A. Herpes: Transmission and viral shedding. Dermatol Clin 1998; 16: 795-7.
9. Mertz G, Coombs R, Ashley R, et al. Transmission of genital herpes in couples with one symptomatic and one asymptomatic partner:

a prospective study. J Infect Dis 1988; 157: 1169-77.
10. Langenberg AGM, Corey L, Ashley RL, et al. A prospective study of new infections with herpes simplex virus type 1 and type 2. N Engl J Med 1999; 341: 1432-8.
11. Koutsky LA, Ashley RL, Holmes KK, et al. The frequency of unrecognized type 2 herpes simplex virus infection among women: implications for the control of genital herpes. Sex Transm Dis 1990; 17: 90-4.
12. Wald A, Zeh J, Selke S, et al. Reactivation of genital herpes simplex virus type 2 infection in asymptomatic seropositive persons. N Engl J Med 2000; 342: 844-50.
13. Benedetti JK, Zeh J, Corey LK. Clinical reactivation of genital herpes simplex virus infection decreases in frequency over time. Ann Intern Med 1999; 131: 14-20.
14. Krone MR, Wald A, Tabet SR, et al. Herpes simplex virus Type 2 shedding in human immunodeficiency virus-negative men who have sex with men: frequency, patterns, and risk factors. Clin Infect Dis 2000; 30: 261-7.
15. Mertz GJ, Benedetti J, Ashley R, et al. Risk factors for the sexual transmission of genital herpes. Ann Intern Med. 1992; 116: 197-202.
16. Brown ZA. Genital herpes complicating pregnancy. Dermatol Clin 1998; 16: 805-9.
17. Mindel A, Taylor J, Tideman RL, et al. Neonatal herpes prevention: a minor public health problem in some communities. Sex Transm Inf 2000; 76: 287-91.
18. Hensleigh P, Andrews W, Brown Z, et al. Genital herpes during pregnancy: inability to distinguish primary and recurrent infections clinically. Obstet Gynecol 1997; 89: 891-5.
19. Fleming DT, McQuillan GM, Johnson RE, et al. Herpes simplex virus type 2 in the United States, 1976 to 1994. N Engl J Med. 1997; 337: 1105-11.
20. Austin H, Macaluso M, Nahmias A, et al. Correlates of herpes simplex virus seroprevalence among women attending a sexually transmitted disease clinic. Sex Transm Dis 1999; 26: 329-34.
21. Wald A, Koutsky L, Ashley RL, et al. Genital herpes in a primary care clinic: demographic and sexual correlates of herpes simplex type 2 infections. Sex Transm Dis 1997; 24: 149-55.
22. Brown ZA, Selke S, Zeh J, et al. The acquisition of herpes simplex virus during pregnancy. N Engl J Med. 1997; 337: 509-15.
23. Brown ZA, Benedetti J, Ashley R, et al. Neonatal herpes simplex virus infection in relation to asymptomatic maternal infection at the time of labor. N Engl J Med 1991; 324: 1247-52.
24. Brown ZA, Wald A, Morrow RA, et al. Effect of serologic status and cesarean delivery on transmission rates of herpes simplex virus from mother to infant. JAMA 2003; 289: 203-9.
25. Sizemore Jr JM, Lakeman F, Whitley R, et al. Historical correlates of genital herpes simplex virus type 2 infection in men attending an STDs clinic Sex Transm Infect 2005; 81: 303-5.
26. Aoki FY. Management of genital herpes in HIV-infected Patients. Herpes 2001; 8: 41-5.
27. Nair SP, Moorty KP, Suprakasan S. Clinico-epidemiological study of HIV patients in Trivandrum. Indian J Dermatol Venereol Lepr 2003; 69: 100-3.
28. Sayal SK, Gupta CM, Sanghi S. HIV infection in patients of sexually transmitted disease. Indian J Dermatol Venereol Lepr 1999; 65: 131-3.
29. Schacker T. The role of HSV in the transmission and progression of HIV. Herpes 2001; 8: 46-9.
30. Ashly RL. Genital herpes: Type specific antibodies for diagnosis and management. Dermatol Clin 1998; 16: 789-93.
31. Goldman BD. Herpes serology for the dermatologist. Arch Dermatol 2000; 136: 1158-61.
32. Gorander S, Mbwana J, Lyamuya E, et al. Mature glycoprotein g presents high performance in diagnosing herpes simplex virus type 2 infection in sera of different Tanzanian cohorts. Clin Vaccine Immunol. 2006; 13: 633-9.
33. Burrows J, Nitsche A, Bayly B, et al. Detection and subtyping of Herpes simplex virus in clinical samples by Light Cycler PCR, enzyme immunoassay and cell culture. BMC Microbiol 2002; 2: 2-12.
34. Aldea C, Alvarez CP, Folgueira L, et al. Rapid detection of herpes simplex virus DNA in genital ulcers by real-time PCR using SYBR green I dye as the detection signal. J Clin Microbiol 2002; 40: 1060-2.

35. Van Doornum GJ, Guldemeester J, Osterhaus AD, et al. Diagnosing herpesvirus infections by real-time amplification and rapid culture. J Clin Microbiol 2003; 41: 576-80.
36. Wald A, Huang ML, Carrell D, et al. Polymerase chain reaction for detection of herpes simplex virus (HSV) DNA on mucosal surfaces: comparison with HSV isolation in cell culture. J Infect Dis 2003; 188: 1345-51.
37. Ramaswamy M, McDonald C, Smith M, et al. Diagnosis of genital herpes by real-time PCR in routine clinical practice. Sex Transm Infect 2004; 80: 406-10.
38. Geretti AM, Brown DW. National survey of diagnostic services for genital herpes. Sex Transm Infect 2005; 81: 316-7.
39. Centers for Disease Control and Prevention (CDC). Sexually transmitted diseases treatment guidelines, 2006. MMWR Recomm Rep 2006; 55: 1-94.
40. Leone PA, Trottier S, Miller JM. Valacyclovir for episodic treatment of genital herpes: a shorter 3-day treatment course compared with 5-day treatment. Clin Infect Dis 2002; 34: 958-62.
41. Wald A, Carrell D, Remington M, et al. Two day regimen of acyclovir for treatment of recurrent genital herpes simplex virus type 2 infection. Clin Infect Dis 2002; 34: 944-8.
42. Aoki FY, Tyring S, Dias-Mitoma F, et al. Single-day patient initiated famcyclovir therapy for recurrent genital herpes: a randomized double-blind, placebo-controlled trial. Clin Infect Dis 2006; 42: 8-13.
43. Whitley R, Diaz-Mitoma F, Hamed K. Single-day famcyclovir therapy for recurrent genital herpes Curr Med Res Opin 2006; 22: 1307-10.
44. Goldberg LH, Kaufman R, Kurtz TO, et al. Long-term suppression of recurrent genital herpes with acyclovir: a 5-year benchmark. Arch Dermatol 1993; 129: 582-7.
45. Handsfield HH, Warren T, Werner M, et al. Suppressive therapy with valacyclovir in early genital herpes: a pilot study of clinical efficacy and herpes-related quality of life. Sex Transm Dis. 2007; 34: 339-43.
46. Spruance SL, Tyring SK, Smith MH, et al. Application of a topically applied immune response modifier, resiquimod gel, to modify the recurrence rate of recurrent genital herpes: a pilot study. J Infect Dis 2001; 184: 196-200.
47. Mark KE, Corey L, Meng TC, et al. Topical resiquimod 0.01% gel decreases herpes simplex virus type 2 genital shedding: a randomized, controlled trial. J Infect Dis 2007; 195: 1324-31.
48. ACOG Practice Bulletin. Clinical management guidelines for obstetrician-gynecologists. No. 82 June 2007. Management of herpes in pregnancy. Obstet Gynecol 2007; 109: 1489-98.
49. Holmes A, McMenamin M, Mulcahy F, et al. Thalidomide therapy for the treatment of hypertrophic herpes simplex virus-related genitalis in HIV-infected individuals. Clin Infect Dis 2007; 44: 96-9.
50. Nagot N, Ouédraogo A, Foulongne V, et al. ANRS 1285 Study Group. Reduction of HIV-1 RNA levels with therapy to suppress herpes simplex virus. N Engl J Med 2007; 356: 790-9.
51. Ouedraogo A, Nagot N, Vergne L, et al. Impact of suppressive herpes therapy on genital HIV-1 RNA among women taking antiretroviral therapy: a randomized controlled trial. AIDS 2006; 20: 2305-13.
52. Perfect MM, Bourne N, Ebel C, et al. Use of complementary and alternative medicine for the treatment of genital herpes. Herpes 2005; 12: 38-41.
53. Wald A, Langenberg AG, Link K, et al. Effect of condoms on reducing the transmission of herpes simplex virus type 2 from men to women. JAMA 2001; 285: 3100-6.
54. Wald A, Langenberg AG, Krantz E, et al. The relationship between condom use and herpes simplex virus acquisition Ann Intern Med. 2005; 143: 707-13.
55. Rana RK, Pimenta JM, Rosenberg DM, et al. Sexual behaviour and condom use among individuals with a history of symptomatic genital herpes. Sex Transm Infect. 2006; 82: 69-74.
56. Casper C, Wald A. Condom use and the prevention of genital herpes acquisition. Herpes 2002; 9: 10-14.
57. Stanberry LR, Cunningham AL, Mindel A, et al. Prospects for control of herpes simplex virus disease through immunization. Clin Infect Dis 2000; 30: 549-566.

58. Zeitlin L, Whaley KJ. Microbicides for preventing transmission of genital herpes. Herpes 2002; 9: 4-9.
59. Fife KH, Warren TJ, Ferrera RD, et al. Effect of valacyclovir on viral shedding in immunocompetent patients with recurrent herpes simplex virus 2 genital herpes: a US-based randomized, double-blind, placebo-controlled clinical trial. Mayo Clin Proc. 2006; 81: 1321-7.
60. Corey L, Wald A, Patel R, et al. Valacyclovir HSV Transmission Study Group. Once-daily valacyclovir to reduce the risk of transmission of genital herpes. N Engl J Med 2004; 350: 11-20.
61. Wald A, Selke S, Warren T, et al. Comparative efficacy of famcyclovir and valacyclovir for suppression of recurrent genital herpes and viral shedding. Sex Transm Dis 2006; 33: 529-33.

26 | ANOGENITAL WARTS

N Usman

In this chapter

- Definition
- Prevalence
- Aetiology
- Transmission of the Virus
- Immunology of Warts
- Clinical Features
- Diagnosis
- Differential Diagnosis
- Treatment Modalities for Anogenital Warts
- Complications
- Anogenital Warts and Pregnancy
- Anogenital Warts in Children
- Anogenital Warts and HIV
- Mechanisms of Interactions between HIV and HPV
- Anogenital Warts and Malignancy
- Vaccine

DEFINITION

Wart is a viral infection caused by human papilloma virus (HPV). It can affect both the skin and the mucosa. Anogenital warts refer to the infection of the anal and genital mucosa and theif adjoining area. Many authors use the term "Anogenital Warts" synonymously with "Condylomata Acuminata", although the latter is described with a characteristic histology.[1]

PREVALENCE

Prevalence of genital HPV infection and distribution of specific HPV types appears to be similar in different regions of the world. Current evidence suggests that over 50% of sexually active adults have been infected with one or more HPV types. In United States, the estimated prevalence among men and women between 15-49 years of age with genital warts is 1.4 million, and 19 million have subclinical infections.[2] In Britain and Ireland 80,000 new cases of anogenital warts are reported yearly.[3] The prevalence of genital warts in India has been reported to be 5.1% to 25.2% of patients with sexually transmitted diseases (STD).[4-6] In a report by Arora et al, the incidence of anogenital warts had increased from 7.2% to 8.8% among the HIV-infected patients over a period of five years.[7]

AETIOLOGY

The causative agent of anogenital warts is HPV, which is a naked, double-stranded DNA virus **(Fig. 26.1)**. There are at present more than 100 different genotypes of HPV. Of these, 45 genotypes have been found to infect the genital epithelium.

HPV belongs to the family Papovaviridae along with polyoma virus. They are non-enveloped and are composed of 72 pentameric capsomers forming the outer coat. This coat consists of major and minor capsid proteins and these are arranged on a skewed icosahedral lattice. The capsids are approximately 60 nm in diameter. The genome consists of circular double stranded DNA, which encodes for overlapping genes and a single control region. The genes are distributed into early (E_1-E_7) and late (L_1 and L_2) regions. The early genes encode for proteins that are involved with regulation of viral DNA replication and transcription, whereas the late region encodes as L_1 and L_2 for major and minor capsid proteins, respectively. Early genes (E_6, E_7) are involved in oncogenic transformation in high-risk HPV types.[8,9]

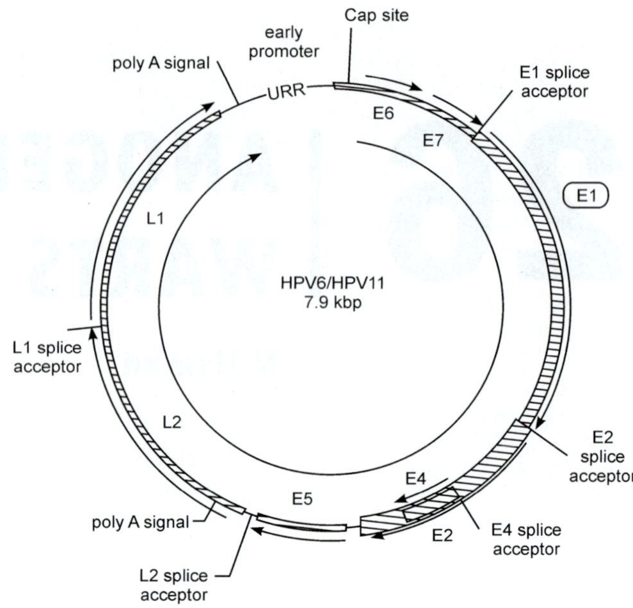

Fig. 26.1 HPV - Structure

HPV are epitheliotropic, and their replication depends on the presence of differentiating squamous epithelium. Viral DNA, but not structural (capsid) protein, can be detected in the lower layers of the epithelium. Capsid protein and infectious virus are found in the superficial differentiated cell layers. The different types of HPV cannot be differentiated serologically like other virus groups, because of the lack of antigen available to produce antibodies for testing, and these viruses cannot be grown in vitro. So far, no HPV type has been shown to transform cells in vitro. The use of raft culture system, which forms a stratified squamous epithelium, has now produced limited amounts of infectious HPV.

Several types of HPV can co-exist in the same wart. Some common types of genital HPV and their associations are shown in Table 26.1.[10]

Table 26.1 HPV Types and Clinical Disease

Clinical diseases	*HPV Types (frequent)*	*HPV Types (less frequent)*
Condylomata acuminata	6, 11	1-5, 10, 16, 18, 30, 31, 33, 35, 39-45, 51-59, 70, 83
Cervical intraepithelial neoplasia (CIN/CIL)		
Low-grade	6, 11	16, 18, 26, 27, 30, 31, 33-35, 40, 42-45, 51-58, 61, 62, 67-69, 71-74, 82
High-grade	16, 18	6, 11, 31, 33, 35, 39, 42, 44, 45, 51, 52, 56, 58, 59, 61, 64, 66, 68, 82
Bowenoid papulosis	16	34, 39, 40, 42, 45
Cervical cancer	16, 18	31, 33, 35, 39, 45, 51, 52, 56, 58, 59, 66
Giant condyloma of Buschke and Lowenstein and other verrucous carcinomas	6, 11	57, 72, 73
Oral/laryngeal papilloma (Recurrent respiratory papillomatosis)	6, 11	2, 16, 30, 32, 40, 57
In HIV patients	7, 72, 73	

TRANSMISSION OF THE VIRUS

Genital HPV infections are transmitted primarily through sexual contact. The infectivity of HPV among sexual partners is estimated to be 60%. During the sexual act, micro abrasions occur in male and female genitalia and anus in homosexuals. It is believed that these micro abrasions permit the transfer of HPV virions from the epithelial cells of the infected partner to the basal layer of recipient. It is a thought but still not proven that moisture and abrasions of the epithelial surface enhance HPV transmission. Transfer by fomites is not a known factor in transmission of genital HPV. Digital transmission has been reported. Perinatal transmission has been observed in infants born to women with genital warts during pregnancy. These infants developed laryngeal papillomas and congenital condylomas. This type of transmission is rare.[2]

IMMUNOLOGY OF WARTS[2]

Inability to propagate HPV in the laboratory has hampered investigation of the immunology of warts. Both cell-mediated immunity (CMI) and humoral response have been demonstrated in patients with genital warts.

Humoral Immunity

Almedia et al, showed "one way cross reactivity" between cutaneous and anogenital warts.[11] The cutaneous warts are auto-inoculable on to the genital mucosa, wheres the genital warts are not able to produce any lesion on the glabrous skin. The aetiological difference between cutaneous and genital warts is also seen in their serological behaviour. The serum from patients with cutaneous wart interacts with antigen from cutaneous as well as anogenital warts, whereas the serum from patients with anogenital warts interacts with the antigen of anogenital wart only.

Various studies have shown that human sera have antibodies that react to HPV proteins. The earlier studies used HPV expressing fusion proteins or synthetic peptides and used antibody assays that recognized only linear epitopes. Thus, the heterogeneity of the virus particles was not taken into account. Almedia[12] analyzed the sera of 42 patients with warts and only half of these patients had demonstrable antibody. No particular correlation between presence of antibody types and duration of the lesions had emerged, though recurrence did seem to be associated with lack of antibody. HPV capsids are the new generation of antigen targets. These antigen targets have defined specificity, which are obtained from recombinant vaccinia virus or baculovirus expressing L_1 and L_1 plus L_2. Using capsids in an ELISA, type specific antibodies to L_1 protein had been detected, and these antibodies strongly correlate with history of HPV-associated disease. Experimentally infected animals generated similar antibodies that have been shown to be neutralizing. It has been also noted that the tempo for developing serum anticapsid antibodies is slow. The median time to seroconversion is approximately one year, and antibodies persist for decades.[2] Though circulating antibodies are detected in patients with warts, they do not help in the elimination of the lesion or in the prevention of recurrences.

In patients with regressing warts, IgM (100%), IgG (97%) and IgA (80%) classes of antibodies to HPV antigens were detected. In 83% of these patients, IgM class of antibodies to virus-infected cells was also seen. Only 12% of the patients with non-regressing warts showed antibodies (IgM) to the infected cells. Pyrhonen[13] showed that when complement-fixing (CF) antibodies (IgG) were present, the cure rate was high. In 75% of such patients cure was observed during first 2 months. The cure rate was high in those with CF antibodies and warts of short duration (less than one year). In contrast, absence of CF antibodies correlated with slow healing process. Increase in the circulating antibodies has been demonstrated in regressing warts. Whether this increase in antibodies is the result of regression of the wart or it is responsible for regression of the warts is not known.

Cell Mediated Immunity

Increase in the CMI has been shown to be effective both in elimination and in the prevention of recurrence of warts. Evidence for the involvement of CMI in wart regression has come from observations that patients with immunodeficiency have an increased incidence of warts. It was noted that those patients with a predominantly cell-mediated defect or a mixed antibody and cell-mediated defect were susceptible, in contrast to those with only antibody defects. A study on the immunocompetence of patients with warts revealed a relative deficiency of cell-mediated immunity which appeared to be related to the duration of infection,[14] thus confirming the observations of Brodersen, Genner and Brothagen that children with warts showed reduced tuberculin reactivity when compared to unaffected controls. In addition to the observation that a marked dermal infiltrate of mononuclear cells present around spontaneously resolving warts, the role for CMI in wart regression is suggested.

The lack of detectable local immunological response may be due to the fact that (i) the virus producing cells are away from the basement membrane as far as the immune response is concerned,(ii) inadequate production of viral particles and viral antigens. This is supported by the smaller number of mature particles seen in genital warts either by immunoperoxidase staining or by electron microscopic studies and (iii) the infected cells may exhibit insufficient histocompatibility antigen display on their surface as seen with other virus induced tumors.

The primary infected cells in a wart are not recognized by the immune system because of the local inhibitory effect of these cells. This is evidenced by the absence of Langerhans cells and T cells in the epidermis surrounding the wart in comparison to the normal epidermis. The antigen of HPV is situated in the granular layer of epidermis, therefore exposure of the antigen to the immune system is hampered, and thus there is delay in development of CMI against warts. Regression of warts due to increase in CMI in wart patients was demonstrated by Viac et al.[15] Cytotoxic T lymphocytic response seems to play an important role in the elimination of warts.[2]

Although neutralizing antibodies may be useful in preventing infection, the cell–mediated immune response is likely to be important in controlling reactivation and regression of infection.[16]

CLINICAL FEATURES

HPV after entry may remain dormant without producing any lesions[16] or may produce symptomatic or asymptomatic lesions.

Symptomatic

The lesions appear after the incubation period of 1-8 months with an average of three months. Rarely, they may resolve after some time without any treatment. Anogenital warts may be single or multiple. In men, genital warts most commonly appear first on the inner lining of the prepuce (subprepucial region) and the frenulum followed by the glans, coronal sulcus, urinary meatus, penile shaft, and the scrotum. In women, the common sites involved are posterior part of the introitus, labia, perineum and perianal area. Lesions can also involve the vagina and cervix, but more commonly it is a subclinical infection. The common presentation is a verrucous papules or pedunculated lesions that may coalesce to form verrucous plaques or cauliflower like growths. Generally the lesions are pink and painless. Depending upon the clinical appearance, warts can be classified as condylomata acuminata, papular wart, keratotic wart, and flat topped papular warts.

1. *Condylomata Acuminata*

The lesions are pedunculated masses (cauliflower like) with fissures and irregular surface **(Fig. 26.2, 26.3, 26.4, 26.5, 26.6)**. The colour of the lesion varies from red to pink or white with characteristic warty digitations. Such lesions are usually seen in the moist partially keratinized epithelium.[2]

2. *Papular Wart*

These are non-pedunculated, hemispherical or dome shaped masses, 1-4 mm in diameter, located on fully keratinized epithelium.[2]

3. *Verruca Vulgaris Type or Keratotic*

These are firm papular lesions with slightly rough horny surface with no pedicle; size ranging from few millimeters to few centimeters in diameter **(Fig. 26.7)**. They are usually seen on dry areas like shaft of penis, outer aspect of prepuce, labia majora, and perineum.[2]

Sessile warts are tiny lesions with no horny surface. They are usually detected on fully keratinized epithelium.

4. *Flat-topped Papules*

These appear macular to slightly raised. They are detected on either partially or fully keratinized epithelium.[2]

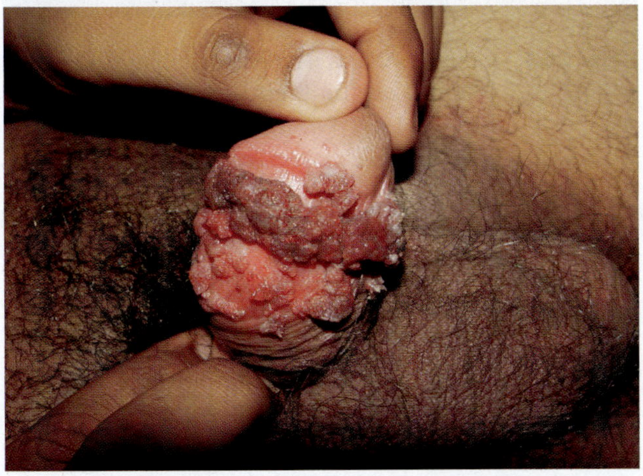

Fig. 26.2 Genital Warts - Exuberant Fleshy Cauliflower like Growth on the Prepuce and Glans.

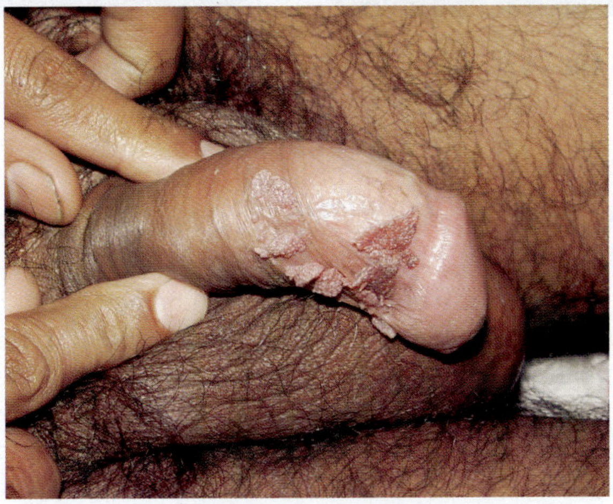

Fig. 26.3 Genital Warts - Fleshy Plaques on the Inner repuce.

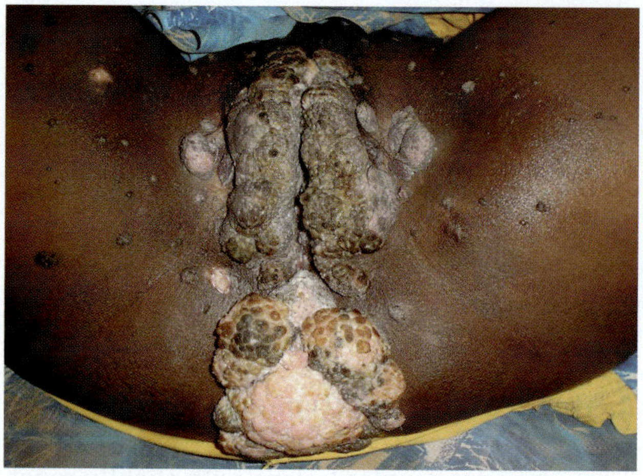

Fig. 26.4 Genital Warts - Buschke Lowenstein Tumor –Verrucous hyperkeratotic exophytic rowth in the genital and perineal area.

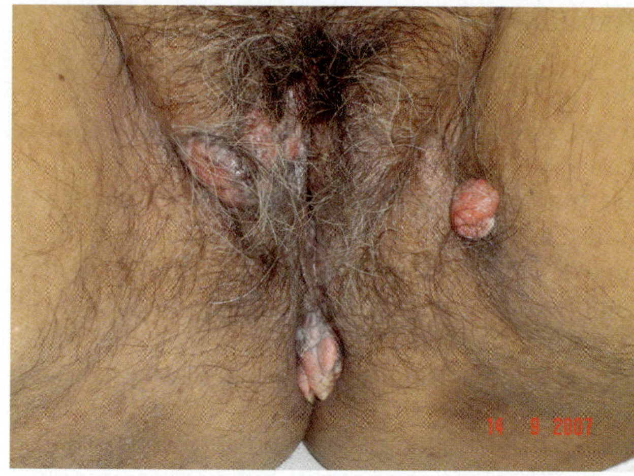

Fig. 26.5 Genital Warts - Verrucous laques on the Genitals and Thigh.

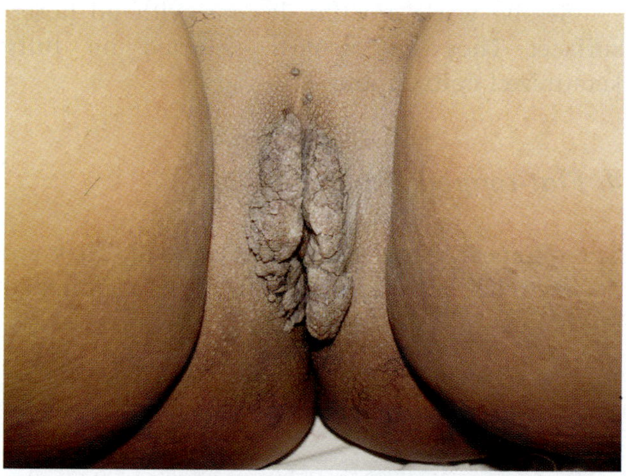

Fig. 26.6 Genital Warts - Verrucous Plaques on the Vulva.

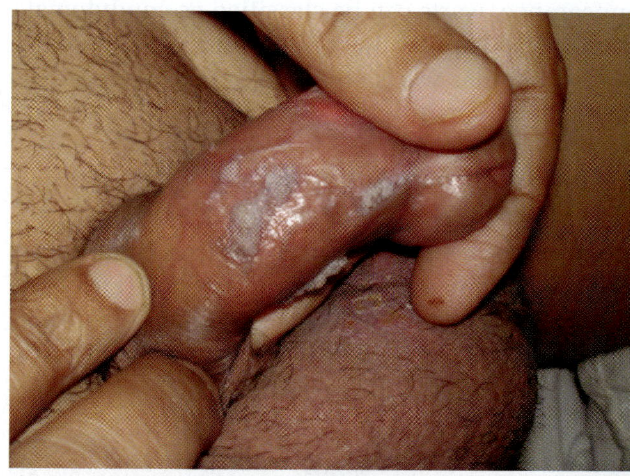

Fig. 26.7 Genital Warts - Keratotic Papules and Plaques on the Prepuce.

5. Bowenoid Papulosis

It is a variant of papular wart characterized by hyperpigmented, dome-shaped, smooth and flat-topped papules, the size of which is around 7 mm in diameter **(Fig. 26.8)**. Histologically, it shows high grade squamous intraepithelial neoplasia and is positive for HPV 16 DNA. In men, it appears on the penile shaft or glans penis and in women around the labia majora and minora, inguinal folds and perianal region.[2] Recurrence rates of upto 20% have been reported. Recently HPV 16/11,16/18, 31/33/51 has been demonstrated in Bowenoid papulosis by in situ DNA hybridization technique.[17] The viral typing and clinical variation of anogenital lesions have no correlation. The clinical presentation at the anogenital region is dependent on the anatomical site of occurrence, abundance of moisture, concomi-tant infections and immune status of the patient.

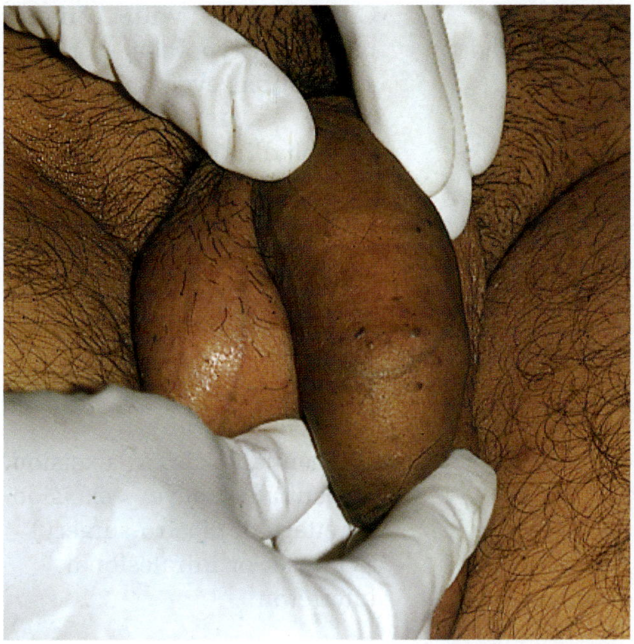

Fig. 26.8 Genital Warts - Bowenoid Papulosis.

Subclinical HPV Infections

Subclinical HPV infections together with latent infections are probably the most likely outcome after exposure to HPV. They may present with symptoms such as burning, fissuring and dyspareunia in some patients. Only these patients should be offered treatment. Predominantly, subclinical infections are asymptomatic. Aceto-white test with 3-5% acetic acid has been described to detect the same but with variable specificity, and this procedure is commonly not recommended.[9]

DIAGNOSIS

Diagnosis of warts in the anogenital region is based on the history of the exposure, clinical appearance, epidemiological proof of the warts in the sexual contact, and the histological appearance. The most sensitive method for detection of HPV DNA is PCR. This technique is able to detect latent infection, but has little benefit in routine diagnosis and management of condyloma and is primarily used as a research tool. Gel electrophoresis and restriction endonuclease cleavage are other methods employed in the detection of viral warts.[18]

Histopathological Features

Gross et al, studied warts of different clinical types and correlated them histologically and virologically.[19] The histological characteristics of the 'classical' protuberant growth-type of condyloma acuminatum in the anogenital region are:

1. Mainly parakeratotic hyperkeratosis of varying degree.
2. Moderate granulomatosis.
3. Pronounced acanthosis and sometimes marked papillomatosis.
4. Marked perinuclear vacuolization with marginal nuclei of sickle form, partially intra-nuclear oedema and basophilic inclusions in the malphigian and granular layer.
5. Increase in the mitotic activity in the basal layers.
6. Koilocytes, which are mature squamous cells with a large, clear perinuclear zone, scattered throughout the outer cell layers. The nuclei of koilocytes may be enlarged and hyperchromatic and double nuclei are often seen. Ultrastructural studies show virus in some of the cell nuclei. Although koilocytes are thought to represent a specific cytopathic effect of HPV, koilocytic features are often subtle, and other cellular changes may mimic koilocytic changes. Thus, detection of koilocytes is not a sensitive or reliable predictor of cervical HPV infection.[4]
7. Viral antigen can be demonstrated in the nuclei of cells in the stratum granulosum by peroxidase-antiperoxidase test, indirect immunofluorescence and indirect immuno-alkaline phosphatase reaction.

The variations occurring in histopathology of plane warts versus genital wart is that plane wart would reveal basket weave orthokeratosis, while hyperkeratosis would be demonstrated by genital wart.

DIFFERENTIAL DIAGNOSIS

Genital warts are to be differentiated clinically from the other verrucous lesions of the genitalia, like condyloma lata of syphilis, non-venereal treponematoses, hypertrophic verrucous type of granuloma inguinale, tuberculosis verrucosa cutis, skin tags and malignancy. Small warts are most often confused with pearly penile papules, others being herpes progenitalis, molluscum contagiosum and hirsutoid papillomas, Fordyce's spots, urethral caruncle, capillary angioma, lichen planus, foreign body granuloma, schwannoma[20] and focal dermal hypoplasia (Goltz syndrome)[21]. The complication of lymphogranuloma venereum and filariasis (due to lymphatic obstruction) may mimic genital warts. Benign tumors like neurofibroma, lipoma, and certain cysts are other genital conditions to be considered in the differential diagnosis of genital warts. Normal physiological glands, like Tyson's, may look like early warts. In multiparous women, mucous tags due to trauma may give misleading appearance of vaginal warts. Around the anus, prolapsed & sentinel piles and anal tags are the important clinical entities to be excluded. In unhygienic persons, dry smegma may appear like warts, and hence cleaning the sub-prepucial region is emphasized before the examination of warts in the male genitalia.

TREATMENT MODALITIES FOR ANOGENITAL WARTS[22]

The preference of patient, the available resources, and the experience of the health care provider should guide treatment of genital wart. No definite evidence suggests that any of the available treatment is superior to others. The treatment modality should be changed if a patient has not improved substantially after three provider administered treatments or if the warts have not cleared after 6 treatments.

(a) Extragenital/Perianal warts

Recommended regimens

Patients applied	Imiquimod 5% cream Podofilox 0.5% solution/gel
Provider administered	Cryosurgery with liquid nitrogen/(Cryoprobe repeat applications every 1-2 weeks.) or Podophyllin resin (10-25%) or Trichloro acetic acid (TCA)/ Bichloro acetic acid (BCA) 80-90%. Small amounts are applied on warts till frosting develops. or Surgical removal (Tangential scissor excision, tangential shave excision, curettage or electro-surgery)
Alternative regimens	CO_2 laser or intralesional interferon

(b) Cervical Warts

(Management of exophytic cervical wart should include consultation with specialist, and should rule out high grade squamous intra epithelial lesions (SIL).

(c) Vaginal Warts

Recommended regimen
Cryosurgery with liquid nitrogen
Cryoprobe not recommended due to risk of vaginal perforation and fistula formation.
or
TCA/BCA (80-90%)

(d) Urethral Meatal Warts

Recommended regimen	Cryosurgery with liquid nitrogen or Podophyllin 10-25%

(e) Anal Warts

	(Rectal mucosal involvement should be managed with consultation of a specialist).
Recommended regimen	Cryosurgery with liquid nitrogen or TCA/BCA (80-90%) or Surgical removal

(f) Oral Warts

	Cryosurgery with liquid nitrogen (Recommended regimen) or Surgical removal

Podophyllin was introduced in the treatment of warts in 1942. It is a complex resinous material containing podophyllotoxin, alphapeltatum and betapeltatum, obtained from American plant *Podophyllum peltatum* and *P. emodi*, an Indian plant that grows in Himalayas (May apple or Mandrake).[23] Podophyllin inhibits mitosis and causes swelling and necrosis of cells. It is used as dry powder or by making solutions with mineral oil, linseed oil, rectified sprit, liquid paraffin, propylene glycol and tincture of benzoin (20% to 50%), which is the usual form used worldwide. Podophyllin is contraindicated in pregnancy. It may produce foetal deaths and abortions. Systemic absorption of podophyllin can rarely result in renal toxicity, neuropathy, coma, hepatotoxicity, granulocytopenia and thrombocytopenia. Prolonged use of podophyllin is not to be advocated for the fear of its oncogenic potential. Podophyllin is applied to the warts by clinicians using cotton tipped swab once or twice a week for upto six weeks. Applications are limited to less than 0.5 ml or 10 cm^2 per treatment session. One to 4 hours after application, it is completely washed off. After 6 sittings if the warts persist, other treatment modalities need to be considered.

Podofilox is 0.5% solution or gel purified from podophyllin. Podofilox has stable shelf life, does not need to be washed off after application and less likely to cause systemic toxicity. The solution or gel is applied with cotton swab or finger respectively, over the condylomas (also on normal appearing skin between the lesions) twice daily for three days, followed by 4 days of no therapy. Such treatment is given for a total of 4 cycles. The total area of treatment should not exceed 10 cm^2 and total volume should not exceed 0.5 ml. The initial application is by health care provider to demonstrate proper application and subsequently by patients themselves.

Imiquimod is a new immune response modifier for local application that induces the release of cytokines including interferon gamma, tumour necrosis factor, and certain interleukins by peripheral mononuclear blood cells and lymphocytes. There is no direct antiviral activity. 5% cream is applied to warts with fingers three times per week (every other night) upto sixteen weeks. The area is washed with mild soap and water 6 to 10 hours after application.[24] The most commonly reported side effect is local irritation.

Imiquimod and Podofilox have not been approved for treatment of perianal, rectal, urethral, vaginal, or cervical warts. Safety in pregnancy has not been established for both the agents.[2]

Cryotherapy is very useful for treatment of warts. It is particularly suitable for internal warts, especially meatal warts and does not require anaesthesia. The cryoprobe, which depends on a supply of nitrous oxide, is manufactured with a number of probes of different sizes (including a cervical cone that may also be used for treating cervical erosions). The tip of a suitable probe or the surface of wart should be sparingly covered with KY jelly before freezing. Two short freeze-thaw cycles are probably just as effective as a single one minute freeze, which is time consuming when multiple warts are present.

Liquid nitrogen is applied by pressing cotton wool swabs on orange sticks dipped in liquid nitrogen on the warts and holding for a minute; adherence to the warts is better if before use, the cotton wool tips are teased to make the ends ragged before application.[9]

All patients are offered a follow up evaluation at 3 months after treatment. Women with genital warts or whose husband has genital warts should be counselled about the need for regular cytological screening.

The comparative efficacy of different modalities of therapy is given in Table 26.2.[25]

Table 26.2 Clearance and Recurrence Rates with Different Treatment Modalities for Genital Warts

Treatment	*Clearance Rates (%)*		*Recurrence Rates*
	End of Treatment	*3 Months or More*	
Cryotherapy	63-88	63-92	0-39
Electrocautery	93-94	78-91	24
Interferon intralesional	19-62	36-62	0-33
Systemic	7-15	18-21	0-23
Topical	6-90	33	6
Laser therapy	27-89	39-86	<7-45
LEEP	<=90	——	——
Podophyllin*	32-79	22-73	11-65
Podophyllotoxin (Podofilox)	42-88	34-77	10-91
Surgical/scissors excision	89-93	36	0-29
Trichloroacetic acid	50-81	70	36
5-fluorouracil	10-71	37	10-13

*Studies using more than one treatment strength have been grouped together.
LEEP = loop electrocautery excision procedure.

Polyphenon (R) E 15% ointment, a mixture of different polyphenols/catechins from green tea extracts (*Camilla sinesis*) which are known to have antioxidant, antiinflammatory ,antiproliferative and anticancer activities is a new topical therapy for genital warts. In a large study of 1400 patients, it was found to obtain total healing in 54.9% patients compared with 35.4% on place bo ($p < 0.01$). Recurence rate was 6.2%. It is safe and has minimal local irritation.[26]

COMPLICATIONS

Warts may resist most of the treatment modalities and persist for as long as ten years and cause embarrassment to the patient. They may increase in number and size. In men, urethral meatal lesion may cause obstruction to the flow of urine. This types of wart after cauterization are liable to produce meatal stenosis. In women, larger warts may cause cervical dystocia. Ulcerations, secondary infection and haemorrhage are the other complications of anogenital warts. Giant condyloma described by Buschke and Lowenstein is histologically benign (intact basal layer) and clinically manifest as large, foul smelling, cauliflower like masses, locally invasive, destructive and non-metastasizing lesions. They are usually positive for HPV6 DNA. Malignant transformation of genital warts has also been reported. A constant problem of warts for both patients and clinicians are their recurrences.[4]

ANOGENITAL WARTS AND PREGNANCY

Warts flourish in pregnancy and there is increase in both size and number **(Fig. 26.9)**. This may be due to the influence of increased hormone level, vascularity and immuno-deficiency, which are seen in pregnancy. Larger warts may cause dystocia. Even without treatment, warts may resolve after delivery. The newborn may pick up infection during labour. Cryotherapy and TCA are ideal for warts in pregnant women. Larger warts can be surgically excised. Podophyllin, podofilox, imiquimod are not advocated in pregnancy. Some clinicians prefer elective caesarian section to prevent transmission of the infection to the neonate.[4]

ANOGENITAL WARTS IN CHILDREN

The mode of infection in children is uncertain. Infants can acquire warts from maternal genital condyloma, at the time of delivery with resulting genital or laryngeal disease. Laryngeal papillomatosis occurs predominantly in infants and young children. There may be an increased risk of laryngeal papillomas in children whose mothers have had genital warts at the time of delivery, but the processes involved in their pathogenesis are unknown. There have been several reports, of condyloma acuminata in young children, which may be the result of sexual abuse. It is believed that infection may also occur through close non-sexual contact within a family.[2,27]

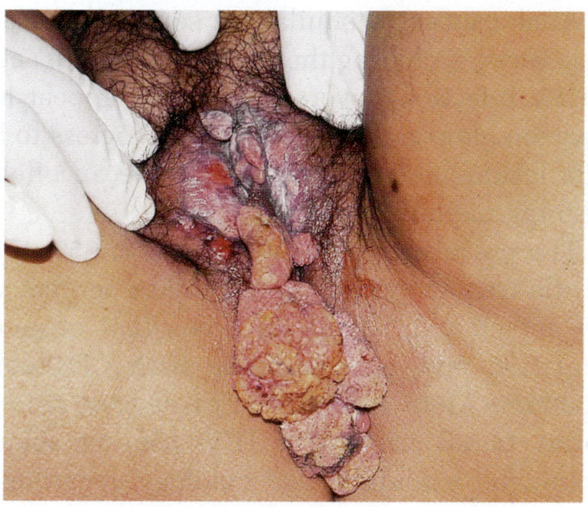

Fig. 26.9 Genital Warts - Keratotic Exuberant Genital Warts in Pregnant Woman.

ANOGENITAL WARTS AND HIV (FIG. 26.10)

Before the acquired immunodeficiency syndrome (AIDS) epidemic, it was well documented that immunosuppressed patients were at increased risk for the benign and malignant manifestations of HPV infection. Iatrogenic immunosuppression such as that of transplantation patients, confers an increased risk for HPV associated neoplasms. The risks of carcinoma in situ of the cervix, vulva, and anus are estimated to be from 14 to 100-fold higher in renal transplantation patients than in normal women.

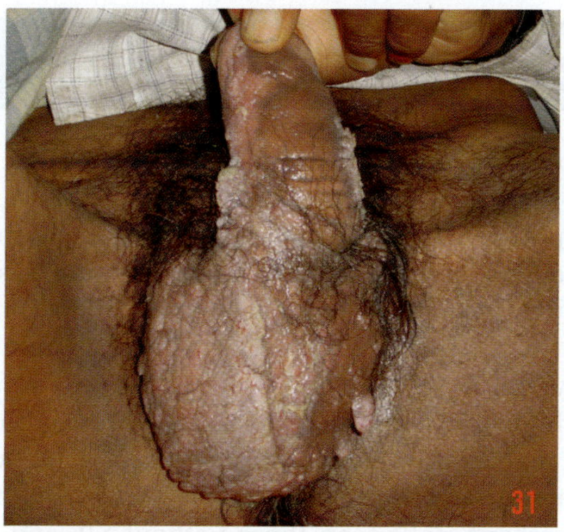

Fig. 26.10 Genital Warts - Keratotic Verrucous Plaques in Sheets on the Scrotal and Penile Skin a in HIV Positive Patient.

The HPV types detected in immunosuppressed patients have been found to be similar to those associated with warts in immunocompetent persons. Although at least one investigator found a selective increase of high-risk HPV types among transplantation patients, another investigator reported "nononcogenic" HPV viruses, such as HPV types 6 and 11 to be associated with cancers in immunosuppressed patients. A few studies suggested that intraepithelial neoplasia develops into cancer at an accelerated rate and that the natural history of cancers is altered by immunosuppression. Given such data, it was expected that similar changes would be seen in the natural history of HPV infection among those with HIV induced immunosuppression. It was reported that the incidence of venereal warts was 8.2 compared with 0.8 per 100 person years of follow up for HIV 1 seropositive and HIV 1 seronegative women, respectively. Studies examining HIV infected women in the United States, Europe, East Africa and West Africa found genital HPV DNA in 8% to more than 50% of HIV seronegative women and 37% to 78% HIV seropositive women[28]. Smaller studies have reported that 26% to 60% of HIV seropositive men and 15% to 29% seronegative men have anal HPV DNA. Among women in whom cervical HPV DNA was detected,

HIV seropositive women were more likely to harbour high risk HPV types 16 and 18 than were HIV seronegative women. Cervical cancer is now considered as AIDS defining illness in women.[28] Increasing HIV induced immunosuppression, as measured by CD4+ counts correlates with increased likelihood of detecting HPV DNA in men and women. It was found low CD4+ counts (200/cm^3) to be a risk factor for detection of anal HPV DNA. HIV infection and immunosuppression play an important role in modulating the natural history of HPV infection.[29] HIV infection influences local immunity by altering HPV transcription and by systemic immunodeficiency.[30]

MECHANISMS OF INTERACTIONS BETWEEN HIV AND HPV

Alterations in the natural history of HPV infection and of HPV related neoplasia among HIV seropositive individuals are probably the result of general or local HIV induced immune system dysfunction. It is possible, for example, that control of HPV is impaired when large numbers of lymphocytes or Langerhans' cells in the area are infected with HIV. Some small studies found that among HIV seronegative women, those with squamous intraepithelial lesions (SIL) had fewer Langerhans' cells than those without SIL and that HIV seropositive women with cervical SIL had even fewer Langerhans' cells than HIV seronegative women with SIL. It is also possible that HIV acts directly on HPV. In vitro studies have shown that intracellular HIV-1 tat m-RNA can transactivate HPV type 16, E6 and E7, a step that is important in development of squamous cell neoplasia. In vitro studies have also shown that extracellular HIV-1 tat protein can enter HPV infected cells and upregulate HPV type 16 E6 and E7. The HIV-1 tat protein enhances E2 dependent HPV type 16 transcription. It is possible that extracellular tat migrates from Langerhans' cells or other HIV infected mononuclear cells that abut HPV infected epithelial cells and upregulates HPV. However, although several in vitro studies suggest that HIV could enter and establish infection in epithelial cells, the mechanisms remain controversial.[28]

ANOGENITAL WARTS AND MALIGNANCY

Role of the HPV in the aetiology of anogenital cancers has been firmly established based on large number of molecular and epidemiological studies. Predictions of the role of HPV in neoplasia induced by experimental studies are consistent with the natural history of cervical cancers. The genital HPV have been grouped into high and low risk types, based on the potential of the infected cells to progress to carcinoma. HPV types 16, 18, 31, 33, 35, 39, 45, 51, 52, 54, 56, 66 and 68 are associated with cancers.[31] CDC recommends that a gynecological evaluation (with pelvic examination and Pap smear) should be performed at base line, and repeated at 6 months and annually thereafter.

Anal cancer is similar to cervical cancer in many ways, including the fact that both are caused by HPV infection, several HPV types appear to be oncogenic, low grade lesions often progress to high grade lesions and Pap smear may be an effective screening method.

The prevalence of HPV in MSM is 65% to75% and the frequency of anal carcinoma in men with HPV infection is about 80 times that of general population and rates increase with CD4 counts <500/mm. More recent studies suggest this risk applies to all men with HIV, leading some to recommend a routine anal cytology, regardless of a history of receptive anal intercourse, especially those with lower CD4 counts.

VACCINE

Prophylactic Vaccine

Several human phase-I trials have established the safety and immunogenicity of candidate prophylactic vaccines. All these preparations are based on virus-like particles (VLP), which are recombinant versions of the major capsid protein (L1) of the relevant HPV types. The individual L1 molecules self assemble into empty viral capsids that assume correct information and induce type specific neutralizing antibodies. The VLP lack nucleic acids and are thus incapable of replication and are noninfectious.

In models using animals and their corresponding papilloma viruses, vaccines based on VLP have been protective. In humans, phase-I trials have shown that neutralizing antibodies are present in sufficient titer in genital secretions to block infection in model system. Thus large scale trials are being mounted to determine clinical efficacy in phase-III trials which are planned for HPV-16 VLP vaccine developed through the National Cancer Institute. HPV-16 is the most common HPV type associated with cervical cancer and dysplasia. The outcome studied in this placebo controlled trial will be on HPV-16 induced SIL (squamous intraepithelial lesion), with a planned 4-year follow-up. Another planned phase-III study is that of a quadrivalent VLP based preparation containing VLP from HPV types 6, 11, 16 and 18. HPV types 6 and 11 are the most common types associated with condyloma acuminata, and types 16 and 18 are the most common types associated with cervical cancer.

Therapeutic Vaccines

Although production of neutralizing antibody may eventually prove to be sufficient to prevent disease; antibodies alone will not suffice to alter the course of established disease. A variety of strategies are being tested to produce a cellular immune response that is thought to be necessary to eliminate an established intracellular viral infection. The strategies that have proven immunogenic are the use of DNA based vaccines and the use of VLP that have proteins other than the L1 protein included in the vaccine. Some of the preparations are now in phase-II and III trials, in patients with established pre-existent cervical, vulval, or anal intraepithelial neoplasia due to target HPV types, mainly HPV-16. Outcomes measures in the study would be stabilization and progression or regression of lesions.

HPV Vaccine[32]

On June 8, 2006, the Food and Drug Administration (FDA) licensed the first vaccine developed to prevent cervical cancer and other diseases in females caused by certain types of genital human papillomavirus (HPV). The quadrivalent vaccine protects against four HPV types (6, 11, 16, 18), which are responsible for 70% of cervical cancers and 90% of genital warts. The Advisory Committee on Immunization Practices (ACIP) voted to recommend use of this vaccine in females, ages 9-26 years.

This prophylactic vaccine, made from non-infectious HPV-like particles (VLP), offers a promising new approach to the prevention of HPV and associated conditions.

Provisional HPV Vaccine Recommendations

- The HPV vaccine is recommended for 11-12 year-old girls but can be administered to girls as young as 9 years of age. The vaccine also is recommended for 13-26 year-old females who have not yet received or completed the vaccine series.
- Ideally, the vaccine should be administered before onset of sexual activity. However, females who are sexually active also may benefit from vaccination. Females who have not been infected with any vaccine HPV type would receive the full benefit of vaccination. Females who already have been infected with one or more HPV type would still get protection from the vaccine types they have not acquired. A Few young women are infected with all four HPV types in the vaccine.

HPV Vaccine Safety

- The HPV vaccine has been tested in over 11,000 females (9-26 years of age) in many countries around the world, including the United States (U.S).
- These studies found that the HPV vaccine was safe and caused no serious side effects. Adverse events were mainly injection site pain. This reaction was common but mild.

HPV Vaccine Efficacy

- The efficacy of this vaccine has mainly been studied in young women (16-26 years of age) who previously had not been exposed to any of the four HPV types in the vaccine. These clinical trials have demonstrated 100% efficacy in preventing cervical precancers caused by the targeted HPV types, and nearly 100% efficacy in preventing vulvar and vaginal precancers and genital warts caused by the targeted HPV types.
- The vaccine has no therapeutic effect on HPV-related disease.
- While it is possible that vaccination of males with the quadrivalent vaccine may offer direct health benefits to males and indirect health benefits to females, there are currently no efficacy data available to support use of HPV vaccine in males.

Duration of Vaccine Protection

- The duration of vaccine protection is unclear. Current studies (with five-year followup) indicate that the vaccine is effective for at least five years.

HPV Vaccine Delivery (Provisional Recommendations)

- The vaccine should be delivered through a series of three intra-muscular injections over a six-month period. The second and third doses should be given 2 and 6 months after the first dose.
- The HPV vaccine is not recommended for use in pregnancy.

Other Vaccines in Development

- A bivalent HPV vaccine is in the final stages of clinical testing in females. This vaccine would protect against the two types of HPV (16,18) that cause 70% of cervical cancers.

REFERENCES

1. Oriel JD. Genital Papilloma Virus Infections; clinical manifestations. In: Morten RS, Harris JRW, Eds. Recent advances in sexually transmitted diseases. New York: Churchill Livingstone; 1988. p. 127-45.
2. Koutsky LA, Kiviat NB. Genital human papilloma virus. In: Holmes KK, Sparling PF, Mardh PR, et al. eds. Sexually transmitted Diseases. 3rd Edn. New York: McGraw Hill; 1999. p. 347-59.
3. Maw RD. Genital Warts – approaching rational treatments. Indian J Sex Trans Dis 1999; 20: 30-32.
4. Kura MM, Hira S, Kohli M, et al. High occurrence of HBV among STDs clinic attendees in Bombay, India. Int J STDs AIDS 1998; 9: 1101-3.
5. Chopra A, Dhalival RS, Chopra D. Pattern and changing trend of STDs at Patiala. Indian J Sex Transm Dis 1999; 20: 22-25.
6. Aggarwal K, Jain VK, Brahma D. Trends of STDs at Rohtak. Indian J Sex Transm Dis 2002; 23: 19-21.
7. Arora R, Rawal RC, Bilimoria FE. Changing pattern of STDs and HIV prevalence among them at five year interval. Indian J Sex Transm Dis 2002; 23: 22-5.
8. Brentjens MH, Yeung-Yue KA, Lee PC, et al. Human papilloma virus: a review. Dermatol Clin 2002; 20: 315-31.
9. Saunders NA, Frazen IH. Simplifying the molecular mechanisms of human papilloma virus. Dermatol Clin 1998; 16: 823-7.

10. Nebesio Cl, Mirowski GW, Chuang TY. Human papilloma virus: Clinical significance and malignant potential. Int J Dermatol 2001; 40: 373-9.
11. Almedia JD, Oriel JD, Stannard LM. Characterization of the virus found in Human genital warts. Micro bios 1969; 3: 225-32.
12. Almedia JD, Goffe AP. Antibody to wart virus in human sera demonstrated by electron microscopy and precipitin tests. Lancet 1965; 2: 1205-7.
13. Pyrhonen S, Johansson E. Regression of warts. An immunological study. Lancet 1975; 1(7907): 592-6.
14. Morison WL. Viral warts, herpes simplex and herpes zoster in patients with secondary immune deficiencies and neoplasms. Br J Dermatol 1975; 92: 625-30.
15. Viac J, Thivolet J, Chardonnet Y. Specific immunity in patients suffering from recurring warts before and after repetitive intradermal tests with human papilloma virus. Br J Dermatol 1977; 97: 365-70.
16. Bunny MH. Viral warts: a new look at old problem. Br Med J 1986; 293: 1045-6.
17. Pala S, Poleva I, Vocatura A. The presence of HPV types 6/11, 6/18, 31/33/51 in Bowenoid papulosis demonstrated by DNA in situ Hybridization. Int J STDs AIDS 2000; 11: 823-4.
18. Strand A, Rylander E. Human papilloma virus subclinical and atypical manifestation. Dermatol Clin 1998; 16: 817-22.
19. Gross G, Pfister H, Hagedorm M, et al. Correlation between human papilloma virus (HPV) type and histology of warts. J Invest Dermatol 1982; 78: 160-4.
20. Ghaly AF, Orange GV. Not every penile lump is a wart! Schwannoma of the penis. Int J STDs AID 2000; 11: 199-200.
21. Singh S, Singh A, Gupta S, et al. Perianal papillomas in focal dermal hypoplasia (Goltz Syndrome) mimicking Condyloma acuminata. Indian J Sex Trans Dis 2000; 21: 87-9.
22. Centers for Disease Control and Prevention. Guidelines for treatment of sexually transmitted diseases. MMWR 2006; 55 (RR-11): 1-94.
23. Bhargava RK, Joshi R. Viral STDs In: Valia RG, Valia AR, Eds. IADVL Textbook and Atlas of Dermatology. Mumbai: Bhalani publishing house, 2001. p. 1476-91.
24. Mohany CO, Law C, Gollnick HPM, et al. New patient applied therapy for anogenital wart is rated favourably by patients. Int J STDs and AIDS 2001; 12: 565-70.
25. Beutner KR, Wiley DJ. Recurrent external genital warts: A literature review. Papillomavirus Report 1997; 8: 69-74.
26. Gross G. Polyphenon E. Aneus topical therapy for condylomata acuminata. Hautarzt 2008, 59: 31-50.
27. Usman N, Shakir FH, Gajendiran K. Anal condylomata acuminata in eleven months old Infant. Indian J Sex Transm Dis 1985; 6: 61-2.
28. Kiviat MB. Human papilloma virus and hepatitis viral infections in human immuno deficiency virus infected persons. In: Devita Jr VT, Hellman S, Rosenberg SA, et al. Eds. AIDS Aetiology, Diagnosis, Treatment and prevention. New York: Lippincott – Raven: 1997. p. 281-91.
29. Ahdieh L, Klein RS, Burk R, et al. Prevalence, incidence and type-specific persistance of human papilloma virus in human immuno deficiency virus (HIV)-positive and HIV- negative women. J Infect Dis 2001; 184: 682-90.
30. Arany I, Tyring SK. Systemic immuno suppression by HIV infection influences HPV transcription and this local immune responses in condyloma acuminatum. Int J STDs and AIDS 1998; 9: 268-71.
31. Galloway DA. Biology of Genital human papilloma virus, In: Holmes KK, Sparling PF, Mardh PA, et al, Eds. Sexually Transmitted Diseases. 3rd New York: Mc Graw – Hill; 1999. p. 335–46.
32. HPV and HPV Vaccine - Information for Healthcare Providers. http://www.cdc.gov/std/hpv/STDFact-HPV-vaccine-hcp.htm

27 | BALANOPOSTHITIS

PN Arora, S Arora

In this chapter

INTRODUCTION

Balanoposthitis is a disease of multifactorial etiology and is characterized by red glistening inflammation of the glans penis and prepuce, often accompanied by thick, foul smelling, subpreputial discharge and phimosis. If left untreated, it leads to complications. Treatment of balanoposthitis depends on treatment of the cause.

DEFINITION

Balanitis is defined as inflammation of the glans penis and posthitis is inflammation of mucosal surface of the prepuce. It may occur individually or in combination i.e. balanoposthitis.

INCIDENCE

The overall incidence of balanoposthitis reported is less than 2 percent.[1] However in the recent years, the incidence has gone up to 20 percent.[2]

AETIOLOGY

Balanoposthitis is a disease confined to uncircumcised males. The warm, humid and relatively anaerobic environment of the preputial sac predisposes to the growth of aerobic and anaerobic organisms. Balanitis alone is far less seen in circumcised males. Balanoposthitis occurring for the first time in elderly males is highly suggestive of diabetes mellitus[3] whereas in younger age group it commonly results from sexually transmitted diseases. The various predisposing and aetiological factors are given below.

PREDISPOSING FACTORS

(a) Poor personal hygiene
(b) Long prepuce
(c) Congenital or acquired phimosis
(d) Failure to dry the glans and prepuce after a bath
(e) Hot and humid climate

Systemic diseases like diabetes mellitus[3], candidiasis, Reiter's disease, Crohn's disease[4], ulcerative colitis[5], HIV infection and other diseases or drugs leading to immunosuppression also predispose to balanoposthitis.

CLASSIFICATION OF BALANOPOSTHITIS[6]

Infections

1. Fungal

(a) *Candida albicans* (commonest cause of infective balanoposthitis[7,8])
(b) Pityrosporum orbiculare[9]

2. Anaerobic Organisms (recorded in 76% of cases[10])

(a) Diphtheria
(b) Diphtheroids
(c) Fusospirochetes

3. Spirochaetal

(a) *Treponema pallidum*

4. Viral

(a) Herpes simplex Virus (HSV)[11]
(b) Human papilloma virus (HPV)

5. Mycobacterial

(a) *Mycobacterium tuberculosis*[12]
(b) *Mycobacterium leprae*[13]

6. Aerobic Organisms[14]

(a) *Gardnerella vaginalis*
(b) Group B streptococcus

(c) *Staphylococcus aureus*
(d) *Calymmatobacterium granulomatis*
(e) Mycoplasma
(f) Pseudomonas
(g) *N. gonorrhoeae*
(h) *Haemophilus ducreyi*
(i) Chlamydia

7. Protozoal

(a) *Trichomonas vaginalis*[15]
(b) *Entamoeba histolytica*

8. Parasitic

(a) Scabies
(b) Pediculosis
(c) Creeping eruptions[16]

Irritants

(a) Smegma
(b) Perfumed soaps
(c) Retention of soaps or detergents in preputial sac
(d) Persistent moisture
(e) Contraceptives
(f) Irritation from infected urine and faeces
(g) Irritants from vaginal secretions
(h) Podophyllin
(i) Vaginal spermicides
(j) Spermicidal lubricants
(k) Condoms

Trauma

(a) Postcoital or post masturbation trauma
(b) Sharp cuts inflicted by pubic hair
(c) Laceration of prepuce by fasteners
(d) Frictional trauma
(e) Teeth bites
(f) Pin pricks
(g) Excoriations
(h) Self inflicted

Fixed Drug Eruptions (Fig. 27.1)

(a) Sulfonamides
(b) Barbiturates
(c) Tetracycline
(d) Carbamazepine
(e) Salicylates
(f) Oxyphenbutazone
(g) Dapsone
(h) Griseofulvin[17]
(i) Chlordiazepoxide
(j) Phenolphthalein
(k) Morphine
(l) Codeine
(m) Quinine
(n) Phenacetin
(o) Erythromycin
(p) Metronidazole[18]

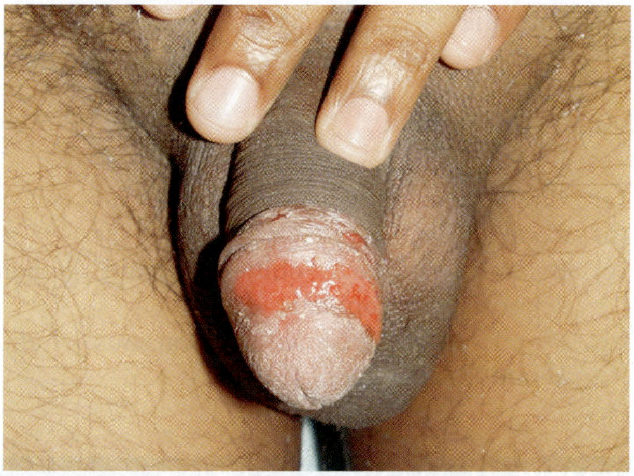

Fig. 27.1 Fixed Drug Eruption - Erythematous Well-defined Erosion.

Premalignant Conditions

(a) Erythroplasia of Queyrat (Bowen's disease of glans penis)
(b) Leukoplakia
(c) Extramammary Paget's disease

Malignant Diseases

(a) Squamous cell carcinoma

(b) Basal cell carcinoma
(c) Basisquamous or metastatic basal cell carcinoma
(d) Melanoma

Cutaneous and Mucocutaneous Disorders

(a) Pemphigus
(b) Dermatitis herpetiformis
(c) Erythema multiforme
(d) Stevens' Johnson syndrome
(e) Toxic epidermal necrolysis
(f) Lichen planus
(g) Psoriasis
(h) Behçet's disease
(i) Aphthae
(j) Porokeratosis of Mibelli
(k) Herpes zoster
(l) Varicella

Miscellaneous

(a) Circinate balanitis
(b) Zoon's balanitis
(c) Balanitis xerotica obliterans and lichen sclerosus et atrophicus
(d) Pseudoepitheliomatous micaceous and keratotic balanitis of Civatte

CLINICAL MANIFESTATIONS

Balanoposthitis is a spectral disorder, varying from an insignificant localized lesion to gangrenous ulceration. There is invariable overlap of clinical presentation of one disease and manifestation of others. It is important to rule out the underlying diseases or to investigate the basic etiopathogenic factors.

The natural course of the disease is that of the predisposing factors and the etiological factors mentioned above, leading to the inflammation. There may or may not be a break in the continuity of the surface of the glans or undersurface of the prepuce. This is followed by preputial oedema, phimosis, and copious, thick, offensive subpreputial discharge accompanied by pain, pruritus, meatal inflammation, burning micturition, feeling of pricking or of insect crawling or sense of stretching of the affected parts. Occasionally, if left untreated, painful lymphadenopathy develops and may progress to extensive ulceration, perforation of prepuce, and even sloughing gangrenous ulceration (phagaedena) of the glans and or prepuce, particularly when infected with fusospirochetes. The progress of the disease is arrested once the symptomatic treatment is started and the underlying cause is dealt with.

Manifestations of balanoposthitis irrespective of etiology are much more severe when associated with HIV infection, particularly so in the advanced stage.[19,20]

The clinical manifestations of different etiological factors leading to balanoposthitis are described under respective headings in different chapters. However, distinctive features of some of the conditions deserve special mention.

Candidal Balanoposthitis

It is the commonest type, and two distinct types of clinical patterns have been described. The first one is due to the presence of *C. albicans* and manifests as small papules or fragile papulopustules on the glans or in the coronal sulcus which break open and leave behind superficial erythematous erosion having a collarette of whitish scales or a thrush like membrane. It may also present as longitudinal fissures on the undersurface of the prepuce. Preputial oedema leads to phimosis and anaerobic infection with offensive purulent curdy discharge from the preputial sac. The second type is due to a hypersensitivity reaction to *C. albicans* and presents with transient erythema and burning, shortly following intercourse wih partners having candidal vaginitis. Healing in these cases may be rapid with topical application of corticosteroids rather than with antifungals.[7,8,21,22]

Anaerobic Balanoposthitis

It is thought to be caused by non-sporing anaerobic bacteria. It presents as erosive balanoposthitis, ulceration and as foul smelling discharge. In a study of 104 patients with above signs, 29 of the culture positive infections were due to mixed anaerobes and 8 due to single anaerobes. A rapid response to treatment with metronidazole also confirmed the anaerobic cause of the infection.[23]

Non-Syphilitic Spirochaetal Balanoposthitis

It has been described from many tropical countries including from India.[24,25] Clinically it is characterized by the presence of extensive tender ulceration of the glans accompanied by a foul smelling purulent discharge. The foul smelling discharge is often due to the associated anaerobic infection. It is caused by *T. refrigens*, *T. phagedenis*, *T. balanitidis* and *T. vincenti*. These organisms have characteristic eel-like movements and few coils on DGI. Treatment with penicillin and metronidazole may prevent the progression to phagedenic complications.

Herpetic Balanoposthitis

Genital herpes presents as grouped small circular erosions lasting for less than a week in recurrent genital herpes but for more than three weeks in a primary infection. Necrotizing balanitis has been described with primary HSV infection.[26,27]

Balanoposthitis due to HPV Infection

HPV infection may present as balanoposthitis. A careful examination and penoscopy with acetowhite test may be needed.[28] High power magnification can illustrate warty balanitis or balanoposthitis.

Trichomonal Balanoposthitis

It is distinguished by invariably accompanying history of urethritis and associated vaginitis in sexual partner. The discharge is copious, mucopurulent, greenish, frothy and has a fishy odour.[29]

Gonococcal Balanoposthitis

It follows sexual exposure to an infected partner. Clinical features include pain, burning, urgency and frequency of micturition, and thick, creamy, greenish yellow purulent urethral discharge. Demonstration of intracellular diplococci on Gram's stain and culture of gonococci and biochemical tests confirm the diagnosis.[30]

Syphilitic balanitis

Syphilis is considered a great imitator and primary[33] or secondary[34] syphilis may present as balanitis.

Behçet's Syndrome (Fig. 27.2)

It is a chronic relapsing disease of unknown cause and usually starts with oral ulcers followed by genital lesions, which commonly heals with scarring. Fibrosis may be seen under magnification. Occasionally eye lesions may precede cutaneous lesions. Recurrent arthritis and other systemic features may occur.[31]

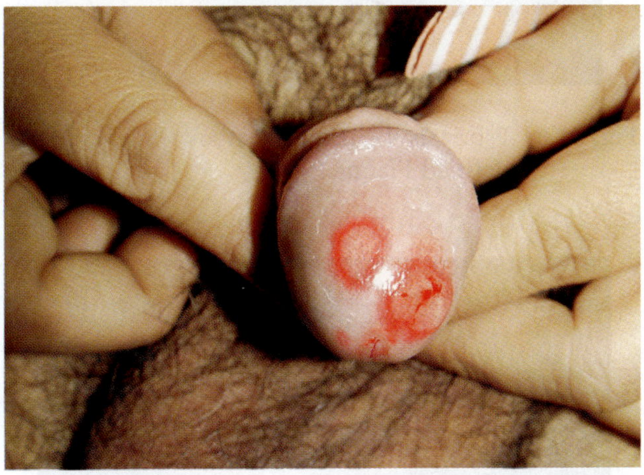

Fig. 27.2 Behcet's Syndrome - Annular Erythematous Moist Plaques.

Penile Psoriasis (Fig. 27.3)

It manifests as bright red coloured plaque of variable severity covered with silvery white scales in circumcised patients. Moist erythematous plaques without scaling occur in uncircumcised males. It usually has an annular or circular morphology. Presence of psoriatic lesions elsewhere supports the diagnosis.

Circinate Balanitis

It is characteristic of Reiter's disease which presents as classical painless, serpiginous geographic dermatitis **(Fig. 27.4)** of the glans penis in uncircumcised men, whereas in circumcised men, it manifests as hyperkeratotic papules.[32] Other features of Reiter's disease are invariably associated and discussed in the respective chapter.

Bowen's Disease (Fig. 27.5)

Bowen's disease of glans may be confused with psoriasis but is gradually progressive in size whereas psoriasis is variable in its course. Histopathology is characteristic.

Lichen Sclerosus

It is also called balanitis xerotica obliterans and it is characterized by a chronic inflammation followed by atrophic sclerosis, depigmentation, induration, urethral stricture and phimosis **(Fig. 27.6)**.[33]

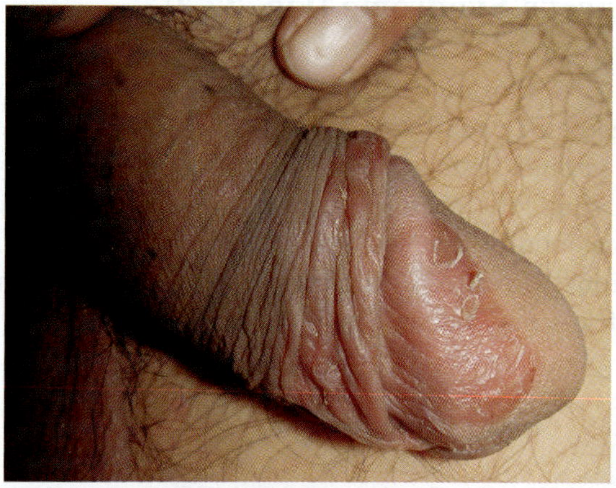

Fig. 27.3 Psoriasis - Erythematous Scaly Well-defined Plaque.

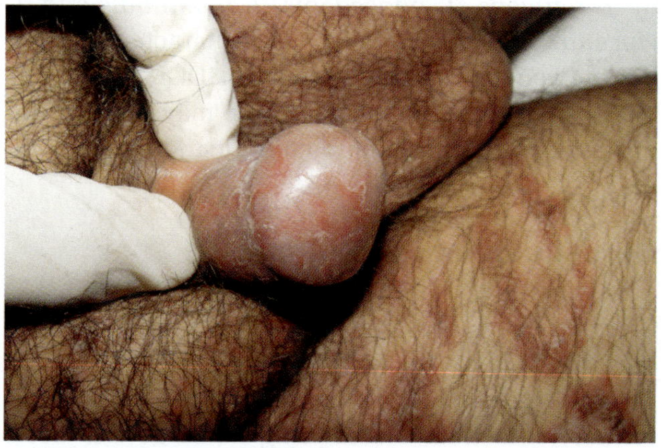

Fig. 27.4 Reiter's Disease - Multiple Annular to Geographic Erythematous Scaly Plaques.

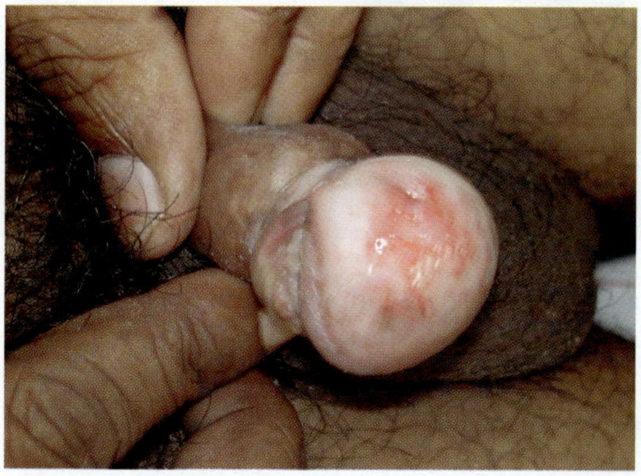

Fig. 27.5 Bowen's Disease - Erythematous Plaque with Biopsy Scar.

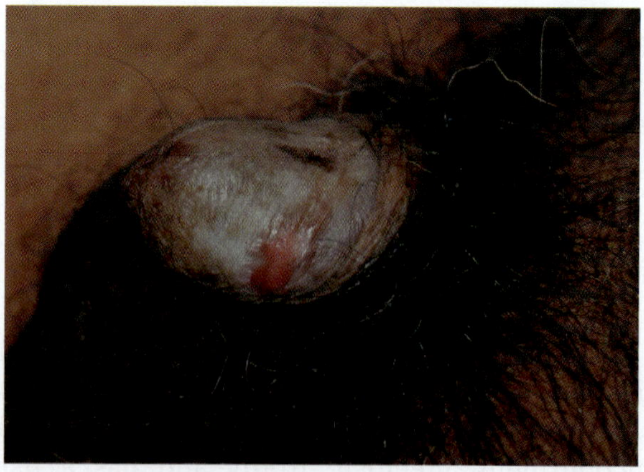

Fig. 27.6 Lichen Sclerosus - Ivory White Atrophic Plaque with Erosion.

Zoon's Balanitis

Chronic benign circumscribed plasma cell balanoposthitis of Zoon **(Fig. 27.7)** is usually seen in middle aged or elderly patients. Classically it presents as shiny red velvety thin plaques often with characteristic 'cayenne pepper' stippling due to hemosiderin. The lesion is usually solitary, asymptomatic or mildly pruritic. Erosive and vegetative types have also been described. Etiology is unknown. Usual sites are glans penis and/or inner surface of the prepuce. The characteristic histopathological features include a thin epidermis showing 'lozenge' keratinocytes, occasional dyskeratotic cells and mild spongiosis with dermal lichenoid infiltrate.[34]

Pseudoepitheliomatous Micaceous and Keratotic Balanitis of Civatte (PMKB) (Fig. 27.8)

It was first described by Lortat-Jacob and Civatte in 1961. Clinically it presents as crusted hyperkeratotic plaques on the penis. The term micaceous refers to the white scaly appearance of the lesion. The lesions tend to progress slowly and recur locally. Some authors suggest that it is a premalignant condition or locally aggressive low-grade malignancy, which has been associated with the development of a verrucous carcinoma.[35,36] Histologically, PMKB reveals hyperplastic epidermis with massive hyperkeratosis and elongated rete ridges, at times surrounded by dense polymorphonuclear infiltrate. Few atypical cells and mitoses may also be seen.

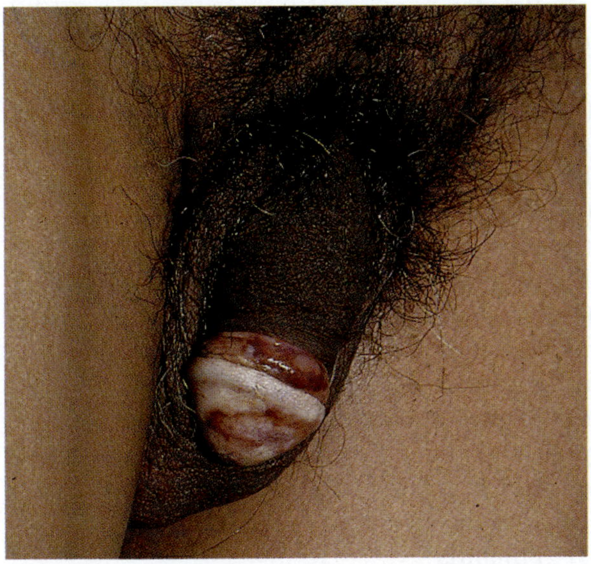

Fig. 27.7 Zoon's Balanitis – Shiny Erythematous Plaque.

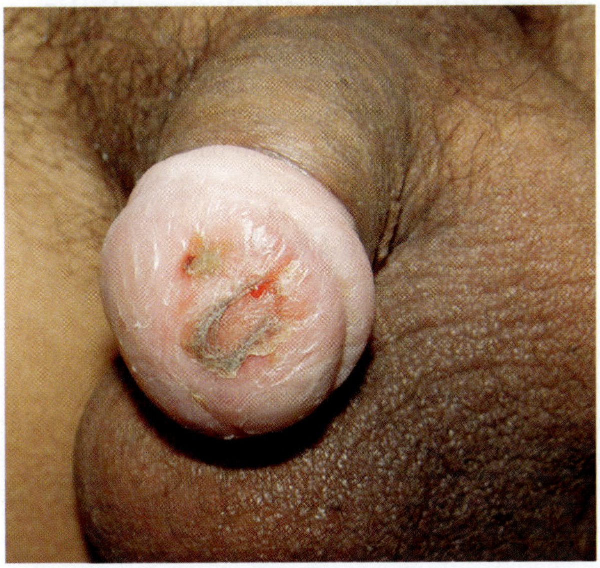

Fig. 27.8 Pseudoepitheliomatous Micaceous and Keratotic Balanitis (PKMB).

Balanoposthitis Associated with Leukemia

Rarely ulcerative balanoposthitis has been described as initial presentation of acute promyelocytic leukemia.[37]

Granulomatous Balanoposthitis

Intravesical bacillus-calmette-guerin (BCG) instillation therapy for vesical cancer leading to granulomatous balanoposthitis[41] is documented **(Fig. 27.9)**.

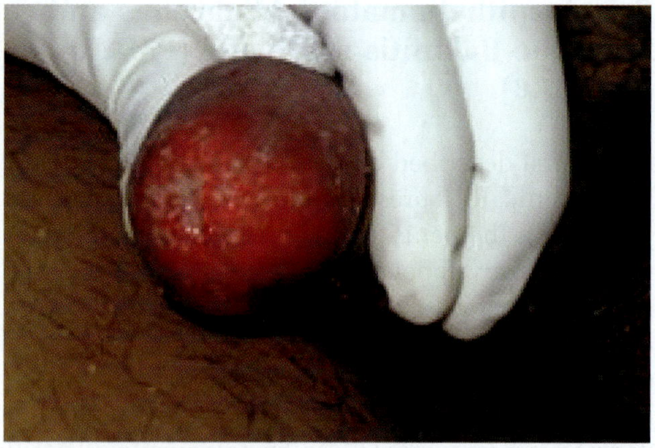

Fig. 27.9 Granulomatous Balanitis, BCG-induced Peri-urethral Erythematous Plaque Studded with Papules and Pustules.

Foreign Body Induced Balanoposthitis

Preputial calculi[42] or foreign bodies like beads introduced in subpreputial region for sexual gratification may rarely lead to balanoposthitis.

Balanoposthitis in Children

Balanitis in children is not uncommon[43]. It often remains undiagnosed in uncircumcised boys. Most of the cases result from irritant balanitis, and infections with Candida, Gardnerella, anaerobic infections and rare infective causes. Biopsy is mandatory in persistent balanitis of obscure aetiology.

Balanoposthitis in Geriatric Age Group

Diabetes mellitus is the commonest underlying cause leading to candidal, bacterial and other infections. In Balanoposthitis which persists and in which the cause remains unclear, biopsy may be warranted.

BALANOPOSTHITIS AND CIRCUMCISION

The presence of prepuce predisposes to collection of microorganisms that contribute to inflammation presenting as balanoposthitis. In a study of 305 patients, all cases of Zoon's balanitis, Bowenoid papulosis, and nonspecific balanoposthitis were observed in uncircumcised males. Lichen sclerosus et atrophicus was diagnosed in only 1 circumcised patient. Most patients with psoriasis (72%), lichen planus (69%) and seborrheic eczema (72%) were uncircumcised males.[38]

COMPLICATIONS

(a) Recurrence
(b) Chronicity
(c) Relapse
(d) Re-infection from the sexual partner
(e) Phimosis
(f) Paraphimosis
(g) Balanitis xerotica obliterans
(h) Depigmentation of glans or prepuce
(i) Hyperpigmentation of the affected parts
(j) Preputial adhesions
(k) Perforation of prepuce
(l) Gangrene (phagaedena)
(m) Scarring
(n) Meatitis
(o) Meatal stricture
(p) Carcinoma of penis in long standing cases
(q) Lymphangitis
(r) Lymphoedema
(s) Phlebitis[45]

DIAGNOSIS

The clinical diagnosis of balanitis, posthitis or balanoposthitis is not difficult due to the presence of signs of inflammation of the affected part. Subpreputial wash followed by naked eye examination of urine for haze will clinically differentiate it from urethritis. The importance of comprehensive and detailed history cannot be overemphasized for etiological diagnosis. A thorough examination of the glans penis, coronal sulcus, urethral meatus, undersurface of the prepuce and frenulum must be done to establish a clinical diagnosis. Prepuce, if present, must be examined and retractility should be assessed. Dorsal slit may be mandatory where retraction of prepuce is not possible. Investigations may be required to confirm the diagnosis and must be individualized in each case. Laboratory tests like complete blood count, urine examination for glucose, subpreputial discharge in normal saline for *T. vaginalis*, KOH preparation for *C. albicans*, dark ground microscopy for *T. pallidum*, Gram's or Giemsa staining and culture for aerobes and anaerobes particularly for mixed infections, blood for VDRL, HIV, patch testing (for condom and contraceptive allergic tests), skin biopsy for histopathological tests and other relevant investigations like examination of vaginal secretions of sexual partners, particularly when trichomonal vaginitis is suspected, may be required to establish the etiological diagnosis. The diagnostic criteria of genital ulcer diseases, premalignant and malignant conditions and other disorders involving the cutaneous and mucocutaneous regions are discussed in the respective chapters. However, in patients who fail to respond promptly, candidal superinfection of an underlying dermatosis or neoplastic process should be considered.

TREATMENT

The general treatment of balanoposthitis irrespective of aetiology remains almost the same, depending on the stage of the disease. Subpreputial wash or irrigation with normal saline or 1:10000 potassium permanganate solution, 1% boric acid solution, 0.6% magnesium sulphate solution or 1% lead acetate solution for 15-20 minutes thrice daily for fifteen minutes each after voiding urine helps in reducing the inflammation.

Specific treatment depends on the aetiology and is discussed in the relevant chapters. Aggressive treatment is warranted when balanoposthitis is associated with HIV infection.

Preventive treatment includes (a) Personal hygiene, (b) Circumcision for phimosis (congenital or acquired), chronic circumscribed balanitis of Zoon, and recurrent relapsing chronic persistent, intractable balanoposthitis, (c) Examination of sexual partner for candidal, trichomonal, or other STDs induced balanoposthitis whenever indicated, and (d) Management of systemic diseases, if any.

Topical corticosteroids have been used with variable efficacies in treatment of balanoposthitis due to psoriasis, lichen planus, fixed drug eruption, plasma cell balanitis and allergic contact dermatitis.

For treatment of PMKB, topical application of 5% 5-FU has been used with encouraging results, but definitive therapy is Moh's microsurgery.

Surgical treatment e.g. meatoplasty, meatotomy, repair of perforation, dorsal slit or circumcision may be required for complications of balanoposthitis after the medicinal treatment is over.

Post treatment surveillance is essential for a variable period depending on the aetiological cause.

REFERENCES

1. Arora PN, Chaterjee RG. Changing patterns of sexually transmitted diseases (Thirty years retrospective study), Indian J Sex Transm Dis 1993; 14: 24-37.
2. Rajnarayan, Kar HK, Gautam RK, et al. Pattern of sexually transmitted diseases in a major hospital in Delhi. Indian J Sex Transm Dis 1996; 17: 76-8.
3. Waugh MA, Evans EGV, Nayyar KE, et al. Clotrimazole (Castren) in the treatment of candidal balanitis in men. Br J Venereal Dis 1978; 54: 184-6.

4. Wijesurenda CS, Singh G, Manuel ARG, et al. Balanoposthitis-An unusual feature of Crohn's disease. Int J STDs AIDS 1993; 4: 184.
5. Lytde P H. Ulcerative Colitis and balanoposthitis. Int J STDs AIDS 1994; 5: 72-3.
6. Waugh MA. Balanitis. Dermatol Clin 1998; 16: 757-62.
7. Oriel JD, Partridge BM, Denny MJ, et al. Genital yeast infection. Br Med J 1972; 4: 761.
8. Sharma VK, Kumar B, Ayyagiri A, et al. Microbial flora in balanoposthitis: study of 100 cases. Indian J Sex Transm Dis 1990; 11: 19-22.
9. Smith EL. Pityriasis versicolour of the penis. Br J Vener Dis 1978; 54: 441.
10. Masfari AN, Kinghorn GR, Duerden BI. Anaerobes in genitourinary infection in men. Br J Vener Dis 1983; 59: 255-9.
11. Chakraborty AK, Dutta AK. Herpetic balanoposthitis. Indian J Dermatol 1981; 26: 15-23.
12. Pavithran K. Papulonecrotic tuberculids on the glans penis. Indian J Dermatol Venereol Leprol 1982; 48: 42-4.
13. Chaudhury DS, Chaudhury MA case report of gangrenous balanitis In progressive reaction in leprosy. Lepr Rev 1966; 37: 225-6.
14. Bhargava RK, Thin RNT. Subpreputial carriage of aerobic micro organisms and balanoposthitis. Br J Vener Dis 1983; 59: 131-3.
15. Cruz-Rojo J , Martíne Z, García MM, et al. A beta-hemolytic streptococcus as a cause of perianal dermatitis, fissures and balanoposthitis. Pediatr. 2005: 483-4.
16. Dal S, Barua MC, Padiyar NV. Ulcerative balanoposthitis due to *Trichomonas vaginalis*. Indian J Sex Transm Dis 1982; 3: 72-4.
17. Pavithran K. Creeping eruptions on the genitals. Indian J Sex Transm Dis 1990; 11: 33-4.
18. Arora PN, Aggrawal SK. Drug eruptions. Indian J Dermatology 1989: 34: 75-80.
19. Arora SK. Metronidazole causing fixed drug eruptions. Indian J Dermatol Venereol Leprol. 2002; 68: 108-9.
20. Franca I, Mansinho K, Claro C, et al. Isolated hyperplastic balanitis. Int Conf AIDS 1994: Aug 7-12; 10: 183.
21. Potekayev N, Yurin O, Potekayev S, et al. Chancriform pyodermia as an indicator for HIV-infection. Int Conf AIDS 1992: Jul 19-24; 8: 124.
22. Martin AG, Kobayashi GS. Yeast infections; candidiasis, pityriasis (tinea) versicolor. in: Freedberg IM, Eisen AZ, Wolf K, Eds. Dermatology in general medicine. 5th Ed. New York: Mc Graw-Hill; 1999: P. 2358-71.
23. Kumar B, Sharma VK, Malhothra S, et al. Balanoposthitis – contribution of women. Indian Sex Transm Dis 1991; 21: 66-8.
24. Cree GE,Willis A T, Phillips K D, et al. Anaerobic balanophosthitis. Br Med J. 1982; 284: 859-60.
25. Piot P, Duncan M, Dyck EV, Ballare RC. Ulcerative balanoposthitis associated with non-syphilitic spirochete infection. Genitourin Med. 1986; 62: 44-6.
26. Chakraborthy AK. Clinicopathological study of balanoposthitis in male. Indian J Dermatol 1982; 27: 105-8.
27. Peutherer JF, Smith IW, Robertson DH. Necrotizing balanitis due to a generalized primary infection with herpes simplex virus type 2. Br J Vener Dis 1979; 55: 48-51.
28. Powers R D, Rein M F, Hayden F G. Necrotizing balanitis due to herpes simplex type 1. JAMA 1982; 248: 215-6.
29. Wikstrom A, Van Krogh G, Hedblad M A, et al. Papilloma virus associated balanoposthitis. Genitourin Med 1994; 70: 175-81.
30. Arumainayagam JT, Sumathipala AH, Smallman LA, et al. Flat condylomata of the penis presenting as patchy balanoposthitis. Genitourin Med 1990 ; 66: 251-3.
31. Michalowski R. Balano Posthites À Trichomonas. A Propos de 16 Observations. Ann Dermatol Venereol 1981; 108; 731-8.
32. Landergren G. Gonorrhoeal ulcer of the penis; Report of a case. Acta Derm Venereol 1961; 41: 320-3.
33. Babu CS, Vitharna S, Higgins SP. Primary syphilis presenting as balanitis. Int J STDs AIDS. 2007; 18: 497-8.
34. Jorizzo J L. Behçet's syndrome. Arch Dermatol 1986; 122b: 556-8.
35. Rice PA, Handsfield HH. Arthritis associated with sexually transmitted diseases. In: Holmes K, Mardh PA, Sparling PF, et al. Eds. Sexually Transmitted Diseases. 3rd Ed. New York: Mc Graw Hill; 1999: P. 921-35.

36. Stühmer A. Balanitis xerotica obliterans. Arch. Dermatolsypholol. 1928; 156: 613-23.
37. Souteyrand P, Wong G, Macdonald D M. Zoon's balanitis (Balanitis Circumscripta Plasmacellularis). Br J Dermatol 1981; 105: 195-9.
38. Read SI, Abell E. Pseudoepitheliomatous, keratotic balanitis. Arch Dermatol 1981; 117: 435-7.
39. Beljaards RC, Vandijk E, Hausman R. Is pseudoepitheliomatous, micaceous and keratotic balanitis synonymous with verrucous carcinoma? Br J Dermatol 1987; 117: 641-6.
40. Steinbach F, Essbach U, Florschutz A, et al. Ulcerative balanoposthitis as initial manifestation of acute promyelocytic leukemia. J Urol 1998; 160: 1430-1.
41. Yusuke H, Yoshinori H, Kenichi M, et al. Granulomatous Balanoposthitis After intravesical Bacillus-Calmette-Guerin instillation therapy. Int J Urol 2006, 13: 1361-3.
42. Hinyokika K. Preputial calculi: A case report. PMID 2001, 47: 513-5.
43. Edwards S. Balanitis and balanoposthitis: A Review. Genitourinary Med, 1996. 72, 155-9.
44. Mallon E, Hawkins D, Dinneen M, et al. Circumcision and genital dermatoses. Arch Dermatol 2001; 737: 503-4.
45. Agrawal SK, Singal A, Pandhi D. Mondor's phlebitis of penis following recurrent candidal balanoposthitis. Int J Dermatol. 2005; 44: 83-4.

28 MISCELLANEIOUS SEXUALLY TRANSMITTED DISEASES

Vinod K Sharma, Manish Bansal

In this chapter

- Molluscum Contagiosum
- Viral Hepatitis
- Cytomegalovirus Infections
- Epstein-Barr Virus Infection
- Scabies
- Pediculosis Pubis
- Genital Mycoplasmas
- Enteric Bacterial Pathogens
- Candidiasis

INTRODUCTION

A large number of infections besides the traditional sexually transmitted diseases (STDs) are now recognized as being sexually transmitted. Their role in the causation of STDs is undisputed since several studies have shown that they are present in significant proportion of patients in association with the traditional STDs. Moreover, the causative organisms are isolated with equal frequency in both the sex partners. They are described under miscellaneous STDs (Table. 27.1).

Table 27.1 Miscellaneous Sexually Transmitted Diseases

Viral Infections
Molluscum contagiosum
Hepatitis A, B, C and D
Cytomegalovirus
Epstein Barr virus
Parasitic Infestations
Scabies
Phthirus pubis
Bacterial Infections
Ureaplasma and Mycoplasma
Bacterial vaginosis
Enteric Pathogens
Protozoal and Fungal Infections
Trichomoniasis
Candidiasis

MOLLUSCUM CONTAGIOSUM[1-10]

Molluscum contagiosum (MC) is caused by a poxvirus which produces cutaneous lesions which appear as small, firm, umbilicated papules. There are three clinical presentations of MC: the childhood variety due to casual contact, the sexually transmitted variety in adults, and the aggressive form seen in patients infected with the human immunodeficiency virus (HIV).

Epidemiology

MC virus occurs worldwide but is more prevalent in tropical areas. It mainly affects children, sexually active adults, and individuals with impaired cellular immunity. There are four main subtypes of molluscum contagiosum: MCV I, MCV II, MCV III and MCV IV. All subtypes cause similar clinical lesions in genital and nongenital regions. Studies show MCV I to be more prevalent (75%–90%) than MCV II, MCV III, and MCV IV, except in immunocompromised individuals. Skin-to-skin transmission is presumed to be the method of spread, including autoinoculation, as well as contact with fomites.

Aetiology

MCV is a brick shaped approximately 100 nm, 200 nm, 300 nm sized virus, with a biconcave viral core enclosed by an inner membrane and an outer envelope. MCV cannot be grown in tissue culture or egg yolk. However it has been shown to produce typical changes on human keratinocytes culture in immuno-incompetent mice.

Clinical Features

Incubation period of molluscum contagiosum is 2 to 3 months, though the range varies from 2 weeks to 6 months. The onset is gradual and most patients are asymptomatic. Some may complain of itching or tenderness. The typical MC lesion is a small firm, dome shaped umbilicated papule with a smooth waxy or pearly surface. The base may or may not be erythematous and varies in size from 1 mm to 1 cm or more. The patient has between 10 and 20 lesions. Individual papules last 2 months or more. Solitary lesions can last for years, but the average case clears in less than 2 years. Rarely some lesions become very large reaching upto 1 to 2 cm or larger in size and are called as *giant molluscum contagiosum*.

In adults, the lesions most often occur on the thighs, inguinal region, buttock, lower abdominal wall, external genitalia **(Fig. 28.1, 28.2)** and perianal region **(Fig. 28.3)**,especially mucosal surfaces. In contrast, in children the lesions are usually distributed on exposed areas of the limbs, face and neck. However, 10 to 50% of children may have lesions on the genital area.

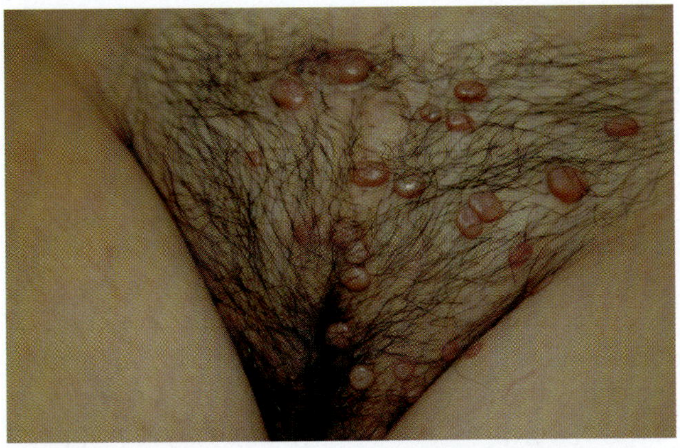

Fig. 28.1 Molluscum Contagiosum - Umbilicated Papules on Vulva.

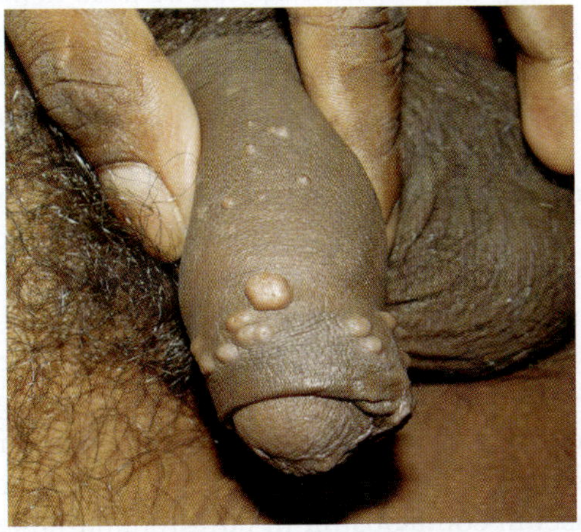

Fig. 28.2 Molluscum Contagiosum - Umbilicated Papules on Penis.

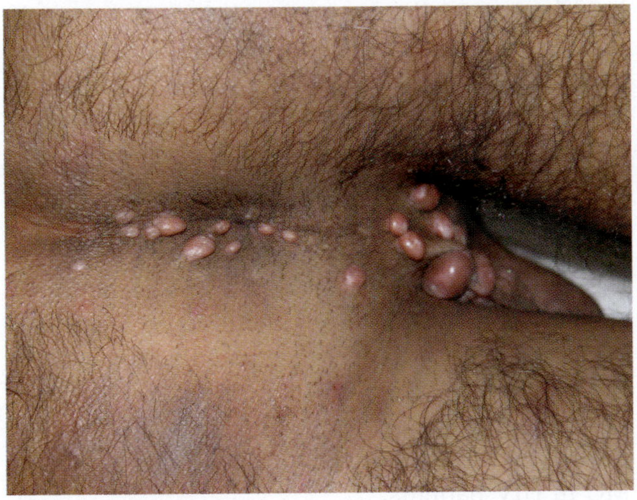

Fig. 28.3 Molluscum Contagiosum - Umbilicated Papules in Perianal Area.

MCV is a common cutaneous pathogen in HIV infection. MCV tends to appear when CD-4 cell count is below 200/mm^3 and the severity of infection tends to parallel with the stage of HIV disease with a prevalence of 5 to 18% among the HIV infected patients. The distribution of lesions of molluscum contagiosum in HIV infected individuals is usually over the face **(Fig. 28.4)**, neck and trunk rather than the genitalia. The lesions may be in hundreds and of larger size ranging from 1 cm to 5-10 cm. These may be follicular. Mucosal lesions are seen when the CD 4 cell count is less than 50/mm^3. Extensive molluscum contagiosum has been seen as a part of immune constitution restoration response which resolves with continuation of the antiretroviral therapy.

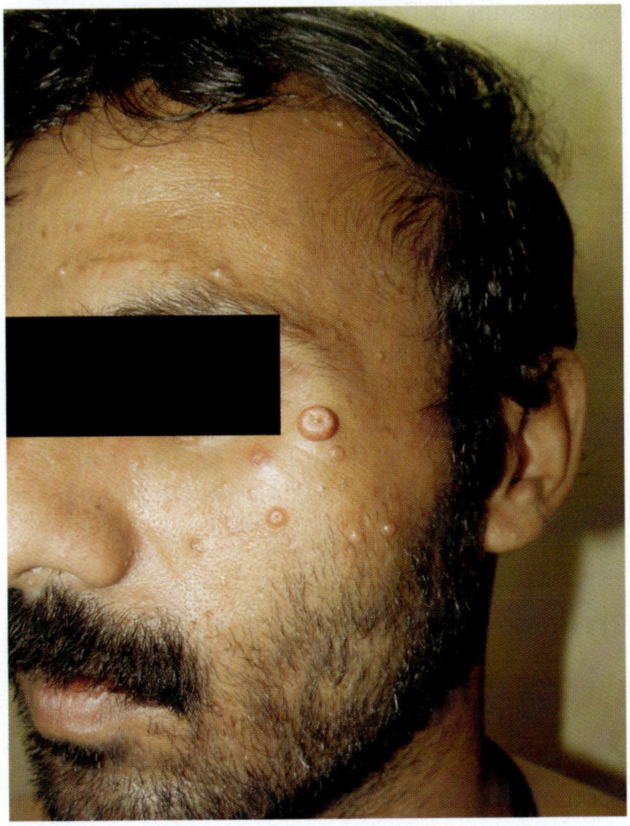

Fig. 28.4 Molluscum Contagiosum - Umbilicated Papules on Face in a HIV Positive Patient.

Diagnosis

The clinical appearance of molluscum contagiosum is in most cases diagnostic. Though molluscum cannot be cultured in the laboratory, histological examination of a curetted or biopsied lesion can also aid in the diagnosis in cases that are not clinically obvious and show typically brightly eosinophilic cytoplasmic inclusion bodies -"molluscum bodies" otherwise known as Henderson-Paterson bodies in lower epidermis. The thick white central core can be expressed and smeared on a slide and stained with Geimsa, Gram, Wright, or Papanicolaou stains to demonstrate the large brick-shaped inclusion bodies. Electron microscopy has also been used to demonstrate the poxvirus structures. Immunohistochemical method using a polyclonal antibody allows recognition of molluscum contagiosum in fixed tissue. In-situ hybridization for MCV DNA has also been utilized. Antibodies were demonstrated in both HIV positive and negative persons and there was no correlation with number of lesions and duration. There is upcoming evidence that dermoscopy facilitates the in vivo diagnosis of skin infections and infestations like viral warts, molluscum contagiosum, scabies, pediculosis. Molluscum contagiosum lesions must be differentiated from verruca vulgaris, condyloma accuminata, varicella, herpes simplex, papillomas, epitheliomas, pyoderma, cutaneuos cyptococcosis, epidermal inclusion cyst, basal cell carcinoma, papular granuloma annulare, keratoacanthoma, lichen planus, and syringoma or other adenexal tumors.

Treatment

Molluscum cantagiosum is a self-limited disease, which, left untreated, will eventually resolve in immunocompetent hosts but may be protracted in atopic and immunocompromised individuals. However, to prevent auto-inoculation and spread to others, therapy is needed. Most of the common treatments are destructive in nature and are described below. In treating children, care should be taken not to put the patient through a traumatic treatment regimen for a benign, self-limited condition. Recently antiviral and immune-modulating treatments have been tried, especially in immunocompromised hosts whose infections are difficult to eradicate.

The simplest and most widely used technique is expression of contents of papules with forceps followed by cauterization of base of the lesion with electrodessication or a chemical agent such as silver nitrate, trichloroacetic acid or iodine. A topical anesthetic such as a eutectic mixture of local anesthetics (EMLA containing 25 mg lidocaine and 25 mg prilocaine per gram) may be applied to the lesions to decrease the pain involved in the procedure. Cryotherapy is effective.

For tiny lesions, which may be difficult to curette, topical preparations can be used to produce an inflammatory response. These preparations are 10 – 20% phenol, tretinoin, 5% imiquimod cream, 5–10% potassium hydroxide, cantharidin and 0.5% podophyllotoxin cream. One author reports the use of 10% iodine solution on MC lesions. This is allowed to dry, then 50% salicylic acid plaster is cut into small pieces and placed on each lesion and repeated for many days till resolution. In a prospective randomized trial comparing the efficacy and adverse effects of four recognized treatments (curettage, cantharadin, combination of salicylic acid and lactic acid, imiquimod) of molluscum contagiosum in children, curettage was found to be the most efficacious treatment and had the lowest rate of side effects.

A course of oral cimetidine has been found to be effective. Molluscum contagiosum is not a self-limited disease in the HIV-positive patient, but rather is an infection refractory to treatment modalities that are successful in the immunocompetent individual. Interferon alpha has been used to treat molluscum contagiosum in immunodeficiency. In HIV patients, HAART may lead to regression of lesions. The antiviral agent cidofovir has been shown to be effective (used either intravenously or 1 – 3% ointment topically). It should be considered for treatment of extensive molluscum contagiosum in HIV disease. Trichloroacetic acid peel, electron beam therapy, and the 585 nm pulsed dye laser have also been reported as treatment options for MC in HIV patients.

VIRAL HEPATITIS[11-18]

Hepatitis viruses are important cause for acute and chronic liver diseases. Liver disease is currently the second leading cause of death in HIV-infected patients in Western countries. In heterosexual relationships, hepatitis B is readily transmitted sexually and hepatitis C and D less so, with no evidence for sexual transmission of hepatitis A. Hepatitis A to D all are transmissible sexually in male homosexuals under some conditions. Recently, a cross sectional study evaluating the role of sexual activity and sexually transmitted diseases showed the higher prevalence of hepatitis G virus (HGV/GBV-C) in the STD clinic group patients compared with the group who never had received treatment for an STDs. Viral sexually transmitted infections (STIs), like bacterial STIs, are preventable, but unlike bacterial STIs, viral STIs often are difficult to treat and the person may harbour the virus for the rest of her or his life. The epidemiology, risk factors, clinical features and management of hepatitis viruses are discussed separately

Hepatitis A

HAV is a non-enveloped 27nm, heat, acid and ether resistant RNA virus in the hepatovirus genus of the picornavirus, known to cause only acute and not chronic hepatic disease. There are four polypeptide capsids VP1 – VP4 in HAV. The virus is inactivated by boiling for 1 minute, by contact with formaldehyde, chlorine and by ultraviolet light.

Prevalence

HAV is transmitted almost exclusively by faeco-oral route. Person-to-person spread is enhanced by poor personal hygiene and overcrowding. Hepatitis A, like other enteric infections can be transmitted during sexual activity especially involving oroanal or digital-rectal intercourse. In-apparent fecal contamination is commonly present during sexual intercourse. Measures like condom use to prevent other STDs do not protect from HAV. HAV transmission through sexual activity may play a major role in the developed countries with good public health system. In developing countries, with inadequate sanitary and water system, water borne infection is so prevalent that sexual mode of transmission becomes insignificant. Outbreaks of hepatitis A have occurred among homosexual men. Some studies have associated the various risk factors like having a greater number of sex partners, frequent oro-anal contact, insertive anal intercourse or serologic evidences of other STDs with HAV. Parenteral spread can occur in intravenous drug users, haemophiliacs using contaminated factor VIII, and other recipients of blood products, but this route is very rare.

HAV replicates in the hepatocytes and appears in bile. It is shed in high concentration in faeces from 2 weeks before to 1 week after the onset of illness. Viremia roughly parallels shedding of virus in faeces and can persist for several weeks after the onset of symptoms.

Clinical Features

The incubation period from the time of exposure to the onset of symptoms is approximately 4 weeks (range 15 – 50 days). It starts with a prodromal illness which will last for about 2 weeks, followed by icteric hepatitis that lasts for a few weeks, sometimes longer than 3 months. There is no prolonged carrier state and infection with HAV produces immunity and hence symptomatic re-infections rarely occur. Chronic infections usually do not occur. Fulminant liver failure develops in about 0.1 % of cases and there is an overall mortality rate of 0.3% in persons under age of 49. The mortality rate increases to 1.8% in persons over the age of 49.

Antibodies to HAV (anti HAV) can be detected concurrent with the clinical onset of hepatitis. The early antibody response is predominantly IgM and persists for several months. Anti HAV IgG appears shortly after the appearance of symptoms and during convalescence and may remain detectable lifelong.

Diagnosis

A specific diagnosis of viral hepatitis-A requires the demonstration of IgM anti HAV, which is virtually present in the serum of all patients. Rheumatoid factor may be false-positive. Absence of anti-HAV IgM is strong evidence against current infection with HAV. Anti-HAV IgG persists for life and is not useful for acute illness. Tests can also be positive after hepatitis-A vaccination.

Treatment

Patients with hepatitis-A infection usually require only supportive care. Patients developing dehydration due to nausea and vomiting or patients with signs and symptoms of acute liver failure may require hospitalization.

Prevention

Both passive vaccination with immunoglobulin (IG) and active vaccination with formalin inactivated cell-cultured-derived HAV are available. HAVRIXR contains inactivated Hepatitis A virus HM 175 strain. It is not recommended for children under 2 years. Adults (older than 18 years) should receive two 1.0 ml injections containing 1440 enzyme linked immunoassay units (ELU) 6 to 12 months apart. Children aged 2 to 18 years should receive 0.5-ml injections containing 360 ELU at 0,6,12 months or two 0.5-ml injections containing 72 ELU, 6 to 12 months apart. Another vaccine manufactured by Merck is also available for prevention.

A combined hepatitis-A and B vaccine has been developed for adults. When administered at 0, 1 and 6 months schedule, the vaccine has equivalent efficacy to that of the monovalent vaccines.

Immunoglobulin (IG) when administered before or within 2 weeks of exposure is 80 to 90 percent effective in protecting against Hepatitis A. Previously unvaccinated persons exposed to patients with HAV (e.g. through household or sexual contact or sharing needle with a person who has hepatitis A) should be administered a single dose of IG (0.02 ml/kg) as soon as possible but not more than 2 weeks after exposure. Hepatitis A vaccine can be administered simultaneously at different sites. Adverse drug reactions to IG are minimal and occur in about 1% of all recipients.

Hepatitis B

HBV is a double-stranded DNA virus in the Hepadnaviridae family. It has been cultivated on different cell lines. The HBV genome has four genes: pol, env, precore and X that encode for viral DNA polymerase, envelope protein, pre-core protein (which is processed to viral capsids) and protein X, respectively. HBV has three antigens – HBsAg and HBcAg and HBeAg present in the surface envelope and in the core protein of virus, respectively. They are also produced by infected hepatocytes. HBcAg is obtained on vigorous disruption of the virus core.

Presence of HBsAg in blood is diagnostic of HBV infection. The core antigen HBcAg is not seen in blood and is detected in hepatocytes. Estimation of HBeAg, which is also present in the core of the virus, is useful to assess the infectivity of the patient, especially in long-term carriers.

Prevalence

Hepatitis B infection is present worldwide and is a significant cause of morbidity and mortality particularly in Asia. Number of new infections per year has declined from an average of 260,000 in the 1980s to about 60,000 in 2004. Highest rate of disease occurs in 20-49 year olds. Greatest decline has happened among children and adolescents due to routine hepatitis B vaccination. Estimated 1.25 million Americans have chronic infection, of whom 20-30% acquired their infection in childhood. Adults chronically infected with hepatitis B virus remain a significant potential source of sexually transmitted hepatitis B.

HBV is a hepatotropic, found in the highest concentration in blood and in lower concentration in other body fluids (e.g. semen, vaginal secretion and wound exudates). The major route of transmission is percutaneous. At present, as a result of screening of the blood and blood products for HBV, transmission by blood transfusion is very rare.

The other routes are sexual contact and perinatal transmission especially in endemic countries. Both homosexual and heterosexual exposure may transmit HBV. Recent data from Moscow showed that during the last two years up to 40% cases of HCV and HBV were sexually transmitted. Sexual transmission can be prevented by use of condom. Health care providers and patients receiving haemodialysis are also at increased risk of acquiring infection.

Various Indian studies have shown high prevalence of HBV antigens among STDs patients. High (59%) serological prevalence of HBV was observed among male homosexuals. The most common risk factors for heterosexual transmission include multiple sex partners, unprotected sexual act or a recent history of STDs. Changes in sexual practices to prevent HIV infection have resulted in lower risk for HBV. HBV infection is more prevalent among HIV infected population.

Clinical Features

The incubation period from the time of exposure to the onset of symptoms is 6 weeks to 6 months. It may be shorter with large inoculum and parenteral exposures and may be prolonged by administration of globulin preparations. HBV infection may be self limited or chronic. In adults, 50% have silent infection resulting in permanent and solid immunity. The remaining develop symptomatic, acute HBV infections and about 1% of these cases result in acute liver failure and death.

Approximately 15 to 20 % of patients develop a transient serum sickness like illness during the prodromal or early acute stage of hepatitis B. Acute hepatitis B infection has clinical picture similar to that of HAV infection. About 90 to 95% of the acutely infected adults recover without any sequelae and about 2 to 6% develop chronic infection. Risk for chronicity is associated with age at infection. About 90% of infected neonates and 60% of infected children develop chronic infection in contrast to 2 to 6% of adults. Approximately 5% of persons with HBV infection become chronic carriers of which two-thirds have a benign form of the diseases, and one-third of chronic HBsAg carriers develop chronic active hepatitis, which can be either "replicative" with virus production or "non-replicative". The "replicative" chronic HBV infection is defined by the presence of detectable HBeAg, has worse prognosis and a increased risk of developing cirrhosis and or hepatocellular carcinoma. The risk of death due to cirrhosis and or hepatocellular carcinoma is 15% to 20% among persons with chronic HBV infection.

Diagnosis

The diagnosis of acute or chronic HBV infection cannot be made on clinical grounds but requires serologic testing. Almost 90 percent of individuals with acute hepatitis B have HBsAg detectable in the serum when presenting to clinician for the first time. The remaining 10 percent HBsAg negative individuals will have antiHBc uniformly present in the sera while antiHBs may be found in some. HBsAg is detectable several weeks after infection and its appearance coincides with the onset of clinical infection. The presence of IgM antibody to hepatitis B core antigen (IgM anti-HBc) is specific and diagnostic of acute HBV infection. It persists for 6 to 24 months. Antibody to HBsAg (anti-HBs) is produced following a resolved infection and is the only HBV antibody marker present following immunization. The presence of HBsAg with a negative test for IgM anti-HBc is indicative of chronic HBV infection. The presence of anti-HBc may indicate acute, resolved or chronic infection. Diagnosis of hepatitis B is confirmed and prognosis is assessed by liver histopathology.

Treatment

Laboratory testing should be used to confirm suspected acute or chronic HBV infection. In acute hepatitis, recovery occurs in 99% of the previously healthy adults. No specific treatment is available for persons with acute HBV infection. Adefovir dipivoxil, interferon alfa-2b, pegylated interferon alfa-2a, lamivudine, entecavir and telbivudine are six drugs used for the treatment of persons with chronic hepatitis B. These drugs should not be used by pregnant women. Drinking alcohol can make your liver disease worse. Interferon alpha is administered by subcutaneous or intramuscular injection at a dose of 5,000,000 units daily for a period of 16 weeks. The patient must be monitored carefully during the treatment for side effects, like flu-like symptoms, depression, rashes and abnormal blood counts.

Prevention

Hepatitis B vaccine is the best protection. The efficacy of latex condoms in preventing infection with HBV is unknown, but their proper use might reduce transmission. Two products are available for hepatitis B prevention; hepatitis B immunoglobulin (HBIG) and hepatitis B vaccine.

HBIG is indicated for post exposure prophylaxis in the following situations: sexual contact of previously unvaccinated person with a patient who has active hepatitis B or who developed hepatitis B, or sexual contact with an HBV carrier (blood test positive for HbsAg) and household contacts. HBIG should be administered within 14 days after the most recent sexual contact. Passive immunization with HBIG provides temporary protection. Simultaneous administration of HBIG and hepatitis B vaccine should be considered.

For perinatal exposure of infants born to HbsAg positive mothers, a single dose of HBIG 0.5 ml should be administered in the thigh immediately after birth followed by the complete course of recombinant Hepatitis B vaccine within 12 hours of life. For persons with direct percutaneous inoculation or transmucosal exposure to HbsAg positive blood or body fluids, a single dose of HBIG 0.06 ml/kg should be administered as soon after exposure as possible followed by the complete course of recombinant hepatitis B vaccine within 1 week.

Pre-exposure Immunization

Pre-exposure immunization is recommended for all persons who attend the STDs clinics and have not been previously vaccinated, including pregnant women with STDs. Hepatitis B vaccination is offered to all persons who have not been vaccinated, universally to neonates, persons with a history of STDs, persons who have had multiple sex partners, those who have had sex with injection drug user, active male homosexuals, household contacts, drug sharing partners of person with chronic HBV infection and persons on haemodialysis, receiving blood products or occupational exposure to blood products.

There are two recombinant hepatitis B vaccines available: Recombivax-HB containing 10 µgm of HBsAg, Engerix-B contains 20 µgm of HBsAg.

Schedule of Vaccination

Three intramuscular (deltoid, not gluteal) doses at 0, 1 and 6 months

Dosage of Vaccine

Engerix-B

- 10 µgm in children under 10 years
- 20 µgm for immunocompetent children older than 10 years and adults
- 40 µgm for dialysis patients and immuno-comprised patients

Recombinant Vax-HB

- 2.5 µgm for children less than 11 years of age of HBsAg negative mothers
- 5 µgm for infants of HBsAg positive mothers and for children and adolescents 11 to 19 years of age
- 10 µgm for immunocompetent adults
- 40 µgm for dialysis and other immuno-suppressed patients

HIV infection can impair the response to hepatitis B vaccine. Therefore, vaccinated HIV infected person should be tested for anti-HBsAg, 1 to 2 months after the third dose. Re-vaccination with three additional doses should be considered for those who do not respond to initial vaccination.

Safe sexual practices, rigorous screening of blood and blood products can lead to reduced transmission of HBV infection.

Hepatitis D Virus Infection (HDV)

It is a unique RNA virus that is replication defective, causing infection only when it is encapsulated by HBsAg. It is fully dependent on the genetic information provided by the hepatitis B virus for its multiplication. It has the same the sources and modes of transmission as that of HBV and can be sexually transmitted. HDV infection occurs in two forms:

1. Acute co-infection develops after exposure to the serum containing both HBV and HDV. It results in hepatitis ranging from mild to fulminant hepatitis. Fulminant hepatitis occurs more frequently with co-infection than with HBV alone.
2. Super infection of a chronic HBV carrier with a new inoculum of HDV and it results in either one of the following clinical situations:
   a. Mild HBV may become fulminant hepatitis
   b. Acute severe hepatitis
   c. Chronic progressive disease leading to cirrhosis (80%)

IgM anti HDV is the most reliable indicator of recent HDV infection along with markers of acute/ chronic HB infection. HDV antigen and HDV RNA can also be detected.

Hepatitis C virus Infection

Hepatitis C virus, previously called as "non A, non B" hepatitis, is a single stranded RNA virus, in the family flaviviridae. HCV is transmitted by blood products and other body fluids. Until 1986, when routine testing of donated blood began, blood transfusions were responsible for the greatest number of HCV cases. Now, the virus is rarely transmitted through that route: Injection drug use—specifically, sharing contaminated needles and other paraphernalia—is the new leading cause, accounting for 60 percent of HCV cases. The virus also can be transmitted in other ways: perinatally, by kidney dialysis, and by organ transplantation. HCV is less frequently transmitted by sexual intercourse (15%), although people with other sexually transmitted infections, including HIV, appear to be at increased risk of contracting the disease in this way.

Heterosexual spread of HCV has been reported from Thailand, Argentina and Egypt. However reports from Malaysia, Jamaica and Tanzania did not show significant evidence for the heterosexual spread. These studies suggest that sexual transmission may occur in resource poor countries but at a lower rate compared with other modes of transmission. Homosexual spread of HCV infection has also been reported from European countries and USA.

Clinical Features

The average incubation period is 150 days. Acute infection is largely asymptomatic (80%). Only 20% of patients develop icteric hepatitis. Fulminant hepatitis may occur with hepatitis A super infection. Chronic infection develops in about 80% of the patients (mostly asymptomatic). Symptomatic chronic infection with cirrhosis develops only in about 20% after 20 years. Coinfection with HIV may accelerate the natural course of the disease resulting in progressive liver disease, which is the major cause of morbidity and mortality. Hepatitis C infection in AIDS patients may increase the risk of hepatotoxicity due to HAART.

Diagnosis and Management

Detection of IgG anti-HCV antibody by screening test - ELISA and RIBA test is confirmatory for both acute & chronic infections. The test will become positive 3 months after exposure to HCV but sometimes after 9 months. PCR assay can also be used to detect viral proteins. Treatment with combination of pegylated IFN (3 million units subcutaneously three times weekly) and ribavirin 1000-1200 mg PO daily is safe in both HIV infected and non-infected patients. The treatment should be provided with no restrictions at the start and reassessed at week 4 and 12, considering virologic responses. Patients with low CD4 counts (15%) should be deferred for treatment and HAART prioritized in order to improve CD4 counts. When possible, nucleoside analogs such as zidovudine, stavudine, and abacavir should be replaced by others having no deleterious interactions with ribavirin (e.g. tenofovir, lamivudine, or emtricitabine). Didanosine should never be co-administered with ribavirin due to potential life-threatening complications. Serious neuropsychiatric or cardiovascular history are contra-indications for interferon therapy.

Hepatitis G virus infection

Hepatitis G virus is a transfusion transmitted agent and do not cause hepatitis. Sexual activity and, possibly, the presence of an STDs increase the risk of HGV/GBC-V transmission. Male to male sex is associated with a high prevalence of exposure to GB virus C.

CYTOMEGALOVIRUS INFECTIONS[19-24]

Cytomegalovirus (CMV) belongs to Herpesviridae family and is termed as Betaherpes-viridae. CMV is a double stranded DNA virus consisting of icosahedral capsids, surrounded by an outer envelope of lipid bilayer. It is the largest member of herpes virus family, and the size is 150-200 nm. The structure is like that of other herpes viruses. Of all the herpes viruses described to date, infection with CMV arguably is the most important cause of morbidity and mortality. In addition to inducing severe birth defects, CMV causes a wide spectrum of diseases in older children and adults, ranging from an asymptomatic, sub-clinical infection to a mononucleosis syndrome in healthy individuals to disseminated disease in immuno-compromised patients. Primary infection is followed by life long carriage of this virus with intermittent shedding in various secretions. The shedding may increase in conditions of immuno-suppression by diseases or by therapy and in pregnancy.

In clinical specimens, one of the classic hallmarks of CMV infection is the cytomegalic inclusion cells, first described by Ribbert in 1904. These cells are markedly enlarged with large purple intranuclear inclusions surrounded by a clear halo and smaller basophilic cytoplasmic inclusions producing "owl's eye" appearance.

Prevalence

CMV infections occur worldwide and are usually inapparent. In a review and meta-analysis of the epidemiology of congenital cytomegalovirus (CMV) infection, the overall birth prevalence of congenital CMV infection was 0.64. About 11% of live-born infants with congenital CMV infection were symptomatic. Non-white race, low socioeconomic status (SES), premature birth, and neonatal intensive care unit admittance were risk factors for congenital CMV infection. Birth prevalence increased with maternal CMV seroprevalence. Maternal seroprevalence accounted for 29% of the variance in birth prevalence between study populations. The rate of transmission to infants born to mothers who had a primary infection or a recurrent infection during pregnancy was 32% and 1.4%, respectively. Possible maternal primary infections (i.e. seropositive mother with CMV IgM) resulted in congenital infections about 20% of the time, but are likely to represent a mixture of primary and recurrent infections. When an infected child introduces CMV into a household, 50% of the susceptible family members seroconvert within 6 months.

The prevalence of CMV infection in the adult population ranges from 40% in Europe to 100% in Africa and Far East. The age at which an individual acquires CMV depends greatly on geographic location, socio-economic status, cultural factors and child rearing practices. Acquisition of CMV in the newborn period is common – either transplacental or perinatal. More than 50% infants become infected with CMV infected breast milk. Others, not infected in infancy may acquire CMV in day care centres.

Poor personal hygiene and communal living facilitate the spread of infection. Virus is present in saliva, urine, semen, breast milk, blood, transplanted donor organs and cervical and vaginal secretions and may be acquired from these sources. In adulthood, sexual activity is the most important route of CMV transmission. Kissing may transfer CMV from toddlers to adults. CMV may also be transmitted by blood transfusion and solid organ transplant.

Clinical Features

Congenital cytomegalovirus (CMV) infection is one of the most common viral causes of congenital infections in high resource countries and a leading cause of hearing loss as well as an important contributor to neurodevelopmental disabilities in children. Congenital CMV disease may be symptomatic or asymptomatic. In the most severe forms, it leads to hepato-splenomegaly, jaundice and purpura. Most infants die within two months and survivors usually (90%) suffer from some neurological damage. Purple or red papules or nodules develop in the skin because of erythropoietic tissue collection in the dermis and lasts for 4 to 6 weeks. Asymptomatic congenital CMV may cause sensorineural hearing loss in 15 to 20% of the cases.

Typical CMV mononucleosis is a disease of young adults. There are fever and lymphocytosis. The lymphadenopathy and splenomegaly may not be striking. Transfusion acquired CMV disease presents as CMV mononucleosis. The incubation period is 20 to 60 days. CMV infection in the immunocompromised patients can be severe and even be fatal. Infection may occur because of reactivation of latent viral infection or may be newly acquired. Viral dissemination leads to multiple organ system involvement with pneumonitis, hepatitis, gastrointestinal ulceration, retinitis and super infection with other opportunistic pathogens. Neurological complications include encephalitis, myelitis and myeloradiculitis when the peripheral nerve roots are infiltrated with lymphocytes in AIDS.

CMV produces a necrotic, rapidly progressing retinitis with characteristic white perivascular infiltrates with haemorrhage (bush-fire retinitis). It was the most common cause of blindness in adult patients with AIDS before the advent of highly active anti-retroviral therapy (HAART) for HIV infection. It occurs in 90% of the affected individuals. In contrast to adults, CMV associated retinitis in children is rare. CMV retinitis is less common in transplant patients also.

In AIDS, CMV infection manifests with severe pain, loss of weight, weakness, remitting fever. Gastrointestinal lesions were erosive-ulcerous or ulceronecrotic. The following pathogenetic chain of CMV infection course in the gastrointestinal tract was established: vasculitis → microcirculatory disorders → segmental ischemia → necrosis with inflammatory infiltration and CMV transformation of the cells → fibrosis → cicatricial transformation of the organ wall. Developing sclerosis due to CMV involvement of the intestine may promote cancer, but this should be proved in further studies. True CMV pneumonia may occur.

Diagnosis

Virus culture from throat washings, urine, bronchoalveolar lavage fluid, cervico-vaginal secretions, CSF, blood or biopsy material is carried out in human embryo fibroblast, and the cell culture is monitored for the development of the characteristic CMV associated cytopathic effect. It takes 5 to 28 days to produce cytopathic effect. Looking for CMV early antigen after 24 to 48 hours of culture (shell-vial assay) can make the diagnosis earlier. A positive blood culture is almost always diagnostic. Urine and saliva may be positive due to routine viral shedding. Newer diagnostic tools like PCR and direct detection of CMV antigenemia are useful rapid methods with greater sensitivity and can be used to monitor CMV disease in immunocompromised host. Assays for CMV DNA or antigen in blood are superior to culture for documenting viremia and pneumonia. Genotypic assays have largely replaced phenotypic assays for CMV resistance to antivirals. Lymphocyte responses to CMV antigen(s) may identify patients at risk for CMV disease. Demonstration of CMV antibody is diagnostic of primary CMV infection. Congenital CMV may be diagnosed by virus isolation or the presence of CMV IgM antibody within 3 weeks of birth. CMV load has limited clinical utility, because of its low positive predictive value. Its high negative predictive value for occurrence of resistant CMV suggests that it may have utility as a screening tool to exclude resistance.

Treatment

CMV infection in a normal host rarely requires treatment. However, in life threatening situations such as AIDS or other immunocompromised situations like recipients of stem cell (HSCT) or solid organ (SOT) transplants, therapy is often required. There are three systemic drugs approved for CMV treatment: ganciclovir, or its prodrug valganciclovir, foscarnet, and cidofovir. An anti-sense therapeutic, ISIS 2922, is also approved specifically as in intravitreal treatment for CMV retinitis. Ganciclovir, and more recently, valganciclovir, have been useful in proactive approaches of CMV disease management; in both prophylactic and preemptive regimens in HSCT and SOT populations. The major anti-herpes agent valacyclovir has also been approved for prophylaxis of renal transplant recipients, or SOTs outside of the US. These drugs have provided major advances in CMV disease management, although they are limited by intolerable toxicities, oral bioavailability and efficacy, and risk of drug resistance with extended use. Several drugs are in early clinical development which may address these limitations.

Prevention

Vaccines are under trial. Although, after 30 years of intensive study, a clinically licensed vaccine is still not available, significant progress has been made in the field of HCMV vaccine development, along with greater understanding of HCMV immunology, molecular biology and pathology. In recent years, new vaccine strategies have been developed that have shown promising results in preclinical studies and are able to induce HCMV-specific immune responses in clinical studies, although efficacy data are not yet available. Until the goal of a CMV vaccine is realized, educating women of child-bearing age about the risk of CMV and modes of prevention are the only control strategies available.

EPSTEIN-BARR VIRUS INFECTION[25-29]

Epstein-Barr virus (EBV) is a DNA virus and is named after Tony Epstein and Yvonne Barr who first described the virus in patients with Burkitt's lymphoma. It is a gamma virus, a member of Herpesviridae family with icosahedral nucleocapsids and envelope. Following primary infection EBV establishes life long latency in the B-lymphocytes in the host.

Prevalence

EBV infections occur worldwide. These infections are most common in early childhood, with a second peak during late adolescence. EBV spreads by close contact especially kissing and can be sexually transmitted. During the dormant state of the virus there is a periodic activation and shedding of viruses in the oropharyngeal secretions. More than 90% of the asymptomatic sero-positive individuals shed the virus in oro-pharyngeal secretions. Transmission of the virus through air or blood does not usually occur. However transmission by blood transfusion and bone marrow transplantation has been described. Usually the infections in children are asymptomatic or present with mild pharyngitis with or without tonsillitis, but with poor hygiene and socioeconomic status, the infection in children may be symptomatic. In contrast, up-to 75% of infections in adolescents present as infectious mononucleosis (IM).

Pathogenesis

The virus is transmitted by saliva and infects the epithelium of the oral cavity. The B-lymphocytes are the target cells and they become infected after contact with the epithelial cells. The virus is attached to the EBV receptors CD21 present on the surface of the B cells and also epithelial cells and is internalized by cell. Inside the cell the viral DNA forms a loop of DNA and enters the cell nucleus. The viral DNA is then integrated into the host DNA. The viral proteins are expressed with the formation of new virus. EBV remains latent in few cells in the throat and in the B cells. They persist in the form of an episome. Six viral genes termed EBNA 1-6 are expressed and they transform the B cell into an immortal continuous dividing cell.

Clinical Features

Primary Syndromes
- Infectious mononucleosis
- Chronic EBV infection
- X linked lymphoproliferative syndromes

Reactivation Syndromes
- Lymphoproliferative disorders in immunocompromised patients
- Burkitt's lymphoma
- Nasopharyngeal carcinoma
- Oral hairy leucoplakia
- Hodgkins lymphoma

Infectious Mononucleosis (IM)

Infectious mononucleosis (IM) is a disease of young adults. In lower socioeconomic groups, EBV tends to infect children at an early stage, and asymptomatic IM is uncommon. In areas with higher standards of hygiene, infection with EBV is often delayed until adulthood, and IM is more prevalent. The incubation period is 4 to 7 weeks. Clinically it is characterized by a prodrome of fatigue, malaise, and myalgia which will last for about 1-2 weeks and is followed by fever, pharyngitis and generalized lymphadenopathy. The cutaneous manifestations are morbilliform rash, sometimes erythema nodosum and erythema multiforme. Other features are splenomegaly, hepatomegaly, abnormal liver function tests and atypical lymphocytosis in the peripheral blood. Usually the disease is self-limiting but sometimes the convalescence may be prolonged.

When neurological Complications (meningitis, encephalitis, Guillaine Barre syndrome, acute transverse myelitis and peripheral neuritis) develop they usually do within first two weeks of EBV infection. Autoimmune haemolytic anaemia (2%), splenic rupture (0.5%), upper airway obstruction, bacterial super-infections and rarely hepatitis, myocarditis, pericarditis and vasculitis are other complications.

Chronic EBV infections

Chronic EBV infections are very rare and patients have an illness lasting for more than 6 months with marked increase in the EBV antibody titre. There is usually systemic involvement in the form of hepatomegaly, lymphadenopathy, pneumonitis, uveitis and neurologic disease.

Lymphoproliferative Disorders

It has been described in immunosuppressed patients (both congenital and acquired immunodeficiency). There is a polyclonal proliferation of EBV transformed B cells in the lymph nodes and multiple organs and patients present with fever and lymphadenopathy and gastrointestinal symptoms.

X linked Lymphoproliferative Syndrome (Duncan's Syndrome)

It is a rare disorder of young boys who have a normal response to childhood infection but develop fatal lymphoproliferative disorders after infection. Most of the patients die of severe IM. The other complications are hypogammaglobulinemia, malignant B cell lymphoma, aplastic anaemia and agranulocytosis.

The other diseases, which are associated with EBV are OHL, Burkitt's lymphoma, nasopharyngeal lymphoma, Hodgkin's lymphoma and leiomyosarcoma.

EBV related malignancies

The Epstein-Barr virus (EBV) has been detected in the tumour cells of a range of diverse neoplasms. In addition to Burkitt's lymphoma (BL) and nasopharyngeal carcinoma (NPC), the list of EBV-associated tumours now includes Hodgkin's disease (HD), post-transplant lymphoproliferative disorders (PTLD), T-cell non-Hodgkin lymphomas (NHL), gastric carcinomas, possibly breast and hepatocellular carcinomas, and smooth muscle cell-derived tumours in immunodeficient individuals.

EBV related oral diseases

Studies have also implicated EBV in the pathogenesis of advanced types of periodontal disease. EBV DNA is detected in 60–80% of aggressive periodontitis lesions and in 15–20% of gingivitis lesions or normal periodontal sites. The periodontal presence of EBV is associated with an elevated occurrence of periodontopathic anaerobic bacteria. Moreover, EBV active infection occurs in 70% of symptomatic and large-size periapical lesions. EBV and cytomegalovirus often co-exist in marginal and apical periodontitis. Periodontal therapy can markedly suppress the EBV load in periodontal pockets as well as in saliva, which has the potential to reduce the risk of viral transmission between close individuals.

Oral Hairy Leucoplakia (OHL)

OHL is a white corrugated lesion normally seen along the lateral borders of the tongue on both sides. It may extend over to the ventral surface or the adjacent buccal mucosa. It usually occurs in HIV infected individuals with the CD4 count of <300 mm^3 and occasionally in organ transplant patients. Most often it is confused with oral candidiasis in which the whitish lesions can easily be removed with a spatula. OHL is not a premalignant lesion. Histologically OHL shows hyperkeratosis, parakeratosis, acanthosis and large vacuolated cells in the prickle layer. The specific diagnosis depends on the demonstration of EBV in the sample by electron microscopy, in situ hybridization, immunohistochemical staining or PCR.

Diagnosis

In IM, the white blood cell count is usually elevated and peaks at 10,000 to 20,000 cells per microlitre during the second or third week of illness. Lymphocytosis is usually found with >10% atypical lymphocytes. Paul-Bunnel test (Heterophil test) is positive in 70-80% of patients with acute IM. Heterophil antibodies agglutinate sheep or horse erythrocytes but do not react with EBV antigens directly. Heterophil antibody titre of 1: 40 is highly diagnostic of acute IM. EBV specific IgM antibody to viral capsid antigens (VCA) is also very useful in the diagnosis of IM. IgG antibody to VCA is elevated in the past infection and it persists for life. Anitbodies to early antigens (EA) are seen either as diffuse pattern in the nucleus and the cytoplasm of the affected cell (EA-D) or as a restrictive pattern in the cytoplasm (EA-R). EA-D antibodies are elevated in acute illness and also in nasopharyngeal carcinoma or chronic active EBV infection. Elevated EA-R antibodies are often seen with Burkitt's lymphoma or chronic active EBV infection. IgA antibodies to EBV antigens may be useful for the diagnosis of nasopharyngeal carcinoma. EBV DNA, RNA or proteins can be detected in tissues from patients with OHL or other malignancies. The monitoring of Epstein-Barr virus viral loads in different tissue compartments is currently being effectively used to assess the treatment response or prognosis in patients with oncological diseases or immunosuppression. For the diagnosis of primary infections, EBV PCR could lead to an increase of >16% in the number of positive diagnoses by confirming a positive IgM VCA in the absence of heterophilic antibodies. Furthermore, EBV PCR is positive in only 3% of sera with elevated antibodies against EA, raising doubt as to the utility of EA titers for diagnosing EBV reactivation.

Treatment

Treatment of IM is usually symptomatic. A short course of steroids may be useful in severe disease with airway obstruction, auti-immune hemolytic anaemia and thrombocytopenia. Patients with severe pharyngitis are treated with appropriate antibiotics. Splenectomy is advised in case of splenic rupture. For the treatment of OHL, oral acyclovir (400-800 mg five times a day) or topical tretinoin or podophyllin may be used. Acyclovir has no significant clinical impact on IM in controlled trials. Therapy for EBV lymphoproliferative disorders is directed towards the reduction of immunosuppressive medication. Newer therapies that are being tried are interferon-alpha or infusion of donor T cells or EBV specific cytotoxic T cells. Vaccines against the major EBV glycoproteins have been effective in animal studies and are undergoing small scale clinical trials.

SCABIES[30-33]

Scabies is one of the first diseases with a known cause. The itch mite *Sarcoptes scabiei var-hominis* was first described in 1687. Scabies affects all races and socioeconomic classes. Both sexes are affected equally although earlier studies have described a male preponderance.

Transmission of scabies occurs through intense physical contact e.g. during playtime in young children, sharing of bed or prolonged handholding. Transmission may also occur through fomites like bed linen, towels, though it is less likely. Sarcoptes scabiei mites are often immobile and rarely survive for more than 1 to 2 days away from the skin of host. Transmission of scabies during sexual contact particularly in sexually active young adults is not uncommon. Patients with scabies attending Genito-urinary medicine (GUM) clinic had comparable number of STDs, as were seen in other GUM clinic population. The diagnosis of scabies in the sexually active age group particularly when genital lesions are present should prompt a search for co-existing STDs especially gonorrhoea and syphilis.

In primary infections, the symptoms appear after 2 to 5 weeks. Clinically, the following features suggest diagnosis of scabies in a patient.

1. Types of lesions: papules **(Fig. 28.5)**, nodules, **(Fig. 28.6)** vesicles, pustules, ulcers, secondary eczematization, excoriation and infection
2. Distribution – in finger web spaces, hands, wrist, elbows, anterior axillary folds, areola in female, abdomen, genitals and buttocks.
3. Burrow, especially when present in finger web space or penis is pathognomonic.
4. Severe pruritus with nocturnal exacerbations.
5. Presence or history of scabies or pruritus in family members.

Besides the classical sites, erythema and scaling may occur on face, neck, scalp, and trunk and may generalize. Nails may become dystrophic. The disease occurs also with great severity in mentally retarded or physically debilitated persons.

In immunocompromised patients, the mite replicates uncontrolled, so that millions can be found on the skin. The presence of HIV disease in patients may modify scabies. Crusted or Norwegian scabies results with its widespread psoriasiform lesions or even erythroderma with fine to lamellar scaling and hyperkeratotic plaques especially on palms, soles and side of fingers. Norwegian scabies is highly contagious with large number of mites in

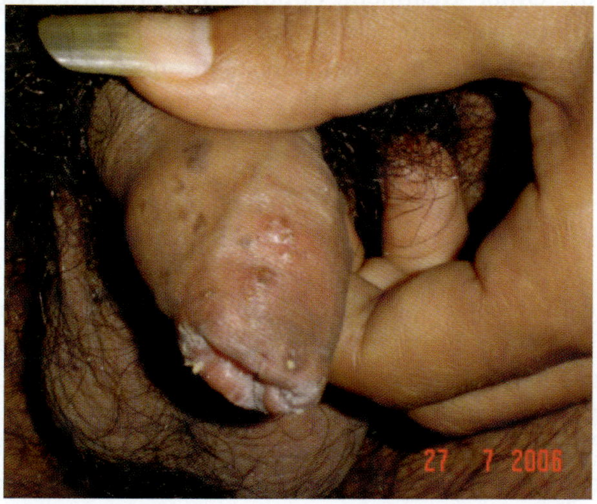

Fig. 28.5 Scabies - Excoriated Papules on Prepuce.

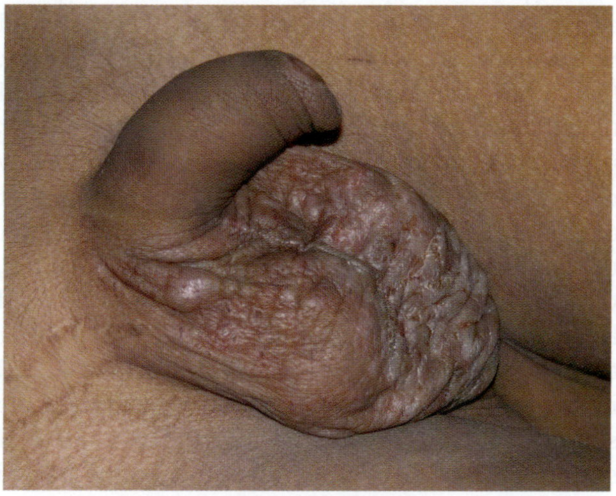

Fig. 28.6 Scabies - Nodules on Scrotum.

the exfoliating scales. Itching is minimal or absent. Patients undergoing immunosuppressive therapy or with immuno-suppression can also develop crusted scabies with bizarre lesions.

Scabies incognito is seen in those patients whose symptoms and signs are modified with topical or systemic use of corticosteroids. There are unusual clinical manifestations, atypical distribution and usually extensive involvement.

Diagnosis is most often clinical. But absolute diagnosis is made with the identification of mite with skin scrapings or other techniques. A burrow is gently scraped off with a blunt scalpel, care is taken to include the blind end. The scraped material is placed on a microscopic slide and a drop of 10-20% potassium hydroxide or mineral oil (xylol) is added. Finding of mites, eggs or fragments of egg shells or faeces (scybala) on examination confirm the diagnosis. Concentration techniques for high yields have been described. Recently dermoscopy has been utilized and recommended as a diagnostic bed side tool for the diagnosis of scabies.

Skin biopsy may also reveal section of mite or pellets of faeces. Epidermal shave biopsy may also help in the demonstration of mite.

Treatment

General: For successful treatment, it is essential that the patient applies antiscabetic medicines properly. Detailed instructions should be given to the patients explaining the treatment regimen and warning against excessive use. They should be explained that following effective therapy, the itching may persist for a few days but will usually resolve within 2 weeks. The antiscabetic preparation is applied to the entire body below neck after a good scrub bath with soap and water and after drying the skin preferably at night. After the contact period of 12 hours (next day morning), the patient should take a bath and change the bed linen. Disinfection of clothing and bedding, other than by ordinary laundering is not required. All members of the family and close physical contacts should be treated, whether having evidence of scabies or not; the symptom free incubation period may be 1 to 2 months.

Different antiscabetic preparations available are:

1. 5% permethrin is the drug of choice because it has excellent activity and low toxicity. Clinical trials show that 5% permethrin is more effective than lindane and crotamiton with toxic effects 40 times lower than 1% lindane.
2. Gamma benzenehexachloride (GBHC) – A single 6 hour application of 1% lindane effectively treats scabies. Some clinicians use a second application after one week. It should not be used in a widespread manner on damaged skin to prevent the cerebral toxicity or aplastic anaemia.
3. 10% crotamiton cream, applied for 24 hours on five consecutive days.
4. Oral ivermectin, which interrupts GABA – induced neurotransmission, has shown good effect as a single dose (200 μg/kg) and can be used in patients with highly eczematous or erosive skin due to the danger of increased absorption and of further irritation by topical scabicidals and also in mentally or physically handicapped patients, where application is difficult.
   Ivermectin is contraindicated in children under 15 kg of body weight and pregnancy. As it is not ovicidal, oral dose should be repeated after 10 to 14 days.
5. A preliminary open study of 0.8% ivermectin lotion has also shown good results.
6. Other treatment options are allethrin with piperonyl butoxide, sulphur(10%).
   Permethrin, benzyl benzoate and crotamiton have no age restriction after the second month of life, in contrast to lindane. Lindane is also contraindicated in pregnancy. Resistance towards permethrin, benzyl benzoate, lindane, and crotamiton has been reported.

Scabies not responding to conventional treatment may be presenting feature of HIV infections. Crusted scabies is treated with repeated applications of permethrin followed by lindane and sulfur if necessary. In case of resistance to topical scabicidals, oral ivermectin can be administered. Pretreatment with keratolytics (3-5% salicylic acid in petrolatum) may be useful.

PEDICULOSIS PUBIS[31,34]

Pediculosis pubis is an infestation of hair bearing areas, most commonly pubic region and is sexually transmitted. The incidence of infestation is related to promiscuity and poor hygiene. The disease occurs throughout the world. Many of the patients infested with *P. pubis* had other sexually transmitted diseases. The population with the highest incidence of pubic lice is similar to that of gonorrhoea and syphilis. Pediculosis pubis is rare in persons older than 35 years.

The Organism

The pubic or 'crab louse' – *Phthirus pubis* has squat body **(Fig. 28.7)**. The female pubic louse is 1 mm in length, the male is slightly smaller. It has 3 pairs of legs. The first set of legs terminate in slender claws, while the second and third pair of legs have well developed claws, perfectly adapted for grasping the hair. They move upto 10 cm a day. The legs are light brown in colour cemented to the hair of host. Eggs are laid in batches of 20 or 30 and hatch in a week time. Development of adult, since the laying of eggs, takes 22 to 27 days. *Pthirus pubis* is a strict human parasite, but infestation among dogs has also been reported.

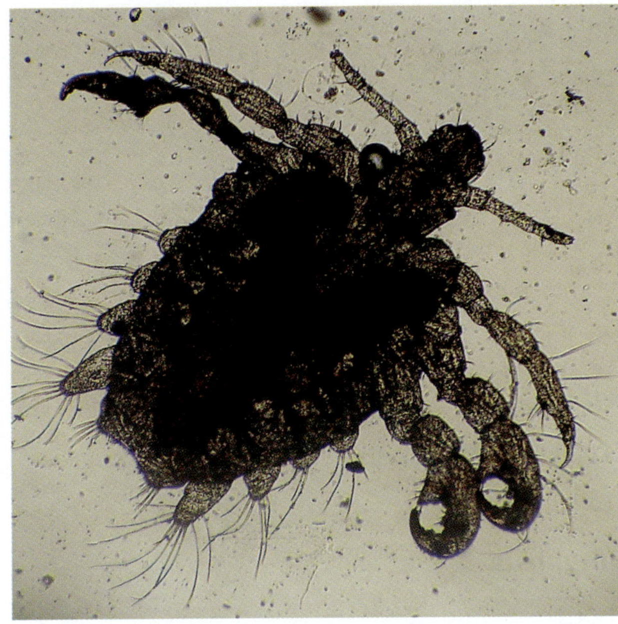

Fig. 28.7 Phthirus Pubis.

Clinical Features

The commonest site is the pubic region. However in hairy individuals, the thighs, trunk, perianal area and occasionally the axilla, beard and moustache may get involved **(Fig. 28.8)**. Involvement of sites other than pubic areas in 60% of homeless population group was observed. Infestation of the eye lashes and scalp hair occurs mainly in children. It is not indicative of sexual abuse though this may occasionally be the case. Children may acquire infection from infected parents or shared beds or other fomites.

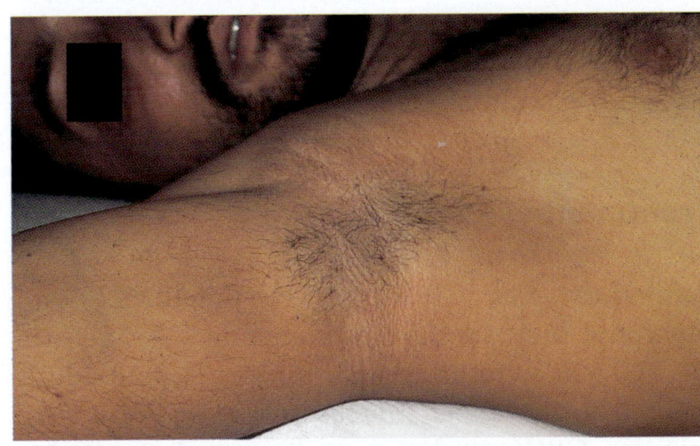

Fig. 28.8 Pediculosis Pubis – Axilla.

Patients who have pediculosis pubis usually seek medical attention because of pruritus or because they notice lice or nits on their pubic hair. Itching occurs mainly in the evening and night. A complete body examination is important in all patients. Excoriation may lead to secondary pyoderma and eczematization. Blue-grey macules (maculae caeruleae) are occasionally seen on the skin of lower abdomen and upper thighs **(Fig. 28.9)**. Their exact pathogenesis is unknown, probably they develop as a response to altered blood pigment or a reaction to the louse's saliva. These persist for several days.

Pediculosis pubis was reported in 26% among 1161 HIV 1 positive patients over a period of 38 months. Infestation may be severe with extensive colonization in HIV positive individuals.

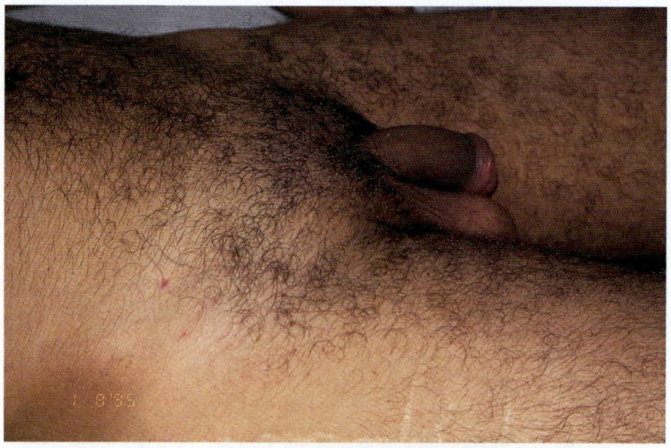

Fig. 28.9 Pediculosis Pubis – *Maculae caeruleae.*

Diagnosis

A careful history and examination for lice or nits confirms the diagnosis. Lice are observed as yellowish brown specks clinging closely to the base of hair. Nits on the hair are cemented at an oblique angle. Blood tests and a thorough examination for concomitant STDs, including HIV infection should be considered in a young sexually active patient.

Treatment

Permethrin 1%, GBHC 1% or pyrethrins with piperonyl butoxide are recommended. Permethrin 1% rinse or pyrethrins with piperonyl butoxide is applied to the affected areas and washed after 10 minutes. GBHC 1% lotion or shampoo is applied to affected area and washed after 4 minutes. GBHC is not recommended for pregnant or lactating women and for children under 2 years.

Permethrin, GBHC or Pyrethrins should not be applied to the eyes. Pediculosis of the eyelashes should be treated by applying occlusive ophthalmic ointment to the eyelid margins twice a day for 10 days. The remaining nits may be removed mechanically with forceps. Application of freshly prepared 10-20 percent flourescein eye drops is also said to be effective.

Isopropyl myristate, an ingredient commonly used in cosmetics, is currently under trial. Oral ivermectin has also been recommended by some authors.

Pediculosis pubis patient with HIV should receive the same treatment regimens. Bedding and clothing should be decontaminated.

Follow Up

Patients should be evaluated after 7 to 10 days if the symptoms persist. A second application of same or alternative pediculicide is given if lice or nits are observed at the hair skin junction.

Management of Sexual Partners

Sex partners of the patient within the last month should be treated. The patient should avoid sexual contact with their sex partner(s) until patients and partners have been treated and re-evaluated to rule out persistent disease.

GENITAL MYCOPLASMAS[35-48]

Mycoplasmas belonging to class named Mollicutes (mollis, soft; cutis, skin, in Latin) are the smallest free-living organisms. They are widespread in nature as parasites of humans, mammals, reptiles, fish, arthropods and plants. Mycoplasmas are distinguished phenotypically from other bacteria by their minute size and total lack of a cell wall because of which they exhibit cellular pleomorphism and resistance to cell wall active antimicrobial such as penicillin and cephalosporins. Mycoplasmas usually colonize mucous surfaces of the respiratory and urogenital tracts, the eyes, alimentary canal and joints. Frequently isolated organisms from the urogenital tract are mycoplasma and the ureaplasma. There are eight genera, five namely mycoplasma, ureaplasma, acholeoplasma, anaeroplasma and astreoleplasma, which collectively form 120 species.

Infections with pathogenic mycoplasmas are rarely of the fulminant type but follow a chronic course. Several virulence factors have been associated to mycoplasmas. The mildly toxic byproducts of mycoplasma metabolism, such as hydorgen peroxide and superoxide radicals, have been incriminated as causing oxidative damage to host cell membranes. Most mycoplasmas adhere to the epithelial linings of the respiratory or urogenital tract, so they may be considered surface parasites. While mycoplasmas such as *M. penetrans* and *M. genitalium* appear to enter the cells through their specialized tip structure, other mycoplasmas internalize, such as *M. fermentans* and *M. hominis*, have no tip structures. *M. hominis* metabolizes arginine, with the production of potentially cytotoxic ammonia. Data indicate that pathogenic mycoplasmas reside and replicate intracellulary over extended periods in human cells. Intracellular location may protect mycoplasmas against the effects of the host immune system and antibiotics.

The clinical picture of mycoplasma infections in humans and animals is more suggestive of damage due to host immune and inflammatory responses rather than to direct toxic effects by mycoplasma cell components. Non-specific immunomodulatory effects may contribute to their pathogenic properties, enabling them to evade or suppress their host defense mechanisms and establish a chronic, persistent infection.

Epidemiology

Several mycoplasma species (16 in total) have been isolated from humans such as. *M. genitalium, M. spermatophilum* and *M. penetrans*. The genital tract is the main site of colonization. Some of them are considered as not having pathogenic potential (*M. primatum, M. spermatophilum*). The most recently discovered, *M. penetrans*, has been isolated from the urine of HIV 1 positive homosexual men. *M. genitalum* and *M. pneumoniae* share several structural properties and a significant antigenic relationship between two species has hampered diagnostic serology. Recently ureaplasma has been divided into *ureaplasma parvum* (biovar 1) and *ureaplasma urealyticum* (biovar 2).

Infants may become colonized with one or both genital mycoplasma during passage through a colonized birth canal, but this does not persist. In adults, colonization following puberty occurs primarily as a result of sexual contact, colonization increases in relation to the number of sex partners for both *Mycoplasma hominis* (*M. hominis*) and *Ureaplasma urealyticum* (*U. urealyticum*). A recent case control study (men and their female partners) revealed that for *M. genitalium,* couples had concordant status, pertaining to the sexual transmission of *M. genitalium* and it was concluded that it behaves in a similar way as *C. trachomatis*. The various clinical syndromes that are associated with genital mycoplasmas are given in Table 28.2. The list includes both causal role and association effect on different clinical syndromes of genital mycoplasma.

Non-gonoccocal Urethritis (NGU)

NGU is the most common STDs syndrome that occurs in men. Collected data support that M. hominis on its own is not a cause of NGU, and it has been found more frequently in men who did not have NGU than those who did.

U. urealyticum have been isolated from 0-56% of healthy men, and from 5.6-42% of men with urethritis. Results of an experiment suggest that *U. urealyticum* may cause disease the first time it gains access to the urethra but subsequent invasion result in colonization without disease. This finding may explain the frequent isolation of ureaplasmas from the urethras of healthy men.

M. genitalium prevalence amongst urethritis patients varies from 8% amongst urology patients to 29% amongst STD patients. The prevalence amongst asymptomatic patients varies from 0% amongst urology patients to 9% amongst STD patients. Men with NGU tend to harbour *C. trachomatis* or *M. genitalium* separately rather than together. *M. gentalium* was found more often in *C. trachomatis*-negative NGU (NCNGU) patients than in those with chlamydial urethritis. In a recent study from Sweden, involving 51 men with urethritis, no co-infection with *M. genitalium* and *C. trachomatis* was detected. According to these studies *M. genitalium* could be considered an important cause of NGU, constituting 13-45% of *C. trachomatis*-negative NGU cases. *M. genitalium* seems to cause more severe urethritis and more often lead to symptomatic urethritis/cervicitis than non-chlamydia-non-gonococcal urethritis/cervicitis that is not associated with *M. genitalium*.

Table 28.2 Clinical Syndromes and Genital Mycoplasma

Clinical Syndromes	*Mycoplamsa*
Nongonococcal urethritis	*U. urealyticum* (20-40%) *M. genitalium* (24-26%)
Nongonococcal nonchlamydial urethritis (acute)	*U. urealyticum* (26-50%) *M. genitalium* (12-19%)
Nongonococcal nonchlamydial urethritis (chronic)	*U. urealyticum* (12-19%), *M. hominis* (4%), *M. genitalium* (1%)
Prostatitis	*U. urealyticum* (13-47%), *M. hominis* (10-12%), *M. genitalium* (4%)
Epididymitis	*U.urealyticum, M. hominis,* ? *M. genitalium*
Reiter's disease	? *M. genitalium*
Bacterial vagnosis	*M. hominis, U. urealyticum*
Pelvic inflammatory disease	*M. hominis*
Post partum/post abortal fever	*M. hominis*
Urinary calculi	*U. urealyticum*
Pyelonephritis and urinary tract infection	*M. hominis,* ? *U. urealyticum*
Involuntary infertility	? *U. urealyticum*
Habitual spontaneous abortions and still birth	? *Mycoplasmas*
Low birth weight	? *M. hominis,* ? *U. urealyticum*

The association of *M. genitalium* with persistent or recurrent urethritis (PRU) is also noted by some authors. *M. genitalium* was detected in 19-27% of men with PRU, suggestive of the aetiological role. *M. gentialium* patients were more likely to have had a previous urethrits in comparison to other patients with non-chlamydial NGU. This could indicate that *M. genitalium* urethritis may have a tendency to recur. There is recent evidence showing that *M. genitalium*-related PRU is more likely associated with persistent or recurrent infection rather than with immunologically mediated inflammation.

Coinfection with *M. genitalium* or *U. ureaplasma* biovar 2 in men with gonococcal urethritis was significantly associated with post gonococcal urethritis (PGU), independent of *C. trachomatis*. Men with GU should be treated presumptively with antibiotics that are active against *C. trachomatis*, *M. genitalium*, and *U. urealyticum* biovar 2.

M. genitalium has been associated with chronic 'abacterial' prostatitis. In one study, 135 patients with chronic abacterial prostatitis underwent transperineal prostatic biopsies to detect microorganisms by PCR, 10 (8%) harboured a STD pathogen in their prostate (*M. genitalium* was detected in 4%).

Bacterial Vaginosis

Genital mycoplasmas are amongst the major aetiological agents currently believed to be part of a synergisitc mixture in bacterial vaginosis (BV), but the particular organism in this mixture essential for the developing and maintenance of the condition is not known.

A number of works have shown *M. hominis* to be asociated with BV in pregnant women and in non-pregnant women. *M. hominis* has been reported in 58-76% of women with BV and from significantly fewer patients with a normal vaginal examination. The connection between *U. urealyticum* and BV is less obvious: *U. urealyticum* is isolated from a high percentage of patients (62-92%) who have a diagnosis of BV, higher apparently than that from control patients.

In a study of role of male partner in the lower genitourinary tract infection of females, 93 consecutive patients in the reproductive age group with symptoms of vaginal discharge along with their sex partners were evaluated microbiologically. The predominant pathogen isolated was *Ureaplasma urealyticum* seen in 43.01% of females and 24.7% of males. Female genital-tract HIV load correlates inversely with Lactobacillus species but positively with bacterial vaginosis and Mycoplasma hominis. Data suggest that the bacterial flora associated with BV influence genital-tract HIV shedding.

Keane et al. studied 15 women with BV and did not find *M. genitalium* in any of the patients and in only two (12%) of 17 women without BV attending an STDs clinic

Cervicitis

The controversial role of gential mycoplasmas is particularly true for cervicitis. *M. hominis* and *U. urealyticum* seem not be have a role in the aetiology of mucopurulent cervicits. There are much fewer studies published on *M. genitalium* infections on women than in men. The connection of *M. genitalium* with cervicits has been suggested. The prevalence of *M. genitalium* is significantly greater in *C. trachomatis*-negative women with genital infections (cervicits, adnexitis) than in asymptomatic pregnant women. Manhart et al. found that *M. genitalium* was strongly associated with cervicitis. After exclusion of women infected with *N. gonorrhoeae* and *C. trachomatis*, women with mucopurulent cervicitis were 3.1 times more likely to have *M. genitalium* detected than were those without cervicitis, and the magnitude of the increase in risk associated with *M. genitalium* was comparable with that observed for *C. trachomatis* and *N. gonorrhoeae*.

The other manifestitations have been enumerated in the above table.

Pelvic Inflammatory Disease

Mycoplasma genitalum is a commonly sexually transmitted pathogen frequently identified among women with pelvic inflammatory disease, the infection and inflammation of a woman's upper genital tract. Although *Chlamydia trachomatis* and Neisseria gonorrhoeae frequently cause pelvic inflammatory disease, up to 70% of cases have unidentified etiology. PCR studies have demonstrated that *M. genitalium* is associated with clinically suspected pelvic inflammatory disease, acute endometritis, and adnexitis, independent of gonococcal and chlamydial infection. Most studies have been cross-sectional, although one prospective investigation suggested that *M. genitalium* was associated with over a 13-fold risk of endometritis.

Adverse Pregnancy Outcomes and Infertility

Mycoplasma and ureaplasma species can adversly affect pregnancy outcome and affect the fertility of a women. In a study, ureaplasma urealyticum and mycoplasma hominis constitutes 20.1% and 1.3%, when tested by cervical swabs in an initial infertility evaluation. In a study documenting the association between preterm birth and vaginal colonization by mycoplasmas in early pregnancy, vaginal colonization with *U. parvum*, but not *U. urealyticum*, is associated with late abortion or early preterm birth.

Diagnosis

In men, the diagnosis is made by collecting and testing the urethral swab or the first void urine sample, and in women high vaginal smear or endocervical swabs. The collected swabs are to be immediately instilled in the transport media, and the swab is not allowed to dry. The culture is done on a beef heart infusion broth (PPLO broth) with 10% fresh yeast extract, 20% horse serum. The culture colonies on the media would look like classical 'fried egg' appearance and the size (200-300μ) in case of *M. hominis* and smaller (10-30μ) without the fried egg appearance in case of ureaplasma. Commercial kits for detection of *M. hominis* and ureaplasma are available. Recently PCR-microtiter plate hybridization assay can be considered an effective tool for the diagnosis of genitourinary infections with mycoplasmas or ureaplasmas. Comparison of multiplex PCR assay with culture for detection of genital mycoplasmas, multiplex PCR offers a rapid, sensitive, and easy method to detect genital mycoplasmas. Serological tests have also been described, and in combination with identification of the organism it can enhance the specificity of the diagnosis.

Treatment

In a controlled clinical trial to evaluate the microbiological cure rate after treatment with tetracyclines or azithromycin in patients infected with *M. genitalium*, Azithromycin (1 gram stat) was more effective than doxycycline (100 mg bid for 9 days) in treating patients infected with *M. genitalium*. It has been shown that *M. genitalium* is a common cause of persistent or recurrent urethritis among men treated with doxycycline. Considering the slow growth of *M. genitalium*, which may require a longer duration of treatment, an azithromycin regimen comprising 500 mg in a single dose on day 1 followed by 250 mg od for 4 days, which has provided excellent cure rates has been recommended . Considering the diversity in the dosage of tetracyclines and azithromycin that has been used in the published studies, a randomized controlled trial should include at least two arms comparing doxycycline 100 mg bd for 7 days and azithromycin 1 g stat, as recommended in the clinical effectiveness guidelines. Tetracyclines are active against many strains of *M. hominis*. In resistant cases clindamycin should be good alternative. Around 10% of ureaplasma exhibit resistance for tetracyclines and 40% cross resistance with erythromycin.

ENTERIC BACTERIAL PATHOGENS[49-54]

Enteric infections traditionally have not been viewed as sexually transmitted diseases. The sexual practices that predispose to acquisition of these infections are anilingus (rimming or active oral-anal sex) and faecal-oral contact occurring indirectly when oral-genital sex (fellatio) following anal genital intercourse. These practices are more common among homosexuals than heterosexuals. The group of diseases affecting the lower intestinal tract of homosexual men were labeled "gay bowel syndrome".

The bacterial pathogens that are sexually transmitted are salmonella, shigella, campylobacter species and *Helicobacter pylori* (*H. pylori*). In a study from South Africa, potential enteric bacterial pathogens in 69 HIV-positive patients with chronic diarrhea were identified using standard microbiological methods. The diarrhoeagenic bacterial agents were isolated from 48 (80%) of the 60 HIV positive patients with diarrhea. The pathogens isolated comprised Campylobacter species (20%), Plesiomonas shigelloides (16.6%), Aeromonas species (13.3%) and Escherichia coli, Shigella and Salmonella (10.0% each). All these infections have become sexually transmitted, because only a small inoculum is needed to cause the disease (shigella 10-100 organisms, campylobacter 500 organisms).

Shigellosis

Shigellosis is caused by Shigella species of enteric bacteria, which are non-motile, short, gram negative rods that ferment lactose slowly or not at all. Fifty serotypes have been grouped into four serogroups A-D. Several population based incidence studies have demonstrated disproportionately higher rates in homosexuals.

The usual incubation period is 1-7 days. Clinically it presents as bacillary dysentery characterized by bloody mucoid stool accompanied with abdominal pain, tenesmus and fever. *Shigella dysentriae* type I cause the most severe infection. Cutaneous shigellosis, in the form of furuncle over the penis had been reported in a 22-year-old homosexual. Other manifestations are haemolytic uraemic syndrome. Diagnosis is made by culture, by taking direct rectal stool swab and plated on Hektoen and or MacConkey agar. Further biochemical and serological identifications are unnecessary for routine purposes, but may be useful for outbreak investigations. Stool microscopy can help in differentiating shigellosis from amoebic dysentery as the former have abundant polymorphonuclear leucocytes.

Treatment is by newer fluoroquinolones, ciprofloxacin 500 mg bid for up to 3 days or trimethoprim sulfamethoxazole bid for 3 days. (TMP 160 mg and SMX 800 mg). Other drugs are nalidixic acid 1 g qid for 5 days and pivemecillinam 400 mg qid for 5 days. Parentral ceftriaxone is a highly effective alternative. Patients with AIDS who develop chronic carriage may require prolonged treatment with a quinolone. Due to wide spread development of resistance, selection of antibiotics should be based on regional antibiotic sensitivity. An oral live attenuated *Shigella flexneri* hybrid vaccine has been used in field trials but its efficacy could not be assessed because of the low incidence of cases in the study population.

Salmonellosis

They belong to the family Enterobacteriaceae. They are anaerobic facultative, gram negative rods, do not ferment lactose or sucrose, but they are motile and always produce H_2S. They have four serogroups A-D, 75-80% of infections are caused by only 10 sterotypes.

The clinical manifestations that are produced by salmonella are acute gastroenteritis, enteric fever, septicemia and focal invasive infections. Salmonella diarrhoea is generally watery, containing mucous and very occasionally blood. Endoscopic examination would reveal colonic mucosal oedema, hyperaemia, friability and petechial hemorrhages. Salmonella septicemia is a well described entity in a HIV infected hosts and recurrent salmonella septicemia has become a CDC surveillence definition of AIDS-defining illness. Focal central nervous system involvement in HIV/AIDS patients has been reported. The usual incubation period is 1-7 days. Chronic carrier state is described in adult population. Diagnosis is by stool culture using a highly selective media. (Potassium tellurite, Wilson Blair). No antimicrobial therapy is advised in gastroenteritis with non-bloody, non-mucoid diarrhoeal stool and mild to moderate dehydration. On the contrary, patients has bloody or mucoid stools, severe illness, severe dehydration requires hospitalization. The first line of treatment is ciprofloxacin 500 mg BID for 3-5 days. Alternative regimens include aminopencillins, ceftriaxone or cefotaxime.

Campylobacter Enteritis

This infection is caused by *Campylobacter jejuni* and campylobacter like organisms (CLO). They are small, curved motile, gram negative rods microaerophilic and non-fermenting. They are isolated from 4-8% of patients with acute diarrhoea. Sexual transmission of these organisms has been documented in animals and humans. The atypical form CLO are more frequently isolated from homosexual men with or without intestinal symptoms, and rarely from heterosexual men and women. In a study CLO were recovered from the stool of 26 of 158 symptomatic homosexual men, 6 of 75 asymptomatic homosexual men and 0 of 150 heterosexual men and women. Two of there CLO are identified as *C. cinaedi* and *C. fennelliae*.

Clinical manifestation runs a broad range from that compatible with mild viral gastroenteritis to severe diarrhoea with blood and pus. In around 10% of patients, abdominal pain and tenderness persists, or recurrent fever or diarrhoea occurs. Otherwise they resolve within 2-3 days. Proctocolitis is evident by endoscopic examination, associated with anal discharge, pain and fever. Faecal leucocytosis is usually present and the diagnosis is confirmed by isolating the organisms from the stool by culture on selective media with microaerophilic atmosphere. For CLO, PCR amplification of 23s rDNA sequences has been used to identify these isolates. Benefit from using antibiotics is not clear, especially if the start of treatment is delayed. Erythromycin 500mg qid for 1 week has been recommended for severe symptoms.

Helicobacter Pylori

A recent review of literature has reported that Helicobacter infection could be transmitted sexually via oral-anal intercourse. Sexual practices where there is contact with faeces may be an important risk factor for the transmission of *H. pylori*, clinically characterized by chronic gastritis.

CANDIDIASIS[55-61]

Syn.: Candidosis; Moniliasis; Thrush.

Candidiasis is an infection caused by the yeast *Candida albicans*, or occasionally by other species of candida like *C. glabrata*, *C. parapsilosis*, C. tropicalis, *C. guilliermondi*, *C. kefy* and *C. krusei*.

Aetiopathogenesis

C. albicans is an oval yeast 2-6 μm to 9 μm in size which can produce budding cells, hyphae and psuedohyphae. There are over 200 species. These species can be differentiated by their colony morphology, microscopy and biochemical properties. Among the non-Candida albicans infections, *C. glabrata* (69%) was most commonly isolated besides *C. parapsilosis*, *C. krusei*, *C. tropicalis*, *C. cerevisae*. Hyphae are usually produced during the process of tissue invasion, though yeasts without hyphae may also occur during the phase of tissue invasion. *C. albicans* is a common commensal of gastrointestinal tract. Candida yeasts are found in the mouth and gut in around 50% of the population and colonize the vagina in up to 20% of asymptomatic females. They are rarely isolated from the healthy skin.

The candidal infection often causes opportunistic infections as these yeasts exist as commensals that colonize the various mucosal surfaces with the exception of genital candidiasis which is often sexually acquired and oral candidiasis in infants. Candidal transmission probably occurs via yeast form which is asymptomatic and changing into pseudomycelial form associated with invasion and symptoms. Yeast develops into a hypha with the expression of virulence genes with cyclic AMP playing a role in *C. albicans* mediated gene expression.

C. albicans has the greatest affinity for adhering to vaginal epithelial cells. The integrity of a mucosa depends upon many factors such as local pH, the presence of glycogen and increased sugar levels. Other factors like physical trauma with increased moisture, occlusion, loss of normal microflora can also affect the local environment. Systemic factors include pregnancy, glycosuria and the administration of broad spectrum antibiotics, cortico-steroids and other immunosuppressive drugs. In HIV positive population, oral candida carrier rates are generally high and can extend to oesophagus resulting in painful swallowing. Besides the role of IgA antibodies in the initial local defence, humoral immunity has no role in protection. Cell mediated immunity is the most important host defence mechanism against mucosal candidiasis.

Clinical Features

Candida can cause superficial infections of skin and mucous membranes. Systemic infections are more serious with involvement of internal organs including septicemia, endocarditis and meningitis. In this chapter we will be describing only the genital candidiasis.

Candidiasis in the Males

Candidal balanoposthitis **(Fig. 28.10)** is the commonest presentation. Asymptomatic colonization of the glans penis occurs both in circumcised and uncircumcised males although the uncircumcised are more likely to develop symptoms, since the internal milieu of preputial sac often favours the growth of microorganisms. Sexual contact of a patient of candidal balanitis may have either abundant vaginal candida carriage or frank vulvovaginitis. Singhi et al. isolated *C. albicans* in 21% of patients with balanoposthitis. The organism was more commonly isolated from married than unmarried individuals. Pathogenic staphylococci were seen in 25% of *C. albicans* positive cases. Sharma and colleague also isolated *C. albicans* among 23% of patients with balanoposthitis, though staphylococci were more commonly isolated in their study. Two types of clinical presentations have been described.

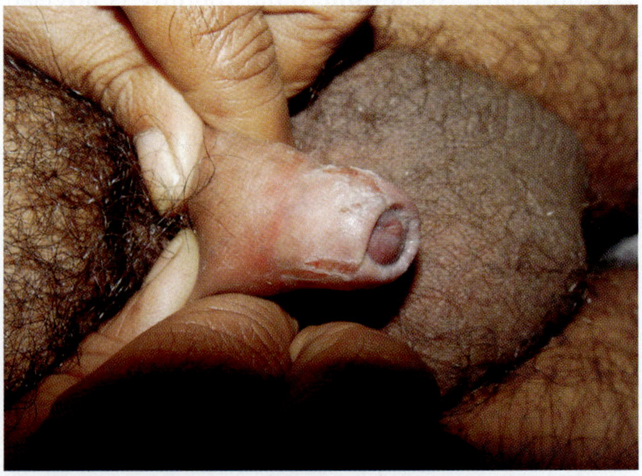

Fig. 28.10 Candidal Balanoposthitis – Maceration and Fissuring of Prepuce.

The first one is due to the presence of *C. albicans* and manifests as small papules or fragile papulopustules on the glans or in the coronal sulcus which breaks open and leave behind superficial erythematous erosions having a collarette of whitish scales with eroded satellite pustules or a thrush like membrane. It may also present as longitudinal fissures on the undersurface of the prepuce. Preputial odema leads to phimosis and superadded anaerobic infection can produce offensive purulent discharge. The second type is due to hypersensitivity reaction to *C. albicans* and presents as transient erythema and burning, shortly after intercourse with infected partner.

Involvement of the penile shaft, scrotal skin and the groins coexists often in hot weather. Diabetes mellitus is frequently associated with candidal balanoposthitis. Florid persistent lesions spreading beyond the genitalia are more likely to be associated with glycosuria.

The differential diagnoses include balanoposthitis due to other causes–trichomonal, bacterial, allergic, psoriasis, lichen planus, etc.

Candidiasis in Females

Many women with candidiasis are asymptomatic or have minimal symptoms. Typical symptoms of vulvo vaginal candidiasis (VVC) include pruritus and vaginal discharge. Other symptoms are vaginal soreness, vulvar burning, dyspareunia and external dysuria. None of these symptoms is specific for VVC. On examination, there is typical dusky red erythema of vaginal mucous membrane and vulval skin with oedema associated with curdy whitish discharge, fissures and erosions **(Fig. 28.11)**. The discharge is typically thick creamy white or 'cheese like'. Generally the pH of the discharge is below 5. The rash may extend to the perineum and groins. The perianal area is often affected. Subcorneal pustules at the periphery may develop in extensive cases. Clinical manifestations of VVC are aggravated during pregnancy. Recurrent VVC (RVVC) is defined as four or more episodes of symptomatic VVC each year and affects less than 5% of women. Vaginal mucosa becomes glazed and atrophic in recurrent chronic VVC. Predisposing factors for VVC are prolonged use of antibiotics, conditions which increase estrogen levels such as pregnancy and hormonal replacement therapy. About 10% of the women in the first trimester and 36-50% in the third trimester have symptomatic disease. Atopy has been associated with VVC as allergic rhinitis was found more (74%) in patients of VVC when compared with controls (42%).

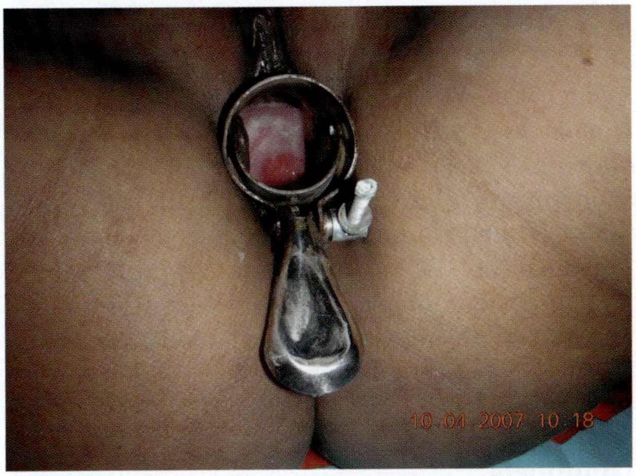

Fig. 28.11 Vulvovaginal candidiasis – White Curdy Discharge on the Vaginal Wall.

VVC has been classified into the following 2 types based on the clinical presentation, microbiology, host factors and response to therapy.

1. **Uncomplicated VVC**
   a. Sporadic or infrequent VVC, or
   b. Mild to moderate vulvovaginal Candidiasis, or
   c. Likely to be *C. albicans*, or
   d. VVC in nonimmuno compromised women.
2. **Complicated VVC**
   a. Recurrent VVC, or
   b. Severe VVC, or
   c. Non *C. albicans* Candidiasis, or
   d. Women with uncontrolled diabetes, debilitation or immuno-suppression or those who are pregnant.

Approximately 10 to 20 percent of women will have complicated VVC, suggesting diagnostic and therapeutic considerations.

VVC in HIV seropositive women

Incidence of VVC is increased in HIV seropositive women. A prospective study on 205 HIV positive patients showed that the risk of developing symptomatic VVC increased 6.8 times for women with CD4 cell count less than 200 cells/microlitre. Treatment of VVC resulted in a 3.2 fold reduction in the concentration of HIV in vaginal secretions and a 3 fold decrease in the likelihood of detecting HIV-1 infected cells.

Diagnosis

Diagnosis of VVC depends upon the demonstration of the yeast by simple microscopic examination of vaginal secretions in 10% KOH or by Gram staining. A wet mount or saline preparation should routinely be done not only to identify yeast cells and mycelia, but also to exclude the presence of "clue cells" and motile trichomonads. The visualization of psuedohyphae strengthens the diagnosis. Vaginal secretion culture on Sabouraud's agar should be performed in the presence of negative microscopic findings. Fifty percent of patients with culture positive symptomatic VVC, have negative microscopic findings. A positive culture also does not always indicate that the yeast is responsible for the vaginal symptoms.

Treatment

The general principles include that all local topical preparations should be applied to all involved skin and mucosal surfaces. Any predisposing factor like diabetes mellitus, or HIV infection should be treated. Most women with uncomplicated VVC have no precipitating factor. VVC can occur concomitantly with other STDs and the latter has to be investigated and treated. The various treatment guidelines are given in Appendix IV.

Treatment of Complicated VVC

Clinical diagnosis should be confirmed by culture, which also helps to identify unusual species including *Candida glabrata*. Each individual episode of RVVC responds to short duration of initial therapy. A longer duration 7-14 days of topical therapy or a repeat dose of oral fluconazole 150 mg at 3 days is recommended to achieve mycological remission before initiating a maintenance antifungal regimen.

Maintenance therapy with antifungal agents includes clotrimazole (500 mg) vaginal suppository once weekly, ketoconazole 100 mg once daily, fluconazole (100-150 mg) once weekly and itraconazole 400 mg once monthly or 100 mg once daily). All maintenance regimens should be continued for 6 months. Recurrence may occur in 30% to 40% women on cessation of maintenance therapy.

During pregnancy only topical azoles should be used. Therapy for VVC should not differ in HIV infected women. Recurring vulvo-vaginal candidiasis is not on indication to test for HIV.

Prevention of Vulvovaginal Candidiasis

Vulvovaginal candidiasis after antibiotic treatment is a common problem, and women often resort to probiotic Lactobacillus spp to prevent such an occurrence. However neither oral nor vaginal lactobacillus administration prevents vulvovaginal candidosis after antibiotic treatment. Many practitioners recommend one dose of prophylactic oral fluconazole 150 mg with onset and another dose on completion of antibiotics. Aimed at susceptible women only, maintenance fluconazole prophylaxis is effective in idiopathic recurrent vulvovaginal candidosis and other categories of secondary recurrent vulvovaginal candidosis—eg, lichen sclerosus and topical oestrogen application. Possible future treatments include topical vaginal use of recombinant mannose-binding lectin to enhance innate defence mechanisms in the vagina.

REFERENCES

1. Scholz J, Rosen-Wolff A, Burgert K et al. Epidemiology of molluscum contagiosum using genetic analysis of the viral DNA. J Med Virol 1989; 27: 87-90.
2. Porter CD, Archard LC. Characterization by restriction mapping of three subtypes of molluscum contagiosum virus. J Med Virol 1992; 38: 1-6.
3. Gottlieb SL, Myskowki PL. Molluscum contagiosum. Int J Dermatol 1994; 33: 453-61.
4. Yamashita H, Uemura T, Kawashima M. Molecular epidemiologic analysis of Japanese patients with molluscum contagiosum. Int J Dermatol 1996; 35: 99-105.
5. Pereira B, Fernandes C, Nachiambo E, et al. Exuberant molluscum contagiosum as a manifestation of the immune reconstitution inflammatory syndrome. Dermatol Online J 2007; 13: 6.
6. Zalaudek I, Giacomel J, Cabo H et al. Entodermoscopy: a new tool for diagnosing skin infections and infestations. Dermatology 2008; 216: 14-23.
7. Hanna D, Hatami A, Powell J. A Prospective Randomized Trial Comparing the efficacy and Adverse Effects of Four Recognized treatments of Molluscum Contagiosum in Children. Pediatric Dermatology 2006; 23: 574-9.
8. Zabawski EJ Jr. A review of topical and intralesional cidofovir. Dermatology Online J 2000; 6: 3.
9. Zabawaski EJ Jr, Cockerell CJ. Topical cidofovir for molluscum contagiosum in children [letter] Pediatr Dermatol 1999; 16: 414-5.
10. Chatproedprai S, Suwannakarn K, Wananukul S, et al. Efficacy of pulsed dyed laser (585 nm) in the treatment of molluscum contagiosum subtype 1. Southeast Asian J Trop Med Public Health 2007; 38: 849-54.
11. Soriano V, Barreiro P, Martin-Carbonero L, et al. Update on the treatment of chronic hepatitis C in HIV-infected patients. AIDS Rev. 2007; 9: 99-113.
12. Brook MG. Sexually acquired hepatitis. Sex Transm Infect. 2002; 78: 235-40.
13. Frey SE, Homan SM, Sokol-Anderson M, et al. Evidence for probable sexual transmission of the hepatitis Gvirus. Clin Infect Dis. 2002; 34: 1033-8.
14. Edwards S, Carne C. Oral sex and the transmission of viral STIs. Sex Transm Infect. 1998;7 4: 6-10.
15. Atkins M, Nolan M. Sexual transmission of hepatitis B. Curr Opin Infect Dis. 2005; 18: 67-72.
16. Mikhailov MI, Gomberg MA, Dolzhanskaya NA, et al. Significance of sexual route of transmission of hepatitis B and C in Russia. Int J STDs AIDS 2002; 13 (Suppl 2): 9-11.
17. Clarke A, Kulasegaram R. Hepatitis C transmission – where are we now? Int J STDs AIDS. 2006; 17: 74-80.
18. Berzsenyi MD, Bowden DS, Bailey MJ, et al. Male to male sex is associated with a high prevalence of exposure to GB virus C. J Clin Virol. 2005; 33: 243-6.
19. Kenneson A, Cannon MJ. Review and meta-analysis of the epidemiology of congenital cytomegalovirus (CMV) infection. Rev Med Virol. 2007; 17: 253-76.
20. Shagil'dian VI, Tishkevich OA, Parkhomenko IuG, et al. Cytomegalovirus infection of the gastrointestinal tract in patients with HIV-infection. Ter Arkh. 2005; 77: 14-20.
21. Drew WL. Laboratory diagnosis of cytomegalovirus infection and disease in immunocompromised patients. Curr Opin Infect Dis. 2007; 20: 408-11.
22. Halwachs-Baumann G. Recent developments in human cytomegalovirus diagnosis. Expert Rev Anti Infect Ther. 2007; 5: 427-39.
23. Biron KK. Antiviral drugs for cytomegalovirus diseases. Antiviral Res. 2006; 71: 154-63.
24. Zhong J, Khanna R. Vaccine strategies against human cytomegalovirus infection. Expert Rev Anti Infect Ther. 2007; 5: 449-59.
25. Cohen JI. Ebstein Barr virus infections including Infectious Mononucleosis. In: Fauci As, Braunwald E, Isselbacher KJ,eds. Harrison's Principles of Internal Medicine. 16th edn. New York: McGraw Hill; 2005. p. 1046-9.

26. Niedobitek G, Meru N, Delecluse HJ. Epstein-Barr virus infection and human malignancies Int J Exp Path 2001; 82: 149-70.
27. Slots J, Saygun I, Sabeti M, et al. Epstein–Barr virus in oral Diseases. J Periodont Res 2006; 41; 235-44.
28. Häusler M, Scheithauer S, Ritter K, et al. Molecular diagnosis of Epstein-Barr virus. Expert Rev Mol Diagn. 2003; 3: 81-92.
29. Luderer R, Kok M, Niesters HG, et al. Real-time Epstein-Barr virus PCR for the diagnosis of primary EBV infections and EBV reactivation. Mol Diagn. 2005; 9: 195-200.
30. Sunderkötter C, Mayser P, Fölster-Holst R, et al. Scabies. JDDG 2007; 424-30.
31. Wendel K, Rompalo A. Scabies and pediculosis pubis: an update of treatment regimens and general review. Clin Infect Dis 2002; 35 (Suppl 2): S146-51.
32. Dupuy A, Dehen L, Bourrat E, et al. Accuracy of standard dermoscopy for diagnosing scabies. J Am Acad Dermatol 2007; 56: 53-62.
33. Hamm H, Beiteke U, Höger PH, et al. Treatment of scabies with 5% permethrin cream: results of a German multicenter study. JDDG 2006; 4: 407-13.
34. Burkhart CG, Burkhart CN. Oral ivermectin for Phthirus pubis. J Am Acad Dermatol 2004; 51: 1037-8.
35. Jensen JS. *Mycoplasma genitalum*: the etiological agent of urethritis and other sexually transmitted diseases. JEADV 2004; 18: 1-11.
36. Yokoi S, Maeda S, Kubota Y et al. The role of *Mycoplasma genitalium* and Ureaplasma urealyticum biovar 2 in postgonococcal urethritis. Clin Infect Dis 2007; 45: 866-71.
37. Sha BE, Zariffard MR, Wang QJ et al. Female genital-tract HIV load correlates Inversely with Lactobacillus species but positively with bacterial vaginosis and *Mycoplasma hominis*. J Infect Dis 2005; 191: 25-32.
38. Keane FE, Thomas BJ, Gilroy CB et al. The association of *Mycoplasma hominis, Ureaplasma urealyticum* and *Mycoplasma genitalium* with bacterial vaginosis: observations on heterosexual women and their male partners. Int J STDs AIDS 2000; 11: 356-60.
39. Dutro SM, Holmes KK et al. *Mycoplasma genitalium* is associated with mucopurulent cervicitis. Int J STDs AIDS 2001; 12 (Suppl 2, Abstracts International Congress of Sexually Transmitted Infections, 24 – 27 June): 69.
40. Manhart LE, Critchlow CW, Holmes KK et al. Mucopurulent cervicitis and *Mycoplasma genitalium*. J Infect Dis 2003; 187: 650-7.
41. Haggerty CL. Evidence for a role of *Mycoplasma genitalium* in pelvic inflammatory disease. Curr Opin Infect Dis 2008; 21: 65-9.
42. Imudia AN, Detti L, Puscheck EE, et al. The prevalence of Ureaplasma urealyticum, *Mycoplasma hominis, Chlamydia trachomatis* and Neisseria gonorrhoeae infections, and the rubella status of patients undergoing an initial infertility evaluation. J Assist Reprod Genet 2008; 25: 43-6.
43. Kataoka S, Yamada T, Chou K et al. Association between preterm birth and vaginal colonization by mycoplasmas in early pregnancy. J Clin Microbiol 2006; 44: 51-5.
44. Taylor-Robinson D. The role of mycoplasmas in pregnancy outcome. Best Pract Res Clin Obstet Gynaecol 2007; 21: 425-38.
45. Yoshida T, Maeda S, Deguchi T, et al. Rapid detection of *Mycoplasma genitalium, Mycoplasma hominis*, Ureaplasma parvum, and Ureaplasma urealyticum organisms in genitourinary samples by PCR-microtiter plate hybridization assay. J Clin Microbiol 2003; 41: 1850-5.
46. Stellrecht KA, Woron AM, Mishrik NG, et al. Comparison of multiplex PCR assay with culture for detection of genital mycoplasmas. J Clin Microbiol 2004; 42: 1528-33.
47. Björnelius E, Anagrius C, Bojs G et al. Antibiotic treatment of symptomatic *Mycoplasma genitalium* infection in Scandinavia: a controlled clinical trial. Sex Transm Infect 2008; 84: 72-6.
48. Wikström A, Jensen JS. *Mycoplasma genitalium*: a common cause of persistent urethritis among men treated with doxycycline. Sex Transm Infect 2006; 82 :276-9.
49. Obi CL, Bessong PO. Diarrhoeagenic bacterial pathogens in HIV positive patients with diarrhea in rural communities of Limpopo Province, South Africa. J Health Popul Nutr 2002; 20: 230-4.

50. Eslick GD. Sexual transmission of *Helicobacter pylori* via oral-anal intercourse. Int J STDs AIDS 2002; 13: 7-11.
51. Quinn TC. Clinical approach to intestinal infections in homosexual men. Med Clin North Am 1986; 3: 611-34.
52. Thorpe CM, Keusch GT. Enteric bacterial pathogens: shigella, salmonella, campylobacter. In: Holmes KK, Mardh PA, Sparling PF, eds. Sexually transmitted diseases. 3rd edn. New York: Mc-Graw Hill; 1999. p 549-62.
53. Sack DA. Acute infectious diarrhoea. In: Rakel RE, Bope ET, eds. Conn's Current therapy. 54 edn. Philadelphia. W.B Saunders: 2002. p. 12-8.
54. Sobel J, Swerdlow DL. Salmonellosis. In: Acute infectious diarrhoea. In: Rakel RE, Bope ET, eds. Conn's Current therapy. 54 edn. Philadelphia. W.B Saunders: 2002. p. 163-6.
55. Holland J, Young ML, Lee O, et al. Vulvovaginal carriage of yeasts other than Candida albicans. Sex Transm Infect 2003; 79: 249-50.
56. Bahn YS, Molenda M, Staab JF, et al. Genome-wide transcriptional profiling of the cyclic AMP-dependent signaling pathway during morphogenic transitions of Candida albicans. Eukaryot Cell 2007; 6: 2376-90.
57. Runeman B, Faergemann J, Larkö O. Experimental Candida albicans lesions in healthy humans dependence on skin pH. Acta Derm Venereol 2000; 80: 421-4.
58. Moraes PSA. Recurrent vaginal candidiasis and allergic rhinitis: a common association. Ann Allergy Asthma Immunol 1998; 81: 165-9.
59. Singhi NK, Bhagava RK, Mangal HN, et al. Micro-organism and balanoposthitis. Indian J Sex Transm Dis 1986; 7; 75-80.
60. Sharma VK, Kumar B, Ayyagiri A, et al. Microbial flora in balanoposthitis; a study of 100 cases. Indian J Sex Transm Dis 1990; 11: 19-22.
61. Sobel JD. Vulvovaginal candidosis. Lancet 2007; 369: 1961-71.

29 TRICHOMONIASIS AND OTHER PROTOZOAL DISEASES

Vinod K Sharma, Jyoti Dhawan, Trilokraj Tejasvi

In this chapter

INTRODUCTION

An increasing number of diseases are currently being recognized as sexually transmitted. Bacterial and viral diseases comprise the vast majority of sexually transmitted diseases (STD), however several protozoa, nematodes and arthropods are also included in this group. It was recognized by the 1960s that enteric protozoan infections may be related to sexual behaviour, and today there is increasing concern that several protozoan infestations may be sexually transmitted.

The protozoa can be classified into major and minor protozoa and according to their primary infection site into intestinal, urogenital tract and blood and tissue protozoa. The current chapter discusses the former two groups, which are sexually transmitted. The other important protozoan infections like *toxoplasmosis* and *Pneumocystis carinii* (now considered as a fungus) pneumonia are opportunistic infections and are covered in Chapter 5.

The major and minor pathogenic protozoa implicated in STDs are listed in Table 29.1 and important morphological features of major protozoa (except cryptosporidium, which is discussed under coccidian, later in the chapter.) are outlined in Table 29.2

Table 29.1 Major and Minor Pathogenic Protozoa[1]

	Species	*Disease*
Major protozoa		
Intestinal tract	*Entamoeba histolytica*	Amoebiasis
	Giardia lamblia	Giardiasis
	Cryptosporidium parvum	Cryptosporidiosis
Urogenital tract	*Trichomonas vaginalis*	Trichomoniasis
Minor protozoa		
Intestinal tract	*Balantidium coli*	Dysentery
	Isospora belli	Isosporiasis
	Enterocytozoon bienusi	Microsporidiosis
	Septata intestinalis	Microsporidiosis
	Cyclospora cayetanensis	Cyclosporiasis

Table 29.2 Morphological Features of Major Protozoa[2]

Protozoan	*Size* (μ)	*Motility*	*Nucleus*	*Others*
T. vaginalis				
Trophozoite	7-23	'jerky rapid'	1	Presence of undulating membrane.
Cyst	No cyst stage			
G. Lamblia				
Trophozoite	10-20	'Falling leaf'	2('owl eyed')	Sucking disc prominent on the ventral side
Cyst	8-19	–	4	–
E. histolytica				
Trophozoite	12-60	Progressive, directional, rapid	One	RBCs in cytoplasm diagnostic of *E histoytica*
Cyst	10-20	–	Mature-4 Immature 1-2	–

The other classification is (1) Protozoa for which the principal route of transmission is sexual intercourse i.e. trichomoniasis, (2) Those for which the primary route of transmission is non-sexual but are transmitted by male homosexual activity and less commonly by heterosexual activity (amoebiasis, giardiasis, etc.).

TRICHOMONIASIS

Trichomoniasis is caused by *Trichomonas vaginalis* (*T. vaginalis*), a protozoan belonging to the order trichomonads. Three species are found in humans: *T. vaginalis* is a parasite of the genitourinary tract, while *T. tenax* and *Pentatrichomonas hominis* are nonpathogenic trichomonads that are found in the oral cavity and large intestine respectively. Donne in 1936 first described the species from a freshly made vaginal discharge smear.[3]

Biology[3]

The shape and size of *T. vaginalis* vary depending on the vaginal microenvironment or culture conditions. It is 15 mm in length, and fusiform in shape and has a characteristic erratic, twitching motility. It has four anterior flagella that originate from the anterior kinetosomal complex, and a fifth flagellum attached to the undulating membrane, that arises from the kinetosomal complex and extends till half the length of organism **(Fig. 29.1)**.

The other components are anterior nucleus with 5 chromosomes, golgi complex, parabasal apparatus and axostyle which runs along to form the tail or projection posteriorly. Three rows of large chromatin granules are arranged parallel to the axostyle which are hydrogenosomes. Reproduction is by mitotic division and longitudinal fission, which occurs every 8-12 hours under optimal conditions. They are present in 2 forms: the smaller form which is more virulent, and the larger form, which is more dormant. The latter are found in asymptomatic infection, while the former in symptomatic disease.

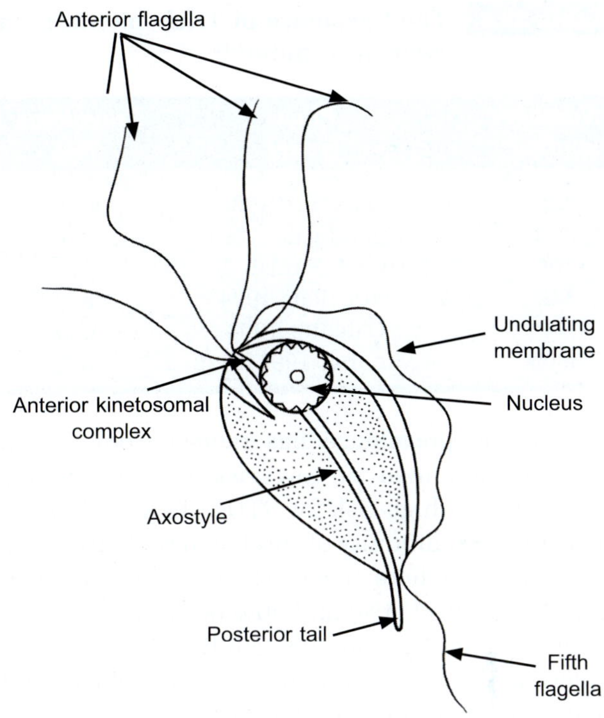

Fig. 29.1 Trichomonas Vaginalis

Prevalence

The World Health Organization (WHO) has estimated that this infection accounts for almost half of all curable sexually transmitted infections worldwide.[4] and approximately one-fourth of all cases of clinically evident vaginal infection. The prevalence ranges from 2-5% in middle class women, 56% in women attending sexually transmitted disease clinics; 50% of them are asymptomatic, while 30% develop symptoms within a period of 6 months of follow up.[5] A study of women with vaginal discharge at STDs clinic in Mumbai, reported a prevalence of 5.9% with trichomoniasis, and a significant association between sexual habits and prevalence of gonorrhoea, trichomoniasis and HIV was observed.[6] The prevalence of trichomoniasis varies from 2 to 60.6% in different parts of India (Table 29.3).

Table 29.3 ThePrevalence of Trichomoniasis in Women in India[7-12]

Number studied	*Place (year)*	*Prevalence (%)*
92	Meerut 1990	60.6
350	Chandigarh 1991	9.4
100	Faridkot, Punjab 2003	2
142	Port Blair 1994	8.4
74	Calcutta 1994	11.1
8900	Mumbai 1991-1999	5.7

In men the prevalence has ranged from 0% in asymptomatic men at low risk to 58% among adolescents at high risk for STDs.[3] In a study from Tanzania, a community of rural men with urethritis was studied, where the most prevalent pathogen was *T. vaginalis* (11%) and 50% of these men were asymptomatic.[13] In another study, 17%[14] of men attending the STDs clinic had trichomoniasis, and men older than 30 years had a higher prevalence of *T. vaginalis* infection.[15] In one Indian study, the prevalence of trichomonas infection was 6.6% in men with STDs.[11] In a study from USA, *T. vaginalis* infection was detected in 71.7% of 256 male partners of women infected with trichomoniasis, of whom 136 (77.3%) were asymptomatic.[16] Trichomoniasis is often associated with a bacterial vaginosis. In one study, *T. vaginalis* was significantly associated with the presence of clue cells on wet mount.[17] *T. vaginalis* was speculated recently to alter normal vaginal ecology contributing to *bacterial vaginosis*[18] Co-infection with other organisms like *Ureaplasma urealyticum* and or *Mycoplasma hominis* in over 90%, *Neisseria gonorrhoeae* in 30%, *yeasts* in 15% and *C. trachomatis* in about 15% has been reported.[3]

Risk factors for acquiring trichomoniasis studied in various studies were low socio-economic and educational status, use of alcohol or marijuana, being separated, older sex partners, multiple partners, having a partner who had children with other women, history of delinquency and other STIs.[19,20]

Transmission[2]

T. vaginalis is almost exclusively transmitted by sexual intercourse. The organisms are isolated from vagina, cervix, urethra, bladder, Bartholin glands and Skene glands in females, whereas in males, organisms have been isolated from the anterior urethra, external genitalia, prostate, epididymis and semen. Transmission rates seem to be high from men to women: a rate of 70% was seen among men having sexual contact with infected women in the previous 48 hours. This compares with a prevalence of 80% to 100% in female partners of infected men.[21,22] Rarely, transmission by contaminated fomites has been reported. *T. vaginalis* survives upto 45 minutes on toilet seats, wash clothes, clothing and bath water.

Perinatal transmission occurs to 2-17% of female children of infected mothers.[22] Reports have also documented *T. vaginalis* as a cause of neonatal pneumonia.[23]

Pathogenesis[3]

Due to lack of animal models, very little information is available on the pathogenesis of trichomoniasis. Studies have implied that various virulence-associated characteristics are important for infection with *T. vaginalis*. The presence and absence of complement and iron also play a role in pathogenesis. The findings of different studies suggest that cyto-adherence, which ultimately leads to cytotoxicity, which is a dynamic and complex process involving a cascade of reactions may be responsible for *T. vaginalis* infection. Few studies have shown role of proteinases in cyto-adherence[24]. It was also observed in one study that molecular mimicry of one of the adhesion molecules with malic enzyme could be responsible for evasion of host immune defenses by the parasite.

Clinical Manifestations

T. vaginalis commonly infects the vaginal epithelium. Other sites affected are the urethra, Bartholin glands and Skene glands and rarely endocervix. In men, it most commonly involves the urethra, others being epididymis and prostate. Infection of extragenital sites like fallopian tubes, perinephric abscess, meningitis and perianal ulcers has also been reported.[3]

Manifestations in Women

The incubation period for *T. vaginalis* infection has been reported to be between 4-28 days. About 50% of women are asymptomatic, but about 30% of this group develop symptoms when they are observed for 6 months.[5]

In symptomatic women, most studies showed that vaginal secretions were usually copious, homogenous, malodourous with a pH of 4.5, and a yellow-green colour. Gardner and Dukes described the colour of discharge as gray in 46% of cases, yellow-green in 36% cases and yellow in 10%.[5] Punctate mucosal haemorrhages with ulcerations over the cervix are referred as colpitis macularis, flea-bitten or strawberry cervix, and is better visualized on colposcopy. The positivity of this finding on naked eye examination is only 2.5%, as compared to 52% on colposcopy. In another study, it was observed that vaginal fluid from women with colpitis macularis had a mean of 18 *T. vaginalis* compared to that of 7 *T. vaginalis* per 400 × microscopic field in women without colpitis macularis.[3]

Twelve percent of patients complained of abdominal pain, which could reflect the presence of severe vaginitis, regional lymphadenopathy, endometritis or salpingitis. Rarely postmenstrual and post-coital spotting are observed.[9] An overview of signs, symptoms and clinical findings in women is given in Table 29.4.

Reproductive complications in women include

- Risk factor for transmission of HIV
- Associated with PID
- Greater risk for tubal infertility
- Associated with preterm birth and low birth weight
- Increased risk of posthysterectomy infection
- Risk factor for cervical neoplasia

Table 29.4 Symptoms, Signs and Clinical Findings in Women with Trichomoniasis[22]

Symptoms	%	*Signs*	%	*Findings*	%
None	9-56	None	15	pH>4.5	66-91
Discharge malodourous	50-75	Diffuse vulval erythema	10-37	Positive whiff test	~50
		Excessive discharge	50-75	Wet mount:	
Pruritus	23-82	Yellow, green	5-42	Excess PMNs	~75
Dypareunia	10-50	Frothy	8-50	Motile trichomonas	40-80
Dysuria	30-50	Vaginal wall inflammation	20-75	Fluorescent antibody	80-90
Lower abdominal pain	5-12	Strawberry cervix:		Acridine orange	50-90
		Naked eye	1-2	Giemsa	50-90
		Colposcopy	45-90	Papanicolau	56-70
				Culture	95-97

Trichomoniasis is associated with higher risk of HIV transmission. Leroy et al. found a significant difference between the prevalence of trichomoniasis among a cohort of HIV infected and non-infected pregnant women in Rwanda.[25] In a prospective study by Laga et al., incident trichomoniasis was significantly associated with HIV seroconversion (OR = 1.9) among a cohort of women in Zaire in multivariate analysis.[26] The associations between HIV and trichomoniasis, similar to other STDs, may relate to (1) increased shedding of HIV as a result of the local inflammation produced by the STDs, (2) increased susceptibility to HIV as a result of the macroscopic or microscopic breaks in mucosal barriers caused by the STDs, or (3) STDs may be more prevalent among HIV infected individuals as a result of common risk factors for both infections.

Studies have shown *T. vaginalis* to be an important factor in infertility among both women and men.[27-34] Trichomonads attach easily to mucous membranes and may also serve as vectors for spread of other organisms, carrying pathogens attached to their surface into the fallopian tubes.[31-34] Grodstein et al. stated that women with *T. vaginalis* infection had a 1.9-fold increased risk (95% CI 1.3-2.8) of tubal infertility compared with control subjects. Women with multiple episodes (2-4) of trichomoniasis had an even higher increased risk.

Moodley et al. demonstrated a significantly higher rate of PID among women with trichomoniasis compared with uninfected women.[35]

Among pregnant women, trichomoniasis is associated with adverse outcomes such as preterm delivery, premature rupture of membranes (PROM), and lowbirth- weight infants in several studies.[36,37]

Trichomoniasis has been associated with post hysterectomy infection.[38] In the puerperal period, *T. vaginalis* was associated with a risk of febrile mortality. There was also an association between postabortal infection and trichomonas colonization.[39]

Trichomoniasis may be a risk factor for development of cervical neoplasia.[40,41] A meta-analysis of 22 cohort and 2 case-control studies found a significant positive association between trichomoniasis and CIN.

Clinical Manifestations in Men

The most common manifestation of *T. vaginalis* infection in men is urethral discharge, or symptoms of urethritis. They may also complain of dysuria, urgency, and post-coital burning. They also may have asymptomatic urethritis. *T. vaginalis* has been reported to cause 1-17% of cases of nonchlamydial nongonococcal urethritis (NCNGU). The urethral discharge in *T. vaginalis* infection is less profuse and purulent compared to that of gonococcal or chlamydial urethritis.[42] In one large study of 447 men attending an STDs clinic, it was observed that the majority of the patients had symptoms of urethritis, and both spontaneous resolution (33%) and prolonged asymptomatic carrier states were observed.[3]

The other less known presentations are: balano-posthitis, inflammation of external genitalia, urethral stricture, epididymitis and infertility. A study on aetiology of chronic prostatitis reported that second commonest cause of chronic prostatitis was *T. vaginalis* (52/276 patients), next only to *C. trachomatis*.[43]

Complications associated with trichomoniasis in men[31-34]

- Common cause of nongonoccocal urethritis, may be a cause of prostatitis, epididymitis
- Risk factor for HIV transmission
- Associated with significant decrease in sperm motility and viability,associated with infertility

Trichomoniasis may contribute to male factor infertility by altering sperm motility and viability.[31-34] Trichomonads have been isolated from approximately 10% of infertile men in some series. In a study trichomonas positive men when treated with metronidazole (400 mg three times a day for 10 days), showed a significant improvement in sperm motility, viability, viscosity, and particulate matter after therapy.[33]

The association of trichomoniasis with HIV amplification is also seen among men. A study suggests that symptomatic inflammatory trichomoniasis may increase HIV excretion in semen. HIV-seropositive men with symptomatic urethritis caused by trichomoniasis had a 6-fold higher concentration of HIV RNA in their seminal plasma compared to HIV-positive men without trichomoniasis.[44]

Diagnosis

Diagnosis based solely on clinical signs and symptoms is unreliable, and it has to be confirmed by laboratory investigations.

Direct Microscopic Examination[3]

Making a wet mount of vaginal discharge and examination of urine in males can be used in making the diagnosis in clinical practice. The detailed methodology for these is described in chapter 13. The sensitivity of detection ranges from 42-92% depending on the experience and expertise of the examiner and specificity upto

98%.[21] Various staining methods have been described to improve the sensitivity of microscopic evaluations. The use of acridine orange, Giemsa, fluorescein and periodic acid-Schiff, among other techniques, have been shown to be more sensitive in some investigators' hands.[45,46] Other stains include, Papanicolaou, neutral red and peroxidase stains. Routine Papanicoloau stained smears have demonstrated *T. vaginalis* on cytological examination in asymptomatic women. Direct fluorescent antibody technique is rapid, easy to perform, and relatively inexpensive as compared to culture.

Culture

Culture is the 'Gold standard' for diagnosis of trichomoniasis. It is especially of use when the organism load is low e.g. in asymptomatic women and men with chronic disease. The inoculum size required is only in the range of 10^2 organisms/mL and the growth of the organism is easy to interpret.

Various media have been used to detect trichomonas, such as Diamond (tripticase, yeast and maltose), modified Diamond, Kupfurberg, Lash, NIH and Feinberg-Whettington media. In one study, it was found that with Diamond and modified Diamond media, detection rate was 90-97% compared to other media.[3] In another study, which compared broth culture to that with modified Columbia agar, showed that the latter was more sensitive (98.5%) than broth (92.1%).[47] The yield on culture usually takes 3-7 days. *T. vaginalis* is an anaerobic organism that grows more slowly under aerobic conditions. Thus, CO2 incubation has been recommended for optimal recovery. The disadvantages of culture techniques are the delay in diagnosis, culture media are not readily available, are more expensive and organisms often die in transit. Cultures are seldom used for diagnosis in routine situations. To improve the acceptability of culture for diagnosis, a two-chambered plastic bag culture system or InPouch TV was developed, which allows direct inoculation, transport and culture, and results are obtained earlier than the routine culture.[2] Its sensitivity has been found to be more than Diamond's medium in one of the study.[48]

Cultivation on cell cultures is more sensitive, enabling the observation of *T. vaginalis* from an inoculum containing as few as 3 organisms/mL. However, cell culture is expensive, inconvenient and even more prone to vaginal bacterial contamination. This technique requires pretreatment of the specimen with antibiotics using Diamond's TYI medium as a transfer medium, followed by subsequent passage onto the cell cultures.

Despite its high sensitivity, this method has not been used outside a limited number of studies.[49]

Immunological Methods

Various serological assays with good sensitivities have been described, but they are less specific than culture and sometimes even wet mount. A variety of techniques, including complement fixation, hemagglutination, gel diffusion, fluorescent antibody and ELISA, have been used to determine the presence of trichomonal antibodies. However, these are certainly not specific in determining recent from remote infection. As well, in low incidence populations, positive antibody could reflect interaction with nonpathogenic trichomonads.[50]

Other detection methods are antigen-detection technique using monoclonal antibody against *T. vaginalis* in vaginal secretions. In a study, ELISA using monoclonal antibodies for the detection of 65-kilodalton surface polypeptide of *T. vaginalis* revealed a sensitivity and specificity of 89% and 97% respectively, versus the culture technique with sensitivity of 97.2% and specificity of 100%.[51]

These serological techniques have essentially been abandoned for PCR-based technology.

Molecular Methods

Other diagnostic techniques are molecular methods based on nucleic acid detection like PCR and DNA hybridization techniques. In an observational study of 337 women with a new PCR test for *T. vaginalis*, it was found that the sensitivities of wet preparation and culture were 52% and 78% respectively, compared to that of the PCR which was 84% sensitive and 94% specific on the same specimens. It was concluded that women with high risk and asymptomatic infection would be benefited with this PCR.[52] In another study, 5′ nuclease assay for detection of *T. vaginalis* DNA from female genital specimens showed that sensitivity and specificity were 97.8% and 97.4% respectively, compared to those of broth culture. It was also reported to have advantage of detection, among large clinical samples in a short time compared to culture.[53]

A commercially available DNA-based test called the Affirm VP system (Becton Dickinson) uses synthetic oligonucleotide probes for detection of *T. vaginalis*, *Gardnerella vaginalis*, and *Candida sp* from a single vaginal swab.[54] Affirm VP had a sensitivity of 92% and a specificity of 98% compared with wet mount and a sensitivity of 92% and a specificity of 99% compared with culture in a study.

A new in-office, antigen-based diagnostic test is currently being developed for detection of trichomoniasis in women.[55] By using a vaginal swab sample, mixing it with a special buffer, and placing a drop of the resulting mixture on a test strip, a positive or negative result can be obtained in 10 minutes. This test has shown sensitivity and specificity of 95%.[55]

Diagnosis in Males

Diagnosis of this infection is much more difficult in males, with the best culture results yielded by combining urethral swabs and urine sediment for culture[56]. PCR appears to have far greater sensitivity in this setting. Among 300 men attending an STDs clinic, culture of urethral swab and urine sediment detected *T. vaginalis* in 5%, in contrast to 17% detected by PCR of urine and urethral swab specimens. The sensitivity of PCR with urine specimens in this study was 100%, in contrast to a sensitivity of 80% for swab specimens[57].

Treatment (CDC 2006)[58]

Recommended Regimen
Metronidazole 2 g orally in a single dose
OR
Tinidazole 2 g orally in a single dose
Alternative Regimen
Metronidazole: 500 mg twice a day for 7 days.
The nitroimidazoles comprise the only class of drugs useful for the oral or parenteral therapy of trichomoniasis. Of these, only metronidazole is readily available and approved by the FDA for the treatment of trichomoniasis. In randomized clinical trials, the recommended metronidazole regimens have resulted in cure rates of approximately 90%-95%; ensuring treatment of sex partners might increase the success rate. Treatment of patients and sex partners results in relief of symptoms, microbiologic cure, and reduction of transmission.

Follow Up

Follow up is unnecessary for men and women who become asymptomatic after treatment or who are initially asymptomatic. Certain strains of *T. vaginalis* can have diminished susceptibility to metronidazole; however, infections caused by most of these organisms respond to higher doses of metronidazole. If treatment failure occurs with metronidazole 2 g single dose and reinfection is excluded, the patient can be treated with metronidazole 500 mg orally twice daily for 7 days or tinidazole 2 g single dose. For patients failing either of these regimens, clinicians should consider treatment with tinidazole or metronidazole at 2 g orally for 5 days.

If these therapies are not effective, further management should be discussed with a specialist; evaluation of such cases should ideally include determination of the susceptibility of *T. vaginalis* to metronidazole.

Management of Sex Partners

Sex partners of patients with *T. vaginalis* should be treated. Patients should be instructed to avoid sex until they and their sex partners are cured i.e., when therapy has been completed and patient and the partner(s) are asymptomatic (in the absence of a microbiologic test of cure).

Special Considerations

Allergy, Intolerance and Adverse Reactions

Patients with an immediate-type allergy to metronidazole can be managed by desensitization. Topical therapy with drugs other than nitroimidazoles can be attempted, but cure rates are low (<50%).

Pregnancy

Vaginal trichomoniasis has been associated with adverse pregnancy outcomes, particularly PROM, preterm delivery, and low birthweight. Data have not indicated that treating asymptomatic trichomoniasis during pregnancy lessens the risk of adverse outcome. Women who are symptomatic with trichomoniasis should be treated to ameliorate symptoms.

Women may be treated with 2 g of metronidazole in a single dose. Multiple studies and meta-analysis have not demonstrated a consistent association between metronidazole use during pregnancy and teratogenic or mutagenic effects in the infants.

HIV positive patients should receive the same treatment regimen as those who are HIV-negative.

Other Therapies

Active immunization against trichomoniasis is done in Europe. Other therapies which have proved useful are metronidazole gel, clotrimazole pessary, nonoxynol-9 and povidine iodine douches.

Metronidazole Resistance

An emerging problem is the development of metronidazole-resistant strains of *T. vaginalis*. Metronidazole resistance has been reported both in vitro and clinically, with increased failures to even high doses of metronidazole.[59,60] The CDC estimates that 2.5% to 5% of *T. vaginalis* isolates display some level of resistance to metronidazole.[59] The mechanism of development of anaerobic resistance to metronidazole also controlled by hydrogenosomes, in that metronidazole competes for H+ as an electron acceptor. In metronidazole-resistant *T. vaginalis*, the expression levels of the hydrogenosomal enzymes pyruvate ferredoxin oxidoreductase, ferridoxin, malic enzyme, and hydrogenase are reduced dramatically, which probably eliminates the ability of the parasite to activate metronidazole.[61]

Resistance of *T. vaginalis* isolates to metronidazole can be overcome by retreating with increased doses of 2 g per day for 2 to 5 days or as much as 3 g per day for 14 days when high-level resistance is encountered.[59,62,63] Intravenous formulations offer no advantage over the oral drug. Some authorities have recommended higher doses of oral medication in combination with pharmacy- prepared intravaginal preparations. Furazolidone and sulphimidazole are effective in vitro against metronidazole resistant *T. vaginalis*.[63] There are limited anecdotal reports of success with paromomycin cream; however, there may also be a high incidence of local side effects associated with this therapy. Another in vitro study showed that the combination of dipyridamole and allopurinol could be useful in treatment of trichomonaisis, and also against other parasites which use de novo purine synthesis for their metabolism.[64]

Tinidazole is a second-generation nitroimidazole with activity against protozoa and anaerobic bacteria, which is found to be effective in metronidazole resistant cases. Tinidazole has a plasma elimination half-life twice that of metronidazole (12-14 hours vs 6-7 hours)[65] and also penetrates better into male reproductive tissues than metronidazole. Several literature reports describe the successful use of tinidazole for treating metronidazole-resistant trichomoniasis.[63,66-70] The largest series of patients was reported by Sobel et al.[63] In this study, 20 patients with clinically refractory trichomoniasis (failure to respond to therapy with oral metronidazole at least 500 mg twice a day for 7 days) were treated with high doses of oral and vaginal tinidazole (2 to 3 g orally plus 1 to 1.5 g intravaginally for 14 days). The cure rate was 92% (22 of 24); no patients discontinued therapy due to side effects[63] Tinidazole was extremely well tolerated at these high doses. Many studies have also demonstrated a lower incidence and severity of side effects after tinidazole therapy compared with metronidazole.

INTESTINAL PROTOZOAL INFECTIONS

Intestinal infections with a wide variety of pathogens now occur as sexually transmitted diseases, and as opportunistic infection in HIV/AIDS population. Protozoa are important enteric pathogens in patients with HIV infection. The spectrum of disease associated with each of these infections depends on a variety of factors which include immunological competence of the individual, the pathogenicity of the microbe and the duration of infection.

Epidemiology

The intestinal protozoal infections are now well recognized in especially risk group population like homosexuals, HIV/AIDS and bisexuals. The first published observation was in 1968 that giardiasis and amoebiasis could be sexually transmitted.[71] The initial studies concentrated on homosexual populations. The comparative studies of the prevalence of intestinal protozoal infection among the homosexual and heterosexual populations were done, where the prevalence of *E. histolytica* was 20%, *G. lamblia* 3%, *E. coli* 20%, *Endolimax nana* 24%, *E. hartmanii* 14% and other *nonpathogenic amoebae* 8% in homosexuals compared to the other group (heterosexuals) where it was as follows: *E. histolytica* 0%, *G. lamblia* 2%, *E. nana* 5% and other *amoebae* 9%.[72] Various studies have put prevalence of *E. histolytica* 21-32% and *giardiasis* at 12-18% among homosexual populations.[72-74] In another study which examined the prevalence of enteric protozoal infection and their associations between the gender, sexual preference and practices in 180 consecutive patients at STDs clinic, 19.6%, 3.9% and 23.5% of homosexuals were infested with *E. histolytica*, *G. lamblia* and other *non-pathogenic entamoeba* respectively, whereas bisexuals were infected with 2.1%, (*E. histolytica*) 4.2% (*G. lamblia*) and 10.4% (*non-pathogenic entamoeba*), and heterosexuals had no *E. histolytica* or *G. lamblia* infection and 9.4% had *non-pathogenic entamoeba* in their stools. Homosexuality and oral anal sex were the most important risk factors.[75] In an another study in homosexual men with or without gastrointestinal symptoms, *E. histolytica* was observed in 29% of symptomatic men and in 25% of asymptomatic men; *G. lamblia* was found in 14% symptomatic and 4% asymptomatic men. On the whole, the initial studies which were done in homosexual population showed that there was definite association between sexual practices and higher prevalence of *E. histolytica* and *G. lamblia* infection.

With HIV/AIDS population increasing, various other exotic protozoal infections have become common. These are referred as new or emerging protozoal infections. In a recent study in Africa where aetiology of acute, persistent and dysenteric diarrhoea was evaluated, *E. histolytica* was found in both HIV positive and HIV negative individuals, where as *microsporidium species* and *Blastocystis hominis* were found only in HIV positive patients.[76] In an another study from Africa, among 50 AIDS patients, 57% had a variety of intestinal protozoa; *isosporiasis* was detected in 7 and *cryptosporidiosis* in 2 patients.[77] In another comparative study between HIV positive and negative individuals *Cryptosporidium parvum* was found exclusively in HIV positive patients where as *G. lamblia* was found in both the groups.[78]

In the current scenario of HIV/AIDS, the opportunistic protozoal infections have outnumbered the major protozoal infections. Various studies have documented prevalence of new or emerging protozoal infections: *cryptosporidiosis* (7.2-30%), *isosporiasis* (1.2-12%), *cyclosporiasis* (11.1%), *microsporidiosis* (9-20%), *blastocystosis* (10-51%) and *nonpathogenic entamoeba* (16-25%). These parasitic infections were either found exclusively or in majority of HIV/AIDS patients compared to that of infection caused by *E. histolytica* and *G. lamblia* which were of prevalence 0-25% and 2.2-6.2% respectively.[77,79-81] Recent studies from North India on prevalence of intestinal pathogens in HIV positive patients have been reported and are given in Table 29.5.

Transmission of Intestinal Protozoal Infection[81]

Transmission of giardiasis, amoebiasis, cryptosporidiosis and other coccidian intestinal protozoa infections is primarily by the faecal-oral route. Drinking faecal contaminated water and having sexual contact with an infected individual appear to be the most frequent causes of infection.

Table 29.5 Prevalence of Protozoal Infections in HIV Positive Patients[82,83]

	Lucknow (n=26)	*Chandigarh (n=120)*
E. histolytica	11.5%	1.6%
G. lamblia	3.8%	8.3%
Cryptosporidium	11%	10.8%
B. hominis	8%	3.3%
Isospora belli	31%	2.5%
Cyclospora	–	3.3%
Enterocytozoon	–	2.5%

It has been estimated that 500-1000 cysts of *G. lamblia* and 2000-4000 cysts of *E. histolytica* can infect an individual. The primary infectious form is the mature quadrinucleate cyst. In most parts of the world, the usual source of infectious material is faecal contaminated water. Food handlers, flies or cockroaches, and poor hygiene in institutionalized individuals can also spread this disease.

E. histolytica is the most common intestinal parasite seen in gay communities throughout the world, with an average prevalence of 25% noted for this group of individuals. High risk behaviour found in this group that would easily predispose individuals to infection includes analingus (anal-oral contact) or fellatio (oral-genital contact) after anal-genital intercourse. Digital anal manipulation or poor hygiene after anal intercourse can easily result in generalized faecal contamination and subsequent infection. It is believed that direct rectal inoculation of trophozoites can occur, but this is thought to be an uncommon method of transmission. It has been shown that cleaning of the anus prior to intercourse does reduce the prevalence of infection, but sharing cleansing equipment among groups of individuals can, in fact, promote infection. It appears that the rate of amoebiasis in homosexual men has decreased during the last 5 years. This decrease may be because of safe sex practices that have been adopted in an attempt to decrease the incidence of AIDS in the gay community.

Despite the high prevalence of *E. histolytica* among homosexual men, it has been well documented that relatively few cases of invasive amoebiasis have occurred in this group. In addition, amoebiasis has only rarely been reported as a cause of morbidity in patients with AIDS. Analyzes has shown that the isolates of *E. histolytica* taken from several populations of homosexuals in the United States and Europe almost always belong to nonpathogenic zymodemes. This apparently is not the case in Japan, where 15% of gays in large cities appear to have pathogenic organisms on the basis of serologic studies.

Heterosexual transmission of *E. histolytica* has also been described. Women can develop genital disease due to poor perineal hygiene. Heterosexuals practising anal intercourse or oral-genital sex in a manner similar to homosexuals can also be infected through the faecal-oral route.

Transmission of *Giardia lamblia* by sexual contact is almost exclusively seen in male homosexuals. Sexual behaviour that is responsible for the transmission of this organism is similar to that responsible for the spread of amoebiasis. There have been rare reports of proctitis and vaginitis caused by *Giardia lamblia*, which indicate the possibility of direct trophozoite transfer as an initiating factor in the development of infection.

It has been proposed that because of the compromized gut immunity in patients of HIV/ AIDS, infection with the coccidian intracellular parasites like *cryptosporidium, isospora* etc have increased.

GIARDIASIS

Giardiasis is the human infection caused by the flagellated protozoan *Giardia lamblia*. Loeuwenhoek described the organism in 1679 and in 1859, Lambl re-described it. In 1915, Stiles renamed it as *Giardia lamblia*. The prevalence of *G. lamblia* is 2.9% in general population,[84] and in homosexuals it is as high as 12-18%.[73] A study among the HIV positive patients attending the AIDS clinic, reported a prevalence of 55% and giardiasis was associated significantly with penoanal sex.[85]

Biology[84]

G. lamblia is a flagellated protozoan belonging to the phyllum sarcomastigophora. It has two distinct life forms, the trophozoite and the cyst. The trophozoite stage is responsible for colonization in man. It is pear shaped and of length 10-20μ (average 14μ), 6-15μ wide and 1-3μ thick with an ovoid sucking disk occupying the anterior ventral surface.

The dorsal surface provides an area for diffusion of nutrients as the adults line the upper jejunal sections of the small intestine. The sucking disk appears to be a rigid structure connected to the exterior by a canal containing flagella. It is hypothesized that the beating of the flagella produces a negative pressure in the concavity of the ventral surface causing its attachment to the microvilli of the small intestine. Eight large flagella are present in four symmetric pairs, and there are two distinct nuclei responsible for the characteristic "monkey-face" appearance on light microscopy **(Fig. 29.2)**. *G. lamblia* multiplies by binary fission; therefore, as long as host nutrition and immediate environmental conditions are satisfactory, the parasite can maintain itself within the host indefinitely.

It is generally believed that the trophozoite stage interferes with the integrity of the brush border of the upper small intestine. The exact mechanism has not been defined, but it has been proposed that it may obstruct absorption by direct microvillous attachment and associated factors, such as fungal or bacterial overgrowth, or the production of an enterotoxin by *Giardia lamblia* itself. In fact, it is a combination of all factors responsible for the pathologic activity.

The cyst state is responsible for the environmental contamination and transmission of this parasite. The cysts are oval, 8 to 14μ long (average 12μ) and 6 to 10μ wide. Four nuclei are present, usually positioned near one end of the cyst. Once passed in faeces, the cysts survive best in wet, cool conditions. They are capable of surviving standard concentrations of chlorine used routinely for water purification systems. Oral contact with the cysts through contaminated water food, hands, or other body contact then reintroduces the cysts into the human host. Once ingested, the cysts apparently need the acidic environment of the stomach to signal excystation. The excystation is completed in the alkaline environment of the upper duodenum where a mature cyst releases a four-nucleated trophozoite. Once the trophozoite has established

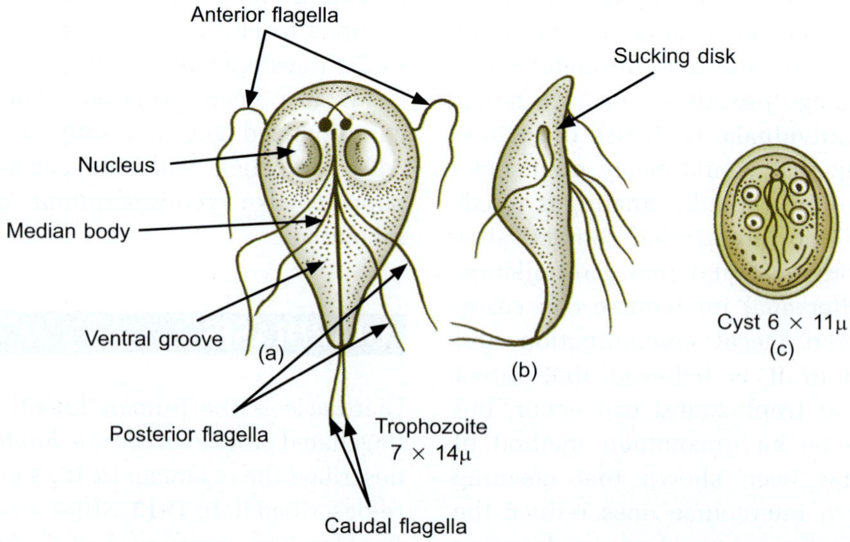

Fig. 29.2 Giardia Lamblia (a) Trophozoite (b) Side View of Trophozoite (c) Cyst

itself, it can multiply by binary fission every 5 hours, thus rapidly establishing its presence in great numbers. From ingestion to the appearance of symptoms it takes approximately 21 days but may as short as 3 days (range 3 to 41 days).

Clinical Features[84]

The most characteristic early phase of giardiasis is an acute diarrhoeal illness of brief duration. The diarrhoea usually lasts 2-3 days. The infection can be acute or chronic. In acute giardiasis, the manifestations are diarrhoea (95%), fatigue (93%), abdominal pain (74%), foul stool (77%), bloating (71%), weight loss (65%), nausea (60%), greasy stool (56%), flatulence (56%), anorexia (60%), frothy stool (48%), vomiting (23%), fever (19%), belching (26%) and constipation (9%). Acute giardiasis generally resolves in 1 to 4 weeks, but may persist for months in children, leading to malabsorption and malnutrition.

The chronic phase of giardiasis is generally milder and may or may not have been preceded by an acute episode. It is manifested by intermittent bouts of diarrhoea over 2-3 years, and flatulence (94%), upper abdominal pain (84%), epigastric gnawing (75%), nervousness (72%), weight loss (53%), constipation (47%), diarrhoea (41%), anorexia (38%), dizziness (34%), pruritus ani (28%), mucous in stool (25%), palpitation (22%), irregular fever (22%), urticaria (19%), nausea (16%), blood in stool (6%) and vomiting (6%). Children infected with giardia who do not have diarrhea should be observed for evidence of malabsorption, impaired growth or failure to thrive, and otitis media with a history of repeated antibiotic treatment failures.

Modes of Transmission

The transmission of giardia to humans is dependent upon the ingestion of cysts excreted in the faeces of infected persons or animals. The principal mode of transmission to humans appears to be person-to person, although indirect transmission from contaminated water and food, originating from humans and animals has been described.

Diagnosis[71]

Identifying the characteristic cyst or trophozoite of the parasite can establish the diagnosis of giardiasis. This is accomplished by obtaining appropriate samples of stool or duodenal fluid. The fresh stool is concentrated by flotation in 33% zinc sulfate or by formalin ether sedimentation. The concentrate is then stained with 1% potassium iodide. On microscopy, motile trophozoites are looked for. The sensitivity is better with active diarrhoea and is specific in experienced hands, but finding trophozoites does not prove disease causation. Microscopy of duodenal aspirate or jejunal biopsy or imprint is used, where the sensitivity is 34-98% and approaches 100% by latter method.

Serological tests like IFA using patients cysts/ trophozoites have 89% sensitivity in symptomatic patients and 71-100% specificity. Immunodiffusion with sonicated cysts and IFA (with cultured trophozoites) have 91-97% sensitivity and 85-100% specificity, while ELISA (cultured trophozoites) has sensitivity of 87% and specificity of 88%.

Treatment[71]

In many healthy, immunocompetent individuals *G. intestinalis* will be eradicated by host defense mechanisms without the need for specific antimicrobial chemotherapy. Administration of an antigiardial drug will generally reduce the severity of symptoms and the duration of the illness.[86,87]

Various antibiotics have been used for treatment of giardiasis. They include acridine derivatives like quinacrine 100 mg tid for 5-7 days with 63-100% cure rates. Metronidazole 250-750 mg tid for 3-10 days has been used with cure rates of 56-95%. Highest cure rate (95%) is obtained with metronidazole 750 mg tid for 3-10 days. Tinadazole 2 g single dose or 125 mg bid for 7 days yields cure rates of 93-97%. Furazolidone at 100 mg tid for 7 days has 72-92% cure rates. Albendazole and paromomycin are the other drugs used with variable efficacy. A recent meta-analysis involving 34 trials performed by the Cochrane collaboration indicates that the preferred treatment regimen is an ultra-short course (i.e. a single dose regimen taken on 1 day) of a nitroimidazole derivative.[88]

Although symptomatic patients with giardiasis are usually offered antimicrobial chemotherapy, the question as to whether asymptomatic patients (particularly those in an endemic area) should be treated remains controversial.

AMOEBIASIS

Amoebiasis is caused by the protozoan *Entamoeba histolytica*. Timothy Richard Lewis first described amoebae in human stools in 1869. In 1893, Quincke and Roos first described amoebic cysts. In 1903 Fritz Schandinn named the parasite *Entamoeba histolytica*.[71]

The majority of cases occur in tropical countries, the prevalence ranging from 15 to 40%; published reports place the prevalence of *E. histolytica* in homosexual men at 7-30%.[81] In patients with AIDS, *E. histolytica* is rare, but still should be considered as a cause of diarrhoea in addition to cryptosporidiosis and isosporiasis. Other high-risk groups include immigrants from countries of high endemicity, and travellers to such countries.

Biology[81]

E. histolytica is a protozoan. Of the seven species that make up the genus entamoeba, it is the only known human pathogen. *E. histolytica* primarily exists in two forms, trophozoites and cysts. The trophozoite, motile by means of its pseudopodia, is approximately 25 to 50µm in diameter. It has a single nucleus with a distinct, central nucleolus, its cytoplasm consists of a clear, outer ectoplasm and a more central, finely granular endoplasm **(Fig. 29.3)**. The organism multiples by simple binary fission within the intestinal lumen. Unless diarrhoea is present, trophozoites become rounded and develop into cysts within the intestinal lumen before being excreted in the stool. In becoming cysts, trophozoites go through a precyst and a cyst maturation process. Trophozoites can no longer encyst after stool evacuation from the host. They are fragile and do not survive long outside the host.

Mature cysts are spherical, approximately 12µm in diameter, and generally contain 4 nuclei. When a susceptible host ingests a mature cyst, its wall degenerates in the small intestine, releasing a single amoeba, which divides into eight uninucleated amoebae. These amoebae migrate to the large intestine and develop into trophozoites, which then encyst and complete the life cycle. Mature cysts can survive upto 3 months in water. They are destroyed by hypercholorination or iodination of drinking water, temperatures higher than 55°C, and prolonged exposure to carbolic acid or warm vinegar.

Pathology[81]

It is apparent that not all *E. histolytica* infections result in clinical disease exhibited by signs or symptoms of tissue invasion. It is proposed that there are distinct pathogenic and nonpathogenic

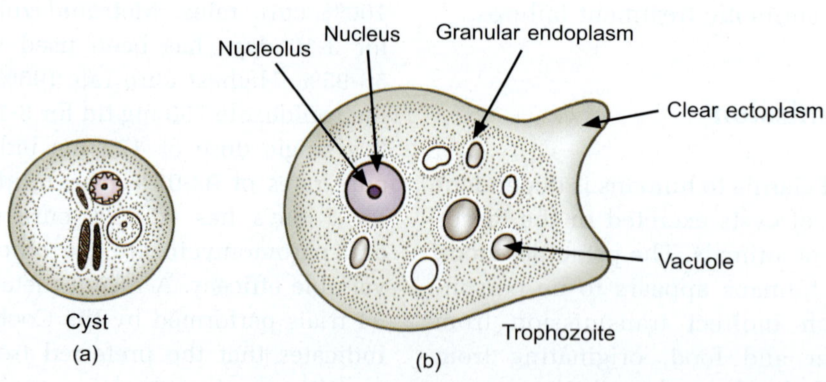

Fig. 29.3 *Entamoeba Histolytica* (a) Immature Binucleate Cyst (b) Trophozoite

strains or zymodeme groups of *E. histolytica* based on the electrophoretic motility of 4 of its basic enzymes, and certain zymodemes appear capable of causing invasive amoebiasis. It is estimated that only 10% of individuals with asymptomatic infection will have isolates that belong to a zymodeme predictive of invasive disease.

On the other hand others think that all *E. histolytica* are capable of invasion, but pathogenicity is the result of a complex interaction between host bacterial flora and the organism. Mirelman has recently demonstrated that an isolate of *E. histolytica*, obtained from an asymptomatic patient and thought to be nonpathogenic, could become pathogenic after contact with bacteria from a patient with invasive amoebiasis.[89]

E. histolytica causes local tissue injury by several bio-chemical mechanisms. Virulent strains are often resistant to both leukocytes and lysis by complement. Diets high in protein and low in iron restrict the growth of trophozoites and may help protect against invasive disease.

Clinical Presentation[81]

The incubation period from ingestion of mature cysts until infection is evident, which ranges from days to months, but averages 2 to 4 weeks. Infected individuals can be totally asymptomatic, have symptoms primarily related to the gastrointestinal tract, or have extraintestinal manifestations of amoebiasis. The majority of patients, 50 to 90%, are believed to be asymptomatic. In one study of homosexual men infected with *E. histolytica*, 50 to 60% had mild gastrointestinal symptoms, but symptoms were also present in a similar percentage of uninfected controls. Gastrointestinal symptoms may be mild or severe in intensity. Generally, asymptomatic patients never become symptomatic. They may excrete cysts for a short period of time, but the majority of these patients will clear the infection within 12 months.[90]

Individuals with nondysenteric colitis may complain of intermittent diarrhoea or constipation, mild abdominal cramping, flatulence and fat intolerance. These symptoms may begin insidiously and fatigue may also be a common complaint. Physical examination at this stage may be fairly unremarkable except for colon tympani and mild tenderness over the caecal area. Some patients may exhibit signs and symptoms of severe amoebic dysentery. Dysenteric amoebiasis, rarely seen in homosexual men, presents with the passage of large numbers of watery stools containing clearly visible blood or mucous. In 50% of cases, the onset of illness is sudden, and fever, severe abdominal cramps, and tenesmus occur. On examination, there is usually generalized abdominal tenderness and signs of dehydration. Toxic megacolon is a complication in about 0.5% of patients, and may be a consequence of inappropriate corticosteroid treatment. Progression to fulminant or necrotising colitis occurs in 0.5% of patients and is associated with a high mortality rate (40%) secondary to perforation, peritonitis or massive bleeding.[90] Tender hepatomegaly occurs in 25% of cases and is due to a toxin released from infected colonic mucosa. Uncommon manifestations include amoebomas, amoebic liver abscess, rectovaginal fistulas and cutaneous involvement.[90]

A palpable mass and tenderness in the right lower quadrant can result from excessive production of granulation tissue in the caecum or rectosigmoid. This mass is known as an amoeboma. Although amoebomas occur very infrequently, they have been known to cause death.

Amoebic liver abscess is seen in fewer than 10% of patients infected with pathogenic *E. histolytica*, and its presence in homosexual men is extremely rare. In approximately 20% of cases, a history of prior amoebiasis is obtained. (Patients initially present most (80%) of the time, with acute onset of fever and continuous, right, upper quadrant pain, temperature higher than 39°C (102.2°F), pallor and tender hepatomegaly). Intercostal and subcostal tenderness is present in 80% of patients and is a useful finding in suggesting the possibility of this diagnosis. If detected and treated early, the fatality rate for hepatic amoebic abscess is less than 1%; however, if rupture into the thoracic cavity occurs, the mortality rate increases to 6 to 30%.

Amoebic involvement of the penis or cervix typically results in ulceration and significant tissue destruction. Clinically, these lesions closely resemble squamous cell carcinoma. Penile amoebiasis has been described in both homosexual and heterosexual men.

Occasionally, usually in immunosuppressed individuals, infection might be widely disseminated and affect other organs, including bone and the brain.[91] The complications are summarized in Table 29.6.

Table 29.6 Possible Complications of Entamoeba Histolytica Infection

Intestinal disease
Fulminant colitis
Toxic megacolon
Perianal disease with fistula formation

Extraintestinal disease
Liver abscess-rupture:

- Pleuropulmonary disease (the most common complication, especially with right lobe abscesses)
- Intraperitoneal rupture
- Pericardial rupture (uncommon; usually associated with left lobe abscesses)

Other manifestations:

- Cerebral amoebiasis
- Genitourinary amoebiasis (rare; more common in women than men), e.g. vaginal fistulae
- Primary cutaneous amoebiasis
- Amoeboma

Diagnosis[71]

A diagnosis of amoebiasis should be strongly considered in male patients with diarrhoeal symptoms who are homosexuals. Demonstrating either the cyst or trophozoite of *E. histolytica* in stool generally makes a definitive diagnosis of intestinal amoebiasis. Three stool specimens, or one purged specimen should be examined for maximum yield as shedding of the organism is intermittent. Differentiation of *Entamoeba* species requires permanent stains (trichrome or iron hematoxylin) after fixation with 10% formalin. The stool examination is positive in 90% cases of invasive amoebic colitis. If stool is negative, proctoscopy followed by colonoscopy may be required. Examinations of scrapings and biopsies for trophozoites have a higher sensitivity than examinations of faecal specimens. *E. histolytica* cysts and trophozoites are rarely found in the stools of patients with liver abscess, the majority of patients having no intestinal symptoms or history of dysentery.[90]

In vitro cultivation of the organisms may be carried out by numerous culture media including the liver extract, egg infusion media or alcohol egg extract of Nelson. Both cysts and trophozoites can be cultured. Zymodeme determination using starch gel electrophoresis of in vitro cultivates can be utilized to differentiate entamoebas. However, culture methods are time-consuming, laborious and often unrewarding, with a sensitivity of only about 50%.[90] Thus, culture methods are restricted to specialised parasitology research laboratories.

Serology[71]

Serological techniques are quite sensitive in detection of patients with amoebic liver abscess and invasive colitis. One hundred percent positivity can be obtained by using ELISA in liver abscess and cellulose acetate membrane precipitation in rectocolitis. The other serological methods used for the diagnosis are indirect agglutination, indirect immunofluorescence, agar gel diffusion, complement fixation and immunoelectrophoresis. Latex agglutination and thin layer immunoassay demonstrates positivity of 1-52%, 55-100%, 83-100% in cyst passers, rectocolitis and liver abscess respectively. The main advantages of these tests is that they are rapid (same day) and their interpretation is less subjective than microscopy.

Molecular Methods

Molecular methods using the polymerase chain reaction amplify *E. histolytica* genes from extracted faecal DNA. Sensitivity and specificity are high (80%–100% and 100%, respectively).[92,93] The advantage of molecular detection is that it is extremely sensitive (able to detect < 1 parasite) and reliably able to differentiate non-pathogenic *Entamoeba* species from *E. histolytica*. Drawbacks of this method are the high level of expertise required, high cost and limited availability of the test.[90]

Treatment[71]

Appropriate drug therapy of ameobiasis must take into account, the drug distribution and sites of amoebicidal activity. Asymptomatic carriers of *E. histolytica* should be treated with a luminal agent to minimise the spread of disease and the risk of developing invasive disease.[90] For cyst passers, diloxanide furoate 500 mg tid for 10 days has 87-96% cure rate, diiodohydroxyquin followed by tetracycline 650 mg tid for 20 days has 95% cure rate, and paramomycin 300 mg/kg/day for 5-10 days has 80-90% cure rate. In patients with invasive disease, metronidazole should be used in conjunction with a luminal agent to eradicate the organism. In invasive colitis, metronidazole 750 mg tid for 5-10 days or 2.4 g qd for 2-3 days has more than 90% cure rate. Tetracycline and dihidroemetine 250 mg qd for 14 days and 1-1.5 mg/kg/day IM for 7 days have 80-90% cure rates. In cases of liver abscess, metronidazole 750 mg for 5-10 days or 2.4 g qd for 1-2 days has 99% cure rate.

New oral vaccines and DNA-based vaccines against *Entamoeba histolytica* are being tried and tested in animals but their safety and efficacy in human beings is still not established.

CRYPTOSPORIDIASIS

Cryptosporidia are tiny (4-5μ) protozoan parasites that primarily inhabit the microvillous region of epithelial cells. Tyzzer in 1907 described the organism. However, the first instance of symptomatic human disease was recorded in 1976. With recognition of AIDS, multiple cases of cryptosporidium enteritis have been identified in immunocompromised homosexual men. In a study the prevalence of cryptosporidiasis in AIDS patients was reported to be 8.3%.[94] In an Indian study, cryptosporodium oocysts were detected in 46.7% of 75 immunocompromised patients which included both cancer and AIDS patients.[95] Salient features of all the coccidian protozoa and microsporidia are given in Table 29.7.

Table 29.7 Salient Features of Coccidian Protozoan and Microsporidia[99]

Features	*C. parvum*	*C. cayetanensis*	*I. belli*	*Microsporidium*
Size (μ)	4-6	8-10	20-30	1-4
No. of sporocyst/oocyst	0	2	2	10-12 coils
No. of sporozoite/sporocyst	4/oocyst	2	4	-
Sporulation time after excretion	0*	7-14 days	24-48 hours	-
Stain(modified acid fast)	Yes	Variable, light pink- red	Yes (whole cyst stains pink)	Chromotope stains (bright pinkish red)

* already sporulated.

Biology[71]

The primary mammalian species causing diarrhoeal disease is *Cryptosporidium parvum*. They belong to the coccidian family. Genotyping of *C. parvum* isolates from waterborne outbreaks has revealed two major, distinct genotypes: bovine and human, respectively. These two genotypes have now been designated as distinct species, *C. parvum* and *C. hominis*, the latter predominantly infecting humans whereas the former has a broader host spectrum.

The estimated ID50 for humans is 132 oocytes. The life cycle of *cryptosporidium* is excystation of oocyte to trophozoite in the intestinal mucosa, then the trophozoite, transformed to type 1 meront, which develops into a merozoite. The merozoite can become a trophozoite again or becomes a type 2 meront, the type 2 meront divides itself into macro and microgamont and after fertilization of the micro with macrogamont an immature cyst is formed, which finally becomes a mature oocyst. (The oocyst sporulate in situ and either release sporozoites for autoinfection or pass from the body in the faeces).

The mechanism by which *cryptosporidium* causes diarrhoea has not been elucidated. It brings about non-inflammatory diarrhoea. Ultrastructural studies show the intestinal mucosa is intact but the microvilli are displaced at the sites of attachment to the parasite and the enterocyte may be elongated at this attachment. The type of diarrhoea caused by cryptosporidiasis is both secretory and malabsorptive.

Mode of Transmission

Since oocysts are infectious when passed in faeces, person to person transmission takes place in day-care centres, or household contacts in immunocompetent patients. In homosexuals and occasionally in heterosexuals oral-anal intercourse and fellatio after anal intercourse are common modes of transmission.

Clinical Manifestation[71]

Asymptomatic infections can occur in both immunocompetent and immunocompromised hosts. The incubation period is usually 3-14 days. In the immunocompetent host the clinical features are febrile symptoms, malaise, anorexia, vomiting, abdominal pain and cramps. Blood and pus do not occur in the stool. Diarrhoea may last as long as 4 months, but usually subsides within 6-12 days.

In immunocompromised hosts, especially in AIDS, diarrhoea can be chronic, persistent and profuse. Stool volume ranges from 1-25L/d. Weight loss, wasting, and abdominal pain may be severe. Biliary tract involvement can manifest as mid epigastric or upper quadrant pain. The intensity and duration of diarrhea in cryptosporidiosis cases is closely associated with the CD4+ T cell counts.

Extraintestinal manifestations have been clearly described in the literature, especially in the gall bladder, biliary ducts and pancreas, leading to conditions such as papillary stenosis, sclerosing cholangitis and acalculous cholecystitis. The respiratory tract can also be affected with manifestations of chronic bronchitis.[100,101]

Diagnosis

Faecal examination for oocytes is done by modified acid fast stain of diarrhoeal stool after sugar floation technique or the detection of reddish-stained *Cryptosporidium* via auramine-rhodamine methods.[102]

In addition, the diagnosis can be established from histologic examination of jejunal biopsy or rectal mucosa for oocytes.

A direct immunofluorescent antibody stain is sensitive and specific and may require less time. ELISA for cryptosporidial antigen in stool with 83-95% sensitivity has been developed, and ELISA for IgM or IgG antibodies to *cryptosporidium* with 90% positivity rate has been described.[71] In a recent study, immuno-chromatographic dip-strip test for cryptosporidium oocysts in stool showed 92% sensitivity and 100% specificity.[103]

Treatment

To date, no chemotherapeutic agent is effective for cryptosporidiosis. In immunocompetent hosts, treatment is not recommended because the disease is self-limited. Although in limited studies spiromycin,[81] paromomycin (500-750 mg qid) have shown modest benefit. Studies have been conducted with hyperimmune bovine colostrum,letrazuril and diclazuril (veterinary medicine drugs), spiramicyn and more recently azithromicyn, octreotide and roxithromycin.[104] Adequate fluid and electrolyte balance and supportive therapy are necessary.[105]

EMERGING PROTOZOAL INFECTIONS

The emerging protozoal infections are isosporiasis, cyclosporiasis, microsporidiasis and blastocystis infection. These protozoal infections have become prevalent as they cause opportunistic infections in HIV/AIDS patients.

For prophylaxis refer to appendix IIc.

ISOSPORIASIS

It is caused by *Isospora belli*, another coccidian parasite frequently seen in homosexual men with enteritis. It is most commonly acquired by consumption of oocysts after which the parasite, invades the intestinal epithelial cells. In immunocompetent individuals it causes self-limited disease. But in immunocompromised individuals especially in AIDS, infection is not self-limited. The reported prevalence of isosporiasis in AIDS patients is 9.7%.[94] *I. belli* infection is indistinguishable from cryptosporidiasis. Eosinophilia which was not found in other enteric protozoal infections has been documented. *I. belli* infect the entire intestine and produce severe intestinal disease. Symptoms include diarrhoea, nausea, steatorrhoea, abdominal pain, headache and weight loss. Disease may persist for months to years. Deaths from fulminant infections have been reported.[99] Isosporiasis can also show extraintestinal dissemination affecting the mesenteric, periaortic, mediastinal and tracheobronchial lymph nodes.[106,107] It may also be related to biliary disease, causing manifestations of acalculous cholecystitis.[108]

The diagnosis is usually made by detection of the large oocysts (25μ) in stool by modified acid fast staining. Sampling of duodenal contents by aspiration, string test or small bowel biopsy may help if the stool microscopy is negative.

Isospora belli differs morphologically from *Cryptosporidium* sp not only because of its intrinsic morphology (elliptical oocyst measuring 22 × 15 μm in diameter, containing two sporocysts with four sporozooites), but also for the intracellular location in the absorptive cell, while *Cryptosporidium* is restricted to the brush borders, immediately under the apical membrane of absorptive cells.[102]

In contrast to cryptosporidiosis, isosporiasis responds to trimethoprim sulfamethoxazole (160/800 mg) qid for 10 days and then bid for 3 weeks. Other alternatives include pyrimethamine (50-75 mg/day)[105] and in another report a combination of pyrimethamine and sulfadiazine for 8 weeks resulted in complete clinical and parasitological cure.[109] In recurrent situations or in non-responding patients it is necessary to administer other drugs such as pyrimethamine, in isolation or in association with sulfadiazine,[110] roxithromycin[111] and metronidazole.[112] Drugs such as tetracycline, ampicillin, nitrofurantoin, quinacrine and furazolidone have already been used but showed no therapeutic success.

CYCLOSPORIASIS

The protozoan is another coccidian species, which is present globally, *Cyclospora cayetanensis* has been reported from the United States, Asia, Africa, Latin America and Europe. It is usually water-borne, but is also transmitted among homosexuals, and enteric infection is more common in HIV positive individuals. In a study of 450 HIV patients with diarrhoea, the prevalence of cryptosporidiosis was 30%, *Isospora belli* 12%, cyclospora species 11%, *G. lamblia* 13% and *E. histolytica* 1%.[113] The cyclospora infection studied in this group had clinical manifestations indistinguishable from cryptosporidiosis or isosporiasis. In all these patients disease manifested with profuse diarrhoea.[113] In a study from Mumbai, India, 50% of HIV patients in the study group had mixed protozoal infections and 6.6% had cyclospora species exclusively out of 334 faecal specimens.[114] It causes persistent diarrhoea in both immunocompetent and immunocompromised individuals. The disease is characterized by non bloody profuse diarrhoea and concomitant weight loss, anorexia, bloating, abdominal cramping, malaise and fatigue. Symptoms tend to be more severe in patients of AIDS, and may persist as long as 70 days.[99]

Diagnosis is made by detection of spherical 8-10μ oocyst in stool. These refractile oocysts are acid fast variable and are fluorescent when viewed under ultraviolet light microscopy.

Cyclosporiasis is effectively treated with trimethoprim sulfamethoxazole (160/180 mg bid for 7 days).[105] The study, quoted above, found 48% recurrence after 1 week of TMP/SMZ, and retreating with TMP/SMZ tid for 1 week resulted in cure.[113] But patients with HIV experience relapses and may require long-term suppressive maintenance therapy. Ciprofloxacin is another alternative which is less effective, but is suitable for patients who cannot tolerate co-trimoxazole.[115]

MICROSPORIDIOSIS[105]

These are obligate intracellular spore-forming protozoa. It has been detected recently as a human disease-causing protozoan especially in AIDS population. Currently six genera have been recognized to cause human disease: encephalitozoon, pleistophora, nosema, vittaforma, septata and enterocytozoon.

Microsporidiosis is most common among patients with AIDS. In these patients; *Enterocytozoon bieneusi* and *Encephalitozoon intestinalis* are increasingly recognized as causes of chronic diarrhoea and wasting. These infections are found in 10-40% of patients with chronic diarrhoea. The other manifestation described with microsporidiasis are AIDS cholangiopathy, acalculous cholecystitis, pneumonitis, chronic sinusitis, myositis, keratoconjuntivitis, nephritis, hepatitis and encephalitis.[99]

Microsporidia are small, gram positive with mature spores 0.5-2μ × 1-4μ. Diagnosis requires electron microscopy, although intracellular spores can be identified on routine microscopy with H&E, Giemsa and tissue Gram's stain. For the diagnosis of intestinal microsporidiosis, chromotrope 2 R-based staining and Uvitex 2B or calcofluor fluorescent staining reveal spores in faeces or duodenal aspirates. For enteric infection of *E. bieneusi* and *E. intestinalis* in HIV infected patients, therapy with albendazole 400 mg BD for 4 weeks may be efficacious.[105]

Fumagillin is a new drug which inhibit angiogenesis, also has been shown to inhibit growth of *microsporidia in vitro.*[116] A randomized, placebo-controlled trial of fumagillin 60 mg daily for 14 days in AIDS patients with *E. bieneusi* infection showed that treated patients had symptomatic improvement and parasite clearance.[116]

BLASTOCYSTOSIS

It is caused by *Blastocystis hominis*, another protozoan, which is classified as an indeterminate form, and was initially considered nonpathogenic. Recently a study on protozoan infection on intestinal permeability using 99 m technetium (99mTc labeled DTPA) assay showed that *B. hominis* is also pathogenic.[117] Various studies have shown high rate of prevalence among HIV/AIDS population ranging from 10-51%.[77,79-81] They have two forms-trophozoite and cystic form. The cyst is considered infectious. They are nonmotile, 5-30μ, spherical, with 2-4 nuclei, and the cell contains a large vacuole with a thin rim of cytoplasm.[118]

They cause both asymptomatic and symptomatic infections. The spectrum of illness includes watery diarrhoea, abdominal pain, perianal pruritus and excessive flatulence.[118] Diagnosis is based on finding the cyst like stage in the stool with special stains. Indirect fluorescent antibody assay (IFA) has been found to be strongly positive in chronic infection as well as in 70% of asymptomatic patients.[119]

Blastocystosis can be treated with metronidazole and iodoquinol.[105] A study of 18 patients with blastocystosis treated with metronidazole 2 g/day for 5 days showed complete clearance in 11 and recurrence and relapse in 7 patients.[120] Co-trimoxazole in standard doses (sulfamethoxazole

800 mg and trimethoprim 160 mg, twice daily for 7 days) is, however, reported to eradicate the organism in more than 90% of infected, symptomatic individuals.[121] Another promising new drug is nitazoxanide. A placebo-controlled trial of nitazoxanide 500 mg twice daily for 3 days reported a clinical and parasitological cure rate of 86%.[122]

THE IMPACT OF AIDS ON ENTERIC INFECTION

Following the recognition of endemic enteric infections among homosexual men, cases of AIDS were reported in New York City, Los Angeles and San Francisco. AIDS which is characterized by an underlying cellular immune deficiency, has frequent multiple opportunistic infections and malignancies. The disease is primarily seen among homosexual men (73% of the total cases), and gastrointestinal complaints are often evident among homosexual men with AIDS. (It is unclear what relation these enteric infections have with the development of AIDS, but besides the coincidence of these two epidemics and the frequent identification of these infections in patients with AIDS, case-control studies on AIDS in homosexual men have demonstrated that faecal exposure during sex and treatment for enteric parasites were significant variables for developing AIDS).

In one limited study, promiscuity, and anal intercourse were major risk factors for infection with HIV. One hypothesis relating these two syndromes includes production of a suppressor substance from *E. histolytica*, which results in alteration of the immune response, rendering a patient more susceptible to HIV which may be acquired during anal intercourse. An alternative hypothesis suggests that multiple intestinal infections, which are commonly seen in the homosexual men, result in an altered immunologic status, including activated T and B cells that are more permissive than nonactivated cells for HIV infection. In this latter hypothesis, frequent exposures to enteric infections among homosexual men would produce a more "susceptible" immunosuppressed state for HIV infection. Obviously, more research is required to explore these possible relations between multiple enteric infections and AIDS in homosexual men.

REFERENCES

1. Levinson W, Jawetz E. Intestinal and Urogenital protozoa. In: Levinson W, Jawetz E, eds. Medical microbiology and immunology. 6th edn. New York: Lange Mc-Graw Hill; 2002: p. 298-304.
2. Leber AL, Novak SM. Intestinal and urogenital amoebae, flagellates and ciliates. In: Murray PR, JoBaron E, Pfaller MA, et al., eds. Manual of Clinical Microbiology. 7th edn. Washington DC: ASM Press; 1999. p. 1391-1403.
3. Kreiger JN, Alderete JF. *Trichomonas vaginalis* and Trichomoniasis. In: Holmes KK, Mardh P-A, Sparling PF, et al. eds. Sexually Transmitted Diseases. 3rd edn. New York: Mc-Graw Hill 1999. p. 587-604.
4. Cates WJr. Estimates of the incidence and prevalence of sexually transmitted diseases in the United States. American Social Health Association Panel. Sex Transm Dis 1999; 26: 52-7.
5. Sweet RL, Gibbs RS. Infective vulvovaginitis. In: Sweet RL, Gibbs RS, eds. Infectious disease of the female genital tract. 4th edn. Philadelphia: Lippincott Williams and Wilkins; 2002. p. 337-54.
6. Divekar AA, Gogate AS, Shivkar LK, et al. Disease prevalence in women attending the STDs clinic in Mumbai, India. Int J STDs AIDS 2000; 11: 45-8.
7. Kumar P, Sharma NK, Sharma U, et al. Trichomoniasis and candidasis in consorts of female with vaginal discharge. Indian J Sex Transm Dis 1990; 11: 54-6.
8. Sokhey C, Dhar K, Vaishnavi C, et al. Isolation of pathogens from clinically suspected vaginitis. Indian J Sex Transm Dis 1991; 12: 59-62.

9. Chopra A, Mittal RR, Kanta S, et al. Vaginitis and vaginal flora - study of 100 cases. Indian J Sex Transm Dis 1993; 14: 52-4.
10. Sharma PK. A profile of sexually transmitted diseases in Port Blair. Indian J Sex Transm Dis 1994; 15: 21-2.
11. Gogte A. Reproductive tract infections in women of child bearing age from Dharavi slums, Mumbai. Indian J Sex Transm Dis 1999; 20: 11-5.
12. Puri KJ, Madan A, Bajaj K. Incidence of various causes of vaginal discharge among sexually active females in age group 20-40 years. Indian J Dermatol Venereol Leprol. 2003; 69: 122-5.
13. Watson Jones D, Mugeye K, Mayaud P, et al. High prevalence of trichomoniasis in rural men in Mwanza, Tanzania: results from a population based study. Sex Transm Infect 2000; 76: 355-62.
14. Schwebke JR, Hook EW 3rd. High rates of *Trichomonas vaginalis* among men attending a sexually transmitted diseases clinic: implications for screening and urethritis management. J Infect Dis 2003; 188: 465-8.
15. Joyner JL, Douglas JM Jr, Ragsdale S, et al. Comparative prevalence of *Trichomonas vaginalis* among men attending a sexually transmitted diseases clinic. Sex Transm Dis 2000; 27: 241-2.
16. Seña AC, Miller WC, Hobbs MM, et al. *Trichomonas vaginalis* infection in male sexual partners: implications for diagnosis, treatment, and prevention.Clin Infect Dis 2007; 44: 13-22.
17. Schneider H, Coetzee DJ, Fehler HG, et al. Screening for sexually transmitted diseases in rural South African women. Sex Transm Dis 1998; 74 (1 Suppl): S147-52.
18. Moodley P, Connolly C, Sturm W. Interrelationships among HIV type 1 infection, bacterial vaginosis, trichomoniasis and the presence of yeasts. J Infect Dis 2002; 185: 69-73.
19. Crosby R, DiClemente RJ, Wingood GM, et al. Predictors of infection with *Trichomonas vaginalis*: a prospective study of low income African-American adolescent females. Sex Transm Infect 2002; 78: 360-4.
20. Klinger EV, Kapiga SH, Sam NE, et al. A community-based study of risk factors for *Trichomonas vaginalis* infection among women and their male partners in Moshi urban district, northern Tanzania. Sex Transm Dis 2006; 33: 712-8.
21. Al-Zanbagi NA, Al-Jehani EF. Recent diagnostic study for the flagellate protozoan *Trichomonas vaginalis*. J Egypt Soc Parasitol 2007; 37: 361-70.
22. Heine P, Mc Gregor JA. *Trichomonas vaginalis*: A reemerging pathogen. Clin Obstet Gynecol 1993; 36: 137-44.
23. McLaren L, Davis L, Healy G, et al. Isolation of *Trichomonas vaginalis* from the respiratory tract of infants with respiratory diseases. Paediatrics 1983; 71: 888-90.
24. Arroyo R, Alderete JF. *Trichomonas vaginalis* surface proteinase activity is necessary for parasite adherence to epithelial cells. Infect Immun 1989; 57: 2991-7.
25. Leroy V, De Clercq A, Ladner J, et al. Should screening of genital infections be part of antenatal care in areas of high HIV prevalence? A prospective cohort study from Kigali, Rwanda, 1992–1993. Genitourin Med 1995; 71: 207–11.
26. Laga M, Manoka A, Kivuvu M, et al. Non-ulcerative sexually transmitted diseases as risk factors for HIV-1 transmission in women: results from a cohort study. AIDS. 1993; 7: 95-102.
27. Sherman KJ, Daling JR, Weiss NS. Sexually transmitted disease and tubal infertility. Sex Transm Dis 1987; 14: 12-6.
28. Sherman K, Chow W, Daling J, et al. Sexually transmitted diseases and the risk of tubal pregnancy. J ReprodMed 1988; 33: 30-4.
29. Grodstein F, Goldman M, Cramer D. Relation of tubal infertility to history of sexually transmitted diseases. Am J Epidemiol 1993; 137: 577-84.
30. El-Shazly AM, Al-Naggar HM, Soliman M, et al. A study on trichomoniasis and female infertility. J Egypt Soc Parasitol 2001; 31: 545-53.
31. Martinez-Garcia F, Regardera J, Mayer R, et al. Protozoan infections in the male genital tract [review]. J Urol 1996; 156: 340-9.
32. Gopalkrishnan K, Hinduja I, Kumar A. Semen characteristics of asymptomatic males affected by *Trichomonas vaginalis*. J In Vitro Fertil Embryo Transfer 1990; 7: 165-7.

33. Jarecki-Black J, Lushbaugh W, Golosov L, et al. *Trichomonas vaginalis*: preliminary characterization of sperm motility inhibiting factor. Am Clin Lab Science 1988; 18: 484-9.
34. Tuttle J, Holbrook T, Derrick F. Interference of human spermatozoal motility by *Trichomonas vaginalis*. J Urol 1977; 118: 1024-5.
35. Moodley P, Wilkinson D, Connolly C, et al. Trichomonas vaginalis is associated with pelvic inflammatory disease in women infected with HIV. Clin Infect Dis 2002; 34: 519-22.
36. Klebanoff M, Carey C, Hauth J, et al. Failure of metronidazole to prevent preterm delivery among pregnant women with asymptomatic *Trichomonas vaginalis* infection. N Engl J Med 2001; 345: 487-93.
37. Minkoff H, Grunebaum AN, Schwartz RH, et al. Risk factors for prematurity and premature rupture of membranes: a prospective study of the vaginal flora in pregnancy. Am J Obstet Gynecol 1984; 150: 965-72.
38. Soper DE, Bump RC, Hurt WG. Bacterial vaginosis and *trichomonas vaginalis* are risk factors for cuff cellulitis after abdominal hysterectomy. Am J Obstet Gynecol 1990; 163: 1016-21.
39. Carey JC, Yaffe SJ, Catz C. The vaginal infections and prematurity study: an overview. Clin Obstet Gynecol 1993; 36: 809-20.
40. Zhang Z, Begg C. Is *Trichomonas vaginalis* a cause of cervical neoplasia? Results from a combined analysis of 24 studies. Int J Epidemiol 1994; 23: 682-90.
41. Viikki M, Pukkala E, Nieminen P, et al. Gynecological infections as risk determinants of subsequent cervical neoplasia. Acta Oncol 2000; 39: 71-5.
42. Schwartz MA, Hootar TM. Aetiology of non gonococcal nonchlamydial urethritis. Dermatol Clin 1998; 16: 727-33.
43. Skerk V, Schonwald S, Krhen I, et al. Aetiology of chronic prostatitis. Int J Antimicrob Agents 2002; 19: 471-4.
44. Hobbs MM, Kzembe P, Reed AW, et al. *Trichomonas vaginalis* as a cause of urethritis in Malawian men. Sex Transm Dis 1999; 26: 381-7.
45. Perazzi B, Menghi C, Coppolillo E, et al. Investigation of *Trichomonas vaginalis* through different methodologies during pregnancy.Rev Argent Microbiol 2007; 39: 99-104.
46. Bickley LS, Krisher KK, Punsalang A Jr, et al. Comparison of direct fluorescent antibody, acridine orange, wet mount, and culture for detection of *Trichomonas vaginalis* in women attending a public sexually transmitted diseases clinic. Sex Transm Dis 1989; 16: 127-31.
47. Stary A, Kuchinka-Koch A, Teodorwicz L. Detection of *Trichomonas vaginalis* on Modified Columbia agar in the routine laboratory. J Clin Microbiol 2002; 40: 3277-80.
48. Borchardt KA, Zhang MZ, Shing H, et al. A comparison of the sensitivity of the InPouch TV, Diamond's and Trichosel media for detection of *Trichomonas vaginalis*. Genitourin Med 1997; 73: 297-8.
49. Garber GE, Sibau L, Ma R, et al. Cell culture compared with broth for detection of *Trichomonas vaginalis*. J Clin Microbiol 1987; 25: 1275-9.
50. GE Garber. The laboratory diagnosis of *Trichomonas vaginalis*. Can J Infect Dis Med Microbiol 2005; 16: 35-8.
51. Lisi PJ, Dondero RS, Kwiatkoski D, et al. Monoclonal-antibody-based enzyme-linked immunosorbent assay for *Trichomonas vaginalis*. J Clin Microbiol 1988; 26: 1684-6.
52. Wendel KA, Erbelding EJ, Gaydos CA, et al. *Trichomonas vaginalis* polymerase chain reaction compared with standard diagnostic and therapeutic protocols for detection and treatment of vaginal trichomoniasis. Clin Infect Dis 2002; 35: 576-80.
53. Jordan JA, Lowery D, Trucco M. TaqMan-based detection of *Trichomonas vaginalis* DNA from female genital specimens. J Clin Microbiol 2001; 39: 3819-22.
54. Petrin D, Delgaty K, Bhatt R, et al. Clinical and microbiological aspects of *Trichomonas vaginalis*. Clin Microbiol Rev 1998; 11: 300-17.
55. Xenostrip-Tv package insert. San Antonio (TX): Xenotype Diagnostics; 2002.
56. Krieger JN, Verdon M, Siegel N, et al. Natural history of urogenital trichomoniasis in men.J Urol 1993; 149: 1455-8.
57. Schwebke J, Lawing L. Improved detection by DNA amplification of *Trichomonas vaginalis* in males. J Clin Microbiol 2002; 40: 3681-3.

58. Centre for Disease Control. Sexually transmitted Diseases Treatment Guidelines, MMWR 2006; 55: 52-5.
59. Schmid G, Narcisi E, Mosure D, et al. Prevalence of metronidazole resistant *Trichomonas vaginalis* in a gynecology clinic. J Reprod Med 2001; 46: 545-9.
60. Sobel JD, Nagappan V, Nyirjesy P. Metronidazole resistant vaginal trichomoniasis an emerging problem. N Engl J Med 1999; 341: 292-3.
61. Land K, Delgadillo-Correa MG, Tachezy , et al. Targeted gene replacement of a ferredoxin gene in *Trichomonas vaginalis* does not lead to metronidazole resistance. Mol. Microbiol 2004; 51: 115-22.
62. Lossick JG, Muller M, Gorrell TE. In vitro drug susceptibility and doses of metronidazole required for cure in cases of refractory vaginal trichomoniasis. J Infect Dis 1986; 153: 948-55.
63. Sobel JD, Nyirjesy P, Brown W. Tinidazole therapy for metronidazole resistant vaginal trichomoniasis. Clin Infect Dis 2001; 33: 1341-6.
64. Afifi MA, el-Wakil HS, Abdel-Ghaffer MM. A novel chemotherapeutic combination for *Trichomonas vaginalis* targeting purine salvage pathways of the parasite. J Egypt Soc Parasitol 2001; 30: 735-46.
65. Sawyer PR, Brogden RN, Pinder RM, et al. Tinidazole: a review of its antiprotozoal activity and therapeutic efficacy. Drugs 1976; 11: 423-40.
66. Hamed KA, Studemeister AE. Successful response of metronidazole- resistant trichomonal vaginitis to tinidazole. Sex Transm Dis 1992; 19: 339-40.
67. Voolmann T, Borcham P. Metronidazole resistant *Trichomonas vaginalis* in Brisbane. Med J Aust 1993; 159: 490.
68. Saurina G, DeMeo L, McCormackWM.Cure of metronidazole and tinidazole resistant trichominasis with use of high dose oral and intravaginal tinidazole. Clin Infect Dis 1998; 26: 1238-9.
69. Dan M, Sobel JD. Trichomoniasis as seen in a chronic vaginitis clinic. Infect Dis Obstet Gynecol 1996; 4: 77-84.
70. Gillette H, Schmid GP, Mosure D, et al. Metronidazole-resistant *Trichomonas vaginalis*, a case series, 1985-1998 [abstract 067]. Proceedings of the 13th meeting of the International Society of Sexually Transmitted Disease Research; 1999 July 11-14; Denver, Colo. Denver: The Society; 1999.
71. Guerrant RL, Sears CL, Ravdin JI. Intestinal protozoa: Giardia lamblia, Entameoba histolytica, cryptosporidiosis and new and emerging protozoal infection. In: Holmes KK, Mardh PA, Sparling PF, et al., eds. Sexually Transmitted Diseases. 3 edn. New York: Mc Graw Hill; 1999. p. 605-27.
72. Ortega HB, Borchardt KA, Hamilton R, et al. Enteric pathogenic protozoa in homosexual men from San Fancisco. Sex Transm Dis 1984; 11: 59-63.
73. William DC, Shookhoff HB, Felman YM,et al. High rates of enteric protozoal infections in selected homosexual men attending a venereal disease clinic. Sex Transm Dis 1978; 5: 155-7.
74. Law CL, Walker J, Qassim MH. Factors associated with the detection of Entameoba histolytica in homosexual men. Int J STDs AIDS 1991; 2: 346-50.
75. Phillips SC, Mildvan D, William DC, et al. Sexual transmission of enteric protozoa and helminths in a venereal-disease-clinic population. N Engl J Med 1981; 305: 603-6.
76. Germani Y, Minssart P, Vohito M, et al. Etiologies of acute, persistent and dysenteric diarrhoea in adults in Bangui, Central African Republic, in relation to human immunodeficiency virus serostatus. Am J Trop Med Hyg 1998; 59: 1008-14.
77. Hunter G, Bagshawe AF, Baboo KS, et al. Intestinal parasites in Zambian patients with AIDS. Trans R Soc Trop Med Hyg 1992; 86: 543-5.
78. Gomez Morales MA, Atzori C, Ludovisi A, et al. Opportunistic and non-opportunistic parasites in HIV-positive and negative patients with diarrhoea in Tanzania. Trop Med Parasitol 1995; 46: 109-14.
79. Mendez OC, Szmulewicz G, Menghi C, et al. Comparison of intestinal parasite infestation indexes among HIV positive and negative populations. Medicina 1994; 54: 307-10.
80. Manatsathit S, Tansupasawasdikul S, Wanachiwanawin D, et al. Causes of chronic

diarrhoea in patients with AIDS in Thailand: a prospective clinical and micro-biological study. J Gastroenterol 1996; 31: 533-7.
81. Levine GI. Sexually transmitted parasitic diseases. Prim care 1991; 18: 101-28.
82. Prasad KN, Nag VL, Dhole TN, et al. Identification of enteric pathogens in HIV-positive patients with diarrhoea in northern India. J Health Popul Nutr 2000; 18: 23-6.
83. Mohandas, Sehgal R, Sud A, et al. Prevalence of intestinal parasitic pathogens in HIV-positive individuals in Northern India. Jpn J Infect Dis 2002; 55: 83-4.
84. Jones JE. Giardiasis. Prim Care 1991; 18: 43-52.
85. Esfandiari A, Jordan WC, Brown CP. Prevalence of enteric parasitic infection among HIV-infected attendees of an inner city AIDS clinic. Cell Mol Biol 1995; 41: S19-S23.
86. Adam RD. The biology of Giardia spp. Microbiol Rev 1991; 55: 706-732.
87. Davidson RA. Issues in clinical parasitology: the treatment of giardiasis. Am J Gastroenterol 1984; 79: 256-61.
88. Zaat JO, Mank T, Assendelft WJ. Drugs for treating giardiasis. The Cochrane Database of Systematic Reviews, 2000; Issue 2, Art. No CD000217.
89. Mirelman D. Effect of culture condition and bacterial associate on the zymodemes of Entameoba histolytica. Parasitol Today 1987; 3: 37-43.
90. van Hal SJ, Stark DJ, Fotedar R, et al. Amoebiasis: current status in Australia. Med J Aust. 2007; 186: 412-6.
91. Farthing MJ. Treatment options for the eradication of intestinal protozoa. Nat Clin Pract Gastroenterol Hepatol 2006; 3: 436-45.
92. Troll H, Marti H, Weiss N. Simple differential detection of *Entamoeba histolytica* and Entamoeba dispar in fresh stool specimens by sodium acetate-acetic acid-formalin concentration and PCR. J Clin Microbiol 1997; 35: 1701-5.
93. Lebbad M, Svard SG. PCR differentiation of *Entamoeba histolytica* and Entamoeba dispar from patients with amoeba infection initially diagnosed by microscopy. Scand J Infect Dis 2005; 37: 680-5.
94. Dieng T, Ndir O, Diallo S, et al. Prevalence of Cryptosporidium species and Isospora belli in patients with acquired immunodeficiency syndrome (AIDS) in Dakar (Senegal). Dakar Med 1994; 39: 121-4.
95. Ballal M, Prabhu T, Chandran A, et al. Cryptosporidium and Isospora belli diarrhoea in immunocompromised hosts. Indian J Cancer 1999; 36: 38-42.
96. Ochiai Y, Takada C, Hosaka M. Detection and discrimination of Cryptosporidium parvum and C. hominis in water samples by immunomagnetic separation-PCR. Appl Environ Microbiol 2005; 71: 898-903.
97. Baishanbo A, Gargala G, Delaunay A, et al. Infectivity of *Cryptosporidium hominis* and *Cryptosporidium parvum* genotype 2 isolates in immunosuppressed Mongolian gerbils. Infect Immun 2005; 73: 5252-5.
98. Schindler AR, Abs El-Osta YG,Stevens M, et al. Capillary electrophoretic analysis of fragment length polymorphisms in ribosomal markers of Cryptosporidium from humans. Mol Cell Probes 2005; 19: 394-9.
99. Ortega YR. Cryptosporidium, cyclospora and isospora. In: Murray PR, JoBaron E, Pfaller MA, Tenover FC, Yolken RH, eds. Manual of clinical microbiology. 7th edn. Washington DC: ASM Press; 1999. p. 1406-12.
100. Salvador Grande F, Saizmonzón L, De La Torre P, et al. Colecistitis alitiasica y cryptosporidiasis intestinal: associación frecuente en pacientes VIH. Rev Esp Enferm Dig 1995; 87: 593-6.
101. Vakil NB, Schwartz SM, Buggy BP, et al. Biliary cryptosporidiosis in HIV infected people after the waterborne outbreak of cryptosporidiosis in Milwaukee. N Engl J Med 1996; 334: 19-23.
102. Cimerman S, Cimerman B, Lewi DS. Enteric parasites and AIDS.Sao Paulo Med J Rev Paul Med 1999; 117: 266-73.
103. Llorente MT, Clavel A, Varea M, et al. Evaluation of an immunochromatographic dip-strip test for the detection of cryptosporidium oocysts in stool specimens. Eur J Clin Microbiol Infect Dis 2002; 21: 624-5.
104. Martins CAP, Guerrant RL. Cryptosporidium and cryptosporidiosis. Parasitol Today 1995; 11: 434-6.

105. Weller PF. Protozoal intestinal infection and trichomoniasis. In: Braunwald E, Fauci AS, Kasper DZ, et al., eds. Harrison's Principles of Internal Medicine. 15 edn. New York: Mc-Graw Hill; 2001. p. 1227-30.
106. Restrepo C, Macher AM, Radany EH. Disseminated extraintestinal isosporiasis in a patient with acquired immune deficiency syndrome. Am J Clin Pathol 1987; 87: 536-42.
107. Michiels JF, Hofman P, Bernard E, et al. Intestinal and extraintestinal Isospora belli infection in an AIDS patient: a second case report. Pathol Res Pract 1994; 190: 1089-93.
108. Benator DA, French AL, Beaudet LM, et al. Isospora belli infection associated with acalculous cholecystitis in a patient with AIDS. Ann Intern Med 1994; 121: 663-4.
109. Ebrahimzadeh A, Bottone EJ. Persistent diarrhoea caused by Isospora belli: therapeutic response to pyremethamine and sulfadiazine. Diagn Microbiol Infect Dis 1996; 26: 87-9.
110. Musey KL, Chidiac C, Beacauire G, et al. Effectiveness of roxithromycin for treating Isospora belli infection. J Infect Dis 1988; 158: 646.
111. Forthall D, Guest SS. Isospora belli enteritis in three homosexual men. Am J Trop Med 1984; 116: 840-2.
112. Pape JW, Verdier RI, Boncy M, et al. Cyclospora infection in adults infected with HIV. Clinical manifestations, treatment, and prophylaxis. Ann Intern Med 1994; 121: 654-7.
113. Deodhar L, Maniar JK, Saple DG. Cyclospora infection in acquired immunodeficiency syndrome. J Assoc Physicians India 2000; 48: 404-6.
114. Verdier RI, Fitzgerald DW, Johnson WD jr, et al. Trimethoprim–sulfamethoxazole compared with ciprofloxacin for treatment and prophylaxis of Isospora belli and Cyclospora cayetanensis infection in HIV-infected patients. A randomized, controlled trial. Ann Intern Med 2000; 132: 885-8.
115. Molina JM, Tourmeur M, Sarfati C, et al. Fumagillin treatment of intestinal microsporidiosis. N Engl J Med 2002; 346: 1963-9.
116. Dagci H, Ustun S, Taner MS, et al. Protozoan and intestinal permeability. Acta Trop 2002; 81: 1-5.
117. Weber R, Canning EV. Microsporidia. In: Murray PR, JoBaron E, Pfaller MA, Tenover FC, Yolken RH, eds. Manual of clinical microbiology. 7th edn. Washington DC: ASM Press; 1999. p. 1413-20.
118. Kaneda Y, Horiki N, Cheng X et al. Serologic response to Blastocystis hominis infection in asymptomatic individuals. Tokai J Exp Clin Med 2000; 25: 51-6.
119. Garavelli PL. The therapy of blastocystosis. J Chemother 1991; 3: 245-6.
120. Ok UZ, Girginkardesler N, Balcioglu C, et al. Effect of trimethoprim/sulfamethoxazole in Blastocystis hominis infection. Am J Gastroenterol 1999; 94: 3245-7.
121. Rossignol JF, Kabil SM, Said M, et al. Effect of nitazoxanide in persistent diarrhea and enteritis associated with Blastocystis hominis. Clin Gastroenterol Hepatol 2005; 3: 987-91.

30 | PELVIC INFLAMMATORY DISEASE

Devinder M Thappa, Sowmya Kaimal

In this chapter

- Definition
- Prevalence
- Risk Factors
- Aetiology
- Pathogenesis
- Clinical Features and Diagnosis
- Treatment
- PID and HIV Infection

DEFINITION

Pelvic inflammatory disease (PID) as described by the Centres for Disease Control and Prevention (CDC) is a spectrum of upper genital tract inflammatory disorders including a combination of endometritis, salpingitis, tubo-ovarian abscess and pelvic peritonitis with salpingitis being the most important component of the spectrum.[1] Acute PID, in general, refers to an infection involving the upper genital tract that is caused by the upward spread of microorganisms from lower genital tract. Chronic PID is a term used to refer to the sequelae of the acute process. PID is one of the most frequent and important infections seen in non-pregnant reproductive age women and is associated with major clinical and public health problems. In women, an increase in the prevalence of sexually transmitted diseases (STDs) is associated with an increase in prevalence of acute PID and its sequelae.[2]

PREVALENCE

(The incidence and prevalence of acute PID is very difficult to determine precisely as it is not a reportable disease in most areas and the wide spectrum of its clinical presentation and lack of accurate clinical diagnostic criteria). In addition, it has been estimated that up to two-thirds of cases of PID go unrecognized.[3] Westrom and Eschenbach noted that the incidence of PID is influenced by multiple factors, including prevalence of STDs, demography, economics, health care characteristics of a population, sexual attitudes, douching, smoking and drug habits and contraceptive practices.[3]

In a community based study in rural areas of Haryana, India, 61% of women of reproductive age had reported symptoms of reproductive tract infection with 41% of those who had on pelvic examination, evidence of PID in the form of cervical discharge and other signs like pelvic or lower abdominal tenderness.[4] A community based study of 859 women in Rajasthan, India revealed that 471 (55%) were symptomatic for reproductive tract infection (RTI), and PID constituted 22% of the 263 confirmed cases of RTI.[5] In a study of 798 women screened in Shahjahanpur (Uttar Pradesh), 272 (34%) were symptomatic for reproductive tract infection (RTI), 54% women with vaginal discharge were found to have PID.[6] Awareness regarding the cause of RTI is very poor and none of the women in Karachi, Pakistan considered vaginal discharge as a symptom of STDs.[7] In developed countries, various sources such as patient surveys, hospital discharge rates, private physician office visits, emergency room visits and retrospective self reporting have been used to calculate incidences of PID. There was an increase in the incidence of acute PID in 1970s and 1980s, as a result of STDs epidemic and widespread use of intrauterine contraceptive device (IUD).[8-12] Since the peak in early 1980s, the hospitalisation rates for acute PID declined with the office visits rates remaining relatively unchanged.[12] According to the CDC report, there was a 57% decline in the number of hospitalised cases of PID from 1981 to 1996. Hospitalizations for PID have declined steadily throughout the 1980s and early 1990s, but have remained relatively constant between 1995 and 2005.[13] In addition to this, with change to less expensive ambulatory treatment, there was a significant decrease in the direct medical costs for PID and its sequelae.[14] This decline in the number of PID cases in USA was attributed to a parallel decrease in the incidence of gonorrhoea and a significant decline in the use of intrauterine devices as a method of contraception. An apparent decline in the incidence of PID was also attributed to more patients being shifted to ambulatory treatment to cut down the costs of health care by Health Maintenance Organizations.

In the U.S., however, reported gonorrhea incidence rates have been either declining or stable since 1996, although, in 2005, the national rate (115.6 cases per 100,000 population) increased for the first time since 1999. Causes for these increases remain unclear; however, data suggest they likely resulted from a combination of increases in the number of tests performed, trends in the types of test performed, and actual increases in disease occurrence.[15] Following a 74 percent decline in the rate of reported gonorrhea from 1975 through 1997, overall gonorrhea rates plateaued, then increased for the past two years. In 2006, the gonorrhea rate was 120.9 cases per 100,000 population, an increase of 5.5 percent since 2005 and an increase for the second consecutive year. Like chlamydia, gonorrhea is substantially under-diagnosed and under-reported, and approximately twice as many new infections are estimated to occur each year as are reported.[16]

Recently, increasing attention has been focussed on what is discussed as 'silent' or 'atypical' PID, a term used for the condition in which women with documented infertility, secondary to tubal scarring and adhesions provided no past history of PID despite the fact that scarring suggested that pelvic infection had occurred in an asymptomatic or unrecognized form.[17] Such an unrecognized PID is probably as common, if not more common than clinically apparent disease.

RISK FACTORS

Knowledge of risk factors is required in order to prevent the significant economic impact and sequelae of PID and this has been emphasized by CDC and others.[18,19]

Besides demographic and social indicators, important roles of sexual behaviours, contraceptive practice, health care behaviour have been stressed.[18-21]

Demographic Factors

Age

Age is an important risk marker for PID and is inversely related to PID rates.[9,18] Adolescent girls are at significant risk of developing acute salpingitis. In a report by Westrom,[9] nearly 70% of women with acute salpingitis were younger than 25 years, 33% experienced their first infection before the age of 19 and 75% were nulliparous. The risk of developing acute PID in the sexually active 15 year old age group was 1: 8, falling to 1: 80 in women 24 years or older.[9,22] It has been suggested that the adolescent population is at greater risk because this population has a high prevalence of STDs, has multiple sexual partners, tends not to use contraceptives which also protect against development of PID and in addition, in this age group estrogen dominance with the resulting cervical ectopy provides a better target for attachment of microorganisms. Socioeconomic factors such as low level of education, unemployment and low income may be indirectly related to prevalence of STDs and sexual and health behaviour.[19] No studies have compared PID rates in urban and rural population.

Sexually Transmitted Diseases

There is a strong correlation between exposure to STDs organisms and PID, with gonorrhoea, chlamydial infection and bacterial vaginosis (BV) being the most important risk factors. In an analysis of risk factors associated with PID of different microbial etiologies among 589 hospitalised patients with PID, Jossens et al[23] reported that an STDs organism was present in 65% of PID cases and *N. gonorhoeae* and *C. trachomatis* were recovered from 55% and 22% of the patients respectively. Eschenbach et al[8] reported that a history of prior uncomplicated cervical gonococcal infection was present more often among patients with acute PID compared with controls. In the United States, *C. trachomatis* has been recovered from the cervix of 5%-39% of women diagnosed as having PID and from the fallopian tubes among zero to 10% of patients with PID. Serologic evidence of *C. trachomatis* infection has been found among 20%-40% of women with a history of PID. *N. gonorrhoeae* has a particularly wide range of recovery rates among women with PID, with isolation rates from the cervix ranging from 27% to 80% and from the fallopian tubes ranging from 13% to 18%.[24]

Sexual Behaviour

Several aspects of sexual behaviour have been proposed to be associated with an increased risk of PID. These include multiple sex partners, high frequency of sexual intercourse and early age at first sexual intercourse. In a recent case control study of PID risk factors, Jossens et al[23] identified more than one sex partner in the previous 30 days as a significant risk factor, whereas lifetime number of partners was not associated with an increased risk for PID. Coitus during menstruation has also been suggested as a risk factor for PID.[25]

Contraceptive Use

Use of different contraceptive methods has a major impact on the risk of acquiring STDs, PID and their sequelae.[2,18,19,26] Non users of contraceptives are at increased risk for PID.[25] Barrier methods, mechanical and chemical, decrease the risk of STDs and PID. Condoms when used appropriately are highly effective in decreasing the risk of acquiring and transmitting STDs organisms associated with PID[27-31] and are associated with decreased risk of tubal factor infertility and ectopic pregnancy.[29,30] It has been suggested that vaginal spermicides decrease the risk of acquiring STDs and consequently may decrease the risk of PID.[31]

IUD is an additional predisposing factor for PID with most studies reporting an increase in the risk of PID and its sequelae. The World Health Organization has reported that in most objective studies comparing IUD use with no contraceptive use, the increase in PID is in the range of 15 to 26 times.[32] Among different IUD, Dalkon Shield users had a maximum (13 fold) risk, with Copper T and Copper 7 having a 4 fold risk. Fairley[33] reported an increased risk of PID in the first 1 to 3 months after insertion of the device and this was related to the introduction of microorganisms into the uterus with insertion. IUD users with PID had significantly more *Fusobacteria spp.* and *Peptostreptococcus spp.* than non-IUD users with PID.[34]

One study showed that IUD use was not associated with PID in low-risk younger women, but in women > 35 years, IUD use was associated with an increased risk of PID. The study also demonstrates an association between IUD use and complicated PID in women > 35 years.[35]

However, an increased risk of PID was not demonstrated with increased duration of use of IUD. Recently results from the PID evaluation and Clinical Health (PEACH) study comparing contraceptive use in 290 women with histologic endometritis with 253 women without it, demonstrated that IUD users had an increased risk of PID with an odds ratio of 13.1 (95% CI, 1.6-109.3).[36]

In contrast, most studies have demonstrated that oral contraceptives reduce the risk for symptomatic and clinically apparent acute PID by 40 to 60%.[37,38] Changes in cervical mucous, preventing ascent of vaginal and cervical microorganisms into the upper genital tract or modification of the immune response are believed to decrease the risk of PID in pill users.

Health Care Behaviour

Health care seeking behaviour influences the risk of PID.[18] Early detection and effective treatment of STDs and PID in women and their partners decreases the risk of PID and its sequelae.[19]

Douching

An increased incidence of acute PID is associated with history of vaginal douching[25,39,40] with the risk significantly related to frequency of douching. Douching was found to be independently related to PID even after adjusting for age, marital status, lifetime partners, STDs history and age at first intercourse[39]. Some case control studies have also demonstrated that vaginal douching is associated with increased incidence of ectopic pregnancy, a major sequelae of PID.[41,42]

Other Risk Factors

Cigarette smoking,[43,44] substance abuse[45] and menstruation[46] are additional risk factors for PID.

AETIOLOGY

PID is a polymicrobial infection and is caused by ascent of microorganisms from the lower genital tract. The STDs agents *Chlamydia trachomatis, Neisseria gonorrhoeae, genital mycoplasmas,* the *facultative anaerobic* and *aerobic bacteria* present in the normal endogeneous flora of the vagina and cervix are the microorganisms most frequently isolated from the upper genital tract of women with PID.[18,23,47-54] Although most proven cases of PID are associated with *N. gonorrhoeae* or *C. trachomatis* in 30% of cases, only anaerobic and facultative bacteria are isolated such as *Bacteroides, Peptostreptococcus* species, *Gardnerella vaginalis,*

Escherichia coli, *Haemophilus influenzae* and *aerobic streptococci*.[23,55] Many of the non STDs organisms are similar to those found associated with BV.[56,57]

Neisseria Gonorrhoeae

Gonococcus as the causative agent is implicated in 33% to 81% of the cases of acute PID when endocervical cultures are used to make a diagnosis.[50,58-60] When specimens are obtained from the abdominal cavity or fallopian tubes, *N. gonorrhoeae* is recovered in 18% compared to 39% from endocervix of total patients and 43% of patients with *N. gonorrhoeae* isolated from the cervix.[61] Generally, the proportion of acute PID associated with *N. gonorrhoeae* depends upon the endemic rates of gonorrhoea infection in a population. Recently, the PEACH study, a large prospective study of acute PID in United States, reported isolation of *N. gonorrhoeae* in only 4% of 274 patients where diagnosis was confirmed by histologic endometritis.[62]

Chlamydia Trachomatis

C. trachomatis is now well established to be the major aetiologic agent in acute PID. The incidence of the isolation rates of *C. trachomatis* in cases of PID depends upon several factors such as the patient population studied (mild disease or severe disease in admitted patients), cultures obtained from biopsy/needle aspiration or from peritoneal fluid or tubal exudate. The isolation rates therefore vary from 10% to 47% in the endocervix and 2% to 51% from upper genital and peritoneal cavity.[63] A 4 fold rise in levels of serum antibody to *C. trachomatis* has been seen in 19 to 62% of cases of acute PID.[63] It has been suggested that patients with milder forms of PID are more likely to have *C. trachomatis* as the causative agent.[64] The two major sequelae of PID, tubal infertility and ectopic pregnancy have been found to be associated with prior chlamydial infection.[41,65-69] The PEACH study found that antibodies to *C. trachomatis* were independently associated with reduced rates of pregnancy and elevated rates of recurrent PID among women with mild to moderate PID.[70] The seroprevalence of chlamydial infection in patients with pelvic inflammatory disease and infertility was found to be 82.7% in patients and 32% in controls by Enzyme Linked Immuno Sorbent Assay (ELISA) in one Indian study.[71] Recently subclinical PID was demonstrated by endometrial biopsy in 27% of women with lower genital tract infections with *Chlamydia trachomatis*.[72]

Genital Tract Mycoplasmas

The genital tract mycoplasmas such as *Mycoplasma hominis*, *Ureaplasma urealyticum* and *Mycoplasma genitalium* have been suggested as potential pathogens in the aetiology of acute salpingitis.[73,74] However, their role remains controversial as some studies have shown no difference between the rates of isolation from the cervices of these patients and sexually active control patients.[50] The frequency of isolation of the mycoplasmas is low from the peritoneal cavity or fallopian tubes of patients with salpingitis (2 to 20%).[50,75] It has been suggested that mycoplasmas may be commensals rather than pathogens in PID[76] and on the other hand, failure to recover mycoplasmas from fallopian tubes in PID cases may be due to the reason that these organisms cause parametritis rather than acute salpingitis.[77] More recently another genital tract mycoplasma, *M. genitalium* has attracted attention as a causative agent for PID in animal models although its role in acute PID in women remains undetermined.[78,79] Data from case-control studies, looking at men with non-gonococcal urethritis and women with cervicitis, have revealed that *M. genitalium* behaves similarly to *Chlamydia trachomatis,* and the carriage of *M. genitalium* and *C. trachomatis* is usually independent of one another.[80] It is feasible that *M. genitalium* may also be an etiologic agent in nongonococcal, nonchlamydial PID, as it has been found to induce salpingitis experimentally in monkeys, has been shown to adhere to human fallopian tube epithelial cells in organ culture, and has been detected in fallopian tube tissue in a woman with salpingitis. Further, *M. genitalium* has been shown to adhere to human spermatozoa, and therefore may potentially be carried by motile sperm to the female upper genital tract.[81] Few studies have examined reproductive sequelae attributed to *M. genitalium* upper genital tract infection, but *M. genitalium* antibodies have been identified more frequently (22% versus 6%) among women with tubal factor infertility compared to women with nontubal factor infertility.[82]

Anaerobic and Facultative Bacteria

Nongonococcal and nonchlamydial bacteria such as *Bacteroides spp, Peptostreptococcus spp, Gardnerella vaginalis, Escherichia coli,* aerobic streptococci and coagulase negative staphylococci are the predominant isolates found in acute PID cases (up to 70%) in addition to *N. gonorrhoeae* and *C. trachomatis*.[25] In nearly one third of hospitalised cases of PID, these anaerobic and aerobic bacteria were found to be the only isolates recovered from upper genital tract.[23] Many of these nongonococcal, nonchlamydial microogranisms have been implicated in BV and several investigators have demonstrated an association between BV and PID.[52,53,57,68-79,83-85] Bukusi et al. have observed that women with PID who are infected with human immunodeficiency virus (HIV) are more likely to have BV than HIV 1 seronegative women whereas *N. gonorrhoeae* and *C. trachomatis* infections were more common in the HIV 1 seronegative group.[54] In another study coagulase negative staphylococcus, coagulase positive staphylococci and *E. coli* were isolated in acute PID.[86]

PATHOGENESIS

Intracanalicular spread of microorganisms from endocervix and vagina to the endometrium and fallopian tubes must occur for PID to develop.[3,18,55,87] CDC has listed 4 factors that might contribute to the ascent of bacteria from the lower genital tract and that might be associated with the pathogenesis of PID. These include uterine instrumentation, hormonal changes during menstruation leading to loss of the mechanical barrier of the cervical mucosa, retrograde menstruation and potential virulence factors of microorganisms associated with the development of PID.

An additional condition that might facilitate the ascending infection is damage to the normal clearance mechanism by the ciliated epithelial cells in the endometrium and fallopian tube.[55] Cervical ectopy occuring more frequently in adolescents and young women results in a larger area for attachment to microorganisms.[87] In chlamydial PID tubal scarring is thought to be due to an immune mediated delayed hypersensitivity type reaction, possibly involving heat shock proteins.[88]

CLINICAL FEATURES AND DIAGNOSIS

Acute PID can present with a broad spectrum of manifestations that include unrecognized subclinical infection to overt infection which may be mild to severe. The most effective strategy for establishing an early accurate diagnosis of PID has not yet been identified. The specificity of any single clinical or laboratory diagnostic finding is low as no symptom or sign is pathognomonic of acute PID.[3] Nearly two-thirds of patients with post PID sequelae report no history of infection[67,89] and on the other hand one third of patients presenting with abdominal or pelvic pain suggestive of PID are found to have other conditions such as appendicitis or ectopic pregnancy or no disease.[3,90,91]

Silent PID

Many women with PID demonstrate vague or subtle symptoms that are not diagnosed as PID suggesting a concept of 'silent' PID.[3,17,18] Such patients in retrospective studies of post PID sequelae do not give any history of having been diagnosed or treated for PID.[17] Many studies have demonstrated the presence of inflammation or microorganisms in the endometrium and fallopian tubes of women with no symptoms of overt acute PID.[92-94] *C. trachomatis* has been recovered from endometrium by culture in 25% of infertile women and in 15% of infected women from fallopian tubes with no clinical or laparoscopic evidence of PID.[94,95] Chlamydial infection is known to persist in the tubes and endometrium in the absence of symptoms after treatment of acute PID.[96] (Although the concept that ascending infection in the absence of clinical signs and symptoms can result in damage to the tubal function is widely accepted, it has been suggested recently by Wolner-Hanssen,[97] that these women with 'silent' or subclinical infection have had symptoms that were unrecognized as being associated with PID with nearly 60% of women with tubal occlusion with no history of PID having sought treatment for symptoms like abdominal pain).

Overt PID

Clinically apparent PID can present with mild to severe symptoms. The classical presentation includes symptoms and signs such as lower abdominal pain, purulent cervical discharge, cervical motion tenderness, adnexal tenderness, fever and leukocytosis. In mild to moderate cases, patient's general condition is good.[3] The onset of symptoms with gonococcal and chlamydial PID is often at the end of or just after menstruation.

Severe disease is seen only in 5 to 10% of overt PID cases[3] and its clinical presentation is more characteristic with fever, chills, nausea and vomiting, abdominal guarding and rebound tenderness suggestive of peritonitis. The white blood cell count, ESR and the C-reactive proteins are raised in most of the cases. However, the accuracy of clinical diagnosis is questionable as only 65% of women with presumed clinical diagnosis of PID could be confirmed on laparoscopic visualisation with 23% having normal pelvic findings and 12% having other pelvic pathology such as appendicitis, endometriosis, ruptured ovarian cyst and ectopic pregnancy.[98] Recent studies have suggested a higher accuracy (80-90%) of clinical diagnosis of acute PID.[53,99] However, the overlap between the visually normal and the acute salpingitis group is so large that it precludes reliance on the clinical factors to differentiate the individual patient with acute salpingitis from the patient with normal pelvis.[98] In an analysis of the prevalence of clinical or laboratory findings in women with laparoscopic confirmation of PID according to aetiologic agent, gonococcal PID was found to be associated with a shorter symptom duration, fever and palpable adnexal mass more often than chlamydial PID which was more frequently associated with abnormal uterine bleeding and an elevated ESR.[100]

A wet mount of vaginal secretions showing increased numbers of leukocytes is a very useful sign of acute PID as is the presence of mucopurulent cervicitis of chlamydial and gonococcal infection of cervix.[3,53,98,100] However in populations with a high prevalence of *C. trachomatis* and *N. gonorrhoeae*, cervicitis has a low positive predictive value for acute PID.[3] The absence of mucopurulent cervicitis and inflammatory cells in the wet mount of genital secretions has a good negative predictive value for ruling out PID. Although laparoscopy is currently the accepted 'gold standard' for diagnosis of acute PID, it is impractical to undertake this investigation in all patients.

Endometrial biopsy demonstrating endometrial inflammation has a good sensitivity and specificity rate for diagnosis of PID with a 90% correlation for histologic endometritis and laparoscopically confirmed salpingitis.[52,91,101] However, the clinical applicability of endometrial biopsy for diagnosis of PID is limited with its results not available for 2-3 days.

The role of sonography as a non-invasive diagnostic test for PID remains to be elucidated. Its clinical use is limited by its poor sensitivity (32%) although the specificity is excellent (97%). Thickened fluid filled tubes with or without free pelvic fluid are the suggestive features of acute PID on sonography.[102]

Laboratory tests such as antichymotrypsin, CA 125, tumour associated trypsin inhibitor and specific genital isoamylases are investigational and have not been shown to have a good positive predictive value.[3,91,100,103]

The clinician has to base the diagnosis of acute PID on clinical grounds in most situations. CDC has recommended a 'low threshold for diagnosis' of PID because of the potential damage to the reproductive health of women, if treatment is not instituted in time. The CDC recommends that in mild cases, treatment should be instituted on the basis of the minimum criteria with all three criteria being present i.e. lower abdominal tenderness, adnexal tenderness and cervical motion tenderness.[18] When more severe clinical findings are present, additional criteria which are more expensive and more invasive need to be looked at in order to avoid making an incorrect diagnosis and unnecessary morbidity. These additional criteria include (a) oral temperature > (101°F) 38.3°C, (b) presence of white blood cells on saline microscopy in vaginal secretions, (c) elevated ESR (d) elevated C-reactive protein (e) laboratory documentation of cervical infection with *N. gonorrhoeae* or *C. trachomatis*, (f) abnormal cervical or vaginal discharge. CDC in 2006 guidelines, recommends following criteria as most specific for diagnosing PID:

1. Histopathologic evidence of endometritis,
2. Transvaginal sonography or magnetic resonance imaging techniques showing thickened, fluid filled tubes with or without free pelvic fluid or tubo-ovarian complex or doppler studies suggesting pelvic infection (e.g. tubal hyperemia), and
3. Laparoscopic evidence of PID.[104]

Diagnosis of a tubo-ovarian abscess (TOA) may be difficult to make on clinical examination alone. Sonography and computed tomographic (CT) scanning and magnetic resonance (MR) imaging increases the diagnostic accuracy for a TOA and may be indicated if there is lack of response to antimicrobial therapy in the first two to three days.[105]

Sequelae of PID

Acute PID is associated with significant sequelae that have an adverse effect on the general and reproductive health of young women.[3,14,18,22,89,106-111]

The short term consequences are perihepatitis (Fitz-Hugh and Curtis syndrome) which may occur in 7 to 16% of hospitalised cases of acute PID.[105] Mortality due to acute PID is not such a major problem in developed countries although it may be significant in countries where health care is not easily accessible. Rupture of a TOA with resultant generalized peritonitis is the most frequent cause of mortality (3 to 8%) associated with PID.[113]

The long term sequelae which develop in approximately 25% of women with acute PID are of more concern and these include infertility, ectopic pregnancy and chronic pelvic pain.[114-116] Unrecognized or 'silent' PID can also result in similar sequelae.[17]

Infertility

Tubal factor infertility (TFI) is the most common long term complication of acute PID.[9,106,109] In a large prospective study by Westrom et al.[106], the reproductive events of patients with a laparoscopic diagnosis of PID were compared with controls. An infertility rate of 16% was found in those with PID whereas only 2.7% in control group failed to become pregnant. TFI was confirmed in 10.8% in the PID group as compared to none in control group. The rate of infertility was found to be directly associated with number of episodes and severity of PID. Similar observations have been made by Lepine et al.[117] more recently, however their data indicated disease severity at initial episode to be more important than the actual number of episodes. Poor outcome regarding fertility was observed in those cases where treatment of PID was delayed. Retrospective seroepidemiologic studies have demonstrated a strong and consistent association between previous chlamydial infection and TFI.[109] The relative risk of TFI is 3 to 8 in cases with past infection with *C. trachomatis*.[66,67,118,119] Most women with TFI and antichlamydial antibodies report no history of a diagnosis or treatment of PID, highlighting the concept of 'silent' PID resulting in tubal damage.[17] There is limited data relating to other organisms such as *N. gonorrhoeae*, mycoplasmas and BV associated anaerobic-aerobic bacteria in their role in TFI.

Ectopic Pregnancy

Damage to the fallopian tube following PID is a well established cause of tubal pregnancy. An eight to ten-fold increase in the rate of ectopic pregnancy has been reported in those with PID.[106,108,110] A direct relationship between the number of episodes of PID and ectopic pregnancy has also been observed.[106] A significant association between ectopic pregnancy and previous chlamydial infection has also been demonstrated similar to TFI.[41,120-123] Role of nonchlamydial infections in ectopic pregnancy is not well studied although few studies have shown an association between *N. gonorrhoeae* and mycoplasmas and ectopic pregnancy.[124,125]

Chronic Pelvic Pain

The cause of chronic pelvic pain is usually due to the presence of pelvic adhesions which result from the inflammatory response to acute PID. This entity is not as extensively studied. Chronic pelvic pain was found to be present in 18% of laparoscopically confirmed cases of PID versus 4% of controls by Westrom et al.[90] The severity and number of episodes of PID were found to be directly proportional to the rate of chronic pelvic pain. Chronic pelvic pain is also highly correlated with the extensive post PID adhesions.[126]

TREATMENT

Early diagnosis and treatment are crucial to the prevention of sequelae of PID. The effectiveness of therapy in prevention of these sequelae depends upon the interval between the onset of symptoms and the institution of treatment. It is important, therefore, not to rely on very strict criteria for the diagnosis of acute salpingitis and to institute early treatment based on a more flexible and realistic approach to diagnosis.

The aetiology of acute PID is polymicrobial and therefore for antibiotic therapy to be effective, a broader cover with antibiotics is required. Whether it is necessary to cover all the organisms implicated in the aetiology of PID, is not proven. The clinician who diagnoses acute PID is often faced with the question of hospitalisation and oral versus parenteral therapy and the controversy in those aspects still exists. However CDC has recommended treatment schedules for acute PID and these are based on the premise that it is appropriate to cover all the major etiologic agents involved in acute PID including *N. gonorrhoeae*, *C. trachomatis*, anaerobes, gram negative enterococci, *G. vaginalis* and anaerobic streptococci.[104] No prospective data exists to address the issue of the clinical efficacy of oral (outpatient) versus parenteral (in patient) therapy of acute PID.

Indications for hospitalization of patients with acute PID as suggested in the guidelines by CDC[104] include the following:

1. Surgical emergencies eg. appendicitis clinically cannot be ruled out.
2. Patient is pregnant
3. Patient does not respond clinically or to oral antimicrobial therapy.
4. Patient unable to follow or tolerate outpatient oral regimen.
5. Patient with severe illness, nausea, vomiting or high fever.
6. Presence of TOA

In addition to the above, women using IUD should be treated on an in-patient basis because of a high co-existent rate of adnexal inflammation.

The major emphasis has been to use combinations of agents to provide empiric broad-spectrum coverage of the polymicrobial aetiology.

The CDC[104] recommends the following treatment schedules for treatment of acute PID:

Parenteral Treatment

Parenteral and oral therapy appear to have similar clinical efficacy treating women with PID of mild or moderate severity. Clinical experience should guide decisions regarding transition to oral therapy, which usually can be initiated within 24 hours of clinical improvement.

Recommended Parenteral Regimen A

Cefotetan 2 g IV every 12 hours
or
Cefoxitin 2 g IV every 6 hours
plus
Doxycycline 100 mg orally or IV every 12 hours

Recommmended Parenteral Regimen B

Clindamycin 900 mg IV every 8 hours
plus
Gentamicin loading dose IV or IM (2 mg/kg of body weight), followed by a maintenance dose (1.5 mg/kg) every 8 hours. Single daily dosing may be substituted.

Alternative Parenteral Regimens

Ampicillin/Sulbactam 3 g IV every 6 hours
plus
Doxycycline 100 mg orally or IV every 12 hours

Oral Treatment

Oral therapy can be considered for women with mild-to-moderately severe acute PID, as the clinical outcomes among women treated with oral therapy are similar to those treated with parenteral therapy. Women who do not respond to oral therapy within 72 hours should be reevaluated to confirm the diagnosis and should be administered parenteral therapy on either an outpatient or in-patient basis.

Recommended Oral Regimen

Ceftriaxone 250 mg IM in a single dose
plus
Doxycycline 100 mg orally twice a day for 14 days
with or without
Metronidazole 500 mg orally twice a day for 14 days
or
Cefoxitin 2 g IM in a single dose and Probenecid, 1 g orally administered concurrently in a single dose
plus
Doxycycline 100 mg orally twice a day for 14 days
with or without
Metronidazole 500 mg orally twice a day for 14 days
or
Other parenteral third-generation cephalosporin (e.g., **ceftizoxime** or **cefotaxime**)
plus
Doxycycline 100 mg orally twice a day for 14 days
with or without
Metronidazole 500 mg orally twice a day for 14 days

Alternative Oral Regimens

If parenteral cephalosporin therapy is not feasible, use of fluoroquinolones (levofloxacin 500 mg orally once daily or ofloxacin 400 mg twice daily for 14 days) with or without metronidazole (500 mg orally twice daily for 14 days) may be considered if the community prevalence and individual risk of *gonorrhoea* is low. Tests for *gonorrhoea* must be performed prior to instituting therapy and the patient managed as follows if the test is positive:

- If nucleic acid amplification test (NAAT) test is positive, parenteral cephalosporin is recommended.
- If culture for *gonorrhoea* is positive, treatment should be based on results of antimicrobial susceptibility. If isolate is quinolone resistant *Neisseria gonorrhoeae* (QRNG), or antimicrobial susceptibility cannot be assessed, parenteral cephalosporin is recommended.

Although information regarding other outpatient regimens is limited, amoxicillin/clavulanic acid and doxycycline or azithromycin with metronidazole has demonstrated short-term clinical cure. No data has been published regarding the use of oral cephalosporins for the treatment of PID.[104]

There are very few microbiologically controlled prospective studies comparing the various antibiotic regimens. Walker et al.[127] performed a meta analysis of antimicrobial regimen efficacy for the treatment of acute PID with 21 studies meeting the criteria regarding appropriate system for making diagnosis of PID and assessment of clinical outcome. The pooled clinical cure rates ranged from 75% to 94% and pooled microbiological cure rates ranged from 71% to 100%. To ensure the best possible prognosis for fertility and to prevent other serious long-term sequelae, vigorous parenteral treatment with careful follow up of the patient is essential.

In those cases where TOA develops, but a rupture is not suspected, hospitalization and vigorous medical management with broad-spectrum antibiotics is instituted. A ruptured TOA is a surgical emergency, which may occur in 3 to 15% of all TOA.[128] Aggressive surgical intervention with hysterectomy and bilateral salpingo-oopherectomy results in more than 95% recovery rate. In unruptured TOA, if patients do not improve within 48 to 72 hours of antimicrobial therapy, surgical intervention needs to be undertaken and it may be possible to conserve reproductive function by aspiration and drainage of intra-abdominal abscesses.[129,130]

The role of steroids in preventing the subsequent adhesions, sterility and chronic pain is controversial. Although advocated by some in the past, no difference in the end results has been observed in a prospective study.[131]

Treatment of Sexual Partners

Appropriate management of acute PID includes examination and treatment of sexual partners of affected women, as the risk of additional episodes of PID will increase, if the male partner with asymptomatic *N. gonorrhoeae* and *C. trachomatis* infection is not treated. These partners should be treated with one of the regimens for uncomplicated gonorrhoeal or chlamydial infections, ceftriaxone 250 mg stat followed by doxycycline 100 mg bid for 7 days or azithromycin 1 gm single dose.

PID AND HIV INFECTION

The seroprevalence of HIV among women with PID is higher than that in women without PID.[132] It has been suggested that the clinical course of PID may be altered by symptomatic HIV infection and that these patients have blunted local mucosal immune responses leading to inadequate response to medical therapy.[133,134] HIV infected women with PID have been observed to have a more severe clinical illness with occurrence of TOA associated with microorganisms other than *N. gonorrhoeae* and *C. trachomatis*.[135,136] However the clinical response to CDC recommended antibiotics was the same in HIV infected and non-infected women.[136] Whether HIV infected women with acute PID require some aggressive interventions (e.g,, hospitilization or parenteral antimicrobial regimens) has not been determined.[104]

In conclusion, PID needs to be diagnosed early so that appropriate treatment can be instituted in order to prevent its medical and economic sequelae. A high index of clinical suspicion of acute PID has to be maintained. In cases of acute salpingitis, hospitalization and use of parenteral antibiotics, which have a broad-spectrum cover for the polymicrobial aetiology of the disease is of vital importance. Further, prevention of repeated infections is equally essential by treating the sexual partners of such women.

Acknowledgement

The authors acknowledge the contribution of Dr Jaswinder Kalra and Dr Sarla Gopalan who were authors of this chapter in the first edition

REFERENCES

1. Centres for Disease Control and Prevention. 1993 Sexually transmitted diseases treatment guidelines. MMWR 1993; 42: 75.
2. Eschenbach DA. Epidemiology of pelvic inflammatory disease. In: Landers DV, Sweet RL, eds. Pelvic inflammatory disease. New York: Springer-Verlag 1997. p. 1-20.
3. Westrom L, Eschenbach DA. Pelvic inflammatory disease. In: Holmes KK, Sparling PF, Mardh PA et al., eds. Sexually transmitted diseases. 3rd ed. New York: McGraw-Hill; 1999. p. 783-809.
4. Aggarwal AK, Kumar R. Study of reproductive tract infections and sexually transmitted diseases among ever married rural women aged 15-44 years. Integrated women Environment and Development project Report, Haryana 1997; 1-2.
5. Rathore M, Vyas L, Bhardwaj AK. Prevalence of reproductive tract infections amongst ever

married women and sociocultural factors associated with it. J Indian Med Assoc. 2007; 105: 71-2, 74, 78.

6. Nandan D, Gupta YP, Krishnan V, et al. Reproductive tract infection in women of reproductive age group in Sitapur/Shahjahanpur district of Uttar Pradesh. Indian J Public Health 2001; 45: 8-13.
7. Bhatti LI, Fikree FF. Health seeking behaviour of Karachi women with reproductive tract infections. Soc Sci Med 2002; 54: 105-17.
8. Eschenbach DA, Harnisch JP, Holmes KK. Pathogenesis of acute pelvic inflammatory disease: role of contraception and other risk factors. Am J Obstet Gynecol 1977; 128: 838-50.
9. Westrom L. Incidence, prevalence and trends of acute pelvic inflammatory disease and its consequences in industrialized countries. Am J Obstet Gynecol 1980; 138: 880-92.
10. Jones OG, Saida AA, St. John RK. Frequency and distribution of salpingitis and pelvic inflammatory disease in short stay in hospitals in the United States. Am J Obstet Gynecol 1980; 138: 905-8.
11. Washington AE, Cates W, Zaidi AA. Hospitalizations for pelvic inflammatory disease. Epidemiology and trends in the United States, 1975 to 1981. JAMA 1984; 251: 2529-33.
12. Rolfs RT, Galaid E, Zaidi AA. Epidemiology of pelvic inflammatory disease: trends in hospitalizations and office visits, 1979-1988. Paper presented at: Joint Meeting of the Centres for Disease Control and Prevention and the National Institutes of Health about Pelvic Inflammatory Disease Prevention, Management and Research in the 1990s; September 4-5, 1990; Bethesda, MD.
13. Centers for Disease Control. Sexually Transmitted Diseases > Surveillance & Statistics > 2006 Reports > 2006 National Report > Special Focus Profiles - Women and Infants- Surveillance 2006. http://www.cdc.gov/stds/stats/womenandinf.htm
14. Rein DB, Kassler WJ, Irwin KL, et al. Direct medical cost of pelvic inflammatory disease and its sequelae: decreasing but still substantial. Obstet Gynecol 2000; 95: 397-402.
15. Centers for Disease Control and Prevention (CDC). Increases in gonorrhea--eight western states, 2000—2005. MMWR 2007; 56(10): 222-5.
16. Centers for Disease Control. Sexually Transmitted Diseases > Surveillance & Statistics > 2006 Reports > Trends in Reportable Sexually Transmitted Diseases in the United States, 2006, http://www.cdc.gov/stds/stats/trends2006.htm.
17. Wolner-Hanssen P, Kiviat NB, Holmes KK. Atypical pelvic inflammatory disease: subacute, chronic or subclinical upper genital tract infection in women. In: Holmes K, Mardh PA, Sparling PF, et al., eds. Sexually transmitted diseases. New York: McGraw-Hill; 1990. p. 615-20.
18. Centres for Disease Control and Prevention. Pelvic inflammatory disease: guidelines for prevention and management. MMWR 1991; 40: 1-25.
19. Washington AE, Aral SO, Wolner–Hanssen P, et al. Assessing risk for pelvic inflammatory disease and its sequelae. JAMA 1991; 266: 2581-6.
20. Padian N, Hitchcock PJ, Fullilove RE. Issues in defining behavioural risk factors and their distribution. Sex Transm Dis 1990; 7: 200-4.
21. Aral SO, Holmes KK. Descriptive epidemiology of sexual behaviour and sexually transmitted diseases. In: Holmes KK, Mardh PA, Sparling PF, et al. eds. Sexually transmitted diseases. New York: McGraw-Hill; 1990. p. 19-36.
22. Westrom L, Mardh PA. Pelvic inflammatory disease: epidemiology, diagnosis, clinical manifestations and sequelae. In: Holmes KK, Mardh PA, Sparling PF eds. International perspectives on sexually transmitted diseases. Impact on venereology, fertility and maternal and infant health. Washington: Hemisphere Publishing; 1982. p. 251-68.
23. Jossens MOR, Schachter J, Sweet RL. Risk factors associated with pelvic inflammatory disease of differing microbial etiologies. Obstet Gynecol 1994; 83: 989-97.
24. Centers for Disease Control and Prevention. Pelvic Inflammatory Disease: Guidelines for Prevention and Management. MMWR 1991; 40(RR-5): 1-25.

25. Jossens MO, Eskenazi B, Schachter J. Risk factors for pelvic inflammatory disease: a case control study. Sex Transm Dis 1996; 23: 239-47.
26. Kani J, Adler MW. Epidemiology of pelvic inflammatory disease. In: Berger GS, Westrom LS, eds. Pelvic inflammatory disease. New York: Raven Press; 1992. p. 7-22.
27. Centres for Disease Control and Prevention. Condoms for prevention of sexually transmitted diseases. MMWR 1988; 37: 133-7.
28. Darrow WW. Condom use and use-effectiveness in high risk populations. Sex Transm Dis 1989; 16: 157-60.
29. Cramer DW, Goldman MB, Schiff I, et al. The relationship of tubal infertility to barrier method and oral contraceptive use. JAMA 1987; 257: 2446-50.
30. Li DK, Daling JR, Stergachis AS, et al. Prior condom use and the risk of tubal pregnancy. Am J Public Health 1990; 80: 864-6.
31. Louv WC, Austin H, Alexander WJ, et al. A clinical trial of nonoxynol-9 for preventing gonococcal and chlamydial infections. J Infect Dis 1988; 158: 518-23.
32. World Health Organization. Mechanism of action, safety and efficacy of intrauterine devices. Geneva, Switzerland: World Health Organization; 1987. Technical report series 753.
33. Fairley TMM. Intrauterine devices and pelvic inflammatory disease: an international perspective. Lancet 1992; 339: 785.
34. Viberga I, Odlind V, Lazdane G, et al. Microbiology profile in women with pelvic inflammatory disease in relation to IUD use. Infect Dis Obstet Gynecol. 2005; 13: 183-90.
35. Viberga I, Odlind V, Berglund L. "Older" age is a risk factor for pelvic inflammatory disease in intrauterine device users. Acta Obstet Gynecol Scand. 2005; 84: 1202-7.
36. Ness RB, Soper DE, Holley RL. Contraception and risk of PID in the PID evaluation and clinical health (PEACH) study. Am J Obstet Gynecol 2002; 186: 929-37.
37. Svensson L, Westrom L, Mardh P-A. Contraceptives and acute salpingitis. JAMA 1987; 251: 2553-5.
38. Wolner-Hanssen P, Svensson L, Mardh PA, et al. Laparoscopic findings and contraceptive use in women with signs and symptoms suggestive of acute salpingitis. Obstet Gynecol 1985; 66: 233-9.
39. Wolner-Hanssen P, Eschenbach DA, Paavonen J, et al. Association between vaginal douching and acute pelvic inflammatory disease. JAMA 1990; 263: 1936-41.
40. Scholes D, Daling JR, Stergachis A, et al. Vaginal douching as a risk factor for acute pelvic inflammatory disease. Obstet Gynecol 1993; 81: 601-6.
41. Chow JM, Yonekura L, Richwald GA, et al. The association between *Chlamydia trachomatis* and ectopic pregnancy: a matched-pair, case-control study. JAMA 1990; 263: 3164-7.
42. Daling JR, Weiss NS, Schwart SM. Vaginal douching and the risk of tubal pregnancy. Epidemiology 1991; 2: 40-8.
43. Marchbanks PA, Lee NC, Peterson HB. Cigarette smoking as a risk factor for pelvic inflammatory disease. Am J Obstet Gynecol 1990; 162: 639-44.
44. Scholes D, Daling JR, Stergachis AS. Current cigarette smoking and risk of aute pelvic inflammatory disease. Am J Public Health 1992; 82: 1352-5.
45. Fullilove RE, Fullilove MT, Bowser BP, et al. Risk of sexually transmitted diseases among black adolescent crack users in Oakland and San Francisco, CA. JAMA 1990; 263: 851-5.
46. Sweet RL, Blankfort-Doyle M, Robbie MO, et al. The occurrence of chlamydial and gonococcal salpingitis during the menstrual cycle. JAMA 1986; 255: 2062-4.
47. Mardh P-A, Lind I, Svensson L et al. Antibodies to *Chlamydia trachomatis*, *Mycoplasma hominis* and *Neisseria gonorrhoeae* in serum from patients with acute salpingitis. Br J Vener Dis 1981; 57: 125-9.
48. Sweet RL, Schachter J, Robbie MO. Failure of beta-lactam antibiotics to eradicate *Chlamydia trachomatis* in the endometrium despite apparent clinical cure of acute salpingitis. JAMA 1983; 250: 2641-5.
49. Wasserheit JN, Bell TA, Kiviat NB, et al. Microbiological causes of proven pelvic inflammatory disease and efficacy of clindamycin

and tobramycin. Ann Intern Med 1986; 104: 187-93.
50. Eschenbach DA, Buchanan T, Pollock HM, et al. Polymicrobial aetiology of acute pelvic inflammatory disease. N Engl J Med 1975; 293: 166-71.
51. Sweet RL, Draper DL, Schachter J, et al. Microbiology and pathogenesis of acute salpingitis as determined by laparoscopy: what is the appropriate site to sample? Am J Obstet Gynecol 1980; 138: 985-9.
52. Paavonen J, Teisala K, Heinonnen PK, et al. Microbiological and histopathological findings in acute pelvic inflammatory disease. Br J Obstet Gynaecol 1987; 94: 454-60.
53. Soper DE, Brockwell NJ, Dalton HP, Johnson D. Observations concerning the microbial aetiology of acute salpingitis. Am J Obstet Gynecol 1994; 170: 1008-17.
54. Bukusi EA, Cohen CR, Stevens CE, et al. Effects of human immunodeficiency virus 1 infection in microbial origins of pelvic inflammatory disease and on efficacy of ambulatory oral therapy. Am J Obstet Gynecol 1999; 181: 1374-81.
55. Rice PA, Schachter J. Pathogenesis of pelvic inflammatory disease. JAMA 1991; 266: 2587-93.
56. Sweet RL. Role of bacterial vaginosis in pelvic inflammatory disease. Clin Infect Dis 1995; 20 (Suppl 2): S276-S285.
57. Hillier SL, Kiviat NB, Hawes SE, et al. Role of bacterial vaginosis-associated microorganisms in endometritis. Am J Obstet Gynecol 1996; 175: 435-41.
58. Eschenbach DA. Epidemiology and diagnosis of acute pelvic inflammatory disease. Obstet Gynecol 1980; 55 (Suppl): 142-53.
59. Cunningham FG, Hauth JC, Gilstrap LC, et al. The bacterial pathogenesis of acute pelvic inflammatory disease. Obstet Gynecol 1978; 52: 161-4.
60. Thompson SE, Hager WD, Wong KH, et al. The microbiology and therapy of acute pelvic inflammatory disease in hospitalized patients. Am J Obstet Gynecol 1980; 136: 179-86.
61. Westrom L, Eschenbach DA. Pelvic inflammatory disease. In: Holmes KK, Sparling PF, Mardh PA et al., eds. Sexually transmitted diseases. New York: Mc Graw- Hill; 1999. p. 783-809.
62. Rabe LK, Hillier SL, Wiesenfeld HC. Endometrial microbiology in women with pelvic inflammatory disease. In: Programme and abstracts of the International Society of Sexually Transmitted Diseases Research; Denver, CO; July 11-4, 1999. Abstract 182.
63. Sweet RL, Gibbs RS. Infectious Diseases of the female genital tract, 4th ed. Philadelphia: Lippincott Williams and Wilkins; 2002. p. 368-412.
64. Svensson L, Westrom L, Ripa KT, Mardh PA. Differences in some clinical laboratory parameters in acute salpingitis related to culture and serologic findings. Am J Obstet Gynecol 1980; 138: 1017-21.
65. Henry-Suchet J, Loffredo V, Sarfaty D. *Chlamydia trachomatis* and mycoplasma research by laparoscopy in cases of pelvic inflammatory disease and in cases of tubal obstruction. Am J Obstet Gynecol 1980; 138: 1022-5.
66. Jones RB, Ardery BR, Hui SL, Cleary RE. Correlation between serum antichlamydial antibodies and tubal factor as a cause of infertility. Fertil Steril 1982; 38: 553-8.
67. Moore DE, Spadoni LR, Foy HM, et al. Increased frequency of serum antibodies to *Chlamydia trachomatis* in infertility due to tubal disease. Lancet 1982; 2: 574-7.
68. Brunham RC, MacLean IW, Binns B, Peeling RW. *Chlamydia trachomatis*: its role in tubal infertility. J Infect Dis 1985; 152: 1275-82.
69. Hartford SL, Silva PD, diZerega GS, Yonekura ML. Serologic evidence of prior chlamydial infection in patients with tubal ectopic pregnancy and contralateral tubal disease. Fertil Steril 1987; 47: 118-21.
70. Ness RB, Soper DE, Richter HE, et al. Chlamydia antibodies, chlamydia heat shock protein, and adverse sequelae after pelvic inflammatory disease: the PID Evaluation and Clinical Health (PEACH) Study. Sex Transm Dis. 2008; 35: 129-35.
71. Vidhani S, Mehta S, Bhalla P, et al. Seroprevalence of Chalmydia trachomatis infection amongst patients with pelvic inflammatory diseases and infertility. J Commun Dis 2005; 37: 233-8.

72. Wiesenfeld HC, Hillier SL, Krohn MA, et al. Lower genital tract infection and endometritis: insight into subclinical pelvic inflammatory disease. Obstet Gynaecol 2002; 100: 456-63.
73. Moller BR. The role of mycoplasmas in the upper genital tract of women. Sex Transm Dis 1983; 10 (Suppl): 281-4.
74. Mardh P-A, Lind I, Svensson L, Westrom L, Moller BR. Antibodies to *Chlamydia trachomatis*, *Mycoplasma hominis* and *Neisseria gonorrhoeae* in serum from patients with acute salpingitis. Br J Vener Dis 1981; 57: 125-9.
75. Mardh PA, Westrom L. Tubal and cervical cultures in acute salpingitis with special reference to *Mycoplasma hominis* and T-strain mycoplasmas. Br J Vener Dis 1970; 46: 179-86.
76. Taylor-Robinson D, Carney FE. Growth and effect of mycoplasmas in fallopian tube organ cultures. Br J Vener Dis 1974; 50: 212-6.
77. Moller BR, Freundt EA, Black FT, Frederiksen P. Experimental infection of the genital tract of female Grivet monkeys for *Mycoplasma hominis*. Infect Immun 1978; 20: 248-57.
78. Palmer HM. Detection of *Mycoplasma genitalium* in the genitourinary tract of women by the polymerase chain reaction. Int J STDs AIDS 1991; 2: 261-3.
79. Taylor-Robinson D. The history and rote of *Mycoplasma genitalium* in sexually transmitted diseases. Genitourin Med 1995; 71: 1-8.
80. Uusküla A, Kohl PK. Genital mycoplasmas, including Mycoplasma genitalium, as sexually transmitted agents. Int J STDs AIDS. 2002; 13: 79-85.
81. Haggerty CL, Totten PA, Astete SG, Ness RB. *Mycoplasma genitalium* among women with nongonococcal, nonchlamydial pelvic inflammatory disease. Infect Dis Obstet Gynecol. 2006; 2006: 30184.
82. Clausen HF, Fedder J, Drasbek M, et al. Serological investigation of *Mycoplasma genitalium* in infertile women. Human Reproduction. 2001; 16: 1866-74.
83. Korn AP, Bolan G, Padian N, et al. Plasma cell endometritis in women with symptomatic bacterial vaginosis. Obstet Gyecol 1995; 85: 387-90.
84. Peipert JF, Montagno AB, Cooper AS, Sung CJ. Bacterial vaginosis as a risk factor for upper genital tract infection. Am J Obstet Gynecol 1997; 177: 1184-7.
85. Korn AP, Hessol NA, Padian NS, et al. Risk factors for plasma cell endometritis among women with cervical Neisseria gonorrhoeae, cervical *Chlamydia trachomatis* or bacterial vaginosis. Am J Obstet Gynecol 1998; 178: 987-90.
86. Baveja G, Saini S, Sangwan K, et al. A study of bacterial pathogens in acute pelvic inflammatory diseases. J Commun Dis. 2001; 33: 121-5.
87. Rice PA, Westrom LV. Pathogenesis and inflammatory response in pelvic inflammatory disease. New York: Raven Press, 1992: 35-47.
88. Paavonen J, Lehtinen M. Immunopathogenesis of chlamydial pelvic inflammatory disease: The role of heat shock proteins. In: infectious Diseases in Obstetrics and Gynaecology. New York: Wiley-Liss 1994: 1-6.
89. Westrom LV, Berger GS. Consequences of pelvic inflammatory disease. In: Berger GS, Westrom LV eds. Pelvic inflammatory disease. New York: Raven Press, 1992. 101-14.
90. Paavonen J, Westrom LV. Diagnosis of acute pelvic inflammatory disease. In: Berger GS, Westrom LV eds. Pelvic inflammatory disease. New York: Raven Press, 1992. p. 49-78.
91. Kahn JG, Walker CK, Washington AE, et al. Diagnosing pelvic inflammatory disease. A comprehensive analysis and considerations for developing a new model. JAMA 1991; 266: 2594-604.
92. Sellors JW, Mahony JB, Chemesky MA, et al. Tubal factor infertility: an association with prior chlamydial infection and asymptomatic salpingitis. Fertil Steril 1988; 49: 451-7.
93. Paavonen J, Kiviat N, Brunham RC, et al. Prevalence and manifestations of endometritis among women with cervicitis. Am J Obstet Gynecol 1985; 152: 280-6.
94. Cleary RE, Jones RB. Recovery of *Chlamydia trachomatis* from the endometrium in infertile women with serum antichlamydial antibodies. Fertil Steril 1985; 44: 233-5.
95. Henry-Suchet J Catalan F, Loffredo V, et al. *Chlamydia trachomatis* associated with chronic inflammation in abdominal specimens from women selected for tuboplasty. Fertil Steril 1981; 35: 599-605.

96. Patton DL, Askienazy-Elbhar M, Henry-Suchet, et al. Detection of *Chlamydia trachomatis* in fallopian tube tissue in women with post infectious tubal infertility. Am J Obstet Gynecol 1994; 171: 95-101.
97. Wolner-Hanssen P. Silent pelvic inflammatory disease: is it overstarted? Obstet Gynecol 1995; 86: 321-5.
98. Jacobson L, Westrom L. Objectivized diagnosis of acute pelvic inflammatory disease. Am J Obstet Gynecol 1969; 105: 1088-98.
99. Eschenbach DA, Wolner-Hanssen P, Hawes SE, et al. Acute pelvic inflammatory disease: association of clinical and laboratory findings with laparoscopic findings. Obstet Gynecol 1997; 89: 184-92.
100. Westrom L. Diagnosis, aetiology and prognosis of acute salpingitis (Thesis). Lund, Sweden: Student literature; 1997.
101. Paavonen J, Aine R, Teisala K, et al. Compairson of endometrial biopsy and peritoneal fluid cytology with laparoscopy in the diagnosis of acute pelvic inflammatory disease. Am J Obstet Gynecol 1985; 151: 645-50.
102. Boardman LA, Peipert JF, Brody JM, et al. Endovaginal sonography for the diagnosis of upper genital tract infection. Obstet Gynecol 1997; 90: 54-7.
103. Pavonen J, Meittinen A, Heinonen PK, et al. Serum CA 125 levels in acute pelvic inflammatory disease. Br J Obstet Gynaecol 1989; 96: 574-9.
104. Centers for Disease Control and Prevention. Guidelines for treatment of sexually transmitted diseases. MMWR 2006; 55 (RR-11): 1-94.
105. Landers DV, Sweet RL. Tubo-ovarian abscess: contemporary approach to management. Rev Infect Dis 1983; 5: 876-84.
106. Westrom LV, Joesoef R, Reynolds G, et al. Pelvic inflammatory disease and fertility. A cohort study of 1,8444 women with laparoscopically verified disease and 657 control women with normal laparoscopic results. Sex Transm Dis 1992; 19: 185-92.
107. Westrom LV. Sexually transmitted diseases and infertility. Sex Transm Dis 1994; 21 (Suppl): 532-7.
108. Safrin S, Schachter J, Dahrouge D, et al. Long term sequelae of acute pelvic inflamma-tory disease. Am J Obstet Gynecol 1992; 166: 1300-5.
109. Chow JM, Schachter J. Long term sequelae of pelvic inflammatory disease: Infertility, ectopic pregnancy and chronic pelvic pain. In: Landers DC, Sweet RL eds. Pelvic inflammatory disease. New York, 1997: 152-169.
110. Buchan H, Vessex M, Goldacre M, Fairweather J. Morbidity following pelvic inflammatory disease. Br J Obstet Gynecol 1993; 100: 558-62.
111. Soper D, Ness RB. Pelvic inflammatory disease and involuntary infertility: prospective pilot observations. Infect Dis Obstet Gynecol 1995; 3: 145-8.
112. Fitz-Hugh T. Acute gonococcal peritonitis of the right upper quadrant in women. JAMA 1934; 102: 2984.
113. Pedowitz P, Bloomfield RD. Ruptured adnexal abscess with generalized peritonitis. Am J Obstet Gynecol 1964; 88: 721-9.
114. Westrom L, Wolner-Hanssen P. Pathogenesis of pelvic inflammatory disease. Genitourin Med 1993; 69: 9-17.
115. Mardh PA. Pelvic inflammatory disease and related disorders; novel observations. Scan J Obstet Gynecol 1990; 69 (Suppl): 83-7.
116. McCormack WM. Pelvic inflammatory disease. N Engl J Med 1994; 330: 115-9.
117. Lepine LA, Hillis SD, Marchbanks PA, et al. Severity of pelvic inflammatory disease as a predictor of the probability of live birth. Am J Obstet Gynecol 1998; 178: 977-81.
118. Bjercke S, Purvis K. Chlamydial serology in the investigation of infertility. Hum Reprod 1992; 7: 621-4.
119. Reiners J, Collet M, Frost E. Chlamydial antibodies and tubal infertility. Int J Epidemiol 1989; 18: 261-3.
120. Walkers MD, Eddy CA, Gibbs RS. Antibodies to *Chlamydia trachomatis* and ectopic pregnancy. Am J Obstet Gynecol 1998; 259: 1823-7.
121. Coste J, Job Spira N, Fernandez H, et al. Risk factors for ectopic pregnancy: A case-control study in France, with special focus on infectious factors. Am J Epidemiol 1991; 133: 839-49.
122. Sheffield PA, Moore DE, Voight LF, et al. The association between *Chlamydia trachomatis* serology and pelvic damage in women with

tubal ectopic gestations. Fertil Steril 1993; 60: 970-5.
123. Odland JO, Anestad G, Rasmussen S, et al. Ectopic pregnancy and chlamydial serology. Int J Obstet Gynecol 1993; 43: 271-5.
124. Miettinen A, Heinonnen PK, Teisala K, et al. Serologic evidence for the role of *Chlamydia trachomatis, Neisseria gonorrhoeae* and *Mycoplasma hominis* in the aetiology of tubal factor infertility and ectopic pregnancy. Sex Transm Dis 1990; 17: 10-4.
125. Robertson JN, Hogston P, Ward ME. Gonococcal and chlamydial antibodies in ectopic and intrauterine pregnancy. Br J Obstet Gynecol 1988; 95: 711-16.
126. Westrom L, Svensson L. Chronic pain after acute pelvic inflmmatory disease. In: Belfort P, Piotti JA, Eskes TKAB eds. Advances in gynaecology and obstetrics: Proceeding of the XII the World Congress of Gynaecology Obstetrics, Rio de Janeiro, October, 1988, vol 6: 265-72.
127. Walker CK, Kahn JG, Washington AE, et al. Pelvic Inflammatory Disease: metaanalysis of antimicrobial regimen efficacy. J Infect Dis 1993; 168: 969-78.
128. Collins CG, Nix FC, Cerrha HT. Ruptured tubo-ovarian abscess. Am J Obstet Gynecol 1956; 72: 820.
129. McNeeley SG, Hendrix SL, Mazzoni MM, et al. Medically sound, cost effective treatment for pelvic inflammatory disease and tubooovarian abscess. Am J Obstet Gynecol 1998; 178: 1272-8.
130. Gerzof SG, Robbins AH, Johnson WC, et al. Percutaneous catheter drainage of abdominal abscesses. N Engl J Med 1981; 305: 653-7.
131. Falk V. Treatment of acute nontuberculous salpingitis with antibiotics alone and in Combination with glucocorticoids. Acta Obstet Gynecol Scand 1965; 44: 3-18.
132. Sweet RL, Landers DV. Pelvic inflammatory disease in HIV-positive women. Lancet 1997; 349: 1265-6.
133. Barbosa C, Macaat M, Brockman S, et al. Pelivic inflammatory disease and human immunodeficiency virus infection. Obstet Gynecol 1997; 89: 65-70.
134. Korn AP, Landers DV. Gynecologic disease in women infected with human immunodeficiency virus-1. Acquir Immuno Defic Syndr 1995; 9: 361-70.
135. Kamenga MC, De Cock KM, St. Louis ME, et al. The impact of human immunodeficiency virus infection on pelvic inflammatory disease: a case control study in Adidjan, Ivory Coast. Am J Obstet Gynecol 1995; 172: 919-25.
136. Cohen CR, Sinei S, Reilly M, et al. Effect of HIV-1 infection upon acute salpingitis: a laparoscopic study. J Infect Dis 1998; 178: 1352-8.

31 | EPIDIDYMITIS AND PROSTATITIS

Nitin S Walia, AK Jaiswal

In this chapter

- Epididymitis
- Aetiopathogenesis
- Diagnosis
- Complications of Acute Epididymitis
- Treatment
- Chronic Epididymitis
- Prostatitis
- Clissification
- Acute Bacterial Prostatitis
- Chronic Bacterial Prostatitis
- Chronic Pelvic Pain Syndrome
- Inflammatory CPPS/Non-Bacterial Prostatitis
- Non-Inflammatory CPPS/Prostatodynia
- Asymptomatic Inflammatory Prostatitis
- Granulomatous Prostatitis

EPIDIDYMITIS

Acute epididymitis is the clinical syndrome consisting of pain, swelling, and inflammation of the epididymis of usually less than 6 weeks while chronic epididymitis is defined as long-standing pain/discomfort in the epididymis and testicle, usually without swelling. Regardless of aetiology, the pain associated with both the acute and chronic condition can cause significant morbidity with as many as six million cases occurring annually in the United States.[1] Researchers have reported that the incidence of epididymitis may range from 1-4 cases per 1000 men per year.[2]

AETIOPATHOGENESIS

Until recently, this condition was considered idiopathic in at least 50 % of patients.[3] Indeed, even with the current state of research into the causes of epididymitis, specific infectious agents have been identified in only 80% of patients. Since the majority of epididymitis are attributed to an ascending infection from the urethra, prostate, and bladder (to the epididymis), the same considerations in the pathogenesis and clinical evaluation apply as to urethritis, prostatitis or cystitis.

The sexually transmitted organisms *N. gonorrhoeae* and *Chlamydia trachomatis* have been clearly established to be the most common etiologic agents in sexually active heterosexual men under the age of 35 years (Table 31.1).[4] Although a history of sexual exposure can usually be elicited in men with *Chlamydia trachomatis* or *N. gonorrhoeae*, this exposure may be more than 30 days before the onset of symptoms. Watson found that half of the patients with epididymitis attributable to *N. gonorrhoeae* did not have urethral discharge.[5] *C. trachomatis* was isolated in approximately two thirds of the NGU patients. In a small series of homosexual men under the age of 35 years with concomitant cystitis, the most common etiologic agent identified was *E. coli*.[6]

Coliform bacteria and pseudomonas (which are not primarily sexually transmitted organisms) account for the aetiology of the majority of cases in men over 35 and in prepubertal boys. These patients often have either congenital or acquired structural urologic abnormalities. Reports implicating the following organisms in epididymitis have also been noted: *Trichomonas vaginalis, Schistosomia haematobium, Coccidioidis imitis, Haemophilus influenzae, Neisseria meningitidis, Brucella* species and *Salmonella species*.[7-10]

Table 31.1 Aetiology of Acute Epididymitis

1. Non-sexually transmitted pathogens:
   (a) *Coliforms or Pseudomonas aeruginosa*
   (b) *Mycobacterium tuberculosis*
   (c) *Miscellaneous*
       Schistosoma haematobium
       Coccidioides immitis
       Haemophilus influenzae
       Neisseria meningitidis
       Brucella species
       Salmonella species
2. Sexually Transmitted pathogens:
   (a) *Neisseria gonorrhoeae*
   (b) *Chlamydia trachomatis*
   (c) *Trichomonas vaginalis*

Before the availability of cultures for *Chlamydia trachomatis*, most epididymitis was thought to be caused by the reflux of sterile urine down the vas deferens while straining against a closed urethral sphincter. Voiding cystourethrography in the non-obstructed non-infected urinary tract has failed to show urethro-vasal reflux, even when straining caused intravesical pressure to exceed 70 cm H_2O pressure.[11] However, an inflamed or physically injured verumontanum may cause alterations in the vasal-urethral "valve", permitting bacterial entry into the vas.[12] In such cases, straining may cause retrograde bacterial spread from an infected seminal vesicle into the vas and epididymis. Candidal epididymitis in immunocompromised (AIDS and transplant) patients has been documented. Epididymitis can also occur due to certain non infective etiologies like polyarteritis nodosa.[13]

DIAGNOSIS

Inflammation of the epididymis causes pain and swelling which is almost always unilateral and usually acute in onset. There may be a history of symptoms suggestive of urinary tract infection. Frequency of micturition, urgency and dysuria are common. On examination the scrotum on the affected side is erythematous, oedematous and tender.[14] The tail of the epididymis at the lower pole of the testis swells up first and later the swelling spreads to the head of the epididymis. The groove between the epididymis and testicle is maintained, unless concomitantly involved.

Gram stain, urine and urethral cultures will demonstrate the causative organism in the majority of cases of epididymitis. Serum micro immunofluorescence antibody titres to *Chlamydia trachomatis* will show a four-fold rise in titres when paired sera are tested, and they are more sensitive than culture. Cultures of epididymal aspirates should be used in only unusual circumstances e.g. patients with indwelling Foley's catheter who have polymicrobial flora present in the urine, patients found at surgical exploration for torsion of testes to have epididymitis, and in patients who fail to respond or develop recurrent epididymitis with uncertain aetiologic agents.[15]

Conditions easily confused with epididymitis include torsion of the spermatic cord or the appendages, testicular infarction, abscess or tumor and traumatic rupture. None of these, except testicular abscess, will usually demonstrate pyuria or bacteriuria. Moreover, in 15% of patients with early torsion, there is swelling only in the epididymis. Diagnosis can be confirmed by Doppler ultrasound or technetium 99 m radionuclide flow scan.[16,17] Colour coded Doppler ultrasonography has a sensitivity of 70% and specificity of 88%.[18] Since epididymitis is rare in prepubertal boys and torsion is relatively common, prompt surgical exploration is recommended to rule out torsion. Similarly, Doppler or radionuclide scan should always be done in men under the age of 35 years as both torsion and epididymitis are common. MRI has also been found to be accurate in the differential diagnosis of epididymitis and torsion in a small series.[19]

In men or boys found to have coliform epididymitis, radiographic and cystoscopic evaluation should be performed to find a structural reason for the patient to have a urinary infection. Intravenous urography will disclose urologic abnormalities in 42 to 54 per cent of men with coliform epididymitis.[20] There may be prostatic calculi, benign prostatic hypertrophy, chronic bacterial prostatitis, neurogenic bladder or a history of recent urinary instrumentation. Intravenous urography in prepubertal children has shown colovesical fistula, reflux of urine into ejaculatory ducts, ectopic ejaculatory ducts, posterior urethral valves, bulbous urethral stricture, and neurogenic bladder.[21]

COMPLICATIONS OF ACUTE EPIDIDYMITIS

The most serious local complications are testicular infarction and abscess formation. Testicular infarction probably results from thrombosis of the spermatic vessels secondary to severe inflammation.[22] Infertility is a known complication of epididymitis as it may lead to bilateral occlusion of vas deferens. Decreased spermatogenesis, delayed sperm maturation and sperm antibodies may in addition cause infertility.[23]

TREATMENT

Therapy may be based on the clinical examination of urinary sediment and urethral swab. Treatment is directed to the specific etiologic organism suspected on initial evaluation and started immediately after collection of culture specimens. Therefore, when urethritis is associated with epididymitis, the treatment of choice is injection ceftriaxone 250 mg IM followed by doxycycline 100 mg PO bid or tetracycline 500 mg PO qid for 10 days. When bacteriuria is present, treatment must be guided by sensitivity testing of the organisms. For epididymitis caused by enteric organisms, for patients allergic to cephalosporin and/or tetracycline or for epididymitis in patients aged > 35 years, either ofloxacin 300 mg orally bid or levofloxacin 500 mg orally once daily for 10 days is recommended.[24]

Supportive measures should include bed rest, scrotal elevation, and oral non-steroidal anti-inflammatory drugs. Elevation improves lymphatic drainage and relieves the sensation of pressure and hence the Prehn sign is unreliable in distinguishing epididymitis from torsion. Injection of the spermatic cord with a local anesthetic may be of symptomatic benefit. In patients in whom the etiologic agent is a sexually transmitted pathogen, treatment is not complete without treatment of the sexual partner.

Patients who have uncomplicated acute epididymitis and also are infected with HIV should receive the same treatment regimen as those who are HIV negative. Fungi and mycobacteria, however, are more likely to cause acute epididymitis in immunosuppressed patients than in immunocompetent patients.

CHRONIC EPIDIDYMITIS

Chronic epididymitis is defined as "symptoms of discomfort and/or pain at least 3 months in duration in the scrotum, testicle, or epididymis, localized to one or each epididymis on clinical examination."[25]

Classification

Inflammatory Chronic Epididymitis

- Idiopathic
- Secondary
  - Infective-Chlamydia, Brucellosis, and Schistosomiasis
  - Post infective (after acute bacterial epididymitis)
  - Tuberculosis
  - Drug induced (amiodarone)
  - Associated with a known syndrome (eg, Behçet's disease)[26]

Obstructive Chronic Epididymitis

It is due to the congenital, acquired or iatrogenic obstruction of the epididymis or vas deferens.

Chronic Epididymylgia

It is characterized by pain or discomfort in the normal epididymis associated with no identifiable pathology. Epididymitis secondary to treatment with the antiarrhythmic drug amiodarone appears to be due to the selective concentration of the drug in the head of the epididymis.[27] This disorder is not associated with urethral or urinary inflammation; antibiotics have no role and responds favorably to a decrease in the dosage of amiodarone.

It is mandatory to treat all other cases of chronic epididymitis with a course of antibiotics. Epididymectomy should be considered if there is no resolution after 4-6 weeks of conservative management. Tubercular infection is invariably bilateral, concomitant with involvement of other genitourinary organs and has higher prevalence in HIV setting. In cases of chronic tuberculous epididymitis, a course of anti-tuberculous therapy should be given but is less effective. If the lesions do not revolve by 2 months, epididymectomy is advised.[28]

PROSTATITIS

Introduction

Prostatitis syndromes represent a common clinical entity grouped together to encompass symptoms and clinical signs associated with disorders of the prostate gland. These diverse symptoms include increased urinary frequency, feeling of incomplete emptying, difficulty in urination, perineal pain or discomfort, low back pain and lower abdominal pain.

Prostatitis and related syndromes are still regarded as an obscure ill-understood condition. This is due to a number of factors: the organ is deeply placed and poorly accessible to clinical examination, the etiology and pathology is unclear, investigation is complex and therapy is time-consuming and unsatisfactory.[29] This is unfortunate because prostatitis is the most common urologic diagnosis in men younger than 50 years and the third most common urologic diagnosis in men older than 50 years, representing 8% of urologic office practice.[30] Recent interest on the subject has lead to a new consensus clinical and histopathological classification and symptoms score index for better clinical management and therapeutic outlook.[31]

Anatomy

The prostate consists of acini draining into ducts, which in turn drain into the prostatic urethra and these are set in a stroma of collagen and muscle tissue. The gland can be divided into a small central zone around the prostatic urethra, and a larger peripheral zone forming 75% of the parenchyma of the gland. An important difference between the zones is that the ducts draining the central zone enter the prostatic urethra at an acute angle compared with the ducts draining the peripheral zone. Urine can thus, enter the peripheral zones more readily than the central zone ducts. Furthermore, contraction of the internal sphincter muscle will tend to compress the ducts of the central zone rather than those of the peripheral zone. During ejaculation, when the internal sphincter muscle is contracted, the intra-urethral pressure rises dramatically and semen enters the peripheral zone ducts more easily than the central zone ducts **(Fig. 31.1)**. Thus, the inflammatory process mainly affects the peripheral zone while the central zone around the urethra is relatively unaffected.[32,33]

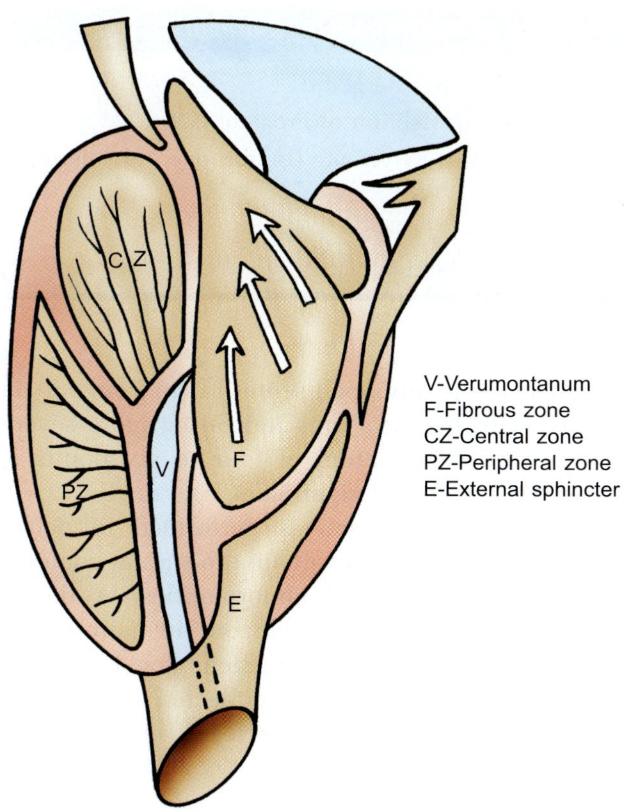

Fig. 31.1 Prostate-Sagittal Section

Pathogenesis

The possible routes of infection in prostate include:

(a) Ascending urethral infection
(b) Reflux of infected urine into prostatic ducts that empty into the prostatic urethra
(c) Invasion by rectal bacteria through direct extension or by lymphatic spread
(d) haematogenous spread

Kirby et al. showed direct evidence of reflux into the prostate.[34] Anatomic or neuro-physiological obstruction resulting in high pressure dysfunctional flow patterns may be the cause of the reflux. This explains the observation that the organisms found in bacterial prostatitis do not differ significantly in type and prevalence from those causing other urinary tract infections.[35]

It is also well established that bacterial prostatitis can develop in men who have phimosis, indwelling urethral catheter or condom drainage system and immediately after transurethral prostatic resection. In addition, the refluxing urine by causing a chemical prostatitis may initiate and perpetuate the chronic inflammatory process in abacterial prostatitis and prostatodynia.[36] The constituents of the refluxing urine contribute towards the formation of prostatic stones by precipitation of minerals upon existing corpora amylacea. Bacterial colonization in protective aggregates or biofilms in these prostatic calculi may lead to recalcitrant chronic prostatitis and recurrent UTI despite antibiotic therapy.[37]

The prostate may be secondarily involved from another primary infection. Lymphatic drainage from nearby sources of infection such as the bladder, urethra or the rectum may influence inflammation of the prostate. There are reports of the involvement of the prostate with procto-colitis especially in homosexual males. Rarely, infection may be haematogenous, consequent upon septicemia or pyaemia; prostatitis is then a complication of another acute illness.[38]

HIV has given a new dimension to the frequency and spectrum of opportunistic infections. The prevalence of bacterial prostatitis among HIV-infected patients was reported to increase from 3% in asymptomatic carriers to 14% in patients with AIDS.[38] Both B and T-cell dysfunction and local immuno-deficiency of prostatic fluid can explain the abnormal susceptibility of patients to infections and favors prostatic abscess formation. Typical and atypical bacteria as well as viral and fungal agents have been recognized as the cause of prostatitis. HIV-infected patients often have persistent sub-clinical foci causing relapsing prostatitis due to the ability of the prostate to harbor organisms and the poor penetration of antimicrobials in prostate tissue.[39]

Sensory or motor dysfunctions of the lower urinary tract or a pelvic musculature abnormality have been held responsible for the symptomatology of chronic pelvic pain syndrome. These may be triggered by urogenital infections, surgery, trauma, abnormal sexual activities and psychological factors.[40]

CLASSIFICATION

Drach, Meares, Fair and Stamey described the first accepted classification separating prostatitis into four groups: Acute bacterial prostatitis (ABP), Chronic Bacterial Prostatitis (CBP), Chronic Abacterial Prostatitis (CAP) and Prostatodynia (PD) according to the cytological and micro-biological findings in both the urine and expressed prostatic secretions.[41] Unfortunately , many patients could not be classified correctly despite persisting symptomatology as it was strictly based on the 4-glass urine test. This has been replaced by the recent NIH classification (Table 31.2).[42]

Table 31.2 Classification of Prostatitis

Meares and Stamey (Traditional)	*National Institute of Health (NIH) – Category*
Acute Bacterial Prostatitis (ABP)	I – Acute Infection of Prostate gland
Chronic Bacterial Prostatitis (CBP)	II – Chronic/Recurrent Infection of Prostate gland
	III – Chronic Pelvic Pain Syndrome (in absence of bacteria)
Non Bacterial Prostatitis (NBP)	III A – Inflammatory CPPS
Prostatodynia (PD)	III B – Non-Inflammatory CPPS
N/A	IV – Asymptomatic Inflammatory Prostatitis

According to this classification, Category III (Chronic Pelvic Pain Syndrome) is based on symptomatology and a new group of asymptomatic patients with significant leukocytes/bacteria in prostate-specific specimens (EPS, semen or biopsy) are classified as category IV.

Evaluation of Prostatitis

The NIH Chronic Prostatitis Collaborative Research Network followed up with a reproducible and valid symptom index (Appendix 31.1) based on three parameters – pain, urinary symptoms and quality of life to assess the patient's baseline status and response to therapy (total scores range from 0 to 43 points, with higher scores indicating more severe symptoms). A reduction of four to six points is generally considered significant.[43]

Genital examination is performed to detect urethral discharge, to evaluate the scrotal contents and to assess perineal abnormalities. A digital rectal examination is carried out in conjunction with the collection of specimens for laboratory evaluation. The specimen is collected sequentially in sterile containers to perform microbiologic studies **(Fig. 31.2)**.

(a) Collect the first 10 ml (VB1: voided bladder 1) of urine as it represents the urethral specimen.

(b) Collect midstream urine (VB2) after passing 100–200 ml as a representative of bladder urine.
(c) Examine the prostate and then massage (except in acute prostatitis) the prostate in an attempt to express prostatic secretions (EPS) for direct microscopy to evaluate for polymorphonuclear leukocytes, motile trichomonas and culture. More than 10 polymorphonuclear leukocytes per HPF are considered abnormal. Clumping of polymorphonuclear cells and a reduction in the number of lecithin bodies also indicates inflammation of the prostate. An additional finding is the presence of macrophages containing fat droplets, also called oval fat bodies.
(d) Collect the next 10 ml of urine (VB3) voided immediately after prostatic massage as it includes EPS left in the prostatic urethra.

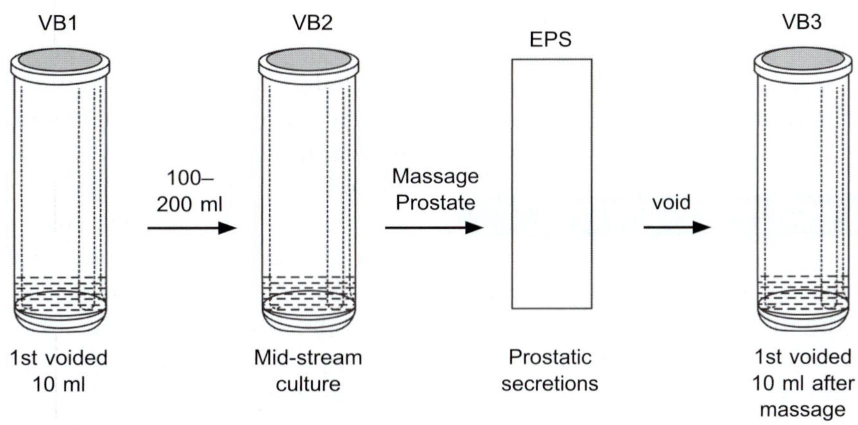

Fig. 31.2 Segmental Cultures of Lower Urinary Tract in Men

The urine specimens are centrifuged and sediment examined under HPF for leukocytes, macrophages, oval fat bodies, erythrocytes, bacteria and fungal hyphae. For the culture, the laboratory should be requested to inoculate media that will detect classical urinary tract pathogens and to use a 0.1 ml inoculum as well as the standard 0.001 ml inoculum. The former sample facilitates the detection and quantification of organisms in low numbers. The specimens must be processed as soon as possible because prostatic fluid contains antibacterial substances that may inhibit their growth.[44]

In conjunction with the urine specimens, some investigators prefer to have the patient provide a semen ejaculate rather than only obtaining expressed prostatic secretions.[45] Bacterial concentrations 10 times higher in the post massage urine or prostatic secretions than in the midstream urine (bladder bacteriuria) provide proof that the prostate is infected. If high numbers of organisms are present in the midstream urine (bladder bacteriuria), localization cannot be done. Non- inflammatory CPPS is diagnosed when no uropathogenic bacteria are cultured and there are insignificant leukocytes in EPS/VB3. Shoskes and colleagues, from the NIH Chronic Prostatitis Collaborative Network, recently reported that by culturing EPS or semen for 5 days rather than the conventional 2 days, an additional 7.5% of CPPS patients would be found positive for bacteria that actually localize to the prostate gland.[46]

This gold standard urologic evaluation has been replaced by a simpler 2-glass pre-(VB2) and post-massage (VB3) urine test in clinical practice. If acute bacterial prostatitis is a possibility, blood culture specimen is obtained and the midstream urine sample alone is adequate.[47]

Another promising approach is to investigate cytokine and oxidative stress levels in EPS and prostate specific secretions. IL-1β and TNF-α levels appeared higher in men with CPPS- IIIA than in those with CPPS-IIIB and healthy controls.[48] Recombinant RNA reverse transcriptase polymerase chain reaction (PCR) for the detection of bacterial genomic fragments in the prostate secretions could also provide further evidence of infection. Gram-positive bacteria identified by the use of this protocol were associated with increased markers of inflammation in prostate specific secretions.[49]

Transrectal ultrasonography is extensively used to evaluate the prostate but is unable to conclusively provide evidence of prostatitis.[50] Urethroscopy or prostate biopsy is not by itself useful in the evaluation of prostatitis.[51] A wide variety of abnormalities have been demonstrated in urodynamic studies, particularly in patients of CPPS. However, these are more useful in excluding other disorders of the urogenital tract.[52]

ACUTE BACTERIAL PROSTATITIS

ABP is rare, probably the easiest to diagnose, as well as to treat, among the different clinical entities in prostatitis. It is dramatic in its manifestations and presents the signs and symptoms of an acute septic process. This entity is characterized by the sudden onset of high fever up to 40°C, chills, marked malaise and sometimes myalgia or arthralgia.

Irritative micturition symptoms of frequency, urgency and dysuria soon develop and there may appear an associated urethral discharge. Difficulty in micturition or acute retention of urine may occur. There is usually a dull aching pain in the perineum, rectum or sacrococcygeal region.

Rectal examination reveals a swollen, very tender and warm prostate; sometimes the prostate feels indurated with scattered soft areas. Prostatic massage will produce a thick purulent discharge full of white blood cells and oval fat bodies, which will grow large numbers of pathogens on culture. However, prostatic massage is both painful and dangerous to the patient as it may induce bacteremia in the acute stages of the disease. It is also unnecessary, as acute bacterial prostatitis is usually associated with a bladder infection by the same organism that is in the prostate, allowing for identification of the pathogen by culture of the voided urine, the urine obtained by supra-pubic needle aspiration of the bladder, or the urethral discharge whenever present.[53]

The organisms causing acute bacterial prostatitis are usually those commonly found in urinary tract infections including the Gram-negative enteric bacteria or *Pseudomonas aeruginosa* as well as Gram-positive *staphylococci* and *streptococci*. Occasionally salmonella and anaerobic bacteria such as *Bacteroides fragilis* or *Clostridium perfringens* can also cause prostatitis.[54]

Therapy

At the beginning, the patient will require bed rest, adequate hydration, antipyretics, analgesics or spasmolytic drugs to alleviate the perineal or rectal pain and stool softeners. Urethral instrumentation should be avoided. Parenteral broad-spectrum antibiotics should be instituted immediately after collection of urine and blood specimens for culture. A combination of aminoglycoside and β-lactam antibiotic is the first choice. However, fluoroquinolones or third generation cephalosporin's are alternative single drug therapies. The intense diffuse inflammation enhances the passage of antimicrobial agents from plasma into the prostatic ducts and acini and the patient usually responds dramatically to therapy.

Acute bacterial prostatitis is a self-limiting disease and only rarely will it develop into a chronic infection. Some patients may continue to experience a certain degree of irritative micturition symptoms in spite of the bacteriological cure of the acute inflammatory process. Rectal examination may still reveal a hard prostate and several months may pass before the prostate returns to a normal consistency.

Prostatic abscess is a rare complication of acute prostatitis seen in immunocompromised or diabetic individuals in the past. It has now become increasingly rare since the advent of effective antibacterial therapy.[55] It should be suspected if a patient of acute bacterial prostatitis or urinary tract infection develops a spiking fever and fluctuation of the prostate in spite of adequate antibacterial therapy. These are caused mainly by *E. coli*. Sometimes metastatic abscess to the prostate may develop from a septic focus elsewhere and is caused mainly by Gram-positive organisms such as *Staphylococcus aureus*.[56] In rare instances, anaerobic bacteria or *Blastomyces dermatitidis* may cause an acute prostatic abscess.[57] Transrectal ultrasound and computerized tomography are helpful in early detection of prostatic abscess.[58] The main and definite treatment of an acute prostatic abscess is adequate surgical drainage by transurethral unroofing or perineal incision as soon as possible after adequate antimicrobial coverage.

CHRONIC BACTERIAL PROSTATITIS

The clinical picture of chronic bacterial prostatitis is quite variable and is typified by recurrent episodes of irritative voiding symptoms such as frequency, urgency and dysuria, occasionally associated with perineal discomfort, low back pain, myalgia or arthralgia and is sometimes complicated by epididymitis. Chills and fever are unusual, although post-ejaculatory pain and haemospermia occasionally occur. No findings on physical examination, rectal examination of the prostate, cystoscopy or urography are specifically diagnostic of chronic bacterial prostatitis. However, it is characterized by two basic features (a) recurrent urinary tract infections and (b) persistence of pathogenic bacteria in the prostatic fluid. These are mainly Gram negative enterobacteria (*E. coli, Proteus* or *Klebsiella*) or *Pseudomonas aeruginosa* and are found only in small numbers in the prostate. Sterilization of urine generally affords relief of symptoms; however, the objective of therapy should be alleviation of symptoms.[59] Chronic bacterial prostatitis may be associated with abnormalities of prostatic architecture like prostatic calculi or fibrosis.[60]

Therapy

Chronic bacterial prostatitis poses a real therapeutic challenge to the treating physician constituting about 5-15% of the prostatitis cases. Trimethoprim-sulphamethoxazole (TMP-SMX) seemed promising but even long-term (4-16 weeks) therapy in full dosage affected a cure in only 33-55% of cases.[61] Other agents with reported efficacy include carbenicillin, erythromycin, minocycline, doxycycline and cephalexin. Stamey et al. revealed that most of these drugs are unable to cross the electrically charged lipid membrane of the prostatic epithelium to reach therapeutic levels within the prostatic acini.[62]

Newer fluoroquinolones reach high concentrations in the prostatic secretions and have proved very effective in prospective comparative studies. Recommended dosage is ciprofloxacin 500 mg PO bid or norfloxacin 400 mg PO bid for 4-12 wks. Direct injection of antimicrobial agents into the prostate has also been proposed but has not become an accepted mode of administration. Studies have shown that only 40% of patients have symptomatic improvement with antimicrobial therapy despite the pathogens being highly sensitive to the antibacterials. Patients not cured by medical therapy can usually be managed satisfactorily by use of continuous suppressive therapy using low dose medication. Preferred regimens include TMP-SMX (one single-strength tablet daily), or nitrofurantoin 100 mg once or twice daily. Suppressive therapy generally controls symptoms and prevents bacteriuria.[63] In Patients with HIV, a prolonged therapy and follow up is required so as to avoid complications.[55]

Table 31.3 Clinical Features of Common Prostatitis Syndromes

Syndrome/NIH Category	*H/O UTI*	*EPS Culture Positive*	*WBCs in EPS*	*Response to Antibiotics*
ABP/I	Yes	Yes*	Yes	Yes
CBP/II	Yes	Yes	Yes	Usually Yes
NBP/IIIA	No	No	Yes	Usually No
PD/IIIB	No	No	No	No

* Prostatic massage is contraindicated in ABP

Patients with persistent symptoms are managed similar to CPPS with other drugs and therapies. Complete excision of the prostate, seminal vesicles and ampulla of vas deferens should uniformly cure all patients of refractory chronic bacterial prostatitis; however, the potential complications and consequences of this radical surgery seldom makes this a reasonable choice unless associated pathologic conditions like prostatic calculi, benign prostatic hyperplasia, or adenocarcinoma of the prostate are also present.[64]

CHRONIC PELVIC PAIN SYNDROME

Chronic prostatitis/chronic pelvic pain syndrome (category III) accounts for 90%-95% of all prostatitis cases.[65] Patients with CPPS have a large variety of symptoms referable to the genitalia (pain along the penis and in the testicles and scrotum, painful ejaculation), the musculoskeletal system (low back pain, perineal pain or discomfort, rectal pain, pain along the inner aspect of the thighs), the lower urinary tract (irritative: frequency, urgency, burning on micturition, suprapubic discomfort) or have obstructive (hesitancy, decreased urinary stream) and psychosexual symptoms (decreased libido, impotence). The symptoms tend to wax and wane over time and have a significant impact on the individual's health. Physical examination is usually unremarkable, and the prostate is normal on rectal examination.[66]

INFLAMMATORYCPPS/NON-BACTERIAL PROSTATITIS

Non-bacterial prostatitis (syn. abacterial prostatitis, prostatosis), the most common type of prostatitis syndrome, is an inflammatory condition of unknown cause. The findings of Schaeffer and co-workers suggest that the incidence of non-bacterial prostatitis exceeds that of bacterial prostatitis by eight-fold.[67]

Although many clinical features of chronic bacterial prostatitis and non-bacterial prostatitis are similar, one important difference bears emphasis-the patient with non-bacterial prostatitis has no history of documented urinary tract infection or positive culture localizing a causative agent to the prostate. Like patients with chronic bacterial prostatitis, however, patients with non-bacterial prostatitis have excessive number of leukocytes and fat laden macrophages in their prostatic fluids.

The etiology of non-bacterial prostatitis is unclear. Extensive microbiologic studies by different investigators have excluded *Neisseria gonorrhoeae*, *Trichomonas vaginalis*, *Gardnerella vaginalis* and *Mycoplasma genitalium* in playing any role in the etiology. Other studies evaluated potential organisms like *Chlamydia trachomatis*, *Ureaplasma urealyticum* in addition to a host of fungi, viruses and anaerobic bacteria in men with persistent chronic non-bacterial prostatitis with no conclusive results. Recent molecular and specialized cultural findings designed to detect fastidious and difficult-to-culture bacteria in prostatic tissue and fluids point to a possible etiologic role for cryptic micro-organisms like *Coagulase-negative Staphylococci* and *Corynebacterium group*. Some workers have proposed prostaglandins, autoimmunity, neuromuscular dysfunction and psychological abnormalities as etiological factors. It thus appears that either non- bacterial prostatitis is an infectious disease caused by yet unidentified pathogens or it is a non-infectious inflammation of the prostate.[68]

Therapy

In view of the fact that the cause of NBP is unknown, no specific therapy for this condition is available. The patient should be reassured, that in spite of unpleasant symptoms that would continue for an indefinite period, no serious condition is present and no complications are expected in the future-primarily no impairment in sexual ability or fertility.

A clinical trial of fluoroquinolones orally for 2-12 wks is indicated. Antibiotics may benefit patients of CPPS in 3 ways: a placebo effect, effect on non-cultured microorganisms, or the anti-inflammatory effect of some antibiotics. Unless the clinical response is definitely favorable, additional treatment using antimicrobial agents is unwarranted.[69]

The main treatment plan should be to control symptoms. Normal sexual activity is encouraged and dietary restrictions imposed only if spicy foods or alcoholic beverages appear to cause or aggravate the symptoms. General relaxant measures such as hot Sitz baths and spasmolytics are indicated to relieve symptoms. Prostatic massage is probably therapeutic only in men who have congested prostates related to infrequent sexual activity. Pain and discomfort often respond to short courses of anti-inflammatory agents; irritative voiding dysfunction usually responds to the use of anticholinergics. In case of proven or suspected functional obstruction of the bladder neck, treatment with alpha-receptor blockers may be of help.[70] Allopurinol has been reported to be effective in small trials but which has not been widely adopted.[71] The efficacy of oral zinc preparations and megavitamins remains unproven.[72]

NON-INFLAMMATORY CPPS/ PROSTATODYNIA

In their classification of prostatitis, Drach and his associates applied the term 'Prostatodynia' to men in whom there were symptoms of urinary irritation or voiding dysfunction in addition to impotence and painful ejaculation. Typically, genitourinary examination reveals no specific abnormality. Bacterial culture is negative and microscopy of prostatic fluids is normal. Such cases require a full urological evaluation, both of the prostate and the outflow tract.

These patients are difficult to treat and in most, there is a neurotic overlay of variable degree. This is easy to understand, as most would have undergone a multiplicity of antibiotic courses, invasive investigations and perhaps a transurethral resection during the course of their illness. Before concluding that the symptoms are entirely psychological, consideration should be given to the findings of Segure et al. who observed that involuntary contractions of the pelvic floor might account for the pain and discomfort and the obstructive urinary symptoms.[73]

When there is functional disturbance in urinary flow, improvement may be obtained with alpha-adrenergic blocking agents in a dose sufficient to allow relaxation of the autonomic component of external sphincter without producing effects on the cardiovascular system. Rectal diathermy, physiotherapy, acupuncture, biofeedback, yoga and neuro-muscular re-education of the muscles of the pelvic floor may be useful in some patients to reduce the hypertonicity of the pelvic floor muscles. Transurethral microwave thermotherapy also appears to be a promising therapeutic approach in refractory patients.[74]

Anti-inflammatory agents, gabapentin, quercetin and antidepressants have proved to be of value in small studies. Although the mechanism of its effect is still unclear, finasteride has been shown to provide relief in a double-blind placebo-controlled trial. Prostatic massage is regaining popularity without any scientific evidence to support it.[75]

ASYMPTOMATIC INFLAMMATORY PROSTATITIS

The patients usually present with other urogenital pathologies - BPH, infertility, haemospermia, elevated PSA, or prostate cancer. Histopathology or microbiological investigations have shown evidence of prostatic inflammation.[76]

GRANULOMATOUS PROSTATITIS

Granulomatous prostatitis is a characteristic reaction of the prostate to a variety of insults. On rectal examination, the prostate appears indurated and nodular. The histopathology shows a granulomatous reaction of lipid-laden histiocytes, plasma cells and scattered giant cells. A prominent eosinophilic infiltrate is apparent in some cases.

A number of specific infections cause granulomatous reactions. Tuberculous prostatitis is usually secondary to tuberculosis elsewhere in the genital tract. Similarly, mycotic prostatitis is secondary to systemic involvement. Rare causes include actinomycosis, candidiasis and syphilis.[77] Recent reports suggest that HIV infection may be associated with an increased risk of granulomatous prostatitis and that the aetiology may include Mycobacterium avium complex. Rarely, granulomatous prostatitis has been associated with rheumatoid disorders, particularly Wegener's granulomatosis[78].

The differentiation from other causes of a hard nodular prostate especially prostatic carcinoma is most important. Therapy is generally the specific treatment of the primary disease.

Conclusion

Several distinct types of prostatitis or prostatitis syndromes are now recognized. Accurate diagnosis is important to differentiate and identify the specific therapy for them. In contrast, urologic procedures and antimicrobials need to be judiciously used in the large number of men suffering from Chronic Pelvic Pain syndrome. Reassurance and general supportive measures will often alleviate the condition remarkably in many of these patients.

REFERENCES

1. Sufrin G. Acute epididymitis. Sex Transm Dis 1981; 28: 132-9.
2. Drotman DP. Epidemiology and treatment of epididymitis. Rev Infect Dis 1982; 4 (S): 788-92.
3. Wolin LH. On the aetiology of epididymitis. J Urol 1971; 105: 531-3.
4. Berger RE, Alexander ER, Harnisch JP, et al. Aetiology, manifestations and therapy of acute epididymitis: prospective study of 50 cases. J Urol 1979; 121: 750-4.
5. Watson RA. Gonorrhoea and acute epididymitis. Milit Med 1979; 144: 785-7.
6. Kessler DK, Berger RE, Holmes KK. Epididymitis in heterosexual and homosexual men. In: 5th meeting of International Society of STDs Research; 1983 August; Seattle, Washington.
7. Fisher I, Morton RS. Epididymitis due to *Trichomonas vaginalis*. Br J Vener Dis 1969; 45: 252-3.
8. Gottesman JE. Coccidioidomycosis of prostate and epididymitis with urethrocutaneous fistula. Urology 1974; 4: 311-4.
9. Thomas D, Simpson K, Ostojich H. Bacteremic epididymo-orchitis due to *H. influenzae* type B. Br J Urol 1981; 126: 832-3.
10. Al-Obeid K, Al Khalifan NN, Jamal W et al. Epididymo-orchitis and testicular abscess caused by Salmonella enteritidis in immuno-compromised patients in Kuwait. Med Princ Pract 2006; 15: 305-8.
11. Kohler PF. An inquiry into the aetiology of acute epididymitis. J Urol 1962; 87: 918.
12. Furness G, Kamat MH, Kaminski Z, et al. The relationship of epididymitis to gonorrhoea. Invest Urol 1974; 11: 312-4.
13. Matsushita T, Adachi H, Watanabe H et al. Classic polyarteritis nodosa presenting rare clinical manifestations in a patient with hemophilia A. Int J Hematol. 2006; 83: 420-5.
14. Berger RE. Acute epididymitis. In: Holmes KK, Mardh PA, Sparling et al., Ed. Sexually Transmitted diseases. 3rd Eds. New York McGraw Hill; 1999. 847-58.
15. Berger RE, Holmes KK, Mayo ME, et al. The clinical use of epididymal aspiration cultures in the management of selected patients with acute epididymitis. J Urol 1980; 124: 60-1.
16. Perri AJ, Slachta GA, Feldman AE, et al. The Doppler stethoscope and the diagnosis of the acute scrotum. J Urol 1976; 116: 598-600.
17. Abu Sleiman R, Ho JE, Gregory JC. Scrotal scanning: Present value and limits of interpretation. Urology 1979; 13: 326-330.
18. Wilbert DM, Schaerfe CW, Stern WD, et al. Evaluation of the acute scrotum by colour-coded doppler ultrasonography. J Urol 1993; 149: 1475-7.
19. Trambert MA, Mattrey RF, Levine D, et al.: Sub acute scrotal pain: Evaluation of torsion versus epididymitis with MR imaging. Radiology 1990; 175: 53-6.

20. Gislason T, Noronha RF, Gregory JG. Acute epididymitis in boys: a 5-year retrospective study. J Urol 1980; 124: 533-4.
21. Bullock KN, Hunt JM. The intravenous urogram in acute epididymo-orchitis. Br J Urol 1981; 53: 47-9.
22. Eisner DJ, Goldman SM, Petronis J, et al. Bilateral testicular infarction caused by epididymitis. Am J Roentgenol 1991; 157: 517-9.
23. Caldamone AA, Cockett AT. Infertility and genitourinary infection. Urology 1978; 12: 304-12.
24. Centre for disease control and prevention. Sexually Transmitted Diseases. Treatment guidelines. MMWR. 2006; 55: 1–94.
25. Nickel JC. Chronic epididymitis: a practical approach to understanding and managing a difficult urologic enigma. Rev Urol. 2003; 5: 209-15.
26. Kaklamani BG, Vaiopoulos G, Markomichelakis N et al. Recurrent epididymal–orchitis in patients with Behçet's disease. J Urol. 2000; 163: 487-9.
27. Gasparich JP, Mason JT, Greene HL, et al.: Amiodarone-associated epididymitis: Drug-related epididymitis in the absence of infection. J Urol 1985; 133: 971-2.
28. Nickel JC, Siemens DR, Nickel KR, et al. The patients with chronic epididymitis: characterization of an enigmatic syndrome. J Urol 2002: 167; 1701-4.
29. Thin RN. The diagnosis of prostatitis: A review. Genitourin Med 1991; 67: 279-83.
30. Collins MM, Stafford RS, O'Leary MP et al. How common is prostatitis? A national survey of physician visits. J Urol 1998; 159: 1224-8.
31. Krieger JN. Prostatitis revisited: new definitions, new approaches. Infect Dis Clin North Am. 2003; 17: 395-409.
32. Blacklock NJ. The Prostate: Surgical Anatomy. In: Chisholm G D, Fair W R, eds. Scientific Foundation of Urology. 3rd ed. London: Heinemann; 1990. p. 340-50.
33. Blacklock NJ. The Anatomy of the prostate: relationship with prostatic infection. Infection 1991; 19: S111-4.
34. Kirby RS, Lowe D, Bultitude MI et al. Intra-prostatic urinary reflux; an etiological factor in abacterial prostatitis. Br J Urol 1982; 54: 729-31.
35. Weidner W, Schiefer HG, Krauss H, et al. Chronic prostatitis: a thorough search for etiologically involved microorganisms in 1461 patients. Infection 1991; 19 Suppl. 3: S119-25.
36. Kaplan SA, Ikeguchie F, Petal SR. Etiology of voiding dysfunction in men less than 50 years of age.Urology 2000; 55: 186-92.
37. Ekyn S, Bultitude MI, Mayo ME, et al. Prostatic calculi as a source of recurrent bacteriuria in the male. Br J Urol 1974; 46: 527-32.
38. Schaeffer AJ. Etiology, pathogenesis, and inflammatory reactions in chronic bacterial prostatitis. In Weidner W, Madsen PO, Schiefer HG, eds, Prostatitis: Etiopathology Diagnosis and Therapy. Berlin: Springer-Verlag, 1994: 151-7.
39. Leport C, Rousseau F, Perronne C, et al. Bacterial prostatitis in patients infected with HIV. J Urol 1989; 141: 334-47.
40. Berghuis JP, Heiman JR, Rothman I et al. Psychological and physical factors involved in chronic idiopathic prostatitis. J Psychosom Res 1996; 41: 313-25.
41. Drach GW, Fair WR, Meares EM et al. Classification of benign diseases associated with prostatic pain: Prostatitis or Prostatodynia? J Urol 1978: 120: 266-9.
42. Nickel JC, Nyberg LM, Hennenfent M. Research guidelines for chronic prostatitis: consensus report from the first National Institutes of Health International Prostatitis Collaborative Network. Urology 1999; 54: 229-33. A summary of the 1997 Guidelines for the new NIH prostatitis classification.
43. Litwin MS, McNaughton-Collins M, Fowler FJ Jr, et al. The National Institutes of Health Chronic Prostatitis Symptom Index: development and validation of a new outcome measure. Chronic Prostatitis Collaborative Research Network. J Urol 1999; 162: 369-75.
44. Kreiger JN, Jacobs R, Ross SO. Detecting urethral and prostatic inflammation in patients with chronic prostatitis. Urology 2000; 55: 186-92.
45. Mobley DF. Semen cultures in the diagnosis of bacterial prostatitis. J Urol 1975; 114: 83-5.
46. Shoskes DA, Mazurick C, Landis R, et al. Bacterial cultures of urine, prostatic fluid

and semen of men with chronic pelvic pain syndrome: role of culture for 2 vs. 5 days. J Urol 2000; 163 (Suppl.): 24.

47. Bonadio M, Meini M, Spitaleri R et al. Current microbiological and clinical aspects of urinary tract infections. Eur Urol 2001; 40: 439-44.
48. Shahed AR, Shoskes DA. Oxidative stress in prostatic fluid of patients with chronic pelvic pain syndrome: correlation with gram positive bacterial growth and treatment response. J Androl 2000; 21: 669-75.
49. Hochreiter WW, Duncan JL, Schaeffer AJ. Evaluation of the bacterial flora of the prostate using a 16S rRNA gene based polymerase chain reaction. J Urol 2000; 163: 127-30.
50. Doble A, Carter SS. Ultrasonographic findings in prostatitis. Urol Clin North Am 1989; 16: 763-72.
51. True LD, Berger RE, Rothman I, et al. Prostate histopathology and the chronic prostatitis/ chronic pelvic pain syndrome: a prospective biopsy study. J Urol 1999; 162: 2014-8.
52. McNaughton M, MacDonald R, Wilt TJ. Diagnosis and treatment of chronic abacterial prostatitis: a systematic review. Ann Intern Med 2000; 133: 367-81.
53. Meares EM Jr. Acute and chronic prostatitis: diagnosis and treatment. Infect Dis Clin North Am 1987; 1: 855-72.
54. Bowie WR. Men with urethritis and urologic complications of STD's. Med Clin North Am 1990; 74: 1551-7.
55. Santillo VM, Lowe FC. The management of chronic prostatitis in men with HIV. Curr Urol Rep 2006; 7: 313-9.
56. Weinberger M, Cytron S, Servadioc, et al. Prostatic abscess in the antibiotic era. Rev Infect Dis 1988; 10: 239-49.
57. Bergner DM, Kraus SD, Duck GB et al. Systemic blastomycosis presenting with acute prostatic abscess. Urol 1981; 126: 132-3.
58. Chia JK, Longfield RN, Cook DH et al. Computed axial tomography in the early diagnosis of prostatic abscess. Am J Med 1986; 81: 942-4.
59. Krieger JN. Prostatitis, epididymitis and orchitis. Mandell GL, Bennett JE, Dolin R, eds. In: Mandell, Douglas and Bennet's Principles and practice of infectious diseases. 4th ed. New York: Churchill Livingstone; 1995. p. 1098.
60. Luzzi GA. Chronic prostatitis and chronic pelvic pain in men: aetiology, diagnosis and management. JEADV 2002; 16: 253-6.
61. Baert L, Leonard A. Chronic bacterial prostatitis: 10 years of experience with local antibiotics. J Urol 1988; 140: 755-7.
62. Stamey TA, Meares EM Jr, Winningham DG. Chronic bacterial prostatitis and the diffusion of drugs into prostatic fluid. J Urol 1970; 103: 187-94.
63. Anderson RU. Management of chronic prostatitis-chronic pelvic pain syndrome. Urol Clin North Am 2002; 29: 235-9.
64. Smart CJ, Jenkins JD. The role of transurethral prostatectomy in chronic prostatitis. Br J Urol 1973; 45: 654-62.
65. Habermacher GM, Chason JT, Schaeffer AJ. Prostatitis/chronic pelvic pain syndrome. Ann Rev Med. 2006; 57: 195-206.
66. Nickel JC. Clinical evaluation of the man with chronic prostatitis/chronic pelvic pain syndrome. Urology 2002; 60: 20-3.
67. Schaeffer AJ, Wendel EF, Dunn JK, et al. Prevalence and significance of prostatic inflammation. J Urol 1981; 125: 215-9.
68. Luzzi GA. Chronic prostatitis and chronic pelvic pain in men: aetiology, diagnosis and management. JEADV 2002; 16: 253-6.
69. Domingue GJ: Cryptic bacterial infection in chronic prostatitis: Diagnostic and therapeutic implications. Curr Opin Urol 1998; 8:45–9.
70. Wagenlehner FM, Naber KG. Therapy of prostatitis syndrome. Urologe A. 2001; 40: 24-8.
71. Persson BE, Ronquist G, Ekblom M. Ameliorative effect of allopurinol on nonbacterial prostatitis: a parallel double-blind controlled study. J Urol 1996; 155: 961-4.
72. Nickel JC, Downey J, Johnston B, et al. Predictors of patient response to antibiotic therapy for the chronic prostatitis/chronic pelvic pain syndrome: a prospective multicenter clinical trial. J Urol 2001; 165: 1539-44.
73. Segura JW, Opitz JL, Greene LF. Prostatosis, prostatitis or pelvic floor tension myalgia. J Urol 1979; 122: 168-71.
74. Osborn DE, George NJ, Rao PN, et al. Prostatodynia- physiological characteristics and

rational management with muscle relaxants. Br J Urol 1981; 53: 621-3.

75. Ludwig M, Schroeder-Printzen I, Ludecke G et al. Comparison of expressed prostatic secretions with urine after prostatic massage a means to diagnose chronic prostatitis/inflammatory chronic pelvic pain syndrome. Urology 2000; 55: 175-7.
76. Nickel JC, Downey J, Young I, et al.: Asymptomatic inflammation and/or infection in benign prostatic hyperplasia. Br J Urol 1999; 84: 976-81.
77. Mohan H, Bal A, Punia RP, et al. Granulomatous prostatitis–an infrequent diagnosis. Int J Urol 2005; 12: 474-8.
78. Murty GE, Powell PH. Wegener's granulomatosis presenting as prostatitis. Br J Urol 1991; 67: 107-8.

Appendix 21.1 NIH – Chronic Prostatitis Symptom Index (NIH–CPSI)

Pain or Discomfort

1. In the last week, have you experienced any pain or discomfort in the following areas?
   a. Area between rectum and testicles (perineum)
   b. Testicles
   c. Tip of the penis (not related to urination)
   d. Below your waist, in your pubic or bladder area.
2. In the last week, have you experienced?
   a. Pain or burning during urination?
   b. Pain or discomfort during or after sexual climax (ejaculation)?
3. How often have you had pain or discomfort in any of these areas over the last week?
   0 Never 1 Rarely 2 Sometime 3 Often 4 Usually 5 Always
4. Which number best describes your AVERAGE pain or discomfort on the days that you had it, over the last week?
   0 1 2 3 4 5 6 7 8 9 10
   No Pain Pain As Bad As You Can Imagine

Urination

5. How often have you had a sensation of not emptying your bladder completely after you finished urinating, over the last week?
   0 Not at all 1 Less than 1 time in 5 2 Less than half the time 3 About half the time
   4 More than half the time 5 Almost always
6. How often have you had to urinate again less than two hours after you finished urinating, over the last week?
   0 Not at all 1 Less than 1 time in 5 2 Less than half the time 3 About half the time
   4 More than half the time 5 Almost always

Impact of Symptoms/Quality of life

7. How much have your symptoms kept you from doing the kinds of things you would usually do, in the last week?
   0 None 1 Only a little 2 Some 3 A lot

8. How much did you think about your symptoms, over the last week?
   0 None 1 Only a little 2 Some 3 A lot
9. If you were to spend the rest of your life with your symptoms just the way they have been during the last week, how would feel about that?
   0 Delighted 1 Pleased 2 Mostly satisfied 3 Mixed 4 Mostly dissatisfied
   5 Unhappy 6 Terrible

Scoring the (NIH –CPSI) Domains

Pain: Total of items 1a, 1b, 1c, 1d, 2a, 2b, 3, and 4 =
Urinary Symptoms: Total of items 5 and 6 =
Quality of life Impact: Total of items 7, 8 and 9 =

32 SEXUALLY TRANSMITTED DISEASE ASSOCIATED ARTHRITIS

Ashok Kumar

In this chapter

- Sexually Acquired Reactive Arthritis (SARA)
- Gonococcal Arthritis
- Syphilitic Arthritis
- HIV-Associated Arthritis
- HBV and HCV Arthritis
- Lymphogranuloma Venereum (LGV) and Arthritis

INTRODUCTION

STDs-associated arthritis is part of the broad category of 'Infection-related arthritis'. The latter can be divided into 3 categories[1]:

1. Septic or invasive arthritis
2. Para-infectious arthritis
3. Post-infectious arthritis or 'Reactive' arthritis (Re A)

By definition, organisms can be demonstrated in the joint in the first category only. In the second category, organisms may be demonstrable in the blood or some extra-articular focus but not in the joint, concurrently with the arthritis. In reactive arthritis, on the other hand, the infective episode is supposed to have occurred in the recent past at a remote site. Organisms can no longer be isolated from the joint fluid or synovium. However, it is possible to demonstrate evidence of recent infection in most instances using serological tests.

The following arthritides may be associated with STD:

1. Reactive arthritis (Reiter's syndrome)
2. Gonococcal arthritis
3. Syphilitic arthritis
4. HIV-associated arthritis
5. HBV and HCV arthritis
6. LGV and arthritis

1. SEXUALLY ACQUIRED REACTIVE ARTHRITIS (SARA)

Some recent evidence suggests that infectious particles or material derived from the pathogens may be present in the affected joint even in patients with reactive arthritis.[2] This has challenged the very concept of reactive arthritis. This is discussed further under aetiopathogenesis. In spite of the controversy raised by these new findings, the entity of reactive arthritis still exists. ReA can be considered both as an infection related arthritis and as a member of the seronegative spondyloarthropathies.

ReA is divided into 2 types based on the mode of acquiring the infection: sexually acquired or 'SARA' and enteric or 'enterically acquired reactive arthritis'. The latter is outside the scope of this chapter.

Nomenclature

Reactive arthritis is the new name for the old term Reiter's syndrome. The reasons in favour of this change in terminology are as follows.[3]

1. Hans Reiter was not the first to describe the syndrome,
2. The classical triad of arthritis, conjunctivitis and urethritis is not seen in the majority of patients.

Moreover, this eponymic honour is most inappropriate for a staunch supporter of Nazi regime.[4]

Aetiopathogenesis

The Pathogens

The pathogens associated with SARA include chlamydia and ureaplasma. It appears that the bacteria or their products reach the synovium and then incite a specific immune response. There is definite evidence that live Chlamydia persists in the joint.[5-7] Chlamydia has also been demonstrated in the joint by PCR in 21% of patients with rheumatoid arthritis (RA) and 14% of patients with osteoarthritis (OA). The organisms are presumably transported to the joint by monocytes.

There is no study from India, focussing on the role of chlamydia in SARA. However, two studies have looked at the bacterial triggers involved in the pathogenesis of sporadic reactive arthritis. Aggarwal et al.[8] found antibodies to *Chlamydia trachomatis* in 2 out of 14 patients and none in the controls. Similarly, Joseph et al.[9] did not find any sample positive for *Chlamydia trachomatis* antigen in the synovial fluid of 11 patients with reactive arthritis and 20 patients with undifferentiated arthritis. There is clearly a need to perform studies on microbiology of SARA.

Role of HLA B27

While the HLA B27 association in ankylosing spondylitis is very strong (~90%), it is much lower in the case of ReA. The frequency of B27 is only about 50% in chlamydia induced ReA. There are 38 different subtypes or variants of HLA B27 that have been given the designations B*2701 to B*2738. The most widespread subtype in the world is B*2705. In northern India, the predominant subtypes are B*2705 (50%) and B*2704 (40%).[10]

Most of the current data suggest that HLA B27 functions as an antigen presenting molecule of a yet-unknown arthritogenic peptide. It is now known that a heterozygous state for the B27 gene is sufficient for the disease to develop. The susceptibility to disease is predominantly genetically determined (> 90%). However, HLA B27 gene contributes only about 36% to the genetic risk. Obviously other genes are involved. X chromosome does not appear to be involved in pathogenesis at all.

Cytokines in Reactive Arthritis

The Th1 cytokines such as IL-1, IFN-γ and TNF-α are crucial for the elimination of the bacteria implicated in the causation of ReA. A relatively low production of Th1 cytokines has been documented in ReA.[11] This might partly contribute to the bacterial persistence in the synovium. Quite paradoxically, however, anti-TNF-α therapy is beneficial in spondyloarthropathies. Study and interpretation of cytokine pattern in ReA is an area of active research.

Role of Autoimmunity

Reactive arthritis (ReA) is a T cell mediated inflammatory process. The immune response is primarily directed against a triggering organism, although autoimmunity has been invoked to explain the long-lasting disease. Sharing of conserved immunodominant proteins between different disease triggering microorganisms could explain the shared clinical picture in reactive arthritis. Autoimmunity in reactive arthritis might be mediated by antigen mimicry between evolutionarily conserved epitopes of ribosomal proteins and their host analogues.[12]

Epidemiology

No epidemiological data are available on SARA in India. In the southern part of Africa, reactive arthritis and undifferentiated spondyloarthropathies have become common only after the advent of AIDS epidemic.[13] It is not known what impact HIV has had on these disorders in India. A study has been reported from the armed forces wherein only 2 cases of SARA were identified out of 102 HIV patients.[14] In another study from Mumbai, 12/300 (4%) patients with HIV infection, had arthralgias/ bone pain but no definite arthritis.[15] The same study also reported HIV positivity in 8/150 high risk individuals attending a rheumatology clinic. The diagnosis of the rheumatic disease in these 8 patients included: rheumatoid arthritis-1, ankylosing spondylitis-1, SARA-1, reactive arthritis in the remaining 5 patients.

Clinical Features

Classical picture consists of a sterile oligoarthritis involving large joints, 1-3 weeks following an infection in the urogenital tract (chlamydia, ureaplasma). As mentioned before, the typical triad of urethritis, conjunctivitis and arthritis (Reiter's syndrome) is rarely seen. Urethritis is often symptomatic in male patients, usually with a mucopurulent discharge, but sometimes presents as gross hematuria secondary to hemorrhagic cystitis. In female patients, nonspecific cervicitis may occur. However, in either sex, urethritis may be asymptomatic also.

The arthritis preferentially involves the lower extremities, is asymmetric. The knee, tarsal joints and the sacroiliac region are preferentially involved. The presence of enthesitis (inflammation of the ligaments and tendons at the sites of their insertion into the bone) is a helpful distinguishing characteristic. It causes heel pain, Achilles tendonitis or pain at the insertion of the patella tendon into the tibial tubercle. Low back pain is common and is often secondary to inflammatory sacroiliitis. Conjunctivitis is frequently mild, transient and easily missed. Iritis is characteristic of more persistent and chronic disease. Helpful diagnostic skin lesions include keratoderma blennorrhagica, balanitis circinata and painless oral ulcers. Fever and weight loss may be associated. Although urethral and gut infections are common in India and HLA B27 gene is prevalent in the population to the tune of 6%[16], there are limited published data on ReA. One possible reason may be under reporting of cases. The author, however, believes that clinically recognisable cases of classical ReA are uncommon. On the other hand, evidence of subclinical infections can be obtained with serology for the putative bacteria amongst patients labelled with undifferentiated spondyloarthropathy, as has been shown in a study from northern India.[8]

Prakash et al.[17] described a series of 36 cases (29 men and 7 women, ratio 4:1) of Reiter's syndrome. The mean age of onset was 23.8 years. Clinical manifestations included non-specific urethritis (53%), dysentery and diarrhoea (33%), low back pain and stiffness (69%), heel pain (44%), conjunctivitis (39%), anterior uveitis (19%), mucosal ulcerations (17%), kidney disease (14%), and keratoderma blenorrhagicum (8%). Peripheral arthritis was mono or oligoarthritis in 58% of patients, mainly affecting the large joints of lower extremities, and it was often asymmetric (mean degree of asymmetry = 0.37). Radiographic sacroiliitis was seen in 42%. HLA-B27 antigen was detected in 83% of 36 patients compared with 5.9% of 118 controls (relative risk 79).

The dermatologists in India often see cases of 'Reiter's syndrome' presenting with the hyperkeratotic skin lesions called keratoderma blenorrhagicum **(Fig. 32.1, 32.2)** and an oligoarthritis. Sometimes, a previous history of sexual contact is also available. However, no sizeable series from India is published in the indexed literature. Only a few case reports have been published on balanitis **(Fig. 27.4)** in Indian journals.[18] There is a need to systematically study ReA in India and report it. Clinical documentation of SARA in India is really scant.

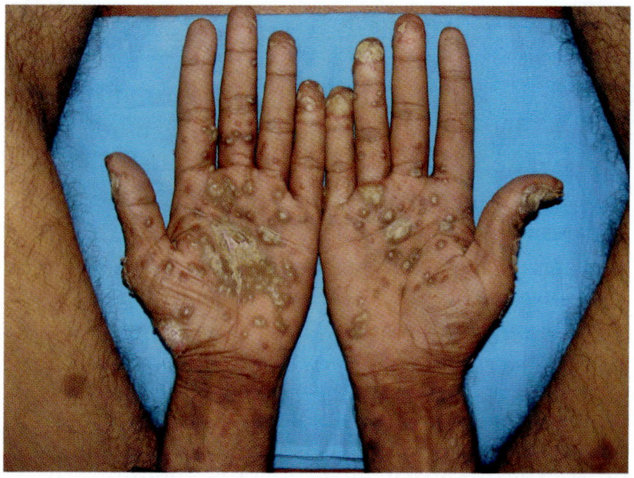

Fig. 32.1 Reiter's disease - Keratoderma blenorrhagicum showing keratotic papules and pustules.

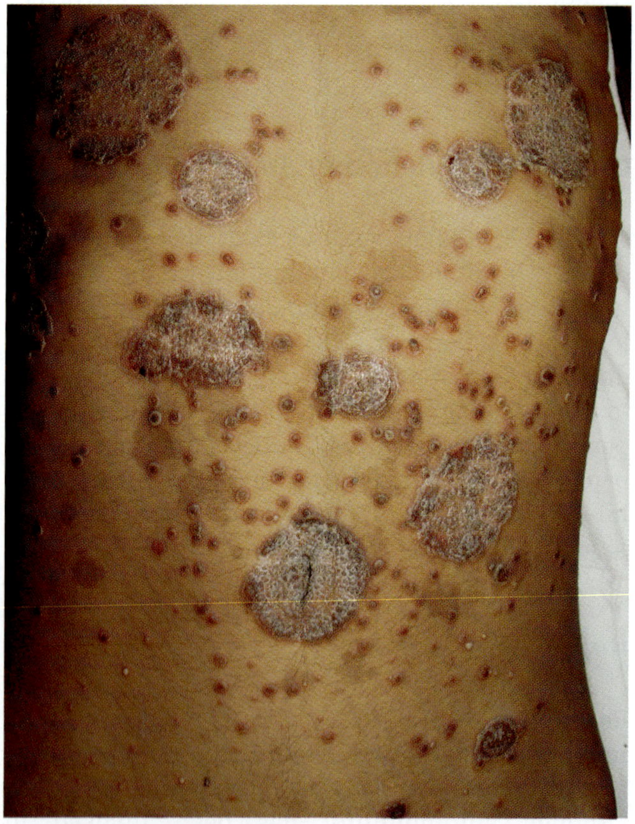

Fig. 32.2 Reiter's disease - Erythematous scaly papules and annular plaques.

Diagnosis

The criteria for diagnosis of reactive arthritis has been given by third International workshop on reactive arthritis (Table 32.1)

Table 32.1 Diagnostic Criteria for Reactive Arthritis

Typical peripheral arthritis
Predominantly lower limb, asymmetric oligoarthiritis
Plus

Evidence of preceding infection

a) Where clear clinical diarrhoea or urethritis within preceding four weeks, laboratory confirmation is desirable but not essential
b) Where no clear clinical infection, laboratory confirmation of infection is essential

Exclusion Criteria

Patients with other known causes of mono/oligoarthiritis, such as other defined spondyloarthropathies, septic arthritis, crystal arthritis, Lyme disease, and streptococcal ReA, should be excluded.

The diagnosis of ReA does not require the presence of HLA B-27 or extra-articular features of Reiter's syndrome (conjunctivitis, iritis, skin lesions, noninfectious urethritis, cardiac and neurological features) or typical spondyloarthropathic features (inflammatory back pain, alternating buttock pain, enthestitis, iritis) but these, if present should be recorded.

There is no established method of testing for the identification of the causative bacteria. For chronic cases, IgA and IgG antibody is estimated. For chlamydia, both serological tests and PCR are available. The latter is useful only on synovial fluid or tissue and is insensitive on blood.

Treatment

Role of Antibiotics

Since bacterial persistence is such a major issue in SARA, the role of antibiotics has been explored in its treatment. In case of *Chlamydia trachomatis* genital infection, antibiotic may prevent pelvic inflammatory disease, scarring, infertility, chronic pelvic pain and passage of the organism to the baby. There is no evidence that antibiotics even when administered in the long term modify the course of ReA. There is, rather, a theoretical concern that antibiotics may render the chlamydia dormant, leading to a change in surface protein expression that enhance the arthritis. Thus, there is no established role of antibiotics in the treatment of SARA.

Symptomatic Therapy

NSAID should be used for symptomatic relief. Splinting of joints should be discouraged in patients with SARA as they have a tendency to develop contractures and ankylosis of splinted joints. Intraarticular steroid injections and injections placed near sites of enthesitis are very helpful. Systemic steroids including dexamethasone pulse are also employed in severe or refractory cases. Hyperkeratotic skin lesions and balanitis respond to coal tar or topical steroid applications. Disease modifying anti-rheumatic drugs such as methotrexate and sulphasalazine have been used with good effect but no controlled trials are available to prove their efficacy in ReA. Physiotherapy plays a pivotal role in the management.

2. GONOCOCCAL ARTHRITIS[20]

Gonococcal arthritis occurs as part of the syndrome of disseminated gonococcal infection (DGI). It is the commonest form of acute bacterial arthritis in adults. About 1% of gonococcal infections are estimated to develop DGI.

Typical presentation comprises a 5-7 day history of fever with chills in a sexually active person who develops multiple skin lesions and fleeting polyarthralgias and tenosynovitis, finally resulting in a persistent, mono or oligoarthritis. The skin lesions include petechiae, papules, pustules, haemorrhagic bullae and necrotic lesions. Typically, the lesions begin as an erythematous macule which progresses to a papule and then a pustule with necrosis or ulceration. At any time, lesions may be present at different stages. They are distributed on the trunk and extremities, including palms and soles but spare the oral mucosa. Septic arthritis can occur in the small joints of hands, wrists, elbows, knees, ankles and rarely, the axial joints. Symptoms of genitourinary tract infection are generally absent in DGI. Women are often menstruating or pregnant.

Cultures of synovial fluid from joints with purulent gonococcal arthritis are usually positive. Similarly, fluid from skin lesions is also positive. Other suitable materials for culture include blood and swabs from urethra, cervix, rectum and pharynx. Culture can take about 24 hours but treatment must be started immediately on empirical basis. Initial treatment with ceftriaxone 1 gram daily is recommended. If the strain is sensitive to penicillin, one can shift to Inj. crystalline penicillin 10-20 million units daily for 7 days. Otherwise ceftriaxone can be continued for 7 days. Ampicillin 1g qid for 7 days is a good alternative. Synovial fluid may have to be frequently drained if it rapidly accumulates. Generally, gonococcal arthritis does not lead to permanent joint damage and complete recovery is the rule.

3. SYPHILITIC ARTHRITIS

Treponema pallidum can cause joint disease. Arthritis is rare in primary and secondary syphilis. In tertiary syphilis, gummatous deposits can occur in the juxta-articular tissue, cartilage and bone. Large, painless effusions are characteristic of this condition. Charcot's joints are the result of neuropathic arthritis resulting from tabes dorsalis, primarily involving weight bearing joints (knee, hip and ankles). Since tertiary syphils is quite rare now, syphilitic arthritis has become a very rare entity.

Congenital syphilis is associated with two important syndromes: Parrot's pseudoparalysis, which is osteochondritis affecting the epiphysis and articular cartilage of the humerus or the tibia of neonates and infants within first 3 months of life. The other one is Clutton's joints, which is a late sequelae of congenital syphilis presenting with chronic hydrarthrosis of one or both knees in children between the ages of 6 and 16 years.

4. HIV-ASSOCIATED ARTHRITIS[21]

A number of musculoskeletal syndromes have been described in patients with HIV infection. Whether HIV itself causes any arthritis is debatable. Psoriatic arthritis and reactive arthritis, particularly SARA, may occur more often in patients with HIV infection. SARA may occur in as many as 11% of patients with HIV. In the presence of HLA B27, this figure mounts to 75% in HIV positive men. These patients may not have uveitis or sacroiliitis. Incomplete forms rather than the classical triad are more commonly seen. Interestingly, the prevalence of HLA B27 appears to be lower in HIV associated SARA than in ordinary SARA. The spectrum of HIV associated joint manifestations vary in different populations; implicating the role of co-factors. Thus, 40% of HIV patients with joint symptoms in Zimbabwe have classical SARA and another 40% have a pauci-articular presentation without the extra-articular manifestations of SARA. In the United States, psoriatic arthritis limited to oligoarticular pattern may occur in one-third of patients with HIV and psoriasis. However, the overall incidence of psoriasis does not appear to be increased.

Acute HIV 'seroconversion illness' may be associated with transient arthralgias. The concurrence of rheumatoid arthritis and HIV is thought to be rare. A picture of polyarthritis can occur with HIV but this is associated with periosteal new bone formation, which is not a feature of RA. A subacute oligoarthritis involving knees and ankles may cause severe arthralgias and disability but it is transient and peaks in intensity in 1-6 weeks and responds well to NSAID. The synovial fluid is non-inflammatory. About 10% of HIV patients suffer from 'painful articular syndrome' which lasts less than a day and involves shoulders, elbows and knees. The pain tends to be intense and incapacitating, requiring short term narcotic analgesics. The prevalence of fibromyalgia is reported to be as high as 29% in HIV patients.

The treatment of reactive arthritis in the setting of HIV infection poses special problems. But immunosuppressive therapies (eg, cyclosporine, methotrexate, PUVA) have been used in some cases, with variable success and without great risk of severe complications

5. HBV AND HCV ARTHRITIS[19]

These 2 viruses may get transmitted sexually. HBV infection may cause immune complex mediated arthritis. This occurs early in the disease when significant viremia is present and anti-HBsAg antibodies are being produced. Usually, the clinical picture consists of an acute symmetrical polyarthritis but it can be migratory at onset. Hand and knee joints are most often involved. Urticaria may accompany. In general, arthritis is confined to the pre-icteric phase of hepatitis. Sometimes, it may persist even after icterus appears. Patients with chronic active hepatitis or those with chronic HBV viremia may have recurrent arthralgias or arthritis. Polyarteritis nodosa may be associated with chronic HBV viremia in 10-30% of cases. Hepatitis C virus is the commonest cause of essential mixed cryoglobulinemia, which classically presents with arthritis, palpable purpura and cryoglobulinemia.

6. LYMPHOGRANULOMA VENEREUM (LGV) AND ARTHRITIS

LGV is described in the 1940s with a syndrome resembling serum sickness including polyarthritis, rash, cryoglobulinemia and circulating rheumatoid factor. Such presentation is rare these days.

REFERENCES

1. Kumar A, Chirkupalli R, Pande I, et al. Infectious arthritis. A new perspective. JIRA 1994; 2: 32-4.
2. Beutle AM, Hudson AP, Whittum-Hudson JA, et al. *Chlamydia trachomatis* can persist in joint tissue after antibiotic treatment in chronic Reiter's syndrome/reactive arthritis. J Clin Rheumatol 1997; 3: 125-30.
3. Siegal LH. Update on reactive arthritis. Bull Rheum Dis 2002; 50: 1-4.
4. Panush RS, Wallace DJ, Dorff RE, et al. Retraction of the suggestion to use the term "Reiter's syndrome" sixty-five years later: the legacy of Reiter, a war criminal, should not be eponymic honor but rather condemnation. Arthritis Rheum. 2007; 56: 693-4.
5. Bas S, Griffais R, Kvien TK, et al. Amplification of plasmid and chromosome Chlamydia DNA in synovial fluid of patients with reactive arthritis and undifferentiated seronegative oligoarthropathies. Arthritis Rheum 1995; 38: 1005-13.
6. Branigan PJ, Gerard HC, Hudson AP, et al. Comparison of synovial tissue and synovial fluid as the source of nucleic acids for detection of *Chlamydia trachomatis* by polymerase chain reaction. Arthritis Rheum 1996; 39: 1740-6.
7. Wilkinson NZ, Kingsley GH, Sieper J, et al. Lack of correlation between detection of *Chlamydia trachomatis* DNA in synovial fluid from patients with a range of rheumatic diseases and the presence of antichlamydial immune response. Arthritis Rheum 1998; 41: 845-54.
8. Aggarwal A, Misra R, Chandrasekhar S, et al. Is undifferentiated seronegative spondyloarthropathy a forme fruste of reactive arthritis? Br J Rheumatol 1997; 36: 1001-4.
9. Joseph J, Rodrigues C, Joshi VR. Bacterial DNA detection in spondyloarthropathies. In: CN Ramchand, Madhavan PN Nair, Bonny Pillo Eds. Recent advances in molecular biology, allergy and immunology. New Delhi: Allied Publishers Ltd, 2001; p. 26-37.
10. Kanga U, Mehra NK, Larrea CK, et al. Seronegative spondyloarthropathies and HLA B27 subtypes: A study in Asian Indians. Clin Rheumatol 1996; 15 (Suppl 1): 13-8.

11. Yin Z, Braun J, Neure L, et al. Crucial role of interleukin-10/interleukin-12 balance in the regulation of the type 2 T helper cytokine response in reactive arthritis. Arthritis Rheum1997; 40: 1788-97.
12. Mertz AK, Daser A, Skurnik M, et al. The evolutionarily conserved ribosomal protein L23 and the cationic urease beta-subunit of Yersinia enterocolitica O:3 belong to the immunodominant antigens in Yersinia-triggered reactive arthritis: implications for autoimmunity. Mol Med. 1994; 1: 44-55.
13. Khan MA. Epidemiology of HLA-B27 and arthritis. Clin Rheumatol 1996; 15 (Suppl): 10-2.
14. Achuthan K, Uppal SS. Rheumatological manifestations in 102 cases of HIV infection. JIRA 1996; 4: 43-7.
15. Swati V, Samant RS, Nadkar MY, et al. HIV infection and rheumatological disorders. JIRA 1996; 4: 83-7.
16. Mehra NK, Taneja V, Kailash S, et al. Distribution of HLA antigens in a sample of the North Indian Hindu population. Tissue Antigens 1986; 27: 64-74.
17. Prakash S, Mehra NK, Bhargava S, et al. Reiter's disease in northern India. A clinical and immunogenetic study. Rheumatol Int 1983; 3: 101-4.
18. Singh M, Kaur S, Kumar B, et al. Reiter's disease-clinical profile of six cases. Indian J Dermatol Venereol Leprol. 1987; 53: 108-11.
19. Kingsley G, Sieper J. Third International Workshop on Reactive Arthritis. September 23-26, 1995, Berlin, Germany. Report and abstracts. Annals Rheum Dis 1996; 55: 564-70.
20. Mahowald ML. Infectious disorders: A. Septic arthritis. In: Klippel JH, Weyand CM, Wortmann RL eds. Primer on the rheumatic diseases. 11th ed. Atlanta: Arthritis Foundation; p. 196-200.
21. Calabrese LH. Human immuno deficiency virus (HIV) infection and arthritis. Rheum Dis Clin North Am 1993; 19: 477-88.

Part 5

Sexually Transmitted Diseases in Special Situations

33 SEXUALLY TRANSMITTED DISEASES IN CHILDREN AND ADOLESCENT

S Murugan, Amit K Malhotra, Vinod K Sharma

In this chapter

- Epidemiology
- Sexual Behaviour in Children and Adolescent
- Bacterial STDs
- Viral STDs
- Sexual Abuse in Children and Adolesent
- Post Exposure Prophylaxis Against Pregnancy and STDs After Sexual Abuse
- Treatment Protocol for STDs in Children and Adolescent
- Chlamydia
- Trichomoniasis and Bacterial Vaginosis
- Gonorrhoea
- Anogenital Warts
- Genital Herpes
- Anogenital Candidiasis
- Syphilis
- Scabies
- Pediculosis Pubis
- Presumptive Treatment
- Prevention of STDs in Children and Adolescent

INTRODUCTION

Sexuality is an integral component in the lives of all human beings (including children and adolescents) but when the sexual behaviour goes unplanned, uncontrolled and unchecked, it leads to dreadful consequences on the sexual health of an individual in the form of sexually transmitted diseases (STDs) and unwanted pregnancy.

WHO defines children as persons between the ages of 0 and 9 years. Adolescents are defined as persons in the 10-19 years age group. Youth has been defined as the 15-24 years age group. 'Young people' are a combination of adolescents and youth i.e. 10-24 years.[1]

STDs in children and young adults (up to age 24 years) deserve special attention as they comprise 50% of all newly acquired STDs but make up only 25% of the sexually active population.[2] Besides legal implications, the etiopathogenesis, clinical manifestations, management, treatment outcomes and long term complications of STDs in this age group differ from that of adults. The sexual development of children and young adults is immature and evolving; therefore any STDs can produce a long lasting negative impact on the sexual health, psychosocial development and overall personality of the individual. Therefore it is imperative for the care providers to study and understand the basic concepts of sexuality and sexual behaviour of children, adolescents, and young adults. Acquisition of STDs by children is either the result of sexual abuse and or due to nonsexual transmission during pregnancy and delivery (perinatal); and rarely due to accidental exposure such as breast feeding and handling. When a child of less than 3 years tests positive for an STIs, vertical transmission should be considered as a possible cause and sexual abuse should be ruled out, Where as when a pre-pubertal young child more than 3 years tests positive for an STDs, then sexual abuse should be considered as a more likely cause and vertical transmission should be ruled out.

EPIDEMIOLOGY

It is estimated that reported cases of STDs represent only 50%–80% of reportable STDs, which may be due to the limited screening or low disease reporting as many STDs are asymptomatic.[3] Up to 60% of patients who have one STDs will concurrently harbour another.

Global Epidemiology of STDs in Children and Young Adults

Adolescents and young adults comprise 50% of all new acquired STDs although they make up only 25% of the sexually active population.[2] As per the CDC estimates, approximately 19 million new infections occur each year and almost half of them develop among young adults.[2] A possible explanation for this behaviour in young people is that they do not have enough information about the transmission of STDs and ignore the precautions required for safe sex. There is an increasing trend in the prevalence of *Chlamydia trachomatis* infection in young females and males who attended STDs clinics in 1997 and 2005 from 12.2% to 15.4%, and 15.7% to 20.5%, respectively.[4] The magnitude of the problem is further complicated as approximately 60% of new HIV infections worldwide are occurring in the young people.[3]

In a study from Cape Town, South Africa, of the 107 patients (aged 2-15 years) who were identified to have STDs *Neisseria gonorrhoeae* was the commonest isolate, followed by *Gardnerella vaginalis*, *Chlamydia trachomatis*, *Trichomonas vaginalis*, and *Treponema pallidum*.[5]

Epidemiology of STDs in Children and Young Adults in India

STDs are among the first ten causes of diseases in young adult males and the second major cause of diseases in young adult women in developing countries.[3] Over all, bacterial STDs (syphilis, gonorrhoea and chancroid) appear to be more frequent than viral STDs in children (herpes genitalis and genital warts). (Table 33.1)

In a hospital based study from a STDs clinic in New Delhi, a prevalence rate of 0.82% over a period of six years from January 1995 to February 2001 was found.[6] There were in all 127 cases of which 66.1% were in the age group of 10-14 years. Up to two-third of them were illiterate and from low socio-economic backgrounds. Notably, 17.3% were from remand homes. The predominant STDs observed among these children were syphilis (25.2%) including six cases of congenital syphilis, vulvo-vaginal candidiasis (11.8%), condyloma-acuminata (14.2%), herpes progenitalis (8.7%) and traumatic lesions (7.9%). Histories or signs of abuse were present in 74% of the patients. Only two cases turned out to be HIV positive.

In another hospital based study from New Delhi, 58 out of 362 patients were younger than 14 years.[7] 93.1% were from lower socioeconomic strata, lived in slums and had not studied beyond the third class. Syphilis was identified in 27.6%, gonorrhoea in 24.1%, chancroid in 22.4%, candidiasis in 10.3%, condylomata acuminata in 6.9%, and herpes genitalis in 6.9%. These children most likely con-tracted the observed STDs as a result of sexual assault, early sexual maturity, sexual promiscuity, and sexual contact with prostitutes.

In one more hospital based study from New Delhi, 50 (3.4%) out of 1418 patients who attended the STDs clinic between January 1996 to December 2000, were children below 14 years of age, with predilection for the boys.[8] Syphilis was the most common STDs (46.8%), followed by vulvo-vaginal candidiasis (19.2%), condylomata acuminata (10.6%), gonorrhoea (8.5%), herpes progenitalis (6.4%), chancroid (4.3%), perianal candidiasis and perianal molluscum contagiosum (2.1% each). Three children had more than one STDs. A history of sexual abuse was elicited in 30 children (60%); none of the children were positive for HIV.

Table 33.1 **Profile of STDs in Children <14 Years from STD Clinics in New Delhi**

Period of Study	*1991 – 2001*[6]	*1988 – 1989*[7]	*1996 – 2000*[8]
Total cases (<14yrs)	127	58	50
Syphilis	25.2 %	27.6 %	46.8 %
Candidiasis	11.8 %	10.3 %	21.3 %
HPV infection	14.2 %	6.9 %	10.6 %
Chancroid	-	22.4 %	4.3 %
Gonorrhoea	-	24.1 %	8.5 %
Herpes genitalis	8.7 %	6.9%	6.4 %
Molluscum	-	-	2.1 %
Traumatic	7.9 %	-	-

SEXUAL BEHAVIOUR IN CHILDREN AND ADOLESCENTS

During the first 3 years of life, sexual exploration such as handling of one's own genitalia, kissing and stroking and touching other children's genitalia, observing toileting and bathing and exposing one's own genitalia are very common, ranging from 10-60%.[9] During 3 to 6 years of age, children engage in frankly seductive behaviour with the opposite sex parent and occasionally with other adults as well that makes them vulnerable for sex abuse and STDs.

Adolescence is a lengthy period of transition from childhood to adulthood with distinct physiological, sexual and psychological life stages associated with an emerging awareness of sexuality and an age-specific drive to experiment with sex.[10] In many societies the gap between the age of sexual maturity and that of legitimate sexual relation (marriage) has widened. During this period, young adults are kept relatively uninformed regarding the sexual matters while life style and social attitudes of the young adults are changing fast due to globalization and liberalization of the society and the impact of media and internet. The situation is further complicated by the gradual breakdown of traditional family life (such as hostel life), diminishing role of parents and the large family unit, and an increasing role of media especially television and internet.

The large number of street children and informally employed adolescents, including those employed as sex workers in urban centers and child labour among non-school going children, are vulnerable for bonded labour and commercial or forced sexual exploitations especially of girls. In the Indian cities of New Delhi, Mumbai and Calcutta, around 1,00,000 children either do "informal" jobs such as washing cars and pushing hand carts, cleaning gutters or survive by begging or collecting edibles from garbage dumps. In Thailand, an estimated 8,00,000 girls under the age of 20 are earning their living as sex workers. In Eastern Europe, tens of thousands of these non school-going children are engaged in drug trafficking and consumption, prostitution or a range of criminal activities. All the above activities are associated with increased risk of STI and HIV.

The following factors influence the occurrence of STDs in children, adolescents and young adults:

1. **Age at first intercourse:** Earlier age at first intercourse poses increased risks to the health and well-being of adolescents, as the initiation of sexual intercourse marks the beginning of exposure to the risk of unintended pregnancy and STDs. In 1979, 50% of women between 15-19 years of age and 70% of men between 17-21 years of age living in metropolitan areas of the U.S. reported that they had sexual intercourse.[11] Average age of 1st sexual experience was 16.2 for women and 15.7 for men. Age at 1st coitus was generally younger among blacks. Indian studies reveal that more than 51% of males and 60% females, of STDs clinic attendees had their first coitus before their 20th birthday.[11] In US, nearly 17% of women and 25% of men plan their 1st intercourse.
2. **Use of condom (consistent/inconsistent):** Factors that influence adolescents' contraceptive behaviours include personal characteristics, family context, social support, knowledge and access to contraception. Only about half of the men and women use contraception at 1st intercourse and those 18 or older are more likely to use it.
3. **Age of the partner:** Sex at a young age with an older partner has been linked to poor reproductive health outcomes during adolescence.[12] Females who engage in early sexual activity with older partners are especially at high risk of experiencing adverse reproductive health consequences. On an average, women tend to have partners nearly 3 years older, men less than 1 year older.
4. **Number of partners:** The more the number of partners, the higher is the risk of acquiring STDs.[13]
5. **Frequency of high risk behaviour:** Indulgence in abuse of substances such as alcohol, marijuana, tobacco and cocaine predispose young adults into risk taking behaviours such as exchange of sex for drugs.[14] The frequency of high-risk behaviour among youths is influenced by the opportunity to engage in them, particularly the amount of time that they are unsupervised by adults. It is found that boys who were unsupervised for more than 5 hours per week after school were twice as likely to have chlamydia or gonorrhoea as boys who were unsupervised for 5 or fewer hours.[15]

During the course of formation of sexual identity adolescents form romantic relationships and engage in a variety of sexual behaviours that includes oral and anal sex. Almost half of the adolescents engage in vaginal sexual intercourse by the end of high school.[9] Biological and psychosocial factors such as exposure to violence at home and early pubertal development increase an adolescent's risk of being in an unhealthy relationship or engaging in sex at an early age.

The change in the pattern of adolescent's sexual activity due to the pressure of media, films, and pornographic website and their easy accessibility also contribute to the increase in the prevalence of STDs in this age group.[16] Myths and misconceptions about sex and sexuality passed on to the teenagers from their colleagues, neighbours, parents or teachers increase their curiosity about opposite sex and predispose them to initiate early sexual activity, which exposes them to the risk of STDs.

The outcomes of sexual activity at young age are teenage pregnancy, infertility, impaired sexual health due to acquisition of STDs & HIV, psychosocial impact and impact on academic performance. The complications of STDs in children and young adults include pelvic inflammatory diseases (PID) and its sequelae (ectopic gestation and infertility), genital cancers and death due to infections such as HIV.

BACTERIAL STDs

Syphilis: Syphilis in children may either be congenital or acquired. Congenital syphilis is caused by the transmission of *Treponema pallidum* by the pregnant women to her foetus through the placenta. It is quite common in developing countries and parallels the incidence of early syphilis in women. Based on the severity of infection various organs may be involved that usually manifest as osteochondritis, periostitis, jaundice, hepatosplenomegaly, and cutaneous lesions. The common cutaneous manifestations include desquamation of palms and soles, papular lesions, periorificial rhagades, bullae on the palms and soles, paronychia and condyloma lata.[17]

The transmission of acquired syphilis is almost always associated with sexual abuse especially in younger children, except when transmission is through breast-feeding and rarely due to blood transmission infused during pediatric surgeries. Clinical features in children are almost similar to that of adults. Initial presentation being primary chancre **(Fig. 33.1)** followed by secondary stage, latent stage and few of them develop tertiary syphilis. The incubation period is the same as that of adults ranging from 9-90 days (average 3 weeks). In children, the chancres are said to be smaller and less likely to be recognized. Most of the children are found to be in latent stage or in secondary syphilis with muco-cutaneous moist lesions either over vulva or anus. Atypicality and multiplicity of ulcers have also been reported in literature. Secondary syphilis develops from 2 weeks to 6 months after primary chancre. All classical features like papular, papulo-squamous with involvement of palms and soles, moist verrucous plaques in and around genitalia and mucous patches **(Fig. 33.2, 33.3)** have been described. Most common lesion in children is erythematous maculopopular rash. The common differential diagnosis for chancre would include impetigo. Secondary syphilis is commonly confused with Pityriasis rosea.

Diagnosis is by demonstration of spirochaete under dark ground microscopy, non-treponemal tests (VDRL, RPR), and treponemal tests (TPHA, TPI, FTA-ABS, MHA-TP) as done in adults. Non-treponemal test, if positive, should be confirmed by treponemal tests like FTA-ABS, MHA-TP, IgG and IgM enzyme immunoassays (to rule out biological false positivity and also to ascertain the mode of transmission).

The presence of genital ulcer facilitates the transmission of HIV among teenagers. Out of 763 young adults with STDs in a study, 11 had both HIV and ulcerative syphilis.[18] So, all patients who have syphilis should be tested for HIV infection. The rate of primary and secondary syphilis in Unites States of America declined by 89.7% between 1990 and 2000 where as the same increased from 2001 to 2005. This trend seems to be universal.

Gonorrhoea: Apart from the perinatal transmission, gonococcal infection in children and young adults are acquired through sexual abuse and increased promiscuity. Accidental infection is comparatively rare. The rate of gonorrhea among teenagers (15-19 years) is high in girls when compared to young men.[19] 90-100% of cases of gonorrhoea below 12 years is acquired by sexual contact. The prevalence of *N. gonorrhoeae* in abused or sexually active adolescents was reported to be 2.8% to 20% from various surveys.[20]

The clinical spectrum of gonococcal infection in children and young adults consists of conjunctivitis, pyuria, urethritis, vaginitis, proctitis, pharyngitis, rhinitis, scalp abscess, arthritis and pelvic inflammatory disease (PID).

In case of prepubertal girls, the most common (75%) form of manifestation of gonorrhoea is vulvovaginitis **(Fig. 33.4)**. It is manifested as labial redness, swelling, itching and vaginal discharge.[21] This is due to the reduced estrogen load, non-stratified epithelial mucosa and alkaline vaginal PH of vaginal mucosa. Non-stratified epitheliium is more vulnerable to bacterial infections compared to stratified squamous epithelium. It most commonly presents with profuse, purulent vaginal discharge and vulval erythema with dysuria and pruritus. Rarely, it can be asymptomatic. Very rarely ascending infection leading to salpingitis or peritonitis had been reported.

The frequency of infection in prepubertal boys is less and usually presents with urethral discharge, asymptomatic pyuria, penile edema (occasional), epididymitis, testicular swelling and conjunctivitis.

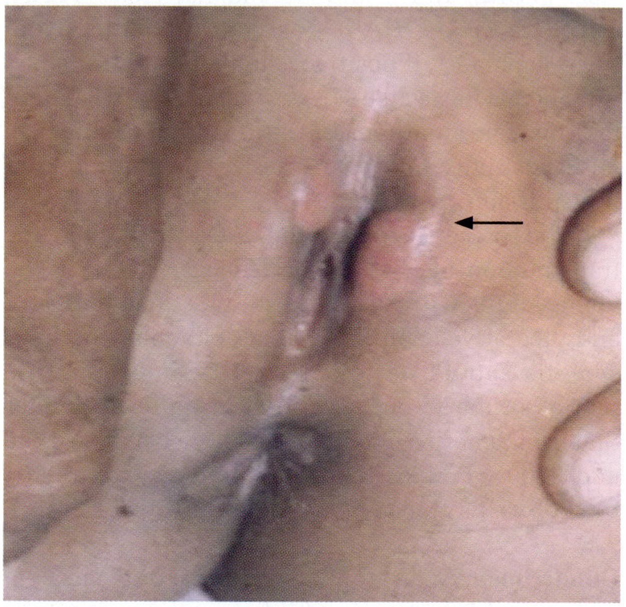

Fig. 33.1 Primary chancre – indurated ulcers on the vulva.

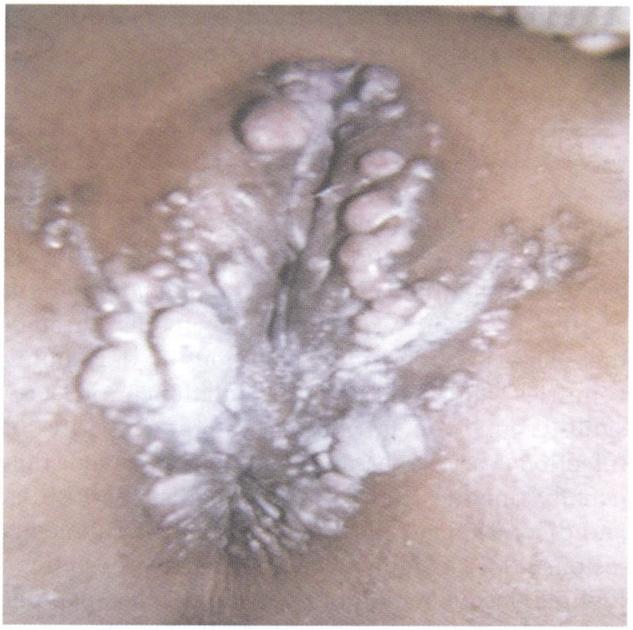

Fig. 33.2 Condyloma lata – moist erythe-matous plaques over vulva and perianal area.

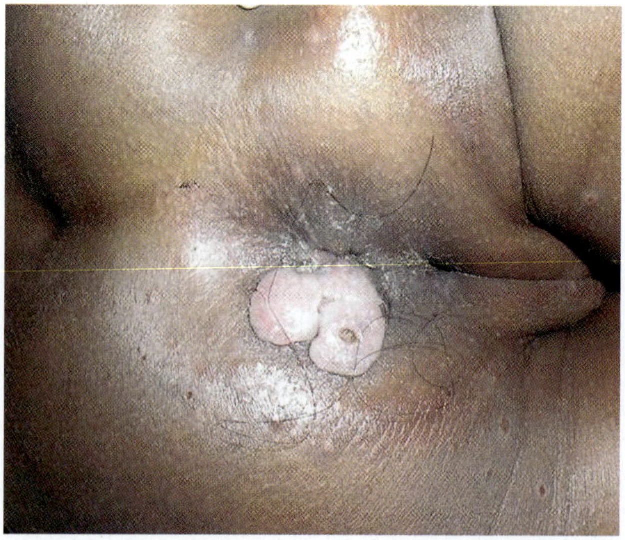

Fig. 33.3 Condyloma lata – moist plaques over perianal area.

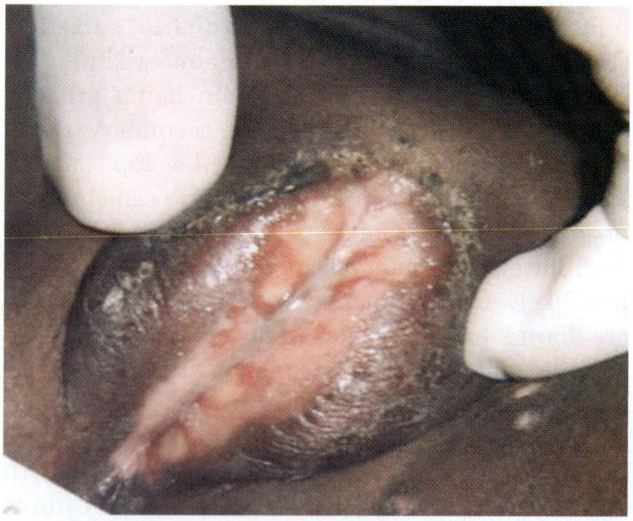

Fig. 33.4 Gonorrhoea – purulent vaginal discharge with erosions on labia minora.

Pharyngeal and rectal infections are common in both sexes. The pharyngeal and rectal infections are mostly asymptomatic and diagnosed only with thorough examinations and investigations. Gonococcal proctitis in girls results either from the spread of infection from the genital discharge or by anal intercourse. When there is a profuse vaginal discharge, it may dribble over the perineum to the anal orifice and by the sphincter action of anal canal; the organisms reach the rectum and produce gonococcal proctitis in the girls. Among boys, it almost always occurs through anal coitus. The proctitis is usually asymptomatic. Some children may complain of discomfort and soreness or pain in the anus during defecation. The discharge is either mucoid or purulent and blood stained. Smears and cultures taken with platinum loop from rectum with the help of a proctoscope establish the diagnosis. Repeated examinations may be necessary for the diagnosis.

Disseminated infection among children is rare. Most commonly it follows genitourinary tract infection and would present with polyarthritis associated with systemic manifestations. The joints commonly affected are ankles, knees, elbows and wrists (mostly larger joints). The other manifestations of disseminated disease include meningitis and pseudo-paresis of involved joints.

Gonococcal infection among teenagers above 15 years resembles that of adults. Because of poor health seeking behaviour, tendency to suppress the facts and inability to spend money for full course of investigations and treatment, they are vulnerable to permanent damage of their reproductive system. Pelvic inflammatory disease, ectopic gestation and infertility among both sexes are the common regular sequelae especially in young adults.

Chlamydial Infections: It is the most commonly reported infectious disease in the United States. Women, especially young women, are hit hardest by chlamydia. Young females aged 15 to 19 have the highest chlamydia rate, followed by females aged 20 to 24. Adolescent girls have a physiologically increased susceptibility to *Chlamydia trachomatis* infection due to increased cervical ectopy. Data from chlamydia screening in family planning clinics across the United States indicate that approximately 7 percent of 15- to 24-year-old females in these settings are infected. Studies have also found that chlamydia is three times more common among adolescent females than adolescent males, and the long-term consequences of untreated disease are much more severe for females.

In women, chlamydia infections, which are usually asymptomatic, may result in pelvic inflammatory disease (PID) which is a major cause of infertility, ectopic pregnancy and chronic pelvic pain. Pregnant young women infected with Chlamydia, can pass the infection to their infants resulting in neonatal ophthalmia and pneumonia. Premature rupture of membranes leads to earlier manifestation of this disease.

The clinical features of chlamydial infections in sexually abused children are: proctitis, pharyngeal infection in both sexes, vaginitis in female children and urethritis in boys. Epididymitis and infertility also can occur due to chlamydial infections in male teenagers who are sexually active.

Other syndromes caused by *C. trachomatis* include lymphogranuloma venereum with sero types of L_1, L_2, and L_3. Clinically it may be compatible with one or more tender fluctuant inguinal lymphadenitis and characteristic of proctogenital lesions. This STDs is relatively rare in many parts of India and accounts for 0.13%.[18]

The facility for the isolation of chlamydia is not available widely in India and the serological tests are available only in sophisticated referral laboratories and are cumbersome costly. So the definite incidence of Chlamydial infection is not available in India.

Because chlamydia is most common among young women, CDC recommends annual chlamydia screening for all sexually active women under age 26, as well as older women with risk factors such as new or multiple sex partners. Data from one study in a managed care setting suggest that chlamydia screening and treatment can reduce the incidence of pelvic inflammatory disease (PID) by over 50 percent.

Other bacterial STDs: Diseases like bacterial vaginosis and granuloma venereum are rare among children. In teenagers the symptoms & treatment are on the same line as adults. Chancroid a bacterial STDs, even though has a declining tendency, still is one of the commonest genital ulcerative condition next only to genital herpes infection. In prepubertal children, it is almost always due to some sort of sexual abuse or assault. It can manifest with acute retention of urine with distended bladder due to severe dysuria in female children following painful genital ulcerations and may present as an acute emergency. In teenagers, the incidence of chancroid is low, but behaves like that of their adult counterpart. Mycoplasma infection has not been reported quite often because of poor availability of diagnostic facilities.

Vulvovaginitis: It is a common manifestation in prepubertal girls. This may be due to nonvenereal cause such as:

(a) Worm infestation (especially *Enterobius vermicularis*): Female adult worm migrates to the anal orifice for egg laying during night hours and produce intense itching and they likely to produce vulvovaginitis due to repeated scratching.
(b) Candidal infection: Long hours of retention of diapers, repeated diarrhoeal diseases, poor and faulty genital washing habits, malnutrition, debilitating diseases, cancers, cytotoxic drugs, radiation, immune deficiency, endocrinopathies and long term anti microbial therapy are some of the factors that induce the vaginal candidiasis in children **(Fig. 33.5)**. Moreover, mother's candidal vaginitis also has a definite role as a cause for the cross infection to the infants. Wet hands and nail bed infection of mothers after toileting, passes the infection to the genitals of these children.
(c) Poor Hygiene: Children playing with the soil without wearing undergarments are prone for bacterial vaginitis.
(d) Foreign bodies: Foreign bodies such as pebbles, stones, grains, peas, beans, beads and small onions may be left inside the vagina unattended during their play.
(e) Trichomonal Infection: *Trichomonas vaginalis* infection is observed in teenaged girls or due to sexual abuse in prepubertal children also. Though Trichomonas can survive in fomites, transmission through fomites has not been reported in children. *Trichomonas vaginalis* infection in children above 1 year of age is mostly due to sexual contact and the rate possibly is 0.4% because it is rarely seen before puberty. Hypertrophic epithelium, absence of glycogen inside the cells and the alkaline environment prevent the growth of Trichomonas.

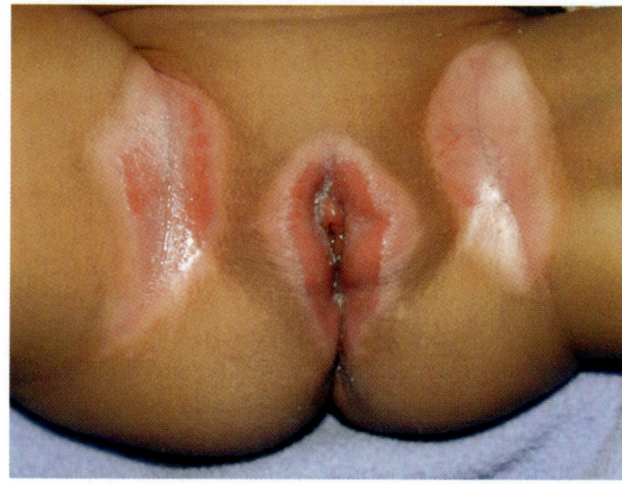

Fig. 33.5 Candidal vaginitis and intertrigo.

Symptoms in teenagers with *Trichomonas vaginalis* vaginitis are greenish white, frothy and offensive discharge from the vagina, but this appears to be rare event. Where the discharge is profuse, excoriations and vulval dermatitis may be noticed. Organisms can easily be demonstrated by mounting a saline preparation from the discharge when examined under the high power objective of light microscope.

VIRAL STDs

Pediatric HIV infection is discussed in a separate chapter.

Herpes Virus Infection: Herpes simplex virus type 2 (HSV 2) and cytomegalo virus can be transmitted through sexual route. HSV 2 infections in children above 1 year and among teenagers are common due to sexual abuse or sexual activities. The HSV 2 infection is one of the common cause of genital ulcer disease. Recurrence is the rule in most of the occasions. Clusters of tiny vesicles are present on the presenting part of the body, which was in direct contact with the virus. Vesicles usually erupt from an erythematous base and are 1-2 mm in diameter. Vesicles will rupture subsequently and produce tiny, grouped, superficial ulceration. These ulcers heal spontaneously, even without treatment, within 10-14 days in the case of primary lesions and within 4-7 days in the case of recurrent lesions. Lesion are usually painful. Tissue smears stained with Leishman's stain will reveal giant epithelial cells and serological test reveals IgM or IgG antibodies.

Cytomegalo virus (CMV) can also be transmitted through transplacental route, perinatal route, sexual contact and non-sexual contact. CMV infection in immuno-competent individuals is usually sub clinical. Rarely it presents as mononucleosis like picture with mild grade fever, malaise, lymphadenopathy and hepatomegaly. Source of the virus includes urine, oropharyngeal secretions, cervical and vaginal secretions, semen, milk, tears, blood and transplanted organs. Higher rates of seropositivity have been observed in males and females with multiple sex partners and history of STDs. Sexual transmission plays a minimal role as a mode of primary CMV infection in children. In fact, no primary CMV infection in children due to sexual abuse had been reported from India.

Human Papilloma Virus Infection: Infection with high-risk human papilloma virus (HR-HPV) can lead to development of anogenital cancers and cervical cancer. Overall HR-HPV prevalence is 22.5% with serotypes of 16, 18, 31, 33, 35, 39, 45, 51, 52, 56, 58, 59 and 68. Prevalence among the teenagers (14-19 years) is 35%. HPV types 6 or 11 are commonly found. Genital warts are usually flat, papular, or pedunculated type of growths on the genital mucosa **(Fig. 33.6)**. Usually visual inspection will be sufficient for the diagnosis. In addition to external genitalia, genital warts can also occur on uterine cervix, inside the vagina, urethra, anus and mouth. Intraanal warts are observed predominantly in patients who have had receptive anal intercourse.

Hepatilis B Infection: HBV is efficiently transmitted by percutaneous or mucous membrane exposure to infectious blood or body fluids that contain blood.

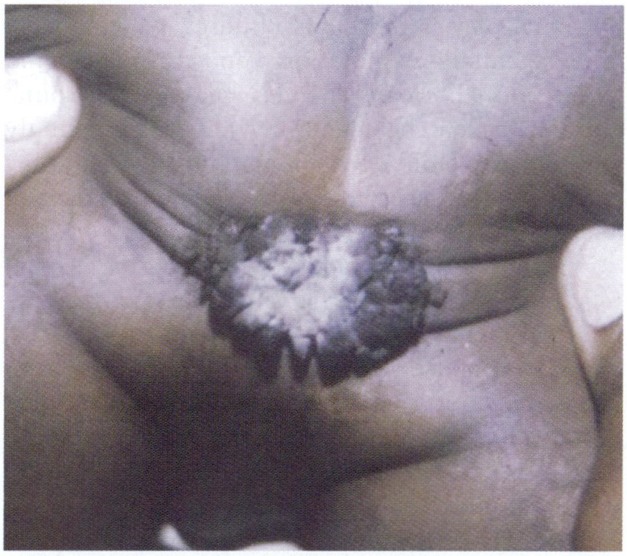

Fig. 33.6 Genital warts – Perianal.

The primary risk factors that have been associated with infection among teenagers are unprotected sex with more than one partner, MSM, history of other STDs and injecting drug use. Majority of the new infections occur in these high-risk groups. Only approximately half of them are symptomatic and approximately 1% of reported cases result in acute liver failure and death. Hepatitis C virus infection is the most common chronic blood borne infection in United States, although HCV is not efficiently transmitted sexually. Intravenous drug users are often highly susceptible for HCV infection along with HIV infection.

SEXUAL ABUSE IN CHILDREN AND ADOLESENT

Definition: Sexual abuse is defined as any sexual activity that a child cannot comprehend or give consent to, or that violates the law.[22] This sexual act may include attempted or successful penetration of any of the child's orifices (oral-genital, genital and anal contact), genital fondling, as well as exhibitionism, voyeurism, photographing and exposure to pornography. It is essential to differentiate sexual abuse from "sexual play" or age-appropriate behaviour where the developmental level of the participants is similar, and the activity occurs without coercion. The common example of sexual play is preschool children viewing each other's genitalia without force and it is considered to be normal. However, engagement of a young child in sexual behaviour by a developmentally more mature child does not amount to sexual play and certainly needs to be investigated for sexual abuse.

Sexual assault (rape) is defined as sexual relations with another person obtained through physical force, threat, or intimidation.

Sexual abuse needs to be differentiated from congenital and acquired conditions that may mimic physical findings caused by sexual abuse and from the nonsexual transmission of STDs, which is rare.

Epidemiology: In 2002, more than 88000 children were confirmed victims of sexual abuse in the United States. Studies indicate that each year approximately 1% of children experience some form of sexual abuse, resulting in the sexual victimization of 12% to 25% of girls and 8% to 10% of boys by 18 years of age.[23] The pattern of childhood sexual abuse appears to depend on the sex and age of the victim. About 80% to 90% of abused children are female, with mean ages of 7–8 years.[24]

The prevalence of sexual abuse have shown increasing trend; it has increased from 12% to 28%[25] and include a wide range of molestations such as kissing, fondling, genital manipulation, oral-genital contact, anal contact, and vaginal or rectal penetration.[26] In two studies of 409 and 532 victims under 14 years of age, genital manipulation and vaginal penetration were the most common complaints, 32.7% in one study and 66.2% in the other. Anal penetration and orogenital contacts followed in frequency in both studies.[27,28]

According to 1987 US national data, 7% of women and men aged 18–22 had experienced forced intercourse, and almost half of all women's nonvoluntary experiences had occurred before age 14. A study from Los Angeles showed that 18% of adolescent females reported having had an unwanted sexual experience, which suggests that these experiences are not uncommon. Moreover, of the experiences reported in the survey, 39% had occurred before the age of 13, and half had occurred between 13 and 16.

Most (75% to 85%) are abused by a male assailant, adult or minor known to the child. Perpetrators may be relatives or nonrelatives and are most frequently male. This individual is most likely to be a family member, especially the father or father substitute (stepfather, mother's boyfriend), uncles, and other male relatives. Adolescents are perpetrators in at least 20% of reported cases, and many have a personal history of sexual and/or physical abuse. Women may be perpetrators, but only a small minority of sexual abuse allegations involve women.

Consequences of Abuse and Forced Intercourse: Transmission of STDs pathogens occurs in 2% to 10% of abused children, and it is presumed that when penetration occurs, the risk is higher. Besides the trauma of the experience of nonvoluntary sexual intercourse, other negative outcomes of forced intercourse include higher frequency of subsequent adolescent sexual activity and a greater number of partners. It may increase the likelihood of teenage pregnancy, early first sex, contraceptive nonuse and multiple partners. Sexual abuse, particularly at early ages, has also been linked to involvement in prostitution, impairments to psychological well-being and mental health, alcohol abuse and suicidal ideation. A recent study showed that women who as children experienced sexual intercourse with adults had lower overall well-being than did women who had experienced childhood sexual contact with adults that only included fondling or who did not experience any such sexual contact.

Sexual victimization results in perceptions of powerlessness, diminished capacity for academic work and other tasks of adolescence, heightened vulnerability to males, an increased salience of sexual issues, misconceptions about sexual norms and the equation of sex with love and care giving. The more intrusive forms of sexual abuse, more violent assaults, longer periods of sexual molestation, and closer relationship of the perpetrator to the victim indicate poor prognosis.

Evaluation of Sexual Abuse: Sexual abuse often leads to significant psychologic, social and legal implications.[29] The physical examination of sexually abused children should not result in additional physical or emotional trauma. Evaluation of a child for sexual abuse often provokes anxiety in the patient and their family members. The parents of the victim also need treatment and support to cope with the emotional trauma of their child's abuse.

A confidential relationship should be established with the patient to explore sensitive issues such as number of sexual partners, sexual orientation, sexual abuse, history of pregnancy, sexually transmitted diseases and drug or alcohol use.[30]

When to Suspect Sexual Abuse: A clinician should suspect sexual abuse in a child when there are behavioural changes along with anogenital or other medical problems. Behavioural changes include sexual acting out, aggression, problems in school, regression (e.g., return to thumb sucking, use of a security blanket), sleep disturbances, depression and eating disturbances. Sexual acting-out behaviour is the most specific indicator of possible sexual abuse. Medical problems include anogenital trauma, bleeding, irritation or discharge, dysuria, frequent urinary tract infections, encopresis, enuresis (especially after continence has been achieved), pregnancy, diagnosis of a sexually transmitted disease (STDs) and oral trauma. Children may present with somatic complaints such as recurrent abdominal pain or frequent headaches resulting from the psychologic stress.

The child's disclosure is often the most important piece of information in determining the likelihood of abuse. Therefore the child should be interviewed alone keeping a neutral tone of voice and using open ended questions in a nonleading manner. The child should be encouraged to respond and elaborate freely.

Physical Examination in a Suspected Case of Sexual Abuse: With a gentle and considerate attitude towards the apprehensive child, complete physical examination, should be carried out to document any lacerations, ecchymoses or petechiae. The oral cavity should be examined to look for bruises or petechiae on the hard and soft palate. The frenulum should be inspected for any lacerations that usually result from forced oral penetration.

Magnification and illumination are essential when examining the genitalia and it can be achieved either by using an otoscope or a colposcope. Demonstration of the instruments before use can be helpful in alleviating a child's fears about the examination. Photographic documentation of the findings and abnormalities should be done either with the help of a colposcope or with a sketch diagrams.

The genital examination of prepubertal girl should be best performed in the frog-leg, position while sitting on the caretaker's lap or prone knee-chest position. In the frog-leg position, the child is supine with the knees apart.[31] If the child is anxious, the examination may be performed while the child is sitting on the caretaker's lap. In the knee-chest position, the child is prone, with knees, chest and head in contact with the table, and the back is in lordosis. It is necessary to perform an examination in the prone knee-chest position to confirm or exclude abnormalities of the posterior aspect of the hymen. Pubertal girls can be examined in the lithotomy position.

Locations of abnormalities should be described as on a clock face with the urethra in the 12-o'clock position and the anus at the 6-o'clock position. In prepubertal girls, use of the speculum is reserved for unexplained bleeding and may require an examination with sedation. In pubertal girls, estrogen causes the hymenal tissue to become thicker and more compliant; therefore, detection of trauma can be more challenging. The use of a moistened cotton swab to gently move the hymen may be helpful in viewing all aspects of a fimbriated or redundant hymen. Another method of improving visualization of the pubertal hymen requires the use of a Foley catheter. The catheter is inserted into the vagina, the balloon is inflated and, with mild retraction, the hymen is stretched. This method allows better visualization of the redundant areas of the hymen. The most common hymenal configurations are crescentic, annular, cuff-like, septate and fimbriated.

The genital examination of boys may be performed with the patient in the sitting, supine or standing position. The physician should examine the penis, testicles and perineum for bite marks, abrasions, bruising or suction ecchymoses.

Evaluation of the anus may be performed with the patient in the supine, lateral recumbent or prone position with gentle retraction of the gluteal folds.

Results of physical examination will be within normal limits in 80 percent of child victims of sexual abuse.[32] The absence of physical findings can be explained by several factors. Many forms of sexual abuse do not cause physical injury. Although the lay public and law enforcement representatives may be fixated on vaginal penetration, sexual abuse may be nonpenetrating contact and may involve fondling, oral-genital, genital or anal contact, as well as genital-genital contact without penetration. Mucosal tissue is elastic and may be stretched without injury, and damage to these mucosal surfaces heals quickly. Finally,many victims of sexual abuse do not seek medical care for weeks or months after the abuse, and superficial abrasions and fissures can heal within 24 to 48 hours.

Physical findings that are concerning but not diagnostic of sexual abuse include the following: (1) notches or clefts in the posterior half of the hymen extending nearly to the vaginal floor, confirmed in all positions, (2) condylomata acuminata in a child older than two years who gives no history of sexual contact, (3) immediate, marked anal dilatation and (4) anal scarring.

Physical findings that are diagnostic of penetration include: (1) acute laceration or ecchymosis of the hymen, (2) absence of hymenal tissue in the posterior half, (3) healed hymenal transection or complete cleft, (4) deep anal laceration and (5) pregnancy without a history of consensual intercourse or sexual assault in children and young adults.

POST EXPOSURE PROPHYLAXIS AGAINST PREGNANCY AND STDs AFTER SEXUAL ABUSE (NACO 2007)[33]

Emergency Contraception (EC) is advised to prevent unwanted pregnancy should be given within 72 hrs of unprotected sexual intercourse **(Table 33.2)**.

Table 33.2 **Post Exposure Prophylaxis with Emergency Contraceptives**

Type of Emergency Contraception	*Dose and Schedule*
Levonorgestrel-only pills (contains 0.75 mg of levonorgestrel per pill)	Levonorgestrel to be taken in 2 doses First dose- to be taken within 72 hours after unprotected intercourse Second dose- same dose to be taken after 12 hrs of first dose

Post exposure prophylaxis of STDs

STDs prophylaxis should be started as early as possible, although the doses should be spread out (and taken with food) to reduce side-effects such as nausea.

A. Post exposure prophylaxis of STDs for adults and older children and adolescents weighing more than 45 kg

1. **For protection against syphilis, chancroid, gonorrhea and chlamydia**
   - Tab. Azithromycin 1gm orally on empty stomach, single dose under supervision

   PLUS
   - Tab. Cefixine 400mg orally after food single dose
2. **For protection against *T. Vaginalis* and *B. vaginosis***
   - Tab Metronidazole 2gm orally after food single dose

   OR
   - Tab Tinidazole 2gm orally after food single dose

B. Post exposure prophylaxis of STI for children

1. **For protection against syphilis and chlamydia**

- Erythromycin 12.5 mg/kg of body weight orally 4 times a day for 14 days

2. **For protection against gonorrhoea**
   - Cefixime 8 mg/kg of body weight as a single dose,
     OR
   - Ceftriaxone 125 mg by intramuscular injection, single dose
3. **For protection against *T. Vaginalis***
   - Metronidazole 5 mg/kg of body weight orally 3 times a day for 7 days

Post Sexual Exposure Prophylaxis of HIV

Refer to district hospital and follow NACO guidelines for the same.

Post Sexual Exposure Prophylaxis Against Hepatitis B

If not vaccinated earlier, it is recommended. If vaccine is not available, refer to the centre where Hepatitis B vaccination facilities are available.

An evaluation of the person's personal safety should be made by a protective services agency or shelter, if available, and arrangements made for protection if needed.

Psychosocial support (both at time of crisis and long-term): Psychosocial management includes counselling and supportive services, which should be available on-site or by referral. Women or children who have been sexually abused may need shelter and legal protection. Adolescents in particular may need crisis support, as they may not be able or willing to disclose the assault to parents or care takers.

Follow-up Services

It is essential to explain the importance of follow-up appointments and services during the first visit itself. The woman should be clearly told whom to contact if she has other questions or subsequent physical or emotional problems related to the incident.

TREATMENT PROTOCOL FOR STDs IN CHILDREN AND ADOLESCENT (U.K. NATIONAL GUIDELINES 2003)[34,35]

CHLAMYDIA

Child < 12 years: Erythromycin 12.5 mg/kg orally qds x 10 - 14 days (maximum dose 500 mg orally qds)

Child > 12 years: Doxycycline 100 mg orally bd × 7 days
or
Erythromycin 500 mg orally qds × 7 days
or
Erythromycin 500 mg orally bd × 14 days
or
Azithromycin 1 g orally in a single dose

TRICHOMONIASIS AND BACTERIAL VAGINOSIS

Child 1-3 years: Metronidazole 50 mg orally tds × 7 days

Child over 3 – under 7 years: Metronidazole 100 mg orally bd × 7 days

Child over 7 – under 10 years: Metronidazole 100 mg orally tds × 7 days

Child > 10 years: Metronidazole 400 mg orally bd × 7 days
or
Metronidazole 2 g orally in a single dose
Metronidazole gel 0.5% and clindamycin cream 2%, are not licensed for use in children.

GONORRHOEA

Gonoccocal Ophthalmia

Ceftriaxone 25-50 mg/kg IV or IM as a single dose up to a maximum dose of 125 mg
or
Cefotaxime 100 mg/kg IM as a single dose.

Child < 2 years: Amoxicillin 50 mg/kg/day orally in a single dose
or
Ceftriaxone 125 mg intramuscularly in a single dose in children who weigh less than 45 Kg
or
*Spectinomycin 40 mg/kg intramuscularly in a single dose [unreliable in pharyngeal infection]

Child 2-12 years: Amoxicillin 50 mg/kg/day orally in a single dose (maximum dose 2 g orally in a single dose) and probenecid 500 mg orally in a single dose
or
Ceftriaxone 125mg intramuscularly in a single dose in children who weigh less than 45 Kg
or
*Spectinomycin 40 mg/kg intramuscularly in a single dose (maximum dose: 2 g) [unreliable in pharyngeal infection]

Child > 12 years: Amoxicillin 2 g orally in a single dose and Probenecid 1 g orally in a single dose
or
*Spectinomycin 2 g intramuscularly in a single dose [unreliable in pharyngeal infection]
or
Ciprofloxacin 500 mg orally in a single dose if growth has ceased (although it has been used extensively in the treatment of pseudomonal infections in children with cystic fibrosis aged 5–17 years without adverse effects).

ANOGENITAL WARTS

Observation period for minimum of 2 months unless symptoms of pain, bleeding or irritation. Consider excision/electrosurgery/cryotherapy under general anaesthesia. Other treatment modalities [eg podophyllotoxin, imiquimod] are not licensed for use in children.

GENITAL HERPES

First episode: Treat if within 5 days of start of episode or while new lesions are still developing.

Child < 2 years: Aciclovir 100 mg orally five times a day for 5 days

Child > 2 years: Aciclovir 200 mg orally five times a day for 5 days

Recurrence

If episodic or suppressive therapy is required see adult guideline.
Valaciclovir and famciclovir are not licensed for use in children.

ANOGENITAL CANDIDIASIS

Child < 16 years: Clotrimazole cream 1% topical application 2 – 3 × daily
Oral imidazoles are not recommended in this age group.

SYPHILIS

Congenital

IV Benzyl penicillin sodium 100,000 to 150,000 units/kg/day (50,000 units/kg every 8-12 hours) for 10 days.

Intramuscular (IM) Procaine penicillin G 50,000 iu/kg daily in a single dose for 10 days up to a maximum daily dose of 750,000 units. Children should not be subjected to more than one IM Procaine penicillin G injection per day: IV Benzyl penicillin sodium treatment is the preferred option if there is necessity to divide the dose of procaine penicillin G.

Acquired

Child < 12 years: IV Benzyl penicillin sodium 200,000 to 300,000 units/kg/day (50,000 units/kg every 4-6 hours) for 10 days.

IM Procaine penicillin G 50,000iu/kg daily in a single dose for 10 days up to a maximum daily dose of 750,000 units

Child > 12 years: IV Benzyl penicillin sodium 200,000 to 300,000 units/kg/day (50,000 units/kg every 4-6 hours) for 10 days.

IM Procaine penicillin G 50,000iu/kg daily in a single dose for 10 days up to a maximum daily dose of 750,000 units

Penicillin Allergy

Doxycycline 100mg orally bd × 14 days or Erythromycin 500 mg orally qds × 14 days

SCABIES

Malathion liquid 0.5% in aqueous base: Apply over whole body [including face, neck, scalp and ears in children aged > 2 years]; wash off after 24 hours. Do not use more than once per week for three consecutive weeks.

Permethrin 5% dermal cream: Apply over whole body [including face, neck, scalp and ears in children aged > 2 years]; wash off after 8 – 12 hours. Do not use more than once a week for three consecutive weeks.

Medical supervision of treatment is required in children aged two months to two years.

PEDICULOSIS PUBIS

Malathion liquid 0.5% in aqueous base: Apply over whole body, allow to dry naturally, wash off after 12 hours or overnight. Do not use more than once per week for two consecutive weeks.

Permethrin 5% dermal cream: Apply over whole body, wash off after 12 hours or overnight. Do not use more than once per week for two consecutive weeks.

Medical supervision of treatment is required in children aged two months to two years.

PRESUMPTIVE TREATMENT

The presumptive treatment of children who have been sexually assaulted or abused is not widely recommended if the regular follow up is assured. However, it may be indicated in a setting when children or their parents/guardians are excessively concerned about the possibility of contracting an STI, even if the risk perceived by the health care practioner is low.

HIV post exposure prophylaxis (PEP) in a child following sexual abuse should be considered especially in a resource poor setting where the prevalence of HIV infection is very high.[36]

PREVENTION OF STDs IN CHILDREN AND ADOLESCENT

Prevention can be achieved through education of the population, identification of symptomatic and asymptomatic people, and effective diagnosis and treatment of the patients and their partners.

Anticipatory guidance should be provided to the adolescents to help them in developing a healthy sexual development while reducing negative aspects of human sexuality. Comprehensive sexuality education should be provided, with emphasis on avoiding unwanted sexual advances (including internet dangers), bullying, pregnancy, and STDs. Adolescents, particularly young adolescents, should be made aware of the potential risks associated with having older sexual partners.

Counselling techniques are useful such as the "helping skill" model, in which the clinician states the problem, identifies options for the patient, identifies consequences of each option, helps the patient make a plan, and develops a plan for check back and follow-up.

Immunization with the hepatitis B vaccine and the human papillomavirus vaccine should be promoted and practiced.

Sexually active patients should be informed, encouraged and guided to use effective contraception and condoms for STDs protection. To date, the condom is the most effective method available for males for protection against STDs. Male circumcision is associated with lower risk of STDs as well as HIV transmission

Physical examination of the reproductive organs and screening for STDs should be performed annually. Teens should be informed of the signs and symptoms of common STDs, the risks and benefits of the various contraceptive options, and the importance of risk-reduction behaviours.

Overview of the Adolescent Reproductive and Sexual Health Strategy (NACO 2007)[33]

The Govt. of India has realized that the health situation of adolescent and youth will be central in determining India's health, mortality, morbidity and population growth scenario. Investment in adolescent reproductive and sexual health will yield dividends in terms of delaying age at marriage, reducing incidence of STDs and reducing the proportion of HIV positive cases in 10-19 age group. This will also help India in realizing its demographic bonus, as healthy adolescents are an important resource for the economy.

The 10th five year plan recognizes adolescents as a distinct group for policy and programme attention. The national population policy 2000 identifies adolescents as an undeserved group for which health specifically reproductive and sexual health interventions are to be designed.

The national youth policy 2003 recognizes 13-19 yrs as a distinct age group which is to be covered in progammes of all sectors including health, education, science and technology etc. In this regard the youth ministry has devised special programmes for adolescent health and empowerment.

Accordingly a national strategy for adolescent reproductive and sexual health (ARSH) has been developed and in the National Rural Health Mission (NRHM) ARSH strategy has been approved as a part of the Reproductive and Child Health Phase II (RCH II). Various States as a part of their State and District RCH II plans have adopted this national strategy. This strategy is now to be implemented in the districts in the primary health care setting.

Youth Friendly RTI/STI services

The key "friendly" characteristics of services for adolescents are at the levels of the user, provider, and health system. Health services must be:

(i) Accessible - ready access to services is provided
(ii) Acceptable - that is, healthcare meets the expectations of adolescents who use the services. e.g. Convenient and confidential services, special hours (after school, evenings, weekends, drop-ins) and comfortable for young men and young couples.

From the provider's and manager's perspective, services must be:

1. **Appropriate**-required care is provided and unnecessary and harmful care is avoided
2. **Comprehensive**-care provision covers aspects from prevention through to counselling and treatment with emphasis on communication skills for young people.
3. **Effective**-healthcare produces positive change in the health status of the adolescents. The health system must focus on efficiency in service delivery that a high quality care provided at the lowest possible cost. Providers who want to work with youth, have special training, are non-judgmental and provide privacy during examination .
4. **Equitable**-that is, services are provided to all adolescents who need them, the poor, vulnerable, marginalized and difficult-to-reach groups/areas.

Services are to be made available for all adolescents, married and unmarried girls and boys. Focus is to be given to the vulnerable and marginalized sub-groups. The package of services is to include promotive, curative and referral services.

Proposed package of STI/RTI services for youth

1. **Promotive Services**
   - Counselling and provision for emergency contraceptive pills

- Counselling and provision for reversible contraceptives
- Information/advice on SRH issues

2. **Preventive services**
   - Provision of condoms
3. **Curative Services:**
   - Treatment of common RTI/STI
   - Treatment and counselling for sexual concerns of male and female adolescents.
   - Management of sexual abuse among girls.
4. **Referral Services:**
   - Voluntary Counselling and Testing Center
   - Prevention of Parent to Child Transmission.
5. **Outreach Services:**
   - Periodic health check ups and community camps.
   - Periodic health education activities.
   - Co-curricular activities.

Outreach Strategy could focus on school-based/peer education programmes, target out-of-school and married youth, use entertainment to gather youth and disseminate health messages (concerts, movies, theatre, etc.) and encourage clinic attendance and organize or link with sports programmes and Red Ribbon club.

Involvement of Adolescents in Prevention

Young people should have information about and be encouraged to:

1. Delay onset of sexual activity. Abstain from sexual activity until married.
2. Learn how to use condoms.
3. Use condoms. These may be discontinued when pregnancy is desired.
4. Limit the number of partners. Avoid multiple partners and stick with one partner.
5. Avoid high-risk partners.
6. Recognize symptoms of RTI/STI: If burning with urination and/or discharge from the penis/vagina, or there are genital sores, young persons and their partners should not have sex, but both should come to the clinic for treatment.

REFERENCES

1. A picture of health? A review and annotated bibliography of the health of young people in developing countries. Geneva, World Health Organisation, 1995 [WHO/FHE/ADH/95.4]
2. Weinstock H, Berman S, Cates W Jr. Sexually transmitted diseases among American youth: incidence and prevalence estimates, 2000. Perspect Sex Reprod Health 2004; 36: 6-10.
3. Carlos T Da Ros, Caio da Silva Schmitt. Global epidemiology of sexually transmitted diseases. Asian J Androl 2008; 10: 110-4.
4. Sexually Transmitted Diseases Surveillance 2005. Appendix 139-50.
5. Argent AC, Lachman PI, Hanslo D, et al. Sexually transmitted diseases in children and evidence of sexual abuse. Child Abuse Negl 1995; 19: 1303-10.
6. Pandhi D, Kumar S, Reddy BS. Sexually transmitted diseases in children. J Dermatol. 2003; 30: 314-20.
7. Pandhi RK, Khanna N, Sekhri R. Sexually transmitted diseases in children. Indian Pediatr 1995; 32: 27-30.
8. Bhogal CS, Chauhan S, Baruah MC. Pattern of childhood STDs in a major hospital of East Delhi. Indian J Dermatol Venereol Leprol 2002; 68: 210-2.
9. Auslander BA, Rosenthal SL, Blythe MJ. Sexual Development and behaviours of adolescents. Pediatr Ann 2005; 34: 785-93.
10. Karl L, Dehni E, Gabriel, et al. Sexually Transmitted infections among adolescents. WHO publications. http://www.who.int/child adolescent health.

11. Zelnik M, Shah FK. First intercourse among young Americans. Fam Plann Perspect 1983; 15: 64-70.
12. Ryan S, Franzetta K, Manlove JS, et al. Older sexual partners during adolescence: links to reproductive health outcomes in young adulthood. Perspect Sex Reprod Health 2008; 40: 17-26.
13. Santelli JS, Brener ND, Lowry R, et al. Multiple Sexual Partners Among US Adolescents And Young Adults. Family Planning Perspectives 1998; 30: 271–5.
14. Yan AF, Chiu YW, Stoesen CA, et al. STDs-/HIV-related sexual risk behaviours and substance use among US rural adolescents. J Natl Med Assoc 2007; 99: 1386-94.
15. Cohen DA, Farley TA, Taylor SN, et al. When and where do youths have sex? The potential role of adult supervision. Pediatrics 2002; 110: 66–72.
16. Fonseca H, Greydanus DE. Sexuality in the child, teen, and young adult: concepts for the clinician. Prim Care. 2007; 34: 275-92; abstract vii.
17. Lowy G. Sexually transmitted diseases in children. Pediatr Dermatol 1992; 9: 329-34.
18. Kavina BK, Billimoria FE, Rao MV. Pattern of STDs & HIV seropositivity in young adults attending STDs clinic of civil hospital, Ahamedabad, Indian J Sex Transm Dis 2005; 26: 60-3.
19. Sexually Transmitted Diseases surveillance 2005. Dept of Health and Human services. CDC Nov. 2006.
20. Gutman LT. Gonococcal diseases in infants and children. In: Holmes KK, Mardh PA, Sparling PF et al, Eds. Sexually Transmitted Diseases 3rd Edn. Mc Graw Hill New York .1999; p: 1145-53.
21. Shapiro RA, Schubert CJ, Myers PA. Vaginal discharge as an indicator of gonorrhea and Chlamydia infection in girls under 12 years old. Pediatr Emerg Care 1993; 9: 341-5.
22. Krugman SD, Wissow LS, Krugman RD. Facing facts: child abuse and pediatric practice. Contemp Pediatr 1998; 15: 131-44.
23. Hymel KP, Child JC. Child sexual abuse. Pediatr Rev 1996; 17: 236-50.
24. Rimsza ME, Niggermann EH. Medical evaluation of sexually abused children: a review of 311 cases. Pediatrics 1982; 69: 8-15.
25. Leventhal JM. Have there been changes in the epidemiology of sexual abuse of children during the 20th century? Pediatrics 1988; 82: 766-73.
26. Emans SJ, Wood ER, Flagg NT, et al. Genital findings in sexually abused symptomatic and symptomatic girls. Pediatrics 1987; 79: 778.
27. White ST, Loda FA, Ingram DL, et al. Sexually transmitted diseases in sexually abused children. Pediatrics 1983; 72; 16-21.
28. De Jong A. Sexually transmitted diseases in sexually abused children. Sex Transm Dis 1986, 13: 123-6.
29. Lahoti SL, Macclain N, Girardet R, et al. Evaluating the Child for Sexual Abuse. Am Fam Physician 2001; 63: 883-92.
30. Guidelines for the evaluation of sexual abuse of children: subject review. American Academy of Pediatrics Committee on Child Abuse and Neglect. Pediatrics 1999; 103: 186-91.
31. Bays J, Chadwick D. Medical diagnosis of the sexually abused child. Child Abuse Negl 1993; 17: 91-110.
32. Adams JA, Harper K, Knudson S, et al. Examination findings in legally confirmed child sexual abuse: it's normal to be normal. Pediatrics 1994; 94: 310-17.
33. National guidelines on prevention, management and control of reproductive tract infections including sexually transmitted infections, Maternal Health Division, NACO, Ministry of Health and Family Welfare, Government of India, August 2007.
34. Thomas A, Forster G, Robinson A et al. National guideline for the management of suspected sexually transmitted infections in children and young people. Sex. Transm. Inf. 2002; 78; 324-31.
35. U.K. National guidelines for the management of suspected sexually transmitted infections in children and young people 2006. http://sti.bmj.com/cgi/data/78/5/324/DCI/6.
36. Ellis JS, Ahmad S , Molyneux EM. Introduction of HIV post-exposure prophylaxis for sexually abused children in Malawi. Arch Dis Child. 2005; 90; 1297-9.

34 SEXUALLY TRANSMITTED DISEASES IN PREGNANCY & NEONATE

Usha Gupta

In this chapter

- Syphilis
- Gonorrhoea
- Chlamydial Infection
- Lymphogranuloma Venereum (LGV)
- Chancroid
- Group B Streptococcal Infection (GBS)
- Donovanosis
- Bacterial Vaginosis
- Genital Herpes
- Neonatal Herpes
- Human Papilloma Virus
- Cytomegalovirus Infection
- Congenital CMV Infection
- Hepatitis B
- Candidiasis
- Trichomoniasis
- HIV Infection
- Safe Drugs to Treat STI in Pregnancy
- Summary Clinical Features of Neonatal STI

INTRODUCTION

Sexually transmitted diseases (STDs) can affect women in the same way as they affect men. As the number of STDs continues to emerge especially in the HIV era, it is increasingly important that the women should be aware of the harmful effects of these diseases and how to protect themselves. Firstly, if the woman acquires the infection prior to pregnancy it can give rise to salpingitis and tubal blockage which can cause ectopic pregnancy or infertility. Secondly, immunological changes occurring during pregnancy can result in change in the severity of the disease e.g. viral warts may overgrow in size and shape. Thirdly, with untreated STDs, the puerperal infections may be more severe.

Women who are pregnant may become infected with the same STDs as non-pregnant women. The consequences of STDs are more serious, even life threatening for a woman and her baby if she becomes infected during pregnancy. The outcome of pregnancy may also be affected as the newborn can get infected in utero via blood e.g. cytomegalovirus infection and syphilis. Chlamydia infection may also cause pneumonia and ophthalmia neonatorum in neonate. Herpes virus can also infect the neonate during the passage through birth canal. STDs may also cause premature rupture of membrane (PROM), still birth, low birth weight, neonatal sepsis, neurological damage (brain damage or motor disorders) and congenital abnormalities (including blindness, deafness and other organ damage). Acute hepatitis, meningitis, chronic liver disease and cirrhosis may also develop.

HIV infection is another cause of concern as it can be transmitted from mother to child. HIV infection may modify the course and treatment of other STDs. Hence all pregnant women must undergo screening test for HIV.

The various STDs syndromes and their complications in women are discussed in a separate chapter. The complications of STDs pathogens in pregnant women and the prevalence of various STDs in women in India are given in Table 34.1 and 34.2 respectively.

Table 34.1 **Complications of STDs and Causative Organisms in Pregnant Women**

Complication	*Pathogen*
Pregnancy associated	
Chorioamnionitis	*N. gonorrhoeae, M. hominis*, Bacterial vaginosis-associated organisms
Spontaneous abortion/foetal wastage	*Herpes Simplex Virus* (HSV), *T. pallidum*, Bacterial vaginosis-associated organisms
Prematurity/PROM	Group B-streptococcus (GBS), *C. trachomatis, N. gonorrhoeae, T. pallidum*, Bacterial vaginosis-associated organisms
Postpartum endometritis	GBS, *N. gonorrhoeae, M. hominis*(?), *C. trachomatis*(?), Bacterial vaginosis associated organisms
Congenital/perinatal infections	
TORCH syndrome	GBS, HSV, Cytomegalovirus (CMV), *T. pallidum*,
Sepsis/death	*C. trachomatis, N. gonorrhoeae*
Conjunctivitis	*C. trachomatis*, GBS, *T. pallidum, Ureaplasma urealyticum*
Neurological involvement	CMV, HSV, *T. pallidum*, GBS.

Table 34.2 Prevalence of STDs in Women in STD Clinics of India

Diseases	*Kurnool*[1] *1992-6 (%) (n = 770)*	*Pondicherry*[2] *1982-90 (%) (n = 1884)*	*New Delhi*[3] *2002-4(%) (n=617)*
Non gonococcal urethritis	18.0	—	1.9
Gonorrhoea	14.8	4.1	1.5
Syphilis	9.0	22.4	29.0
Herpes genitalis	13.0	12.3	11.5
Genital warts	4.2	10	17.2
Non venereal dermatoses	6.5	—	—
LGV	0.9	3.6	0
Molluscum contagiosum	2.2	60.3	—
HIV positive	0.5	—	—
Vulvovaginitis	28.3	12.3	37.1
Donovanosis	0.4	7.3	0
Chancroid	2.2	2.4 1.8	
Psychosexual	2.6	—	—
Scabies	—	0.6	—

The prevalence of STDs in women was found to be 18.1% in a community based study done in Tamil Nadu (Table 34.3).[4]

Table 34.3 Prevalence of STDs in Women in General Population in Tamil Nadu (n = 1105).

Disease	Percent Affected
Any STD	18.1
Classical STDs	12.6
Gonorrhoea	3.9
Syphilis	0.2
Chalmydia	5.1
Trichomonas	5.1
HBsAg	4.8
HIV	2.0

It is apparent that syphilis, vulvovaginitis, herpes genitalis and gonorrhoea are common STDs in women. The common clinical features of STDs are similar in men and women and are described elsewhere and only the special features in women are emphasized in this chapter.

SYPHILIS[5,6]

Syphilis can affect the outcome of pregnancy depending upon the stage. Fimura et al.[7] in their observations regarding the outcome of pregnancy in relation to the stage of maternal syphilis, reported that among infants born to mothers with primary and secondary syphilis, half of them were premature, still born or died in the neonatal period and rest of them had congenital syphilis. With early latent syphilis, the transmission rate decreased to 40%, while 20% were premature, 4% died in the neonatal period and 10% were still born, 20% of them were normal and born at full term. In case of late latent syphilis – 9% premature births, 11% still births, and only 10% congenital syphilis were observed. With longer duration of untreated maternal syphilis the severity of effect in foetus will decrease. The mother who had congenital syphilis can hardly transmit the disease to the foetus.

The severity of disease in the foetus also varies, it is more severe in more recent infections and less so in long-standing disease (Kassowitz's law). However a patient who has had several miscarriages, still births and congenitally syphilitic children may give birth to healthy non infected child and again have a baby with congenital syphilis. Usually the last infant has fewer signs and symptoms of the disease.[7]

All women should be screened serologically for syphilis during the early stages of pregnancy. The majority of states mandate screening at the first prenatal visit for all women. Antepartum screening by nontreponemal antibody testing is typical, but in some settings, treponemal antibody testing is being used. If the test is positive, then the possibility of biological false positive (BFP) reactions should be kept in mind. Usually BFP occurs at a titre of 1:8 or less. Pregnant women with reactive treponemal screening tests should have confirmatory testing with nontreponemal tests with titers. In populations in which use of prenatal care is not optimal, RPR-card test screening should be performed at the time a pregnancy is diagnosed. For communities and populations in which the prevalence of syphilis is high or for patients at high risk, serologic testing should be performed twice during the third trimester, at 28 to 32 weeks' gestation and at delivery. Any woman who delivers a stillborn infant after 20 weeks' gestation should be tested for syphilis. No infant should leave the hospital without the maternal serologic status having been determined at least once during pregnancy.[8]

The test for congenital syphilis in a newborn may be positive from the cord blood. This could be due to passive reaginemia. Even a positive FTA-ABS test may be found due to non-specific interference by the production of IgM and IgG antibody by the neonate. Therefore a positive serology at birth does not necessarily indicate the presence of infection. Hence routine screening of the newborn serum or umbilical cord blood is not recommended.

Treatment

Penicillin is effective for preventing maternal transmission to the foetus and for treating foetal infection. Evidence is insufficient to determine specific, recommended penicillin regimens that are optimal.[8]

Recommended Regimen

Treatment during pregnancy should be the penicillin regimen appropriate for the stage of syphilis.

Other Management Considerations

Some specialists recommend additional therapy for pregnant women in some settings (e.g. a second dose of benzathine penicillin 2.4 million units IM administered 1 week after the initial dose for women who have primary, secondary, or early latent syphilis). During the second half of pregnancy, syphilis management may be facilitated by a sonographic foetal evaluation for congenital syphilis, but this evaluation should not delay therapy. Sonographic signs of foetal or placental syphilis (i.e., hepatomegaly, ascites, hydrops, or a thickened placenta) indicate a greater risk for foetal treatment failure[9]; such cases should be managed in consultation with obstetric specialists. Evidence is insufficient to recommend specific regimens for these situations.

Women treated for syphilis during the second half of pregnancy are at risk for premature labour and/or foetal distress, if the treatment precipitates the Jarisch-Herxheimer reaction. These women should be advised to seek obstetric attention after treatment, if they notice any contractions or decrease in foetal movements. Stillbirth is a rare complication of treatment, but concern for this complication should not delay necessary treatment. All patients who have syphilis should be offered testing for HIV infection.

Follow-Up

Coordinated prenatal care and treatment follow-up are vital. Serologic titers should be repeated at 28–32 weeks gestation, at delivery, and following the recommendations for the stage of disease. Serologic titers can be checked monthly in women at high risk for reinfection or in geographic areas in which the prevalence of syphilis is high. The clinical and antibody response should be appropriate for the stage of disease. The majority of women will deliver before their serologic response to treatment can be assessed definitively. Inadequate maternal treatment is likely if delivery occurs within 30 days of therapy, if clinical signs of infection are present at delivery, or if the maternal antibody titer is fourfold higher than the pretreatment titer.

Congenital syphilis[10]

The details are given in the chapter on congenital syphilis.

GONORRHOEA

Gonorrhoea can manifest as cervicitis, urethritis, endometritis, salpingitis and perihepatitis in women. It can also cause conjunctivitis, tonsillitis and proctitis. Chronic asymptomatic infection is common in 50% of women. Almost all patients with gonococcal infection during pregnancy are asymptomatic. In the neonates, the passage through the birth canal of the infected mother can give rise to ophthalmia neonatorum, pharyngitis and proctitis. Meningitis as a complication of ophthalmia neonatorum has also been described.[6] The importance of gonorrhoea in women during pregnancy is that it may ruin the obstetric future by giving rise to complications like tubal blockage and ectopic pregnancy as a result of PID. Disseminated gonococcal infection and oropharyngeal infection (15-35%) are more common during pregnancy. Gonococcal infections may also lead to PROM, chorioamnionitis, septic abortions, intrauterine growth retardation, prematurity and post partum sepsis.

Post abortal gonococcal endometritis and salpingitis are now well recognized complications of termination of pregnancy.[5] Patients undergoing therapeutic abortions who have untreated endocervicitis, have high risk of developing post abortal endometritis.[5] Various studies have shown that the perinatal outcome in mothers with untreated gonorrhoea would result in spontaneous abortion (11-35%), perinatal mortality (8-11%), prematurity (17-67%) and premature rupture of membranes (20-75%).[11] Because of these complications few experts suggest routine cultures at the initial prenatal visit and a repeat culture early in the third trimester.[12]

Risk of developing PID reduces during the first trimester of pregnancy because of cervical mucous plug which forms a barrier and reduces the risk of anterograde transmission of infection. In the later part of pregnancy, chorion fuses with decidua blocking the uterine cavity, hence upward transmission of infection is prevented.

Treatment

Treatment of gonococcal infection is discussed in a separate chapter.

As per WHO 2003 and CDC 2006 Uncomplicated gonococcal infection of urethra, cervix and rectum in pregnant women can be treated with one of the following regimens.[13]

Cefixime 400 mg orally in a single dose or
Ceftriaxone 125 mg IM in a single dose or
Spectinomycin 2 g by IM injection

Pregnant women should not be given quinolones or tetracyclines. They should be treated with recommended or alternative cephalosporin. Women who cannot tolerate cephalosporin can be given spectinomycin 2 g IM single dose. Test for cure is no longer recommended, if they have received any of the CDC recommended regimens for gonorrhoea. Only those patients with persistent symptoms, a subsequent culture and antimicrobial susceptibility is tested after 1-2 months of treatment.[13]

Gonococcal Infections Among Infants

N. gonorrhoeae can be transmitted at birth. Neonatal gonorrhoea can cause opthalmia, neonatorum, scalp abscesses, vaginal, rectal, oral, joint and disseminated infections.[14]

Gonococcal infection among infants usually results from exposure to infected cervical exudate at birth. It is usually an acute illness that manifests 2–5 days after birth. The prevalence of infection among infants depends on the prevalence of infection among pregnant women, whether pregnant women are screened for gonorrhoea, and whether newborns receive ophthalmia prophylaxis. The most severe manifestations of *N. gonorrhoeae* infection in newborns are ophthalmia neonatorum and sepsis, which can include arthritis and meningitis. Less severe manifestations include rhinitis, vaginitis, urethritis, and reinfection at sites of fetal monitoring.[14]

Ophthalmia Neonatorum Caused by N. gonorrhoeae

In the United States, although *N. gonorrhoeae* causes ophthalmia neonatorum less frequently than *C. trachomatis* and nonsexually transmitted agents, identifying and treating this infection is especially important because ophthalmia neonatorum can result in perforation of the globe of the eye and blindness.[14]

Diagnostic Considerations

Infants at increased risk for gonococcal ophthalmia are those who do not receive ophthalmia prophylaxis and those whose mothers have had no prenatal care or whose mothers have a history of STDs or substance abuse. Gonococcal ophthalmia is strongly suspected when intracellular gram-negative diplococci are identified in conjunctival exudate, justifying presumptive treatment for gonorrhoea after appropriate cultures for *N. gonorrhoeae* are obtained. Appropriate chlamydial testing should be done simultaneously. Presumptive treatment for *N. gonorrhoeae* might be indicated for newborns who are at increased risk for gonococcal ophthalmia and who have conjunctivitis but do not have gonococci in a Gram-stained smear of conjunctival exudate.[14]

In all cases of neonatal conjunctivitis, conjunctival exudates should be cultured for *N. gonorrhoeae* and tested for antibiotic susceptibility before a definitive diagnosis is made. A definitive diagnosis is vital because of the public health and social consequences of a diagnosis of gonorrhoea. Nongonococcal causes of neonatal ophthalmia include *Moraxella catarrhalis* and other *Neisseria species* that are indistinguishable from *N. gonorrhoeae* on Gram-stained smear but can be differentiated in the microbiology laboratory.[14]

Recommended Regimen

Ceftriaxone 25-50mg/kg IV or IM in a single dose, not to exceed 125 mg

Topical antibiotic therapy alone is inadequate and is unnecessary if systemic treatment is administered.

Follow-Up

Infants who have gonococcal ophthalmia should be hospitalized and evaluated for signs of disseminated infection (e.g., sepsis, arthritis, and meningitis). One dose of ceftriaxone is adequate therapy for gonococcal conjunctivitis.

DGI and Gonococcal Scalp Abscesses in Newborns

Sepsis, arthritis, and meningitis (or any combination of these conditions) are rare complications of neonatal gonococcal infection. Localized gonococcal infection of the scalp can result from foetal monitoring through scalp electrodes. Detection of gonococcal infection in neonates who have sepsis, arthritis, meningitis, or scalp abscesses requires cultures of blood, CSF, and joint aspirate on chocolate agar. Specimens obtained from the conjunctiva, vagina, oropharynx, and rectum that are cultured on gonococcal selective medium are useful for identifying the primary site(s) of infection, especially if inflammation is present. Positive Gram-stained smears of exudate, CSF, or joint aspirate provide a presumptive basis for initiating treatment for *N. gonorrhoeae*. Diagnoses based on Gram-stained smears or presumptive identification of cultures should be confirmed with definitive tests on culture isolates.[14]

Recommended Regimens

Ceftriaxone 25-50 mg/kg/d IV or IM in a single dose for 7 days, with a duration of 10-14 days, if meningitis is documented

or

Cefotaxime 25 mg/kg IV or IM every 12 hours for 7 days, with a duration of 10-14 days, if meningitis is documented.

Prophylactic Treatment for Infants Whose Mothers Have Gonococcal Infection. Infants born to mothers who have untreated gonorrhea are at high risk for infection and may be given following regimen in the absence of signs of gonococcal infection:

Ceftriaxone 25–50 mg/kg IV or IM, not to exceed 125 mg, in a single dose.

CHLAMYDIAL INFECTION[15-17]

The clinical spectrum and epidemiology of *C. trachomatis* infection is described in chapter 22. The effect of the infection on pregnancy could be post partum endometritis, post abortal endometritis, spontaneous abortion and foetal deaths, prematurity, low birth weight and PROM.[17] It was noticed in a study that pregnant mother infected with chlamydia at or before 18 weeks gestation had higher incidence of prematurity, low birth weight infants and perinatal deaths.[15]

Among babies born of infected mothers about, 60-70% of them have risk of acquiring infection during the passage through the birth canal, among which 20-50% will develop ophthalmia neonatorum in first 2 weeks and 10-20% would develop pneumonia within 3-4 months after birth.[18] The neonate may remain afebrile with paroxysmal cough and chest X-ray shows diffuse infiltration. In utero transmission is not known to occur. There is no evidence that additional therapy with a topical agent provides further benefit.

Treatment

Doxycycline, ofloxacin, and levofloxacin are contraindicated in pregnant women. However, clinical experience and studies suggest that azithromycin is safe and effective.[19-21] Repeat testing (preferably by nucleic acid amplification test [NAAT]) 3 weeks after completion of therapy is recommended for all pregnant women. The frequent gastrointestinal side effects associated with erythromycin might discourage patient compliance with the alternative regimens.

Recommended Regimens: Refer to chapter 22.

Chlamydial Infections Among Infants

Prenatal screening of pregnant women can prevent chlamydial infection among neonates. Pregnant women aged <25 years are at high risk for infection. Local or regional prevalence surveys of chlamydial infection can be conducted to confirm the utility of using these recommendations in particular settings.

C. trachomatis infection of neonates results from perinatal exposure to the mother's infected cervix.

Initial *C. trachomatis* perinatal infection involves the mucous membranes of the eye, oropharynx, urogenital tract and rectum and might be asymptomatic in these locations. *C. trachomatis* infection in neonates is most frequently recognized by conjunctivitis that develops 5–12 days after birth. *C. trachomatis* also can cause a subacute, afebrile pneumonia with onset at ages 1–3 months. *C. trachomatis* has been the most frequent identifiable infectious cause of ophthalmia neonatorum, but perinatal chlamydial infections, including opthalmia and pneumonia, are detected less frequently because of the institution of widespread prenatal screening and treatment of pregnant women.

Ophthalmia Neonatorum Caused by C. trachomatis

A chlamydial etiology should be considered for all infants aged ≤30 days who have conjunctivitis, especially if the mother has a history of untreated chlamydia infection.

Recommended Regimens

Erythromycin base or ethylsuccinate 50 mg/kg/d orally divided into 4 doses daily for 14 days.

An association between oral erythromycin and infantile hypertrophic pyloric stenosis has been reported in infants aged <6 weeks who were treated with this drug. Infants treated with erythromycin should be followed for signs and symptoms of idiopathic hypertrophic pyloric stenosis (IHPS).

Data on use of other macrolides (e.g., azithromycin and clarithromycin) for the treatment of neonatal chlamydia infection are limited. The results of one study involving a limited number of patients suggest that a short course of azithromycin, 20 mg/kg/day orally, 1 dose daily for 3 days, may be effective.

Topical antibiotic therapy alone is inadequate for treatment of chlamydial infection and is unnecessary when systemic treatment is administered.[14]

Follow-Up

The efficacy of erythromycin treatment is approximately 80%; a second course of therapy might be required and, therefore, follow-up of infants is recommended to determine whether initial treatment was effective. The possibility of concomitant chlamydial pneumonia should be considered.

Infant Pneumonia Caused by C. trachomatis

Characteristic signs of chlamydial pneumonia in infants include 1) a repetitive staccato cough with tachypnea and 2) hyperinflation and bilateral diffuse infiltrates on a chest radiograph. Wheezing is rare, and infants are typically afebrile. Peripheral eosinophilia ($\geq$400 cells/mm^3) occurs frequently. Because clinical presentations differ, initial treatment and diagnostic tests should include *C. trachomatis* for all infants aged 1–3 months who possibly have pneumonia (especially with untreated maternal chlamydial infection).

Follow-Up

The treatment and follow up is same as for ophthalmia neonatorum. Follow-up of infants is recommended to determine whether the pneumonia has resolved. Some infants with chlamydial pneumonia have abnormal pulmonary function tests later in childhood.

Infants Born to Mothers Who Have Chlamydial Infection

Infants born to mothers who have untreated chlamydia are at high risk for infection; however, prophylatic antibiotic treatment is not indicated, and the efficacy of such treatment is unknown. Infants should be monitored to ensure appropriate treatment if symptoms develop. Neonatal ocular prophylaxis with silver nitrate solution or antibiotic ointment does not prevent perinatal transmission of *C. trachomatis* from mother to infant. However ocular prophylaxis with these agents does prevent gonococcal ophthalmia and therefore should be continued.[14]

LYMPHOGRANULOMA VENEREUM (LGV)

LGV is caused by *C. trachomatis*, serotypes L1, L2 and L3. The occurrences of acute LGV cases are more common in men than in women, in the ratio of 5:1 or more. On the other hand long term complications like ulceration, genital hypertrophy and rectal strictures are more common in women. Although transplacental congenital infection has not been reported, acquisition of infection during passage through an infected birth canal can occur.[22]

Treatment

Pregnant women should be treated with erythromycin. Azithromycin might prove useful for treatment of LGV in pregnancy, but no published data are available regarding its safety and efficacy. Doxycycline is contraindicated in pregnant women.[14]

CHANCROID

Chancroid is caused by *H. ducreyi*. The most common site for 'soft chancre' is labia, clitoris and fourchette. The symptoms with which women present are dysuria, rectal bleeding, dyspareunia or vaginal discharge. The classic ulcer of a chancroid is superficial and shallow with ragged edge with an erythematous halo. Multiple ulcers are the rule in women in contrast to solitary ulcers in more than 50% of men.[5] Bubo formation classically described in men are rare in women.[23] CDC recommends that a probable diagnosis of chancroid can be made by following criteria.[13]

(a) If the individual has one/more painful genital ulcer.
(b) There is no evidence of syphilis on dark field examination or by serology at least 7 days after the onset of ulcers.
(c) Either the clinical presentation of the genital ulcers and inguinal lymphademopathy are typical for chancroid or tests for HSV are negative.

Treatment of chancroid remains the same as that of men, except in pregnant women where quinolonoes are contraindicated and, the safety of azithromycin has not been established. Ceftrioxone or erythromycin is the preferred regimen for pregnant and lactating women. No adverse affects of chancroid on pregnancy outcome or on fetus have been observed.[5,13]

There is no report of congenital or neonatal infection.[24]

GROUP B STREPTOCOCCAL INFECTION (GBS)

GBS (*Streptococcus Agalactiae*) is known to colonize 5–25% females and rarely associated with vaginitis or cervicitis in non pregnant females. There are reports of GBS related infections in pregnancy e.g. chorioamnionitis, post partum wound infection and post partum endometritis. 1–2% of neonates born to GBS carrier mother develop the disease. The mortality rate is upto 50%. The risk is higher if the baby is premature or with low birth weight. The baby may develop pneumonia or septicemia within the first week. Late onset meningitis can also develop.

Treatment with erythromycin or ampicillin is effective. It is controversial whether treatment during pregnancy can eradicate the organism or prevent neonatal disease. Routine prophylactic treatment for exposed neonate is recommended.[5]

DONOVANOSIS

A chronic progressively destructive infection of the genital area caused by *Klebsiella granulomatis* (formerly known as *Calymmatobacterium granulomatis*)[24] a gram negative bacilli.In women,the usual sites of infection are labia and fourchette. The epithelium overlying the lesion subsequently enlarges to produce beefy, red velvety granulomatous ulcer. Untreated disease may involve groin and perianal area and bone involvement has been described. In long standing cases, squamous cell carcinoma may develop.[25] O'Farrell has reported that during pregnancy donovanosis has a more aggressive course.

Treatment

Pregnancy is a relative contraindication to the use of sulfonamides. Pregnant and lactating women should be treated with the erythromycin regimen, and consideration should be given to the addition of a parenteral aminoglycoside (e.g., gentamicin). Azithromycin might prove useful for treating granuloma inguinale during pregnancy, but published data are lacking. Doxycycline and ciprofloxacin are contraindicated in pregnant women.[14]

Neonatal Donovanosis

Infants born to infected mothers may acquire infection at birth[26-28] and develop lesions of the umbilicus, penis, and vulva as well as disseminated infection.

BACTERIAL VAGINOSIS[29-33]

Bacterial vaginosis may be associated with an increased incidence of adverse pregnancy outcomes (e.g. PROM, pre-term delivery and low birth weight). Rarely it can cause PID, puerperal pyrexia, septic abortion, neonatal bacteremia and cutaneous abscess. A symptomatic pregnant women should be treated, and those with a history of previous pre-term delivery should be screened to detect asymptomatic infections.

Treatment

Recommended Regimens for pregnant women
Metronidazole 500 mg orally twice a day for 7 days
Or
Metronidazole 250 mg orally three times a day for 7 days
Or
Clindamycin 300 mg orally twice a day for 7 days

Whether treatment of asymptomatic pregnant women with BV who are at low risk for preterm delivery reduces adverse outcomes of pregnancy is unclear. One trial in which oral clindamycin was used demonstrated a reduction in spontaneous preterm birth.[29] Several trials have evaluated the use of intravaginal clindamycin during pregnancy to reduce preterm birth and treat asymptomatic BV. One trial in which women were treated before 20 weeks' gestation demonstrated a reduction in preterm birth.[30] In three other trials, intravaginal clindamycin cream was administered at 16–32 weeks' gestation, and an increase in adverse events (e.g., low birthweight and neonatal infections) was observed in newborns.[31-33] Therefore, intravaginal clindamycin cream should be used only during the first half of pregnancy.

GENITAL HERPES

The clinical features and types of genital herpes are described in chapter 25. Pregnancy does not influence the recurrence compared to the general population although it has been noticed that primary episode during pregnancy may be more severe than in non pregnant women.[6] Its importance in pregnancy is due to the devastating obstetric complications and neonatal infection.[34] The risk of transmission to the neonate is high (30-50%) if the women acquire genital herpes at the time of delivery and is low (<1%) among the women who acquire genital herpes during the first half of pregnancy. This may be due to type specific antibodies (maternal) that would protect the neonate.[35]

Babies born to mothers with long-standing herpes infections have a natural protection against the virus. Herpes antibodies in the mother's blood cross the placenta to the foetus. These antibodies help protect the baby from acquiring infection during birth, even if there is some virus in the birth canal. That's the major reason that mothers with recurrent genital herpes rarely transmit herpes to their babies during delivery. Even women who acquire genital herpes during the first two trimesters of pregnancy are usually able to supply sufficient antibody to help protect the foetus.[32]

Babies born prematurely may be at a slightly increased risk, however, even if the mother has a long-standing infection. This is because the transfer of maternal antibodies to the fetus begins at about 28 weeks of pregnancy and continues until birth. Babies delivered at term are protected by antibodies – but premature babies haven't gotten a full load.[36]

Mothers who acquire genital herpes during the last trimester of pregnancy may also lack the time to make enough antibodies to send across the placenta. In addition, newly infected people – whether pregnant or not - have a higher rate of asymptomatic shedding for roughly a year following a primary episode. This higher rate of asymptomatic shedding, plus the lack of antibodies, create the greater risk for babies whose mothers are infected in the last trimester.[36]

Mothers who acquire genital herpes in the last few weeks of pregnancy are at the highest risk of transmitting the virus to their infants. If the mother's infection is a true primary (she has no previous antibodies to either HSV-1 or HSV-2), and she seroconverts (becomes HSV positive) at the end of pregnancy, the risk of transmission can be as high as 50%. The risk is also high if she has prior infection with HSV-1 but not HSV-2.[36]

The foetal infection occurs almost always due to viral shedding from the cervix or lower genital tract infection. The risk of perinatal infection due to asymptomatic shedding was found to be 4%.[38] The virus invades the uterus following the rupture of the membrane or when the foetus comes in contact with lesions during the time of delivery through the birth canal. Infection is rarely transmitted to the placenta, when the membrane is intact. One practice that may contribute to transmission of neonatal herpes is the use of a fetal scalp monitor (scalp electrodes) during childbirth.

This instrument, which is used to monitor the baby's heartbeat, actually makes tiny punctures in the baby's scalp. Several studies have shown that those breaks in the skin may serve as portals of entry for herpes virus. An alternative is the external monitor, which tracks the baby's heartbeat through the mother's abdomen.[36]

During pregnancy HSV may be acquired in utero, intrapartum or postpartum. About 5% of babies with neonatal herpes acquire the infection prior to labour. 85% of neonatal herpes occur due to direct contact with maternal genitalia or secretions during delivery, 10% cases after birth due to direct contact with caretaker.[34,37-38]

Treatment

Acyclovir, valacyclovir and famciclovir are used for the treatment of genital herpes in non-pregnant women. Acyclovir appears to be safe during pregnancy. CDC along with pharmaceutical company manufacturing acyclovir maintains the registry for exposure to this drug during pregnancy. More than 700 fetus were exposed to the acyclovir during the first trimester without any adverse effects. Episodic therapy with acyclovir may be useful in recurrent episodes and daily suppressive therapy with acyclovir may reduce the signs and symptoms but does not completely eliminate the viral shedding. Between 10-14% of the women with genital herpes have active lesion at the time of delivery. According to the American College of Obstetrics and Gynaecology, caeserian delivery is indicated in women with active genital lesions or with typical prodrome. Ceserian delivery is performed only if the active lesions are present at the time of labour or within 4-6 hours of rupture of the membrane.[39]

NEONATAL HERPES

Neonatal herpes is not a reportable disease in most countries, so there are no hard statistics on the number of cases nationwide. However, most researchers estimate between 1,000 and 3,000 cases a year in the United States, out of a total of 4 million births. To put this in greater perspective, an estimated 20-25% of pregnant women have genital herpes, while less than 0.1% of babies contract an infection.

Transmission rates are lowest (0.04%) for women who acquire herpes before pregnancy and have no signs or symptoms of an outbreak at delivery. The chances of transmission are highest when a woman acquires genital herpes late in pregnancy.

Unfortunately, when infants do contract neonatal herpes, the results can be tragic. About half of infants who are treated with antiviral medication escape permanent damage. But others may suffer serious neurological damage, mental retardation or death. It's fear of these terrible consequences, rather than the level of risk, that makes neonatal herpes a concern.

Disseminated Neonatal Herpes Infection

Epidemiology

- Disseminated neonatal herpes is the most common and most lethal form of neonatal herpes.[40]
- 50% of infants with neonatal herpes.

Natural History

- Presents usually at 9-11 days of age, but as late as 4 weeks.
- Widespread disease, including: pneumonitis, hepatitis, disseminated intravascular coagulation, with or without encephalitis, exanthem, or kerato-conjunctivitis.
- Symptoms include: irritability, seizures, respiratory distress, jaundice, bleeding, shock, and a characteristic vesicular rash.
- 10-50% will not develop skin lesions during the course of their illness.[41]
- Encephalitis in 60 to 75%.

Prognosis

- Mortality without treatment is >80%, with treatment 57%[42] all but a few survivors have neurological impairment (abnormal neurologic status at one year 92% in untreated patients and 86% in treated patients with disseminated disease).

Central Nervous System Herpes in the Neonate

Definition

CNS involvement documented by abnormal CSF findings (increased cell count, positive CSF PCR for HSV) or head MRI or CT changes in conjunction with positive surface cultures.

Epidemiology

- 70% of infants with neonatal herpes (including those with disseminated/CNS disease).[40]

Natural History

- Symptoms include: irritability, seizures, poor feeding, bulging fontanel, thermal instability.
- CSF findings: HSV culture positive 25-40%, pleocytosis, and proteinosis.
- May not have mucocutaneous lesions.[41]

Prognosis

- 50% of untreated babies with localized CNS disease die, 10% of treated infants with localized CNS disease die.[42]
- 75% survivors have psychomotor retardation, often with: microcephaly, hydranencephaly, porencephalic cysts, spasticity, blindness, or learning disabilities.
- Abnormal neurologic status at one year decreased from 83% to 50% in patients with local CNS disease.

Mucocutaneous and Ocular Herpes

Definition

Disease limited to skin or mucus membranes only. Normal CSF, CXR, and LFT's. No evidence of CNS or visceral organ involvement. Diagnosis by positive culture or fluorescent antibody for HSV.

Epidemiology

- 30-40% of patients with neonatal herpes have localized disease.

Natural History

- Usually presents at 15-17 days of age (as late as 4 weeks).
- Sites include: skin, mouth, and eyes.

Prognosis

- Progression from local infection with skin lesions to CNS or disseminated disease decreased from ~70% to 5-20% with early treatment.[42]

Cutaneous Herpes

Skin classically with clusters of discrete vesicles on an erythematous base, occur in 90% of infants with skin, eye, or mouth disease, invariably recur in first 6 months of life, many infants have lesions recurring after a year of age.

Oral Herpes

Vesicles (mucoceles have no associated erythema)

Ocular Herpes

Eyes with keratoconjunctivitis, or later, with chorioretinitis (dendritic keratitis is pathognomonic). May lead to corneal ulcers, cataracts, optic atrophy and/or blindness

Management of the Infant Exposed to Herpes

In mother with recurrent infection, who is HSV-2 seropositive
(Note these recommendations are likely to change, consult a pediatric infectious disease specialist or neonatologist for the most recent recommendations).

- Culture nasopharynx, rectum, and conjunctivae after 24 to 48 hours of life, and repeat at 7-10 day intervals until 28 days old.
- If symptoms develop reculture all sites, including CSF, and begin treatment with acyclovir.

Mother with first episode infection of positive preparation prepartum cultures of both vulva and cervix

- Cultures of CSF, nasopharynx, rectum conjunctivae and blood
- Begin treatment with acyclovir, 5-7 days if cultures remain negative and no symptoms develop.

Treatment of Neonatal Herpes

1. For disseminated and CNS disease
   - Acyclovir 20 mg/kg body weight IV every 8 hours for 21 days
2. For disease limited to the skin and mucous membranes
   - Acyclovir 20 mg/kg body weight IV every 8 hours for 14 days

HUMAN PAPILLOMA VIRUS

HPV types 6 and 11 usually cause anogenital warts. The most important sequelae are the development of cervical, vaginal and vulvar neoplasia.

The genital warts frequently increase in size and number during pregnancy sometime filling the entire vaginal canal or covering the perineum and thereby making vaginal delivery or episiotomy difficult. It is possibly the moistness due to constant vaginal discharge throughout the pregnancy which offers favourable condition for the viral growth. Accelerated viral replication with advancing pregnancy has also been hypothesized. Most women with vulvar lesions also have cervical infection and vice versa due to the multifocal involvement and subclinical nature of the disease. Rarely it can cause life-threatening hemorrhage due to increased vascularity during pregnancy. The lesions usually improve after delivery possibly related to less amount of moisture, vascularity, and immunosuppression due to pregnancy.[5] The different treatment modalities during pregnancy include trichloro or dicholoroacetic acid 80 to 90% once a week, cryotherapy, laser ablation, excision and electrocautery. Podophyllin, 5-FU, imiquimod and interferon are contraindicated during pregnancy.[39]

HPV can be transmitted perinataly. Aspiration of infected material at the time of vaginal delivery can cause laryngeal papillomatosis & perianal warts in infants. In a study of 301 pregnant women with HPV infection, 40% transmission of infection to the newborn was observed, and it was higher for those who delivered vaginally (51%) than with caesarian section (27%). Some authors prefer doing caesarian section if the wart is enormous in size and obstructs the vaginal canal.[43]

CYTOMEGALOVIRUS INFECTION[44-47]

Cytomegalovirus (CMV) is double stranded DNA virus, which has ability to remain latent within the host for years. CMV is transmitted through infected body fluids. Only the persons with immunosuppression are prone to get recurring illness. However, CMV infection presents a specific challenge to the pregnant women because of the perinatal infection and mortality. So whenever a pregnant women experiences infectious mononucleosis like symptoms she should be evaluated for CMV infection. Cytomegalovirus infection is the most common perinatal infection and 40-50% infants born to mothers with primary CMV will have congenital infection. Of these 5 to 18% will be overtly symptomatic at birth and 80% of the survivors have severe neurological morbidity. Most of the congenitally infected infants are asymptomatic at birth and 10 to 15% of these children subsequently develop neurological sequelae.

The risk of fetal injury is higher with primary infection and is very low with recurrences or reactivated CMV infection. The virus can present itself in different strains. Boppana et al,[29] examined anti CMV antibodies from 46 pregnant women with preconceptual immunity to CMV. Of these 16 delivered CMV infected infants. They found that 62% of the mothers of infants with congenital CMV infection had acquired antibodies with new specificities as compared with 13% of the mothers whose infants were not infected. Earlier it has been thought that once an individual has been infected with CMV, that person is protected against reinfection. But the current thinking is that even seropositive women can be reinfected with different strains of CMV and can pass the newly acquired strain to the fetus and thereby causing serious injury.

Diagnosis

Serological diagnosis of primary CMV in the mother is difficult because IgM antibodies persist for longer periods of time. For the best diagnostic results paired serum samples are taken for CMV antibodies. First sample is taken upon suspicion of CMV infection and another is taken within 2 weeks. If the tests show a fourfold rise in IgG and a significant level of IgM antibodies then it indicates an active infection.

Virus culture can be performed from the urine and throat.

Serologic testing: ELISA is the most commonly available test for measuring antibody to CMV which can be used to determine acute infection, prior infection or presence of passively acquired maternal antibody in infants. Other tests include various fluorescence assays, indirect haemagglutination and latex agglutinations. ELISA tests for CMV specific IgM are available. CMV specific IgM may be produced in low levels in reactivated CMV infection.

A more reliable diagnostic procedure to assess fetal infection is by polymerase chain reaction (PCR) and CMV culture performed in amniotic fluid at least 6 weeks following presumed maternal infection and past the 21st week of pregnancy.

Treatment

Currently no treatment exists for CMV infection. Ganciclovir is used for patients with immunosuppression. Vaccines are still in the research and developmental stage.

CDC Recommendations for Pregnant Women

1. Throughout the pregnancy, practice good personal hygiene, especially handwashing with soap and water, after contact with diapers or oral secretions (particularly with a child who is in day care).
2. Women who develop a mononucleosis-like illness during pregnancy should be evaluated for CMV infection and counseled about the possible risks to the unborn child.
3. Laboratory testing for antibody to CMV can be performed to determine if a women has already had CMV infection.
4. Recovery of CMV from the cervix or urine of women at or before the time of delivery does not warrant a caesarean section.
5. The demonstrated benefits of breast-feeding outweigh the minimal risk of acquiring CMV from the breast-breeding mother.
6. There is no need to either screen for CMV or exclude CMV-excreting children from schools or institutions because the virus is frequently found in many healthy children and adults.

CONGENITAL CMV INFECTION[48]

It is calculated that 40,000 infants are born each year congenitally infected with CMV; up to 10% of these will have symptoms at birth that are commonly associated with congenital CMV disease, including intrauterine growth retardation, jaundice, hepatosplenomegaly, petechiae or purpura, thrombocytopenia, and pneumonia. Hepatomegaly, splenomegaly and petechiae are the most common. The liver is usually smooth and nontender and commonly measures 5 cm or more below the RCM. Ascites may be present prenatally and persist postnatally for 1-2 weeks. The hepatomegaly usually resolves by 3 months of age, and persistence beyond 1 year is highly unusual. A mild hepatitis is usually present, but the transaminase levels in neonatal hepatitis due to CMV rarely exceeds 300 IU. Hyperbilirubinemia, on the other hand, may be quite striking, with conjugated (direct) bilirubin levels up to 30 mg/dL. The abnormal results of liver function tests gradually resolve over the first few weeks of life. Chronic hepatitis due to a congenital infection with CMV is unusual but can occur. Enlargement of the spleen is very common in congenital CMV infection, and in some cases it may be the only abnormality detectable at birth. Petechiae observed in congenital CMV disease are usually pinpoint and generalized over the infant's trunk and extremities. Present at birth, they can be transient and resolve within 48-72 hours. They can be the only apparent manifestation of CMV infection; however, more commonly, the triad of hepatomegaly, splenomegaly, and petechiae is seen. Petechiae are usually but not always accompanied by thrombocytopenia, and platelet counts in the first few weeks of life range from 2,000/mm^3 to 125,000/mm^3. Usually resolves during the second week of life, but may persist, requiring repeated platelet transfusions. Sometimes the infant may have a generalized purpuric rash, with evidence of extramedullary hematopoiesis, similar to congenital rubella syndrome. Pneumonitis is unusual but usually severe, interstitial pneumonitis occurring in the context of a diffuse, multisystem infection. CNS manifestations are very common and include lethargy and poor feeding, hypertonia or hypotonia, microcephaly, intracranial calcifications, chorioretinitis, and sensorineural deafness.

Ocular involvement with CMV occurs in 10-20% of symptomatic infants. Most commonly it produces a chorioretinitis that is usually old and inactive at birth. This retinitis is usually unilateral but can produce blindness if the macula is involved, as well as strabismus and optic atrophy. Congenital CMV and congenital toxoplasmosis produce similar lesions; however, congenital CMV characteristically does not produce microphthalmia or cataracts, and alternative diagnoses such as congenital rubella or toxoplasmosis or metabolic disorders should be sought if these eye findings are present. Recent reports showed 23% of children with congenital CMV infection had either progression of an existing retinal lesion or delayed development of chorioretinitis between the ages of 1.5-10 years.

Microcephaly defined as a head circumference of less than the third percentile for gestational age, may be present at birth. It may be part of the overall small size of a growth-retarded infant or may be disproportionate and accompanied by normal weight, length, and chest circumferences. This microcephalia is accompanied with intracraneal calcifications, but asymptomatic infants can also have them; characteristically the calcifications are distributed in a linear, periventricular pattern ranging from tiny, punctate lesions to large deposits of calcium that appear to line the entire ventricular system. Calcifications also may involve the cortical and subcortical regions or involve the basal ganglia. Other neuroradiographic abnormalities include periventricular leukomalacia, cortical atrophy, unilateral or bilateral ventricular enlargement, subdural effusions and hemorrhage. Infants with intracranial calcifications are more likely to experience cognitive and audiologic deficits later in life than those infants who do not have detectable abnormalities, but their functional outcome varies widely, and further studies are needed to determine if the pattern or density of the calcifications are predictive of outcome. Approximately half of the infants with symptomatic and 15% of infants with asymptomatic congenital CMV infection will have an associated hearing loss. Infants may also have septal defects, biliary atresias, inguinal hernias, hip dislocation, and other musculoskeletal abnormalities. In addition, infants with toxoplasmosis, herpes simplex, syphilis, and HIV infections may be coinfected with CMV, and infants with metabolic disorders, such as maple syrup urine disease, may have congenital CMV infection as well.[48]

Diagnosis

The diagnosis of congenital CMV infection is established by isolating virus from urine, saliva, or tissue obtained during the first 3 weeks of life. All infants in whom the diagnosis is suspected should have a viral culture performed. The virus is usually present in a very high titer, and cultures are commonly positive within 2-3 days of incubation. It is important the test be performed early in life, because detection of the virus in bodily fluids or tissue after the age of 3 weeks can indicate either a congenital, perinatal, or postnatal infection. Standard serologic tests, such as detection of CMV IgG and IgM antibodies used alone or as part of a TORCH titer panel are commonly used to diagnose congenital CMV infection, but this approach has several drawbacks and should be discouraged. Although the absence of IgG antibodies to CMV in cord or infant blood probably rules out congenital CMV infection in an immune-competent mother-infant pair, its presence has limited value because 50-80% of women of childbearing age will have

CMV IgG antibodies that will be transplacentally transferred to their infant. A significantly higher titer of IgG antibodies to CMV in the infant than in the mother may imply an active congenital infection, but in practice this difference is usually difficult to ascertain. Serologic samples obtained serially at 1, 3, and 6 months, may rule out congenital infection if the level of CMV antibodies gradually declines; if the levels persist, serologic test results alone cannot determine whether the infant was congenitally or perinatally infected. The presence of IgM antibodies at birth, however, is highly suggestive of a congenital CMV infection, provided the test was performed properly, but a confirmatory urine culture for CMV is recommended to definitively establish the diagnosis. Furthermore, a negative CMV IgM antibody does not exclude the diagnosis of congenital infection. The concept of screening newborns for this congenital infection is not new; recently CMV DNA has been detected by PCR in urine. Also, CMV DNA detected in the cerebrospinal fluid and its presence appears to be significantly associated with developmentaldelay.[48] The evaluation of new born with suspected CMV infection is shown in Table 34.3.

Table 34.4 Evaluation of the Neonate with CMV[48]

Clinical	Height, weight, and head circumference; liver/spleen size; ophthalmologic examination
Laboratory	Complete blood count and peripheral smear; platelet count; liver transaminase levels; bilirubin levels (direct and indirect); urine CMV culture; CS Fluid for cell count, protein and glucose levels, CMV DNA if available and patient stable
Other	Unenhanced CT scan of brain; hearing assessment by brain stem-evoked responses

Prevention

Prevention of congenital CMV disease is desirable and urgently needed. Because the majority of symptomatic congenital CMV disease and its sequelae occur in women who have experienced primary CMV infection during pregnancy, pregnant women and their foetuses would benefit greatly if a safe, effective CMV vaccine were licensed. The use of a CMV vaccine also appears to be cost effective. While research continues, alternative options for prevention of primary CMV infection in pregnant women are being considered. Some experts think that because reliable inexpensive serologic tests are now available for CMV, all women of childbearing age should know their CMV serostatus. Those women who are seronegative should be aware that young children are likely sources of CMV infection, and they should practice good hygiene when they are with young children in their home or in group child-care environments. A similar form of behavioural intervention is currently practiced by women who wish to avoid exposure to toxoplasmosis during pregnancy (avoidance of raw meat, cat litter boxes, and sandlots) and was also practiced during rubella epidemics before a vaccine was available.[48]

Treatment

Two antiviral chemotherapeutic agents, ganciclovir and foscarnet, are licensed specifically for treatment of serious, life-threatening or sight-threatening CMV in the immunocompromised patients. It is recommended that ganciclovir not be routinely used to treat infants with congenital CMV disease until the results of ongoing clinical trials establish its safety and efficacy. Anecdotal evidence does suggest, however, that critically ill newborns, especially those who are premature and have CMV pneumonia, may acutely benefit from ganciclovir treatment, and its use should be carefully considered in selected cases.[48]

HEPATITIS B

Hepatitis B is caused by Hepatitis B virus, a DNA virus with three major antigens; surface antigen (Hbs Ag), core antigen (Hbc Ag), and 'e' antigen (Hbe Ag).

The natural course following an acute infection is that 85-90% experience complete resolution and develop protective antibodies, 10-15% would develop chronic infection, of which 15-30% would develop chronic active hepatitis/persistent hepatitis and about 20% of these patients would go on to develop hepatocellular carcinoma. Only less than 1% of patients with acute infection develop fulminant hepatitis leading to death.

The relevance of this infection during pregnancy is that infected mothers would perinatally transmit the infection to neonate, while the baby is traversing the birthcanal or when it comes in contact with genital secretions. Up to 90% of chronic carrier mothers can transmit the infections to the newborn at the time of delivery especially when the women are Hbs Ag and Hbe Ag positive.

Combination of active and passive immunization can prevent both vertical and horizontal transmission of hepatitis B infection. Neonatal immunoprophylaxis is 85-95% effective in preventing the neonatal hepatitis B infection. Thus CDC recommends an universal hepatitis B vaccination for all infants. The available vaccines are DNA recombinant vaccines, so do not carry risk of transmission of blood borne pathogen. All obstetricians must screen their patients for hepatitis B infection, because selective screening might miss out 30-50% of the infection.

All newborns in Hong Kong are now vaccinated against HBV. Baby born to HBsAg positive mother will also receive 0.5 ml hepatitis B immunoglobulins (HBIg) at birth. Three doses of Hepatitis B vaccine are given at a schedule of 0, 1, 3-5 month. Blood tests for antibody response are generally not required. Breast feeding is not contraindicated in HBsAg positive mothers provided that immunoprophylaxis has already been given to the infant.[24]

CANDIDIASIS

Higher glycogen content in the vaginal environment and enhanced adherence of Candida species to vaginal epithelial cells results in an increase risk of symptomatic vaginitis in pregnancy. The problem becomes more severe as pregnancy progresses. Local therapy with nystatin or imidazole vaginal pessaries can be used. Ketoconazole and itraconazole should not be used due to toxicity and risk of teratogenicity. Neonatal infections usually present with perioral or perianal rash or oral thrush. The details are given in relevant chapter.

TRICHOMONIASIS

Trichomoniasis infection in pregnancy is associated with puerperal maternal morbidity (postpartum fever) and a small but statistically significant increased risk of preterm delivery. There is increasing evidence of association between infection with *T. vaginalis* and PROM & low birth weight. Female neonates may acquire infection perinatally but this seems to be transient in most cases.[39] The details are given in relevant chapter.

HIV INFECTION

HIV infection in pregnancy is discussed in a chapter 7.

SAFE DRUGS TO TREAT STI IN PREGNANCY

The safety profile of common drugs used in the treatment of STDs is shown in Table 34.4 and Table 34.5.[49-51]

SUMMARY CLINICAL FEATURES OF NEONATAL STI

The Clinical features of neonatal STI are summarized in Table 34.6.

Appendix 34.5 FDA Pregnancy Categories of Drugs

A	Foetal risk not revealed in controlled studies in humans.
B	Foetal risk not confirmed in studies in humans but has been shown in some studies in animals.
C	Foetal risk revealed in studies in animals but not established or not studied in humans; may use if benefits outweigh risk to fetus.
D	Foetal risk shown in humans; use only if benefits outweigh risk to fetus.
X	Contraindicated; benefit does not outweigh risk.

Table 34.6 Safety Profile of Drugs Used for Treatment of STIs in Pregnancy[56-58]

Drug	*FDA Category*	*Comments*
Penicillins	B	Safe during all trimesters*.
Cephalosporins	B	Safe; however avoid certain cephalosporins (cefaclor, cephalexin, ceftriaxone and cephadrine).[56]
Erythromycin	B	Erythromycin ethylsuccinate is safe; however erythromycin estolate is contraindicated because of hepatotoxicity.
Azithromycin	B	Evidence increasing in favour of azithromycin safety as well as efficacy as an alternative to erythromycin.
Metronidazole	C	Newer meta-analyses refute teratogenic risks,[57] which were suspected in earlier reports.
Tinidazole	C	Not sufficient human data; slight elevated risk in animals.
Fluconazole	C	High-dose or continuous intake has been shown to be associated with various foetal abnormalities. Smaller doses of fluconazole, as used for treatment of vaginal candidiasis, have been associated with minimal or no risk of fetal abnormalities.
Aminoglycosides	D	Hearing defects, vestibular problems, inner ear damage.
Tetracyclines	D	Various malformations (including enamel hypoplasia).
Fluoroquinolones	D	Bone defects in offsprings.
Acyclovir	B	Considered safe in pregnancy.[58]
Local application of TCA/BCA	?	Safe, but podophyllin, 5-FU, imiquimod and interferon are contraindicated in pregnancy.

*There is no absolutely safe drug in pregnancy. Always benefits of treatment have to be weighed against the risks.

Table 34.6 Summary of Clinical Features of Neonatal STIs.

STI	*Important Clinical Manifestations in Neonates*
Congenital syphilis	Vesico-bullous rash, rhagades, syphilitic rhinitis, fever, hepatosplenomegaly, anaemia, jaundice, seizures. Premature or stillbirth or death of newborn.
Gonorrhoea	Ophthalmia neonatorum, scalp abscesses, vaginal, rectal, oral, joint, disseminated infections.

(*Contd.*)

STI	*Important Clinical Manifestations in Neonates*
Chlamydia	Neonatal conjunctivitis, sub acute pneumonitis, nasopharyngeal or rectovaginal infections.
Neonatal Herpes	Vesicular muco-cutaneous exanthem, kerato-conjunctivitis, disseminated herpes hepatitis, disseminated intravascular coagulation. Herpetic encephalitis presents as irritability, seizures, bulging fontanel and thermal instability.
CMV infection	Sub-clinical, hepatosplenomegaly, microcephaly, jaundice, petechie, hydrocephalus, hemolytic anemia and pneumonitis.

REFERENCES

1. Rangnanayakulu B, Ravikumar GP, Bhaskar GV. Patterns of STDs at Kurnool.Indian J Sex Transm Dis 1998; 19: 117-21.
2. Reddy BSN, Garg BR, Rao MV. An appraisal of trends in sexually transmitted diseases. Indian J Sex Trans Dis 1993; 14: 1-4.
3. Ray K,Bala M, Gupta SM, et al. Changing trends in sexually transmitted infections at a regional STDs centre in North India. Indian J Med Res 2006; 124: 559-68.
4. Thomas K, Thyagarajan SP, Jeyaselan I et al. Community prevalence of sexually transmitted diseases and human immunodeficiency virus infection in Tamil Nadu, India: A probability proportional to size cluster survey. Natl Med J India 2002; 15:135-40.
5. Sweet RL, Gibbs RS. Sexually transmitted diseases. In: Sweet RL, Gibbs RS eds. Infectious disease of female genital tract. 4th Edn. Philadelphia: Lippincott Williams and Wilkins; 2002. p. 118-75.
6. Infections in gynaecology In: Campbell S, Monga A eds. Gynaecology by ten teachers. London: ELST; 2000: p. 183-204.
7. Radolf JD, Sanchez PJ, Schulz KF, Murphy FK. Congenital syphilis. In: Holmes KK, Sparling PF, Mardh PA, et al. eds. Sexually transmitted diseases. 3rd edn. New York: Mc-Graw Hill; 1999. p. 1165-89.
8. Walker GJ. Antibiotics for syphilis diagnosed during pregnancy. Cochrane Database Syst Rev 2001; 3: CD001143.
9. Hollier LM, Harstad TW, Sanchez PJ, et al. Fetal syphilis: Clinical and laboratory characteristics. Obstet Gynecol 2001; 97: 947-53.
10. http://www.niaid.nih.gov/factsheets/stdsyph.htm
11. Edwards LE, Barrada MF, Hamman AA, et al. Gonorrhoea in pregnancy. Am J Obstet Gynecol 1978;132: 637-41.
12. Phillips RS, Hanff PA, Wertheimertt, et al. Gonorrhoea in women sense for routine gynaecological care; criteria for testing. Am J Med 1985; 85: 177-82.
13. Centre for disease control. Sexually transmitted diseases: Treatment guidelines. MMWR 2002: 51, 18-29.
14. Centre for disease control. Sexually transmitted diseases: Treatment guidelines. MMWR 2006.
15. Sweet RL, Gibbs RS.Chlamydial infections. In; Sweet RL, Gibbs RS eds. Infectious diseases of female genital tract. 4th Edn. Philadelphia: Lippincott Williams and Wilkins; 2002: p. 57-100.
16. Wolner - Hanssen P, Westrom L, Mardh PA. Perihepatitis in chlamydial salphirgitis. Lancet 1980; 1: 901-4.
17. Gencay M, Koskiniemi M, Saikkn P, et al. *Chlamydia trachomatis* seropositivity during pregnancy is associated with perinatal complications. Clin Infect Dis 1995; 21: 424-6.
18. Alexander ER, Harrison R. Role of *Chlamydia trachomatis* in perinatal infection. Rev infect Dis 1983; 8: 713-9.

19. Kacmar J, Cheh E, Montagno A, et al. A randomized trial of azithromycin versus amoxicillin for the treatment of *Chlamydia trachomatis* in pregnancy. Infect Dis Obstet Gynecol 2001; 9: 197-202.
20. Rahangdale L, Guerry S, Bauer HM, et al. An observational cohort study of *Chlamydia trachomatis* treatment in pregnancy. Sex Transmit Dis 2006; 33: 106-10.
21. Hay P, Ugwumadu AHN, Manyonda IT. Oral clindamycin prevents spontaneous preterm birth and mid trimester miscarriage in pregnant women with bacterial vaginosis. Int J STDs AIDS 2001; 12 (Suppl 2): 70-1.
22. Perine PL, Stamm WR. Lymphogranloma venereum. In: Holmes KK, Sparling PF, Mardh PA, et al. eds. Sexually transmitted diseases. 3rd Edn. New York: Mc Graw Hill; 1999: p. 423-32.
23. Roral Ak, Albritton W. Chancroid and Hemophilus ducreyi. In: Holmes KK, Mardh PA, Sparling PF, et al. eds: Sexually transmitted diseases 3rd edn. NewYork: Mc Graw Hill; 1999: p. 515-23.
24. Ho KM, Lam WS. Handbook of Dermatology & Venereology (Social Hygeine Handbook 2nd edition) STDs in Pregnancy. www.hkmj.org./skin/content.htm.
25. 'O' Farrell N. Donovanosis in pregnancy. Int J Sex Transm Dis AIDS 1991: 2: 447-8.
26. Arnell RE, Potekin JS. Granuloma inguinale (granuloma venereum) of the cervix: an analysis of thirty-eight cases. Am J Obstet Gynecol 1940; 39: 626-35.
27. Scott CW, Harper DM, Jason RS, Helwig EB. Neonatal granuloma venementreum. Am J Dis Child 1953; 85: 308-15.
28. Banerjee K. Donovanosis in a child of six months. J Indian Med Assoc 1972; 59: 293.
29. Hay P, Ugwumadu AHN, Manyonda IT. Oral clindamycin prevents spontaneous preterm birth and mid trimester miscarriage in pregnant women with bacterial vaginosis. Int J STDs AIDS 2001; 12(Suppl 2): 70-1.
30. Lamont RF, Duncan SLB, Mandal D, et al. Intravaginal clindamycin to reduce preterm birth in women with abnormal genital tract flora. Obstet Gynecol 2003; 101: 516-22.
31. McGregor JA, French JI, Jones W, et al. Bacterial vaginosis is associated with prematurity and vaginal fluid mucinase and sialidase: results of a controlled trial of topical clindamycin cream. Am J Obstet Gynecol 1994; 170: 1048-59.
32. Joesoef MR, Hillier SL, Wiknjosastro G, et al. Intravaginal clindamycin treatment for bacterial vaginosis: effects on preterm delivery and low birth weight. Am J Obstet Gynecol 1995; 173: 1527-31.
33. Vermeulen GM, Bruinse HW. Prophylactic administration of clindamycin 2% vaginal cream to reduce the incidence of spontaneous preterm birth in women with an increased recurrence risk: a randomised placebo-controlled double-blind trial. Br J of Obstet Gynaecol 1999; 106: 652-7.
34. Sweet RL, Gibbs RS. Herpes simplex virus. In: Sweet RL, Gibbs RS eds. Infectious disease of female genital tract. 4th Edn. Philadelphia: Lippincott Williams and Wilkins; 2002. p. 101-17.
35. Brown AZ, Voniver LA, Benedetti J, et al. Effects on infants of a first episode of genital herpes during pregnancy. N Engl J Med 1987; 317: 1246-51.
36. Managing Herpes, How to live and love with a chronic STDs. Ebel C, Wald A. American Social Health Association, Triangle Park NC, 27709. www.herpeshealth.com
37. Prober CG, Suependn WM, Xasukawa LL, et al. Low risk of herpes simplex virus infection in neonates exposed to the virus at the time of vaginal delivery to mothers with recurrent genital herpes simplex virus infections. N Engl J Med 1987; 316: 240-4.
38. Nahmias AJ, Josey WE, Naib ZM, et al. Perinatal risk associated with maternal genital herpes simplex virus infection. Am J Obstet Gynecol 1971; 110: 825-37.
39. Sexually transmitted diseases. In: Cunningham FG, Gant NF, Leveno KJ, Gilstrap LC, Hauth JC, Wenstorn KD, eds. Williams Obstetrics. New York: McGraw Hill; 2001. p. 1485-1516.
40. Toltzis, P. Current issues in neonatal herpes simplex virus infection. Clin Perinatol 1991. 18: 193-208.
41. Arvin, AM, Yeager, AS, Bruhn, FW, et al. Neonatal herpes simplex infection in the

absence of mucocutaneous lesions. J Pediatr 1982: 100: 715-21.
42. Whitley RJ, Nahmias, AJ, Soong, S, et al. Vidarabine therapy of neonatal herpes simplex virus infection. Pediatrics 1980; 66: 495-501.
43. Maw DR. Treatment of anogenital warts. Dermatol Clin 1998; 16: 829-34.
44. Brown HL, Abernathy MP. Cytomegalovirus infection. Semin Perinatal 1998; 22: 260-6.
45. Ornoy A. The effects of cytomegalic virus (CMV) infection during pregnancy on the developing human foetus. Harefuah 2002; 141: 565-8, 577.
46. Gaytant MA, Steegers EA, Semmekrot BA, Merkus HM, Galama JM. Congenital cytomegalovirus infection: review of the epidemiology and outcome. Obstet Gynecol Surg 2002; 57: 245-56.
47. Boppana. Pregnant women can pass new CMV strains to foetus. N Engl J Med 2001; 344: 1366-71.
48. Nieves MR. Congenital CMV infection & Disease. The Pediatric Bulletin – Bimonthly reviews of current trends in the filed of pediatrics. www.hawaii.edu/medicine/pediatrics/pedtext/s03c//.html
49. Donders GG. Treatment of sexually transmitted bacterial diseases in pregnant women. Drugs. 2000; 59: 477-85.
50. Burtin P, Taddio A, Ariburnu O, et al. Safety of metronidazole in pregnancy: a meta-analysis. Am J Obstet Gynecol 1995; 172: 525-9.
51. Ratanajamit C, Vinther SM, Jepsen P et al. Adverse pregnancy outcome in women exposed to acyclovir during pregnancy: a population-based observational study. Scand J Infect Dis 2003; 35: 255-9.

35 SEXUAL ASSAULT AND SEXUALLY TRANSMITTED DISEASES

R K Sharma

In this chapter

- Rape
- Incest
- Unnatural Sexual Offences
- Sexual Deviations
- Sexual Harassment
- Medico-Legal Issues In AIDS and STD

INTRODUCTION

Sexual assault is an act of sexual intimacy done without the consent of the victim or where consent has been obtained by means of threat, fear or fraud. In our country sexual assault is a serious offence.

Sexual offence may be described as natural sexual offences like rape or unnatural sexual offences like sodomy, buccal coitus, tribadism, bestiality and certain sexual deviations.

RAPE

Definition: Rape in India is defined (under Section 375 of Indian Penal Code) as unlawful sexual intercourse by a man,

(i) With his own wife under the age of 15 years or
(ii) With any other woman under the age of 16 years with or without her consent or
(iii) With any other woman above the age of 16 years, against her will, without her consent or
(iv) With her consent—when her consent has been obtained by putting her or any person in whom she is interested in fear of death or hurt or
(v) With her consent—when the man knows that he is not her husband and the consent is given because she believes that he is another man to whom she is or believes herself to be lawfully married or
(vi) With her consent—when at the time of giving such consent, by reason of unsoundness of mind or intoxication or the administration of any stupefying or unwholesome substance, she is unable to understand the nature and consequence of that to which she has given consent.

Explanation

Penetration is sufficient to constitute the sexual intercourse necessary to the offence.

Punishment for Rape

Section 376 Indian Penal Code imposes a minimum term of seven years imprisonment and a maximum of life imprisonment for the offence of rape. However, a judge can award less sentence at his discretion.

Custodial Rape

It has been sometimes observed that women are sexually abused in jails, remand homes, hospital or where the woman is in custody and she is not in a position to render sufficient opposition to the act. In such cases, provisions of custodial rape are attracted under Section 376-C, 376-D Indian Penal Code.

Section 376-D IPC—Whoever, being on management of a hospital or being on the staff of a hospital takes advantage of his position and has sexual intercourse with any woman in that hospital, such sexual intercourse not amounting to the offence of rape, shall be punished with imprisonment of either description for a term which may extend to five years and shall also be liable to fine.

So, to constitute the offence of rape it is not necessary that there should be a complete penetration of penis. Partial penetration within labia majora, or even an attempt at penetration is quite sufficient for the purpose of law. So, it may be possible in a rape case that absence of injuries or seminal stains is there. Ideally, doctors should refrain from using the word 'rape' as it is a legal entity, not a medical condition. The doctors should only mention facts and condition of the victim and state that there is an evidence of sexual activity or not.

In cases where rape cannot be proved, it may be tried under less serious charge of indecent assault on a female committed with intent or knowledge to outrage her modesty. It is punishable under section 354 of Indian Penal Code by a term, which may extend upto two years, or fine, or with both. A woman may be accused of an indecent assault on a man but not rape.

Consent

According to law of India, a woman of sixteen years and above is capable of giving consent to the act of sexual intercourse. But the consent must be conscious, free, voluntary and given when she is mentally fit.

In certain sections of custodial rape [under clause (a) to (g) of subsection (2) of section 376 of Indian Penal Code] where sexual intercourse is proved and the question arises whether it was without the consent of the woman alleged to have been raped and she states in her evidence before court that she did not consent, the court shall presume that she did not consent (Section 114A, Indian Evidence Act). Thus the onus of proving consent shifts to accused from victim in such limited cases.

Prevalence of Rape

According to National Crime Records Bureau Report (1998), there were 15031 cases reported in India. Madhya Pradesh reported the highest incidence accounting for 22.3% of total cases. Among the cities, Delhi and Mumbai recorded more crimes numbering 365 and 118 respectively. In rates, Mizoram 9.3% led the table followed by Madhya Pradesh 4.3%, Dadra and Nagar Haveli 3.9% & Delhi 3.4%

Victims of rape were maximum in age group of 16-30 years accounting for 8414 out of 15033 reported cases.

Age

No age is safe for rape. The children are easily abused as they can offer less resistance. Small infants even at the age of 4-6 months have also been abused. Even older women are not safe from rape. For committing rape, the law of India does not presume any limit under which a boy can be considered physically incapable of committing rape. In such cases, the development of child along with development of sexual organs has to be taken into consideration while deciding that he is capable of performing rape or not.

Socio-Economic Status

Incidence of rape is more reported from lower socio-economic status, as they tend to live in unsafe and crowded areas.

Examination of Victim

The examination of victim should be carefully done as per provisions of law as they are different from one state to another in India. As per the recent judgement of Punjab and Haryana High Court, it is mandatory to get the rape victim examined only by a female doctor. In Delhi, only a gynaecologist does the medical examination of rape victims. The examination of rape victim should be under supervision of a female medical practioner.

Consent

The consent to examine rape victim should be taken before commencement. It should be in writing. As per provisions of law, police or court has no power to compel a woman to submit private parts for examination to a medical practitioner, male or female.

Examination

After taking consent, the medical examination should be started in presence of a female attendant or witness while a male doctor examines the patient. No attempt should be made to undress the woman. She should be politely asked to remove clothes. The exact time of examination, name of the person who brought the victim, a short factual summary of incidence should be recorded in medico-legal report in the register, which has been approved by the state administration.

Two marks of identification of the victim should also be noted. A short description of place of occurrence of event, details of act, relative position of parties, whether ejaculation occurred or not, pain during act, loss of consciousness during act or efforts to resist should be recorded. The general behaviour and mental state of the victims should be noted. The detailed examination should begin in the following order.

1. **Clothes:** If clothes are same as those worn by her at the time of sexual assault, they should be carefully examined for the presence of blood or seminal stain or any other discharge. The clothes especially undergarments should be preserved for examination by Forensic Science Laboratory.
2. **Injuries:** The physical examination of body especially forearms, wrist, face, breasts, chest, inner aspects of thighs, and back should be done to look for scratches, abrasions or bruises caused as a result of struggle/compression. Teeth marks if any may be observed on breasts, nipples, lips, or cheeks. Swabs from teeth bite should be taken for the presence of saliva.
3. **Genitals:** The examination should preferably be done in lithotomy position. The pubic hairs should be examined first, if they are found to be matted, they should be cut off with a pair of scissors to look for spermatozoa. They should be preserved in a dry bottle for examination at Forensic Science Laboratory. Dried seminal stains on external genitals/thighs can be scraped carefully or moistened with normal saline and slides may be made for microscopic examination. If bloodstains are present, they should also be preserved in a similar manner. Bruise or laceration if any on external genitalia may be carefully noted. The examination of hymen should be carefully done now. In a case of rape, hymen may have fresh radiate tears (more in posterior half), the edges of which may be red, swollen or painful if the examination of the victim is done within 24 hours. These tears heal within five to six days and looks like small tags of tissue after 10 days. Frequent sexual intercourse/delivery completely destroys hymen. There may be cases where hymen may be found to be intact and not lacerated. In such cases, the distensibility of hymen can be recorded. The fourchette and posterior commissure are not usually injured in cases of sexual assault. The degree of injury is dependent on the force used.

In small children, the hymen usually escapes injury, as it is deep seated but becomes red and inflamed. Sexual assault in children and adolescents is discussed in detail in chapter 33.

The vaginal secretions from the posterior fornix should be taken either by introducing a plain sterile cotton swab or by introducing 1 ml pipette and sucking the contents. The contents should be immediately transferred to a microscopic slide in a form of thin film and should be fixed. The slide can be viewed for spermatozoa. In married women, spermatozoa may be present because of previous sexual intercourse. The spermatozoa can be seen up to 17 days in vagina after last sexual intercourse. Even if spermatozoa is not present, the estimation of acid phosphatase level can be done in fluid obtained from posterior fornix to detect presence of seminal fluid.

Sexually Transmitted Disease

A woman can get venereal disease as a result of sexual assault if the person who committed sexual assault was suffering from such diseases. A discharge may be observed in cases of gonorrhoea. A thin film from the discharge may be made, fixed and stained with Gram's stain to see for gonococci under the microscope. The incubation period of gonorrhoea is about 2-8 days, so in a case of suspicion, another smear may be taken after few days to confirm. If syphilitic sores are seen or suspected, serum for dark ground examination for *Treponema pallidum* and blood for serological examination should be collected. The incubation period of syphilis varies from 9-90 days, so samples at a later date may be taken for confirmation. The sores on genitalia may be due to chancroid, which can also be confirmed by making smears to demonstrate H.ducreyi bacillus, which is Gram-negative strepto-bacillus with rounded ends. The other common infection that is transmitted is chlamydial vaginitis and viral STDs like herpes.

The most important sexually transmitted diseases is AIDS, which can be transmitted by sexual assault. The chances that a victim may get HIV infection in a single encounter are varied (3-5 percent). If it is suspected, relevant tests like ELISA or western blot may be done at repeated interval to confirm. Currently CDC has recommended post exposure prophylaxis after sexual assault according to degree of risk involved. For details refer to appendix III on post exposure prophylaxis.

If sodomy has been attempted or performed, then anal swabs from around the anus and anal canal may be collected and looked for spermatozoa/ seminal fluid.

Examination of the Accused

In India, the examination of the accused is done on a written request of the police. The person is brought under the custody of police to medical officer for examination. As per the law, whenever a person is arrested for committing sexual assault, a doctor should medically examine him as early as possible. In most of the states of India, the examination of the accused is conducted either by medical officers working in emergency services or a dermatologist and venereologist is called upon for examination. In some centres where forensic experts are available, such cases are referred to them.

The examination of the accused should be recorded in medico-legal register duly authorized by state government. The police constable who has brought him should identify the accused. This should be recorded in the report. The consent of the accused is not necessary for examination as per the provisions of the law of India. In fact, a reasonable amount of force can also be applied to collect evidence from his person. The marks of identification should be noted and left thumb impression of the accused may be taken on medico-legal report itself. The medical officer should record preliminary data and then proceed for complete examination. Examination of clothes should be done to detect semen/bloodstain or tears. Undergarments should be especially looked for stains and should be preserved for examination by Forensic Science Laboratory. A complete physical examination involving all systems like cardiovascular, alimentary, respiratory and nervous system should follow. The complete body especially inner aspects of thighs should be examined for mud, blood or seminal stains. The genitalia should be examined. Pubic hair if matted should be cut and preserved. The penis should be examined for injury or some stain, circumcision, presence of smegma or discharge. The cremastric reflex may be elicited to rule out neuronal loss.

If, it is suspected that a person is suffering from STDs, relevant evidence may be collected. After the examination is over, the doctor has to give opinion on two accounts.

1. Whether the person is capable of performing sexual intercourse or not?
2. Whether there is an evidence of recent sexual intercourse?

The capability to perform sexual intercourse depends on erection of the penis. It is naturally assumed that all normal males who have well developed sexual organs are capable of erection, thus can perform sexual intercourse. So, the opinion about capability to perform sexual intercourse is given in a double negative form like "There is nothing to suggest that this person is not capable of performing sexual intercourse".

If it is suspected that person may have some erectile dysfunction, he should be examined for chronic diseases like diabetes, hypertension, chronic alcoholism, neuropathies, or some psychic reasons. The opinion about recent sexual activity can be given if some stain/injury/redness is seen on penis/scrotum. Previously it was thought that absence of smegma could indicate recent sexual activity. Now it is not relied upon, as smegma collection depends on personal hygiene and circumcision.

Samples may be taken of vaginal epithelial cells, which adhere to penis during sexual intercourse, by taking a wet swab around penis and making microscopic slides. These vaginal cells are rich in glycogen and stain readily with iodine and can easily be inspected microscopically.

Previously, it was common to preserve semen in accused for which accused used to be asked to provide sample by masturbation. In non-cooperative accused, it was obtained by doing prostatic massage. Now this is not done. Sample of blood obtained from finger is preserved on a gauze piece and is dried and then sealed for examination by Forensic Science Laboratory.

INCEST

Incest is defined as sexual intercourse between man and woman who are related with blood or by marriage i.e. within forbidden degrees of relationship like a daughter, grand-daughter, sister, step sister, niece, aunt or mother. In India, incest per se is not a crime unless it attracts provisions of rape. However, in many western countries, incest is recorded as a crime and is punishable.

UNNATURAL SEXUAL OFFENCES

Section 377 of Indian Penal Code defines sexual offences relating to carnal intercourse against the order of nature with any man, woman or animal. Penetration is sufficient to prove the offence. The unnatural sexual offences are punishable with imprisonment of life or with a term of ten years and also with fine. These offences are classified as

1. Sodomy
2. Buccal coitus
3. Bestiality

Incidence

In India, unnatural sexual offences as mentioned above are quite less in percentage as compared to western countries.

The sodomy is frequent with small children working in tea stalls, workshop or offices. The sodomy has also been reported in prisoners or in armed forces especially those posted in the hilly areas.

Sodomy

It is also called buggery and is defined as anal intercourse between man and man or between man and woman. If the passive agent is a young child, it is called pederasty. The question of consent does not arise in sodomy, as it is punishable even if it is being done between two consenting adults. Marriage allows only normal intercourse not sodomy. If a couple is caught doing sodomy although they may be married to each other, it is punishable.

Buccal Coitus

It is also called sin of Gommorrah when genitalia are stimulated by mouth or penis is introduced in mouth. Sudden deaths have been reported by impaction of penis into lower part of pharynx or aspiration of semen-ejaculate.

Bestiality

It is defined as when a lower animal is used for sexual gratification. The common animals which are subjected to this cruelty are: dogs sheeps, cats or sometime cows or buffalo. Usually penis is inserted into vagina or rectum of the animal. Cases have been reported when animals especially dogs have been stimulated to perform sexual intercourse by inserting their penises into vagina of woman.

Since these offences are punishable under law, they may be brought for medical examination to the doctor.

Examination of Victim or Passive Agent

Usually the police bring a victim or passive agent of sodomy for medical examination to the doctor. The consent of the victim or passive agent must be taken.

The examination should preferably be done in knee elbow position. Abrasion, contusion or laceration may be seen around anal sphincter and person may complain of severe pain. These injuries are more important if the victim is a small boy or girl as compared to the accused person and a great force has been used to penetrate. Blood or semen stains may be present around anus and they should be lifted as described earlier. Swabs from inside and around anus must be taken and examined microscopically.

In a person who is habituated to sodomy following features may be present:

1. The shaving of anal hair may be seen.
2. A funnel shaped depression of buttocks toward anus may be seen.
3. There may be a complete relaxation of anal sphincter when lateral traction is applied on both buttocks.
4. The anus may be dilated and patulous with disappearance of radial folds. Prolapse of rectal mucosa may be seen.
5. Old lacerations may be seen around anus.
6. A complete absence of injuries may be there.
7. The presence of STDs in form of discharge, chancre or wart may be seen.

Examination of Accused

The examination of accused is quite helpful if done within hours of act as the signs start decreasing with time. The examination of accused must be done on written request of police. Consent is not required. The marks of identifications must be noted. The complete physical examination, as in the case of accused of rape, must be done. There may be abrasion on the prepuce, glans penis or frenulum. Stains of faecal material may be seen on penis. The swabs must be taken from penis and around area to look for faecal material. The blood/ semen stains may also be present and should be lifted as described earlier. There may be marks of struggle on the body. If the person is suspected/ suffering from STDs, the victim should also be examined for the same.

Bestiality is observed in villages in young shepherds who take animals for grazing and remain with them for almost the whole day.

Lesbianism

This is female homosexuality which is practiced between two females and mostly consists in friction of external genital organs by mutually body contact for sexual gratification. In some cases, the clitoris of the woman may be found to be enlarged. In some cases, artificial object may be used for stimulation.

Lesbianism is not punishable as it is not a crime under Section 377 of Indian Penal Code. It is usually found in females who are living together like in hostels or asylums.

SEXUAL DEVIATIONS

The common sexual deviations are described as follows:

1. **Sadism:** This is a sexual perversion where infliction of pain, torture and humiliation to partner, act as sexual stimulation. It may be seen in both sexes but is common in males. Male may inflict injuries by beating with hands or sticks or sometime sexual organs may be targeted, foreign bodies may be inserted in vagina and breast may be contused or sometimes, sadist may get so much excited, that he may murder her (lust murder) or he may eat her body (necrophagia) after raping her corpse (necrophilia).
2. **Masochism:** It is just opposite of sadism where gratification is obtained by getting beaten, tormented or humiliated by sexual partner. It is common in males but occurs in females also. The females may invite males to inflict pain on her or abuse her.
3. **Fetishism:** This perversion is seen in males only. In this male gets sexual gratification just by seeing some part of the woman or her article like undergarment, shoe, clothes etc.
4. **Transvestism:** It is the desire to wear the clothes of opposite sex. It is quite common in homosexuals. Some transvestites may seek medical treatment to change their gender.
5. **Exhibitionism:** It is a deviation in which exhibitionist get pleasure by showing his genitals to women, girls or small children. He may also make some lewd gesture. It is a punishable offence under Sec 294 of Indian Penal Code.

SEXUAL HARASSMENT

Many cases are reported every day of sexual harassment of women at work places done by the superiors; such cases had created a strong public awareness to fight this evil.

Government of India has taken a serious view to fight this evil. A specific provision has been made in CCS (Conduct Rules), 1964, prohibiting sexual harassment of women by Government servants. This provision is Rule 3-C of CCS (Conduct Rules), 1964. Government against its employees can initiate severe penal action against its employees. In private institutions also, rules have been made to deal with this menace. The rules are based on guidelines and norms laid down by Supreme Court, which are as follows.

Guidelines and norms laid down by the Hon'ble Supreme Court in Vishaka and others v State of Rajasthan and others (JT 1997 (7) SC 384].

Having regard to the definition of 'human rights' in Section 2 (d) of the Protection of Human Rights Act, 1993, TAKING NOTE of the fact that the present civil and penal laws in India do not adequately provide for specific protection of women from sexual harassment in work places and that enactment of such legislation will take considerable time.

It is necessary and expedient for employers in work places as well as other responsible persons or institutions to observe certain guidelines to ensure the prevention of sexual harassment of women.

Definition

For this purpose, sexual harassment includes such unwelcome sexually determined behaviour (whether directly or by implication) as:

(a) Physical contact and advances
(b) A demand or request for sexual favours
(c) Sexually coloured remarks
(d) Showing pornography
(e) Any other unwelcome physical, verbal or non-verbal conduct of sexual nature

Where any of these acts is committed in circumstances where under the victim of such conduct has a reasonable apprehension that in relation to the victim's employment or work whether she is drawing salary, or honorarium or voluntary, whether in Government, public or private enterprise, such conduct can be humiliating and may constitute a health and safety problem. It is discriminatory, for instance when the woman has reasonable grounds to believe that her objection would disadvantage her in connection with her employment or work including recruiting or promotion or when it creates a hostile work environment. Adverse consequences might be visited if the victim does not consent to the conduct in question or raises any objection thereto.

Criminal Proceedings

Where such conduct amounts to a specific offence under the Indian Penal Code or under any other law, the employer shall initiate appropriate action in accordance with law by making a complaint with the appropriate authority.

In particular, it should ensure that victims, or witnesses are not victimized or discriminated against while dealing with complaints of sexual harassment. The victims of sexual harassment should have the opinion to seek transfer of the perpetrator or their own transfer.

MEDICO-LEGAL ISSUES IN AIDS AND STD

AIDS and STDs have raised a lot of medico-legal issues in India and abroad.

The issues can be divided into

(a) Medical
(b) Social
(c) Ethical
(d) Legal

Medical Issues

The issue, which often raises controversy, is rights of patients or victims of AIDS and STDs. Every patient or victim has the right to receive treatment for the disease. AIDS testing is not compulsory in India. Nobody can be forced to go for such testing. However, government has the right to enforce it during screening tests for government jobs. It is common knowledge that hospital workers can get infected while treating AIDS patients and can bring lawsuits for compensation. The patients can be referred to designated hospitals in case of AIDS/STDs where adequate facilities are provided to deal with such cases.

Social and Ethical Issues

In our society, carrying of AIDS/STDs is a big stigma and doctors are duty bound to maintain secrecy to protect the identity of patients. They can disclose this information only after express consent of patients or relatives in case of deceased. However, in certain cases information can be divulged and this is called as Privilege Communication.

Privilege Communication

It is agreed that whatever information a doctor has acquired during treatment of that patient has to be kept confidential, but doctor has to perform his duty to society also. In such cases, disclosure of information is called privilege communication. In this regard, we have to understand what is absolute and privilege communication.

(a) Absolute Privilege

It applies to any statement made in court of law or parliament or state assembly. It also extends to statement made to lawyer during preparation for a court hearing as whatever has been said in these cases cannot be a ground for libel or slender.

(b) Qualified Privilege

Outside above any disclosure made by the doctor can be protected if following conditions are met:

1. The statement must not be malicious and must be in good faith to a person who has the right to receive it. Like if a person suffering from STDs intends to use public swimming pool, the doctor can make disclosure about his disease to incharge of swimming pool but not to any other person.
2. Only relevant information needs to be conveyed to appropriate authority, not the whole medical history of the individual.

In 1998, the honourable Supreme Court of India passed an order in a case where a patient has sued the doctor as he has disclosed to his fiancée that he is suffering from AIDS and subsequently his marriage was cancelled on receipt of this information. The honourable Supreme Court observed ‘So long as the person is not cured of the communicable venereal disease or impotency, the right to marry cannot be enforced through a court of law and shall be treated as suspended right and if a person suffering from the dreadful disease like AIDS, knowingly marries a woman and thereby transmits the infection to that woman, he would be guilty of offences under Section 269 IPC [negligent act likely to spread infection/disease dangerous to life] and Section 270 IPC [malignant act likely to spread infection/disease dangerous to life]. Moreover where there is a clash of the fundamental rights, as in this instant case, namely, the doctor’s right to privacy as part of right of life and the bride’s right to lead a healthy life, which is her fundamental right under Article 21, the right which would advance public morality or public interest, would alone be enforced through process of law.

(c) Legal Rights

Affliction of AIDS and STDs raises a lot of legal rights of the victims. The victims may sue the assailant for damages and criminal intention. If a person in full knowledge of the fact that he is suffering from AIDS sexually assaults a woman/man with added intention to infect her/him so that she/he will die can also be booked under Section 307 [attempt to murder] or under Section 302 IPC [murder] if person dies because of that along with different sections likes 269 and 270 IPC.

The presence of STD/AIDS on the sexual partner in case of married couple can be taken by the other spouse as a ground of divorce as it can be granted easily if this plea is taken in court of law.

If a person gets AIDS during discharge of professional duties like as in hospital workers, he can sue hospital authorities if sufficient infrastructure facilities are not available. No worker can be discharged from services only on the fact that he is HIV positive, his other health parameters also have to be taken into consideration, if he is fit otherwise, he cannot be removed from service.

REFERENCES

1. Crime in India 1998. National Crime Records Bureau, Govt.of India, New Delhi. p. 28-30.
2. Franklin CA. Modi's Medical Jurisprudence and Toxicology. 21st edition, Mumbai: N M Tripathi Ltd. 1988; p. 368-97.
3. Sharma R K. Legal aspects of patient care 1st edition, New Delhi: Modern Publishers; 2000. p. 11.

PART 6

Drug Resistance

36 DRUG RESISTANCE IN SEXUALLY TRANSMITTED DISEASES

Meera Sharma, Sunil Sethi

In this chapter

- Neisseria Gonorrhoeae
- Haemophilus Ducreyi
- Herpes Simplex Virus (HSV)
- Human Immunodeficiency Virus (HIV)
- Treponema Pallidum
- Human Papilloma Virus
- Chlamydia Trachomatis
- Trichomonas Vaginalis

INTRODUCTION

In all societies, sexually transmitted diseases (STDs) are among the most common infections. In the developing countries, three bacterial STDs gonorrhoea, chlamydial infections and syphilis rank amongst the top 10 to 20 diseases causing loss of healthy productive life due to major complications such as salpingitis, infertility, ectopic pregnancy and perinatal morbidity. Among the viral STDs, infection with human immunodeficiency virus (HIV) has become the leading cause of death during the last two decades. Two other very important viral STDs are hepatitis B virus (HBV) and human papilloma virus (HPV) infections. Although bacterial STDs remain extremely common in all parts of the world, their incidence is decreasing in most of the developed countries, whereas on the other hand, the global spread of the HIV pandemic in a relentless manner further makes the situation even more grave. The problem has been further compounded by the emergence of drug resistance amongst various agents causing STDs, particularly *Neisseria gonorrhoeae*, *Herpes simplex virus* and HIV. The emerging drug resistance warrants constant monitoring, need to look for the new drugs and change of operative plans to control the spread of STDs.

NEISSERIA GONORRHOEAE

In most parts of the world, gonococci are resistant to penicillins and tetracyclines, and resistance to multiple agents is also becoming very common. In some developed countries, the penicillins are still used effectively but major resistance problems exist in regions where gonorrhoea is most prevalent. Significant quinolone resistance has emerged in the WHO Regions of the Western Pacific and South-East Asia and has spread to countries on the Pacific rim. Although, there is no documented resistance to the third- generation cephalosporin antibiotics (cefixime–oral and ceftriaxone sodium–injectable), but the cost of these agents limit their use in many developing countries.[1]

Penicillin Resistance

Penicillin had been extensively used in the past for the treatment of gonorrhoea, but today in most parts of the world, gonococci are resistant to penicillins and tetracyclines, and resistance to multiple agents is common.[1] Penicillin resistant strains of *N. gonorrhoeae* are more prevalent in developing countries where other effective antibiotics are either not available or are too expensive and contact tracing procedures are not developed. The problem has been further aggravated by appearance of penicillinase producing *N. gonorrhoeae* (PPNG).[2]

PPNG was first reported in 1976 simultaneously from UK and USA, which originated from Africa and South East Asia.[3,4] Most epidemiological investigations have indicated that Far East, Asia and West Africa had been the main foci of PPNG, from where the strains have been imported to other countries.[5] After its first documentation in 1976, it has been extensively reported from Philippines, Singapore and West Africa.[5,6] Presently the PPNG are widely distributed throughout the globe; reports of PPNG from more than 40 countries are available in the literature. Resistance can be as high as 80% in some parts of the developing world. Although the true prevalence of penicillin resistance is unknown in the industrialized world, it is a problem in some parts of USA, whereas it is a major problem in the developing countries.[6]

Data from USA and Australia, where good surveillance programmes exist have shown that the prevalence of PPNG infections was initially increasing slowly but has markedly increased in the recent years.[7] In the WHO Western Pacific Region, according to 1998 data from 16 countries, particularly high levels of resistance have been recorded in China (62%), Hong Kong (69%), Philippines (82%), Vietnam (77%), Singapore (59%), Republic of Korea (74%) and Mongolia (26%).[1]

In South East Asian Region countries also, PPNG are found in high prevalence. Studies from Thailand and Indonesia show high proportions of both PPNG and chromosomal mediated resistant *Neisseria gonorrhoeae* (CMRNG).[8,9] In India, the first case of PPNG was reported from Chennai in 1980[10] and later from Chandigarh in 1984.[11,12]

In Delhi the resistance to penicillin rose from 12.8% in 1973 to 50.5%[13] in 1980 and in Bombay, penicillin resistance was seen in 56% cases in the same period.[14]

Studies from a number of African countries also indicated that a high proportion of isolates were penicillin resistant.[15]

After its first documentation in 1976, extensive research has been carried out on the mechanisms of development of drug resistance amongst *N. gonorrhoeae*. Antibiotic resistance in *N. gonorrhoeae* results from two different mechanisms: either due to mutation in the chromosomal genes or due to plasmid mediated β lactamase production.

In fully sensitive wild strains of *N. gonorrhoeae*, the minimal inhibiting concentration (MIC) for penicillin is <0.06 mg/l but mutation in a series of loci on the chromosome results in small additive increases in penicillin resistance MIC of 1 mg/l or greater. The currently recommended dose of penicillin becomes ineffective with MIC 1 mg/l. The main genetic loci that are involved in chromosomally mediated resistance are: *pen A*, *pen B* and *mtr*.[16] Mutation at pen A locus alone results in 8 fold increase in resistance,[17] *pen B* results in a 4 fold increase in resistance to penicillin and tetracycline. Mutation at *mtr* locus results in 2-4 fold increase in resistance to penicillin. The cumulative effect of these 3 mutations is a 128-fold increase in penicillin resistance.

There are 2 different types of resistance plasmids, viz. endogenous and exogenous plasmids. The endogenous plasmids are considered so because their GC ratio is indistinguishable from the chromosomal DNA of *N. gonorrhoeae*.

Endogenous Plasmids

1. 2.6 megadalton plasmid: No phenotypic character attributed, thus termed 'cryptic'.
2. 7.8 megadalton plasmid: Described in 1983 and is again 'cryptic'.
3. 24.5 megadalton plasmid: It co-exists with the 2.6 megadalton plasmid. It is present only in 7–8% strains, although it may be present in as high as 40% strains from South East Asia. It has conjugative properties and is able to mobilize other plasmids like R plasmid.[6]

   Insertion of the resistance determinant *tetM* into this 24.5 megadalton plasmid results in a plasmid of 25.2 megadalton, thus giving rise to high-level tetracycline resistance.[18]

Exogenous Plasmids

Production of β lactamase (penicillinase) was first shown to be due to exogenous plasmids 3.2 megadalton in strains from Africa and UK and 4.4 megadalton from Asia and USA.[3] Initially, 24.5 megadalton plasmid was found only in 40% of the Asian strains. Because of the conjugative nature of the plasmid, within a very few years, 24.5 megadalton plasmid was found along with 3.2 megadalton plasmid. Another 2.9 megadalton plasmid has been found to code for β lactamase production. Therefore, irrespective of the size of the plasmid, β lactamase enzyme produced is identical and of TEM-1 type. DNA homology studies showed that these plasmids contain 40% of the transposable DNA sequence TnA, which contains the gene Tn2 coding for TEM β lactamase.[6]

Tetracycline Resistance

Although tetracyclines are not recommended for treatment of gonorrhoea, they are widely available and extensively used particularly in many developing countries.

In the WHO Western Pacific study, tetracycline resistant *Neisseria gonorrhoeae* (TRNG) were found to be widely present but unevenly distributed. In 1998, particularly high proportions of TRNG were seen in Singapore (84%), the Solomon Islands (74%) and Vietnam (35.9%).[1]

TRNG are a significant problem in the WHO South East Asia Region (SEAR), particularly in Thailand and Indonesia.[9] In India, 28% of 50 consecutive isolates in New Delhi[19] and 10% of 94 isolates from Bangladesh were reported to be TRNG.[20]

Both chromosomal and plasmid-borne resistance against tetracyclines are found in gonococcal infection, the later being responsible for high level resistance.[16,18] Chromosomal resistance is linked to the *mtr* and *penB* gene alterations.[16] High-level tetracycline resistance in gonococci results from the acquisition of the *tetM* determinant and was first reported in 1986.[18] *tetM* in *N. gonorrhoeae* is located on a self-mobilizing plasmid and exists as 'Dutch' and 'American' types, which differ slightly.[21]

A steady rise in resistance to tetracycline occured from 5.6% in 1973 to 27.8% in 1982[22] and later 48.1% strains resistant to tetracycline were reported from North India.[23]

Spectinomycin Resistance

This injectable agent retains its activity against *N. gonorrhoeae* in most parts of the world. In the Western Pacific Region, 8% of strains from military personnel in the Philippines were spectinomycin-resistant.[24] In 1990, 8.9% strains from Thailand were spectinomycin-resistant, whereas no resistance was detected in 1994–1995.[24-25] In several African studies, all isolates have been reported to be susceptible to spectinomycin.[1] Therefore, although there have been several documented episodes of spectinomycin resistance in *N. gonorrhoeae* but it has not spread possibly because of the limited use of the antibiotic.

In *N. gonorrhoeae*, resistance to spectinomycin or to aminoglycosides usually occurs via a single-step chromosomal mutation, resulting in high-level resistance.[1]

Ciprofloxacin Resistance

As the gonococci were extremely susceptible to quinolones, these drugs were extensively recommended for the treatment of the drug resistant *N. gonorrhoeae*. Ciprofloxacin and ofloxacin are the primary treatment regime in a number of countries. However, gradually, quinolone-resistant gonococci (QRNG) emerged and spread in areas with high burden of gonococcal disease. The development of resistance was mainly due to antibiotic overuse or misuse.[1] Resistance, which is exclusively chromosomally mediated, has developed incrementally. Recently, a number of gonococcal strains have been identified with high level fluoroquinolone resistance. In the Western Pacific regions, the highest proportion of quinolone resistant strains were seen in the Philippines (63%), Hong Kong (48.8%), China (54.2%) and the Republic of Korea (11.2%).[1]

In South-East Asia, both low and high level QRNG have been detected including India, Sri Lanka, Myanmar and Nepal. This severely limits its therapeutic use.[1]

In Africa, quinolones are rarely used because they are generally not available, although there are very few available data of quinolone resistance.[1]

In Japan, prevalence of ciprofloxacin, levofloxacin and gatifloxacin resistant *N. gonorrhoeae* were 69%, 66.7% and 70% respectively.[26]

In 2003, fluoroquinolone- resistant *N. gonorrhoeae* prevalence was 2% in Canada[27], 9% in UK[28], 90.5% in Bangladesh[29], 70% in US,[30] 93.7% in Hong Kong, 78.3% in Korea, and 55.9% in Philippines.[31]

Quinolone resistant isolates have been reported from various parts of our country. In Delhi, 50% of the isolates showed resistance to ciprofloxacin in 1997,[32] 75% in 2000.[33] 77.7% resistance to ciprofloxacin was seen in Chandigarh in 2006.[34] Similarly, ciprofloxacin resistant strains have been reported from Mumbai.[35]

Of new concern is the emergence in Hawaii of multidrug resistance strains that are resistant to penicillin, tetracycline, ciprofloxacin, with decreased susceptibility to cefixime.[36]

The targets of the quinolones are topoisomerases, including DNA gyrase. High-level resistance is mediated by alteration of the target sites, via mutation in the *gyrA* gene. Multiple mutations also occur in the *parC* gene, which codes for the production of topoisomerase IV, a secondary target for quinolones in gonococci. Quinolone resistance is almost exclusively mediated by chromosomal mutations, which affect either the target sites or access of the antibiotic to the cell.[1]

The first step towards diagnosis of drug resistant *N. gonorrhoeae* is clinical suspicion. Then further evaluation is necessary like laboratory tests, and if PPNG is isolated, proper treatment and follow up is necessary. There are various techniques for demonstration of β lactamase production, viz. acidometric test, rapid iodometric test or chromogenic cephalosporin method. With the emergence of PPNG, extensive research work was carried out on the drugs effective on them. Spectinomycin and aminoglycosides had been recommended for treatment of infection with the resistant strains. But with the development of resistance against these drugs as well, the drugs currently recommended are: ceftriaxone or cefixime. The ciprofloxacin is being used only in those areas where quinolone resistance has not yet been reported.[1]

Macrolide Resistance

Erythromycin is sometimes used to treat gonorrhoea if a patient has a cephalosporin allergy or a history of immediate and/or anaphylactic reaction to penicillins.[37] In some parts of the world, azithromycin, a 15-membered macrolide, is used to treat gonorrhoea (1 g orally in a single dose). The increased use of azithromycin in treating other diseases may increase the selective pressure for macrolide-resistant gonococcus.

Macrolides such as erythromycin and azithromycin act by binding to the 50S subunit of bacterial ribosomes and restrain protein synthesis by inhibiting the elongation of peptide chains .The mechanisms of resistance to macrolides include efflux of these antibiotics and modification of the ribosomal target by modification of enzymes or mutations to reduce the affinity of the antibiotics for ribosomes. The first efflux pump described for *Neisseria gonorrhoeae* was the MtrC-MtrD-MtrE system, encoded by the *mtrRCDE* operon, which exports hydrophobic agents including dyes such as crystal violet 38 and macrolides such as azithromycin and erythromycin.[39] A fourth Mtr protein (MtrF) may also be associated with this efflux system.[39] More recently, another macrolide efflux pump, encoded by the *mef* gene, which had originally been described for some of the gram positive organisms[40], has now been found in clinical strains of *N. gonorrhoeae*.[41] In Seattle, 22.7% *N. gonorrhoeae* isolates were erythromycin resistant (MIC $\geq$ 1 mg/L), and the erythromycin and azithromycin susceptibilities were highly correlated.[42]

HAEMOPHILUS DUCREYI

During 1930s, sulphonamides used to be very effective therapy for chancroid. In 1970, drug resistant strains of *H. ducreyi* started emerging leading to clinically significant treatment failures. For several years, *H. ducreyi* infections were treated with trimethoprim sulphamethoxazole combinations but resistance emerged against this regime also (initially in Thailand and subsequently in Kenya and Rwanda).[43] Erythromycin is still an effective treatment with no confirmed reports of emergence of resistance. Fluoroquinolones are now extensively being used for the treatment of chancroid.

Many isolates of *H. ducreyi* possess β lactamase, which is a TEM 1 β lactamase derived from Tn2 transposon. A 6000 kDa plasmid codes for this. Other plasmids 7300, 5700 and 3200 kDa have also been demonstrated. The larger plasmids are same with the 2 types of plasmids of *N. gonorrhoeae*. In Africa, all strains tested have been reported to produce penicillinase. Resistance to other antibiotics is also common. *TetM* resistance factor has been detected in *H. ducreyi*. It is located in a conjugative plasmid of 34000 kDa.[6]

HERPES SIMPLEX VIRUS (HSV)

Drug resistance in viruses is defined as ED50 significantly higher than the normally achievable therapeutic concentration. Mostly, resistance is due to point mutations.

Strains resistant to any of the common drugs, nucleoside analogues or phosphonacetic acid have changes either in thymidine kinase (TK) or DNA polymerase genes.

Herpes virus TK is not essential for replication of the virus and therefore many different kinds of mutations are possible giving rise to lack of functional enzymes and hence to drug resistance. In contrast, DNA polymerase is always essential for replication of the virus and therefore only a few base substitutions leading to subtle changes in a functional protein are allowed, which does not compromise the normal functioning of the enzyme.[44]

It is not yet very clear, why the drug resistant strains are so rare among the clinical isolates. After more than 10 years of widespread use of acyclovir, the incidence of drug resistant strains has remained constant at <3%.[45] The prevalence of resistance to acyclovir in Indian strains of HSV is found to be 5.4%.[46] Approximately, 5% of immunocompromised subjects shed drug resistant virus. All the 3 different mechanisms play a role in development of drug resistance, viz. TK, Tk^r and $DNApol^r$. Foscarnet resistance is selectively due to base substitution at DNA polymerase gene.

Therapy of acyclovir resistant HSV infection includes use of DNA polymerase inhibitors like foscarnet and nucleotide analogues like cidofovir. Bryant et al.[47] reported resistance to both acyclovir and foscarnet in a leukemic child.

HUMAN IMMUNODEFICIENCY VIRUS (HIV)[48-50]

There are mainly three groups of antiretroviral drugs used for the treatment of HIV infection. These are nucleoside analogue reverse transcriptase inhibitors, non-nucleoside analogue reverse transcriptase inhibitors and protease inhibitors. Among these nucleoside analogue reverse transcriptase inhibitors have been extensively studied and used for therapy in HIV infected patients.

Drug resistance was first demonstrated against zidovudine (AZT) and then subsequently it was shown against all other nucleoside inhibitors. Resistance to non-nucleoside reverse transcriptase inhibitors is even more common and the strains are cross-resistant. Resistance against various Protease inhibitors has also been demonstrated.

HIV-1 variants resistant to AZT have been described in many instances. The degree of resistance increases with the duration of treatment. It has been seen that, more than 16 weeks of AZT therapy leads to high-level resistance in 15% of patients. These HIV-1 variants, resistant to AZT are transmissible from person to person and thus the prevalence of resistance in HIV-1 in the population is increasing gradually. HIV-1 isolates resistant to didanosine (nucleoside analogue reverse transcriptase inhibitors) have also been described, especially with didanosine monotherapy. Resistance has been described with other nucleoside analogue reverse transcriptase inhibitors like zalcitabine, lamivudine and also occasionally with stavudine. Recently, HIV-1 variants resistant to multiple reverse transcriptase inhibitors have increasingly been described, particularly with prolonged therapy. HIV-1 isolates resistant to protease inhibitors like saquinavir and indinavir have also been reported. Resistance of HIV-1 to ritonavir has been well documented, both *in vitro* as well as *in vivo*.

Drug resistance in HIV is again due to point mutations giving rise to altered affinity of reverse transcriptase for its inhibitors. Point mutations and sometimes sequences of mutations lead to progressively increasing resistance. For example, resistance mutations during AZT therapy appear in an orderly fashion and mutations at two codons, 41 and 215, are associated with highest levels of resistance and rapid progression of the disease. Resistance against didanosine involves mutation at codon 74. Mutation at codon 69 increases resistance against zalcitabine by almost five fold.[48] The replication of HIV, like any other retroviruses, is characterized by conversion of RNA into complementary single stranded DNA and then into double stranded DNA by the viral enzyme reverse transcriptase. All polymerases make base incorporation errors, but DNA dependant DNA polymerases 'proof read' and correct these errors. On the other hand, reverse transcriptase does not proof read and consequently, the fidelity of replication is low. The estimated error of reverse transcriptase is high, i.e. 10^{-4}/base, i.e. one base pair error per every 10,000 bases incorporated.

Combination chemotherapy (zidovudine plus didanosine; zidovudine plus lamivudine etc.) has been tried in several trials with success. Multi-drug therapy requires the virus to develop multiple separate mutations to develop resistance to all the anti-retroviral agents used and thereby significantly increases the delay period in development of resistance. There is now little doubt about the necessity for use of combination of anti-retroviral drugs to achieve long-term suppression of HIV replication. Combination of different agents have shown to decrease HIV viral load by 2–3 logs and allow suppression of HIV RNA to below the threshold level for detection, for even more than 2 years.

TREPONEMA PALLIDUM

Penicillin is the most effective drug in the treatment of syphilis and resistance is unknown. The co-infection of syphilis with HIV may cause problem in the management of syphilis. Crossen et al.[50] reported two patients with neurosyphilis who failed to respond to penicillin and were successfully treated with ceftriaxone. One of the patient tested positive for CSF VDRL and was treated with weekly benzathine penicillin, 2.4 MU for 4 weeks with good response. The CSF counts improved but CSF VDRL remained positive. The investigations for syphilis were normal but the patient developed psychiatric symptoms and was given injectable ceftriaxone 1000 mg/daily for 14 days with dramatic improvement in symptoms. Second patient of untreated syphilis was given penicillin injection and his psychiatric symptoms improved but after few years, he deteriorated without any sign of infection with syphilis. Because of the previous experience, the patient was treated with ceftriaxone and had dramatic improvement in his condition. The above instances suggest failure of penicillin in neurosyphilis but it would require further studies to demonstrate whether it was due to resistance to penicillin or some other factors.

HUMAN PAPILLOMA VIRUS

The results of treatment of human papilloma virus with antiviral drugs are variable. Recently, the resistance of HPV-6 to interferon-alpha have been suggested. Garcia Millian et al.[51] proposed that HPV-6E_7 almost completely inhibits induction of interferon responsive element that promotes transient transinfection, thereby resulting in ineffectiveness of the drug. They also demonstrated the absence of local immune response in the lesion of HPV by demonstrating absence of mRNA for interleukin-15 and IFN gamma. Further, it was shown that HPV negative patients develop resistance to recombinant IFN-alpha-2b and increased level of antiIFN alpha 2b antibodies but responded to neutral IFN-alpha, suggesting the development of resistance to IFN is a complex phenomenon resulting from host and viral elements. Koonsaeng et al.[52] reported similar drug resistance to IFN and isotretinoin while treating vulval intraepithelial neoplasia-III.

CHLAMYDIA TRACHOMATIS

Tetracycline is the first line drug till today in the most parts of the country for the treatment of chlamydial infection. The widespread and indiscriminate use of tetracycline has given rise to drug resistance. Lenart et al.[53] reported that chlamydial strains of human serovars L2 (LGV-434) in a tissue culture treated with tetracycline developed complete absence of large aberrant reticulate bodies with increased concentration of tetracycline but on stoppage of tetracycline there was regrowth of chlamydia on the tissue culture, suggesting resistance to tetracycline. Somani et al.[54] reported multi-drug resistance to doxycycline, azithromycin and ofloxacin by identifying the identical genotypes of organism and suggested the cause could be widespread use of subtherapeutic doses of antibiotics. Stamm reported[55] antimicrobial resistance in patients who failed to respond to treatment or persistence of pneumonia by *Chlamydia trachomatis*.

TRICHOMONAS VAGINALIS

The widely used antibiotic for treatment of *T. vaginalis* is metronidazole. The resistance to metronidazole seems to be increasing with time. Schmid et al.[56] did in vitro culture of vaginal discharge and correlated with the therapeutic outcome and found resistance of *T. vaginalis* to metronidazole. A Sobel et al.[57] used tinidazole for treatment of 24 cases of metronidazole resistant *T. vaginalis*.

It is apparent from the above description that development of drug resistance is an ongoing process and constant monitoring is essential for treatment and control of all STDs caused by bacterial, viral, chlamydial or trichomonal agents.

REFERENCES

1. Antibiotic resistance in *Neisseria gonorrhoeae*. John T (ed). Antimicrobial resistance in *Neisseria gonorrhoeae*. WHO Collaborating Centre for STDs and HIV, Sydney, Australia 2001.
2. Sethi S, Sharma M, Kumar B. Pencillinase producing strains of *Neisseria gonorrhoeae*. Bull PGI; 1999; 33: 71-4.
3. Phillips I. Beta lactamase producing penicillin resistant gonococcus. Lancet 1976; 2: 656-7.
4. Ashford WA, Golash RG, Hemming VG. Penicillinase-producing *Neisseria gonorrhoeae*. Lancet 1976; 2: 657-8.
5. Reyn A. Drug susceptibility pattern of *Neisseria gonorrhoeae*: A worldwide review. Asian J Infect Dis 1977; 1: 1-14.
6. Jephcott AE. Gonorrhoea, chancroid and granuloma venereum. In: Collier L, Balows A, Sussman M, eds. Topley and Wilson's Microbiology and Microbial Infections. 9th edn. London: Arnold; 1998. p. 623-40.
7. Lind I. Antimicrobial resistance in *Neisseria gonorrhoeae*. Clin Infect Dis 1997; 24: S93-S7.
8. Lind I, Hutapea N. Antimicrobial resistance of *Neisseria gonorrhoeae* in Medan, North Sumatra, 1996. Abstract O145. *Proceedings International* Congress of Sexually Transmitted Diseases, Seville, 1997.
9. Knapp JS, Wongba C, Limpakarnjanarat K, et al. Antimicrobial susceptibilities of strains of *Neisseria gonorrhoeae* in Bangkok, Thailand: 1994-1995. Sex Transm Dis 1997; 24: 142-8
10. Vijayalakshmi K, Gopalan KN, Gopal Krishnan B, et al. The first case of beta lactamase strain of *N. gonorrhoeae* from Madras. Indian J Sex Transm Dis 1982; 3: 13-4.
11. Sharma M, Kumar B, Agarwal KC et al. Penicillinase producing strains of *Neisseria gonorrhoeae* from Chandigarh. Indian J Med Res 1984; 80: 512-5.
12. Sharma M. Agarwal KC, Kumar B, et al. Penicillin resistant gonococci. Indian J Dermatol Venereol Leprol 1985; 51: 22-5.
13. Masshoor K, Bhujwala RA, Pandhi RK, et al. Susceptibility of *Neisseria gonorrhoeae* to penicillin, ampicillin, tetracycline, erythromycin, cotrimoxazole and supristol-An in vitro study Indian J Pathol Microbiol 1980; 23: 171-5.
14. Moses JM, Desai MS, Bhosle CB, et al. Present pattern of antibiotic sensitivity of gonococcal strains isolated in Bombay. Br J Vener Dis 1971; 47: 273-8.
15. Osoba AO, Path FRC. Overview of penicillinase producing *Neisseria gonorrhoeae* in Africa. African J of Sex Transm Dis 1986; 51-64.
16. Cannon JG, Sparling PF. The genetics of gonococcus. Ann Rev Microbiol 1984; 38: 111-3.
17. Spratt BG. Hybrid penicillin binding proteins in penicillin resistant strains of *Neisseria gonorrhoea*. Nature 1988; 332: 173-6.
18. Morse SA, Johnson SR, Biddle JW, et al. High level Tetracycline resistance in *Neisseria gonorrhoeae* is result of acquisition of Streptococcal tet M determinant. Antimicrob Agents Chemother 1986; 30: 664-70.
19. Bhalla P, Sethi K, Reddy BS, et al. Antimicrobial susceptibility and plasmid profile of *Neisseria gonorrhoeae* in India [New Delhi] Sex Transm Inf 1998; 74: 210-2.
20. Bhuiyan BU, Rahman M, Miah NR. Antimicrobial susceptibilities and plasmid contents of *Neisseria gonorrhoeae* isolates from commercial sex workers in Dhaka, Bangladesh: emergence of high-level resistance to ciprofloxacin. J Clin Microbiol 1999; 37: 1130-6.
21. Gascoyne-Binzi DM, Heritage J, Hawkey PM. Nucleotide sequences of the tet(M) genes from the American and Dutch type tetracycline resistance plasmids of *Neisseria gonorrhoeae*. J Antimicrob Chemother 1993; 32: 667-76.
22. Bhujwala RA, Pandhi RK, Bhargava NC, et al. *Neisseria gonorrhoeae* and its sensitivity to penicillin and tetracycline over a decade. Indian J Med Microbiol 1983; 1: 43.
23. Sharma M, Kumar B, Sharma SK, et al. Antimicrobial susceptibility pattern of *N. gonorrhoeae* to penicillin, tetracycline and kanamycin. Indian J Med Microbiol 1986; 4: 111-4.
24. Clendennen TE, Echeverria P, Saengeur S et al. Antibiotic susceptibility survey of *Neisseria*

gonorrhoeae in Thailand. Antimicrob Agents Chemother 1992; 36: 1682-7.

25. Clendennen TE, Hames CS, Kees ES, et al. In vitro antibiotic susceptibilities of *Neisseria gonorrhoeae* isolates in the Philippines. Antimicrob Agents Chemother 1992; 36: 277-82.
26. Shigemura K, Okada H, Shirakawa T, et al. Susceptibilities of *Neisseria gonorrhoeae* to fluoroquinolones and other microbial agents in Hyogo and Osaka, Japan. *Sex Transm Infect* 2004; 80: 105-7.
27. Expert Working Group for the Canadian STI Guidelines. Gonorrhea treatment guidelines in Canada: 2004 update. CMAJ. 2004; 171: 1345-6.
28. GRASP Steering Group. The Gonococcal Resistance to Antimicrobials Surveillance Programme (GRASP) Year 2003 Report. London: Health Protection Agency; 2004.
29. International Centre for Diarrheal Disease Research, Bangladesh. Surveillance Update Health and Science Bulletin. 2003; 1: 17-20.
30. Wang SA, Harvey AB, Conner SM, et al. Antimicrobial Resistance for *Neisseria gonorrhoeae* in the United States, 1988 to 2003: The Spread of Fluoroquinolone Resistance. Ann Intern Med. 2007; 147: 81-8.
31. Tapsall J. Surveillance of antibiotic resistance in *Neisseria gonorrhoeae* in the WHO Western Pacific region, 2003. Commun Dis Intell. 2005; 29: 62-4.
32. Rattan A, Kumari S, Khanna N, et al. Emergence of fluoroquinolones resistant *Neisseria gonorrhoeae* in New Delhi, India Sex Transm Inf 1998; 74: 229.
33. Bhalla P, Vidhani S, Reddy BS, et al. Rising quinolone resistance in *Neisseria gonorrhoeae* isolates from New Delhi. Indian J Med Res 2002; 115: 113-7.
34. Sethi S, Sharma D, Mehta S.D et al. Emergence of ciprofloxacin resistant *Neisseria gonorrhoeae* in north India. Indian J Med Res 2006; 123: 707-10.
35. Divekar AA, Gogate A. Ciprofloxacin resistance in *Neisseria gonorrhoeae* isolated in Mumbai (formerly Bombay). India. Sex Transm Inf 1999; 75: 122.
36. Wang SA, Lee MV, O'Connor N, et al. Multidrug-resistant *Neisseria gonorrhoeae* with decreased susceptibility to cefixime-Hawaii, 2001. Clin Infect Dis. 2003; 37: 849-52.
37. Tapsall JW, Shultz TR, Limnios EA, et al. Failure of azithromycin therapy in gonorrhea and discorrelation with laboratory test parameters. Sex. Transm. Dis 1998; 25: 505-8.
38. Zarantonelli L, Borthagaraya G, Lee EH, et al. Decreased azithromycin susceptibility of *Neisseria gonorrhoeae* due to mtrR mutations. Antimicrob. Agents Chemother. 1999; 43: 2468-72.
39. Shafer WM, Veal WL, Lee E.-H, et al. Genetic organization and regulation of antimicrobial efflux systems possessed by *Neisseria gonorrhoeae* and *Neisseria meningitides*. 2001 J. Mol. Microbiol. Biotechnol. 3: 219-24.
40. Roberts MC, Sutcliffe J, Courvalin P, et al. Nomenclature for macrolide and macrolide-lincosamide streptogramin B resistance determinants. Antimicrob. Agents Chemother. 1999; 43: 2823-30.
41. Luna VA, Cousin Jr. S, Whittington WL, et al. Identification of the conjugative mef gene in clinical *Acinetobacter junii* and *Neisseria gonorrhoeae* isolates. Antimicrob. Agents Chemother. 2000; 44: 2503.[6]
42. Cousin Jr SL, Whittington WLH, Robert MC. Acquired macrolide resistance genes and the 1 bp deletion in the mtrR promoter in *Neisseria gonorrhoeae*. Antimicrob Chemoth 2003; 51: 131-3.
43. Bogaerts J, Kestens L, Tello WM, et al. Failure of treatment for Chancroid in Rwanda is not related to HIV infection: in vitro resistance of *Haemophilus ducreyi* to trimethoprim sulphamethoxazole. Clin Infect Dis 1995; 20: 924-30.
44. Field HJ, Whitley RJ. Antiviral chemotherapy. In: Collier L, Balows A, Sussman M, eds. Topley and Wilson's Microbiology and Microbial Infections. 9th edn. London: Arnold; 1998; p. 989-1010.
45. Collins P, Ellis MN. Sensitivity monitoring of clinical isolates of herpes simplex virus to acyclovir. J Med Virol 1993; 1: 58-66.
46. Abraham AM, Kavitha S, Joseph P et al. Indian Acyclovir resistance among Indian strains of Herpes Simplex virus as determined using a

dye uptake test. J Med Microbiol, 2007; 25: 260-2.
47. Bryant P, Sasadeusz J, Carapetiz J, et al. Successful treatment of forcarnet-resistant herpes simplex stomatitis with intravenous cidofir in a child. Pediatr Infect Dis 2001; 20: 1083-6.
48. Joseph JE Jr, Martin SH. Antiviral therapy of human immunodeficiency virus infection. In: Holmes KK, Mardh PA, Sparling PF, et al. eds. Sexually Transmitted Diseases, 3rd edn. New York: Mc Graw Hill; 1999. p. 1009-1030.
49. Ballard AL, Cane PA, Pillay D. HIV drug resistance: genotypic assays and their possible applications. Sex Transm Inf 1998; 74: 243-8.
50. Crossen WM, Nieku H, Nielson O, et al. Ceftriaxone treatment of penicillin resistant neurosyphilis in alcoholic patients. J Neurol Neurosurg Psychiatry 1995; 59: 194-5.
51. Garcia-Millian R, Santos A, Perea SE, et al. Molecular analysis of resistance of interferon in patients with laryngeal papillomatosis. Cytokines Cell Mol Ther 1999; 5: 79-85.
52. Koonsaeng S, Verschraegen C, Freedman R, et al. Successful treatment of recurrent vulvar intraepithelial neoplasia resistant to interferon and isotretinoin with cidofovir. J Med Virol 2001; 64: 195-8.
53. Lenart J, Andersen AA, Rockey DD. Growth and development of tetracycline – resistant Chlamydia suis. Antimicrob Agents Chemother 2001; 45: 2198-203.
54. Somani J, Bhullar VB, Workowski KA et al. Multiple drug-resistant *Chlamydia trachomatis* associated with clinical treatment failure. J Infect Dis 2000; 181: 1421-7.
55. Stamm WE. Potential for antimicrobial resistance in *Chlamydia pneumoniae*. J Infect Dis 2000; 181: S456-9.
56. Schmid G, Narcisi E, Mosure D, et al. Prevalence of metronidazole-resistant *Trichomonas vaginalis* in gynaecology clinic. J Reprod Med 2001; 46: 545-9.
57. Sobel JD, Nyirjesy P, Brown W. Tinidazole therapy for metronidazole-resistant vaginal trichomoniasis. Clin Infect Dis 2001; 33: 1341-6.

PART 7

Control of Sexually Transmitted Diseases

37 CONTROL OF SEXUALLY TRANSMITTED DISEASES

Neena Khanna, Ajay Khera

In this chapter

- History of STDs Control Programmes in India
- National AIDS Control Programme (NACP) I
- National AIDS Control Programme II
- National AIDS Control Programme III (2006-2011): Overview
- Goals and Objectives of NACP III
- Components of NACP III
- Prevention Strategies
- Linking Prevention to Care, Support and Treatment
- Care, Support and Treatment
- Capacity Building
- Strategic Information Management

INTRODUCTION

Sexually transmitted diseases are considered a major global health problem, with more than 330 million cases being reported every year. Of these, over 80% of patients are believed to be from developing countries. In India, STDs are one of the most prevalent communicable diseases,[1] although the data on the pattern of STDs is likely to be fallacious due to lack of a comprehensive national registry, inefficient reporting and data collection systems, and the fact that patients with STDs seek help not from the public health facility but from the private sector, reporting from where is understandably abysmal. The annual incidence rate of STDs in India is estimated to be about 6%, with 3-4% of rural population being suspected to be infected at any particular time. On an average, 40-50 million new cases of STDs are estimated to occur every year.

STDs pose an enormous public health problem in view of the large number of patients, innumerable, mostly undocumented complications and the long-term suffering. STDs preferentially affect the economically productive sections of the society (20-40 years of age) causing loss of productive life measured as disability-adjusted-life-years (DALYS) lost.[2] The arrival of the HIV pandemic has complicated the situation, especially in the background of amplified transmission of HIV infection in the presence of STDs.

HISTORY OF STD CONTROL PROGRAMMES IN INDIA

Pre-HIV Era (1949–1985)

In 1949, India responded to the problem of venereal diseases (VDs) by launching the National VD Control Programme with emphasis on the control of syphilis **(Fig. 37.1)**. This focus on syphilis shifted in 1981-82 onto teaching, training and research in the various aspects of STDs, and the programme was renamed National STDs Control Programme. To enhance the clinical and para-clinical aptitude of in-service doctors and paramedical staff, two training centres were established, one at Delhi and the other in Madras (now Chennai). Training facilities were augmented by establishing regional training centres in Calcutta (Kolkata), Nagpur and Hyderabad. Surveillance centres (27 in number) and research centres (40 in number) have also been set up to enhance the skills of concerned technical personnel.[4] STD clinics (845 in number) attached either to medical colleges and teaching hospitals or to district hospitals were functioning in various parts of the country.

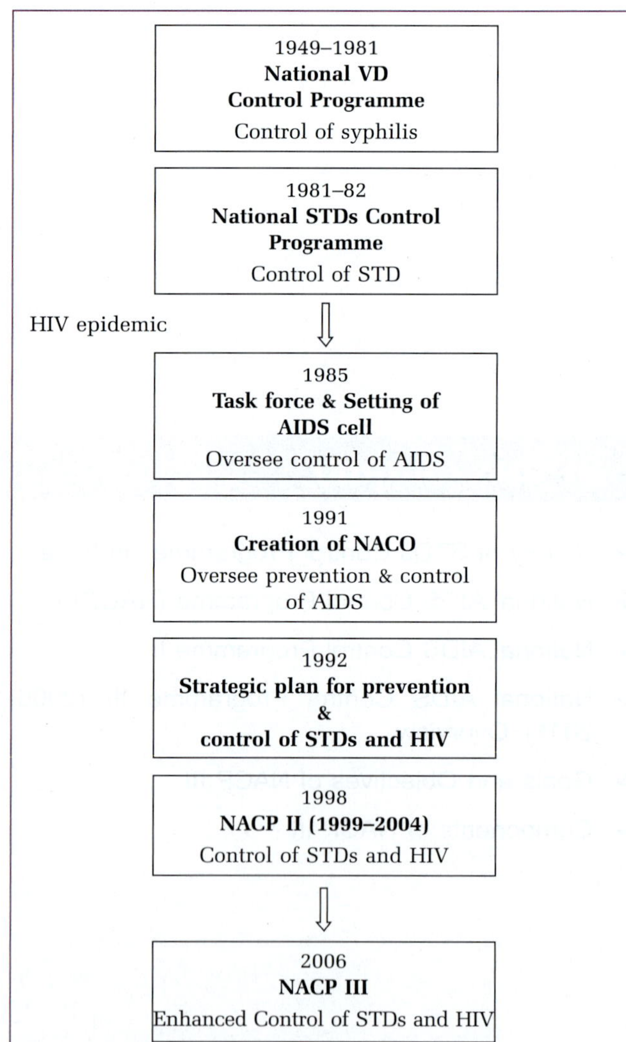

Fig. 37.1 History of VD/STD/HIV Control Programmes in India.

HIV Era

Initial Response

The appearance of the HIV pandemic added a new dimension to STD control programmes. As the first reports of HIV infection began appearing, the initial response of the government and community was almost hysterical, quite similar to other parts of the world.[5] However, since the initial aberrant response, the Government of India in conjunction with ICMR had committed to focus resources and priorities to contain HIV epidemic in the country.[6] Thus, in 1985, the Government of India constituted a Task Force to look into the HIV epidemic, and an AIDS Cell was established in the Directorate of Health Services, New Delhi, to coordinate activities pertaining to AIDS control in the country. In 1991, National AIDS Control Organization (NACO) was officially created as the executive governmental organization to oversee AIDS prevention and control efforts in India through the National AIDS Control Programme (NACP). To meet the onslaught of HIV epidemic, in 1992, the Government of India drew up a "Strategic Plan for Prevention and Control of AIDS" for the period 1992-1997.[7] This strategic plan received support from the World Bank (WB), the World Health Organization (WHO) and other international agencies. The aim of the plan was to establish a comprehensive, multi-sectoral programme for the prevention and control of AIDS in India, which would:

- Prevent HIV transmission
- Decrease morbidity and mortality asso-ciated with the infection
- Minimize the socio-economic impact resulting from HIV infection

Recognizing the close relationship and interaction between HIV and STDs, the National STDs Control Programme was merged with NACP; certain components of the former programme like teaching, training and epidemiology, however, remained independent.

Medium-term Plan (MTP)

- In 1990, an MTP (1990-1992) was launched in four states (Tamil Nadu, Maharashtra, West Bengal and Manipur) and four metropolitan cities (Chennai, Kolkata, Mumbai and Delhi).
- Its objectives were to facilitate targeted IEC campaigns, establish a surveill-ance system and provide safe blood.

NATIONAL AIDS CONTROL PROGRAMME (NACP) I[5]

- In 1992, NACP I (1992-99) was launched with the objective to raise awareness about HIV infection, to slow down the spread of HIV infection, and reduce morbidity, mortality and impact of AIDS in the country.
- To strengthen its management capacity, a National AIDS Control Board (NACB) was constituted and an autonomous National AIDS Control Organization (NACO) was set up for implementing the project.
- The key outcomes of NACP I included:
  - Capacity development at the state level in the form of setting up State AIDS Cells (SACs) in 25 states and 7 union territories.
  - Establishing a well-functioning blood safety programme aimed at reducing HIV transmission through blood.
  - Expansion of HIV sentinel surveillance system.
  - Collaboration with non-government organizations (NGOs) on prevention interventions.
  - Intensified communication campaigns.
  - Launching of focused programmes to contain the epidemic with the help of bilateral partners in Tamil Nadu (with USAID), in Andhra Pradesh, Gujarat, Kerala, Orissa and West Bengal (with DFID), and Karnataka and Rajasthan (with CIDA).

NATIONAL AIDS CONTROL PROGRAMME II[1]

- NACP II was launched with the help of credit from World Bank in 1999.
- ***Focus:*** Based on the experience gained in Tamil Nadu along with evolving trends of the HIV/AIDS epidemic, the focus of controlling AIDS shifted from raising awareness to changing behaviour, decentrali-zation of programme implementation at the state level (and even district level), and greater involvement of NGOs.
- ***Objectives:*** The policy and strategic shift was reflected in the two key objectives of NACP II:
  - Reduce the spread of HIV infection in India
  - Increase India's capacity to respond to HIV/AIDS on a long-term basis
- ***Aims:*** To keep HIV seroprevalence
  - <5% of the adult population in high prevalence states
  - <3% in states where the prevalence was moderate
  - <1% in states where the epidemic was still in a nascent stage
- ***Policy initiatives:***
  - Adoption of National AIDS Prevention and Control Policy (2002)
  - Formulation of National Blood Policy (2002)
  - Encouraging greater involvement of people with HIV/AIDS (GIPA)
  - Launching of the National Rural Health Mission
  - Launching of the National Adolescent Education Programme
  - Limited provision of anti-retroviral treatment (ART)
  - Setting up of the National Council on AIDS (NCA), chaired by the Prime Minister, to provide policy guidelines and political leadership to the response.
- ***Key achievements:***[1] The key achievements of NACP II include:
  - Establishment of 1033 targeted interventions (TIs) for high-risk groups (HRGs) with the help of NGOs, with >50% of these projects being located in high prevalence states and covering >45% of the HRG population. In addition, 875 voluntary counselling and testing centres (VCTCs) and 679 STD clinics were established at the district level.
  - Collection of data from a number of regional and national surveys including HIV sentinel surveillance (HSS) and behaviour surveillance survey (BSS).
  - Expansion of Prevention of Parent-to-Child Transmission (PPTCT) Programmes across states.
  - Introduction of a Computerized Management Information System (CMIS) and a Computerized Project Financial Management System (CPFMS).
  - Increased support from bilateral, multilateral and other partner agencies.
- ***Results:*** HIV prevalence has stabilized in Tamil Nadu, Andhra Pradesh, Karnataka, Maharashtra and Nagaland, showing declining trends indicating that the expected outcomes of NACP II have broadly been accomplished.
- ***Lacunae:*** Areas which required greater focus include:
  - *Understanding complexities in the epidemic:* The understanding of complexities and exact dimension of the epidemic, especially in northern and north-eastern states of the country, was not complete.
  - *Staffing:* Lack of staff at State AIDS Control Societies (SACSs), frequent transfers and unfilled positions have contributed to the uneven implementation of the programme.
  - *Capacity development:* Despite decentralization, results were suboptimal due to lack of capacity development and technical support at the periphery.
  - *Implementation of targeted interventions (TIs):* TIs in HRGs did prevent the spread of infection, but these were not uniformly and extensively implemented as MSM, IDUs and rural population were not given priority in some states, partly due to judgmental attitude towards them and partly due to weak private-public partnership.

- *Suboptimal use of condoms:* Although condom promotion and procurement registered an improvement, it was still suboptimal, emphasizing the need for more aggressive social marketing.
- *Convergence:* Convergence of RCH and NACP II remained a difficult challenge.
- *AIDS reporting:* AIDS mortality and under-reporting was an important lacuna.

NATIONAL AIDS CONTROL PROGRAMME III (2006-2011): OVERVIEW

Preparatory Phase[1]

- The framework of NACP III was based on lessons learnt from and achievements of Phase I and II and after wide-ranging consultations with several organizations.
- The initial guidelines were field-tested in a highly vulnerable state (Uttar Pradesh), a high prevalence state (Andhra Pradesh) and in the north-east (Nagaland).
- For public participation in the planning process, UNAIDS and NACO set up an e-consultation followed by a series of handholding consultations with stakeholders including people living with HIV/AIDS (PLHA) networks, NGOs, community-based organizations (CBOs), national expert groups, development partners at state level for the preparation of state and district level programme implementation plans (PIP).
- In October 2005, a joint pre-appraisal mission led by the World Bank critically appraised the strategic framework document and endorsed it.
- Several studies were initiated to validate programme implementation plans.

Positioning of NACP III *vis-a-vis* Other Programmes[1]

The National Rural Health Mission (NRHM) was launched in April 2005 with the aim of providing accessible, affordable, effective, accountable and reliable health care consistent with outcomes envisioned in the Millennium Development Goals (MDGs). Since many components of the NACP III will be delivered through the health system, the integration with NRHM is important to synergize the delivery of various services especially with the Reproductive and Child Health (RCH) Programme and Revised National TB Control Programme (RNTCP). NACP III also includes services for the management of STIs. At the same time the programmatic response to address prevention, management and control of RTIs/STIs largely falls under the RCH II Programme (2005), which draws its mandate from the National Population Policy (2000). The components of RTI/STI, blood safety, condom promotion, sentinel surveillance and PPTCT have close links with RCH and NACP III.

GOALS AND OBJECTIVES OF NACP III[1]

NACP III (2006-2011) has specific goals and objectives with commitment to achieve the MDG of reversing the spread of HIV/AIDS by 2015. NACP-III envisages:

- Expansion of coverage of HRGs by TIs to 80% (from 45% under NACP II)
- Treatment of all eligible PLHA with ART and targeting them specifically for positive prevention activities
- Integration of care, support and treatment (CST) with prevention
- Reduction of transmission through blood to 0.5%
- Coverage of 80% deliveries of HIV-positive mothers by the PPTCT programme

Goals[1]

The primary goal is to halt and reverse the epidemic in India over the next 5 years by integrating programs for prevention and care, support and treatment (CST) of HIV through a four-pronged strategy:

1. Prevention of new infections in HRGs and general population through:
   - Complete coverage of HRGs with targeted interventions (TIs)
   - Improved interventions in general population
2. Providing greater care, support and treatment to a larger number of PLHA
3. Strengthening infrastructure and human resources at district, state and national levels
4. Strengthening a nation-wide Strategic Information Management System (SIMS)

Objectives[1]

- A specific objective of NACP III is to reduce new infections in the first year of programme by 60% in high prevalence state so as to obtain the reversal of the epidemic, and by 40% in vulnerable states so as to stabilize the epidemic.
- The priorities and thrust areas of NACP III include:
  - Prevention
  - Care, support and treatment (CST)
  - Impact mitigation
  - Decentralization of implementation
  - Monitoring and evaluation

COMPONENTS OF NACP III

Prevention

- Targeted interventions (TIs)
- Sexually transmitted disease services
- Condom promotion
- Blood safety
- Integrated counselling and testing centres
- Prevention of PTCT
- Communication

Care, support and treatment

- Antiretroviral treatment
- Treatment of opportunistic infections
- Centres of excellence
- Care and support
  - Community care centres
  - Providing enabling environment

Capacity building

- Training
- Mainstreaming
- Public-private partnership

Strategic information management

- Monitoring and evaluation
- Surveillance
- Research

PREVENTION STRATEGIES[1]

Prevention is the mainstay of strategic response to HIV/AIDS because 99% of the adult population of India is still uninfected, and there is still scope to reverse the progression of the epidemic and reduce the overall prevalence. The programme aims to reduce new infections in all categories and prevent the spread of infection from HRGs to the general population. A behaviour change strategy based on effective information, education and communication campaigns and supported by appropriate services is being implemented. Timely and accessible service delivery will ensure continuum of care at every level. A package of clearly defined and interlinked services with clarity where they will be available will enhance utilization.

Targeted Interventions

Target Population[1]

Targeted interventions which earlier covered populations with varying risk levels under NACP II will be redesigned to focus on specific populations. The coverage of low or negligible risk groups will be scaled down and funding withdrawn from year 2 of NACP III, and the focus of prevention strategies will be on three groups:

- ***High-risk groups (HRGs):*** They include CSWs, IDUs and MSM and are estimated to be 4 million.
- ***Bridge population:*** Bridge population includes those people who, through close proximity to HRGs, are at higher risk of contracting HIV and includes long-distance

truckers (estimated population of 2.5-3 million and HIV prevalence of 6-11%) and migrant workers (estimated population of 8 million and unknown HIV prevalence) both needing specific and nation-wide interventions. It also includes clients/partners of sex workers (SWs) (both males and females).

- ***Highly vulnerable people of the general population:*** It includes women in the age group of 15-49 years, youth and children and constitute 40% of the country's population.

Implementation of TIs[1]

For the programme to be effective, it is important to prioritize its strategies and to ensure that the programme is sustainable. The implementation of preventive strategies will depend on the endemicity of the district.[4] For category A and B districts, all four strategies discussed will be used, while for category C and D districts, the first three strategies will be used so as to saturate the coverage of all HRGs.

- *Formation of CBOs and peer-led TIs in urban areas*: All towns and cities will be covered with high-intensity TIs with outreach and service provisions for SWs (female, male and Hijra populations) and their clients.
- *NGO-led TIs in rural areas with population >5000*: Since villages are widespread and most have over 10 practising FSWs, an outreach and service delivery plan to access these FSWs in line with the TI approach will be designed, i.e., capacity building among smaller NGOs and subsequently linking them to larger networks for long-term sustainability.
- *Small, scattered villages*: Focus will be on providing an enabling environment and integrating vulnerable persons into the society by providing alternative livelihood opportunities through government machinery by mainstreaming HIV/AIDS in all departments.
- *Mainstreaming interventions in rural areas with population <5000*: Focus will be on creating awareness about HIV/AIDS and STIs, and providing referral services for STI treatment, ICTC/PPTCT, CST with the help of two link workers (1 male, 1 female) per 5000 population. The link worker will be trained in communication on HIV/AIDS and accessing referral services.

NGO vs CBO-delivered Interventions

- CBO-led interventions, as opposed to NGO-led interventions, are based on the principle of community ownership and empowers communities to handle responsibility, analyze issues based on data collected and then work out strategies to reduce their health risks in a non-judgmental way.
- In a CBO-led intervention, all aspects of TIs (including selection of peer educators, monitoring of services, framing of byelaws, financial and administrative aspects, etc.) are managed by the CBO, leading to greater and sustainable change of one's health behaviour.
- The NGO-led TIs cover about 800 persons, while CBO TIs cover about 1200 persons, but these will incur additional contingency costs because more CBOs will be newly established to cover a larger population.
- Under NACP III, it was proposed that 50% of all TIs will be handed over to CBOs, entailing a strategic withdrawal of NGOs.

Core Activities of TIs[1]

TIs will be redesigned to be more comprehensive to ensure that even while upscaling the interventions to achieve saturation in HRGs, the older and more mature TIs will be modified to become CBOs so as to empower the communities.

The core activities of a TI would include:

- Behaviour change communication (BCC) interventions to increase demand for products and services
- Providing access to STI services (including counselling to increase compliance to treatment, provide risk reduction and focus on

partner referral) through NGOs or public-private partnership
- Monitoring access and utilization of condoms
- Providing an enabling environment to motivate practice of safe behaviour
- Increasing programme sustainability through CBOs and building ownership in HRGs
- Linking prevention with care, support and treatment to facilitate access and use of these services.

The number of TIs needed in each state to achieve 80% coverage are:

- >250: Uttar Pradesh and Maharashtra
- 100-200: Bihar, Andhra Pradesh, Tamil Nadu, West Bengal, Madhya Pradesh, Karnataka, Rajasthan and Orissa
- <100: Other 23 states

Differential Strategies Among Various Groups[1]

The prevention strategy will involve saturation of the coverage of three HRGs who will be provided with a comprehensive package of preventive services by SACS in partnership with various NGOs/CBOs, other ministries and support from bilateral and UN agencies along with PLHA networks. Specific prevention strategies to be adopted will depend on the target group.

High-risk Groups (HRGs)

The following principles will guide the implementation of prevention strategies in HRGs:

- *District-level mapping and planning:* Mapping of SWs will help in understanding the concentration and dispersion points of SWs in different geographic areas and provide an insight into the operational aspects of sex trade which has changed from being a brothel-based activity to more being street-based and home-based. This change has increased the probability of infection going unnoticed or unattended.
- *Focus on coverage of clients of SWs and partners of IDUs and MSM:* They are important because they form a bridge between HRGs and general population.
- *Specific TIs for MSM:* The coverage of MSM is low due to difficulty in their recognition, gaps in understanding their behaviour and lack of expertise in designing appropriate interventions for them. Strategies for MSM planned under NACP III are:
  - TIs for MSM mostly operate in NGO mode, but the recent highly successful models of MSM networks has encouraged support for the formation of MSM CBOs. But this will require capacity building among MSM to organize and assume leadership.
  - Specific needs of the community would be addressed, e.g., availability of thicker condoms and lubricants and treatment of anal STIs.
  - Special efforts will be undertaken to bring about behaviour change through innovative communication strategies and materials.
  - Operation research will be carried out to understand sexual practices of bisexual men and provide them access to preventive care, support and treatment.
- *Specific TIs for IDUs:* About 10% of IDUs are HIV-positive, but IDU-driven HIV can quickly escalate to the general population, necessitating a comprehensive response based on robust epidemiological networks. Several strategies are planned under NACP III:
  - *Oral substitution:* Despite scientific evidence that substitution treatment with methadone and buprenorphine improves the physical, psychological and social wellbeing of dependent users, India will need to formulate a national policy on substitution.
  - *Harm reduction package:* Both IDUs and their sex partners will be provided a comprehensive harm reduction package (consisting of primary health care, needle/syringe exchange, substitution, condom provision, etc.) and an enabling environment (provided through

mobilization of social support in collaboration with the Ministry of Social Justice and Empowerment).

Bridge Population[1]

Prevention strategies for the bridge population will involve expansion of coverage by SACS in collaboration with National Highway Authority of India (NHAI), NGOs, truckers' associations and unions and companies having a stake in truckers. The following principles will guide the implementation of prevention strategies in the bridge population.

Truckers

The prevention strategy to cover truckers will consist of:

- Mapping of truckers, their partners and their meeting points.
- Identifying the preferred providers and providing points convenient to truckers for establishing facilities to provide free counselling, testing, treatment and health education services as well as linking primary health facilities to CST centres.
- Increasing the participation of CBOs and trucker's associations, unions, etc., in trucker's HIV intervention programmes. Peer educators would be selected from among the locally stationed peers including dhaba owners, tea shop owners and petrol pump attendants rather than from the mobile population.
- Providing TIs at halt points (highway stretches, business activity areas, check posts or port areas, transhipment centres) consists of a package of three core components:
  - BCC activities for creating awareness about HIV/AIDS/STIs and condoms through peer educational activities, organizing camps and using IEC materials.
  - Improving access to condoms along halt points both through professional social marketing organizations and also distributing them free-of-cost.
  - Treating STIs and providing ICTC services. It is important to provide them with access to appropriate STI treatment close-by, since referring truckers to government clinics is not helpful because the distance and time act as disincentives.
- The focus on SWs involved with truckers will be more at resting halt points and less at commercial halt points.

Migrants[1]

There are over 200 million migrants in India, of which the 8 million temporary migrants are important because of frequent movement between source and destination sites in the absence of migrant-friendly services and living in large cluster formations around industries or cities in unauthorized slums. Specific TIs in migrants will consist of:

- Mapping of hot spots (both source and destination) to identify sites for TI and to develop database on number, routes and types of migration, identifying risk groups among them and establishing partnership with NGOs to facilitate safe migration and reduced vulnerability to HIV.
- Establishing 'safe spaces' and peer support groups for migrants in destination areas to facilitate access to services and information on HIV/AIDS.
- Encouraging employers to undertake preventive education activities preferably replicating volunteerism model of CARE in which one peer educator is identified among migrants to disseminate preventive messages to 250 fellow workers. Employers will be encouraged to establish ICTCs and condom sale outlets.
- Introducing HIV/AIDS modules in the Ministry of Labour's pre-departure training programmes for overseas migrants and MEA's orientation programmes for embassy staff.
- Focusing on women impacted by migration (those who migrate and those whose partners migrate) because of their vulnerability to sexual abuse and HIV infection.

Vulnerable Groups of General Population

The vulnerable group in general population consists of women, youth, children and tribals. Under NACP II, the focus on vulnerable groups was fragmented. Although some measures were taken, there was no evaluation of their impact on arresting the epidemic:

- National Adolescents Education Programme (AEP) was developed (in collaboration with the Ministry of Human Resource Development) to cover secondary and senior secondary schools.
- In five states, peer education clubs were established at school level, and in 16 states, HIV prevention education was integrated into the school curriculum.

Under NACP III, women, youth and children in special settings, viz., young people in high prevalence districts, school drop-outs (especially girls), working children, children of sex workers and orphans of HIV/AIDS infected, shall be focused for TI.

Women

Women in the reproductive age group constitute 40% of India's HIV-positive population, with peak age being around 25 years (10-15 years being peak age in men) with 50% of them being housewives with a single partner. Prevention strategies include:

- Mitigating the impact of HIV infection on the infected and the affected.
- Increased access of women (including widows of positive men, survivors of trafficking and violence, partners/spouses of migrant and mobile population and long-distance truckers, single women, etc.) to accurate information on HIV/AIDS prevention, BCC and condom provision through a cadre of link workers.
- Reducing their risks and vulnerabilities, vulnerability being the degree to which an individual or a section of population has control over their risk of acquiring HIV, or the degree to which those who are infected and affected by HIV are able to access appropriate care and support.
- Increasing access to treatment through PPTCT.

Youth

HIV affects young people especially girls disproportionately, with nearly 1/3rd of reported HIV cases being in the 15-29 years age group. Lack of correct information (73% have misconception about modes of transmission of HIV/AIDS, few know where to access condoms[8]), behaviour of experimentation, biological predispositions and gender imbalances, societal norms, poverty and economic dependence make this group very vulnerable to STIs and HIV infection. Based on their level of vulnerability to HIV infection, NACP III categorizes young people into three groups:

- *A group:* Young people in general population, who will be covered through curricular and mainstreaming efforts initiated by respective the ministries.
- *B group:* Vulnerable young people in high and low vulnerable districts (with a large concentration of CSWs, IDUs, MSM, significant outmigration, high HIV prevalence, etc.) who will be covered through behaviour change and education efforts of dedicated workers (link workers and volunteers).
- *C group:* Young people most at risk of infection (adolescents in sex work, young IDUs, street children, working children, etc.) who will be covered through TIs and community-based efforts through dedicated workers and CBOs.

Children

About 170,000 children <15 years of age are infected with HIV/AIDS in India. Children acquire HIV perinatally or sexually, the latter being more frequent in marginalized population (street children, adolescent sex workers, orphans and migrants) because poverty forces them to the risk of unprotected sex and substance abuse. Prevention strategies for children under NACP III include:

- Increasing the coverage of vulnerable children and strengthening child protection systems.
- Mainstreaming HIV/AIDS in the existing schemes and programmes for children.

Tribals

Tribals who form 8.2% of the population and live in hard-to-reach areas with limited access to health services will receive special attention because of their vulnerability to sex networking, trafficking, drug trade, etc.

STD Services[6,7]

With the prevalence of STIs in general population at 4-6% and upwards of 20% in most clusters of SWs, STI/ RTI prevention and treatment strategies form an important component of HIV containment programmes.

Background

Under NACP II, although 922 STD clinics (in medical colleges and district hospitals) were provided financial assistance, there were several lacunae:

- The utilization of STD clinics was suboptimal because most among the vulnerable population access STD care from private service providers (PSPs) and not from designated STD clinics.
- STD clinics were not linked to TIs in a manner that would provide access to HRGs.
- Validation studies on recommended syndromic treatment guidelines reflect high levels of antimicrobial resistance to major STDs.
- Anal and oral STDs were not covered under the then available syndromic guidelines.
- Diagnostic facilities were limited, and it was difficult to manage some patients with STDs even at referral centres.

Resolutions Under NACP III

- To make STD services accessible to the most vulnerable population and to establish uniform protocols for RTI/STI treatment across programmes, NACP III will be integrated with the RCH II programme.[1]
- Symptomatic patients with STIs in general population and in HRGs, both at the district and sub-district level, will be provided access to treatment through a large network of public health facilities and about 25,000 accredited PSPs (of modern medicine, AYUSH and other systems) franchised by NACO. Appropriate equipment and consumables will be provided to PSPs for STD care, and the types of services provided will depend on the background of the PSP[6]:
  - *Allopathic practitioners:* They will be respon-sible for counselling including condom promotion, providing information on cause and transmission of STIs and performing simple diagnostic tests and providing syndromic treatment of STIs/ RTIs in symptomatic patients as well as partner management.[6]
  - *Non-allopathic practitioners:* They will be responsible for counselling including condom promotion, providing information on cause and transmission of STIs and identification of syndrome and referral in symptomatic patients.[6]
- Standard procedures, flow charts and training modules will be established, and public doctors and PSPs will be trained with focus on revised protocols. Syndromic management protocols will incorporate oral/anal STIs.[7]
- HRGs will be routinely screened for STDs by a designated NGO administering TI and referred for treatment.[6,7]
- The demand for services will be generated through BCC.
- Two national STI prevalence studies will be commissioned. Regular surveillance of STIs in HRGs will be initiated in collaboration with STD network laboratories. About 2% of the subjects who are not responding and a random sample of subjects referred from TIs will have laboratory surveillance of STIs.[1]

- Regional centres will be established for monitoring drug resistance to gonococci and cervical smears collected from random sampling of HRGs coming for check-ups will be transported for monitoring drug resistance and deciding on syndromic management guidelines.

Condom Promotion[1]

Background

- Condom use has been promoted and supplied free-of-cost (through public health channels) and at subsidized rates (through retail channels) under the National Family Planning Programme since 1960s.
- Condom promotion for NACP I and NACP II was done through linkage with the National Family Planning Programme, which led to an increase in the awareness of prevention of HIV infection with consistent condom use. Available data suggest that the use of condoms is variable in different populations, and despite high awareness and increased availability, its use remains suboptimal.
  - *HRGs:* >80%, but varies in different situations, e.g., among SWs, condom use was variable in paying and non-paying clients at 50% and 20% respectively.[8]
  - *General population:* 59% (73% urban vs 54% rural).
- ***Reasons for low condom use:***
  - Lack of self-risk perception is a major reason for low condom use.
  - Disruptive supply because of problems in the supply chain.
  - Promotional initiatives are often limited to mass media, which have limited impact on HRGs and bridge population.
  - Lacunae in social marketing.

Resolutions Under NACP III

Several improved and innovative strategies have been included to increase condom use:

- Introduction of target (HRGs, bridge population, general population, PLHAs)-specific strategies to encourage condom use including making social marketing programmes focus on sexually active men, clients of SWs and MSM.
- ***Channels of supply:*** Better and easy availability of condoms:
  - *Free condoms:* Uninterrupted availability of free condoms by streamlining the supply chain and distribution with minimal wastage in TIs.
  - *Subsidized condoms:* Social marketing of condoms through social marketing organizations (SMOs) especially in unreached urban pockets and rural areas with triple (pregnancy, HIV, STIs) protection message and access creation in non-traditional outlets in high-risk areas. The numbers of SMOs will be increased from the present 5 to 25.
  - *Commercial supply:* Easy availability through retail outlets.
  - *Newer condoms:* Evidence-based programming of female condoms and extra-thick, lubricated condoms for MSM.

The objectives of NACP III are to:

- Increase condom use to 3.5 billion pieces/year by 2009 (from the present 1.6 billion) through intensive demand generation and supply efforts with support from an outsourced agency.
- All three channels of condom supply will work complementary to each other providing products to different target groups. The consumer base for socially marketed condoms will be increased by switching the current users of free supply condoms with appropriate behaviour change strategies and motivating non-users to use condoms in all non-spousal sex acts. Free supply of condoms will be limited to those who cannot afford to buy socially marketed condoms (people below poverty line).

Blood Safety[1]

Background

To ensure access to safe blood, under NACP II, the NACO had financed for modernization of 1230 blood banks including 82 blood component separation centres. Notwithstanding these achievements, 39 districts in the country have no facilities for supply of safe blood.

Resolutions Under NACP III

- Broad objectives of the blood safety programme under NACP III are to ensure provision of safe and quality blood within 1 hour of requirement in a health facility and reduce transfusion-associated HIV transmission to 0.5%.
- This is sought to be achieved by:
  - Ensuring regular voluntary blood donors to constitute the main source of blood supply through donor recruitment and retention. The target is to raise voluntary blood donation to 90% (from present 50%) by end of the programme.
  - Establishing blood storage facilities in PHCs.
  - Promote appropriate use of blood components and blood products.
  - Develop a long-term policy for capacity building to achieve efficient and self-sufficient blood transfusion services.
- NACP III is committed to strengthening quality assurance programmes and accreditation of blood banks, external quality assessment scheme (EQAS) for HIV testing and improving transportation and storage of blood and blood products.

Implementation

- *At the district level:* There should be at least one NACO-supported blood bank in each district and at least one voluntary blood donation camp should be organized in every district.
- *At the state level:* SACS will have dedicated staff, and a State Blood Transfusion Council will be established for blood safety. Blood banks will be supervised every 3 months.
- *At the national level:* There will be three supervisory agencies: Blood Safety Division of NACO, National Blood Transfusion Council (NBTC) and Technical Resource Group (TRG) on blood safety, and the states will be categorized as poor, average and better performing, and remedial steps will be taken in states performing suboptimally.

Integrated Counselling and Testing Centres

Background

The number of ICTCs (earlier VCTCs) has increased from 79 in 1998 to 2815 in 2006. Despite this increase in number under NACP II, access to them by vulnerable groups has been poor, with only 5-7% of HIV infected people knowing their HIV status.

Resolutions Under NACP III

- Existing VCTCs and PPTCT centres will be redesignated as ICTCs and remodelled to integrate all HIV-related services.
- An additional 2140 centres will be established (taking the total to 4955) to cover all districts. These centres will initially be set up in medical colleges and district hospitals but eventually scaled up to sub-district levels in CHCs, in private sector and even in non-health sector. In hard-to-reach areas (e.g., tribal areas), mobile units will be made available.
- *Functions of ICTCs:* ICTCs will be responsible for:
  - Counselling (IEC/BCC, condom promotion, STI treatment linkages, etc.)
  - Making tests available whose quality will be assured by internal and external quality assurance mechanisms.

 - Referrals, e.g., pregnant women will be referred to PPTCT centres, those with STI symptoms to STD clinics, and those with TB symptoms to RNTCP centres.

Prevention of PTCT

Background

- In India, annually about 189,000 pregnancies occur in HIV+ mothers leading to an estimated cohort of 56,700 infected babies.
- Although the PPTCT programme (using nevirapine) was initiated in 2001, by 2004, only 3.94% of all pregnant women received HIV counselling and testing, and only 2.35% of HIV-positive pregnant women received ART prophylaxis.
- Currently, 1,882 PPTCT centres are functioning in India (502 standalone PPTCT centres and 1,380 ICTCs which offer PPTCT services). Of these, 1,600 are in six high prevalence states, and most are in the public sector with only few in the private sector.

Resolution Under NACP III

The aim is to prevent vertical transmission of HIV in an annual cohort of 189,000 HIV-positive pregnant women throughout the country and ensuring that PPTCT reaches 98% from year 4 of NACP III. This will be done by:

- Establishing additional 2140 PPTCT centres as part of ICTCs to provide universal access.
- Scaling PPTCT services through public-private partnerships and extending them upto the level of CHCs (based on the results of a feasibility study in 2000 by NACO and UNICEF to demonstrate the possibility of implementing PPTCT in the public sector with single-dose nevirapine which had an efficacy of 48% in PPTCT).
- Strengthening referrals and linkages by defining a minimum package of services to be provided at different levels of care and developing standard operating procedures for strengthening linkages between PPTCT and ART services for infected parents and children.
- Estimating the CD4 count of all pregnant HIV-positive women.
- Strengthening infant feeding counselling to reinforce mother's decision and to support infant feeding method of their choice.
- Adopting long-term follow-up of mother and child for opportunistic infections and ART and integrate with RCH services.

Communication

Communication is an integral strategic intervention in all components of HIV/AIDS prevention and CST programmes. A communication strategy will:

- Motivate behaviour change in HRGs and bridge populations.
- Raise awareness levels on risks.
- Promote the use of condoms among youth and women in general population.
- Generate demand for health services (with an enabling environment for prevention and for institutional and community care and support).

Background

NACP II included the following communication interventions:

- IEC through TV, radio and print.
- Media campaigns in partnership with the Ministry of Information and Broadcasting.
- Capacity building of SACSs.
- Youth parliament at the national level and legislature sessions at state levels.
- National media summit.

Communication strategies introduced in NACP II had the following impacts:

- Improved awareness about HIV infection especially methods of protection (condom and single partner sex), but the impact on behaviour change towards safe sex practices and utilization of services was suboptimal.

- Good responce to strategies of condom promotion, demand generation for services and reducing stigma.
- Created an enabling environment for PLHAs at the institutional level and in the community but suboptimally.

Resolutions Under NACP-III

NACP III has a Communication Strategy and Implementation Plan to promote behaviour change (in individuals, communities and institutions) through risk reduction, vulnerability reduction, stigma reduction and increased awareness, and increased demand for services and their optimal utilization over 5 years. A set of priority objectives has been defined for various groups:

- *Priority 1: HRGs and bridge population*: Highest priority will be given to motivate behaviour change (consistent use of condoms with all partners and reduce the number of casual partners, use of clean needles, accept needle exchange, etc.) in HRGs and bridge populations.
- *Priority 2*: The next priority groups include:
  - *Vulnerable groups in general population (women, children, youth and tribals):* Priority in this group will be to raise awareness about the risk of HIV infection, avoid experimentation/casual and commercial sex, and to use condoms in all sexual encounters.
  - *PLHAs:* Priority in this group will be to raise awareness about social mobilization efforts and services available to promote the use of condoms and impress upon them the need for greater networking and advocacy within their own community for strength and empowerment. They will be motivated to take advantage of economic and social empowerment being created for them under NACP III.
- *Priority 3*: Service providers and healthcare workers will be sensitized and encouraged to improve their attitude to PLHAs and offer better quality of services and ensure an enabling environment.
- *Priority 4*: Mainstreaming and multisectoral partners will be sensitized to create policies which support programmes on HIV/AIDS.

LINKING PREVENTION TO CARE, SUPPORT AND TREATMENT[1]

Expanding care, support and treatment (CST) and linking them to prevention strategies will not only help reduce AIDS-related mortality but also reduce poverty, stigma and discrimination and increase the number of PLHAs targeted for communication interventions designed to change their high-risk behaviour. Most importantly, this will help achieve the primary objective of controlling the spread of the epidemic. Under NACP III, three categories of services (preventive services, care and support and treatment) will be p rovided as a package (either directly or as referral). All care centres (CCC, TB clinics and ART centres) will focus on preventive strategies (ICTC, PPTCT, STD clinics and TIs on HRGs) because each component of service is relavant.

Components of Care (Tables 37.1 and 37.2)

Level of Delivery

Under NACP II, the focus was on service delivery through tertiary and district level health care institutions, and a significant scale-up was achieved through increase in the number of VCTCs, STD clinics and PPTCT centres. However, it was observed that HIV services provided at the tertiary and district levels were not easily accessible to the target population.

Table 37.1 **General Services Linking Prevention, Care, Support and Treatment in NACP III**

i. Creating awareness about symptoms, spread, prevention and services available
ii. Management of STIs and RTIs
iii. Condom promotion
iv. Promotion of voluntary blood donation and access to safe blood
v. Integrated counselling and testing (ICT)
vi. Prevention of PTCT
vii. Post-exposure prophylaxis
viii. Infection control
• Management of opportunistic infections
• Control of TB in PLHA
• Antiretroviral therapy and related services
ix. Outreach community/home-based care
x. Reducing stigma and discrimination

Table 37.2 **Specific Services for HRGs Linking Prevention, Care, Support and Treatment under NACP III**

i. STI services: programme owned, programme linked and referral
ii. Condoms: free and social marketing
iii. BCC through peer and outreach
iv. Building an enabling environment
v. Community organizing and ownership building
vi. Linking HIV-related care and support services
Additional Components for IDUs
i. Detoxification, deaddiction and rehabilitation
ii. Needle exchange
iii. Substitution therapy
iv. Abscess management
Additional components for MSM
i. Lubricants
ii. Appropriate condoms

Under NACP III, it was proposed to integrate and scale up service delivery to sub-district and community levels through the existing infrastructure in public and private sectors. Services will be delivered at various levels and will be packaged based on needs at different levels of health care so as to improve the efficiency of services delivered and avoid duplication.

- At the district level, the full complement of preventive, supportive and curative services will be made available in all medical colleges and district hospitals. These include a whole spectrum of HIV-related 'core and integrated services' including psychosocial counselling and support, ART, management of infections (OIs, STIs and TB), positive prevention, specialized paediatric HIV care and treatment, palliative care and pain management as well as referral to specialists.
- Linkages of NGOs/CBOs with hospitals will help provide the component of continuum of care and support with outreach, peer support services and home-based care. Community linkages will also provide means to follow up children born to HIV-positive women, and support them at the community level and outreach.

- Testing facility for PPTCT services will be provided in medical colleges and in district hospitals in ANCs for rapid screening of pregnant women.
- At sub-district hospitals and CHCs, the package will be tailored to more basic needs (Table 37.3).

Table 37.3 Differential Package Based on Epidemiological Profile of the District*

Level	*Target Group*	*Services Provided*
Category A districts (High prevalence)		
Medical colleges/ district, block and sub-divisional hospitals, village/community	General population, HRGs, PLHA	All HIV-related services (ICT, PPTCT, STD care, OI management and ART with necessary linkages) made available under one roof. CHC/not-for-profit private health institutions to provide ICT, PPTCT, STDs and OI with necessary linkages to prevention and CST services in PHC/PSPs for STD control, OI and condom promotion Mobile ICTC to reach hard-to-reach areas
Category B districts (Concentrated epidemic)		
District, block and sub-divisional hospitals, village/community	General population, HRGs, PLHA (services curtailed at the periphery)	All HIV-related services as under category 'A' districts but supplies to be adjusted according to patient load. PHCs to function 24 hr as in category 'A' districts
Category C districts (Low prevalence with increased presence of vulnerable population)		
District, block and sub-divisional hospitals, village/community	Vulnerable populations, HRGs	ART clinics will be added in large districts and if not available within 6 hours travel by road. ICTC, will be established in CHCs where the case load for testing is high (>15/day including PPTCT). Where case load is less, existing staff trained for counselling services. Drugs and supplies adjusted according to patient load. PLHA-related services: CCC to be established only if there is a minimum of 50 PLHAs identified in the district
Category D districts (Low prevalence and low/unknown vulnerability)		
District, block and sub-divisional hospitals, village/ community	Basic service package	ART services provided in medical colleges. CHC will provide STD and OI management but not ICTC. Services limited to syndromic management of STDs, IEC and condom promotion

* Refer Tables 4.1 and 4.2.

CARE, SUPPORT AND TREATMENT[1]

Under NACP II, the focus was on low-cost care, support and treatment of common OIs. ART programme was launched in 2004 only in 8 institutions in 6 high prevalence states and in Delhi, and has gradually been upscaled to a total of 54 ART centres treating about 33,000 patients (including 1300 children). However, this constituted only 10% of the estimated eligible patients needing treatment.

Under NACP III, a comprehensive strategy will be adopted to strengthen family and community care, provide psychosocial support to affected individuals (particularly to marginalized women and children) and ensure accessible, affordable and sustainable treatment services. The strategy would include:

- Identification of institutions
- Strengthening referral linkages for CD4 testing
- Capacity building of ART teams
- Procurement of antiretroviral drugs

Antiretroviral Therapy (ART)

Under NACP III, first-line ART will be provided to:

- PLHAs referred from TIs
- Seropositive women particularly those who have participated in the PPTCT programme
- Infected children
- BPL patients

The success of treatment will be improved by:

- Achieving drug adherence of >95% to prevent drug resistance.
- Promoting private-public partnership to deliver care, e.g., identifying NGOs to provide care to PLHAs and providing them free drugs, capacity building and linkages.
- Ensuring regular supply of ART drugs through effective supply chain management.

For pediatric HIV infection, the goals of prevention and CST programme are:

- Provide ART to >90% of children living with AIDS at the end of 5 years of NACP III.
- Prevent transmission of HIV infection to newborns through scaling-up of PPTCT.

Pediatric ART formulations will be made available by end of first year and protocols for paediatric treatment formulated by NACO will be implemented simultaneously with upscaling of PPTCT services:

- In children <18 months, infection will be diagnosed using DNA PCR at 6 weeks of age, to be made available at six national reference centres.
- Children >18 months will be evaluated as adults.

Criteria for ART

The initiation of ART in adults will be determined as per the criteria (Table 37.4).

Table 37.4 NACO Criteria for Initiating ART

CD4 (cells/mm^3)	*Actions*
<200	Always treat with ART
200-350	Offer ART if symptomatic Initiate Rx before CD4 drop <200 cells/mm^3 for asymptomatic patients
>350	Defer treatment in asymptomatic patients

ART Centres

- Based on needs, about 250 ART centres (both in government and private sector) with facilities to perform CD4 counts will be established.

- In category A and B districts (total 228), ART centres will be strengthened by integrating services of manpower (counselors and laboratory personnel) from ICTCs and STD services. A person from PLHA network will be posted at ART centres to facilitate access to care and treatment services. Eligible PLHAs and those initiated on ART will be provided adherence counselling and support.
- Although follow-up at a ART centre will be monthly (or more frequently if required), every week the outreach worker (1/25 PLHAs) will sensitize the patient on drug adherence, compliance and issues related to toxicity and monitoring to ensure 100% adherence.
- Drugs for children will be provided through ART centres to ensure single-point delivery of services both to parents and children. PPTCT centres will also be linked with ART centres for follow-up and early diagnosis in children and mothers.

Capacity Building

- Faculty in medical colleges where ART centres are located, paediatricians at ART centres with >10 children with HIV, paediatric counselors and technical staff at diagnostic testing centres will be trained on the basis of established modules.
- Research centres (10 in number) will be established for testing resistance by the end of first year.
- Ensuring quality in the delivery of ART by
  - Improving infrastructure to deliver care in an enabling manner.
  - Improving environmental conditions.
  - Improving quality of facilities by periodic training of all providers.
  - Ensuring strict adherence to treatment protocols and standards.
  - Supervising delivery of CST services to PLHAs in a manner that is both supportive and proactive.
  - Monitoring through CMIS: In the four high prevalence states of TN, AP, Maharashtra and Karnataka, all patient records will be computerized and patients will be provided SMART cards. Based on the outcome of this initiative, action to upscale it to other states will be undertaken.

Drug Resistance, Surveillance and Monitoring

Resistance to first-line ART is about 4-8% a year, implying that at the end of fourth year 25% of patients will be resistant to it. Although drug resistance to ART is inevitable, the following strategies will be adopted to delay it:

- Build capacity into current monitoring systems for early warning indicators at the level of ART providers.
- Build capacity of referral institutions to manage PLHAs with drug resistance.
- Reinforce adherence through continuum of care.
- Finalize a policy on second-line ART.

Surveillance for drug resistance will be carried out by the National AIDS Research Institute (NARI) as the nodal institute with 10 sentinel sites for collection of specimens from different sites in the country.

Treatment of Opportunistic Infections (OIs)

OIs are responsible for morbidity and mortality of AIDS patients, and treatment of these infections will be an important component of CST. This will be done through:

- Early recognition of the HIV status with access to chemoprophylaxis of OIs especially those with proven preventive strategies (pneumocystis pneumonia and toxoplasmosis).
- Developing standard treatment protocols for management of OIs and making them available at all sites. Tuberculosis, the leading cause of death in PLHAs, will be aggressively addressed by developing standard treatment protocols, setting up ICT services in centres of RNTCP and referral of all HIV-positive

subjects with symptoms suggestive of TB to RNTCP. The treatment of TB will follow RNTCP guidelines and compliance of DOTS ensured.

- Treating common OIs at periphery centres (PHC, CHC, CCCs and by PSPs who treat 40-50% of these infections) and referring only serious infections to district hospitals or medical colleges. Referrals will be assisted by established linkages and guidelines.
- Providing drugs for chemoprophylaxis and treatment of OIs in public and private sector health care facility.
- Upscaling of the smart card system to track infections in individual patients.
- Establishing sentinel surveillance of OIs in each state to detect discernible trends in the prevalence of different infections.

Care and Support

Women and children will be special targets because of feminization of the epidemic. Synergies of the existing programmes under RCH and ICDS will be strengthened with CSOs working on women's and children's issues to provide CST to women and children infected and affected.

Community Care Centres (CCCs)

- Under NACP II, although 122 CCCs were established (to provide treatment for minor OIs, psychosocial support and short stay homes for those ostracized), they were not linked to other activities or programmes.
- Under NACP III, addititional 228 CCCs (each with 30 beds) will be established in partnership with PLHA networks in A, B and in some C districts. These centres will focus on providing four types of services to PLHAs:
  - Counselling, in particular for drug adherence, since ART is now an important component of the programme.
  - Treatment support.
  - Referral and outreach for follow-up.
  - Social support services.

Enabling Environment

Effective prevention, care and support for HIV/AIDS can be provided only in an environment in which human rights of the affected/infected person are respected and where they live in dignity without stigma and discrimination. Several studies have shown a high level of discrimination (70%) against PLHAs and marginalized groups by service providers, at work places, in community and in the family. Providing an enabling environment would necessitate a review and reform of structural constraints, legal procedures and policies that impede interventions aimed at marginalized populations.

Background

- During NACP II, there was a shift in the role of PLHAs from just being beneficiaries of services to becoming important partners of the nation to fight against HIV.

Resolution Under NACP III

The following strategies will be adopted to provide an enabling environment:

- Facilitate the establishment of PLHA networks in most districts and all states by the year 2010. The PLHAs will be accredited for partnership with NACO to create an enabling environment by addressing the issues of stigma, discrimination, legal and ethical concerns.
- **GIPA:** There will be a greater involvement of people with HIV/AIDS (GIPA) with clear guidelines for mobilization and networking among PLHAs and also utilizing them as advocates for prevention and CST.
- Address issues of stigma and discrimination at all levels through evidence-based research and advocacy, capacity development and partnership building.

CAPACITY BUILDING[1]

Capacity building is the development of skilled and competent human resources at all levels of an organization. In the last two phases of NACP, the focus was mainly on the technical aspects of prevention, diagnosis and clinical management. The aim of NACP III is to build capacity at national, state and district levels:

- Of programme managers in leadership and strategic management.
- Of HCPs, CBOs and NGOs in technical and communication skills at all levels of care.
- Of grassroot workers in technical, communication and counselling skills.

Training

- NACO will develop a training policy to identify priorities and needs of training, the location and types of training to be imparted, and monitor quality and effectiveness of training. The emphasis of training will be on skill development for better performance and for behaviour change.
- A comprehensive 5-year training plan has been prepared with special focus on the identification of trainers and trainees, training load in each category, duration of training, training sites, number of batches to be organized, and time frame on an annual basis.

Mainstreaming

Mainstreaming is necessary to achieve the organizational objectives of NACP III. It will also help organizations achieve revenue and efficiency targets.

Categories of Mainstreaming

An organization can mainstream HIV prevention in two ways:

- Internal mainstreaming is the process of reducing the impact of HIV/AIDS on the organization by providing access to knowledge and services.
- External mainstreaming is reducing the spread of HIV in the domain in which the organization operates.

Background

NACP II had a minimal component of mainstreaming except for NCERT which linked up HIV prevention to its population education programmes and university talks on AIDS. Measures to protect the members of the armed forces were instituted and some ministries like labor, railways and steel developed active programmes. Some private sector organizations also integrated HIV in their workplace and outreach programmes.

Resolutions Under NACP III

The strategy of NACP III on mainstreaming will work towards having:

- HIV prevention strategies into the work plan of major government/private organizations.
- Allocating internal resources to such programmes.

The strategies to be adopted will include:

- Commitment of several ministries to mainstreaming. Although in most ministries mainstreaming will be internal (only for its employees), 11 priority ministries including education, home affairs, labour, etc., will be involved in external mainstreaming.
- Shift from direct implementation and funding to advocacy and providing technical support and implementing work place policy both in government and private organizations.
- Ensure mobilization of private sector (through employers' unions/PLHA networks) to upscale interventions.

- Develop projects for workers engaged in small enterprises by carefully mapping them and building partnerships with local associations and CSOs.

Public-Private Partnership (PPP)

It was estimated that >80% of people use the private health sector for outpatient care and >50% for inpatient care, and so their involvement in any health care activity is essential.

Resolutions Under NACP III

- Private sector will be encouraged to offer prevention and treatment services, provide linkages to government services and extend such services to the immediate community. Not all services will be paid for by the government, and the objective of PPP is to ensure the private sector is co-opted as a responsible partner to fight against HIV/AIDS.
- The National Steering Committee will develop a joint operational plan and identify mechanisms for strengthening linkages between the private and government sector. These could include activities to support vulnerable and infected population, mobile VCTCs, BCC through outreach or provision of smart cards or vocational classes for children of SWs.
- ***PPP in health sector:*** Private HCPs through PPP will be used with appropriate safeguards to ensure quality (through training manuals and standard operating protocols made available to all private HCPs) in preventive and treatment services:
  - *STD treatment:* Since 3/4th of STIs are treated in the private sector, co-option of private HSPs in treatment will ensure universal access to STI services. The proposed mapping exercises will include identification of HSPs most frequented for STD care, the quality of treatment being provided, and their competencies to ensure standardized quality after appropriate training. An estimated 15 million STD episodes and an additional 7 million cases to cover persons from HRGs and BPL will be treated in the private sector.
  - *Gynaecological services:* Due to several reasons, women prefer to go to the private sector, including quacks, for gynaecological problems. Private HCPs will be identified and contracted to provide the required package of services, especially where public services are not available.
  - *ICTCs (fixed and mobile):* Private sector facilities will be identified for expanding access to ICTC. Mobile services (to provide IEC about condoms, testing and counselling and preventive care such as ANC services, etc.) will be used to overcome the barrier of distance.
  - *ART centres:* About 100,000 PLHAs will seek private care requiring an additional 126 ART centres across the country. NACO will provide training and, based on feasibility, consider the supply of drugs at government rates. Besides, where government infrastructure is not functioning well, private hospitals will be contracted for providing services to neighbouring populations.
  - Outsourcing laboratory services
  - *Training*: PPP will be encouraged in planning and organizing training on capacity building, as also in technical, managerial, communication components, etc.
  - *Others:* Other areas of PPP will include community care centres and blood banks.

Civil Society Partnership Forums

- The partnership between CSOs and government agencies in planning and implementation of NACP III has been formalized, and the functioning will be facilitated at district and state level by TSUs (in states where they have been established) or NGOs (in states where TSUs do not exist).

- District level forums will be established with CSOs, NGOs, CBOs and Red Ribbon as members. The forum will be informed of the implementation plans and will be provided data to review progress.
- State forums will be established with two members from each district forum, while the national forum will have representatives from the state level fora.

Steering Committee of Development Partners

All agencies (whether private or government) working in the area of HIV/AIDS will need to align their work to the national framework approved by the NCA. They will be members of the Steering Committee of Partners at the national and state level. The committee will ensure no duplication of agenda and a harmonized working relationship so as to move resources to underserved areas.

STRATEGIC INFORMATION MANAGEMENT

Monitoring and Evaluation

Background

The HIV surveillance system in India includes:

- Sentinel- and facility-based HIV sero-prevalence surveys for measuring trends in HIV prevalence and developing state and national prevalence estimates.
- BSS surveys and research studies to track HIV-related risk behaviours.
- Computerized Management Information System (CMIS) established nationwide for providing strategic information on programme monitoring and evaluation.
- Computerized Project Financial Management System (CPFMS).

However, data so collected have not been effectively analyzed and used for planning and implementation because the analytical capacity at the state level (except in Andhra Pradesh and Tamil Nadu) is weak.

Resolutions Under NACP III

To overcome the lacunae, the following steps will be taken under NACP III:

- A single nationwide monitoring and evaluation framework will be established to ensure effective use of existing information.
- ***CMIS:*** CMIS, the three-tier data flow system to collate state and district data for monthly and annual reports, will be revamped to overcome the existing gaps and add features to support decentralization to the district level in the first year.
- ***Strategic Information Management Unit (SIMU):*** SIMU will be established (national and state level) to maximize the effective use of available information, track the epidemic, implement evidence-based planning and assess the effectiveness of the response.
- ***Monitoring systems:*** Monitoring systems and indicators will be modified to be consistent with national needs and international standards and for global comparison.
- ***Evaluation:*** All intervention strategies will incorporate internal evaluation tools (including 130 core evaluation indicators), and midterm and terminal external evaluations will be carried out. Programme reports will be produced on a monthly/ quarterly basis and a quarterly 'dashboard' with information on key indicators will serve as a monitoring tool.

Surveillance

Background

- HIV sentinel surveillance (HSS) was carried out in 2005 at 702 sites (175 clinic based, 268 urban ANC and 128 rural ANC, 30 IDU, 83

FSW and 18 MSM sites). For sentinel survey, HIV testing strategy adopted is anonymous; unlinked and some additional variables are collected with the specimen. There is a well-defined system of external quality assurance for field work and laboratory testing. Sampling is done at select sentinel sites annually for a period of 3 months:
  - *ANC Sites:* 400 consecutive women attending the ANC sites and meeting the inclusion criteria are recruited or until the end of surveillance period, whichever is earlier.
  - *STD Sites:* A total of 250 samples from two sources, STD (150) and Obstetrics and Gynaecology (100) clinics located in the same hospital, are collected. Only consecutive new cases of STDs diagnosed syndromically (i.e., cases of genital ulcer, urethral or cervical discharge and genital warts) are recruited.
  - HRG samples are collected at service points, e.g., deaddiction centers, dropin centers, until a sample size of 250 is reached or until the end of surveillance period, whichever is earlier.
- National BSS conducted in 2001 helped NACP establish a baseline of risk behaviours.

Lacunae

- The second round of BSS was delayed and the programme made certain assumptions until the previous results became available as late as in 2008.
- STD surveillance has been very weak and community-level STI surveillance and health facility surveys have been conducted only once.

Resolutions Under NACP III

- The surveillance system will focus on tracking the epidemic, identifying pockets of HIV infection and estimating the burden of HIV infection and other surrogate markers like STIs, hepatitis B, hepatitis C, etc. Other areas of focus will be AIDS case reporting, HIV-associated morbidity and mortality, ART and STI drug resistance surveillance and sentinel surveillance of OIs. NACP III will explore possibilities of integrating PPTCT surveillance and ANC surveillance systems.
- HSS 2006 was done at 1122 sites to cover all the districts of the country (628 ANCs and 494 sites catering to HRGs).
- Integrating HSS with Integrated Biological and Behavioural Surveillance (IBBS) every 2-3 years among HRGs will be explored.
- Two types of BSS will be conducted at least once in 3 years:
  - Annual risk assessment at the district level
  - Methodologically rigorous BSS at the state level
- Development of guidelines to define high prevalence/vulnerability in districts.

Research

Background

- Since early 1990s, HIV-related research in India has contributed to a much better understanding of the dynamics of the epidemic. However, issues of quality of research, utilization, transfer and management continue to be areas of concern because most data remain unvalidated, scattered and underutilized because of poor documentation and dissemination practice.
- The potential of intervention/action research and interdisciplinary approach to cross-cutting themes have remained underutilized.

Resolutions Under NACP III

- A research wing with a multidisciplinary Research Advisory Committee will be established in NACO with strong linkages with research/academic institutions at regional/state level.
- Critical gaps in existing knowledge and key areas of research especially operation research

will be identified to develop an appropriate research agenda.

- Capacity building of researchers especially for monitoring and evaluating community-based interventions will be encouraged.

Programme Management and Decentralization

Under NACP III, implementation will be decentralized down to the district level by establishing HIV resource units within district health societies.

NACO

NACO provides leadership to the HIV/AIDS Control Programme in India, implementing one national plan within one monitoring system. During NACP III, NACO will continue to work on the decentralized model evolved during NACPII. Under NACP III, the capacity of NACO will be further strengthened for coordinating with a large number of partners within and outside the government, laying down and enforcing technical protocols and operational guidelines on interventions to be undertaken, ensuring quality and assisting SACS to build their technical capacity for managing programme implementation based on evidence. NACO will, however, undertake a more interventionist role in states that fail to deliver till such time their capacity is built. Due to special vulnerabilities of north-eastern states, a sub-office of NACO will be set up to provide programme implementation support to north-eastern states.

The governance structure of NACO will consist of (Fig. 37.2):

- National Council on AIDS (NCA)
  - Under the chairmanship of the Prime Minister, it is the largest body overseeing the NACP. It has members from 31 participating ministries and civil society representatives.
  - It provides political will and support to the implementation of the National Framework on AIDS Control, particularly in the context of mainstreaming HIV prevention within all organs of the government as well as the private sector and civil society.
- National AIDS Control Board (NACB)
  - Under the chairmanship of Secretary of Health.
  - It oversees the programme management of NACO, approves its annual plans and reviews its quarterly performance reports.
- Technical Advisory Groups (TAGs)
  - NACO constitutes Technical Advisory Groups on various thematic areas like public health, surveillance, etc., for guiding and assuring technical monitoring of the programme.
  - TAGs will meet as per need and visit states to review the quality of implementation of interventions and provide guidance.

Decentralization of the Programme

Due to decentralization of the programme, the role of state and district units will be important.

- *State AIDS Control Society (SACS)*
  - During NACP II, decentralized autonomous societies (SACS) with appropriate functional independence, were set up to upscale the programme to the needs of the states under NACP III.
  - SACS will be the main implementing arm of NACO and will have a governance structure at the state level for programme support and oversight (Fig. 37.3).
  - The governing body of SACS is its highest policy-making body and is headed either by the Minister of Health or the Chief Secretary. It will approve its annual action plan, annual budget and new policy initiatives.
  - The executive committee of SACS is headed by the Principal Secretary/Secretary of Health. It will exercise powers as delegated to it by the governing body.
  - Project Director (PD) is a pivotal position in SACS.

- ***Functions of SACS:*** Besides collaboration with NRHM, RCH, RNTCP and other health programmes, it has three broad roles: medical and public health services, communication and social sector services, and administration, planning, coordination, finance and procurement.
- The work load of SACS is contingent on the size and population of the state and the burden of disease.

- *State Council on AIDS (SCA):*
  - SCA will be set in all states and will be headed by the Chief Minister with the Minister of Health as the Vice Chairperson.
  - It will set policy guidelines, review the state's performance including mainstreaming by key departments.
- *Technical Support Units (TSUs):*
  - TSUs will be established to assist in the implementation of prevention strategies.
  - After NGO identification/CBO formation, they will help in capacity building and creating an enabling environment and assisting SACS in the supervision of CST programmes, logistics management, monitoring and evaluation, etc.
- *District AIDS Prevention and Control Unit (DAPCU)*
  - DAPCU will operate within the District Health Society, sharing the administrative and financial structures of NRHM.
  - While the unit will report to and work through the Chief Medical Officer of the district for medical interventions, it will also be responsible for non-health-related activities such as adolescent education programme, supportive supervision of TIs, etc., through the office of District Collector or Zilla Panchayat.

Support to States with Weak Capacities

- During NACP I and II, states varied in scale and quality of their programme delivery, which was partly by political support and partly by technical assistance available in the state.
- During NACP III, NACO will ensure that states perform at the planned level and SACS will have greater accountability. This will be ensured by less frequent changes of senior level functionaries, dedicated staff for the programme and filling up vacant posts.

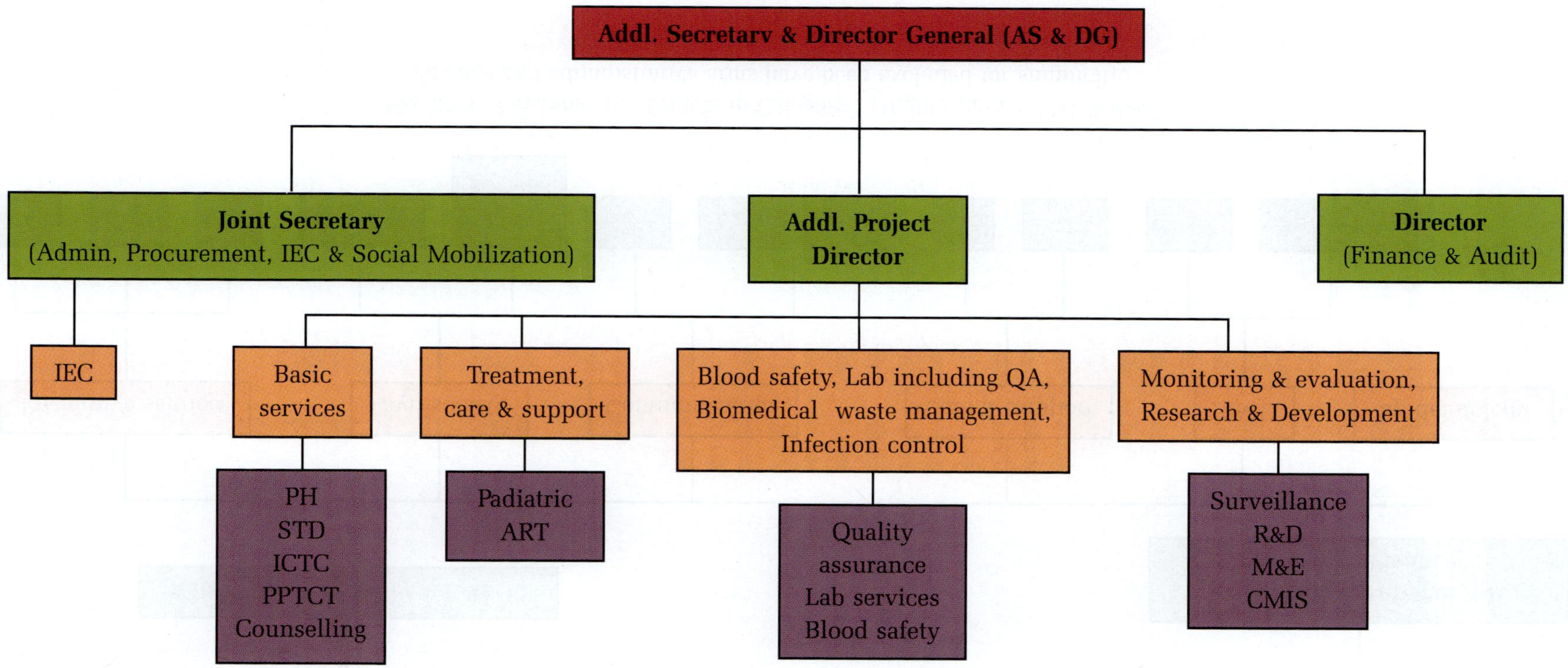

Fig. 37.2 Organogram of NACO.
Finance and administrative arms have been excluded for simplicity.

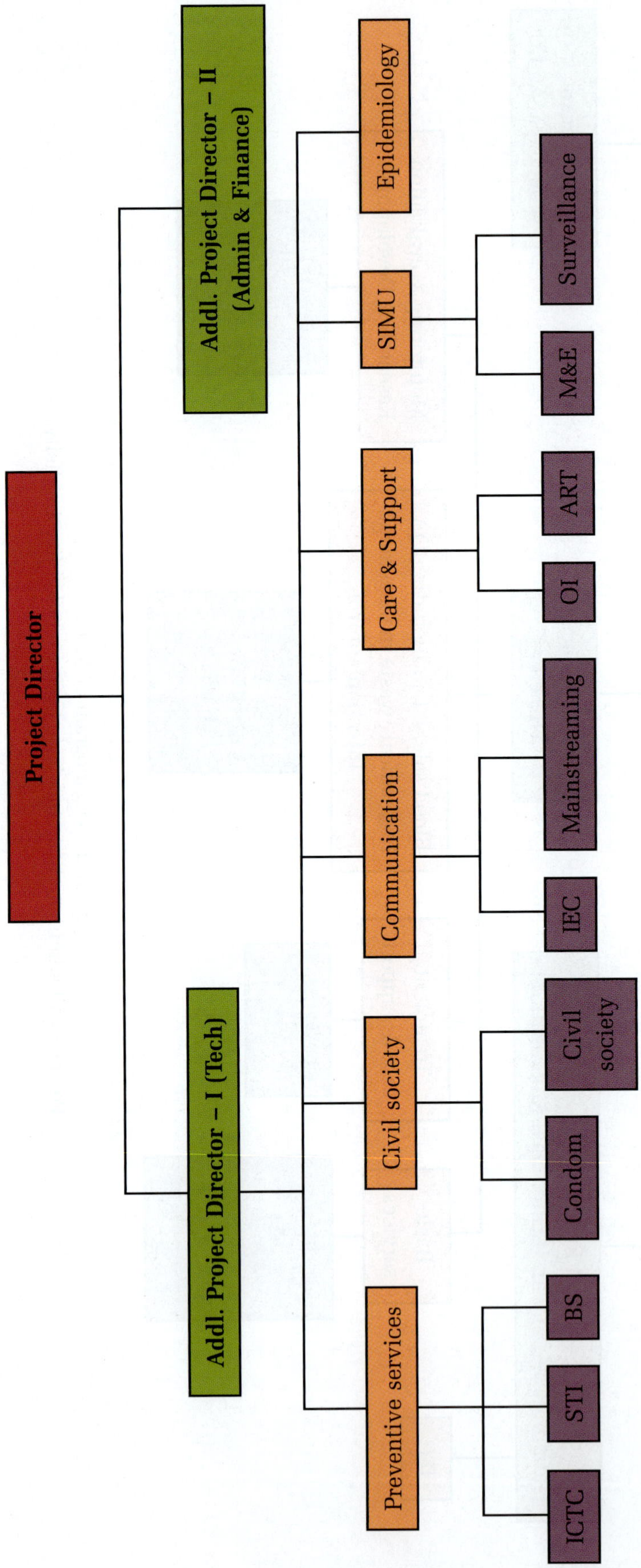

Fig. 37.3 Organogram of SACS in Category I (Highly Vulnerable) States. Finance and administrative arms have been excluded for simplicity.

REFERENCES

1. National AIDS Control Programme Phase III (2006-2011). Strategy and implementation. NACO, Ministry of Health and Family Welfare, Govrnment of India, 2006.
2. Jacob M, John TJ, George S, et al. Increasing prevalence of human immunodeficiency virus infection among patients attending a clinic for sexually transmitted diseases. Indian J Med Research 1995; 101: 6-9.
3. HIV Sentinel Surveillance and HIV Estimation, 2006. NACO, Ministry of Health and Family Welfare, Government of India, 2008, New Delhi.
4. Prioritisation of districts for programme implementation. NACO, Ministry of Health and Family Welfare, Government of India, 2006, New Delhi.
5. Khanna N, Nadkarni V, Bhutani LK. In: Tan B, Chan R eds. Sexually transmitted diseases in Asia and Pacific. Melbourne: Venereology Publishing Inc, 1998: 114-137.
6. Operational Guidelines for Programme Managers and Service Providers for strenghthening STI/ RTI Services NACO, Ministry of Health and Family Welfare, 2007, Government of India, New Delhi.
7. National Guidelines on Prevention, Management and Control of RTIs including STIs. Maternal Health Division. Ministry of Health and Family Welfare, 2007, Government of India, New Delhi.
8. National Behavioural Surveillance Survey (BSS) 2006. NACO, Ministry of Health and Family Welfare, Government of India, 2008, New Delhi.

38 CONDOMS AND MICROBICIDES

R D Mehta

In this chapter

- Historical Overview
- Barrier Methods
- Male Condom
- The Female Condom
- Other Barrier Devices
- Conclusion

INTRODUCTION

The time swift against all odds poses challenges to mankind to combat diseases, but the golden rule 'Prevention is better than cure' stands true even today. With the advent of HIV, one could even say that, 'Prevention is the only cure'. As pharmacotherapy still lacks the punch of being 'viricidal' in nature and having many side effects, the barrier method of contraception 'Condom' has become an important tool of prevention against the spread of STDs and in turn HIV and AIDS. The cyber generation of this modern era finds no social, religious, ethical and moral barriers to uphold the Gandhian norms of forbearance and abstinence. Sex is no more a sanctity practice, the natural way of procreation. It has turned into a 'fad', a status symbol, or a symbol of being anti-orthodox. Thus, premarital and extramarital contacts whether heterosexual or homosexual are rising in number and so are STDs. The alarming increase in the prevalence rate of STDs and HIV has prompted health managers and sociologists to focus on 'Condoms' and other barrier methods to checkmate the transmission of STDs. The fact that STDs facilitate HIV transmission has galvanized the development of newer biomedical preventive tools and improvising the existing methods. The developing world needs barrier methods which are safe, cost effective and acceptable to promiscuous or sexually active persons with high-risk behaviour. The sequential armament of generation next is "Chemical Condom", the microbicides which assure sexual life without latex, prioritizing pleasure with safety. Microbicides are chemical substances which reduce the risk of STDs including HIV when applied to the rectum and vagina.[1] Prevention tops the priorities of managing the pandemic of HIV/AIDS.

HISTORICAL OVERVIEW

The Egyptians were the first to use colourful penile coverings as early as 1000 B.C., but these seem to have been more of decorative nature than as a barrier. Italian anatomist Gabrielle Fellopius described linen sheaths as preventive measures to protect against syphilis. In the 16th century, Dr. Condom, a physician in the Court of King Charles II of England, first prepared the condom from the outer membrane of a sheep's intestine. The widespread use of condom started in 1844, when Goodyear and Hannock began to massproduce vulcanized rubber condoms. Simultaneously, cervical caps and diaphragm became available for use as pioneer female condoms in Germany between 1838 and 1860.

BARRIER METHODS

The physical and chemical barrier methods used as preventive measures include

1. Male condom
2. Female condom
3. Sponge
4. Diaphragm
5. Cervical cap
6. Spermicides
7. Microbicides

These are effective against many STD pathogens including HIV 1 and 2.[2,3]

MALE CONDOM

The word 'Condom' may have been derived either from 'Dr. Condom' the English Physician, or the Latin word 'Colonel Cundum' which means 'receptacle'. It is a protective device put by the male on an erect penis to cover the glans and shaft, the virtual entry or exit point for STD pathogens. It protects both the user and its partner if used prior to genital contact and remains intact during a sexual act. It must be used consistently so as to be efficacious. Different types of male condoms are available commercially, including those made from latex, natural membranes and polyurethane.

Latex Condom

This is the most widely used type of male condom. Latex condoms have been proven in different laboratory experiments and clinical studies to be an effective barrier against various bacteria and viruses including HIV and Hepatitis B virus (HBV).[3] Laboratory testing of latex condom by simulating mechanical friction of coitus is performed to check its barrier effectiveness. In one study, 30% of latex condoms tested allowed detectable leakage of particles of size similar to that of HIV;[4] however, the simulating conditions in the study were criticized for being much harsher than actual sexual intercourse. More recent studies demonstrate the efficacy of latex condoms against the transmission of HIV and other viral and bacterial microorganisms between sex partners.[5,6,7]

It is important to use condoms consistently and correctly for absolute protection. The latex device should cover the organ in such a way that genitoulcerative diseases like syphilis, chancroid, granuloma inguinale, lymphogranuloma venereum (LGV), herpes progenitalis, condyloma acuminata, etc. are prevented, which usually require intimate mucocutaneous contact for transmission. Similarly, the male urethral opening is also protected by the condom against diseases like gonococcal urethritis, NGU, trichomoniasis, HIV and HBV transmitted through seminal, urethral fluid or partner's infected vaginocervical fluid. However, it must be remembered that the pubic region, upper inner thighs and oral cavity are left unprotected and are vulnerable to disease transmission.

The incorporation of spermicides as lubricants in condoms may provide an added advantage, but this still remains to be proved. The efficacy of spermicidals like nonoxynol-9 is questionable as at the quantity of lubricant impregnated into the condom is too low to be effective and could further decrease shelf-life of the condom.[8]

Allergic contact dermatitis to latex condom has been described.[9] Contact dermatitis to latex has been more frequently described in health care workers exposed to latex products in the form of gloves and those working in the latex industry. Condoms prelubricated with spermicides further increase allergenicity, and the prevalence rate of contact dermatitis ranges between 1 and 7%.[10]

Preventive Efficacy of Latex Condoms

Condoms are an effective tool of prevention when used correctly and consistently. The various studies of HIV discordant heterosexual couples conducted in California, Italy and CSWs in Africa conclusively establish that consistent use of condoms may reduce the risk of HIV seroconversion by sevenfold.[11] Various other clinical studies provide the same evidence that consistent condom use protects the person from the acquisition of HIV infection despite regular sexual exposure to their HIV-positive partners. In a study on 123 couples discordant to HIV infection, the healthy partners remained seronegative over a two-year span with regular use of condoms. Among the inconsistent users, 9.8% out of 122 turned seropositive.[12] Another study reported 1.8% seroconversion after consistent use of latex condoms, while 12% became HIV-positive among those who used condoms irregularly.[13] It may be concluded that correct and consistent use of latex condoms virtually provides complete protection to both partners. It has been shown that condom effectiveness in decreasing STD risk is affected by disease infectivity and number of exposures. Generalization from low infectivity to highly infectious STDs or short-term to long-term situations can overestimate the effectiveness.[14]

In underdeveloped countries, the importance of consistent and correct use of condoms with risk reduction education strategies is being highlighted in order to decrease the prevalence and transmission of HIV. It is critical for health managers to realize and incorporate strategies to overcome barriers to condom use. A study of 49 women and 203 men from Mumbai highlighted the problem of privacy regarding condom purchase from stores and social stigma associated with condom use.[15] Various studies emphasize the need to ease the social costs and constraints to safe sexual behaviour through acceptance and promotion of regular use of condoms.

Mechanical failures of condoms may result in the transmission of STDs. In a study conducted in the United States to assess the incidence of mechanical failures of condoms using sex diaries of 892 women, it was estimated that 500 (2.3%) condoms broke during intercourse out of 21,852 condoms used and another 290 (1.3%) slipped during usage. Breakage was more common with young, single or nulliparae, while slippage was found more amongst married and multiparas.[16]

Condom use needs to be popularized as a preventive tool against STDs and HIV. The condom is a popular method of contraception even in the Western world. In one study undertaken to assess planned use of condoms in the prevention of STDs among 2782 women, who were to undergo sterilization, only 646 were using the condom prior to sterilization, and half of them did not intend to use it after the surgical procedure, considering themselves safe against pregnancy. Thus, 11% of the study sample might have experienced high exposure risks to various STD organisms and HIV, if not counseled.[17] In another study of 966 sex workers in China, the promotion of condom use and education regarding the mode of transmission of HIV resulted in an appreciable decrease in the incidence of STDs. After counselling, the consistent use of condoms was found to increase from 30 to 81%, thus decreasing the incidence of STD (gonorrhoea, trichomoniasis and chlamydial) infections from 17.5/100 persons per year to 3.0/100 persons per year.[18] Prevention is important in incurable STDs such as herpes genitalis, and its incidence can be decreased by improving condom use. Regular use of condoms is even more important for the partners of pregnant women to prevent HSV-2 infection.[19]

Condom and Safe Sex

Condoms are a popular means of contraception for the common man.[20] Its use as a barrier for STDs and HIV in sexually active persons needs to be promoted and publicized.[21,22] The National AIDS Control Programme identifies the importance of condom promotion although sociocultural factors may prevent its widespread acceptance.[23] The strengthening of IEC activities through governmental agencies and non-government organizations (NGO) is to create public awareness about safe sex, which is the most important preventive action in curbing the rising incidence of STDs and HIV.[24] Similarly, the most prevalent herpes progenitalis caused by *Herpes simplex virus* type 2 (HSV-2) can be prevented effectively by consistent condom use. A USA study claims aversion of 3.15 lakh cases out of 3.5 lakh new cases if more consistent use of condom is promoted.[25]

The predominant mode of transmission of HIV in India is heterosexual.[26] It is estimated that ulcerative conditions of the genital tract increase the possibility of acquisition of HIV by 10-fold, while STDs presenting with a discharge increase transmission of HIV by fivefold.[27]

Although it may sound simple for community health workers to promote the already publicized method for birth spacing 'NIRODH' (the Sanskrit word for prevention), or condom for prevention of STDs, observations of the author suggest that the acceptability of condom by sexually active persons with high-risk behaviour is an uphill task.

The National AIDS Control Organization (NACO), and different State AIDS Control Societies (SACS) under various public health programmes have started free condom distribution at all STD clinics and health centers as a preventive measure against the spread of STDs and HIV. Condom promotion is being done through wall messages at roadside and public places, posters, video-film shows, radio and television. However, in such campaigns, reservations have been expressed that promotion of condoms to the young generation may promote 'Free Sex' rather than 'Safe sex'. NACO is ensuring easy access to good quality, affordable, acceptable condoms of international standard for safe sex. The government provides condoms at subsidized prices for distribution through retail outlets. In 2000-2001, 465.43 million condoms were distributed through social marketing strategy, while 627.42 million condoms were supplied through free distribution schemes.[28] Condoms are also available at chemist shops, departmental stores, etc. The concept of a 'Condom Club' in which a nurse interacts with teenagers and supplies condoms was also found acceptable to the younger generation.[29] This approach may be used by NGOs in India.

Condom Consistency

Statistics suggest that the target population of the age group of 15-24 years forms more than 35% of

AIDS cases in our country, and the situation remains more or less same in the whole of South-East Asia. The younger generation must be counseled to practice self-control if unwilling to adopt the barrier methods.[30] One of the studies conducted in Mumbai reflects that only 27% of unmarried young men used condom as protective gear during premarital contacts even with CSWs.[31]

The only developing country which achieved declining trends in HIV prevalence was Thailand, which implemented the "100% Condom" programme since 1991, which proves how massive campaigns of consistent condom use may bring down the significant number of new HIV positivity.[32] The CDC Youth Risk Behavioural Survey in USA found that consistent condom use lags behind even amongst the youth of most developed and educated societies of the world, i.e. male students (60.5%), female students (48.6%), Black students (66.14%), White students (52.5%). The prevailing condition is not encouraging and should be considered as a challenge by health managers to hit hard for consistent condom use.[33]

The Myanamar National AIDS Programme (NAP) recommends 100% 'Targeted Condom Promotion' (TCP) as the main combat force to fight against STDs and HIV.[34]

Condom promotion activities happen to be the mainstay of HIV/AIDS prevention by Tamil Nadu AIDS Control Society as part of Targeted Intervention Campaign, where high priority has been given to promote condom use among high-risk people and vulnerable population.[35] In Tamil Nadu, the outlets for sale of condoms has risen to 60,000, with sale rising from 31600 million to 55505 million units in 2000-2004. Similarly, condom use by CSWs has improved from 56 to 86% during the same period. Another study does boast the successful prevention programme in Tamil Nadu where 14% of truckers had unprotected sex in 1996 as against the low 3% by 2002.[36]

Advantages of Latex Condoms

1. Cheap, safe, easy to use and a readily available preventive measure.
2. Effective in preventing not only STDs but also undesired pregnancy, hence making coitus hassle-free.
3. May prolong erection and check premature ejaculation, making the act more enjoyable.
4. Decreases the messiness of intercourse.
5. Semen in the condom is an 'eye evidence' of protection.

Disadvantages of Latex Condoms

1. Many users complain of reduced sensuality and sensitivity and thus the pleasure of intercourse.
2. It may break or slip during the act especially when used with oily lubricants as they cause the latex to deteriorate.
3. Every act requires a new condom.
4. Unpleasant latex odour.
5. It may cause premature ejaculation in some individuals owing to the time taken for wearing the condom over an erect organ.

Social and Psychological Repercussions of Condom Use

Condoms have embarrassing social connotations, as these are often perceived as being associated with promiscuity and venereal disease. At a personal level, condoms are often perceived by both partners as a barrier to natural enjoyment. Even suggesting the use of condom to the male partner has been found insulting and offending. In sharp contrast, among the sexually active generation in the West, the use of condom is now being seen as a measure of concern and care for the partner. Thus, the negative image of latex condom is changing atleast in the West, although it may take somewhat longer in developing countries.

A newer consumer-friendly version of latex condom has become more popular now because it is loose at the tip and snug at the base.[37] It provides more friction and pleasure during coitus.

Failure of Condoms

1. Influence of alcohol may lead to its inadequate or improper use.
2. Improper storage of condom, heat, moisture and sunlight may damage the condom, so storage must be in dry, dark and cool place.
3. Use of expired condoms.
4. Oil or petroleum-based lubricants may cause condoms to slip during the act and also weaken the latex.
5. Breakage during coitus.

Natural Membrane Condom

Undesirable latex sensitivity led to the development of natural membrane condoms or 'lambskin condoms'. These are porous and hence cause easy passage of HIV, HSV, HBV, etc.[38] However, seminal fluid dynamics during intercourse may not be possible to be simulated to test the efficacy of membrane condoms in preventing the transmission of STDs.

The advantage of membrane over latex condoms is that it gives more natural feel and sensuality. They are stronger, less elastic and hence are not likely to break during coitus. However, membranous condoms are considerably more expensive.

Polyurethane Condoms

Recent advances in technology have allowed the development of thinner yet stronger condom. Polyurethane condoms, also know as plastic condoms, allow better sensuality and sensitivity.[39] These are odourless and colourless and have longer shelf-life. Oily lubricants do not damage the condom.

Disadvantages include that these are more expensive, require lubrication, and tend to be noisy during sexual intercourse.

Three newer thermoplastic varieties have been developed which are transparent, odourless and loose-fitting. One may be rolled on like the latex condom and the other one is slipped over the penis. These newer types are gaining popularity. The third variety is made of a synthetic thermoplastic elastomer material used in manufacturing non-allergenic examination gloves.

THE FEMALE CONDOM

The female condom is a pre-lubricated, polyurethane sheath which fits loosely into the vagina. It lines the vaginal walls from labia to cervix. The method of use is same as of the traditional diaphragm. It has two flexible rings at both ends which help positioning the sheath. The first one at the closed end fits behind the pubic bone and second one which is the open end remains against the labia.

Preventive Efficacy of Female Condom

The female condoms expand opportunities against pregnancy and STDs/HIV, i.e. dual protection. The efficacy ranges from 94-98% as compared to male condom (92-96%).[40] So we may consider that 340 million cases of curable STDs annually and 39 million HIV infection every year (50% of which are young women) can be dealt if female condoms are popularized. The fact is substantiated by studies conducted in Kenya, Thailand and USA. The female condom available in market are FC2, V-Amour Female Condom, approved by Indian Drug Controller, Natural Sensation Panty Condom® available in Latin America, PATH Woman's Condom: phase I trial completed, Silk Parasol Female Condom™: phase I trial planned for 2006, and Belgian Female Condom. The female condom has been shown to be an effective mechanical barrier against HIV and other STDs.[41] Consistent use is an important pre-requisite for sustained protection. In a study,[42] 20 consistent users had remained free from *Trichomonas vaginalis*, whereas among inconsistent users, the re-infection rate was 14.7%.

The use of female condom needs to be popularized as a tool of women's empowerment. It helps them negotiate with their sex partners, thus preventing the transmission of HIV and STDs. Its development should receive high priority, more sociopolitical and scientific initiative as an important preventive technology against the dreaded epidemic.[43]

Advantages

1. It provides natural sexual pleasure to both partners as compared to the male condom. The polyurethane material also transmits the body heat unhindered.
2. The introitus is covered 'in toto', thus provides reliable protection.
3. Oil lubricants may be used concomitantly.

Disadvantages

1. Wearing of condom in advance of inter-course may be undesirable.
2. Aesthetic appeal is lost after the insertion of the condom.
3. The act of coitus is often noisy and embarrassing to the couple.
4. Slipping may occur during the intercourse.
5. It is expensive as compared to the male condom.

Female Condom Acceptance

The female condom is greatly acceptable because women find a protective device over which they have control. Many feel that it is stronger than the male latex condom and find it more enjoyable.

Some women find discomfort and difficulty while putting it on. It also gives a messy feel during the coital act and uneasy feel of outer and inner rings. Partner resistance to female condom may dampen its acceptability. Recent studies have shown that in urban Zimbabwe, washing and reuse was also acceptable.[44]

The different condom types and STDs prevented by each (CDC 2006) are given in Table 38.1.

OTHER BARRIER DEVICES

These include sponge, diaphragm and cervical caps. In addition, spermicides and microbicides are chemical barriers to combat microorganism transmission from one partner to the other.

Table 38.1 **STDs Prevented by Condoms**

Type of Condom	*STDs*
Latex	Protective against HIV, chlamydia, gonorrhoea, trichomonas, PID; limited data on HSV-1 and 2, HPV
Natural membrane	Not protective against HIV, bacterial vaginosis and viral STDs. Not to be used for protection against STDs
Polyurethane	Protective against HIV, chlamydia, gonorrhoea, trichomonas, PID; Limited data on HSV-1 and 2, HPV
Female polyurethane condom	Protective against HIV, limited data for other STDs

Sponge

It is a flexible device with in-built grooves for comfortable insertion and removal. It is impregnated with sodium cholate, nonoxynol-9 and benzalkonium chloride. This combination has been found to be effective in inhibiting HIV reverse transcriptase[45] and inactivating microorganisms responsible for STDs.[46]

Advantages

It is cheaper and a user-friendly device and may be inserted prior to the act. Spermicidal impregnation makes it a multi-use device and is disposable unlike cervical cap and diaphragm which are to be washed and stored after each use.

Disadvantages

It needs to be left in position for at least six hours after the intercourse. It is associated with higher vaginal infection rates, unpleasant odour and irritation.

However, the overall preference score is high because most women find it convenient to use, and there is no associated discomfort.

Diaphragm

This barrier device, also known as the 'Dutch Cap', is a shallow cup made of synthetic rubber or plastic with a flexible rim made of spring or metal. This reusable device covers the cervix and can be inserted six hours prior to the intercourse and hence could be used without partner's knowledge. A proper-sized diaphragm (5-10 cm sizes are available) snugly fits between symphysis pubis and sacrum. Spring tension and vaginal muscle tone maintain the position of diaphragm.

It must always be used with a spermicide, which needs to be reapplied prior to each coitus. It provides protection only against those STDs that primarily involve the cervix[47] such as *N. gonorrhoeae*, *Chlamydia trachomatis* and *Trichomonas vaginalis*. Its protective efficacy increases with the use of spermicides.

It is expensive and there is an associated risk of increased incidence of urinary tract infections because of alterations caused in normal vaginal flora owing to the use of spermicides. The male partner may feel uncomfortable with its presence, and the users may find the insertion and removal procedures tedious. Lax vaginal tone and improper fitting may cause its slipping during coital act. The latex device has an unpleasant odour, and it cannot be used with oily lubricants. The acceptability of diaphragm is poor in Indian women because of the skills required for insertion and removal as well as lack of privacy in washing and storing it particularly in rural areas.[48]

Cervical Cap

It is a smaller barrier device as compared to the diaphragm. It is made of silicon and covers the cervix with a suction mechanism. It is to be combined with spermicide and may be left in place for 48 hours after intercourse. It should be changed every third year. Acceptability of cervical cap ranges from 75 to 89%, but unwelcome odour, dislodgment during intercourse and partner discomfort were complained by users. There are no data supporting its efficacy in preventing STDs and HIV.

Spermicides

These are chemical agents used to kill sperms, and in addition they may inhibit STD pathogens. Various spermicides in use include nonoxynol-9, octoxynol, cholorhexidine, benzalkonium chloride and menfegol, gossypol, gramicidin and povidone iodine. These are available as foams, gels, suppositories, foaming tablets and vaginal contraceptive films (VCF).

Preventive Efficacy of Nonoxynol-9 (N-9)

Laboratory animal as well as human studies have assessed the efficacy of N-9 in preventing STD microorganisms including HIV.[49] But Harison found N-9 to be ineffective against HIV 1/2.[50,51] It is a non-ionic surfactant which destroys lipid envelopes, and hence it is more effective against enveloped viruses like HBV. It has cidal effects against HBV, HSV, treponemes, gonococci, *H. ducreyi* and chlamydia.

The adverse effects of N-9 are associated with the frequency, concentration and quantity used. In terms of administration and contraception, negligible side effects are reported. However, the higher concentration of it necessary when used to prevent HIV/STDs may prove it more hazardous. It has been shown that frequent use of large amounts of N-9 may cause vaginocervical ulceration. It is also found to be associated with a change in vaginal flora that may facilitate the transmission of HIV and STDs.

Advantages

It is easy to use, has a lubricant effect and can be used without the knowledge of the male partner. It is usually acceptable to both partners. Sper-micides are devoid of any long-term side effects.

Disadvantages

Planned activity is the pre-requisite, as it requires at least 10 minutes for dissolution. It may be messy especially if it leaks out of the vagina. A sensation of warmth, over-lubrication and irritation may be felt by some users.

The acceptability of spermicide is increasing; N-9 and menfegol foaming tablets are available with tolerable side effects such as burning, stinging and itching.

Microbicides

Microbicides are chemical substances that reduce the transmission of HIV and other STD micro-organisms when applied to the coital orifices, i.e. rectum and vagina. At present, about 75 compounds are undergoing various stages of development and clinical trials, which may turn out to be popular chemical barrier against STD pathogens and HIV. The microbicides under development may have multipronged actions.

1. Killing or inactivating pathogens (e.g. UC-781, Dapivirine-TMC120, Tenofovir/PMPA)
2. Strengthening the body's normal defenses (e.g. ACIDFORM™/Amphora™, Buffer gel®)
3. Inhibiting microorganism entry/fusion (e.g. Vivagel™, SPL-7013, Invisible Condom™, Carraguard® Pro 2000)
4. Combinations of various modus operandi (1-3) (e.g. PC 815, Carraguard® and MIV-150)

Microbicides are evaluated in mouse, pig, rabbit, cat and macaque animal models to assess the efficacy and toxicity of candidate microbicides before these are put forward for human trials.[52]

The 'efficacy of microbicides is questionable if used alone, but concurrent use of condom is the best option'. In case condom use is not possible or if the female partner may find the use of microbicides much easier, the use of condom might be avoided in favour of microbicides. The shift of choice is called 'Condom Migration', and this suspected phenomenon has prevented the widespread endorsement of microbicides alone. If used concurrently, the HIV risk reduction would be 20% or more. Microbicides may be a good alternative for 'Condom' and 'No Condom' dilemma, and at least these can be used for harm reduction which may sound better than 'No Protection'. Additionally, the microbicide provides a standby preventive tool if the condom breaks or leaks.[53]

These chemicals are topically used to kill pathogens of STDs or interfere with the mechanism of infection. Research activities are focused on products that may increase natural host defense mechanisms such as acid buffering agents, lactobacillus preparations and antimicrobial peptides (magainins, protegrins, defensins). Other compounds may interfere with viral entry to the target epithelial cells, such as monoclonal antibodies,[54] sulfated polysaccharides and sulfonated polymers. A suppository made of extract from neem tree, soapnut (Reetha) and quinine hydrochloride is a promising contraceptive and microbicide.

Sulfated polysaccharide, dextrin sulfate, inhibits the adherence of HIV and chlamydia to the epithelial cells. N-docosanol is a potent antiviral, which may inhibit enveloped and non-enveloped virus even when applied topically. Squalamine is a steroid-based compound which has shown inhibitory effect against most STD pathogens including HIV. C31G is a newer surfactant with lower irritancy score as compared to N-9 and also appears to be more effective. The various new microbicides and their mechanism and phase of development are summarized in Table 38.2.

CONCLUSION

Barrier methods originally conceptualized as contraceptive devices are becoming more popular as preventive measures against STDs and HIV.[56] These have not yet gained momentum as the only 'preventive modality' in our country to combat the dreaded HIV and other STDs. A lot needs to be done to promote safe sex through consistent and proper use of condoms, enforcing the fact that preventive modalities are meant for 'SAFE SEX' not for 'FREE SEX'.

Table 38.2 Microbicides – The Present Scenario (March 2007)[55]

Mechanism of Action	*Candidate Microbicide*	*Active Agent*	*Phase*	*In vitro Activity*	*Animal Model Activity*
Vaginal defense enhancers	ACIDFORM™/ Amphora™	Acid buffer	Phase I	*C. trachomatis* HSV, sperm, *N. gonorrhoeae*	*C. trachomatis*, HSV
	BufferGel®	Proton (acidity)	Phase II/III	*C. trachomatis*, HIV, HSV, sperm, *T. pallidum*. *H. ducreyi*	*C. trachomatis*, cell-associated, HIV, HSV, HPV *N. gonorrhoeae*, sperm, *T. vaginalis*
Entry/fusion inhibitors	VivaGel™/SPL 7013		Phase I		
	Invisible Condom™		Phase I/II		
	Carraguard®	Carraeenan	Phase III	*C. trachomatis*, HIV, HPV, HSV-2, *N. gonorrhoeae*, sperm	HIV, HPV, HSV-2, *N. gonorrhoeae*, *H. ducreyi*, sperm
	PRO 2000	Naphthalene sulphonate polymer	Phase III	*C. trachomatis*, HIV, HSV, *N. gonorrhoeae*	HSV, *N. gonorrhoeae*, HIV
Replication inhibitors	UC-781	Cellulose sulphate gel	Phase I	*C. albicans*, *C. trachomatis*, *H. ducreyi*, HIV, HPV, HSV, *N. gonorrhoeae*, sperm, *T. vaginalis*	HSV, *N. gonorrhoeae*, *C. trachomatis*, sperm
	Dapivirine (TMC 120) Tenofovir/ PMPA gel		Phase I/II Phase IIB		

(*Contd.*)

Combinations	PC 815 (Carraguard® and MIV-150)		Phase I		
	PSS	Polystyrene sulphonate	Phase I	HSV, HIV, HPV, *C. albicans*, *C. trachomatis*, *H. ducreyi*, *N. gonorrhoeae*, *T. pallidum*, sperm	*C. trachomatis*, *C. albicans*, HSV, sperm
	Savvy™ (C3IG)	Alkyl amine oxide and alkyl betaine	Phase II/III	*C. albicans*, *T. pallidum*, HIV, HSV, *H. ducreyi*, sperm	*C. trachomatis*, HIV, HSV, sperm

REFERENCES

1. Anna Forbes, Demanding Microbicides: An Invisible Condom in Your Future? 2003, www.thebody.com/columnists/forbes/microbicides.html- site accessed, 5 March, 2007.
2. Conant MA, Hardy D, Sernatinger J, et al. Condoms prevent transmission of AIDS associated retrovirus. JAMA 1986; 255(13); 1706.
3. Judson FN, Ehret JM, Bodin GF, et al. In vitro evaluations of condom with and without Nonoxynol 9 as physical and chemical barriers against *Chlamydia trachomatis, Herpes simplex virus type 2* and *Human immunodeficiency virus*. Sex Transm Dis 1989; 16: 51-6.
4. Carey RF, Herman WA, Retta SM et al. Effectiveness of latex condoms as a barrier to human immunodeficiency virus sized particles under conditions of simulated use. Sex Transm Dis 1992; 19: 230-4.
5. Vassey JT, Larson DB, Lyons JS, et al. Condom safety and HIV. Sex Transm Dis 1994; 26; 59-61.
6. Vail JG, Mercer DJ. Condom safety and HIV Comments from PATH (Letter). Sex Transm Dis 1994; 21. 61.
7. Stone KM, Timyan J, Thomas EL. Barrier methods for the prevention of sexually transmitted diseases. In: Holmes KK, Mardh PA, Sparling PF et al, Eds. Sexually Transmitted Diseases. 3rd Ed. New York: McGraw Hill; 1999. p. 1307-22.
8. Smith N. Nonoxynol-9 in condoms. Int J STDs AIDS 1990; 1: 449.
9. Rekart ML. The toxicity and local effects of the spermicide nonoxynol-9. J AIDS 1992; 5: 425-7.
10. Stratton P. Nonoxynol-9 lubricated condoms may increase release of natural rubber latex protein. XI International conference on AIDS. Vancouver: abstract Th C 433, 1996.
11. Condom efficacy. In Interventions to Reduce the Risk of Sexual-Exposure through Promotion of Condom Use. www.hopkins-aids.edu/prevention/prevention4.html, site accessed on 31 March, 2007.
12. De Vincenzi I. A longitudinal study of human immunodeficiency virus transmission by heterosexual partners. N Eng J Med 1994; 331: 341-6.
13. Saracco A, Musicco M, Nicolosia A et al. Man-to-woman sexual transmission of HIV: Longitudinal study of 343 steady partners of infected men. J AIDS 1993; 6: 497-502.

14. Man JR, Stine CC, Vessey J. The role of disease specific infectivity and number of disease exposures on long term effectiveness of the latex condom. Sex Transm Dis 2002; 29: 350-2.
15. Roth J, Krishnan SP, Bunch E. Barriers to condom use: Results from a study in Mumbai (India). AIDS Educ Prev 2001; 13: 65-77.
16. Macaluso M, Kelaghan J, Artz L, et al. Mechanical failure of the latex condom in a cohort of women at high STDs risk. Sex Transm Dis 1999; 26: 450-8.
17. Sangi-Haghpeykar H, Poindexter AN. Planned condom use among women undergoing tubal sterilization. Sex Transm Dis 1998; 25: 335-41.
18. Ma S, Dukers NH, van den Hoek A et al. Decreasing STDs incidence and increasing condom use among Chinese sex workers following a short term intervention: a prospective cohort study. Sex Trans Infect 2002; 78: 80-1.
19. Casper C, Wald A. Condom use and the prevention of genital herpes acquisition. Herpes 2002; 9: 10-14.
20. Misra RS. Sex, sexually transmitted diseases and AIDS, New Delhi: Vigyan Prasar; 1996: 124.
21. Cates W Jr, Steiner MJ. Dual protection against unintended pregnancy and sexually transmitted infections: what is the best contraceptive approach. Sex Transm Dis 2002; 29: 168-74.
22. Condom for prevention of HIV Transmission. In: NACO Training Module on HIV Infections and AIDS for Medical Officers. National AIDS Control Organization, Ministry of Health and Family Welfare, Government of India. 1999; p. 75-9.
23. Condom Promotion and Provision. In: AIDS-No time for complacency Regional Publication, SEARO No. 26 World Health Organization, Geneva, AITBS Publishers and Distributors, New Delhi. 1999; p. 32.
24. Education on Risk Reduction and Condom Provision. In: Management of Sexually Transmitted Diseases at District and PHC levels. Regional publication, SEARO, No. 25, World Health Organization Geneva, AITBS Publishers and Distributors, New Delhi. 1999; p. 5.
25. Andria Langenberg. Interrupting Herpes Simplex Virus Type 2 Transmission: the Role of Condoms and Microbicides. Herpes 2004; 11 (Suppl 3): 147-54.
26. Health Programmes in India In: Park K, Editor. Park's Text Book of Preventive and Social Medicine.18th Ed. Jabalpur: Banarasi Das Bhanot; 2005. p. 336-9.
27. HIV Infection and Sexually Transmitted Diseases. In: NACO Training Module on HIV infection and AIDS for Medical Officers. National AIDS Control Organization. Ministry of Health and Family Welfare, Government of India 1999, p. 42.
28. Control of Sexually Transmitted Diseases (STDs) and Condom Promotion. In: Combating HIV/ AIDS In India. Ministry of Health And Family Welfare, National AIDS Control Organization, Government of India. 2000-2001, p. 23-4.
29. Thomson C, Smith H. 'Condom Club': an interface between teenage sex and genitourinary medicine. Int J STDs AIDS 2001; 12: 475-8.
30. In Fact Sheet; Young People and HIV/AIDS, Situation in South East Asia. Published by World Health Organisation Regional Office for South East Asia, Mahatma Gandhi Marg, New Delhi-India-2006.
31. Jeejebhoy SJ. ed. Looking back looking forward: a profile of sexual and reproductive health in India. New Delhi: Population Council, 2004.
32. Rajanapithayakorn W. The 100 percent condom use programme: a success story. In AIDS in Asia; The Challenge Ahead. Editor Jai. P Narain, World Health Organization. Sage Publication, New Delhi. 2004, p. 77-90.
33. Prevention-Consistent Condom Use- www.hopkins-aids.edu/prevention/prevention 4.html. site accessed on 29 March, 2007.
34. Prevention. In Review of the Myanamar National AIDS Programme 2006 Publisher: World Health Organization: Regional office for South East Asia. 2006; 47-90.
35. Charles B, Krishnamurthy P. In Preventive Measures: Context of Prevention in Tamilnadu: TAMILNADU RESPONSE TO HIV/AIDS 1986-2005 Conquering a silent epidemic. Editor Dr. Kurien Thomas, Prof. S.P. Thyagarajan – 2006 p. 81-97.
36. AIDS prevention and Control Project, 2003 AIDS epidemic update December 2004, 37-39.

Published by UNAIDS- 20 avenue Appia- 1211 Geneva 27, Switzerland.

37. Roman M. What to wear to bed, Men's Health, July/August: 1994; p. 35.
38. Lytle CD, Carney PG, Vohra S et al. Virus leakage through natural membrane condoms. Sex Transm Dis 1990 ; 17: 58-62.
39. Rosenberg MJ, Waugh MS, Solomon HM, et al. The male polyurethane condom: A review of current knowledge. Contraception 1996; 53: 141-6.
40. Female Condom : A powerful Tool for protection, In Global HIV/AIDS : Moving Forward in 2006. Global Health Council – PATH. www. Global-campaign.org/Engdownload.htm. site accessed on 27 March, 2007.
41. Drew WL, Blair M, Miner RC et al. Evaluation of virus permeability of a new condom for women. Sex Trans Dis 1990; 17: 110-2.
42. Soper DE, Shupe D, Shangold GA, et al. Prevention of vaginal trichomonas by compliant use of the female condom. Sex Trans Dis 1993; 20: 137-9.
43. Gollub EL. The female condom: tool for women's empowerment. (Review) Am J Public Health 2000; 90: 1377-81.
44. Pettifor AE, Beksinska ME, Rees HV, et al. The acceptability of reuse of the female condoms. among Urban South African Women. J Urban Health 2001; 78: 647-57.
45. Psychoyos A, Creatsas G, Hassan E, et al. Spermicidal and antiviral properties of cholic acid: Contraceptive efficacy of new vaginal sponge containing sodium cholate. Hum Repord 1993; 8: 866-9.
46. Cates W, Stone KM. Family Planning, STDs & contraceptive choice: A literature update- PartI Fam Plann Perspect 1992; 24: 75-84.
47. Rosenberg MJ, Davidson AJ, Chen JH, et al. Barrier contraceptives and sexually transmitted disease in women: A comparison of female dependant methods and condoms. Am J Public Health 1992; 82: 669-74.
48. Park K. Demography and Family planning. In: Park K. editor. Park's Text Book of Preventive and Social Medicine. 18thEd. Jabalpur: Banarasi Das Bhanot; 2005. p. 362.
49. Feldblum PJ, Weir SS. The protective effect of nonoxynol-9 against HIV infection. Am J Public Health 1994; 84: 1032-4.
50. Harrison PF. The microbicides research and development "pipeline" a status report. Microbicides 2002; Antwerp, p. 12-5.
51. Nonoxynol-9 ineffective in preventing HIV infection Press release WHO/55. WHO 28 June, 2002. www.who.int/inf/en/pr-2002-55.html.
52. Zeitilin L, Whaley K. Microbicides for preventing transmission of genital herpes. Herpes 2002; 9: 4-9.
53. Foss AM, Peter T, Vickerman P, et al. Shifts in condom use following microbicide introduction: should we be concerned? AIDS 2003; 17: 1227-37.
54. Cone RA, Whaley KJ. Monoclonal antibodies for reproductive health: Part-I Preventing sexual transmission of disease and pregnancy with topically applied antibodies. Am J Reprod Immunol 1994; 32: 144-51.
55. Microbicides in on going and planned clinical trials. In Global Campaign for Microbicides. March 2007. www.global-campaign.org/download.htm. site accessed on 31 March, 2007.
56. Weller S, Davis K.Condom effectiveness in reducing heterosexual HIV transmission. Cochrane Database Syst Rev 2002; (1): CD 003255.

39 VACCINES AGAINST SEXUALLY TRANSMITTED INFECTIONS

Alison Blume, Rajul Patel

In this chapter

- *Chlamydia Trachomatis*
- Neisseria Gonorrhoea
- *Treponema Pallidum*
- Herpes Simplex Virus (HSV)
- Human Immunodeficiency Virus (HIV)
- Human Papillomavirus (HPV)
- Hepatitis B Virus (HBV)

INTRODUCTION

The need for vaccines against STIs has long been seen as an important tool for their prevention. However, developing effective vaccination has been proved difficult, and to-date only vaccines against Hepatitis B and human papillomairus (HPV) have been proved useful. Clinical trials are continuing with vaccines against both HIV and Herpes simplex virus (HSV). Little progress has been made with vaccines against chlamydia, gonorrhoea or syphilis.

Unlike other infectious diseases, repeated exposure to an STI can occur over a prolonged period of time. Consequently, protective STI vaccines must have extremely high efficacy if they are not to merely delay infection. Natural infection in itself, for many STIs, does not confer useful protective immunity against future reinfection despite a full spectrum of humoral and cell-mediated responses. It is, therefore, not surprising that traditional vaccines, using inactivated whole organisms and stimulating principally humoral immune responses alone were not effective.

Once developed, STI vaccines must be voluntarily accepted by a large proportion of the at-risk population. Some view widescale vaccination as an endorsement of risk behaviour sending potentially mixed messages concerning STI prevention, abstinence and dangers of unprotected sex to the youth. These views may greatly hamper the efforts to achieve adequate coverage.

CHLAMYDIA TRACHOMATIS

Recurrent infection by *Chlamydia trachomatis* does provide a degree of immunity; however this is serovar-specific.

Human trials of inactivated whole-cell vaccine were discontinued because of limited protection and significant safety concerns, and the focus has shifted to the development of sub-unit vaccines.[1]

Among sub-unit vaccines, most work has centered around the major outermembrane protein (MOMP), but animal model studies indicate that MOMP vaccines do not afford sufficient protection.[2,3]

Various other known and putative outermembrane proteins (OMP), including cysteine-rich OMP2 and OMP3, are being evaluated as sub-unit antigens.[2,4] Other sub-units have also been proposed, including chlamydia heat shock proteins (HSPs),[5] cytidine triphosphate synthetase,[6] *crpA*[7] and an exoglycolipid.[8] Immune responses to chlamydial HSP-60 antigen have been detected in patients who have chlamydial pelvic inflammatory disease. Because the protein is similar to the human homolog, it has been hypothesized that molecular mimicry may result in autoimmune inflammatory damage that contributes to chlamydial pathogenesis.[9] The *Chlamydia trachomatis* genome encodes over 900 proteins; thus it is likely that many new candidate antigens will be identified in the future.

Experiments have found that antibodies deve-loping after exposure to chlamydial heat shock protein (a component of all cell types expressed in response to stress) can cause a hypersensitivity reaction upon reinfection[10] and are a possible mechanism in the development of pelvic inflammatory disease.[11] This may explain why early vaccine trials carried out in 1950s using inactivated chlamydia found that, while it provided some degree of protection against infection, some subjects developed an exaggerated illness.[12]

Antibodies against MOMP give serovar-specific immunity in mice and do not show hypersensitivity features. One MOMP vaccine, despite giving 80% protection to monkeys challenged to *C. trachomatis* serovars D, E, F and G (responsible for 80% of human genital Chlamydia infection),[13] failed to show adequate protection in human clinical trials.[12] In addition to the search for new antigens, some research has also explored new means of delivering sub-units, including DNA vaccines[6] and vector systems such as *Vibrio cholerae* ghosts and lactobacillus mutants (4).

Current efforts are focusing on recombinant sub-unit vaccines and on DNA plasmid technology.

NEISSERIA GONORRHOEAE

The development of a vaccine against gonorrhoea has encountered many difficulties, and it has been hampered by both limited understanding of what constitutes protective immunity and lack of an animal model.[1]

Gonorrhoea has numerous serotypes, and no naturally occurring protective antibodies have been found. Multistrain variability must be considered in vaccine development to ensure that the proteins selected will afford protection against diverse gonococcal strains.[14] One immune evasion strategy may be induction of antibodies to the reduction-modifiable protein (Rmp) that blocks the function of bactericidal antiporin antibodies.

Gonorrhoea is only infectious in humans, making human trials necessary at all stages of vaccine development. Pili surface proteins can rapidly change to different antigenic forms making vaccine targets almost impossible to identify.[11] Reinfection with gonorrhoea is common but likely to be with a serovar exhibiting a different principal outermembrane protein (POR), making this a potential vaccine target.[15] Little progress has been made in recent years. Currently, research is focussed on transferrin binding, pilin and porin proteins, discovery of new antigens and development of strategies for delivering sub-units that are free of contaminating Rmp.[16,17,18]

There are no candidates currently in clinical trials, although Sanofi-Pasteur has identified gonococcal vaccines as a target for long-term vaccine development.[1]

TREPONEMA PALLIDUM

Subjects with untreated active syphilis have been shown to have some degree of immunity to reinfection (chancre immunity). This correlates with vigorous humoral and cellular immune responses to multiple antigens.[19] Despite this immune response, *T. pallidum* persists in the lymph nodes and is able to evade the immune system. Early vaccine efforts using killed whole *T. pallidum* required large doses given over long periods to induce immunity in animal models.

More recent efforts to develop a syphilis vaccine focus on recombinant *T. pallidum* proteins.[1,10] Three of these show limited efficacy in animals. An antigen designated TpN19 (or previously 4D) elicited partial protection in rabbits. TpN19 is interesting because it assembles into an oligomeric ringlike structure in its native form although its function in pathogenesis or in the physiology of *T. pallidum* is unknown. Vaccination with recombinant endoflagellar protein or another protein designated either TpN36 or TmpB also resulted in partial protection in animals.[10] To-date no vaccines are proceeding into late clinical trails.

HERPES SIMPLEX VIRUS (HSV)

Two separate goals exist for developing a vaccine against HSV. A prophylactic vaccine would protect against HSV acquisition and would need to be given prior to virus exposure. The second goal is for a useful therapeutic vaccine to be given to those with latent infection to prevent clinical recurrences and limit asymptomatic shedding and viral transmission.

Shortly after infection, HSV establishes latency in neurons, an immunologically protected site, giving natural and acquired immune responses a very short time to neutralize infection before latency is established. Many different vaccination strategies (Table 39.1) have been tried, and it is useful to understand some of the earlier attempts before moving on to current trials.

Table 39.1 Types of HSV Vaccines that Have Undergone Clinical Evaluation[20]

Autoinoculation of live HSV
Killed whole virus vaccines
Attenuated live virus vaccines
Modified live virus sub-unit vaccines
Cell culture-derived sub-unit vaccines
Recombinant sub-unit vaccines (glycoprotein vaccines)
Disabled infectious single cycle (DISC) virus vaccines
Nucleic acid (DNA) vaccines

Killed whole virus vaccines were initially developed in 1970s. As there is no viral replication, killed viruses are less immunogenic than live attenuated viruses, necessitating multiple doses of vaccine, including boosters, to maintain the antibody levels.[21] Two of these vaccines remain commercially available in Europe, although no randomized placebo-controlled trials have confirmed their efficacy. The Skinner vaccine consists of formalin-inactivated HSV-1, and the Lupidon vaccine uses heat-inactivated virus. Both claim some prophylactic effect in serodiscordant couples,[21,22] and both have shown a modest effect in reducing the number and severity of clinical episodes in those with recurrent herpes simplex disease over limited follow-up periods.[22,23]

Sub-unit vaccines consisting of preparations of glycoproteins showed some promise in animal models; clinical trials, however, failed to show any benefit either in prevention of infection or in clinical disease.[24] In animal models, vaccines based on HSV-1 show less efficacy in preventing HSV-2 disease than those based on HSV-2.[25]

Recombinant viral protein vaccines use recombinant DNA technology to insert genes encoding for specific viral proteins into a carrier organism (*E. coli* or yeast species) along with promoter genes. Viral proteins produced by the carrier organism are used in the vaccine. Two such vaccines have been evaluated in large clinical trials. The Chiron Corporation (California, USA) used recombinant Glycoprotein B and D from HSV-2 with adjuvant MF59. This was trialled in HSV-2 serodiscordant couples, and although it induced high levels of neutralizing antibodies, the vaccine failed to prevent infection. The vaccinated subjects showed delayed infection with some efficacy during the first five months of the trial, but the overall efficacy rate at one year was not significantly different from placebo.[26] Chiron abandoned further development of this vaccine.

GlaxoSmithKline (GSK) developed a similar vaccine using recombinant glycoprotein D from HSV-2 with a different adjuvant: alum and 3-0-deacylated-monophosphoryl lipid A (MPL). The vaccine was again trialled in HSV-2 serodiscordant couples. Overall the vaccination showed a non-specific trend towards protection; in female subjects who were seronegative to HSV-1 at baseline, however, the vaccine gave 73% protection against clinical disease and 46% protection against HSV-2 seroconversion.[27] Measured antibody response was the same in males and females. This sex-dependant efficacy has yet to be explained. The vaccine also failed to show efficacy in females with antibodies against HSV-1, and results paralleling these have been seen in some natural history studies where prior HSV-1 infection affords limited protection but definite disease modification for HSV-2. The discrepant results obtained from the Chiron vaccine and the GSK vaccine studies may be due to the different adjuvant used, as both vaccines stimulated high levels of neutralizing antibodies. The GSK adjuvant induced higher levels of interferon gamma, and may consequently provoke stronger cell-mediated immune responses than the Chiron vaccine.[21] Follow-up trials are continuing for the GSK vaccine.

No randomized clinical trials have to-date demonstrated a clinically useful benefit from a therapeutic vaccine for HSV-1 or HSV-2 infection although some studies have shown modest efficacy in reducing the number and duration of recurrences.[20]

Other novel vaccine strategies are currently in development. One therapeutic vaccine, using a live attenuated HSV-2 strain with a gene encoding for an essential glycoprotein deleted, recently failed to show any clinical or virological effect in a clinical trial.[28] Other *vaccines using HSV DNA inserted* into plasmids are currently being tested for human safety and immunogenicity – e.g. facilitated gD2 vaccine.[21] Other vaccines under development are vector vaccines using vectors like vaccinia virus, adenovirus and salmonella.

HUMAN IMMUNODEFICIENCY VIRUS (HIV)

Since the identification of the virus responsible for the global pandemic in 1984, vaccine development has been a priority. Despite many differing strategies and several large clinical trials, an effective and safe vaccine is still thought to be some time away. Many factors about HIV itself, and the host immune response to HIV, make the development of vaccines difficult. Many subtypes of HIV exist with dramatically different genetic sequences. As subtypes are clustered geographically, different parts of the world may potentially require different vaccines. Both humoral and cell-mediated immune responses are likely to be necessary to protect against HIV as both free virus and cell-associated virus are involved in transmission.[29] Also despite the high levels of antibodies that develop in response to acute infection, only partial control of HIV replication is seen. Any effective vaccine will need to elicit strong cytotoxic T lymphocyte (CTL) responses in addition to antibody production.[29]

Scientific Obstacles to the Development of AIDS Vaccine[30]

1. Antigenic diversity and hypervariability of the virus
2. Transmission of disease by mucosal route
3. Transmission of the virus by infected cells
4. Resistence of wild type of virus to seroneutralization
5. Integration of the virus genome into the host cell chromosomes
6. Latency of the virus in resting memory T-cells
7. Rapid emergence of virus escape mutants in the host
8. Down-regulation of MHC class I antigens

Candidate HIV Vaccines[31]

1. Live attenuated HIV vaccines
2. Whole inactivated vaccine (inactivated HIV-1)
3. Sub-unit vaccine - recombinant HIV-1 envelope glycoproteins produced from yeast, insect cells, mammalian cells used as sub-unit vaccines (no efficacy in human trials)
4. Synthetic vaccines - synthetic peptide immuno-gens with sequence of part of HIV-1 (unable to induce neutralizing antibodies against primary isolates)
5. Naked DNA vaccines - containing one or more HIV genes (weak immunogens)
6. Live recombinant vector vaccines - live attenuated viral or bacterial strain used as vector to carry HIV genes encoding antigens of interest.
   - Viral vectors: Vaccinia virus
Canarypox
Adenoviruses
Alphaviruses
Flaviviruses
Rhabdoviruses
Myxoviruses
Picornaviruses
   - Bacterial vectors: BCG
Salmonella
Lactobacillus
Streptococcus
Listeria
7. Prime boost combinations - priming with viral vector or nucleic acid vaccine and boosting with another vector or sub-unit vaccine, e.g, canarypox+recombinant sub-unit protein or vector+vector combination

Traditional vaccine methods were used in early studies. Live attenuated vaccines elicited robust immune responses in macaques using simian immunodeficiency virus (SIV); however all developed AIDS after a long period of time and died.[32] Testing of inactivated virus vaccines in the SIV/macaque model has proved disappointing with poor immunogenic responses.

Highly purified viral proteins produced using recombinant DNA technology have also been trialled. Two such vaccines composed of recombinant gp120 have been tested in phase III efficacy trials in subjects at high risk of HIV infection. Both showed no protection against HIV acquisition.[33,34] These vaccines produce a modest humoral immune response, but do not evoke a CTL response, so their failure was not unexpected.[35] Other modifications are being made in this group to increase the efficacy of vaccine, such as mixing gp120 from primary isolates and soluble gp140 glycoprotein trimers, removal of glycosyl moieties to unmask neutralisation epitopes (the site of gp120 CD4 receptor complexes), and deletion of the 1st and 2nd variable loops from gp120. Non-structural protein-based vaccines containing highly conserved protein than envelope proteins, e.g. nef, tat proteins, are being made. Vaccines containing fusion of both structural and envelop proteins are also under development – e.g. gp120 nef-tat fusion sub-unit protein vaccine.

Novel vaccine strategies are currently under development. Many promising vaccine technologies are entering early clinical trials. The first consists of HIV DNA segments formed into plasmids under the control of potent promoter genes. These have been shown to elicit strong CTL responses in animal models.[29] These are preferred to be used as prime vaccines before boosting with a viral vector vaccine in prime boost strategy. Some vaccines based on this stratergy include Advax DNA (DNA vaccine containing gag, env, nef, pol and tat genes from HIV clade C) and GTU multi-HIV.

Vector vaccines are synthesized using vectors which have been genetically modified to reduce their pathogenicity. Examples of vectors being trialled include modified vaccinia virus, canarypox virus, adenovirus 5, adenovirus-associated virus and Venezuelan equine encephalitis virus.[36] Some bacteria are also used as vectors like BCG, salmonella, shigella, lactobacillus and listeria. Genes encoding for HIV proteins are inserted into these vectors, which can then express HIV proteins in vaccinated subjects. It is increasingly being recognized that more than one vaccine approach may be necessary to produce sufficient immune responses.[29] Some of these novel vaccine approaches have been trialled in SIV infected macaques, with some success in delaying the course of infection.[37,38] Some of the vaccines based on this principle include Advax (Venezuelan equine encephalitis virus containing gag gene from HIV-clade C) and Merck d5 (Adenovirus serotype 5 containing gag/pol/nef gene from HIV clade B). Synthetic peptide-based vaccines containing synthetic peptide immunogens (either linear and branched or initially concentrated on V3 loop of gp120) are being synthesized.

Prime Boost Concept

Animal studies found that priming with a viral vector vaccine or a DNA vaccine followed by boosting with either another vector or sub-unit/ peptide vaccine induce a stronger immune response compared to vaccination with either vaccine alone. Several prime boost strategies have been used over the past decade. DNA vaccine for priming and recombinant Ad5 boosting has been tried in human volunteers with good results. Currently, many trials are ongoing based on this concept.

If an effective vaccine is found, there is concern that risky sexual behaviour may increase. A study in Uganda showed that 50% of military recruits would stop using condoms if they received an effective HIV vaccine,[39] although risky sexual behaviour was not shown to increase during a phase III HIV vaccine trial.[40]

HUMAN PAPILLOMAVIRUS (HPV)

HPV is a double-stranded DNA tumor virus of the papovavirus family. The virus infects basal epithelial layers in the transformation zone of the cervix, where the most vulnerable (stem) cells are found. HPV types 16 and 18 account for nearly 70% of cases of cervical cancer, AIS (non-invasive cervical cancer), cervical intraepithelial neoplasia (CIN) grade 3, vulvar intraepithelial neoplasia (VIN) grade 2/3 and vaginal intraepithelial neoplasia (VaIN) grade 2/3, and account for 50% of CIN 2 lesions. HPV 6 and 11 are responsible for approximately 90% of genital wart cases. These four types of HPV also cause approximately 35-50% of all low-grade cervical, vaginal and vulvar lesions (grade 1-CIN, VIN and VaIN). As cervical cancer is associated with infection with high-risk types of HPV, antiviral vaccination strategies have great potential in the prevention of cervical cancers.[41]

HPVs contain a small circular DNA genome that encodes only six early (E) and two late (L) proteins. E1 and E2 proteins are involved in viral DNA replication; E4 and E5 proteins are involved in the amplification of viral genome in the upper layers of the epithelium; E6 and E7 proteins of high-risk HPV types are involved in oncogenic transformation; and L1 and L2 proteins form the viral capsid. The L proteins are capable of self-assembly into empty capsids referred to as virus-like particles (VLPs) that lack HPV viral genome and hence are incapable of causing infection. VLPs are immunogenic, which makes them attractive vaccine candidates; however, because they are type-specific vaccines, they must include various strain-specific VLPs to provide broad protection.[1]

Two vaccines are newly licensed for the prevention of HPV infection. They both employ recombinant DNA technology to produce VLP consisting of the L1 structural protein from HPV which forms part of the viral capsid. VLPs are produced by the expression of L1 protein in a heterologous system (yeast or insect cells). These non-infectious VLPs are empty shells mimicking the structure of HPV virions.[42] Both vaccines incorporate L1 proteins from HPV 16 and 18 – the two HPV types responsible for the majority of cervical dysplasia and cancer. The quadrivalent vaccine produced by Merck also incorporates L1 proteins from HPV 6 and 11, affording some protection against commoner strains causing external genital warts.

The bivalent vaccine produced by GlaxoSmithKline (GSK) uses an MPL alum adjuvant. The phase III efficacy trial was carried out in healthy women aged between 15 and 25 years who were serologically negative for both HPV 16 and 18. Following three doses of vaccine given at 0, 1 and 6 months, more than 98% of women had an antibody response at all follow-up visits, and the titre was higher than that seen after natural infection.[43] Using intention to treat analysis, the vaccine was 86% effective at preventing infection by HPV 16 or 18, and 100% effective at preventing cervical intraepithelial dysplasia 1 (CIN1) and higher grades of dysplasia caused by the same HPV types.[44] The vaccine also showed some protection against HPV 45 and a lesser effect on HPV 31, but there was no cross-protection to other high-risk HPV types.[44]

Merck's quadrivalent vaccine with alum adjuvant has produced similar good results in clinical trials. Gardasil (a quadrivalent vaccine) is currently approved by FDA for prevention of genital warts, cancers and precancerous conditions of cervix and vulva in 9-26-year-old females.[41]

Three doses of either vaccine or placebo were given to over 12,000 women aged 16 to 23 years. Those in the vaccine arm showed 90% reduction in type-specific persistent infection and clinical HPV disease. The vaccine was 100% effective at preventing HPV 16 and 18-related CIN 2/3 and cancer.[45] External warts caused by HPV 6 and 11, and vulval intraepithelial neoplasia caused by HPV 16 and 18 -were reduced by 65-90% in vaccinated subjects.[46] The vaccine was also tested for immunogenicity in younger adolescent boys and girls, and elicited higher antibody titres than those seen in adults.[45] At this stage, it remains unclear as to whether booster doses will be required.

Ideally vaccination will be offered to young women before the onset of sexual activity, as HPV infection is acquired shortly after coitarche.[47] Concerns that vaccination might encourage early onset of sexual activity or reduce condom use may limit the uptake of these vaccines in some settings. Whether recommendations should include vaccinating young males to increase herd immunity is another issue that needs to be resolved. At the current prices, a widespread vaccination programme would be costly, with benefits taking many years to show. Currently the highest burden of cervical cancer is in the developing world where the cost of these vaccines may prove prohibitive.

Important Points about HPV Vaccine

- The quadrivalent HPV vaccine (Gardasil) protects against HPV types 6, 11, 16 and 18.
- HPV types 16 and 18 cause 70% of cervical cancer cases and 50% of high-grade cervical abnormalities.
- HPV types 6 and 11 cause 90% of cases of genital warts and approximately 10% of low-grade cervical abnormalities.
- Vaccination is indicated for females aged 9–26 and males aged 9–15 years.
- Best time to vaccinate: the sooner the better – ideally before onset of sexual activity, although sexually active women will also benefit.
- Women should continue with regular Pap tests as not all oncogenic or high-risk types are covered by the vaccine.
- Vaccination is not a treatment for an existing HPV-related disease – it is preventive of infection with four HPV types.

HEPATITIS B VIRUS (HBV)

Effective vaccines against HBV have been available since 1981. These sub-unit vaccines consist of the small envelope protein of the virus which can assemble as VLPs. The envelope protein contains hepatitis B surface antigen (HBsAg), and elicits a neutralizing antibody response.[48] Earlier vaccines were derived from plasma taken from low infectivity HBV carriers. This practice was changed with the evolution of the HIV epidemic as many HBV carriers were from groups at high risk of HIV. Newer vaccines employ recombinant DNA technology using yeast cells. Hypersensitivity to yeasts is a contraindication to these vaccines.

The WHO recommends that all countries provide a universal Hepatitis B vaccination programme for infants and adolescents. As of 2003, 72% of the 192 member states had implemented universal vaccination.[49] In the United States, the incidence of acute Hepatitis B has fallen by 67% in the first 12 years of such a policy.[50]

Protective levels of anti-HBs antibodies (>10 iu/mL) develop in 95-99% of healthy infants, children and young adults who receive a series of three doses.[48] The efficacy of the vaccine in preventing disease in those who develop an antibody response of at least 10 iu/mL is nearly 100%.[50] Response to the vaccine is limited in those aged over 40 years, and in immunocompromised individuals.[48] In recent years, HBV pre-S mutants have been discovered in endemic areas that, in rare cases, have infected individuals despite adequate anti-HBs levels post-vaccination.[50] Newer vaccines incorporating further HBV surface proteins, or using DNA plasmids, have superior efficacy to traditional vaccines when given to non-responders, and may provide better protection against mutant viruses.[51,52]

REFERENCES

1. Stanberry LR, Rosenthal SL. Progress in vaccines for sexually transmitted diseases. Infect Dis Clin N A 2005; 19: 477-90.
2. Batteiger BE, Rank RG, Bavoil PM. Partial protection against genital reinfection by immunization of guinea-pigs with isolated outer-membrane proteins of the chlamydial agent of guinea-pig inclusion conjunctivitis. J Gen Microbiol 1993; 139: 2965-72.
3. Moore T, Ekworomadu CO, Eko FO. Fc receptor-mediated antibody regulation of T cell immunity against intracellular pathogens. J Infect Dis 2003; 188: 617-24.
4. Eko F O, He Q, Brown T. A novel recombinant multisubunit vaccine against Chlamydia. J Immunol 2004; 173: 3375-82.
5. Hechard C, Grepinet O, Rodolakis A. Molecular cloning of the Chlamydophila abortus groEL gene and evaluation of its protective efficacy in a murine model by genetic vaccination. J Med Microbiol 2004; 53: 861-8.
6. Zhang D, Yang X, Berry J. DNA vaccination with the major outer-membrane protein gene induces acquired immunity to *Chlamydia trachomatis* (mouse pneumonitis) infection. J Infect Dis 1997; 176: 1035-40.
7. Starnbach M N, Loomis W P, Ovendale P. An inclusion membrane protein from *Chlamydia trachomatis* enters the MHC class I pathway and stimulates a CD8 + T cell response. J Immunol 2003; 171: 4742-9.
8. Whittum-Hudson J A, Rudy D, Gerard H. The anti-idiotypic antibody to chlamydial glycolipid exoantigen (GLXA) protects mice against genital infection with a human biovar of *Chlamydia trachomatis*. Vaccine 2001; 19: 4061-71.
9. Beagley KW, Timms P. *Chlamydia trachomatis* infection: incidence, health costs and prospects for vaccine development. J Reprod Immunol 2000; 48: 47-68.
10. Sparling PF, Elkins C, Wyrick PB et al. Vaccines for bacterial sexually transmitted diseases: A realistic goal? Proc Natl Acad Sci. 1994; 91: 2456-63.
11. Wagar EA, Schachter J, Bavoil P, et al. Differential human serologic response to two 60000 molecular weight *Chlamydia trachomatis* antigens. 1990; 162: 922-7.
12. Rupp R, Stanberry LR, Rosenthal SL. New biomedical approaches for sexually transmitted infection prevention: vaccines and microbiocides. Adolesc Med 2004; 15: 393-407.

13. Su H, Caldwell HD. Immunogenicity of a synthetic oligopeptide corresponding to antigenically common T-helper and B-cell neutralising epitopes of the major outer membrane protein of *Chlamydia trachomatis*. Vaccine. 1993; 11: 1159-66.
14. McKnew D L, Lynn F, Zenilman J M. Porin variation among clinical isolates of *Neisseria gonorrhoeae* over a 10-year period, as determined by Por variable region typing. J Infect Dis 2003; 187: 1213-22.
15. Plummer FA, Simonsen JN, Chubb H et al. Epidemiologic evidence for the development of serovar-specific immunity after gonococcal infection. J Clin Invest. 1989; 83: 1472-6.
16. Rokbi B, Renauld-Mongenie G, Mignon M. Allelic diversity of the two transferrin binding protein B gene isotypes among a collection of Neisseria meningitidis strains representative of serogroup B disease: implication for the composition of a recombinant TbpB-based vaccine. Infect Immun 2000; 68: 4938-47.
17. Gulati S, Ngampasutadol J, Yamasaki R. Strategies for mimicking Neisserial saccharide epitopes as vaccines. Int Rev Immunol 2001; 20: 229-50.
18. Zhu W, Thomas CE, Sparling PF. DNA immunization of mice with a plasmid encoding Neisseria gonorrhea PorB protein by intramuscular injection and epidermal particle bombardment. Vaccine 2004; 22: 660-9.
19. Wicher V, Zabek J, Wicher K. Pathogen-specific humoral response in *Treponema pallidum*-infected humans, rabbits and guinea pigs. J Infect Dis. 1991; 163: 830-6.
20. Stanberry L R . Clinical trials of prophylactic and therapeutic herpes simplex virus vaccines. Herpes 2004; 11: 161A-169A.
21. Jones CA, Cunningham AL. Vaccination strategies to prevent genital herpes and neonatal herpes simplex virus (HSV) disease. Herpes. 2004; 11: 12-7.
22. Skinner GR, Turyk ME, Benson CA, et al. The efficacy and safety of Skinner herpes simplex vaccine towards modulation of herpes genitalis; report of a prospective double-blind placebo-controlled trial. Med Microbiol Immunol. 1997; 186: 31-6.
23. Straus SE, Corey L, Burke RL et al. Placebo-controlled trial of vaccination with recombinant glycoprotein D of herpes simplex virus 2 for immunotherapy of genital herpes. Lancet. 1994; 343: 1460-3.
24. Mertz GJ, Ashley R, Burke RL et al. Double blind, placebo-controlled trial of a herpes simplex type 2 glycoprotein vaccine in persons at high risk for genital herpes infection. J Infect Dis. 1990; 161: 653-60.
25. Walz MA, Price RW, Hayashi K, et al. Effect of immunization on acute and latent infections of vaginouterine tissue with herpes simplex types 1 and 2. J Infect Dis 1977; 135: 744-52.
26. Corey L, Langenberg AG, Ashley R et al. Recombinant glycoprotein vaccine for the prevention of genital HSV-2 infection: two randomised controlled trials. Chiron HSV Vaccine Study Group. JAMA 1999; 282: 331-40.
27. Stanberry LR, Spruance SL, Cunningham AL et al. Glycoprotein-D-adjuvant vaccine to prevent genital herpes. NEJM 2002; 347: 1652-61.
28. de Bruyn G, Vargas-Cortez M, Warren T et al. A randomized controlled trial of a replication defective (gH deletion) herpes simplex virus vaccine for the treatment of recurrent genital herpes among immunocompetent subjects. Vaccine 2006; 24: 914-20.
29. Letvin NL. Strategies for an HIV vaccine. J Clin Invest. 2002; 110: 15-20.
30. Girard MP, Mastro TD, Koff W. Human immunodeficiency virus. In: Plotkin SA, Orenstein WA, eds. Vaccines, 4th edn. Philadelphia: Saunders publishing company 2004: 1232-40.
31. Excler JL. AIDS Vaccine development: perspectives challenges and hopes. Indian J Med Research 2005; 121: 568.
32. Baba TW, Jeong YS, Dennick D et al. Pathogenicity of live, attenuated SIV after mucosal infection of neonatal macaques. Science. 1995; 267: 1820-5.
33. rgp 120 HIV Vaccine Study Group. Placebo-controlled phase 3 trial of a recombinant glycoprotein 120 vaccine to prevent HIV-1 infection. J Infect Dis 2005; 191: 654-65.
34. Choopanya K, Tappero JW, Pitisuttithum P et al. Preliminary results of a phase III HIV vaccine

efficacy trial among injecting drug users in Thailand. Int Conf AIDS. 2004 Jul 11-16; 15: abstract no. ThOrA1427.
35. Calarota SA, Weiner DB. Present status of human HIV vaccine development. AIDS. 2003; 17(suppl 4): S73-84.
36. Markel H. The search for effective HIV vaccines. NEJM 2005; 353: 753-7.
37. Amara RR, Villinger F, Altman JD et al. Control of a mucosal challenge and prevention of clinical AIDS in rhesus monkeys by a multiprotein DNA/MVA vaccine. Science 2001; 292: 69-74.
38. Barouch DH, Santra S, Schmitz JE et al. Control of viraemia and prevention of clinical AIDS in rhesus monkeys by cytokine-augmented DNA vaccination. Science. 2000; 290: 486-92.
39. Zimet GD, Mays RM, Fortenberry JD. Vaccines against sexually transmitted infections: Promise and problems of the magic bullets for prevention and control. Sex Transm Dis. 2000; 27: 49-52.
40. McCarthy M. News: HIV vaccine fails in phase 3 trial. Sceptics question analysis that suggests HIV vaccine could be protective in non white people. Lancet. 2003; 361: 755-6.
41. Sharma R, Sharma CL. Quadrivalent human papillomavirus recombinant vaccine: the first vaccine for cervical cancers. J Can Res Ther 2007; 3: 92-5.
42. Villa LL, Costa RLR, Petta CA et al. Prophylactic quadrivalent human papillomavirus (types 6, 11, 16 and 18) L1 virus-like particle vaccine in young women: a randomised double-blind placebo-controlled multicentre phase II efficacy trial. Lancet Oncol. 2005; 6: 271-8.
43. Harper DM, Franco EL, Wheeler C et al. Efficacy of a bivalent L1 virus-like particle vaccine in prevention of infection with human papillomavirus types 16 and 18 in young women: a randomised controlled trial. Lancet. 2004; 364: 1757-65.
44. Harper DM, Franco EL, Wheeler CM et al. Sustained efficacy up to 4.5 years of a bivalent L1 virus-like particle vaccine against human papillomavirus types 16 and 18: follow-up from a randomised controlled trial. Lancet 2006; 367: 1247-55.
45. Block SL, Nolan T, Sattler C et al. Comparison of immunogenicity and reactogenicity of a prophylactic quadrivalent human papillomavirus (types 6, 11, 16 and 18) L1 virus-like particle vaccine in male and female adolescents and young adult women. Paediatrics 2006; 18: 2135-45.
46. Garland SM, Hernandez-Avila M, Wheeler CM et al. Quadrivalent vaccine against human papillomavirus to prevent anogenital diseases. NEJM 2007; 356: 1928-43.
47. Steinbrook R. The potential of human papillomavirus vaccines. NEJM 2006; 354: 1109-12.
48. Wood A. Vaccines to prevent viral hepatitis. NEJM 1997; 336: 196-204.
49. Global progress toward universal childhood hepatitis B vaccination, 2003. MMWR Morb Mortal Wkly Rep 2003; 52: 868-70.
50. Poland G, Jacobson R. Prevention of hepatitis B with the hepatitis B vaccine. NEJM 2004; 351: 2832-8.
51. Bertino JS, Tirrell P, Greenberg RN et al. A comparative trial of standard or high-dose S subunit recombinant hepatitis B vaccine versus a vaccine containing S subunit, pre-S1, and pre-S2 particles for revaccination of healthy adult nonresponders. J Infect Dis 1997; 175: 678-81.
52. Rottinghaus ST, Poland GA, Jacobson RM, et al. Hepatitis B DNA vaccine induces protective antibody responses in human non-responders to conventional vaccination. Vaccine 2003; 21: 4604-8.

Part 8

Non-Venereal Skin Diseases of Genitalia

40 NON-VENEREAL DISEASES OF GENITALIA

Binod K Khaitan

In this chapter

- Dermatologic Diseases Affecting the Genitalia
- Developmental Lesions of Genitalia
- Lesions Due to Trauma
- Non-Venereal Sclerosing Lymphangitis
- Peyronie's Disease
- Lichen Planus
- Plasma Cell Balanitis
- Fixed Drug Eruption (FDE)
- Lichen Sclerosus et Atrophics (LSA)
- Fournier's Gangrene
- Behcet's Disease
- Phimosis and Paraphimosis
- Genital tuberculids

INTRODUCTION

All lesions on genitalia are not sexually transmitted. A dermatovenereologist is usually familiar with diseases which are non-venereal and present on genitalia. There is no strict classification of such diseases. However, one can categorize these into three major groups.

1. Common dermatological diseases with lesions on genitalia either exclusively or along with lesions elsewhere, e.g. vitiligo, psoriasis, lichen planus, etc.
2. Diseases involving genitalia and considered to be physiological abnormalities, e.g. pearly penile papules, Fordyce spots, etc.
3. Non-venereal diseases peculiar to genitalia. Some of the important conditions are as follows:
   (a) Peyronie's disease
   (b) Plasma cell balanitis
   (c) Lichen sclerosus et atrophicus
   (d) Lichen planus of the genitalia
   (e) Fixed drug eruption
   (f) Fournier's gangrene
   (g) Behcet's disease
   (h) Non-venereal sclerosing lymphangitis
   (i) Angiokeratoma of Fordyce
   (j) Phimosis and paraphimosis
   (k) Genital tuberculids

Some of these diseases may also occur elsewhere but have specific presentations on genitalia.

DERMATOLOGICAL DISEASES AFFECTING GENITALIA

Most dermatological diseases generally occur elsewhere and also involve the genitalia. When other sites are involved, the diagnosis is straightforward. When the lesion is present exclusively on genitalia, the venereologist has the task to differentiate it from true STDs. The general principles of treatment in such situations are essentially same as for non-genital lesions.

Vitiligo, particularly acrofacial vitiligo, may have depigmented macules on the glans, prepuce, penile shaft, scrotum, vulva and also in perianal area. These are asymptomatic and usually do not require any treatment. Exclusive involve-ment of lips, nipples, fingertips and penis is also known.

Sometimes, patients with psoriasis, post-kala-azar dermal leishmaniasis, lepromatous leprosy, dermatophytic infection or other common dermatoses have lesions on genitalia, especially in males. The lesions have the same morphology as over the rest of the body, and one should examine for the evidence of disease process elsewhere on the body. Flexural psoriasis is a specific type of psoriasis with exclusive or near exclusive involvement of groins, genitals, umbilicus, perianal area, flexural areas below breasts, popliteal fossae and antecubital fossae and presented as sharply demarcated, erythematous plaques without significant infiltration or scaling. An important differential is Hailey-Hailey disease.

Among vesiculobullous diseases, pemphigus vulgaris involves oral mucosa in a large majority of patients, and genital mucosa, particularly glans penis and labia, are also known to be affected. At the time of presentation, the commonest finding is superficial erosion or ulcer; however occasionally unruptured vesicles or bullae may be seen. The presence of oral ulcers of pemphigus and flaccid bullae, crusts and ulcers in other parts of the body make clinical diagnosis easy. The presence of acantholytic cells on Tzanck smear and the classical histological and direct immunofluorescence findings make a definite diagnosis. Ulcerated vegetative plaques of pemphigus vegetans are rare as compared to ulcerative lesions of pemphigus vulgaris. These are seen characteristically on groins in both sexes and in labial sulci in females.

Bullous pemphigoid rarely may have genital are lesions. In contrast to pemphigus vulgaris, where lesions localized only to genitals are extremely rare, a variant of bullous pemphigoid known as localized vulvar pemphigoid is known to exclusively affect the genitals. Vulvar bullous pemphigoid is also seen in children.

Cicatricial pemphigoid, though a rare disease, may have vesiculobullous lesions on genitalia which heal with scarring. Cicatricial pemphigoid confined to vulva is also extremely rare; only three cases were reported so far. These vesiculobullous diseases sometimes need to be differentiated from ulcerative STDs.

DEVELOPMENTAL LESIONS OF GENITALIA

Like any other part of skin, some developmental defects or malformations may involve or encroach upon genitalia, viz. epidermal naevi, seborrhoeic keratosis, angiomas, lymphangiomas, inclusion cysts, enlarged sebaceous glands and rarely benign appendageal tumours. The morphology of such lesions is similar as in other areas, except that maceration occurs on lesions over the groins, coronal sulcus and subpreputial area. Some of these lesions may lead to venereophobia. Reassurance to the patient after clinical evaluation and histological confirmation when necessary is usually sufficient. The larger lesions need ablative therapy with electrodesiccation, surgical excision, radiofrequency ablation, laser ablation or other appropriate physical modalities of treatment.

Angiokeratoma of Fordyce

It is a distinct entity presenting as tiny erythematous, soft to firm, discrete red to blue-black papules on the scrotal skin **(Fig. 40.1)**. Some lesions become brownish with time. The lesions may bleed intermittently due to friction of undergarment or minor trauma. Angiokeratoma of Fordyce is a benign disease and not a marker of systemic disease. It requires ablative treatment with electrocautery, CO_2 laser, or 585-nm pulsed dye laser.

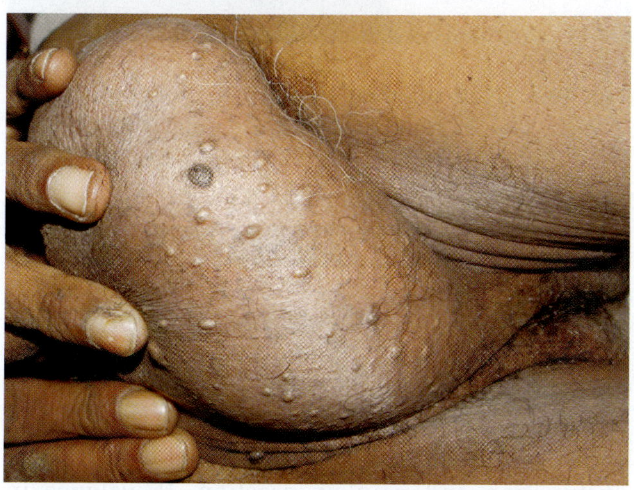

Fig. 40.1 Angiokeratoma of Fordyces – Erythematous Keratotic Papules on Scrotum.

Pearly Penile Papules

Pearly penile papules have also been called hirsutoid papillomas, papilla in corona glandis or corona capilliti.[1] These are anifestations of a harmless non-pathological process which may be the cause of worry to affected persons mainly young adults. These present as tiny 1-2 mm, skin-coloured or shiny papules arranged in a row or sometimes more than one row around coronal sulcus or just proximal to it or as scattered lesions on glans penis **(Fig. 40.2)**. These papules are barely elevated and considered to be physiological as these are prominent dermal papillae with slight hypertrophy. It is found in upto 10% of males and in as high as upto 48% males. Structurally, these are variants of angiofibroma and their histology resembles adenoma sebaceum, subungual and periungual fibromas, fibrous papules of nose and acquired acral angiofibromas. Rarely pearly penile papules need to be differentiated with early lesions of condyloma acuminata, based on the dirty white colour and rough, verrucous or granular surface

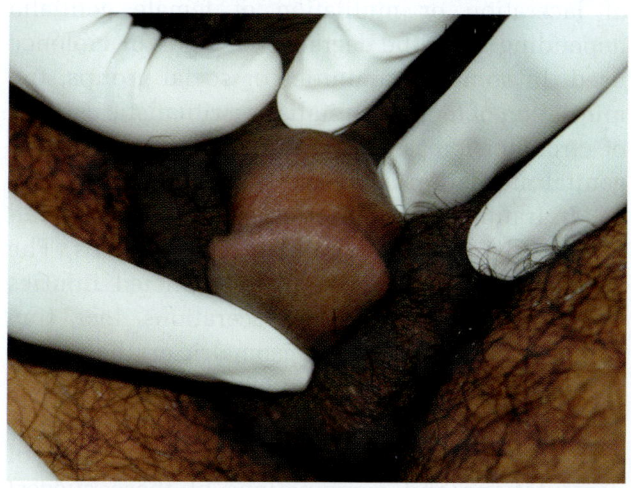

Fig. 40.2 Pearly Penile Papules.

of the latter. Reassurance to the person about the physiological nature of the lesions is the only measure required. If it causes severe psychological distress, then cryotherapy, electrodessication, CO_2 laser and pulse-dye laser may be tried with variable experiences.

Fordyce Spots

These are ectopic sebaceous glands present in the sub-preputial area of penis or on vulva. These present as multiple, asymptomatic, discrete, randomly distributed tiny yellowish barely elevated papules. Similar lesions may be present over the lips. The harmless nature of these lesions needs to be explained to the patient.

LESIONS DUE TO TRAUMA

Self-inflicted traumatic lesions as a result of sexual behavioural aberration or trauma at the time of intercourse in situations such as a reluctant partner, inadequate spontaneous lubrication, inadequate penile erection, etc., are not uncommon. The rupture of hymen leading to some amount of bleeding and sometimes discomfort in a young female either at the time of first intercourse or due to some other gratifying activities like masturbation is well known. Rape is another extreme situation where the trauma may involve extreme degree of laceration or mutilation of female genitalia depending upon the degree of coercion or violence used. In some communities or social groups, the mutilation of female genitalia as a ritualistic activity of circumcision is also practised. This practice of genital mutilation is not prevalent in India.

In traumatic lesions, the diagnosis will depend on the reliable history and pattern of lesions. The lesions may look bizarre in self-inflicted injuries or may present as bruises, lacerations, tear, tiny abrasions, asymmetrical or geometric erythematous sores. Associated oedema in both male and female genitalia, lesions developing within minutes or a few hours of intercourse, and a variety of permutations and combinations of these suggest trauma. The treatment will depend upon the type of trauma and routine principles of prevention of secondary infection and providing rest to the part to promote healing will be applicable. In addition, it is important to look for evidence of any 'real' STDs at the time of examination and follow-up.

NON-VENEREAL SCLEROSING LYMPHANGITIS

It is an uncommon condition related to aggressive or rigorous intercourse leading to diffuse but subtle trauma to penis in young males. It is usually painless and presents as single or grouped cord-like soft to firm lesions arising from coronal sulcus and involving the dorsal part of the penis **(Fig. 40.3)**. It is attributed to thickened and sclerosed lymphatics, but there is some venous component as well. It regresses spontaneously within a few weeks.

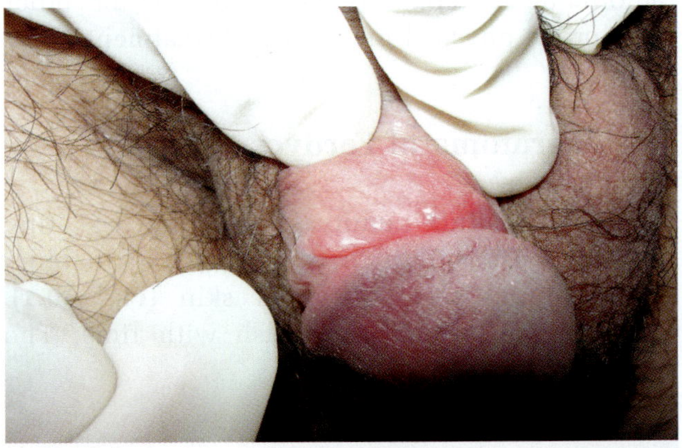

Fig. 40.3 Non-venereal Sclerosing Lymphangitis – Erythematous Cord along the Coronal Sulcus.

PEYRONIE'S DISEASE

Also known as penile fibromatosis or plastic induration of the penis, Peyronie's disease characteristically has one or more indurated fibrous longitudinal cord-like subcutaneous plaques in the penile shaft which may be associated with erectile dysfunction and pain on erection. Prevalence in the population was found to be 3.2%.

Aetiology and Pathogenesis

The exact cause is unknown. In majority of cases it occurs as an isolated abnormality. It may be associated with other fibromatous diseases such as palmoplantar fibromatosis, knuckle pads and keloid. Athero-matous changes are known to be associated as seen with the use of β-blockers. The etiology is multifactorial with genetic predisposition, trauma and tissue ischemia causing the release of fibrogenic cytokines.[2]

The pathological changes are in the form of fibrous infiltration in the connective tissue of corpora cavernosa from the septum between the two corpora cavernosa comprising of fibroblastic tissue with dense collagen. Sometimes calcification and very rarely ossification may occur. The changes may extend into tunica albuginea.

Clinical Features

It presents usually in middle-aged men. Painful erection with varying degree of dorsal or lateral bending of the penis in erection is the main presenting feature. The firm to hard, cord-like longitudinal area or indurated localized area may sometimes be tender. Erectile deformity may lead to intercourse being painful, difficult or even impossible. The course is unpredictable and it may improve or remain unchanged after few months of progression.

High-resolution ultrasonography or MRI of erect penis may help in evaluating the severity.

Treatment

Spontaneous recovery is possible in 20-30% cases. Pain may improve in 35-100%, size of plaque in 11-100% and angulation in 10-82% with time. The milder asymptomatic disease may not require any treatment. However, the persistent lesions with painful erection require treatment. Most cases report to urologists and some treatment modalities are exclusively in their domain. The following modalities have been tried with varying results:

(a) Intralesional corticosteroids
(b) Clostridial collagenase injections
(c) Intralesional injections of Verapamil[3] in deformity <300
(d) Extracorporeal shock wave treatment with standard lithotriptor[4]
(e) Dexamethasone pulse therapy
(f) Nisbet's operation comprising of surgical removal of normal tunica albuginea opposite the point of maximum curvature
(g) Penile prosthesis
(h) Surgical correction of curvature with 16-dot plication technique

Surgical correction should be done after 12 months of disease with stability of symptoms for at least 3 months. For more details refer to Chapter 48.

Procarbazine, vitamin E, paraminobenzoate, tamoxifen, colchicine, radiotherapy, acetyl carnitine have little or no benefit.

LICHEN PLANUS

Lichen planus is a papulosquamous disorder presenting characteristically on skin as violaceous flat-topped pruritic papules. There are several morphological variants of lichen planus. In about 15% cases, lichen planus involves exclusively the mucous membrane, either oral or genital or both. In addition, mucous membrane involvement is seen in upto 30-70% of cases along with cutaneous involvement.[6]

Clinical Features

If the lesion is present on penile skin, it presents as lesions elsewhere, i.e. violaceous flat-topped papules or plaques, with different sizes with minimal scaling **(Fig. 40.4)**. However, annular lesions are seen more frequently on genital skin. On glans penis or preputial skin, the lesions have whitish discoloration, and violaceous hue and hyperpigmentation is not uniform. Rarely the lesions are also seen on scrotal skin. Ulceration of genital lichen planus is rare as compared to oral

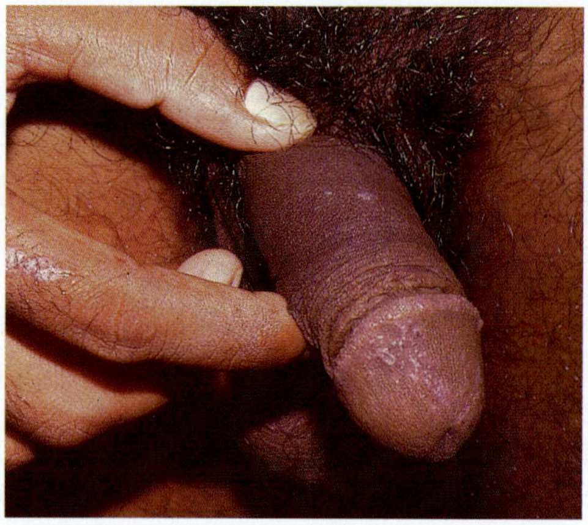

Fig. 40.4 Lichen Planus – Violaceous Papules over the Glans and Hand.

lichen planus. In female, the lesions are present on vulval skin and labia majora or sometimes on the inner aspect of labia minora. Erosive vaginal lichen planus may lead to vaginal adhesions and dyspareunia. The vulvovaginal-gingival syndrome is a variant of mucosal lichen planus characterized by erosions and desquamation of vulva, vagina and gingivae.[7,8] Mild lesions are small, flat papules, usually multiple and grouped, and the severe disease may be erosive with severe itching and pain. If induration is present and the colour is ivory white, a biopsy is required to differentiate from lichen sclerosus et atrophicus. On healing, ulcerative lesions leave behind scarring. Occasionally lesions of secondary syphilis may have a lichenoid presentation, but the lesions are present more on the folds with moist papules; its non-pruritic nature and other clinical evidence of secondary syphilis give the clue. However, in such cases, dark-ground microscopy and serological tests are essential.

In general, the genital lesions of lichen planus tend to last longer than skin lesions, and recurrences are common.

Histology

A classical lesion of lichen planus shows hyperkeratosis and irregular acanthosis. There may be atrophy of the epidermis in late stages. There is damage to basal keratinocytes with presence of cytoid bodies in the upper dermis and pigment incontinence along with predominant lymphohistiocytic infiltrate in a band-like pattern. The histology of genital lesion is similar to cutaneous lesions of lichen planus with certain differences due to the site. Apart from non-keratinized or less keratinized epidermis with parakeratosis, the band-like infiltrate which is otherwise lymphohistiocytic is rich in plasma cells. Cytoid bodies may be present but much less in number.

Treatment

Moderately potent topical corticosteroids are generally helpful in treating few lesions. Topical tacrolimus[9] and pimecrolimus[10] are also effective. If lesions are persistent or recurrent, a course of oral corticosteroid may rarely be required. Symptomatic relief with antihistamines or analgesics is required in some patients. Estrogens are not effective in treating erosive vaginal lichen planus.

PLASMA CELL BALANITIS

Also known as Zoon's balanitis or plasma cell mucositis or balanitis circumscripta plasmacellularis, plasma cell balanitis is an idiopathic, benign disorder of uncircumcised male genitalia.

Clinical Features

This condition presents with characteristic clinical features in middle-aged or elderly uncircumcised men as a solitary, circumscribed, persistent plaque with shiny smooth surface on glans penis **(Fig. 40.5)**.[11] The plaque is moist with a glistening appearance and has minute red specks (cayenne pepper spots). The lesion is usually asymptomatic and single, although multiple lesions have been described. Some patients can have mild pruritus. Plasma cell balanitis most commonly involves glans penis and prepuce. However, it may extend to involve the inner surface of prepuce. Plasma cell balanitis has to be differentiated from erythroplasia of Queyrat [squamous cell carcinoma (SCC) in-situ], which clinically has a velvety surface and shows features of SCC in-situ on histopathology.

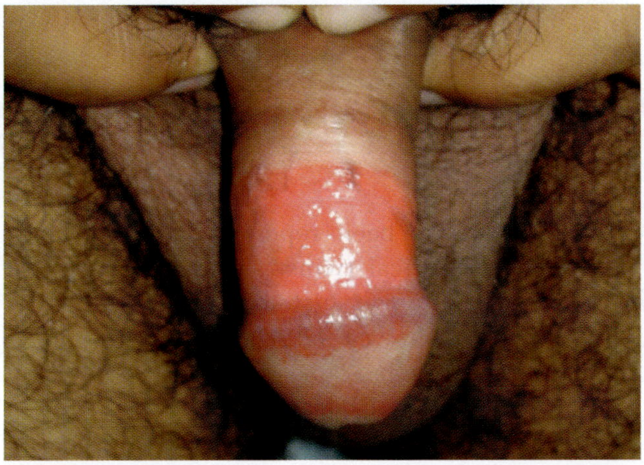

Fig. 40.5 Plasma Cell Balanitis – Erythematous Shiny Well-defined Plaque on Prepuce and Glans.

Several variants of plasma cell balanitis have been described. In one, there is marked dermal oedema and predominantly lymphocytic infiltrate. Others are erosive and hypertrophic variants.

Histopathology

The epidermis is attenuated with absence of horny and granular layers. Suprabasal keratinocytes are diamond shaped which are also called "lozenge keratinocytes". Mild spongiosis with occasional dyskeratotic keratinocytes are observed. In the dermis, there may be dense mixed infiltrate with predominance of plasma cells along with extravasated erythrocytes. Haemosiderin deposits and vascular proliferation are other histological features.

Treatment

Topical corticosteroids cause mild improvement, but the lesion usually recurs following discontinuation of treatment. Sometimes it is frustrating. Superadded candidal infection may occur with prolonged use of topical corticosteroid, and a combination with topical antifungal agents is sometimes helpful. Circumcision is curative.[12] Reports of treatment with CO_2 laser and copper vapour laser have appeared in literature.[13] Topical tacrolimus 0.1% ointment has been found effective in treating Zoon's balanitis with no relapse after one-year follow-up.[14]

FIXED DRUG ERUPTION (FDE)

It is a specific manifestation of drug reaction, where the lesions remain confined to certain areas, and with each exposure of a particular drug, the lesions reappear on the same old sites of reaction, although sometimes new areas may be involved with fresh episodes. Several drugs have been known to be responsible for FDE. Analgesics, NSAIDS, antibiotics, sulphonamides, cotrimoxazole and tetracyclines are among the more frequent causes of FDE.[15]

Clinically there is sharply demarcated, erythematous, oedematous plaques appearing within few hours of ingestion or injection of the offending drug. Sometimes the lesions are so inflamed that bullous changes or ulceration can occur. Once the offending drug is withdrawn, the lesions heal in 5-10 days leaving behind dark-brown to black hyperpigmentation. Although FDE may present on any part of the body, glans penis is a common site either exclusively or along with other sites on the body **(Fig. 40.6)**.[15,16] The acute onset, the temporal relationship with drug intake, the well-cirumscribed nature of the lesion and acute changes occurring on subsequent episodes on a pre-existing hyperpigmented macule strongly

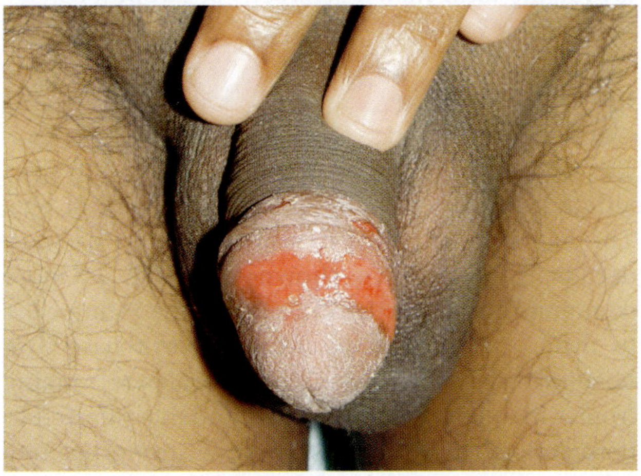

Fig. 40.6 Fixed Drug Eruption.

suggest the diagnosis of FDE. On glans penis, an acute episode presents as a circular or oval superficial erythematous erosion or ulcer with minimal crust, and underneath the crust the raw area is usually tender.

FDE on genitalia needs to be differentiated from other ulcerative STDs as well as other causes of balanitis in male. Once the lesion heals, a provocation with the suspected drug leading to reappearance of the lesion gives the final proof. Usually the application of potent topical corticosteroids for a few days is enough for healing. The residual hyperpigmentation is extremely difficult to treat, and it may take several years for complete clearance.

LICHEN SCLEROSUS ET ATROPHICUS (LSA)

LSA is a chronic inflammatory skin disease that causes substantial discomfort and morbidity, most commonly in adult women, but also in men and children. It is characterized by atrophic papules and plaques, occurring in any part of the skin and commonly in the anogenital skin of both sexes.

The first reported case of lichen sclerosus was by Hallopeau in 1887. The other synonyms are leucoplakia, lichen albus, hypoplastic dystrophy and kraurosis vulvae. The latter two exclusively denote LSA of female genitalia. The International Society for the Study of Vulvovaginal Diseases favours the term lichen sclerosus. Dermatologists favour the term lichen sclerosus et atrophicus.

Epidemiology

The onset of LSA has been reported in all ages, although it is not common under 2 years of age. The mean age of onset in women is fifth or sixth decade. Studies have shown that LSA is more common in women than in men at the ratio of 6:1 to even 10:1. Epidemiological surveys based on hospital referrals showed the prevalence ranging from 1 in 300 to 1 in 1000 of all patients referred to dermatology. One study showed a strong positive relation between risk and age, the highest risk being for 50-59 years and the incidence of LSA was 14 per 100,000/year.[17]

Aetiology

Familial LSA has been reported in identical as well as non-identical twins, sisters, mothers and daughters. A study of histologically proven LSA of 84 patients showed positive correlation with class II antigens, HLA-DQ7, and to a lesser extent to DQ8 and DQ9, but larger series have not found any correlation of class I antigens. The interleukin-1 receptor antagonist gene has been speculated to be a candidate gene for LSA.

The association between autoimmunity and LSA has been described in several studies. In one study, 40% of patients with LSA had thyroid and parietal cell autoantibodies. Other studies have shown association with alopecia areata, vitiligo, pernicious anaemia, diabetes mellitus and cicatricial pemphigoid. The association was more common in females as compared to males. Several infective agents like pleomorphic acid fast bacilli, spirochaetes (borrelia) and human papilloma virus have been implicated, but none have been proved to be causal. Local factors such as trauma, constant friction and radiation treatment have been recognized as triggering factors.[17] It has also been observed that Koebner phenomenon can trigger LSA, like in post-vulvectomy scars and circumcision scars.

Clinical Features in Females

LSA most commonly affects the anogenital region (85-98%), with extragenital lesions in 15-20% of patients. Most commonly affected non-genital areas are inner thighs, submammary area, neck, shoulders and wrists. The plaque may encircle the vagina, and the perianal area appears as hourglass or inverted key hole pattern. Involvement of oral mucosa is rare. The most common symptom on genitalia is intractable pruritus. Other features are soreness of vulva and perianal area, dysuria dyspareunia and tenesmus. It may be totally asymptomatic, and diagnosable at routine examination. Painful traumatic fissures and tear may occur due to defecation and sexual intercourse. The skin changes include hypopigmented or depigmented small, polygonal papules or atrophic plaques with thin cellophane paper-like texture, wrinkled, fragile with telengiectasia, purpura, erosions, or tender fissures in labial sulci and perianal area **(Fig. 40.7)**. Some women may show areas of scaling, hyperkeratosis and sclerosis. The end stage is severe scarring and fusion of labia. Vagina is never involved in LSA.

Complications of LSA include complete fusion or resorption of labia minora, buried clitoris and narrow introitus which makes intercourse impossible.

In prepubertal girls, pruritus and soreness are common symptoms; dysuria and painful anal fissures causing constipation is also observed. Purpura may be occasionally seen. At menarche, the symptoms and signs spontaneously improve in two-third cases.

Clinical Features in Males

It is most common in middle-aged men, but in a study of prepubertal boys who were circumcised for phimosis, 14% had LSA.

Glans penis and prepuce are the most commonly affected sites. The lesions are usually asymptomatic, but presenting symptoms include present are pruritus, dysuria, painful erection, reduced sensation on the glans, and reduction in urinary stream and calibre. In uncircumcised men, a sclerotic constricting band 1-2 cm distal to the prepuce develops to result in phimosis. Examination would initially reveal only erythema, but with time, porcelain white macules, papules and sclerotic plaques are found. Older lesions become depressed. Rarely purpura, ecchymosis and even haemorrhagic bullae within the lesion may develop. Involvement of urethral meatus along with phimosis would result in difficulty in micturition. Most boys would present with meatal stenosis and phimosis and involvement of the glans. Perianal involvement and extragenital lesions in males are rare. The end stage of LSA in men is balanitis xerotica obliterans (BXO) **(Fig. 40.8)**. The onset and evolution of BXO is insidious, characterized by hypopigmented, thickened, contracted and fissured prepuce fixed over the glans and not retractable with moderate force.

Differential Diagnosis

In females, it has to be differentiated from nummular dermatitis, lichen simplex chronics, lichen planus, vitiligo, candidial vulvitis and cicatricial pemphigoid. In prepubertal girls, sexual abuse should be ruled out which may be coexistent and could lead to LSA as a Koebner phenomenon in trauma scar.

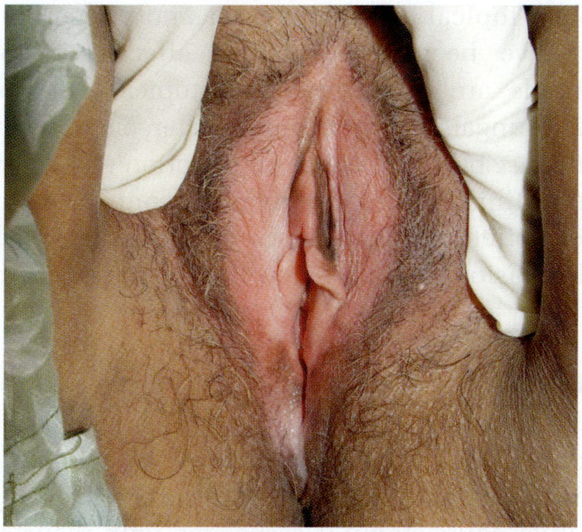

Fig. 40.7 Lichen Sclerosus – Hypopigmentation and Atrophy of the Vulva.

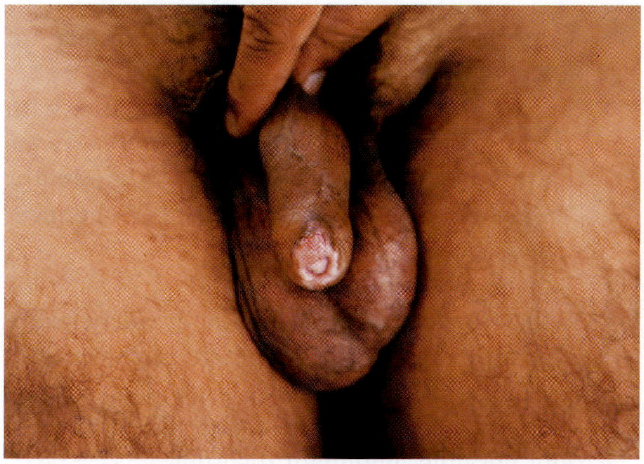

Fig. 40.8 Lichen Sclerosus (Balanitis Xerotica Obliterans) – Sclerosis and Depigmentation of Prepuce with Phimosis.

In males, the differential diagnoses include vitiligo, post-inflammatory hypopigmentation, repeated episodes of genital herpes or other ulcerative, STDs and trauma.

Histopathology

The characteristic histopathological features are epidermal atrophy, basal cell degeneration, pale staining homogenous zone in the papillary and upper dermis due to oedema or sclerosis and a band of inflammatory infiltrate comprising of CD4 and CD8 lymphocytes, in equal proportion, along with macrophages, mast cells and plasma cells **(Fig. 40.9)**.

On hairy areas, follicular plugging is also present. Squamous hyperplasia may be present due to chronic pruritus. Special stains show deposits of acid mucopolysaccharides in homogenous area and basement membrane. Electron microscopy shows structural changes in collagen. Immunohistochemistry reveals fewer elastin, fibrillin and increased expression of tenascin, an anti-adhesion molecule, and reduced expression of fibronectin in the upper dermis.[18]

Management[17]

The following guidelines can be followed in the management of LSA.

- Confirm histology by a punch biopsy of affected area.
- Treat the patient, even if asymptomatic, with very potent topical corticosteroids twice daily for 3 months, then taper off gradually. Treatment may be repeated whenever necessary.
- Advice to avoid local irritants.
- Check for non-healing erosion or warty lesion that may indicate development of carcinoma.
- Patient is advised regarding need of surgery to relieve symptoms of scarring and to treat any possible malignant disorder.
- Long-term follow-up.

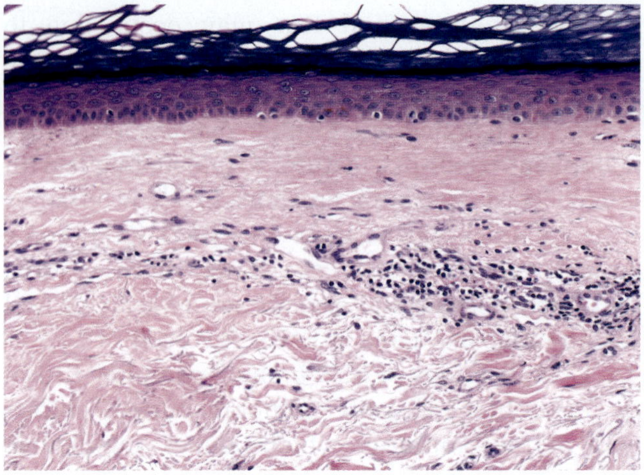

Fig. 40.9 Lichen Sclerosus (late): Photomicrograph showing sclerosis of papillary dermis with atrophy of the overlying epidermis.

Treatment

Potent topical corticosteroids are the mainstay of therapy, e.g. 0.05% clobetasol propionate twice daily for 2-3 months and then gradually tapered as symptoms subside. A similar regimen can also be used in children. Androgens like 2% testosterone have been used in female patients. However, a placebo-controlled trial showed no better results compared to emollients. In another study, 2% progesterone, 2% testosterone and 0.05% clobetasol propionate were compared, and topical corticosteroid was found to be the treatment of choice. Topical tacrolimus 0.1% and pimecrolimus 1% have been found to be effective. Topical retinoids are of no use, and topical antibiotics or antifungals are indicated if there is associated secondary bacterial or fungal infection respectively. Oral antihistamines are given to control pruritus. Stool softening agents may be necessary in girls and occasionally in women with perianal LSA.

Surgical

Circumcision is the treatment of choice for phimosis in male patients and the procedure may be curative. Vulvectomy is associated with recurrence rates as high as 50% and is no longer indicated if no malignancy is present. Surgical management in women may be necessary for dissection of a buried clitoris, division of fused labia and enlargement of narrowed introitus. Other ablative techniques, viz. cryotherapy, pulse dye laser and CO_2 laser, have been used in some cases with severe LSA. Acitretin (20-30 mg/d for 16 weeks) has also been used in women with severe LSA.

In asymptmotic patients, topical treatment may prevent progression of the disease and development of malignancy but side effects are also encountered. Each case has to be individualized and a long-term follow-up should be advised.

Prognosis

Studies of a large group of women with LSA show that 4.5% had risk of developing squamous cell carcinoma (SCC). Therefore, a long-term follow-up is necessary.[19] No median age for development of cancer has been established. Rarely in men the LSA can transform into SCC.[20] Extragenital LSA does not carry any risk of malignant change.

FOURNIER'S GANGRENE

It is also known by other names as idiopathic scrotal oedema, synergistic gangrene and necrotising fasciitis of the perineum **(Fig. 40.10)**.

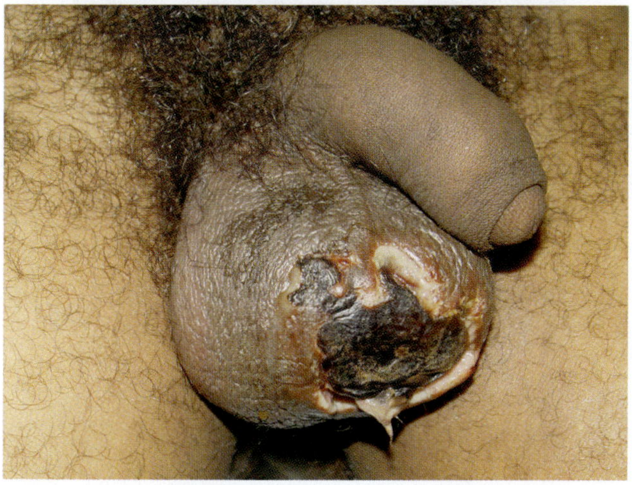

Fig. 40.10 Fournier's gangrene – Large ulcer with necrotic eschar on the scrotum.

It is an uncommon condition due to vascular compromise following bacterial infection. It has been observed to follow minor trauma, some surgical procedures in perineal area, urethral dilatation, injections of haemorrhoids or opening of periurethral abscesses. Surgeons encounter this condition more frequently than do venereologists. Risk factors for developing Fournier's gangrene include alcoholism, diabetes, malnutrition, advanced age and peripheral vascular diseases.

The organisms isolated from gangrene are most commonly streptococcus, occasionally associated with staphylococcus, *E. coli* and *Clostridium welchii*. In about half the cases, definite causative organism is not known. Group A streptococci can also cause, Fournier's gangrene in immunocompetent patients. Clinically the patient presents with sudden pain in scrotum with swelling, and prostration, pallor and pyrexia. Initially only a part of the scrotal skin is involved, and rapidly within few hours or days it may involve the whole of scrotum, and the entire scrotal coverings would slough off to expose the scrotal contents. The testis is healthy and unaffected by the process. Similar necrotizing process sometimes involves the lower abdominal wall, and hence Fournier's gangrene is a surgical emergency. The infection spreads along fascial planes, hence the external skin findings may represent only a small proportion of the underlying necrotic tissue. Histologically a fulminating inflammation in the subcutaneous tissue with necrosis associated with obliterating arteritis of the scrotal skin is seen. X-ray of the genital area or CT may demonstrate gas bubbles within the tissue.

Treatment

A swab from the necrosed area should be sent urgently for culture and antibiotic sensitivity. Usually the organisms are sensitive to gentamycin and cephalosporins, and parenteral antibiotics should be started immediately. Debridement in the form of wide excision of the sloughed/necrosed tissue is to be done. The indications of hyperbaric oxygen therapy remain controversial. Despite adequate management, mortality due to Fournier's gangrene may be as high as 16-40%.

BEHCET'S DISEASE

It is a chronic multisystemic disorder characterized by oral and genital aphthae, arthritis, variety of cutaneous lesions along with ocular, gastrointestinal and neurological manifestations. This condition was first described by the Turkish dermatologist Hulusi Behcet in 1937.

Aetiology

Although the exact cause is unknown, there is strong genetic predisposition with association with HLA-B5 (Bw5I). In addition, there are various immunological abnormalities such as suppressor T-cell dysfunction, increased polymorphonuclear leucocyte motility and abnormal NK-cell activity. Circulating immune-complexes and vasculitis suggest some unknown antigenic trigger.

Clinical Features

The International Study Group criteria for the diagnosis for Behcet's disease are the presence of recurrent oral ulcers; minor, major or herpetiform aphthae that recurred at least 3 times in one year; plus two of the following criteria: recurrent genital ulceration, eye lesions as anterior uveitis, posterior uveitis or retinal vasculitis as observed by ophthalmologist, cutaneous lesions as erythema nodosum, pseudofolliculitis, papulo-pustular lesions or acneform nodules, and a positive pathergy test.[14]

Other cutaneous presentations are pyoderma-like lesions, necrotizing vasculitic ulcers and thrombophlebitis. The gastrointestinal and neurological manifestations include thrombosis of major vessels, gastroinstestinal perforations, meningo-myelitis, brain stem syndrome and dementia.

Oral or genital aphthae are required features for the diagnosis of Behcet's disease, and they are often the presenting manifestations. The most common site for genital aphthae is the scrotum in males and vulva in females **(Fig. 40.11)**. Other sites are shaft of the penis and perineum. A typical ulcer is painful, 1-3 cm in diameter, shallow or deep, and has a yellow fibrous base. The other types of ulcers are major aphthae (large sized with necrotic changes) and herpetiform ulceration. The major aphthae heal with scarring **(Fig 40.12)**. The minor aphthae and herpetiform aphthae subside within 1-3 weeks, whereas the larger ulcers subside over weeks to months.[21]

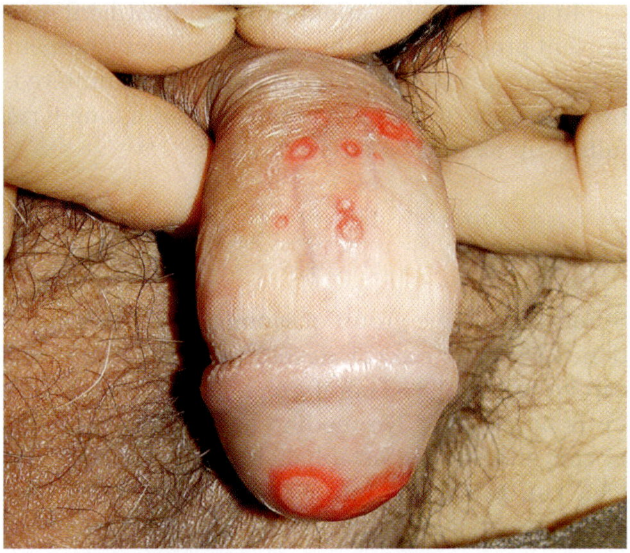

Fig. 40.11 Behcet's Disease – Multiple erythematous ulcers with central yellowish base and surrounding rim of erythema.

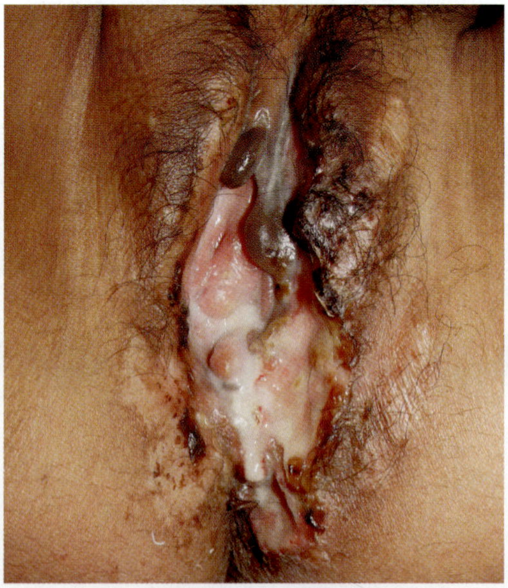

Fig. 40.12 Behcet's Disease – Major aphthous ulcer destroying the vulva with multiple healed scars.

Differential Diagnosis

These ulcers have to be differentiated from common ulcerative STDs like chancre, chancroid and herpes progenitalis. Some authors suggest that the initial presentation of Behcet's ulcer should be differentiated from ulcers of herpes with either culture or PCR. The other cutaneous manifestations associated with Behcet's disease also help in differentiating it from STDs.

Histopathology

Vasculitis and thrombosis characterize the histological features of Behcet's disease. Recent clinicopathological analysis of cutaneous lesions from patients with Behcet's disease gathered from various centres around the world confirmed that neutrophilic vasculitic reaction is a predominant histopathological finding.[21]

Treatment

If only mucocutaneous disease is present, then topical or intralesional corticosteroids are the treatment of choice. Other agents which are used according to severity and availability are colchicine, dapsone, thalidomide, low dose methotrexate, prednisolone, interferon-alpha and combination of the above drugs. Severe disease or systemic involvement would warrant treatment with immunosuppresants like cyclophosphamide, chlorambucil and cyclosporine.

Prognosis of the disease varies as the disease is known for its chronicity. Mortality is low and occurs only in severe cases with pulmonary or central nervous system involvement. Morbidity is high as severe oral and genital ulceration may be debilitating due to its chronicity and recurrence, and ocular involvement may lead to blindness.[21]

PHIMOSIS AND PARAPHIMOSIS

Phimosis is inability to retract the prepuce proximal to the coronal sulcus, and paraphimosis is the inability to cover the glans again with prepuce after retracting it. Phimosis and paraphimosis only occur in uncircumcised males. The incidence of pathological phimosis is 0.4 cases/1000 boys per year.[22]

Phimosis is caused by the adhesion of prepuce over the glans due to a variety of reasons. In young boys, if the smegma is not cleaned periodically and the prepuce is not retracted to clean the glans, then the adhesion develops slowly over the years. This can be prevented by regular cleaning of the glans as part of bathing, or if phimosis is still not too tight then gradual retraction may be done over a few days. A jet of lukewarm water or saline through the nozzle of a syringe helps in gradual correction of phimosis. Several non-venereal inflammatory or neoplastic conditions may lead to phimosis such as LSA, recurrent balanitis or balanoposthitis, candidal balanitis in diabetes, squamous cell carcinoma or genital verrucous carcinoma. Ulcerative STDs such as primary chancre can also lead to phimosis, which is temporally related and is of acute onset. If phimosis is constricting as seen in some cases of LSA or causing discomfort or pain, then circumcision is the teatment of choice. Potent topical corticosteroids are cost effective than surgery in boys less than 12 years of age. Paraphimosis is seen with acute cases of ulcerative STDs or balanoposthitis with some amount of oedema. Once the primary process is dealt with, it can be corrected or emergency circumcision may be required in more severe cases. The cause of paraphimosis can be iatrogenic quite often after penile examination, urethral catheterization or cystoscopy. The glans appears congested and enlarged with a collar of swollen foreskin behind the head of penis. Remainder of the shaft is unaffected. Both phimosis and paraphimosis may be urological emergencies. Manual pressure, ice packs, compressive elastic dressings, intralesional hyaluronidase or puncture by hypodermic needle may be used to reduce edema. If severe constricting band is formed, then emergency dorsal slit should be performed.

GENITAL TUBERCULIDS

Tuberculids are caused due to hypersensitivity reaction to an internal focus of *M. tuberculosis* infection or its constituent parts. Papulonecrotic tuberculid and lichen scrofulosorum are true tuberculids that are known to be associated with *M. tuberculosis*. When they occur exclusively on the penis, it is termed as 'penile tuberculid',[23] and when it occurs exclusively in female genitalia, it is termed as 'vulval tuberculid'[24]. Overall, genital tuberculids are rare. The criteria for diagnosing genital tuberculids are typical clinical features supported by histopathology, positive mantoux and response to antituberculosis therapy and absence of tubercle bacilli from skin biopsy or culture. A focus of tuberculosis is most often found.

Papulonecrotic Tuberculid

Papulonecrotic tuberculid is restricted to male genitalia. It presents as recurrent painless papular lesions over the glans which gradually evolve into ulcers and then heal with depressed scars over a period of 2–3 months. The combination of varioliform scars and firm indurated papules is quite suggestive of the diagnosis **(Fig. 40.13)**. A 'worm-eaten' pattern of the scars has also been described.[25] Occasionally, only a single subcutaneous nodule with scab may be the only finding.[26] Histopathology of a papule shows wedge-shaped area of dermoepidermal necrosis surrounded by epithelioid cell granulomas with Langhan's giant cells, neutrophils and fibrinoid necrosis of blood vessels.

Lichen Scrofulosorum

In lichen scrofulosorum, usually generalized lesions are present, and rarely lesions may occur on genitalia as well.[27,28] However, multiple tiny discrete papules restricted to genitalia have been reported.[24] Underlying tuberculosis can be found in lymph nodes, bones and lung. On biopsy, perifollicular and perieccrine epithelioid cell granuloma with Langhan's giant cell is seen. Caseation is a rare finding.

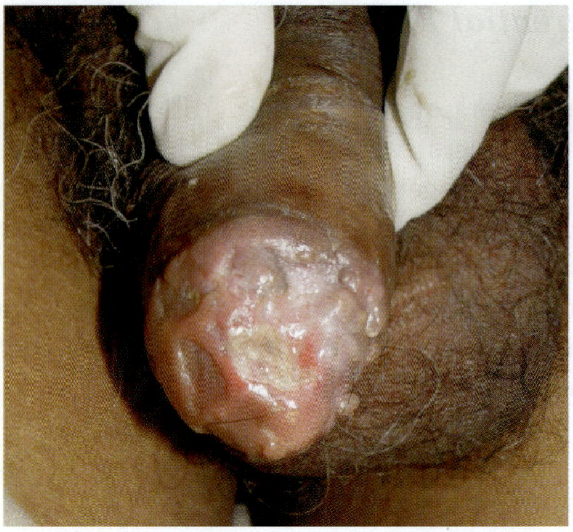

Fig. 40.13 Papulonecrotic tuberculide - Necrotic ulcer with bridging scars on the glans.

Management of Genital Tuberculid

The diagnosis must be confirmed by histopathology, positive mantoux test and absence of *M. tuberculosis* on biopsy and culture. Underlying focus of tuberculosis should be looked for by chest X-ray, raised ESR, urine microscopy for acid fast bacilli and ultrasound abdomen. Tuberculids respond to standard antitubercular therapy which must be started after complete hemogram, hepatic and renal function tests.

REFERENCES

1. Agrawal SK, Bhattacharya SN, Singh N. Pearly penile papules: a review. Int J Dermatol 2004; 43: 199-201.
2. Pryor J, Akkus E, Alter G, et al. Peyronie's disease. J Sex Med 2004; 1: 110-5.
3. Levine LA, Goldman KE, Greenfield JM. Experience with intraplaque injection of verapamil for Peyronie's disease. J Urol 2002; 168: 621-5.
4. Lebret T, Loison G, Herve JM, et al. Extracorporeal shock wave therapy in the

treatment of Peyronie's disease: experience with standard lithotriptor (Siemens- multiline). Urology 2002; 59: 657-61.

5. Gholami SS, Lue TF. Correction of penile curvature using the 16-dot plication technique: A review of 132 patients. J Urol 2002, 167: 2066-9.
6. Ive FA. The umbilical, perianal and genital regions. In, Champion RH, Burton JL, Burns DA, Breathnach SM. eds. Rook/Wilkinson/Ebling Textbook of Dermatology. Sixth edition. Oxford: Blackwell Science; 1998. p. 3163-238.
7. Pelisse M. The vulvo-vaginal-gingival syndrome. A new form of erosive lichen planus. Int J Dermatol 1989; 28: 381-4.
8. Yoshida M, Maeyama Y, Yasumoto S, et al. Vulvo-vaginal-gingival syndrome of lichen planus. Int J Dermatol 2006; 45: 1252-4.
9. Byrd JA, Davis MD, Rogers RS Recalcitrant symptomatic vulvar lichen planus: response to topical tacrolimus. Arch Dermatol 2004; 140: 715-20.
10. Lonsdale-Eccles AA, Velangi S. Topical pimecrolimus in the treatment of genital lichen planus: a prospective case series. Br J Dermatol 2005; 153: 390-4.
11. Sonteyrand P, Wong E, MacDonald DM. Zoon's balanitis (balanitis circumscripta plasma cellularis). Br J Dermatol 1981; 105: 195-9.
12. Ferrandiz C, Ribera M. Zoon's balanitis treated by circumcision. J Dematol Surg Oncol 1984; 10: 622-5.
13. Baldwin HE, Geronemus RG. The treatment of Zoon's balanitis with the carbon dioxide laser. J Dematol Surg Oncol 1989; 15: 491-4.
14. Roé E, Dalmau J, Peramiquel L, et al. Plasma cell balanitis of Zoon treated with topical tacrolimus 0.1%: report of three cases. J Eur Acad Dermatol Venereol 2007; 21: 284-5.
15. Sehgal VN, Gangwani OP. Genital fixed drug eruptions. Genitourin Med 1986; 62: 56-8.
16. Gaffoor PM, George WM. Fixed drug eruption occurring on the male genitalia. Cutis 1990; 45: 242-4.
17. Powell JJ, Wojnarowska F. Lichen sclerosus. Lancet 1999; 353: 1777-83.
18. Fung MA, LeBiot PE. Light microscopic criteria for the diagnosis of early vulvar lichen sclerosus. A comparison with lichen planus. Am J Surg Pathol 1998; 22: 473-8.
19. Carlson JA, Ambros R, Malfetano J, et al. Vulvar lichen sclerosis and squamous cell carcinoma: A cohort case-control and investigational study with historical perspective and sclerosis in the development of neoplasia. Hum Pathol 1998; 29: 932-48.
20. Simonart T, Noel JC, De Dobbeleer, et al. Carcinoma of the glans penis arising after 20 years of lichen sclerosus. Dermatology 1998; 196: 337-8.
21. Ghate JV, Jori JL. Behcet's disease and complex aphthosis. J Am Acad Dermatol 1999; 40: 1-18.
22. Shankar KR, Rickwood AM. The incidence of phimosis in boys. BJU Int 1999; 84: 101-2.
23. Aires NB, Santi CG, Nico MMS. Tuberculid of the glans penis. Acta Derm Venereol 2006; 86: 552-3.
24. Pandhi D, Mehta S, Singal A. Genital tuberculid in a female child: A new entity (Childhood vulval tuberculid). Pediatr Dermatol 2007; 24: 573–5.
25. Srivastava N, Solanki LS, Singh SP, et al. Papulonecrotic tuberculid of the glans: worm-eaten appearance. Int J Dermatol 2007; 46: 1324-5.
26. Yonemura S, Fujikawa S, Su JS, et al. Tuberculid of the penis with a scab on the nodule. Intl J Urol 2004; 11: 931-3.
27. Gandhi V, Vij A, Bhattacharya SN. Lichen scrofulosorum on the genitalia - an unusual presentation. Int J Dermatol 2007; 46: 548-9.
28. Thami GP, Kaur S, Kanwar AJ, et al. Lichen scrofulosorum: a rare manifestation of a common disease. Pediatr Dermatol 2002; 19: 122-6.

41 PREMALIGNANT AND MALIGNANT LESIONS OF GENITALIA

M Ramam, Jyoti Dhawan

In this chapter

INTRODUCTION

Even though STDs are considered synonymous with infections, it is important for students of this discipline to be aware of genital neoplasms for two reasons. First, patients often report with genital malignancies to a STD practitioner and knowledge about these conditions will result in early diagnosis and appropriate management. Second, there is considerable evidence that sexual exposure is related to the development of genital neoplasm,[1-3] and thus these conditions fall within the purview of STDs.

DEFINITION

There is no universally accepted definition of premalignant conditions, and lately some workers have contested the concept and stated that the so-called precancers are in fact cancers that have an indolent course and a low potential for metastasis.[4,5] As a clinical concept, premalignancy is used to denote conditions that, if left untreated, progress to invasive malignancy with the potential for metastasis. Most genital conditions that are widely accepted as premalignant represent intraepidermal or intraepithelial neoplasias. In recent reports, these are referred to as intraepithelial neoplasias with a prefix indicating the site such as cervical, vulvar, vaginal, penile or anal. Older terms for these conditions include bowenoid papulosis, erythroplasia of Queyrat and Bowen's disease. Two other conditions have been included as premalignant conditions in this chapter: Buschke-Lowenstein tumour, a disease whose position between infection and neoplasia is not settled, and lichen sclerosus et atrophicus, an inflammatory condition that may be associated with the development of neoplasia in some cases.

Squamous cell carcinomas are by far the commonest genital malignancy. Other malignant tumours that may develop on the genitals include basal cell carcinoma, malignant melanoma and sarcomas. A list of premalignant and malignant conditions considered in this account is given in Table 41.1.

Table 41.1 Premalignant and Malignant Lesions of Genitalia

Premalignant
Bowen's disease
Bowenoid papulosis
Subclinical (colposcopically visualized) lesions
Extramammary Paget's disease
Buschke-Lowenstein tumour
Lichen sclerosus et atrophicus
Malignant
Squamous cell carcinoma
Basal cell carcinoma
Malignant melanoma
Connective tissue tumours ("sarcomas")

AETIOPATHOGENESIS

The relation between genital malignancies and sexually transmitted agents is strongest in cervical cancer[1] but has also been implicated in the cancer of the anus,[2] vulva[3] and penis.[7] Nuns have low mortality from cervical cancer;[1] there is a strong association between the total number of sex partners and cervical neoplasia[8] and also with the total number of sex partners of the male partner.[9] Similar, but weaker, associations were noted for penile[7] and anal cancer.[2] These associations led to the search for the causative organism, and over the years many agents were considered including *Treponema pallidum*,[10] *Neisseria gonorrhoeae*,[11] *Trichomonas vaginalis*,[12] *Gardnerella vaginalis*[13] and Herpes simplex virus type 2 (HSV 2).[14] In the last two decades, evidence has accumulated linking the human papilloma virus (HPV) to genital neoplasia. HPV DNA has been demonstrated in most patients with invasive cervical cancer in many countries[15] including India.[16-18] The HPV types most frequently found in genital neoplasia are 16 and 18.[19]

It has been recognized that only a small proportion of patients affected with oncogenic HPV types go on to develop invasive neoplasias.[20] The reasons for this are not clear. An association with HIV co-infection has been reported in HPV-induced genital cancers.[21] Different variants of HPV 16 have been described, and it is unclear if some of these variants are more oncogenic than others.[22] The role of host factors has also been investigated and specific HLA class II alleles have been reported to be associated with both increased risk and protection from HPV-associated cervical cancer.[23,24]

PREMALIGNANT LESIONS

An account of morphological variants of precancerous conditions follows. In many conditions, older terminology has been retained because they are familiar to venereologists and dermatologists.

Bowen's Disease

Bowen's disease on the genital mucosa was previously described as erythroplasia of Queyrat. It is characterized by a well-defined, erythematous, crusted plaque **(Fig. 41.1, 41.2)**. On the penis, the lesion is usually situated on the glans. With time, the plaque may spread to involve the preputial skin. Similar lesions have been described on the vulva. The development of induration in the plaque signifies invasive carcinoma. The disease has been found to be associated with infection with HPV-31.[25] Extensive lesions involving penis, scrotum and inguinal canal have been reported in patients with HIV. The chances of malignant transformation increase with HIV coinfection.[26]

A biopsy reveals atypia of keratinocytes extending throughout a thickened epidermis. Keratinocytes are enlarged with large hyperchromatic nuclei and numerous mitotic figures. A number of dyskeratotic cells are seen. In about half the cases, the cells of the basal layer are not enlarged or atypical and form a palisade of small cells below the remainder of atypical keratinocytes, the so-called eyeliner sign. The surface may be eroded or covered with a parakeratotic crust. A dense band of lymphocytes is frequently present in the papillary dermis.

There may be temporary improvement with the application of topical corticosteroids. Other agents such as topical imiquimod,[27] 5-fluorouracil, electrodessication, cryotherapy, photodynamic therapy[28] and radiotherapy have been reported to be useful. Excision of the lesion is the definitive treatment. Invasive carcinoma has been concurrently found in 10% of cases in one series.[29] If invasion develops, the lesion should be treated like a squamous cell carcinoma. Perianal Bowen's disease has a higher risk of invasion and recurrence, and thus a wider excision and prolonged follow-up is required in these lesions.[30,31]

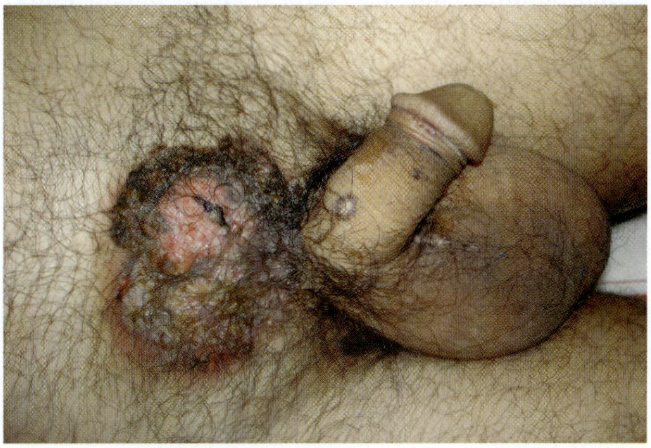

Fig. 41.1 Bowen's Disease – Crusted, eroded plaque involving suprapubic area and the penis.

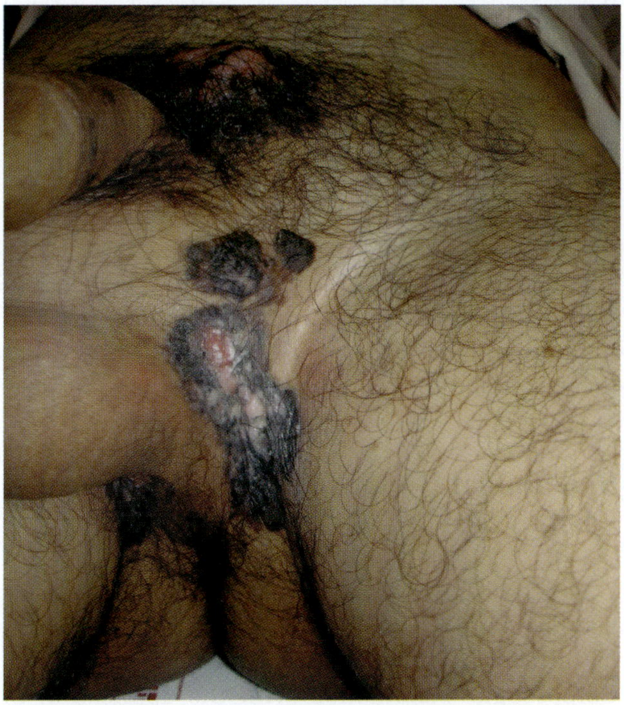

Fig. 41.2 Bowen's Disease – Eroded plaque in the groin.

Bowenoid Papulosis

Bowenoid papulosis is characterized by multiple, brown, small, 2-10 mm, slightly elevated papules. The colour may vary from that of skin colour to brown, erythematous to violaceous **(Fig. 26.7)**. The lesions are asymptomatic and have often been present for long periods of time before the patient comes to medical attention. The surface is slightly verrucous in some papules but may be smooth. Some papules coalesce to form small plaques, and there may be mild scaling on the surface. In men the papules are usually present on the penile shaft and glans, and in women on the perianal area and the vulva. Occasionally lesions may occur on extragenital sites and even oral mucosa.[32,33] DNA of high-risk HPV-16, 18 and 31 may be detected in the lesions.[25]

Biopsy of a papule reveals unexpectedly atypical findings in these banal lesions. The epidermis is thickened and hyperkeratotic with focal parakeratosis. There may be necrotic and dyskeratotic keratinocytes. There is a crowding of the nuclei of keratinocytes which are large, hyperchromatic and pleomorphic. Mitoses are frequent and some are atypical. Koilocytes are uncommon. The histopathological features are identical to erythroplasia of Queyrat and Bowen's disease although some authors have stated that cytologic atypia is less severe in Bowenoid papulosis.[34]

Invasive carcinoma is distinctly rare and spontaneous regression has been reported.[35,36]

The papules may be destroyed by any physical (electrocautery, cryotherapy, laser) or chemical (podophyllin, trichloroacetic acid) modality with equally good results. Recurrence may develop in some patients. The use of topical cidofovir[37] and imiquimod[38] has also been described recently, but these compounds require further evaluation.

Subclinical (Colposcopically Visualized) Lesions

Unaided visual examination of the genital tract has been shown to have little success in the detection of intraepithelial neoplasia especially in women. Colposcopic examination with the application of acetic acid is useful in finding suspicious lesions, which may be further investigated by exfoliative cytology or biopsy. If dysplasia detected is low-grade, no treatment is required and regular follow-up is recommended. If high-grade dysplasia including intraepithelial neoplasia is detected, excision by surgery or laser is the treatment of choice. Other modalities that have been described include application of 5-FU, electrodessication, cryotherapy and radiotherapy.

Extramammary Paget's Disease

This extremely rare condition presents as an itchy, red, scaly plaque in the anogenital region of patients who are usually older than 50. In most cases, the condition represents an intraepidermal adenocarcinoma with no other association; invasive carcinoma was reported in 12% and an associated vulval adenocarcinoma in 4%.[39] About 12% of patients have an associated underlying malignancy.[40]

Biopsy reveals large, pale atypical cells in the epidermis, arranged singly or in clusters. The nuclei of the cells are hyperchromatic, and abnormal mitotic figures may be visible. Neoplastic cells may extend down the hair follicles and sweat glands. These pale cells are called Paget cells and contain mucin, which is not seen in normal epidermis. Mucin immunohistochemistry thus is helpful in the diagnosis and characterization of extramammary Paget's disease.[41]

The standard treatment is wide excision, but recently, conservative vulva-sparing surgery has been recommended although recurrences are more frequent with the latter.[42] Non-surgical modalities like topical imiquimod and photodynamic therapy can be used if no underlying malignancy is detected.[43] A combination of topical retinoids, 5FU and imiquimod was effective in a case resistant to imiquimod alone.[44] The prognosis is excellent in cases that are not associated with an underlying adnexal or visceral tumour.

Buschke-Lowenstein Tumour

Buschke-Lowenstein tumour, otherwise known as giant condyloma accuminatum, presents as asymptomatic, papillomatous growth on the genitalia or perianal area that grows to a large size **(Fig. 41.3, 41.4)**. Most lesions are 5 cm or more in diameter at the time of presentation. The surface and consistency of the lesion is variegated: soft areas have a papillomatous surface while hard areas have a smoother surface. Typical cutaneous and mucosal warts may be present adjacent to the mass. Maceration and secondary infection are frequent in uncircumcised men. Local invasion of the tumour may lead to perforation of the prepuce and extension into the deeper structures of the glans leading to induration. Giant condyloma acuminatum affecting the urinary bladder in a patient with multiple sclerosis on immunosuppressives has been described.[45] Low-risk HPV types 6 or 11 are found in association with this tumour.[46]

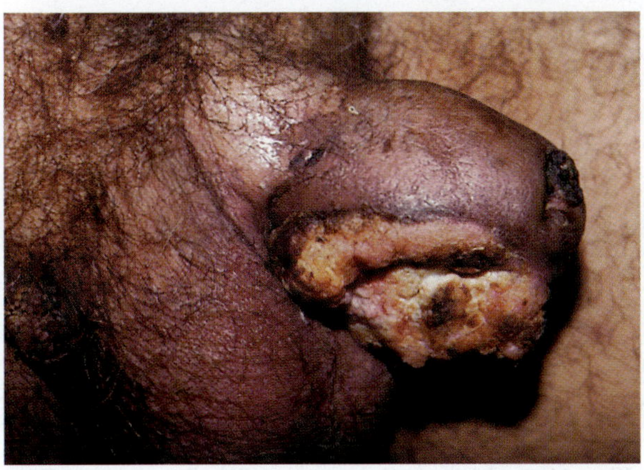

Fig. 41.3 Buschke-Lowenstein Tumour – Penis.

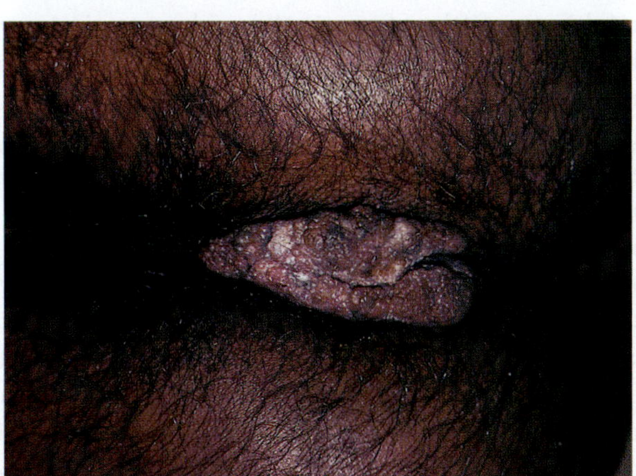

Fig. 41.4 Buschke-Lowenstein Tumour - Perianal area.

Biopsy shows a poorly circumscribed, epidermal growth that is both exophytic and endophytic, and extends deeper into the dermis than adjacent normal epidermis. An important histopathological feature is the absence of significant atypia of keratinocytes. Dense dermal inflammation is usually seen. These patients often undergo multiple biopsies to rule out a malignancy because the clinician sees a large, invasive growth while the pathologist finds no atypia or dysplasia indicative of malignancy. Human papilloma virus-induced changes of vacuolization of the cells of the granular layer with clumping of coarse keratohyaline granules are usually absent in the main lesion, but may be observed in the adjacent, smaller warts.

The exact position of Buschke-Lowenstein tumour in the spectrum of benign and malignant lesions is not established. It grows larger and deeper than typical genital warts and tends to persist for longer. Some authors believe the tumour represents verrucous carcinoma, a locally invasive carcinoma that tends not to metastasize.[47]

In a study of 42 cases of Buschke-Lowenstein tumour affecting the anorectal and perianal region, the tendency for local recurrence was seen in upto 66%. The recurrence was associated with longer duration of the disease. Malignant transformation was reported in 56% and metastasis was rare.[48] Recently it has been proposed that if tumours are confined to the glans, a glansectomy can be carried out in place of amputation to preserve maximal penile length and functional integrity of corpora cavernosa. Patients were able to resume sexual activity one month post-operatively and no recurrence was observed in 18 to 65 months of follow-up.[49] Other workers have administered interferon α post-operatively or into the lesion to prevent recurrence.[50] In our experience and that of others,[51] the lesion may respond partially to podophyllin. The frequency of application may need to be increased above the usual schedule of once-weekly applications and we have used alternate-day application in some patients. However, this course is not advisable for lesions in the perianal area or if the patient is unable to carry out instructions as misuse of the agent can lead to severe oedema and ulceration. There may be a reduction in the size of tumour with this therapy. However, complete clearance with podophyllin alone is uncommon and the residual lesion may require excision or cryotherapy. In our opinion, amputation of the genitalia is unwarranted because of the indolent course of the disease and the response to simpler modalities of treatment. Imiquimod is a newer agent which can be used for debulking of the tumour but requires further evaluation.[52] Regular follow-up is necessary to monitor for recurrences and local invasion.

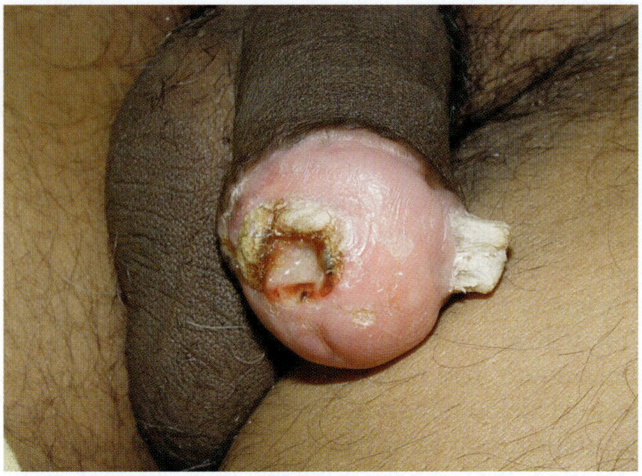

Fig. 41.5 Lichen Sclerosus with Squamous Cell Carcinoma and Cutaneous Horn.

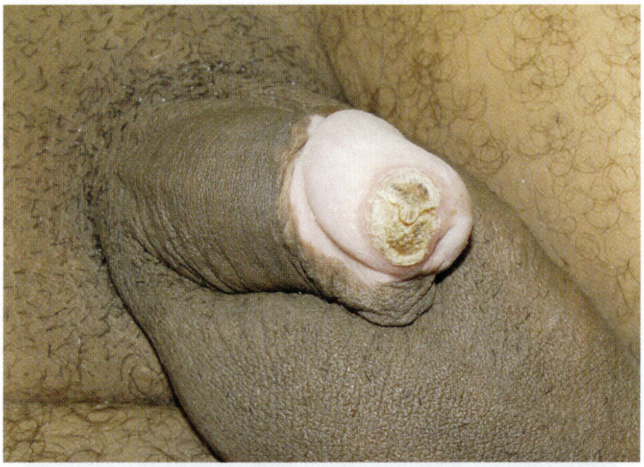

Fig. 41.6 Lichen Sclerosus with Squamous Cell Carcinoma.

Lichen Sclerosus et Atrophicus

Lichen sclerosus et atrophicus is a disease of unknown aetiology with a predilection for genital skin. It occurs in both sexes but appears to be commoner in women. There are two age groups in which the disease is common: prepubertal children and older men and women. The well-developed lesion is a shiny, hypopigmented atrophic plaque with underlying sclerosis. Telangiectasias and purpuras may be visible on the surface. The papules and plaques may enlarge and encircle the vulval orifice in women or the preputial opening in men. In men, this constriction leads to phimosis and predisposes to injury during coitus. There may be meatal stenosis with restriction of the urinary stream. In women, the mucosal surface may show fissuring. The perianal skin may also be affected. Some patients also have lesions at other, non-genital sites. The disease has been associated with HPV infection, and "high-risk" HPV types in patients with genital disease may enhance the risk of penile cancer **(Figs. 41.5, 41.6)**.[53]

A skin biopsy reveals oedema and sclerosis of the papillary dermis. The overlying epidermis shows atrophy and follicular plugging. There is vacuolization of the basal layer. A band-like infiltrate of lymphocytes is seen in the upper dermis just below the zone of oedema and sclerosis. In older lesions, oedema is less prominent, the basal layer is reconstituted, the infiltrate diminishes and sclerosis extends into the reticular dermis. At this stage, the changes may be indistinguishable from morphoea.

Early in disease, clobetasol propionate produces significant softening of the skin and completely reverses the skin changes in the vulva in approximately one-fifth of patients and may improve phimosis in men.[54] Once symptoms and signs are relieved, therapy can be maintained with mild to moderate potent topical steroids. Treatment with topical tacrolimus and pimecrolimus has also led to a significant reduction in itching, erythema and induration in a few trials.[55,56] UVA1 and CO_2 laser therapy may be of benefit in the management of recalcitrant lichen sclerosus poorly responsive to standard therapies.[57,58] There are anecdotal reports of use of testosterone and progesterone in the disease without much benefit.[59,60] If phimosis is unresponsive to treatment, circumcision may be considered so that the glans can be visualized and monitored.

The lesions must be monitored at regular intervals for the development of squamous cell carcinoma. The risk of developing cancer is widely recognized in women, and a cohort study found that invasive carcinoma developed in 21% of women with symptomatic lichen sclerosus.[61] A recent study has suggested that men may also have an increased risk for developing squamous cell carcinoma.[62,63]

MALIGNANT LESIONS

Squamous Cell Carcinoma of Penis and Vulva

Squamous cell carcinoma is the commonest neoplasm of the genital tract in both men and women. The incidence of penile cancer varies considerably from one population to another, and is reported to be highest in Uganda and lowest in Israel.[64] Epidemiological data for India is not available but the disease is not uncommon. The risk factors for developing penile cancer reported in different studies include phimosis, chronic balanoposthitis, lichen sclerosus et atrophicus, condyloma accuminata, multiple sexual partners and smoking.[65] Neonatal circumcision is protective[7,66-70] but circumcision after the first year appears not to provide any significant reduction in risk. Treatments with PUVA and UVB have been associated with penile cancer in Western populations,[51] but it is unlikely that these findings are relevant to Indian patients. HPV DNA has been detected in about 40 to 80% of cases.[6,71]

The condition presents as an asymptomatic, indurated papule or nodule that may be ulcerated. Early lesions may be mistaken for a sexually transmitted infection especially donovanosis, and it is imperative to consider the diagnosis of penile cancer in patients with long-standing ulcers or those recalcitrant to treatment. If neglected, the nodule progresses into an exophytic mass with necrosis and secondary infection **(Figs. 41.7, 41.8)**.

Squamous cell carcinoma of the vulva presents with firm, indurated papules and nodules which may ulcerate. As in men, a high index of suspicion in ulcers that do not behave as expected will prevent misdiagnosis of vulval carcinoma.

Metastasis to regional lymph nodes is common in both penile and vulval carcinoma and has been reported in about 60[72] and 30%[73] of cases respectively.

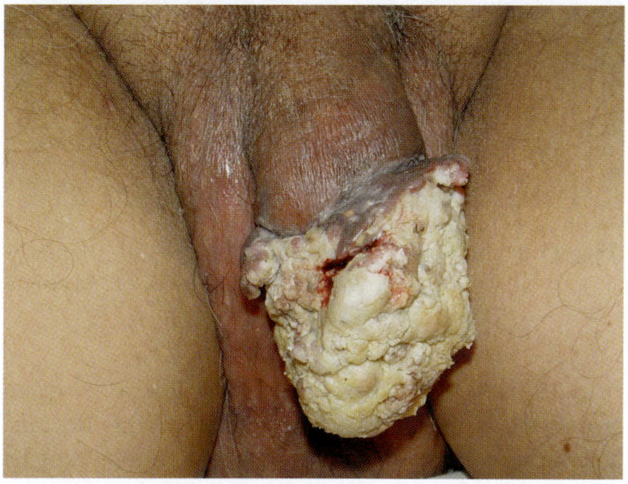

Fig. 41.7 Squamous Cell Carcinoma of Penis – Exophytic Growth.

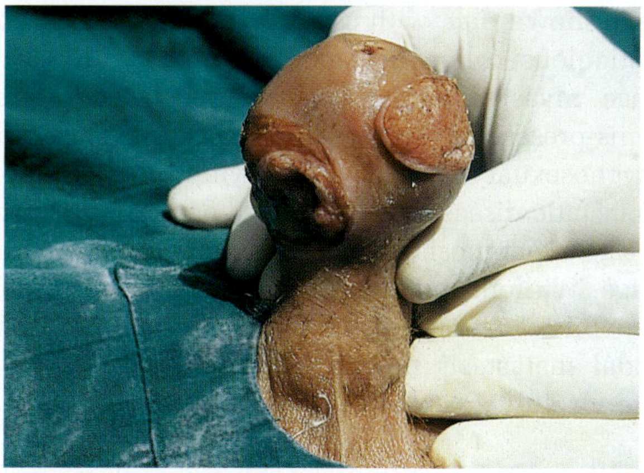

Fig. 41.8 Squamous Cell Carcinoma – Eroding the Glans.

The diagnosis is confirmed by biopsy which demonstrates nests of atypical keratinocytes extending into the dermis **(Fig. 41.9)**. The tumour shows varying degrees of differentiation; well-differentiated tumours show mature keratinocytes with intercellular bridges and multiple horn pearls while undifferentiated tumours show cells with a high nuclear-cytoplasmic ratio, few intercellular

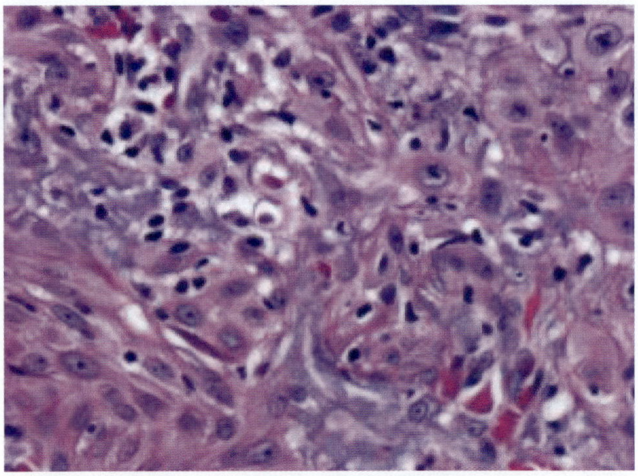

Fig. 41.9 Squamous Cell Carcinoma of Penis – Photomicrograph of Nodules of Atypical Keratinocytes in the Dermis.

bridges and little keratinization. There is often a dense infiltrate of lymphocytes in the dermis. The involvement of regional lymph nodes can be assessed by fine needle aspiration cytology.

The treatment consists of excision of the tumour with a 2 cm margin. On the penis, this implies partial or complete amputation, but recent studies have shown that, with careful patient selection and meticulous follow-up, most patients with early-stage invasive penile carcinoma can be offered penis-preserving surgery to reduce physical and psychosexual morbidity.[74] If lymph nodes show metastatic disease, lymphadenectomy is indicated.

The prognosis depends on tumour size and stage. Without metastasis, the 5-year survival rate in penile cancer is 60-90%, while it is 10-30% when nodal metastasis develops.[72] The 5-year survival rate for vulval carcinoma is about 70%.[75]

Other Malignancies

Malignancies of the genital tract other than squamous cell carcinoma are distinctly uncommon.

Basal Cell Carcinoma

Less than 200 cases of basal cell carcinomas have been reported on the genitals and perianal area, and represent less than 1% of all basal cell carcinomas.[76,77] HPV does not appear to play a role in the development of these tumours.[76,78,79] The carcinoma occurs in older patients in the fifth to tenth decades. At presentation, the lesion is usually large in size and is ulcerated in about a third of patients. Biopsy reveals aggregates of basaloid cells with peripheral palisading and clefts between the aggregates and the stroma. Excision is the treatment of choice, and the 5-year survival rate approaches 100%.[76]

Malignant Melanoma

Melanomas of the penis and vulva are rare and comprise about 1[80] and 4-10%[81] of all malignancies at these sites, respectively. The tumour usually presents as a pigmented macule or nodule; some lesions may be non-pigmented. Biopsy of the nodule reveals a poorly circumscribed lesion with atypical melanocytes within the epidermis and in irregular nests and aggregates in the dermis that vary in size and pigmentation. The melanocytes have large nuclei with prominent nucleoli and do not diminish in size with descent into the dermis. Wide local excision with a clear surgical margin is the treatment of choice. Lymphadenectomy is indicated if there is spread of disease to the lymph nodes. As with other cutaneous melanomas, prognosis depends on the stage of disease. The prognosis is good for stage I lesions with a 5-year survival rate of more than 90% and poor for patients with thick tumours and metastatic disease who have a 5-year survival rate of 30% or less.[82,83]

Sarcomas

Sarcomas of the genitals are extremely uncommon and are beyond the scope of this chapter. The interested reader is referred to a comprehensive account of these tumours.[84]

HIV AND ANOGENITAL MALIGNANCIES

HIV infection predisposes to the development and progression of anogenital neoplasias in both men and women. There is a higher incidence of anal squamous intraepithelial lesions and anal cancer in men infected with HIV. In a cross-sectional study of 211 HIV infected males, 90 (60%) had abnormal anal cytology, including atypical cells of unknown significance in 40 (26%), low-grade squamous intraepithelial lesions in 28 (19%), and high-grade squamous intraepithelial lesions in 22 (15%) patients.[85] Another study has shown that these lesions are also seen in men who do not have receptive anal intercourse and appears to be related to HIV infection, irrespective of the mode of acquisition.[86] In addition, there was a significant correlation of anal squamous intraepithelial lesions with depressed CD4+ cell counts and anal HPV detection.[86] The progression of low-grade to high-grade squamous intraepithelial lesions is higher in HIV-positive homosexual or bisexual men than in HIV-negative men.[87]

Similarly, there is a higher incidence of cervical squamous intraepithelial lesions and cancer in women infected with HIV. Cervical intraepithelial neoplasia was detected by cytological examination in 42% of 273 HIV-positive women and 8% of 161 HIV-negative women; half of the cases found in the HIV-positive group were high-grade lesions.[88] HIV-positive women with severe immunosuppression (defined as CD4+ cell count below 500×10^6/L) are at greatest risk of cervical intraepithelial neoplasia.[89] The presence of these lesions is a significant risk factor for genital HIV shedding.[90] The risk of recurrence or progression of low-grade squamous intraepithelial neoplasia is about 4-5 times higher in women who are HIV-positive.[91] Similarly, vulval intraepithelial lesions are more likely to progress to invasive carcinoma in HIV-positive women.[92] Interestingly, antiretroviral therapy protects against the development of genital dysplasia.[93,94] Therapy also appears to decrease the risk of progression from vulvar intraepithelial lesions to invasive vulvar carcinoma in HIV-1positive women.[95]

REFERENCES

1. Fraumeni JF Jr, Lloyd JW, Smith EM, et al. Cancer mortality among nuns: role of marital status in aetiology of neoplastic disease in women. J Natl Cancer Inst 1969; 42: 455-68.
2. Daling JR, Weiss NS, Hislop TG, et al. Sexual practices, sexually transmitted diseases, and the incidence of anal cancer. N Engl J Med 1987; 317: 973-7.
3. Newcomb PA, Weiss NS, Daling JR. Incidence of vulvar carcinoma in relation to menstrual, reproductive, and medical factors. J Natl Cancer Inst 1984; 73: 391-6.
4. Lober BA, Lober CW. Actinic keratosis is squamous cell carcinoma. South Med J 2000; 93: 650-5.
5. Ackerman AB, Vassallo. Conversion or transformation into cancer. In: Ackerman AB, Mones J. edrs Resolving quandaries in dermatology, pathology and dermatopathology. New York: Ardor Scribendi; 2001. p. 110-3.
6. Rubin MA, Kleter B, Zhou M, et al. Detection and typing of human papillomavirus DNA in penile carcinoma: evidence for multiple independent pathways of penile carcinogenesis. Am J Pathol 2001; 159: 1211-8.
7. Maden C, Sherman KJ, Beckmann AM, et al. History of circumcision, medical conditions, and sexual activity and risk of penile cancer. J Natl Cancer Inst 1993, 85: 19-24.
8. Hulka BS. Risk factors for cervical cancer. J Chronic Dis 1982; 35: 3-11.
9. Buckley JD, Henderson BE, Morrow CP, et al. Case-control study of gestational choriocarcinoma. Cancer Res. 1988; 48: 1004-10.
10. Rojel J. The interrelation between uterine cancer and syphilis: a pathodemographic study. Acta Pathol Microbiol Scand 1953; 97: 1-82.
11. Furgyik S, Astedt B. Gonorrhoeal infection followed by an increased frequency of cervical carcinoma. Acta Obstet Gynecol Scand 1980; 59: 521-4.

12. Zhang ZF, Graham S, Yu SZ, et al. *Trichomonas vaginalis* and cervical cancer. A prospective study in China. Ann Epidemiol. 1995; 5: 325-32.
13. Frega A, Stentella P, Spera G, et al. Cervical intraepithelial neoplasia and bacterial vaginosis: correlation or risk factor? Eur J Gynaecol Oncol 1997; 18: 76-7.
14. Olsen AO, Orstavik I, Dillner J et al. Herpes simplex virus and human papillomavirus in a population-based case-control study of cervical intraepithelial neoplasia grade II-III. APMIS 1998; 106: 417-24.
15. Bosch FX, Manos MM, Munoz N, et al. Prevalence of human papillomavirus in cervical cancer: a worldwide perspective. International biological study on cervical cancer (IBSCC) study group. J Natl Cancer Inst 1995, 87: 796-802.
16. Saranath D, Khan Z, Tandle AT, et al. HPV16/18 prevalence in cervical lesions/cancers and p53 genotypes in cervical cancer patients from India. Gynecol Oncol 2002; 86: 157-62.
17. Gopalkrishna V, Aggarwal N, Malhotra VL, et al. *Chlamydia trachomatis* and human papillomavirus infection in Indian women with sexually transmitted diseases and cervical precancerous and cancerous lesions. Clin Microbiol Infect 2000; 6: 88-93.
18. Chatterjee R, Roy A, Basu S. Detection of type specific human papillomavirus (HPV) DNA in cervical cancers of Indian women. Indian J Pathol Microbiol 1995; 38: 33-42.
19. Wilczynski SP, Walker J, Liao SY et al. M. Adenocarcinoma of the cervix associated with human papillomavirus. Cancer 1988; 62: 1331-6.
20. Helmerhorst TJ, Meijer CJ. Cervical cancer should be considered as a rare complication of oncogenic HPV infection rather than a STDs. Int J Gynecol Cancer 2002; 12: 235-6.
21. Frisch M, Biggar RJ, Goedert JJ. Human papillomavirus-associated cancers in patients with human immunodeficiency virus infection and acquired immunodeficiency syndrome. J Natl Cancer Inst 2000; 92: 1500-10.
22. Da Costa MM, Hogeboom CJ, Holly EA, Palefsky JM. Increased risk of high-grade anal neoplasia associated with a human papillomavirus type 16 E6 sequence variant. J Infect Dis 2002; 185: 1229-37.
23. Odunsi K, Ganesan T. Motif analysis of HLA class II molecules that determine the HPV associated risk of cervical carcinogenesis. Int J Mol Med 2001; 8: 405-12.
24. Odunsi K, Terry G, Ho L, et al. Susceptibility to human papillomavirus-associated cervical intra-epithelial neoplasia is determined by specific HLA DR-DQ alleles. Int J Cancer 1996; 67: 595-602.
25. Hama N, Ohtsuka T, Yamazaki S. Detection of mucosal human papilloma virus DNA in bowenoid papulosis, Bowen's disease and squamous cell carcinoma of the skin. J Dermatol. 2006; 33: 331-7.
26. Schmitz MW, Goldberg LJ, Adler AJ. An extensive case of Bowen's disease in an HIV-positive male. AIDS Patient Care STDS. 2007; 21: 78-80.
27. Peris K, Micantonio T, Fargnoli MC, et al. Imiquimod 5% cream in the treatment of Bowen's disease and invasive squamous cell carcinoma. J Am Acad Dermatol 2006; 55: 324-7.
28. Axcrona K, Brennhovd B, Alfsen GC et al. Photodynamic therapy with methyl aminolevulinate for atypia/carcinoma in situ of the penis. Scand J Urol Nephrol 2007; 21: 1-4.
29. Graham JH, Helwig EB. Erythroplasia of Queyrat. A clinicopathologic and histochemical study. Cancer 1973; 32: 1396-1414.
30. Sarmiento JM, Wolff BG, Burgart LJ, et al. Perianal Bowen's disease: associated tumors, human papillomavirus, surgery, and other controversies. Dis Colon Rectum 1997; 40: 912-8.
31. Marchesa P, Fazio VW, Oliart S, et al, Perianal Bowen's disease: a clinicopathologic study of 47 patients. Dis Colon Rectum 1997; 40: 1286-93.
32. Popadopoulos AJ, Schwartz RA, Lefkowitz A, et al. Extragenital bowenoid papulosis associated with atypical human papilloma virus genotype. J Cutan Med Surg 2002; 6: 117-21.
33. Daley T, Birek C, Wysocki GP. Oral bowenoid lesions:differential diagnosis and pathogenetic insights. Oral Surg Oral Med Oral Pathol Oral Radiol Endod 2002; 90: 466-73.

34. Patterson JW, Kao GF, Graham JH, et al. Bowenoid papulosis. A clinicopathologic study with ultrastructural observations. Cancer 1986; 57: 823-36.
35. Yoneta A, Yamashita T, Jin HY, et al. Development of squamous cell carcinoma by two high-risk human papillomaviruses (HPVs), a novel HPV-67 and HPV-31 from bowenoid papulosis. Br J Dermatol 2000; 143: 604-8.
36. Eisen RF, Bhawan J, Cahn TH. Spontaneous regression of bowenoid papulosis of the penis. Cutis 1983; 32: 269-72.
37. Snoeck R, Van Laethem Y, De Clercq E et al. Treatment of a bowenoid papulosis of the penis with local applications of cidofovir in a patient with acquired immunodeficiency syndrome. Arch Intern Med 2001; 161: 2382-4.
38. Petrow W, Gerdsen R, Uerlich M,et al. Successful topical immunotherapy of bowenoid papulosis with imiquimod. Br J Dermatol 2001; 145: 1022-3.
39. Fanning J, Lambert HC, Hale TM, et al. Paget's disease of the vulva: prevalence of associated vulvar adenocarcinoma, invasive Paget's disease, and recurrence after surgical excision. Am J Obstet Gynecol 1999; 180: 24-7.
40. Chanda JJ. Extramammary Paget's disease: prognosis and relationship to internal malignancy. J Am Acad Dermatol 1985; 13: 1009-14.
41. Smith RF, Stern BH, Smith AA. Mucin immunohistochemistry in the diagnosis and mapping of extramammary paget's disease. J Cell Mol Med 2007 Dec 10. [Epub ahead of print]
42. Louis-Sylvestre C, Haddad B, Paniel BJ. Paget's disease of the vulva: results of different conservative treatments. Eur J Obstet Gynecol Reprod Biol 2001; 99: 253-5.
43. Mirer E, El Sayed F, Ammoury A, et al. Treatment of mammary and extramammary Paget's skin disease with topical imiquimod. J Dermatolog Treat 2006; 17: 167-71.
44. Ye JN, Rhew DC, Yip F et al. Extramammary Paget's disease resistant to surgery and imiquimod monotherapy but responsive to imiquimod combination topical chemotherapy with 5-fluorouracil and retinoic acid: a case report. Cutis 2006; 77: 245-50.
45. Wioedemann A, Diekman WP, Holtmann G et al. Report of a case of giant condyloma(Buschke-Löwenstein tumour) localized in bladder. J Urol 1995; 153: 1222-4.
46. Lévy A, Lebbe C. Buschke-Löwenstein tumour: diagnosis and treatment. Ann Urol (Paris) 2006; 40: 175-8.
47. Steffen C. The men behind the eponym–Abraham Buschke and Ludwig Lowenstein: giant condyloma (Buschke-Loewenstein). Am J Dermatopathol 2006; 28: 526-36.
48. Chu QD, Vezeridis MP, Libbey NP et al. Giant condyloma acuminatum (Buschke-Löwenstein tumour) of anorectal and perianal region. Analysis of 42 cases. Dis Colon Rectum 1994; 37: 950-7.
49. Hatzichristu DG, Apostolidis A, Tzortzis V, et al. Glansectomy: an alternative surgical treatment of Buschke-Lowenstein tumour of the penis. Urology 2001; 57: 966-9.
50. Moreira PM,Perez LA, Colome EM. Giant inguinal condyloma (Buschke-Löwenstein tumour) with clinical aspect of squamous cell carcinoma. Rev Cubana Med Trop 2002; 52: 70-2.
51. Bedi TR, Pandhi RK. Buschke-Lowenstein's tumour presenting with urinary fistula. Br J Vener Dis 1977; 53: 200-2.
52. Heinzerling LM, Kempf W, Kamarashev J et al,. Treatment of verrucous carcinoma with imiquimod and CO_2 laser ablation. Dermatology. 2003; 207: 119-22.
53. Nasca MR, Innocenzi D, Micali G. Association of penile lichen sclerosus and oncogenic human papillomavirus infection. Int J Dermatol. 2006; 45: 681-3.
54. Cooper SM, Gao XH, Powell JJ, et al. Does treatment of vulvar lichen sclerosus influence its prognosis? Arch Dermatol. 2004; 140: 702-6.
55. Hengge UR, Krause W, Hofmann H, et al., Multicentre, phase II trial on the safety and efficacy of topical tacrolimus ointment for the treatment of lichen sclerosus. Br J Dermatol 2006; 155: 1021-8.
56. Nissi R, Eriksen H, Risteli J et al. Pimecrolimus cream 1% in the treatment of lichen sclerosus. Gynecol Obstet Invest 2007; 63: 151-4.

57. Beattie PE, Dawe RS, Ferguson J et al.UVA1 phototherapy for genital lichen sclerosus. Clin Exp Dermatol 2006; 31: 343-7.
58. Peterson CM, Lane JE, Ratz JL. Successful carbon dioxide laser therapy for refractory anogenital lichen sclerosus. Dermatol Surg 2004; 30: 1148-51.
59. Bornstein J, Heifetz S, Kellner Y et al. Clobetasol dipropionate 0.05% versus testosterone propionate 2% topical application for severe vulvar lichen sclerosus. Am J Obstet Gynecol 1998; 178: 80-4.
60. Bracco GL, Carli P, Sonni L, et al. Clinical and histologic effects of topical treatments of vulval lichen sclerosus. A critical evaluation. J Reprod Med 1993; 38: 37-40.
61. Carlson JA, Ambros R, Malfetano J, et al. Vulvar lichen sclerosus and squamous cell carcinoma: a cohort, case control, and investigational study with historical perspective; implications for chronic inflammation and sclerosis in the development of neoplasia. Hum Pathol 1998; 29: 932-48.
62. Powell J, Robson A, Cranston D, et al. High incidence of lichen sclerosus in patients with squamous cell carcinoma of the penis. Br J Dermatol 2001; 145: 85-9.
63. Kanwar AJ, Thami GP, Kaur S, et al. Squamous cell carcinoma in long standing untreated lichen sclerosus et atrophicus of penis. Urol Int 2002; 68: 291-5.
64. Parkin DM, Whelan SL, Ferlay J, et al. editors. IARC Scientific Publications No. 143, Vol. VII, Cancer incidence in five continents. IARC Scientific Publications, Lyon, 1997.
65. Tolstrup J, Munk C, Thomsen BL, et al. The role of smoking and alcohol intake in the development of high-grade squamous intraepithelial lesions among high-risk HPV-positive women. Acta Obstet Gynecol Scand. 2006; 85: 1114-9.
66. Tsen HF, Morgenstern H, Mack T et al. Risk factors for penile cancer: results of a population-based case-control study in Los Angeles County (United States). Cancer Causes Control 2001; 12: 267-77.
67. Maiche AG. Epidemiological aspects of cancer of the penis in Finland. Eur J Cancer Prev 1992; 1: 153-8.
68. Daling JR, Sherman KJ, Hislop TG, et al. Cigarette smoking and the risk of anogenital cancer. Am J Epidemiol 1992; 135: 180-9.
69. Brinton LA, Li JY, Rong SD, et al. Risk factors for penile cancer: results from a case-control study in China. Int J Cancer 1991; 47: 504-9.
70. Hellberg D, Valentin J, Eklund T et al. Penile cancer: is there an epidemiological role for smoking and sexual behaviour? Br Med J (Clin Res Ed) 1987; 295: 1306-8.
71. Senba M, Kumatori A, Fujita S et al. The prevalence of human papillomavirus genotypes in penile cancers from northern Thailand. J Med Virol. 2006; 78: 1341-6.
72. Srinivas V, Morse MJ, Herr HW et al. Penile cancer: relation of extent of nodal metastasis to survival. J Urol 1987; 137: 880-2.
73. Binder SW, Huang I, Fu YS et al. Risk factors for the development of lymph node metastasis in vulvar squamous cell carcinoma. Gynecol Oncol 1990; 37: 9-16.
74. Pietrzak P, Corbishley C, Watkin N. Organ-sparing surgery for invasive penile cancer: early follow-up data. BJU Int 2004; 94: 1253-7.
75. Edwards CL, Tortolero-Luna G, Linares AC, et al. Vulvar intraepithelial neoplasia and vulvar cancer. Obstet Gynecol Clin North Am 1996; 23: 295-324.
76. Gibson GE, Ahmed I. Perianal and genital basal cell carcinoma: A clinicopathologic review of 51 cases. J Am Acad Dermatol 2001; 45: 68-71.
77. Betti R, Bruscagin C, Inselvini E et al. Basal cell carcinomas of covered and unusual sites of the body. Int J Dermatol 1997; 36: 503-5.
78. Nehal KS, Levine VJ, Ashinoff R. Basal cell carcinoma of the genitalia. Dermatol Surg 1998; 24: 1361-3.
79. Kort R, Fazaa B, Bouden S, et al. Perianal basal cell carcinoma. Int J Dermatol 1995; 34: 427-8.
80. Southwick A, Rigby O, Daily M et al. Malignant melanoma of the penis and sentinel lymph node biopsy. J Urol 2001; 166: 1833.
81. Kendall Pierson K. Malignant melanoma and pigmented lesions of the vulva. In: Wilkinson EJ, edr. Pathology of the Vulva and Vagina. Edinburgh: Churchill Livingstone; 1987. p. 155-179.
82. Stillwell TJ, Zincke H, Gaffey TA et al. Malignant melanoma of the penis. J Urol 1988; 140: 72-5.

83. Verschraegen CF, Benjapibal M, Supakarapongkul W, et al. Vulvar melanoma at the M. D. Anderson Cancer Centre: 25 years later. Int J Gynecol Cancer 2001; 11: 359-64.
84. Weiss SW, Goldblum JR, Enzinger FM, eds. Enzinger and Weiss's Soft Tissue Tumours. 4th ed. St Louis: Mosby Inc; 2001.
85. Ciobotaru B, Leiman G, St John T et al. Prevalence and risk factors for anal cytologic abnormalities and human papillomavirus infection in a rural population of HIV-infected males. Dis Colon Rectum 2007; 50: 1011-6.
86. Piketty C, Darragh TM, Da Costa M et al. High prevalence of anal human papillomavirus infection and anal cancer precursors among HIV-infected persons in the absence of anal intercourse. Ann Intern Med 2003; 18: 138-144.
87. Palefsky JM, Holly EA, Hogeboom CJ et al. Virologic, immunologic, and clinical parameters in the incidence and progression of anal squamous intraepithelial lesions in HIV-positive and HIV-negative homosexual men. J Acquir Immune Defic Syndr Hum Retrovirol 1998; 17: 314-9.
88. Conti M, Agarossi A, Parazzini F et al. HPV, HIV infection, and risk of cervical intraepithelial neoplasia in former intravenous drug abusers. Gynecol Oncol 1993; 49: 344-8.
89. Harris TG, Burk RD, Palefsky JM, et al. Incidence of cervical squamous intraepithelial lesions associated with HIV serostatus, CD4 cell counts, and human papillomavirus test results. JAMA 2005; 293: 1471-6
90. Spinillo A, Zara F, Gardella B et al. Cervical intraepithelial neoplasia and cervicovaginal shedding of human immunodeficiency virus. Obstet Gynecol 2006; 107: 314-20.
91. Nappi L, Carriero C, Bettocchi S et al.Cervical squamous intraepithelial lesions of low-grade in HIV-infected women: recurrence, persistence, and progression, in treated and untreated women. Eur J Obstet Gynecol Reprod Biol 2005; 121: 226-32.
92. Conley LJ, Ellerbrock TV, Bush TJ et al. HIV-1 infection and risk of vulvovaginal and perianal condylomata acuminata and intraepithelial neoplasia: a prospective cohort study. Lancet 2002; 359: 108-13.
93. Taylor G, Wolff T, Khanna N et al. Genital dysplasia in women infected with human immunodeficiency virus. J Am Board Fam Pract 2004; 17: 108-13.
94. Minkoff H, Ahdieh L, Massad LS et al. The effect of highly active antiretroviral therapy on cervical changes associated with oncogenic HPV among HIV-infected women. AIDS 2001; 15: 2157-64.
95. Massad LS, Silverberg MJ, Springer G et al. Effect of antiretroviral therapy on the incidence of genital warts and vulvar neoplasia among women with the human immunodeficiency virus. Am J Obstet Gynecol 2004; 190: 1241-8.

PART 9

Psychological Aspects of Sexually Transmitted Diseases

42 SEXUAL BEHAVIOUR AND SEXUALLY TRANSMITTED DISEASES

B M Tripathi, Atul Ambekar

In this chapter

- Sexuality and Sexual Behaviour in Indian Context
- Sexual Knowledge, Attitude and Behaviour
- Sexual Behaviour of High Risk Populations
- Sexual Behaviour and Prevention of STDs/AIDS

INTRODUCTION

Sexual behaviour includes all activities related to the expression and gratification of sexual needs. It is an important component of the expression of one's sexuality. The term 'sexuality' is often used to refer to its various aspects like sexual behaviour, sexual orientation, gender identification and role, social roles, relationships and eroticism. Sexuality is influenced by a number of social, cultural, psychological and biological factors, and developmental experiences throughout the life cycle. Inherent complexities and issues of privacy make the study and understanding of human sexual behaviours more difficult. Sexual behaviours have been studied in the context of sexual relationships and practices, reproductive health, sexually transmitted diseases (STDs) and other reproductive tract infections, birth control and contraceptive decision-making. Sexual behaviour and practices are linked to the acquisition and spread of STDs including HIV/AIDS. In the recent years, a rising trend of STDs and HIV infection has been observed in the country. The incidence rate of STDs in India is estimated to be 5%, which means 40-50 million new infections every year.[1] Not only the number of people suffering but also the pattern of infection seems to be changing as well.[2] Currently India is the country with largest HIV epidemic in South Asia.[3,4] STDs and HIV infection are no longer restricted to the high-risk groups but have spilled over to affect the general population as well.[5] In the current context, the understanding of sexual behaviours in general population as well as in high-risk groups is important in the prevention and treatment of STDs and HIV/AIDS.

In this chapter, our discussion is restricted to the areas of (i) sexual behaviour in the Indian context of cultural and current perspective; (ii) sexual behaviour linked to sexual knowledge and attitude in general population and at-risk groups; (iii) factors associated with/contributing to high-risk sexual behaviour and in turn to the risk of acquiring or spreading STDs/HIV infection; and (iv) prevention of STDs and HIV infection.

SEXUALITY AND SEXUAL BEHAVIOUR IN INDIAN CONTEXT

Ancient Hindu literature is rich in sexual symbolism and eroticism. Vatsyayana's *Kamasutra*, (a practical discourse on aspects of sexuality)[6], erotic sculptures carved on the stone walls of holy shrines of Khajuraho, Konark, and many other Hindu temples of the medieval era beautifully depict the various techniques of sexual acts practiced during those times. Certain indications towards polygamous and polyandrous relationships from famous Indian mythological scriptures indicate a state of extraordinary openness in sexual matters in certain periods of Indian history, contrary to the periods of Muslim and British reigns and contemporary India. Prostitution as a profession has a long history in India and is mentioned in Kautilya's *Arthashastra* (circa 300 BC) and Vatsayana's *Kamasutra*.[7,8]

The *devadasi* (handmaiden of God) system of dedicating unmarried young girls to the Gods in Hindu temples, which often made them objects of sexual pleasure to temple priests and pilgrims, was an established custom in India by 300 AD. Prostitution was prevalent in large Indian cities during the eighteenth and the first half of nineteenth centuries of British rule.[9]

The practice of homosexuality was also not new to India. Vatsayana's *Kamasutra* refers to the practice of eunuchs and male servants giving oral sex to their male patrons and masters.[7-9] Some erotic sculptures of medieval Hindu temples depict lesbian acts. The Muslim rulers in India were reported to have maintained harems of young boys. During the British rule, sodomy (anal intercourse) was made illegal under section 377 of the Indian Penal Code enacted in 1861. Indian homosexual activists thought that male homosexuals are often subjected to undue harassment and blackmail because of this legal provision.

By and large, our society is still rooted in traditions and people's attitude towards sex is influenced by values which are peculiar to the traditional belief system. Marriage is a norm in India. The average age at marriage for both sexes has been rising by about a year per decade.[10] As a result, a substantial proportion of boys and girls have to pass through a long period of heightened sexual desires.[9] Our dominant value system strongly disapproves premarital sexual relations amongst males and females, and fidelity within marriage is the ideal norm. Virginity until marriage is still greatly valued. We find a custom in some communities where young boys and girls are betrothed at young age but are allowed to have sex only after the bride attains menarche, when she is sent to stay with her husband (a practice called '*gauna*'). Although unmarried men may have more opportunities for sexual adventures (often with married women/female sex workers) than unmarried women, no mainstream society in India actually encourages men to have premarital sex.[11] As is the case of premarital sex, sanctions against extramarital affairs and sex are severe against women. The Hindu concept of '*pativrata*' - the ideal for a woman to remain loyal to her husband under all circumstances, has no counterpart for men.[9] Thus, unmarried women for the fear of being called promiscuous find themselves unable to seek reproductive health services.[12] However, women are now getting greater attention towards emancipation of their sexuality. Sexual activity among unmarried adolescent women has been steadily increasing and so is the vulnerability towards STDs including HIV. Many young girls are also at risk of sexual abuse and violence including rape.[13] The issue of teenage pregnancy is of concern and is associated with significant morbidity and mortality of the mother and the child.

Gender relations in marriage are dynamic and continually negotiated. Women tend to use access to sex as a resource, a bargaining chip to reward/punish their husbands.[14] Sexual coercion occurs frequently in marriage.[15] However, women and men tend to differ in their perception of the nature of sexual coercion.[14] Women consider sex to be coerced if sexual relations with their husbands are against their wishes. Men in contrast feel that they have a right to demand sex in marriage.

Engaging in sex frequently, having multiple sex partners, having many children, and impregnating one's wife soon after marriage have been considered significant indicators of masculinity/male characteristics.[16] Women are limited in their ability to control such interactions because of their low social status and economic dependence and also because of the power men have over women's sexuality.[14-16] Women are often discriminated by their own kind.[17] In many cases, the mother-in-law often takes the decision of marriage and first pregnancy.[18]

Diseases of the genitalia are regarded as *gupt rog* (secretive ailments), sex being considered a taboo and not a topic for open discussion in the society. Ignorance about sexual matters and illiteracy foster myths and prejudices towards sex. '*Virya*' (semen) is considered to be the source of physical and spiritual strength. Loss of virya (through masturbation/nocturnal emissions or *swapnadosh*/wet dream) is considered harmful both physically and spiritually, and a cause of weakness.[7,9,19] This could be the reason for guilt feelings associated with pleasure during masturbation.[20] Our traditional systems of medicine, both Ayurveda and Unani, lay emphasis on semen preservation, sexual restraint and diet. According to metaphysical physiology, food is believed to be converted into blood and blood into semen. As a result, many beliefs and practices are prescribed to preserve and enhance the quality and quantity of semen. *Dhat syndrome*, a culture-bound syndrome in India, is characterized by the guilt about loss of semen in young men, often leading to undue concern with its debilitating effect on physical and psychological health.[21]

Social and attitudinal changes and socio-economic developments in the post-independence period have lead to the emergence of consumerist society and development of 'Western' oriented life styles. Western influence is evident in daily living, particularly in urban areas amongst the youth. The youth in major metropolitan cities often frequent pubs, late night parties and discotheques exposing themselves to risky behaviours. Recent years have seen developments in electronic media, and sex entertainment is available through video, X-rated films and internet.

Our society presents a contrasting picture of notions about sexuality, attitudes and sexual behaviour. The society can neither be regarded as rigid, nor permissive with regard to sexuality, making generalization difficult. The behaviour patterns vary across regions and states, gender, sub-populations, tribal and religious groups.

SEXUAL KNOWLEDGE, ATTITUDE AND BEHAVIOUR

Adult Population

There is low level of knowledge about body and reproductive health, including reproduction and contraception, among men and women of all ages, marital status and geographical locations in the country. Young men and adult males, as compared to young women, usually know more about certain matters pertaining to sexuality like masturbation, orgasm, sexual intercourse, oral sex and contraception.

Traditionally sexual problems are known as *gupt rog* (secretive ailments), which refer to culturally defined illnesses of secret parts of the body and are therefore need to be kept secret. Male sexual problems can be broadly categorized into contact problems (STDs), which are referred to as *garmi* in local language, and non-contact problems.[22,23] Men show great concern towards non-contact problems, viz., quality and quantity of semen, impotence/erectile difficulties and premature ejaculation. Masturbation and nocturnal emissions (*swapnadosh*) are also frequently considered to be health problems. These sexual dysfunctions can have deep psychological impact, and can greatly influence the quality of married life, sexual behaviour and reproductive health. Males residing in slums who have non-marital relations and those who spend more time with peers in male organizations and in smoking, drinking and gambling activities more often report non-contact problems. Interestingly, there is some indication that semen loss may be associated with high-risk sexual behaviour.[25] Having a non-contact problem is closely associated with having a contact problem.[25,26]

Women usually find their first sexual experience to be traumatic. Despite this first negative experience, majority of women develop a positive attitude towards sex as years progress. It has also been observed that both rural[27] and urban[28] women communicate their sexual desires through direct physical contact or through various forms of verbal communication. It is quite contradictory to the earlier notion that Indian women do no express their desire for sex. Women are known to deny sex to their husbands if they drink (alcohol) heavily or not support the family. In such cases women often have to bear the consequences including physical violence and sexual coercion.[29,30]

Pre- and extramarital relations, although not socially approved, have been reported in many studies. General population surveys have reported premarital sexual activity among 7-48% of male respondents and 3-10% of female respondents.[28,31,32] Men have numerous premarital sex partners including sex workers, friends, relatives and future spouses.[32] Premarital/extramarital sexual encounters are significantly higher among unmarried, urban males. Almost half of those who have had sex before or outside marriage reported not using a condom during such encounters.[31,32]

Heterosexual relations have also been reported amongst middle-class professionals. In males, premarital sex is observed to increase the likelihood of extramarital sex.[33]

Fondling of breasts, kissing and vaginal penetrative sex are identified as the most common sexual acts of rural men and women. Sexuality and sexual behaviour are expressed and practiced in a variety of contexts in rural areas. Some factors and rituals that provide sexual contexts include (a) *Kumar Purnima* in Orissa which provides a unique opportunity to young and old women alike to share sexual knowledge and transmit certain sexual culture in an acceptable form; (b) *Gauna* (time gap between marriage and consummation of marriage) in North India is particularly a vulnerable period for young men; (c) the practice of *Kudike* (widow remarriage where widow is remarried but does not get the position of wife) adds another dimension to sexual context in rural Karnataka; (d) the practice of commercial sex in a very non-commercial context in certain rural communities in Rajasthan and the practice of *Atta-satta* (marrying on an exchange basis); and (e) pornographic literature and films which provide another explicit sexual context in rural areas. Given the highly selective rural-urban migration and risky sexual behaviour of single migrant men, women in rural areas become vulnerable irrespective of their behaviour.[34,35]

A study on sexual behaviours and risk perceptions among young men in the border towns of Nepal revealed the presence of risk behaviours in the migrant population (viz., Indian truck drivers and transportation workers) and the potential risk of HIV transmission across borders.[36]

The behavioural surveillance surveys (BSS) serve as early warning signals of the potential risk for HIV, can help explain the trends in HIV prevalence in sub-populations at high risk of infection, and reflect the impact of HIV prevention programmes over time. In India, the first rounds of BSS were conducted by APAC (AIDS Prevention and Control) and FHI (Family Health International) and NACO (National AIDS Control Organization).[37] The APAC and FHI surveys in general population included auto-rickshaw drivers, diamond workers, industry workers, fishing industry workers, migrant workers, miners and plantation workers from many states of India. The reports suggest that many young men are involved in unprotected sex with female commercial sex workers (CSWs). The knowledge that consistent condom use prevents HIV/AIDS does not necessarily translate into desired behaviour change. Although BSS have generally been conducted in the context of HIV infection, the findings are relevant in understanding sexual behaviours and prevention of STDs and HIV/AIDS.

The BSS (2001) findings reveal that more than three-fourths of the 84478 respondents across the country had at least heard of HIV/AIDS. More than 70% of the total respondents were also aware of the major routes of HIV/AIDS transmission. However, the potential of mother-to-child transmission is still less known to respondents across the country. Less than one-third of the respondents had heard of STDs and only one-fifth were aware of the linkage between STDs and HIV. There was low awareness about HIV/AIDS and its transmission amongst rural women in Bihar, Uttar Pradesh, Madhya Pradesh and West Bengal. Awareness about condom was less in rural areas, and over one-third of rural females had neither seen nor heard about condom. The median age at first sex was 21 years for males and 18 years for females in the entire country. About 11.8% males and 2% females reported sex with non-regular partners in a 12-month recall period. Less than half of males and about 60% females did not report using condom during the last sex encounter with their non-regular partners. The second round of nationwide BSS ("endline BSS") was conducted in 2006.[38] This was conducted among 97,240 men and women aged 15–49 years in the 25 states/union territories of India. Table 42.1 highlights the findings from nationwide baseline BSS amongst general population conducted in 2001[37] and 2006.[38] As the table indicates, there is improvement on almost all parameters of knowledge of HIV/AIDS, yet there is hardly any change in sex with a non-regular partner in the last 12 months and reporting at least one symptom of HIV. This underscores the fact that improvement in knowledge does not always mean adopting safer practices.

Table 42.1 Sexual Behaviour and Knowledge of HIV/AIDS Among General Population of India

Indicators	*Proportion of Respondents (in %)*	
	BSS 2006	*BSS 2001*
Reporting sex with non-regular partners in the last 12 months	5.8	5.7
Reporting last time condom use with non-regular sex partners	58.3	40.1
Reporting consistent condom use with all non-regular sex partners	41.8	26.5
Reporting easy availability of condoms	90.0	88.5
Ever heard of HIV/AIDS	80.4	67.4
Reporting HIV/AIDS can be transmitted through sexual contact	74.3	61.6
Reporting HIV/AIDS can be transmitted through needle sharing	74.6	62.1
Reporting HIV/AIDS can be transmitted through vertical transmission	66.8	58.3
Having no incorrect belief on the transmission of HIV/AIDS	40.3	16.5

(Contd.)

Reporting HIV/AIDS can be prevented by having one faithful uninfected partner	62.6	49.7
Reporting HIV/AIDS can be prevented through consistent condom use	65.1	50.2
Knowing both methods of HIV prevention	57.1	39.2
Aware of HIV/AIDS testing facility in their area	27.8	9.7
Aware of someone who is infected with HIV/AIDS	16.0	8.4
Ever heard of STDs	37.7	30.8
Aware of linkage between STDs and HIV/AIDS	23.5	18.4
Reporting at least one STD symptom in the last 12 months	5.1	5.4
Reporting STD treatment in a Govt. Hospital/clinic during the last episode	25.7	22.7

Recent data on the knowledge about HIV/AIDS in India are also available from the third round of the National Family Health Survey conducted in 2005–2006. The findings indicate that about 80% ever married men aged 15–49 years have 'heard the term AIDS'. The corresponding figure for women is 57%. The proportion of respondents who had the knowledge that 'consistent condom use can reduce the chances of getting HIV/AIDS' was about 68% among men and about 35% among women.[10]

Adolescent Population

Much of sexual behaviour is learnt, and early sexual experiences, particularly those in puberty and early adolescence, can have an effect on sexual behaviour during the later part of life. Sexual knowledge is often acquired through mass media and friends. Men report that they receive information about sexuality from their sisters-in-law (*bhabhis*), older brothers, 'instinct' and mass media. Other sources include peers, schoolbooks and teachers, and community awareness programmes. Parents are neither considered nor preferred as a source of such information by adolescents. While girls feel masturbation causes weakness, disease, infertility and marital disharmony, boys feel that 'losing semen' leads to weakness.[11] Generally males have more knowledge about sex, and masturbation is a source of sexual release in premarital years.[39] Substantial lacunae in the knowledge of HIV/AIDS, STDs and sexuality have been observed among college students[14,40] as well as amongst girls from rural areas.[41] Although adolescents are somewhat aware of the methods of contraception, they do not know how to use them effectively. Adolescent rural girls, because of their ignorance about sexuality, reproductive health and contraception, are vulnerable to suffer from various negative consequences. At times it has been found that girls are unaware regarding the fact that sexual intercourse could result in pregnancy and STDs; they are also at times unaware about the symptoms of STDs.[37]

There is an increasing trend of risk behaviours among adolescents. More and more young people are becoming sexually active in their mid-teens.[42,43] Sexual activity begins as early as from 10 years of age among street boys to mid- and late-teens among boys and girls in both rural and urban areas. Surveys of adult students indicate that although premarital sexual experience among them is not as common as in Western countries, it is not as rare as perceived widely.[8] Peer group norms have been found to have significant association with intended and actual sexual behaviour. Children of highly educated parents are less likely to engage in sexual activities in their adolescent years.[44] It is observed that boys tend to brag about their sexual experiences in group, while they express fears and insecurities in private.[45] Adolescents especially in urban areas have favourable attitudes towards premarital and extramarital sex.[43] Recreational view of sexuality and sexual adventuring is noted in a considerable number of female college students in Delhi.[46] Interestingly, while students acknowledge deep personal interest in sexual gratification and liberal sexual standards before marriage, they consider monogamy as the cornerstone of marital relationships.

In a study on sexual behaviours and their correlates among college students in Mumbai, it was found that some 47% male respondents and 13%

female respondents had sexual experience with the opposite gender, and 26% and 3%, respectively, had had intercourse. The strongest predictors of sexual behaviour were students' knowledge about sexuality-related issues, attitude towards sex, and levels of social interaction and exposure to erotic materials. For young women, the potential consequences of premarital sex, viz., pregnancy, desertion by one's future husband, domestic discord or loss of honor, often deter premarital sexual activity. Male students who initiate sexual activity appeared to have done so at a young age.[47] A high prevalence of risk behaviours, more or less similar to that of adolescents in other parts of the world, including drug intake, alcohol use, smoking, cannabis and premarital sex, has been observed amongst rural and urban male adolescents in North India. Most risk behaviours are common in urban adolescents.[48] Among predo-minantly unmarried school and college students (mostly in urban centres), premarital sex has been reported in 8-39% of male students and 1-20% of female students.[49] Sexual abuse has also been reported in adolescents. Rural boys are more likely to have experienced coercive sexual intercourse than urban boys, and urban girls are more likely to have experienced any form of sexual abuse than rural girls.[50] Street children in urban areas are particularly vulnerable to sexual abuse[51], as are children in tourism centers. Concerns have been expressed about the growing 'sex tourism' as a risk for children and adolescents.[52] Youth in Goa have been reported to be engaging in various sexual practices with tourists.[53] There is very little information on female sex partners of unmarried male students. Neighbours, relatives, CSWs, friends and fiancées have been mentioned as sex partners. There is an indication that the premarital sex partner of a male student is often a married (older) woman who may be a relative or neighbour.[8] A sizable proportion of unmarried male students visit CSWs. Condoms are seldom used in premarital and extramarital sex, probably because of the mostly unplanned nature of such encounters and also because condoms are considered to interfere with sexual pleasure. Interestingly adolescents residing in rural areas find it difficult to dispose of condoms.[11]

SEXUAL BEHAVIOUR OF HIGH-RISK POPULATIONS

Commercial Sex Workers (CSWs)

Commercial sex is widely recognized as a contributing factor to the spread of STDs and HIV infection. HIV infection is high among sex workers and their clients.[54] Female sex workers can be broadly categorized into four groups: brothel-based, home-based and part time, street-based, and call girls.[55] Both brothel- and street-based sex workers are also referred to as 'direct sex workers'. Some women operate from home or work at stalls, nightclubs, etc. selling sex to supplement their income. This category of women is referred to as 'indirect sex workers'. Brothel-based sex workers tend to have a higher turnover of clients than street-based sex workers, who in turn have more clients than indirect sex workers.[55]

The findings of a few empirical studies in red-light areas of a few large cities in India corroborate the common knowledge that CSWs, particularly those working in brothels, lead a poor standard of life in dilapidated and unhygienic environments.[56] These women are bonded to brothel owners who are unwilling to permit insistence on condoms. Brothel rules and client insistence on sex without condoms are upheld through violence meted out by pimps, police and local mafia. The competitive nature of the trade and resulting insecurity among women is a constraint in adopting behavioural changes.[55] A large proportion of them suffers intermittently from various kinds of STDs.

CSWs who are known as 'call-girls' are usually more educated and attractive than those living in brothels, and are often also engaged in some other occupation. They earn higher incomes and have some freedom in choosing their clients, who mostly belong to middle and upper classes. Many of them had STDs at one time or other and have undergone abortions. A high proportion of their clients prefer oral sex to vaginal intercourse.[57] Alcohol and drug use is also common among CSWs, and has an effect on sexual behaviour and consequent risk to STDs and HIV. In the first round of BSS conducted in India[58], among a total of 5,572 FSW, 22% were daily alcohol users. Overall, around 15% of FSW reported that they drink regularly before sex. About 6% had tried other addictive drugs including injections in the past 12 months. Interface between drug use and sex work has also been examined. In some studies from north-east India, the prevalence of HIV infection among sex workers who were injecting drug users was significantly higher (up to nine times higher) than among non-injecting drug users.[59,60]

There is also some indication that condom use may be increasing among sex workers. Indeed this increase in condom use has been proposed as a factor behind improving HIV situation among sex workers in some parts of India such as Tamil Nadu. In fact data from the first round of BSS showed that a high percentage of direct sex workers reported condom use with their last client. However, condom use with husbands or boy friends was rarely reported, perhaps in part to distinguish these personal partnerships from their professional relations. Lower condom use in non-commercial sex (when practiced by CSWs or their clients with other partners) is potential for HIV spread from higher to lower risk populations.

Clients of CSWs

A few hundred thousand men have sexual relations with CSWs every day in India. In the first round of BSS conducted in India,[58] among a total of 5684 clients of sex workers, a majority (80%) were between 20 and 35 years of age. Nearly half (52%) were married and about a fifth (21%) were transport workers. Earlier studies have also reported that clients who frequently visit CSWs are low-level industrial workers living away from their families, transport workers, traders and customers in transitory markets, visitors to fairs, festivals and pilgrim centres, defense personnel, students, pimps and others who have some control over prostitutes, traders and service providers in red-light areas, and professional blood donors. As in many other countries, Indian truck drivers and their helpers are generally known to visit many CSWs during their stopovers.[8]

The relationship between commercial sex and substance use applies to clients of sex workers as well. In the BSS by NACO[58], about 23% respondents reported drinking daily. Nearly 13% of respondents regularly consumed alcohol before having sex with their commercial partners. Around 22% reported use of other compounds like cannabis and opium. About 10% had injected drugs in the last 12 months.

Men Having Sex With Men (MSM)

The prevalence of MSM has been reported to be 2-12% in different population groups.[48] The 'gay culture' as observed in Western settings has yet to be fully established in South Asia. MSM in India have a great diversity and fluidity in social sexual and gender identities and behaviours as compared to the Western 'gay' experience.[61] There is a certain indication at least in larger cities that there is an increasing acceptance of same-sex relationships. Vast majorities of MSM are married and are living with their wives. Bisexuality tends to be practiced by men irrespective of their marital status.[62] MSM is often practiced without a 'homosexual identity' in covert manner and in discrete surroundings. In India, the percentage of men reporting sex with other men is highly variable and varies between 6 and 60%.[32,64,64,65] The figures for anal sex (with/without specifying gender of the partner) vary between 13 and 42%.[28,63] Use of condom during anal sex is relatively infrequent.[22,48] Situational homosexuality may occur in unequal (exploitative/potentially exploitative) relationships defined by age (older men with adolescent boys, particularly hotel/restaurant workers), occupation (truck drivers with cleaners), or power (jail inmates).[66-69] They all form an important group at risk of STDs/HIV transmission.

Many members of a culturally identifiable group known as '*hijra*' in most parts of India are known to depend at least partly on working as male prostitutes for their livelihood. It has been observed that *hijras* engage in sexual activity with men for money or for satisfying their own homosexual desires.[70] Not much is known about sexual techniques *hijras* practice or are asked to practice when they perform the role of a sex worker. They are often passive partners in anal intercourse without use of condoms, making them vulnerable to HIV and other STD infections.[62] Apart from the *hijra* community, there are many full-time or part-time male sex workers.

Transport Workers and Migrant Population

Migrant workers and truck drivers have a high rate of contact with CSWs.[67,69] Sex partners among married truck drivers vary from 1 to 40 in number. Married men have more sex encounters with CSWs than their wives. The predominant form of sexual activity with non-marital partners is vaginal intercourse, followed by oral sex and anal intercourse. Interestingly, the perceived risk for HIV is virtually non-existent in this high-risk group. There is denial of vulnerability of spreading it to their wives, although three-fourth believe that there is some chance that women they had sex with have HIV/AIDS.[71] Condom use during commercial sex amongst this population has also been low (11-28%).[67,69,71]

Dhaba, an inexpensive eating and drinking point, primarily meant for low-income highway travelers, serves as a halt place for long-distance truck drivers. Commercial sex activities flourish near halt places like dhabas. CSWs living nearby often visit these places in search of clients. Sometimes the truckers pick up such CSWs, and sexual acts take place within the trucks or in roadside bushes. Truck drivers are known to visit villages adjacent to the national highway to obtain alcohol and women. Alcohol and substance use has an effect on sexual behaviours and condom use. Some truck drivers also report their inability to visit a CSW unless inebriated with alcohol or opium. Truck drivers also have homosexual relationship with 'helpers'.[66] Wives and steady sexual partners are at increased risk of contracting HIV/STDs.[69]

Other Risk Groups

A high prevalence of STDs and blood-borne infections, sexual risk behaviours, alcohol/drug abuse and poor knowledge of HIV has been observed among jail inmates.[68]

Social customs and sexual openness of certain Indian tribes makes them freely indulge in premarital and extramarital sex. Outsiders sexually exploit women from these tribes. As a result, the prevalence of STDs is high (8-30%) in some tribal groups.[72]

Populations Attending STD Clinics

Most patients who attend STD clinics in different regions of the country are young males and have a history of contact with CSWs. The first sexual encounter of male STD patients is often with CSWs. However, many male patients attribute their infection to sexual contact with acquaintances, friends, relatives or neighbours. The reason for male preponderance observed in such clinic-based studies could be due to higher attendance to such clinics by males because of social reasons and also because of more painful symptoms of certain STDs in males as compared to females. Thirty to forty percent of male STD patients visiting STD clinics are repeaters, and the majority of them had their first sexual experience during their teenage. It is estimated that only 5 to 10% of people suffering from the disease attend public STD facilities.

Concomitant infection with STDs, particularly those characterized by genital ulcers, increases the chance of HIV infection. STD clinic attendees have a high HIV prevalence (1-64% in major urban areas; 0-45% outside major urban areas).[73,74,75] A person having STDs has a greater risk of acquiring HIV from an infected partner.

High-risk Behaviour in Populations Affected with STDs/HIV

A clinic-based study on a group of STD patients reveals that, although knowledge about condom use is high in this group, the actual use of condom use has been low. Although STD patients are well informed about STDs and know methods to avoid infection, this knowledge has little impact on their behaviour.[76]

Although HIV-1 is still the predominant virus amongst high-risk HIV infected persons in Mumbai, dual HIV-1 and HIV-2 infections are increasing specially amongst the high-risk group of promiscuous heterosexuals and FCSWs. A raise in HIV2 infections was observed later than dual HIV-1 and HIV-2 infections, indicating that HIV-1 infected persons through continued high-risk behaviour got infected with HIV-2. The findings reflect that the high-risk behaviour continues in promiscuous heterosexuals and CSWs.[77] There is little information about the sexual behaviour of HIV infected persons. Recently, however, there have been some studies examining the sexual behaviour of HIV-positive individuals.[78] A recent study on adherence and sexual behaviour among patients on retroviral therapy in India reported that a majority of HIV-positive individuals remained sexually active while on ART. However, a majority of them had sex only with their regular partners; only a minuscule proportion reported having sex with casual partners or sex workers. About one-fourth of HIV-positive individuals do not disclose their HIV status to their spouses.[79]

Sexual Risk Behaviour Linked to Alcohol/Substance Use

Alcohol and sexual behaviour has been studied from ethnographic, sociological and health perspective. Studies have demonstrated direct and indirect linkage between alcohol/substance use and sexual behaviours, but only few studies have specifically examined the nature of linkage and its effect on high-risk behaviours and prevention of related health problems.[80,81] Intoxication has been connected with risky sexual behaviour, and failure to use condoms with STDs and unplanned pregnancies.

It has been observed that consumption of alcohol and visit to sex workers increases manifold during festivals and celebrations. On the contrary, during months of Shravana (observed by Hindus) and Ramzan (observed by Muslims), restraints on such vices help in decreasing/preventing high-risk behaviours. The number of clients visiting CSWs decreases during 'dry' (alcohol free) periods. An absence of or a reduction in alcohol use is associated with a decrease in high-risk sexual behaviours and STDs.[82,83] An observed association between drinking and high-risk sexual activity could imply that these two behaviours are part of a larger risk-taking tendency, or alcohol itself influences sexual risk-taking or both. The larger control of HIV/STDs during festivities could be achieved through an informed policy on dry alcohol days.[80]

Men who have been drinking alcohol report more contact and non-contact sexual problems as compared to those who do not use alcohol.[84] The association between alcohol and substance use and high-risk sexual behaviours is more evident among high-risk groups like CSWs and truckers. The clients of CSWs consume alcohol for sexual excitement. Alcohol use is strongly associated with high-risk sexual behaviours for reasons like 'alcohol increases and sustains sexual drive', 'one can visit a CSW only when alcohol is consumed', 'it is difficult to engage in oral sex without alcohol consumption', 'the CSWs demand alcohol for themselves'.

Condom use is low under the influence of alcohol.[58] In a study on the assessment of risk factors in STDs, alcohol was found to be significantly associated with the acquisition of STDs.[85] Using indepth interviews with men and women to learn about their sexual histories and recent sexual behaviours, a study described the use of alcohol particularly in group sex encounters in Haryana.[86] There is increasing trend towards smoking, alcohol use, late night parties, sexual intercourse, adolescent pregnancies, STDs and violence amongst youth, particularly among those residing in urban metropolitan cities. Media also influences such high-risk behaviour.[47] Alcohol use and sexual experimentation during adolescence and youth are risk factors for acquiring STDs. In a study from Shilong, Meghalaya, among 200 students, sexual behaviour was found to be strongly associated with alcohol use.[87] Similarly, in yet another study among adolescents in the slums of Mumbai, alcohol use was associated with risky sexual behaviour along with the perception that alcohol heightens sexual pleasure and makes it longlasting.[88]

Apart from alcohol, other substance use has also been linked to high-risk sexual behaviours. Substance users including injecting drug users commonly visit CSWs. The average number of sex partners of drug users has been found to be more than that of non-drug users from the same community.[89] Among psychiatric patients also, a history of drug abuse has been found to be strongly associated with engaging in risky sexual behaviours.[90] In some areas, especially the north-eastern part of the country and metropolitan cities, IDUs are reported to have high seropositivity for HIV infection. Some women IDUs are engaged in sex work as well.[59] Thus, many drug users are sexually active and can pass on the HIV infection to their spouses as well as to the general population, fueling the HIV epidemic.[5]

Alcohol and substance use is common among youth and adolescents, high-risk groups like transport workers and migrant workers, commercial sex workers, jail inmates and HIV infected persons. However, few studies have examined the triangular relationship between alcohol us, sexual behaviours and STDs including HIV infection in the high-risk and general population.

SEXUAL BEHAVIOUR AND PREVENTION OF STDs/AIDS

As STDs and HIV prevalence rise in the population, the chance of someone encountering an infected partner close to the beginning of their sexual life also rises. It is therefore crucial to reach people with appropriate preventive interventions before their first sex encounter.[91] Adolescents have poor knowledge about issues related to sexuality. It is important that adolescents receive age-appropriate and adequate information and education about issues related to sexuality from reliable and knowledgeable sources. Sex education should aim to increase knowledge about sex and STDs/HIV, to develop self-assertiveness and to develop positive attitudes towards sexuality. Education imparted in this way will serve the two-fold purpose of satisfying their natural curiosity and protecting them from engaging in high-risk sexual behaviour. Although sex education is a part of university education, the curriculum rarely discusses issues related to reproductive health and sexuality. Many teachers in schools and colleges avoid teaching these topics as they find these too embarrassing.[92] Teaching adolescents about sex is not only an effective way to safeguard the future health of the nation but also results in developing a stable value system and adopting a responsible lifestyle. Young people can be agents of change and spearhead advocacy for sex education among peers, community members and parents.

Apart from students, there is also a need to impart sex education to general population and high-risk groups such as CSWs, truck drivers, migrant workers, jail inmates and drug users. Sex education programmes to these populations need to be tailored according to the specific needs of these groups.

Research has shown that appropriately designed prevention programmes that provide a comprehensive range of coordinated service scan limit the further spread of HIV and other STDs even when the latter are well established in a community. However, in order to be effective, such prevention programmes should be based on a thorough continuing assessment of local population needs and they should involve the local population in planning and implementing interventions and services. Such prevention programmes have been shown to be cost effective.[93] The spread of HIV is influenced in short term by condom use and prevalence of STDs, and these are the factors that can be manipulated to limit the spread of infection.[94]

Some well-designed and well-executed intervention programmes by government and non-government agencies in a few red-light areas of the country have been carried out. One example was the STDs/HIV Intervention Project among sex workers in Sonagachi, Kolkata (Calcutta), initiated in 1992. The programme focussed on the promotion of condom use, AIDS awareness through peer educators, and provision of STD treatment facility in the area. Such intervention programmes have shown increase in condom use, improvement in knowledge about STDs and reduction in the prevalence of STDs among CSWs.[95] One of the key factors of its success is peer-group education in raising AIDS awareness among sex workers and motivating them to use condoms. Even when health education programmes succeed in motivating sex workers to use condoms, their clients who usually have higher bargaining power are often reluctant to use condoms. There is an indication that sex workers can control the behaviour of their clients to some extent by monetary bargaining.[96] The training and recruitment of a few select sex workers as peer educators in the programme served as an important step towards shifting the project's approach from a 'behavioural communication change model' to an 'empowerment model'. Working with and for their own group under the supervision of experts proved to be an effective intervention strategy amongst these vulnerable women. The HIV epidemic has been brought to a halt and maintained at low levels of transmission, even in situations of poverty in Kolkata because of the emergence of organizations among female sex workers which enable them to negotiate successfully for "protected sex".

In a review of published studies that evaluated different approaches to preventing STDs/HIV transmission in heterosexual men (IDUs, STD clinic patients, men in workplace and students), it was found that no single intervention could be identified as more effective than the other in reducing the incidence of STDs/HIV in heterosexual men. In general, the studies had used either group-based or individual interventions. However, successful interventions include localized and national programmes, video-based education programmes, counselling and communication skill development, and long-term peer educators; a single approach is unlikely to be successful in any given setting.[97]

There is also a need to address male sexual health, i.e. masturbation and semen loss concerns in sexual health campaigns in South Asia, keeping in mind the magnitude of these concerns, their potential to confound management of STDs, and their significance as an idiom of psychosocial distress. Addressing such issues leads to immediate identification among young men and provide, an entry point for sexual health and safer sex education.[98]

Among Indian truck drivers, substantial deficits with respect to HIV prevention information, motivation and behavioural skills have been observed, and have been found to be predictive of HIV risk and preventive behaviour. There is a need to focus on higher levels of HIV prevention information, safer sex motivation (consisting of attitudes, social norms and perception of vulnerability to HIV) and safer behavioural skills, paralleling interventions with sex workers.

It has been seen that people tend to have safe sex with high-risk partners and high-risk sex with safe partners (i.e. with spouse), which predisposes general population to the risk of infection.[99,100] Prevention programmes should also focus on steady sexual partners of persons with high-risk behaviours as the former are also at a high risk of acquiring STDs and HIV/AIDS.

Voluntary counselling and testing (VCT) is one of the essential components of various HIV prevention programmes. VCT results in the reduction of risk behaviours amongst the target groups but is not enough as a primary prevention strategy, and other behavioural interventions are needed to bring an observable change.[101]

To convince people to adopt healthy behaviours, what is needed is motivation and skills to translate knowledge into practice. Hence, apart from providing information, it is also important to teach other skills. Sexual intercourse should be discussed displaying affection. Meta-analytic review reveals that service-based prevention interventions have positive effects among population at risk through sexual transmission. The positive effects include both behavioural and biological prevention, such as reduction in STDs.[102] Consistent and correct use of condoms coupled with risk reduction education strategies are vital for the prevention of STDs and HIV transmission.[103] STDs and HIV prevention strategies should target not only individuals but also communities and social policies.[104]

Acknowledgements: Our sincere thanks to Dr. Sameer Malhotra, who was one of the authors of the previous version of this chapter. Our sincere thanks are due to Drs. Peter Kok, Health Advisor, Cordaid; Shalini Bharat, Unit for Family Studies, Tata Institute of Social Sciences, Mumbai; Prabha Chandra, Dept. of Psychiatry, National Institute of Mental Health and Neurosciences, Bangalore; Ravi K. Verma and Avina Sarna, Horizons/Population Council, India, New Delhi; Ravindra Rao, National AIDS Control Organisation, New Delhi. We sincerely thank Dr. Avinash P who has been helpful in the collection of review material.

REFERENCES

1. Ramasubban R. HIV/AIDS in India: Between Rhetoric and Reality. In: Pachauri, S Subramanian S. eds. Implementing a reproductive health agenda in India: the beginning. Population Council, South East Asia-Regional Office; 1999. p. 347-76.
2. Sharma VK, Khandpur S. Changing patterns of sexually transmitted infections in India Natl Med J India. 2004; 17: 310-9.
3. Monitoring the AIDS Pandemic (MAP) AIDS in Asia: Face the facts, 2004, Monitoring the AIDS Pandemic Network. Accessed at http://www.mapnetwork.org/docs/MAP_AIDSinAsia2004.pdf.
4. Ambekar A, Rao S, Lewis G. South Asia Regional Profile: Drugs and Crime, 2005, United Nations Office on Drugs and Crime, Regional Office for South Asia, New Delhi, 2005.
5. Panda S, Chatterjee A, Bhattacharya SK, et al. Transmission of HIV from injecting drug users to their wives in India. Intern J STDs & AIDS 2000; 11: 468-73.
6. Doniger W, Kakar S. Kamasutra by Mallanaga Vatsyayana. Oxford University Press, 2003.
7. Khazanchand (Kaviraj) ed. Indian Sexology: New Delhi: S.Chand & Co. Ltd, 1972.
8. Nag M. Sexual behaviour in India with risk of HIV/AIDS transmission. Health Transit Rev 1995; 5: 293-305.
9. Nag M. Sexual Behaviour and AIDS in India, New Delhi, Vikas Publishing House, 1996.
10. National Family Health Survey – III. India: National Fact sheet. Ministry of Health and Family Welfare, Government of India, 2007.
11. Chandiramani R, Kapadia S, Khanna R, et al. Critical review of studies on sexuality and sexual behaviour conducted in India from 1990 to 2000. Paper presented at the Reproductive health Research Review Dissemination Workshop, Dec. 2001, Mumbai.
12. Rani M, Bonu S. Rural Indian women's care-seeking behaviour and choice of provider for gynecological symptoms. Stud Fam Plann. 2003; 34: 173-85.
13. Sharma BR, Gupta M. Child abuse in Chandigarh, India, and its implications. J Clin Forensic Med. 2004; 11: 248-56.
14. George A. Differential perspectives of men and women in Mumbai, India on sexual relations and negotiations within marriage. Reprod Health Matters, 1998; 6, 87-96.
15. Weiss HA, Patel V, West B, et al. Spousal sexual violence and poverty are risk factors for sexually transmitted infections in women: a longitudinal study of women in Goa, India. Sex Transm Infect 2008; 84: 133-9.
16. Verma RK, Pulerwitz J, Mahendra V et al. Challenging and changing gender attitudes among young men in Mumbai, India. Reprod Health Matters. 2006; 14: 135-43.
17. Thappa DM, Singh S, Singh A. HIV infection and sexually transmitted diseases in a referral STDs centre in South India. Sex Transm Inf 1999; 75: 191.
18. International Centre for Research on Women (ICRW). Adolescent sexuality and fertility in India- Preliminary Findings. Information Bulletin. International Centre for Research on Women, Washington DC, USA, 1997.
19. Kar GC, Varma LP. Sexual problems of married male mental patients. Indian J Psychiat 1978; 20, 365-70.
20. Sharma A, Sharma V. The guilt and pleasure of masturbation: A study of college girls in Gujarat, India. Sex Marit Therap 1998; 13; 63-70.
21. Malhotra HK, Wig NN. Dhat syndrome: A culture bound neurosis of Orient. Arch Sex Behav 1975; 4; 519-28.
22. Pelto P J, Joshi A, Verma RK. Development of sexuality among men in India and its implications for reproductive health programmes: The Population Council, New Delhi, 2000.
23. Research and Intervention in Sexual Health: Theory to Action (RISHTA). Addressing Gupt Rog. Narrative prevention counselling for STI/HIV prevention. International Institute for Population Studies (IIPS), University of

Connecticut Health Center (UCHC), Walden University, Population Council, New Delhi, 2007.

24. Verma R K, Nastasie B, Rama Rao G, et al: Men's Secret Illnesses (Gupt Rog) and its Relationship to Sexual Risk: A Case from India. 2003 accessed at www.jhuccp.org/igwg/presentations/Monday/Plen2/MensSecret.pdf.
25. Rama Rao G, Saggurty N, Verma RK et al. Risky Sexual behaviour, marital relationship and gupt rog ('secret illnesses' in Hindi) in the slums of Mumbai city, India. Accessed at http://paa2004.princeton.edu/download.asp?submissionId=41255.
26. Verma R, Lhungdim H. Perception and practice of sexual acts: Findings based on key informant interviews and case studies in rural India. Paper presented at national conference on sexual behaviour at TISS, Mumbai, 26-27 Dec, 2000.
27. Joshi A, Dhapola M, Kurien E, et al. Rural women's experiences and perceptions of marital sexual relationships. Ford Foundation Working Papers Series 1998.
28. India Today. Women's Sexual Survey. September, 2003, Accessed at: http://www.indiatoday.com/itoday/20040920/cover3.shtml.
29. Martin SL, Kilgallen B, Tsui AO, et al. Sexual behaviours and reproductive health outcomes-Associations with wife abuse in India. JAMA 1999; 282: 1967-72.
30. Chandrasekaran V, Krupp K, George R, et al. Determinants of domestic violence among women attending an human immunodeficiency virus voluntary counselling and testing center in Bangalore, India. Indian J Med Sci. 2007; 61: 253-62.
31. Carolina Population Centre Uttar Pradesh reproductive health survey 1995-1996. North Carolina, Carolina Population Centre, 1997.
32. India Today. Men's sexual survey. September, 2004, Accessed at: http://www.indiatoday.com/itoday/20040920/cover3.shtml.
33. Bhattacharjee J, Gupta RS, Kumar A, et al . Pre and extramarital heterosexual behaviour of an urban community in Rajasthan. India J Commun Dis 2000; 32: 33-9.
34. Verma R, Lhungdim H. Perception and practice of sexual acts: Findings based on key informant interviews and case studies in Rural India. Paper presented at national conference on sexual behaviour at TISS, Mumbai, 26-27 Dec. 2000.
35. Family Health International, STDs prevalence study among women in migrant communities of Kailali District, Nepal. Final report, accessed at www.fhi.org/en/HIVAIDS/pub/survreports/migrantwomen.htm - 37k - 30 Aug 2004.
36. Tamang A, Nepal B, Puri M, et al. Sexual behaviour and risk perceptions among young men in border towns of Nepal. Asia Pacific Population Journal 2000; 16: 195-210.
37. NACO National HIV Sentinel behavioural surveillance survey-2001, New Delhi, NACO. Ministry of Health and Family Welfare, Government of India, 2002.
38. National AIDS Control Organisation (NACO). Endline behavioural surveillance survey -2006, NACO. Ministry of Health and Family Welfare, Government of India, New Delhi, 2007.
39. Collumbien M, Bohidar N, Das R, et al. Male sexual health concerns in Orissa: An Ethnic Perspective, AIMS Research Centre, Bhubaneshwar, Orissa. Continence, ed. WJ Robinson. New York: Critic and Guide Company, 1998.
40. Sharma AK, Sehgal VN, Kant S, et al. Knowledge, attitude, belief and practice (KABP) on AIDS among senior secondary students. Indian J Commun Med, 1997; 22:168-71.
41. Lal SS, Vasan RS, Sarma PS, et al. Knowledge and attitudes of college students in Kerala towards HIV/AIDS, sexually transmitted diseases and sexuality. Natl Med J India 2000; 13: 231-6.
42. Kannan AT: Adolescent health: issues and concerns in India. Health for the Millions 1995; 21: 29-30.
43. Sharma A, In the season of love, let's talk about sex & teens, 2004, accessed at http://www.hindustantimes.com/sexsurvey/teen_story.html.
44. Selvan MS, Ross MW, Kapadia AS, et al. Study of perceived norms, beliefs and intended sexual behaviour among higher secondary school students in India. AIDS Care 2001; 13: 779-88.
45. Amin A, Fatula E , Khanna R. Attitudes and behaviours of men in relation to gender and sexuality: Evidence from qualitative studies conducted in the Santrampur taluka of

Panchmahals district, Gujarat, Working Paper No. 4, SARTHI, 1997.
46. Sachdev P. University students in Delhi, India: Their sexual knowledge, attitudes and behaviour. The J Fam Welfare 1997; 43, 1-12.
47. Abraham L, Kumar KA. Sexual experiences and their correlates among college students in Mumbai City, India. Internat Fam Plann Perspect 1999; 25: 139-46.
48. Kishore J, Singh A, Grewal I, et al. Risk behaviour in an urban and a rural male adolescent population. Natl Med J India 1999; 12: 107-10.
49. Hawkes S, Santhya KG. Diverse realities. STDs and HIV in India. Sex Trans Infect 2002; 78(suppl): 131-9.
50. Patel V, Andrew G. Gender, sexual-abuse and risk behaviours in adolescents: A cross sectional survey in schools in Goa. Natl Med J India 2001; 14: 263-7.
51. Ramkrishna J, Karott M, Murthy RS. Experiences of sexual coercion among street boys in Bangalore, India in Towards adulthood: Exploring the sexual and reproductive health of adolescents in South Asia, Department of Reproductive Health and Research (RHR), World Health Organization, Geneva, 2003.
52. SANLAAP, A situational analysis of child sex tourism in India, SANLAAP and ECPAT, New Delhi, 2003.
53. Ram U, Bhat R. Tourism and sexual behaviour: Experiences of youths in Goa, India. Expanded Abstract Submitted for PAA – 2006, accessed at http://epc2006.princeton.edu/download.aspx?submissionId=60101.
54. National AIDS Control Organisation (NACO). Indian Scene: Overview, 2005, accessed at http://www.naco.nic.in/indianscene/overv.htm.
55. Family Health International. What drives HIV in Asia: A Summary of trends in sexual and drug-taking behaviours. Family Health International, 2001.
56. Gilada IS. AIDS and sex work: An Indian perspective. In: M. Berer and S. Ray (eds.). Women and HIV/AIDS: An Indian Resource Book Information. Action and Resources on Women and HIV/AIDS. Reproductive Health and Sexual Relationship. London: Pandora Press, 1993.
57. Kapur P. The life and world of call girls in India. New Delhi: Vikas Publishing House 1978.
58. National AIDS Control Organisation (NACO). National baseline high risk and bridge population behavioural surveillance survey 2001: PART 1 Female sex workers and their clients, National AIDS Control Organisation, Ministry of Health and Family Welfare, India.
59. Panda S, Bijaya L, Devi N, et al. Interface between drug use and sex work in Manipur. Natl Med J India 2001; 14: 209-11.
60. Agarwal AK, Singh GB, Khundom KC, et al. The prevalence of HIV in female sex workers in Manipur. J Commun Dis 1999; 31: 23-8.
61. Asthana S and Oostvogels R. The social construction of male 'homosexuality' in India: implications for HIV transmission and prevention. Soc Sci & Med 52: 707-21.
62. Khan S. Cultural contexts of sexual behaviours and identities and their impact upon HIV prevention models: An overview of South Asian men have sex with men. Indian J Soc Work 1994; 55: 633-46.
63. Raizada, SB Gupta, A Kumar. Sexual practices other than peno-vaginal sex: Perceptions and practices in an urban community. Indian J Commun Med 2002, XXVII : 4.
64. Durex. Global Sex Survey 2004, accessed at www.durex.com/uk/globalsexsurvey/index.asp.
65. Kamasutra annual sex survey 2004: Research Findings, accessed at http://www.ksontheweb.com/64/category.ift.
66. Rao A, Nag M, Mishra K, et al. Sexual behaviour pattern of truck drivers.and their helpers in relation to female sex workers. Indian J Soc Work 1994; 55: 603-16.
67. Rao. KS, Pilli RD, Rao AS et al. Sexual lifestyle of long distance lorry drivers in India questionnaire survey. BMJ 1999; 318: 162-3.
68. Singh S, Prasad R, Mohanty A. High prevalence of sexually transmitted and blood borne infections amongst the inmates of a district jail in Northern India. Internat J STDs & AIDS 1999; 10: 475-8.
69. The Centre for Development and Population Activities (CEDPA), Knowledge, attitude, behaviour and practices (KABP) Survey of male reproductive and sexual health among truckers and cleaners helpers in three cities of

Jharkhand, 2003, accessed at www.cedpa.org/ publications/ pdf/india_truckerscleaners.pdf.

70. Nag M. Sexual behaviour and AIDS in India: State-of -the-Art. Indian J Soc Work (Special Issues: Sexual Behaviour and AIDS in India) 1994; 55: 503-46.
71. Bryan AD, Fisher JD, Joseph Benziger T. Determinants of HIV risk among Indian truck drivers. Social Sci & Med 2001; 53: 1413-26.
72. Aswar NS, Wahab SN, Kale KM. Prevalence and some epidemiological factors of syphilis in Madia Tribe of Gadricholi District. Indian J of Sex Trans Dis 1998; 19: 53-7.
73. Jacob M, John TJ, George S, et al. Increasing prevalence of human immuno-deficiency virus infection among patients attending a clinic for sexually transmitted diseases. Indian J Med Res 1995; 101: 6-9.
74. Rodriguez JJ, Mehendale SM, Shafhard ME, et al. Risk factors for HIV infection in people attending clinics for sexually transmitted diseases in India. BMJ 1995; 311: 283-6.
75. Kar HK, Jain RK, Sharma PK, et al. Increasing HIV prevalence in STDs clinic attendees in Delhi, India: 6 year (1995-2000) hospital based study results. Sex Transm Infect 2001; 77: 393.
76. Grover V, Kannan AT, Indrayam A, et al. Sexually transmitted diseases awareness and sexual behaviour-A study in clinical setting in an urban area of Delhi. Indian J Sex Trans Dis 1999; 20: 16-20.
77. Kamat HA, Banker DD, Koppikar GV. Increasing prevalence of HIV-2 and dual HIV 1-2 infections among patients attending various out door patient departments in Mumbai. Indian J Publ Health 1999; 43: 85-6.
78. Sr Krishnan AK, Hendriksen E, Vallabhaneni S, et al. Sexual behaviours of individuals with HIV living in South India: A qualitative study. AIDS Education and Prevention 2007; 19: 334-45.
79. Sarna, A, Gupta I, Pujari S, et al. Examining adherence and sexual behaviour among patients on antiretroviral therapy in India. Horizons Final Report. Washington, DC: Population Council, 2006.
80. Tripathi BM, Malhotra S. Alcohol use & sexual risk behaviour: exploring links, drug dependence treatment centre, All India Institute of Medical Sciences, New Delhi, 2002.
81. Ray R, Ambekar A. Drug abuse and HIV/AIDS in South Asia: Vulnerabilities and responses. Draft report submitted to United Nations Office on Drugs and Crime, Regional Office for South Asia, New Delhi, 2005.
82. Ambwani PN, Gilada IS. Dry alcohol days during festivals to prevent HIV/AIDS. XII International Conference on AIDS, Geneva, 1998. AIDSLINE ICA 12/98410386. 1998.
83. Chandra PS, Bengal V, Ramkrishna J, et al. Development and evaluation of a module for HIV/AIDS related risk reduction among patients with alcohol dependence (Project report). Bangalore, National Institute of Mental Health and Neurosciences, 1999.
84. Verma R, Sharma S, Singh R, et al. Beliefs concerning sexual health problems and treatment seeking among mean in an Indian slum community paper presented at the 3rd I ASSCS, 1-3 Oct. 2001, Melbourne, Australia (cited with permission) 2001.
85. Sharma AK, Chaubey D. Risk factors in sexually transmitted diseases. Indian J Sex Transm Dis 1996; 17: 8-10.
86. SWACH (Survival for Women and Children) Foundation: An in-depth study to understand men's reproductive health behaviour and feasibility of special intervention. Progress report. Ford Foundation, New Delhi, India 1998.
87. Longkumer M, Shrivastava HC, Murugesan P. Alcohol abuse and risky sexual behaviour among the indigenous college students in Shillong, India, International Institute for Population Sciences, India, 2005.
88. Singh SK, Schensul JJ, Gupta K. Alcohol use and risky sexual behaviour among adolescents in low income slum communities in Mumbai, India, Int Conf AIDS 2004 Jul 11-16; 15:(abstract no. C11731).
89. Sharma AK, Aggarwal OP, Dubey KK. Sexual behaviour of drug-users: is it different? Preventive Medicine 2002; 34: 512-5.
90. Chandra PS, Krishna VAS, Benegal V, et al, High-risk sexual behaviour & sensation seeking among heavy alcohol users. Indian J Med Res 2003; 117: 88-92.

91. Pisani E. AIDS into 21st century: Some critical consideations. Reprod Health Matters 2000; 8: 63-76.
92. Jejeebhoy SJ. Adolescent sexual and reproductive behaviour. A review of the evidence from India. Social Scheme and Medicine. 1998; 46, 1275-90.
93. UNAIDS, 'Intensifying HIV prevention: UNAIDS policy position paper, UNAIDS, Geneva, 2005.
94. Venkataramana CB, Sarada PV. Extent and speed of HIV infection in India through the commercial sex networks: a perspective. Trop Med Int Health 2001; 6: 1040-61.
95. Nag M: Empowering female sex workers for AIDS prevention and far beyond: Sonagachi shows the way. Indian J Soc Work 2002; 63: 473-501.
96. Bhattacharya S, Senapati SK. Sexual practice of sex workers in a red light area of calcutta, Indian J Soc Work 1994; 55: 547-56.
97. Elwy AR, Hart GJ, Peticerw M. Effectiveness of intervention to prevent sexually transmitted infections and human immune deficiency virus in heterosexual men: A systematic review. Arch Int Med 2002; 162: 1818-30.
98. Lakhani A, Gandhi K, Collumbien M. Addressing semen loss concerns: Towards culturally appropriate HIV/AIDS intervention in Gujarat, India. Reprod Health Matters 2001; 9: 49-59.
99. Peterman TA, Lin LS, Newman DR, et al. Does measured behaviour reflect STDs risk? An analysis of data from a randomized controlled behavioural intervention study. Project RESPECT Study Group. Sex Transm Dis 2000; 27: 446-51.
100. Weiss HA, Patel V, West B, et al. The burden and determinants of reproductive tract infections in India: a population based study of women in Goa, India. Sex Transm Infect 2006; 82: 243–9.
101. Tripathi B M. HIV Counselling and testing, Nat J Inf Dis 1999; 1: 22-6.
102. Neumann MS, Johnson WD, Semaan S, et al. Review and meta-analysis of HIV prevention intervention research for heterosexual adult populations in the United States. J Acquir Immune Defic Syndr 2002; 1; 30 (Suppl 1): S106-17.
103. Roth J, Krishnan SP, Bunch E. Barriers to condom use: Results from a study in Mumbai (Bombay), India. AIDS Edu Prev 2001; 13: 65-77.
104. Deodhar NS. Review of the national HIV/AIDS control programme in India with a view to making it community-oriented, more effective, and sustainable. J Publ Health Policy 2003; 24: 159-80.

43 PSYCHOSEXUAL DISORDERS

Sameer Malhotra, Vinod K Sharma

In this chapter

- Sexual Dysfunctions
- Paraphilias
- Gender Identity Disorder
- Sexual Beliefs and Notions
- Dhat Syndrome
- Homosexuality
- Venereophobia

INTRODUCTION

Sexuality is an important aspect of one's existence and health. Broadly speaking, it is influenced by physical as well as psychosocial factors. Biological factors, life experiences, knowledge, attitude and behaviour, all contribute to the development of one's sexuality. Sexuality is considered abnormal if

a. The sexual behaviour is destructive;
b. It cannot be directed towards the partner;
c. It excludes the stimulation of primary sex organs;
d. It is associated with inappropriate guilt and anxiety.[1]

Sexual disorders carry significant importance. They can have significant psychological, marital, social and legal implications on the individual. They are associated with significant distress and dysfunction in the individual as well as the partner.

The DSM (Diagnostic and Statistical Manual of Mental Disorders) system (American Psychiatric Association, 1994) and the ICD classification of mental and behavioural disorders (World Health Organization, 1992) have described psychosexual disorders.[2,3] Both these systems have discussed sexual disorders under different heads and subheads. A comprehensive list of sexual disorders as described in the two classification systems is shown in Table 43.1.

Table 43.1 Classification of Psychosexual Disorders

DSM-IV Classification	*ICD-10 Classification*

Sexual and gender identity disorders
• Sexual dysfunctions
  Sexual desire disorders (hypoactive sexual desire disorder, sexual aversion)
  Sexual arousal disorders
  Orgasmic disorders (female and male orgasmic disorders, premature ejaculation)
  Sexual pain disorders (dyspareunia, vaginismus)
  Sexual dysfunction due to a general medical condition
  Substance-induced sexual dysfunction
  Sexual dysfunction not otherwise specified
• Paraphilias
• Gender identity disorders
• Sexual disorder not otherwise specified (includes marked feelings of sexual inadequacy, persistent and marked distress about sexual orientation)
	Behavioural syndromes associated with physiological disturbance and physical factors include sexual dysfunctions
	• Sexual dysfunction not caused by organic disorder or disease
	  Lack or loss of sexual desire
	  Sexual aversion and lack of sexual enjoyment
	  Failure of genital response
	  Orgasmic dysfunction
	  Premature ejaculation
	  Nonorganic vaginismus
	  Excessive sexual drive
	  Other sexual dysfunction not due to organic disorder or disease
	  Unspecified sexual dysfunction
	Disorders of adult personality and behaviour
	• Gender identity disorders
	• Disorders of sexual preference (include paraphilias)
	• Psychological and behavioural disorders associated with sexual development and orientation (include egodystonic homosexuality)
	  Other specified neurotic disorders
	• Dhat syndrome

The sexual response cycle consists of phases of sexual desire, excitement, orgasm and resolution. Sexual dysfunction could result from disturbances in one or more of these, or from pain associated with sexual intercourse (sexual pain disorders). Sexual dysfunctions are associated with marked distress and interpersonal difficulty (Table 43.2).[2]

Table 43.2 Sexual-Response Cycle and Associated Disorders

Phase of Sexual Cycle	*Characteristics*	*Disorder*
Desire	Fantasies about sexual activity and desire for sexual activity	Hypoactive sexual desire disorder; sexual aversion disorder
Excitement	Sexual pleasure and associated physiological changes, penile tumescence and erection in males; pelvic vasocongestion, vaginal lubrication and expansion, swelling of external genitalia in females	Male erectile disorder (erectile impotence); female sexual arousal disorder
Orgasm	Peaking of sexual pleasure, release of sexual tension and rhythmic contraction of perineal muscles, anal sphincter and sex organs. In males, sense of ejaculatory inevitability followed by semen ejaculation. In females, contractions of the wall of the outer third of the vagina	Female orgasmic disorder, male orgasmic disorder (including anorgasmia), Premature ejaculation (PME)
Resolution	Sense of muscle relaxation and general wellbeing. Males are physiologically refractory to further erection and orgasm for variable time periods.	Postcoital dysphoria Postcoital headache

Adapted from Sadock VA, 19951 & DSM-IV APA, 19942

Social, ethnic, religious and cultural factors influence sexual desire, attitudes, expectations and behaviour. Individual variations also account for differences in sexual functioning.

The 'psychosexual' disorders are not better accounted for by major psychiatric ailments, general medical conditions and are not exclusively due to physiological effects of substance use. Mostly the definitions and descriptions as recognized by the DSM-IV criteria have been followed in this chapter.[2] An attempt is made to be somewhat over-inclusive so as to provide a glimpse into the broad area of sexual disorders.

Although fewer in number, Indian studies are available on sexual dysfunctions in patients presenting to the psychiatric clinic of general hospital, psychosexual clinics and STD clinics.[4,5] A recent study conducted at the All India Institute of Medical Sciences (AIIMS), New Delhi, examined the clinical profile of psychosexual disorders in a thousand subjects attending a sex therapy clinic. The problems of premature ejaculation (77.6%), nocturnal emissions (71.3%), masturbatory guilt (33.4%), small penile size (30%), erectile dysfunction (23.6%) and venereo-phobia (13%) were prevalent in the study group.[5] The study highlights the relevance of sexual disorders to dermatovenereologists and also the need for timely recognition, careful assessment as well as appropriate referral to relevant specialists like psychiatrists, urologists and endocrinologists. Across various studies, erectile impotence and premature ejaculation are common amongst males; sexual desire and sexual pain disorders are common in females. The areas of female sexuality and associated disorders, sexual disorders other than sexual dysfunctions, the issues pertaining to the management of sexual disorders have not been adequately addressed in literature.

The onset, context and etiological factors associated with sexual dysfunctions may vary. Accordingly sexual dysfunction may be present since the onset of sexual functioning (primary) or may develop after a period of normal functioning (secondary); it may or may not be limited to certain types of stimulation, situations or partners; it may result from psychological factors, general medical conditions, substance abuse or side effects of medication, specific physical deficits or a combination of these factors.

SEXUAL DYSFUNCTIONS

Disorders of Sexual Desire

Hypoactive Sexual Desire Disorder

It is seen in both sexes, more so in females. It is characterized by persistent or recurrent deficiency or absence of sexual fantasies, feelings and desire to indulge in sexual activity, inappropriate to age and personal context. It manifests as decreased frequency and avoidance of sexual intercourse, or with complaints of lack of desire. The disorder manifests around puberty and may remain lifelong. Sexual desire is influenced by biological drive and factors like self-esteem, previous sex experience, availability of partner and appropriate circumstances, interpersonal factors and periods of abstinence. Biologically, hypoactive sexual desire may be associated with neurochemical (central dopaminergic blockade) or hormonal (decreased testosterone levels in males, increased prolactin) disturbance.[6] Psychosocial factors and conditioning are also known to affect desire. Psychodynamically, hypoactive desire may represent a defence against unconscious sexual fears.[1,2]

Sexual Aversion Disorder

It is characterized by persistent or recurrent extreme aversion to and avoidance of all or almost all genital sexual contact with the sexual partner. At times it is difficult to distinguish between hypoactive desire disorder and sexual aversion disorder, and in some cases both may co-exist. Previous traumatic sexual experiences, viz., rape or child abuse, repeated painful experiences with coitus, interpersonal problems with the partner, early developmental conflicts in the unconscious, associating sexual intercourse with guilt, shame, pain and fear, have been implicated as psychological etiological factors.[1,2] The disorder should be carefully assessed and the underlying cause should be appropriately treated. Mental and behavioural therapies are useful tools in the management of such disorders.

Excessive Sexual Drive (Sex Addiction, Satyriasis)

Although not a universally accepted or recognized disorder, it may be encountered in both sexes, usually manifesting in late adolescence and young adulthood. It is referred to as "Don Juanism" in males and nymphomania in females.[1] The term sex addiction has often been used to describe persons who compulsively seek out sexual experiences and whose behaviour becomes impaired if unable to gratify their sexual impulses. Sex addicts are unable to control their sexual impulses and their entire life revolves around sex-seeking behaviour and activities. A longstanding persistent or recurrent pattern of such behaviour and a history of several unsuccessful attempts to stop such behaviour are observed. The disorder manifests as out-of-control, self-destructive or high-risk sexual behaviour with persistence despite adverse consequences (medical, legal and interpersonal domains); repeated attempts to stop or limit such behaviour; sexual fantasies and obsessions; need for increasing sexual activities; severe mood changes associated with sexual activity; substantial amount of time spent in such activities; and interference of sexual behaviour in socio-occupational life. It is commonly associated with impulse control and substance use problems. Behavioural manifestations often include paraphilias and compulsive masturbation. In order to diagnose it as an independent disorder, one should be able to rule out other possible etiologies like bipolar mood disorders and early stages of dementia. Psychotherapies and pharmacotherapies have been used to manage the disorder. Serotonin-specific re-uptake inhibitors (like fluoxetine) are known to reduce libido in some persons, a side effect that can be used therapeutically. Medroxyprogesterone acetate diminishes libido in men. Androgenic compounds contribute to sex drive in women, thus antiandrogens (like cyproterone acetate) can be of benefit in reducing sex drive in female patients.[1]

Sexual Arousal Disorders

These disorders are characterized by persistent or recurrent, partial or complete failure to attain or maintain the sexual excitement response until completion of the sexual act. The sexual excitement response refers to lubrication and swelling response in females, and penile erection in males. Sexual arousal is influenced by testosterone in men and oestrogen in women. Other potential mechanisms include central dopaminergic stimulation, modulation of cholinergic-adrenergic balance, peripheral α1 agonism and nitric oxide.[6] Sexual arousal disorder is associated with marked distress and dysfunction.[2]

Female sexual arousal disorder can lead to painful coitus and associated problems like secondary dyspareunia, vaginismus and sexual desire problems. Vaginal dryness could result from psychological factors, infections, oestrogen deficiency and use of anticholinergic medication.

Erectile dysfunction[1,7] in males can be a cause of non-consummation of marriage, infertility and disruption of marital and sexual relationships. It may present as a primary or lifelong problem (if the male has never been able to attain or maintain an erection sufficient enough for successful sexual intromission or coital connection), or as a secondary or acquired one (following an initial period of normal functioning).

The problem may manifest or can be felt at different periods within the same phase of excitement, viz. inability to attain an erection, inability to sustain an erection till penetration, and inability to sustain an erection for a sufficient time following penetration. Impotence has been defined as the inability to attain and sustain an erection at most attempts. It is often associated with premature ejaculation and may also be associated with sexual desire problems.

The coordination between nervous system, vascular supply and hormonal factors is required for smooth erectile function.[1,7] The disorder may result from a complex interplay of several physiological, biological, psychological, interpersonal and situational factors. Due to physiological reasons, it is difficult to attain erection soon after ejaculation. The quality and frequency of erections may also decline with advancing age.

The problem is likely to be psychogenic if erection occurs normally in certain situations like during masturbation, in sleep or with a different partner. Erectile dysfunction may manifest in a specific situational context or with a particular partner, thereby suggesting the role of external factors, both situational as well as interpersonal. Neurotransmitters like dopamine and β adrenergic transmission have a facilitatory effect on erectile function while α1 adrenergic transmission has an inhibitory effect.[1] Clinically the role of neurotransmitters is reflected by erectile dysfunction or impotence associated with antidopaminergic (antipsychotic) drugs and β-blockers, and enhanced erection with dopaminergic agonists and priapism with trazodone (α1 blocker).

Across different cultures, manliness is equated to virility and sexual potency.[8,9,10] There is considerable stress, even if covert, on males to perform. A vicious cycle therefore sets in, with performance anxiety contributing to sexual dysfunction and the latter contributing or adding to the former. Previous sexual experiences if unpleasant or performed under stress, haste or with guilt or mixed feelings may also contribute. Unconscious fears, conflicts, sexual myths and beliefs also play an important role. Inadequate understanding and fear of stigmatization prevent early and appropriate help-seeking from professionals and may add to the stress and anxiety and to the problem as a whole.

The disorder, like any other psychosexual disorder, requires adequate, careful and appropriate assessment. This requires the clinician to be empathic, reassuring and competent. There is a need to ensure confidentiality and privacy, and to comfort the patient to establish mutual trust and rapport.

Assessment should include patient's understanding about sexuality and the problem; assessment of patient's knowledge, beliefs and attitude, myths, pattern of sexual behaviour; defining the exact nature of the problem, pattern (since when, context), associated problems in other phases of the sexual response cycle; pressure of performance; liking of the sexual partner and attitude towards her; sexual understanding and attitude of the spouse or partner; previous sexual experiences (with spouse, partner, casual, commercial, masturbatory, paraphilias) and the circumstances and the mindset under which performed, viz. under the influence of substance or drugs, attempts to test potency, presence of guilt feelings with respect to masturbation or previous sex experiences; associated psychopathology or feelings of depression and anxiety; and associated comorbid physical ailments, substance abuse, medication history, history of spinal surgery or trauma.

The assessment of functioning should include a history of early morning erections, ability to attain some erection, history of masturbation or previous sexual functioning.

A careful physical examination should include the assessment of secondary sexual characteristics and genitalia (penile shaft, testicular size, etc.). Cremasteric reflex and bulbocavernosal reflex should be checked to assess for neuropathies.

Investigations and medical and surgical aspects of treatment are discussed in detail in a chapter on erectile dysfunction.

Psychological: Psychiatric management also includes sexual counselling, sex education and psychotherapies. The purpose is to allay myths and fears, educate regarding normal human sexual anatomy and physiology, and to teach behavioural skills.

Conjoint marital unit therapy, as advocated by Master and Johnson, is based on the concept of marital unit or a dyad as the object of therapy. Both partners need to actively participate in the therapy as both are considered to be responsible for the sexually distressing relationship. The marital or interpersonal relationship as a whole is treated, and specific emphasis is laid on sexual functioning. Individual sessions focus on understanding their current problem and their life style. Specific suggestions pertaining to sexual acts and lifestyle are followed by the couple. The problem can be effectively approached by a team of male and female therapists.[8]

Behavioural exercises help in ameliorating fear of inadequate performance. Sexual dysfunction is assumed to be a learnt maladaptive behaviour and therefore behavioural regime efforts are made to unlearn maladaptive patterns and to learn adaptive ones. Relaxation exercises help in allaying anxiety. The couple is advised specific sexual play by the therapist. The therapy progresses in a graded fashion beginning with less demanding exercises (sensate focus exercises) that focus on sensory awareness to touch, site, sound and smell and ending up with satisfying sexual intercourse. Mastery of the initial, less demanding assignments instills a sense of confidence and helps in dissociating anxiety from the sexual act.[8]

Depending on the dysfunction, specific exercises can be used for their management.

Other forms of psychotherapy like supportive psychotherapy and insight-oriented psychotherapy can be incorporated in the treatment regime.[1]

Orgasmic Disorders

Orgasmic disorders include male and female orgasmic disorders and premature ejaculation in males.[2] Serotonin and $\alpha 1$ adrenergic transmission mediate orgasm and ejaculation. Drugs with $\alpha 1$ blocking properties may cause impaired ejaculation, and serotonergic agents may inhibit orgasm.[1]

Female orgasmic disorder (inhibited female orgasm, anorgasmia) is defined as recurrent or persistent inhibition of the female orgasm. It manifests as the absence or delay in orgasm after a normal sexual excitement phase, judged to be adequate in focus, intensity and duration. The diagnosis of the disorder should take into account factors like age, sexual experience and adequacy of sexual stimulation.

Male orgasmic disorder (inhibited male orgasm, retarded ejaculation) is characterized by persistent or recurrent delay or absence of orgasm following a normal sexual excitement phase during sexual activity. Before arriving at a diagnosis, the clinician needs to consider factors like the individual's age, focus, intensity and duration of the act.[2]

The condition is different from retrograde ejaculation, which is mostly organic. In retrograde ejaculation, ejaculation occurs but the ejaculate passes backwards into the urinary bladder. Some men may have partial dysfunction or inhibition of orgasm, and may experience a slow dribbling of ejaculate. They do not experience an orgasmic spurt and the pleasure associated with it.

Male orgasmic disorder is seen mostly following genitourinary surgeries (viz., prostatectomy); in elderly persons on drugs with anticholinergic side effects; use of antihypertensive drugs (methyl dopa, guanethidine monosulfate), phenothiazines, SSRIs; in disorders like Parkinsonism and neurological disorders with lumbosacral spinal involvement. It is often associated with obsessive compulsive disorder or temperament. Transient retarded ejaculation is seen following heavy alcohol consumption or with hyperglycemia. Primary inhibited male orgasm may reflect unconscious conflicts or considering genitals and sex as dirty and sinful. Secondary inhibition may arise out of interpersonal difficulties with the partner and reflect a covert hostility towards the partner. Mutual agreement on issues pertaining to pregnancy, contraceptives, type and need for sex and satisfaction should be assessed.[1]

Premature ejaculation (PME) is a condition in which a man recurrently achieves orgasm and ejaculation before he wishes to do so. It is difficult to define the time frame, and no specific time duration has been defined to differentiate normal functioning from dysfunction. The diagnosis is made when a male regularly (on a recurrent or persistent pattern) ejaculates on minimal sexual stimulation before or soon after entering the vagina.[2] Factors like age, novelty of the sexual partner, frequency and duration of coitus may affect the duration of the excitement phase, and should be considered before making this diagnosis. In certain individuals, prolonged stimulation is required to attain an erection, and as a result the effective time interval between satisfactory erection and ejaculation may appear to be short; the primary diagnosis in such cases should be that of delayed erection.

The ICD-10 system of classification and Masters and Johnson have defined the disorder taking into account both partners rather than the individual alone.[3,8] Accordingly, the failure/inability to control ejaculation sufficiently to enjoy sexual interaction is used to define the disorder. The diagnosis is made when a man cannot control ejaculation for sufficient period during intravaginal containment to satisfy the partner in about half of the episodes of coitus. This definition assumes that the female is capable of an orgasmic response. The problem can be related to the concern of partner satisfaction. The disorder is commonly associated with erectile dysfunction and sexual desire problems. In severe cases, ejaculation may occur prior to vaginal entry or in the absence of an erection.

PME is unlikely to be of organic origin; however, it can be a result of a psychological reaction to organic impairment like erectile failure or pain.

Performance anxiety, performance in haste, unconscious fear about the vagina, fear of castration, previous sexual experiences (if performed in haste or under stress/fear of discovery leading to quick orgasm and ejaculation) and negative cultural conditioning are some factors that play an aetiological role in the development of such a dysfunction. Partner role is very important and may exacerbate or help in the management of PME.

Sex counselling, behavioural exercises including relaxation techniques, and adoption of specific postures during sexual play help in management. The squeeze technique is typically used to raise the threshold of penile excitability. In this technique, the penis is stimulated until the initial sensation of impending orgasm and ejaculation is felt by the male. The male signals this to the female partner who then stops penile stimulation abruptly and forcibly squeezes the coronal ridge of the penis for a few seconds. The painful stimulus prevents orgasm and ejaculation in the male, and may lead to decline in erection. This technique is repeated several times during the sexual play.[8] In an alternative stop-start technique, stimulation is interrupted for some time and no squeeze is applied.

SSRIs and clomipramine (a tricyclic antidepressant with serotonergic reuptake blockade) may be used to delay ejaculation, following proper assessment, keeping in mind and discussing the potential benefits and side effects.

Sexual Pain Disorders

Dyspareunia is characterized by recurrent or persistent pain during intercourse and can affect both sexes, mostly females. The pain is real and unbearable and can lead to subsequent avoidance of sexual act. In females it is often associated with vaginismus.[1,2]

The causes are usually psychogenic or local infections or traumatic conditions. Female genital surgeries are often associated with temporary dyspareunia. Anxiety or fear about sex resulting in an involuntary tension of vaginal muscles and previous traumatic sexual history of child abuse or rape could play an aetiological role in its development. It is important to rule out organic etiologies, viz., pelvic inflammatory disease in females, infected hymenal remnants, episiotomy scars, Bartholin's gland infections, vaginitis, cervicitis, endometriosis, dermatological disorders (lichen sclerosis) and other pelvic disorders. Irritation associated with improperly fitted or inadequately lubricated condoms and allergic reactions to the contraceptive method used may also contribute. Postmenopausal women may develop this problem because of atrophy of the vaginal mucosa and diminished lubrication.

The disorder, though uncommon in males, is usually associated with Peyronie's disease, prostatitis, gonorrhoeal and herpetic infections. Post-ejaculatory pain may result from involuntary spasm of the perineal muscles due to psychological conflicts about the sex act or as a side effect of some medicines including some antidepressants.

Vaginismus is the involuntary and persistent constriction of the outer third of the vagina that prevents penile insertion and intercourse.[1,2] It may reflect a general tendency or may be specific to coitus. In the former case, it may be demonstrated during gynaecological examination in which involuntary vaginal constriction prevents introduction of the speculum into the vagina. The disorder is usually seen in educated women of high socioeconomic status. The affected woman may consciously wish to have coitus, but unconsciously prevents penile entry into her body. It may reflect strict religious upbringing equating sex to sin, previous life-traumatic experiences, sexual conflicts, anticipation of pain and dyadic relationship problems with partner. Local causes presenting as vaginismus should be ruled out. Sex education, counselling and behaviour therapy are helpful in managing the disorder. Relaxation techniques help in allaying anxieties. The affected woman is advised to use her fingers or size graduated vaginal dilators to dilate the vaginal opening.

Sexual Dysfunction due to General Medical Diseases

The diagnosis of such a condition is made from clear evidence (from history, physical examination and lab findings) that the distressing sexual dysfunction is due to direct physiological effects of a general medical condition.[2] Clues can be obtained from the temporal association between onset, exacerbation or remission of the general medical condition and that of sexual dysfunction. Sexual dysfunction can affect various phases of the sexual-response cycle ranging from problems of desire to orgasm. The disturbance is not better accounted for by another mental disorder like a major depression. A host of various medical conditions have been found to have direct physiological links with sexual dysfunctions, and some of these have been described elsewhere in this chapter.

Substance-Induced Sexual Dysfunction

Distressing sexual dysfunction is seen shortly after significant substance intoxication or withdrawal and is clearly linked to substance use.[2] Substances like alcohol, opioids, cocaine, amphetamines, and hypnotic-sedatives are known to be associated with the dysfunction. The type of dysfunction depends on the properties of the substance used and patterns of its use. In small amounts, the substances can enhance sexual performance by disinhibiting, anxiolytic and euphorogenic properties. Continued chronic use can cause dysfunction in the various phases of the sexual-response cycle. For example, alcohol can lead to sexual dysfunction through a CNS depressant effect, direct gonadal effect or an indirect hormonal effect following compromised liver functioning. It is known to be associated with erectile disorders in men and tends to decrease testosterone levels in them. Opioid use can also lead to erectile dysfunction and decreased libido.

PARAPHILIAS

Paraphilias are characterized by recurrent and intense sexual feelings, urges, fantasies and behaviours that involve unusual objects, activities or situations.[2] For example, they may involve non-human objects or children or non-consenting partners. These are usually associated with the suffering or humiliation of the self or the partner. The unusual fantasies are at most times gratifying to the ego. These are associated with significant distress and dysfunction (Table. 43.3).

Table 43.3 **Paraphilia and their Characteristic Features**

Type of Paraphilia	*Characteristic Features (manner in which sexual pleasure and excitement is obtained)*
Exhibitionism	Exposure of one's genitals to an unsuspecting stranger
Fetishism	Sexual fantasies and behaviour involving the use of non-living objects (fetish) like the female undergarments, belt and shoes. The sexual activity is directed to the non-living object or the wearing of the inanimate object by the partner. The focus throughout the sexual cycle, from desire to orgasm, is on the inanimate object associated with the human body
Sexual sadism	Real acts involving psychological and physical suffering of the partner/victim; acts of humiliation of the partner or victim, restraint and blindfolding the victim, pinching, beating and inflicting injuries to the victim
Sexual masochism	Intense sexual urges, fantasies or behaviours involving the act (real, not simulated) of being humiliated, beaten, bound or otherwise made to suffer
Frotteurism	Touching and rubbing against a non-consenting person/stranger
Paedophilia	Sexual fantasies and behaviour involves sexual activity with pre-pubescent children. The person is at least 16 years of age and at least 5 years older than the child.
Transvestic fetishism	Cross-dressing: while cross-dressed, the affected person usually indulges in sexual acts like masturbation, imagining himself to be the male subject as well as the female object of his fantasy. The condition is defined specifically for heterosexual males and therefore should not be confused with gender identity disorder
Voyeurism	Act of observing unsuspecting persons/strangers who are naked, removing their clothes or engaging in sexual acts. The observer gains sexual excitement from this observational (peeping) act, often fantasizes sexual experience with the observed person and hardly engages in a sex act with the latter. The observer is also referred to as 'peeping tom'
Others	
Coprophilia	Defaecating/faeces
Klismaphilia	Enemas
Urophilia	Urinating/urine
Telephone scatologia	Obscene phone calls
Zoophilia	Animals
Hypoxyphilia	Hypoxia (hanging, using plastic bag, suffocation)
Necrophilia	Dead or near dead
Partialism	Part of the body (foot)

Unconscious sexual conflicts, child neglect or abuse, past traumatic sexual experiences, underlying personality and impulse contol problems (like borderline personality) and learning can contribute to the development of paraphilias. In this regard, the role of pornographic literature and films cannot be negated. There is also a need to carefully assess and rule out any other major psychiatric disorder.

Psychotherapeutic techniques have been frequently employed to manage such disorders. Behaviour therapy is used with a focus on unlearning of maladaptive patterns and learning of healthy and adaptive sexual patterns and practices. This is done by pairing of noxious (aversive) stimuli with the paraphillic urge, impulse and feelings. Desirable sexual feelings and behaviour are positively reinforced. Insight-oriented psychotherapy is used to deal with unconscious conflicts. Sex therapy can aid in managing associated sexual dysfunctions. Drugs like antipsychotics and antidepressants have also been used. Anti-androgens have been used in hypersexual paraphilias, and SSRIs have been used for impulse control problems.[11]

GENDER IDENTITY DISORDER

It is characterized by a strong and persistent cross-gender identification (not merely a desire for any perceived cultural advantages of being the other sex) and persistent discomfort with one's own sex or sense of inappropriateness in the gender role of that sex.[2] In pure sense, it is not concurrent with physical intersex conditions like androgen insensitivity syndrome, congenital adrenal hyperplasia or ambiguous genitalia; nevertheless, such conditions should be assessed before making a diagnosis. It is associated with significant distress and socio-occupational dysfunction. The cross-gender behaviour of a child is generally apparent to the parents before 3 years of age. The childhood manifestations include repeated fantasies and stated desire or insistence that one is of the other sex, preference for cross-dressing with marked aversion towards normative sex clothing, intense desire to participate in stereotypical games and pastimes of the other sex, preference for playmates of the opposite sex, and assertion that one's genitalia are disgusting and that one would develop genitalia of the other sex. A boy with this disorder may insist to sit for urination and express the desire to get rid of his penis and testes, and a young girl may stand to urinate and insist that she will grow a penis. In adolescents and adults, the manifestations include preoccupation to get rid of the primary and secondary sexual characteristics and requests for hormone and surgical interventions to physically alter their sexual characteristics to simulate the other sex. It is important to differentiate gender identity disorders (transsexualism) from transvestism, homosexuality, psychotic and certain personality disorders.

SEXUAL BELIEFS AND NOTIONS

Sexual myths and prejudices about sex abound. Our society is deep-rooted in traditions, and sex is not to be openly discussed. Disorders of the genitalia are often referred to as "gupt rog" or secretive ailments. Amongst males, anxieties and concerns about semen loss, weakening of semen, loss of sexual vigour (*kamzori* or weakness), nocturnal emissions (*swapnadosh*), masturbation, shape and size of penis are common in the society.[4,10,12,13] Access to pornographic literature and films adds to the confusion.[10]

Masturbation is a common universal practice, more so in males than in females. Culturally and morally speaking, it is often considered a sin and a root cause of sexual, physical and mental ill-health, and nevertheless is associated with significant guilt, worry and depression.[12,13] Despite strong cultural beliefs and irrespective of the frequency or the technique employed, masturbation has not been identified as a direct aetiological factor in sexual dysfunctions.[8] During the pubertal hormonal spurt and the associated physiological changes, masturbation is frequently accompanied by sexual fantasies and serves as a preparatory ground for adult interaction with the partner. Due to the rising age at marriage for both genders, a significant proportion of young males and females have to pass through a long period of heightened sexual desires. Masturbation provides an acceptable release for heightened sexual impulses during this period. Even after a permanent sexual relationship has been established, masturbation remains a healthy sexual activity during non-availability/illness of the partner. It is considered maladaptive, when it becomes compulsive, is performed in public and is preferred over partner interaction.[1]

DHAT SYNDROME

Dhatu rog or shukrameha is a commonly recognized problem in our culture and has been prevalent since ancient times. Dhat syndrome is characterized by vague somatic complaints (like fatigue and loss of appetite) and mental weakness ascribed to the loss of semen in urine as a result of excessive indulgence in masturbation or sexual activities or due to nocturnal emissions.[10,12-19] The primary complaint of the affected person is loss of semen. It is often associated with psychosexual dysfunctions like erectile impotence and premature ejaculation and with features of anxiety or depression. The whitish discharge, although believed to be semen by the patient, is usually related to the presence of oxalates and phosphates in the urine. Ancient scriptures (like the *Charak Samhita*) and traditional systems of medicine (like the Ayurveda) have described this disorder and have laid emphasis on celibacy and avoidance of masturbation. According to a commonly held belief in the society, rich food gets converted into blood and blood gets converted into semen. Semen is regarded as an important *dhatu* (life elixir or vital force), and emphasis is laid on its preservation in order to ensure mental as well as physical health. Such deep-rooted beliefs give us clues to some understanding of the aetiology of the disorder.

The disorder has been subjected to clinical research and now finds acceptance in the current ICD-10 classificatory system in the category of other neurotic disorders under the broad rubric of neurotic, stress-related and somatoform disorders.[3] Strictly speaking it is not a sexual dysfunction, and is a sex-related disorder – sexual neuroses. Sex education, counselling and relaxation exercises are often used to address this problem. In sex education, emphasis is laid on the understanding of the normal human anatomy and physiological processes, particularly pertaining to the sex organs. Myths, prejudices, beliefs and attitudes towards sexuality are addressed. Comorbid psychopathology should be explored, assessed and appropriately treated. The latter may require the use of anxiolytics and or antidepressants.

HOMOSEXUALITY

It refers to sexual activity between persons of the same sex.[20] Sexual orientation is dynamic, and therefore different categories ('homosexual', 'hetero-sexual') are not necessarily mutually exclusive and fixed. Considering homosexuality as a mental illness is subject to significant controversies. Persistent and marked distress about sexual orientation (egodystonic homosexuality) is regarded as morbid.

VENEREOPHOBIA

It is not classified under psychosexual disorders but is an anxiety-related disorder. Venereo-neuroses are those neuroses that manifest with exposure to infection, including overreaction to infection, venereophobias and abnormal disease convictions, and factitious STDs and AIDS.[21] Some individuals may be unusually preoccupied with bodily processes, manifesting a genitally preoccupied hypochondriasis. There is irrational concern about the appearance of genitals or sensation in genitals. The preoccupation may assume an obsessional or delusional quality. The patient may self-manipulate genitals to produce discharge and demand treatment. Demanding treatment in the absence of demonstrable pathology is one indication of venereoneuroses and it is believed that such patients are more seriously disturbed. Syphiliphobia was common in 20th century, and in last 2 decades it was replaced by AIDS/HIV phobia. Many of these patients may have had a single sexual act that makes them phobic of sex for life. Reassurance, counselling, sex education and treatment of underlying hypochondriasis are used for management.

Sex is a basic human instinct and is inseparable from one's life. Sexual health is a very sensitive and important area, but is often ignored, dealt in a casual manner and full of controversies, myths and prejudices. Sexual disorders are a vast group of disorders. These disorders affect the individual's as well as the partner's life drastically and have significant medical, psychological, marital, social and legal implications.

There is a need to raise general awareness about sexual health in the society and to impart correct knowledge in an appropriate and healthy way. Age appropriate and sensitively handled sexual and moral education shall help in the process. This shall help in prevention, early diagnosis and timely treatment of such problems. As clinicians, we need to approach the area sensitively, sensibly and with professional competence and ethics. There is a need for careful assessment and development, modification and utilization of effective interventions to deal with these disorders. Issues of privacy make research into the area difficult. Systematic and careful research shall aid in enhancing the understanding and management of such disorders.

REFERENCES

1. Sadock VA. Normal human sexuality and sexual and gender identity disorders. In: Kaplan HI, Sadock BJ, eds. Comprehensive Text Book of Psychiatry. 6th edn. Baltimore: Williams and Wilkins; 1995. p. 1295-1360.
2. American Psychiatric Association. Diagnostic and statistical manual of mental disorders. 4th edn., Washington DC: APA; 1994.
3. World Health Organization. The ICD-10 Classification of mental and behavioural disorders: Clinical description and diagnostic guidelines, WHO, Geneva; 1992.
4. Avasthi A, Nehra R. Sexual disorders: a review of Indian research. In: Murthy RS, eds. Mental health in India 1950–2000. Bangalore: PAMH; 2001. p. 42-53.
5. Verma KK, Khaitan BK, Singh OP. The frequency of sexual dysfunctions in patients attending a sex therapy clinic in North India. Arch Sex Behav 1998; 27: 309-13.
6. Taylor D, Paton C, Kerwin R, eds. The Maudsley 2005-2006 prescribing guidelines. 8th edition, The South London and Maudsley NHS trust & Oxleas NHS Trust, London & New York: Taylor & Francis, 2005.
7. Vyas JN, Pandey SK Sexual disorders. In: Vyas JN, Ahiya N, eds. Textbook of Postgraduate psychiatry. 2nd edn. New Delhi: Jaypee Brothers; 1999. p. 333-44.
8. Masters WH, Johnson VE, eds. Human sexual inadequacy. London: J and A Churchill Ltd; 1970.
9. Tripathi BM, Malhotra S. Study on determinants of sexual risk behaviours amongst alcohol users in diverse cultural settings, a report submitted to WHO, Geneva. 2002.
10. Tripathi BM, Malhotra S. Sexual behaviour and sexually transmitted diseases. In : Sharma VK, et al. Sexually Transmitted Diseases and AIDS. 1st edn. New Delhi: Viva Books Pvt. Ltd; 2003. p. 431-43.
11. Meyer JK. Paraphilias. In: Kaplan HI , Sadok BJ, rds. Comprehensive text book of psychiatry. 6 th edn. Baltimore: Williams of Wilkins; 1995. p. 1334-47.
12. Kaviraj Khazanchand, edr. Indian Sexology. New Delhi: S. Chand and Co; 1972.
13. Kulhara P, Avasthi A Sexual dysfunction in Indian subcontinent, Intervention. Review of Psychiatry 1995; 7: 231-9.
14. Wig NN. Problems of mental health in India. J Clin Social Psychiat 1960; 17: 48-53.
15. Malhotra HK, Wig NN. Dhat syndrome: A culture bound sex neurosis of orient. Arch Sex Behav 1975; 4: 519-28.
16. Behere PB, Natraj GS. Dhat syndrome: the phenomenology of a culture bound sex neurosis of the orient. Indian J of Psychiatry 1984; 26: 76-8.

17. Sing G. Dhat syndrome revisited. Indian J Psychiat 1985; 22: 119-22.
18. Chadda RK, Ahiya N. Dhat syndrome: a sex neurosis of the Indian subcontinent. Br J of Psychiat 1990; 156: 577-9.
19. Bhatia MS, Malik SC. Dhat syndrome – a useful diagnostic entity in Indian culture. Br J Psychiat 1991; 159: 691-5.
20. Gadpaille WJ. Homosexuality and homosexual activity. In: Kaplan HI, Sadock BJ, eds. Comprehensive Textbook of Psychiatry. 6th edn. Baltimore: Williams and Silkins; 1995. 1321-33.
21. Ross MW. Psychological perspectives on sexuality and sexually transmitted disease. In Holmes KK, Sparling PF, Mardh PA, et al. eds. Sexually Transmitted Diseases. 3rd Edition. New York: Mc Graw Hill; 1999. 107-13.

44 ERECTILE DYSFUNCTION

Prem Nath Dogra, Anup Kumar

In this chapter

FUNCTIONAL ANATOMY OF THE PENIS

The penis is composed of three cylindrical structures, the paired corpus cavernosa and the corpus spongiosum, which houses the urethra covered by a loose subcutaneous layer and skin. The tunica albginea of corpora cavernosa supports corpus spongiosum and glans. It contains and protects the erectile tissue. It provides rigidity to corpora cavernosa and helps in veno-occlusive mechanism. Corpus spongiosum acts as a pressurized narrow chamber to allow the expulsion of semen from urethra. The glans provides sensory input to facilitate erection, increases pleasure and acts as a cushion to lessen the impact of penis on female organs. The smooth muscle regulates blood flow into and out of the sinusoids. The ischiocavernosus muscle pumps blood distally to speed up erection and provides additional penile rigidity during rigid erection phase. The bulbocavernosus muscle also compresses the bulb, thus helping in the expulsion of semen.

Arterial Supply (Fig. 44.1)

The main source of blood supply to the penis is through the internal pudendal artery, a branch of the internal iliac artery. In many instances, however, accessory arteries exist, arising from the external iliac, obturator, vesical and femoral arteries, and may occasionally become the dominant or only arterial supply to corpus cavernosum. The three branches of the penile artery are the dorsal, the bulbourethral and the cavernous arteries. The cavernous artery is responsible for tumescence of corpus cavernosum, and the dorsal artery for engorgement of glans penis during erection. The bulbourethral artery supplies the bulb and corpus spongiosum.[1]

Venous Drainage (Fig. 44.2)

Venous drainage from the three corpora originates in tiny venules leading from peripheral sinusoids immediately beneath tunica albuginea. These venules travel in the trabeculae between tunica and peripheral sinusoids to form subtunical venular plexus before exiting as emissary veins. Outside tunica albuginea, the venous drainage is as follows:

1. The skin and subcutaneous tissue. Multiple superficial veins run subcutaneously and unite near the root of the penis to form a single (or paired) superficial dorsal vein, which in turn drains into saphenous veins. Occasionally the superficial dorsal vein may also drain a portion of corpora cavernosa.

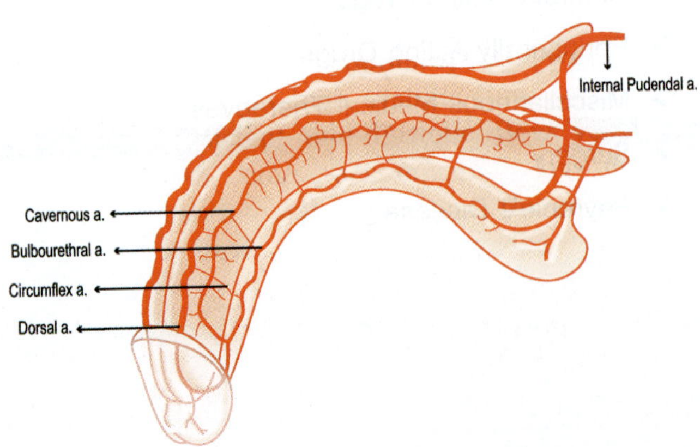

Fig. 44.1 Arterial Supply of the Penis.

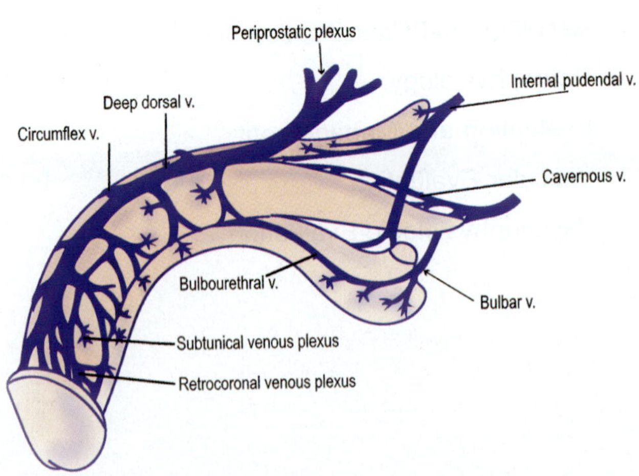

Fig. 44.2 Venous Drainage of the Penis.

2. The pendulous penis. The emissary veins from corpus cavernosum and spongiosum drain dorsally to the deep dorsal, laterally to the circumflex, and ventrally to the periurethral veins. Beginning at coronal sulcus, the prominent deep dorsal vein is the main venous drainage of glans penis, corpus spongiosum and distal two-thirds of corpora cavernosa. Usually a single vein, but sometimes more than one deep dorsal vein, runs upward behind symphysis pubis to join periprostatic venous plexus.
3. The infrapubic penis. Emissary veins draining the proximal corpora cavernosa join to form cavernous and crural veins. These veins join the periurethral veins from the urethral bulb to form the internal pudendal veins.[1]

MECHANISM OF ERECTION

Sexual stimulation triggers the release of neurotransmitters from the cavernous nerve terminals. This results in the relaxation of these smooth muscles and the following events.

1. Dilatation of arterioles and arteries by increased blood flow in both the diastolic and systolic phases.
2. Trapping of the incoming blood by the expanding sinusoids.
3. Compression of the subtunical venular plexuses between tunica albuginea and peripheral sinusoids, reducing the venous outflow.
4. Stretching of tunica to its capacity, which encloses the emissary veins between the inner circular and the outer longitudinal layers and further decreases the venous outflow to a minimum.
5. An increase in intracavernous pressure (maintained at around 100 mm Hg), which raises the penis to an erect state (the full-erection phase).
6. A further pressure increase (to several hundred millimeters of mercury) with the contraction of ischiocavernosus muscles (rigid-erection phase).[1]

Mechanism of Detumescence

Three phases of detumescence have been reported in an animal study. The first entails a transient intracorporeal pressure increase, indicating the beginning of smooth muscle contraction against a closed venous system. The second phase shows a slow pressure decrease, suggesting a slow reopening of the venous channels with resumption of the basal level of arterial flow. The third phase shows a fast pressure decrease with fully restored venous outflow capacity.[1]

Neural Control of Erection[2,3]

1. **Sympathetic innervation:** This innervation originates from T10 to L2 spinal segments, reaching the superior hypogastric plexus, from which they travel in the hypogastric nerve to form pelvic plexus. They cause detumescence.
2. **Parasympathetic innervation:** The parasympathetic pathway arises from neurons in the intermediolateral cell columns of the second, third and fourth sacral spinal cord segments. The preganglionic fibers pass in the pelvic nerves to pelvic plexus, where they are joined by the sympathetic nerves from superior hypogastric plexus. They cause erection.
3. **Somatic innervation:** Pudental nerve (S2-4 spinal segments) innervates ischiocavernosus (produces rigid erection phase) and bulbocavernosus muscle (causes ejaculation). Dorsal nerve of the penis carries sensory afferents from penile skin, glans, urethra and corpus cavernosum.
4. **Supraspinal pathways:** The medial preoptic area (MPOA) and the paraventricular nucleus of the hypothalamus and hippocampus are important integration centers for sexual function and penile erection.[1]

Types of erection: There are three types of erection: psychogenic, reflexogenic and nocturnal. Psychogenic erection is a result of audiovisual stimuli or fantasy. Impulses from the brain modulate the spinal erection centers (T11–L2 and S2–S4) to activate the erectile process. Reflexogenic erection is produced by tactile stimuli to the genital organs. The impulses reach the spinal erection centers; some then follow the ascending tract, resulting in sensory perception, whereas others activate the autonomic nuclei to send messages through cavernous nerves to the penis to induce erection. This type of erection is preserved in patients with upper spinal cord injury. Nocturnal erection occurs mostly during rapid-eye-movement (REM) sleep. PET scanning of humans in REM sleep shows increased activity in the pontine area, the amygdalae and the anterior cingulate gyrus, but decreased activity in the prefrontal and parietal cortex. The mechanism that triggers REM sleep is located in the pontine reticular formation. During REM sleep, cholinergic neurons in the lateral pontine tegmentum are activated, whereas adrenergic neurons in the locus coeruleus and the serotonergic neurons in the midbrain raphe are silent. This differential activation may be responsible for nocturnal erections during REM sleep.[1]

Neurotransmitters

Peripheral Neurotransmitters

Most researchers now agree that NO released from nonadrenergic/noncholinergic (NANC) neurotransmission and from the endothelium is the principal neurotransmitter mediating penile erection. NO increases the production of cGMP, which in turn relaxes the cavernous smooth muscle. Detumescence after erection may be a result of the cessation of NO release, the breakdown of second messengers by PDEs, or sympathetic discharge during ejaculation. During the return to the flaccid state, cGMP is hydrolyzed to GMP by the highly specific cGMP-binding PDE type 5 (PDE5).[1]

Central Neurotransmitters

Dopaminergic and adrenergic receptors may promote sexual function and that 5-HT receptors inhibit it.

AETIOLOGY AND CLASSIFICATION

Prevalence: As reported in the Massachusetts Male Aging Study (MMAS), between the ages of 40 and 70 years, the probability of complete ED increased from 5.1 to 15%, moderate dysfunction increased from 17 to 34%, and mild dysfunction remained constant at about 17%.[4]

Incidence: The crude incidence rate of impotence in White males in the United States was found to be 25.9 cases/1000 man-years.[4]

Risk factors: General health status, diabetes mellitus, cardiovascular disease, concurrence of other genitourinary disease, psychiatric or psychological disorders, other chronic diseases, smoking, medications and hormonal factors.[4,5]

Classification: A classification recommended by the International Society of Impotence Research is shown in the Table 44.1.[6] Various disorders that can be associated with erectile dysfunction are listed in Table 44.2.

Table 44.1 **Classification for Male Erectile Dysfunctions**

Organic
I. Vasculogenic
A. Arteriogenic
B. Cavernosal
C. Mixed
II. Neurogenic
III. Anatomic
IV. Endocrinological

(*Contd.*)

Psychogenic

- I. Generalized type
  - A. Generalized unresponsiveness
    - i. Primary lack of sexual arousability
    - ii. Aging-related decline in sexual arousability
  - B. Generalized inhibition
    - i. Chronic disorder of sexual intimacy
- II. Situational type
  - A. Partner-related
    1. Lack of arousability in specific relationship
    2. Lack of arousability due to sexual object preference
    3. High central inhibition due to partner conflict or threat
  - B. Performance-related
    1. Associated with other sexual dysfunctions (e.g. rapid ejaculation)
    2. Situational performance anxiety (e.g. fear of failure)
  - C. Psychological distress or adjustment-related
    1. Associated with negative mood state (e.g. depression) or major life stress (e.g. death of partner)

Table 44.2 **Disorders Associated with Male Erectile Dysfunction**

Cardiovascular diseases
Atherosclerosis
Venous leakage syndrome
Coronary artery disease
Arteriovenous malformations
Aortic aneurysms
Cardiac failure
Endocrine disorders
Diabetes mellitus
Pituitary-adrenal-testes dysfunction
Acromegaly
Thyroid disturbance
Hyperprolactinaemia
Addison's disease
Cushing's syndrome
Adrenal neoplasia
Neurological disorders
Multiple sclerosis
Transverse myelitis
Parkinson's disease
Stroke
Temporal lobe epilepsy
Spinal cord injuries
Tumours of the CNS
Amyotrophic lateral sclerosis
Sensory neuropathies

(*Contd.*)

Urological disorders
Peyronie's disease (fibrous bands in penile shaft)
Chronic renal failure
Hydrocoele
Varicocoele
Hepatic disorders (cirrhosis)
Pulmonary disorders (COPD, respiratory failure)
Infections (elephantiasis, leprosy, mumps)
Genetic disorders
(Klinefelter's syndrome, congenital penile vascular and structural abnormalties)
Nutritional disorders
Malnutrition
Vitamin and zinc deficiencies
Obesity
Psychiatric disorders
Depression
Anxiety
Substance use disorders (alcohol, opioids, cocaine, amphetamines, barbiturates, tobacco)
Pharmacological agents (drugs)
Antihypertensives
Psychotropics (certain antipsychotics and antidepressants)
Oestrogens and antiandrogens
H-2 receptor antagonists
Digoxin
Cytotoxic drugs
Poisonings (e.g. lead, herbicides)
Surgical procedures (e.g. certain abdominoperineal surgeries)
Others (like radiation therapy, pelvic fracture, severe systemic debilitating disease)

Adapted from Saddock 1995[1]

PATHOPHYSIOLOGY

Psychogenic

Two possible mechanisms have been proposed to explain the inhibition of erection in psychogenic dysfunction: direct inhibition of the spinal erection center by the brain as an exaggeration of the normal suprasacral inhibition[3] and excessive sympathetic outflow or elevated peripheral catecholamine levels, which may increase penile smooth muscle tone to prevent the relaxation necessary for erection.

Neurogenic

The MPOA, the paraventricular nucleus and the hippocampus have been regarded as important integration centers for sexual drive and penile erection. Pathologic processes in these regions, such as Parkinson's disease, stroke, encephalitis or temporal lobe epilepsy, are often associated with ED. In a patient with spinal cord injury, the degree of erectile dysfunction that persists depends largely on the nature, location and extent of the spinal lesion. Reflexogenic erection is preserved in 95% of patients with complete upper cord lesions, whereas only about 25% of those with complete lower cord lesions can achieve an erection. An improved understanding of the neuroanatomy of pelvic and cavernous nerves has resulted in modified surgery for cancer of the rectum, bladder and prostate, producing a lower incidence of iatrogenic impotence. For example, the introduction of nerve-sparing radical prostatectomy has reduced the incidence of impotence from nearly 100% to 30 to 50%.[5,7-9]

Endocrinologic

Hypogonadism leads to decreased serum testosterone levels, causing decreased libido and erectile dysfunction.[10] Hyperprolactinemia, whether from pituitary adenoma or drugs, results in both reproductive and sexual dysfunction. Hyperthyroidism is commonly associated with diminished libido, which may be caused by increased circulating oestrogen levels and less often with ED. In hypothyroidism, low testosterone secretion and elevated prolactin levels contribute to ED. Diabetes mellitus, although the most common endocrinologic disorder, causes ED through its vascular, neurologic, endothelial and psychogenic complications rather than due to hormone deficiency. The proposed mechanisms of ED in diabetic animals include: (1) impaired NO synthesis; (2) increased endothelin B receptor binding sites and ultrastructural changes; (3) increased levels of oxygen-free radicals and oxidative stress injury; (4) NO-dependent selective nitrergic nerve degeneration; and (5) elevated levels of advanced glycosylation end products.[5,11]

Arteriogenic

In a majority of patients with arteriogenic ED, impaired penile perfusion is a component of the generalized atherosclerotic process. The incidence and age at onset of coronary disease and ED are parallel. Common risk factors associated with arterial insufficiency include hypertension, hyperlipidemia, cigarette smoking, diabetes mellitus, blunt perineal or pelvic trauma, and pelvic irradiation. Focal stenosis of the common penile or cavernous artery is most often seen in young patients who have sustained blunt pelvic or perineal trauma. Long-distance cycling is also a risk factor for vasculogenic and neurogenic ED.[12-14]

Cavernosal (Venogenic)

1. The presence or development of large venous channels draining the corpora cavernosa.
2. Degenerative changes (Peyronie's disease, old age and diabetes) or traumatic injury to tunica albuginea (penile fracture) resulting in inadequate compression of the subtunical and emissary veins.
3. Acquired venous shunts—the result of operative correction of priapism—may cause persistent glans/cavernosum or cavernosum/spongiosum shunting.[5]

Drug-Induced

Centrally acting sympatholytics including methyldopa, clonidine (inhibition of the hypothalamic center through α_2-receptor stimulation) and reserpine (depletion of the stores of catecholamines and 5-HT by blocking vesicular monoamine trans-porters I and II) are known to cause sexual dysfunc-tion. Other drugs known to cause ED are oestrogens and drugs with antiandrogenic action such as ketoconazole and cyproterone acetate.[5,15]

EVALUATION AND MANAGEMENT

At the NIH Consensus Conference on Impotence (1992), ED was defined as the inability to achieve and/or maintain erection of sufficient rigidity and duration to permit satisfactory sexual performance. The Second International Consultation on sexual medicine (ICSM) has advocated the management of ED based on a patient-centred and evidence-based principle summarized in **Figs. 44.3 and 44.4**.[5]

Questionnaires

The International Index of Erectile Function (IIEF) is the most widely used self-administered questionnaire (SAQ), and it is statistically validated in at least seven languages. The IIEF is a 15-item SAQ; it addresses and quantifies five domains: erectile function, orgasmic function, sexual desire, intercourse satisfaction and overall satisfaction.[16]

Medical and Psychosexual History (AUA Guideline 2005)

The initial assessment of a sexual problem includes a detailed medical, sexual and psychosocial history.

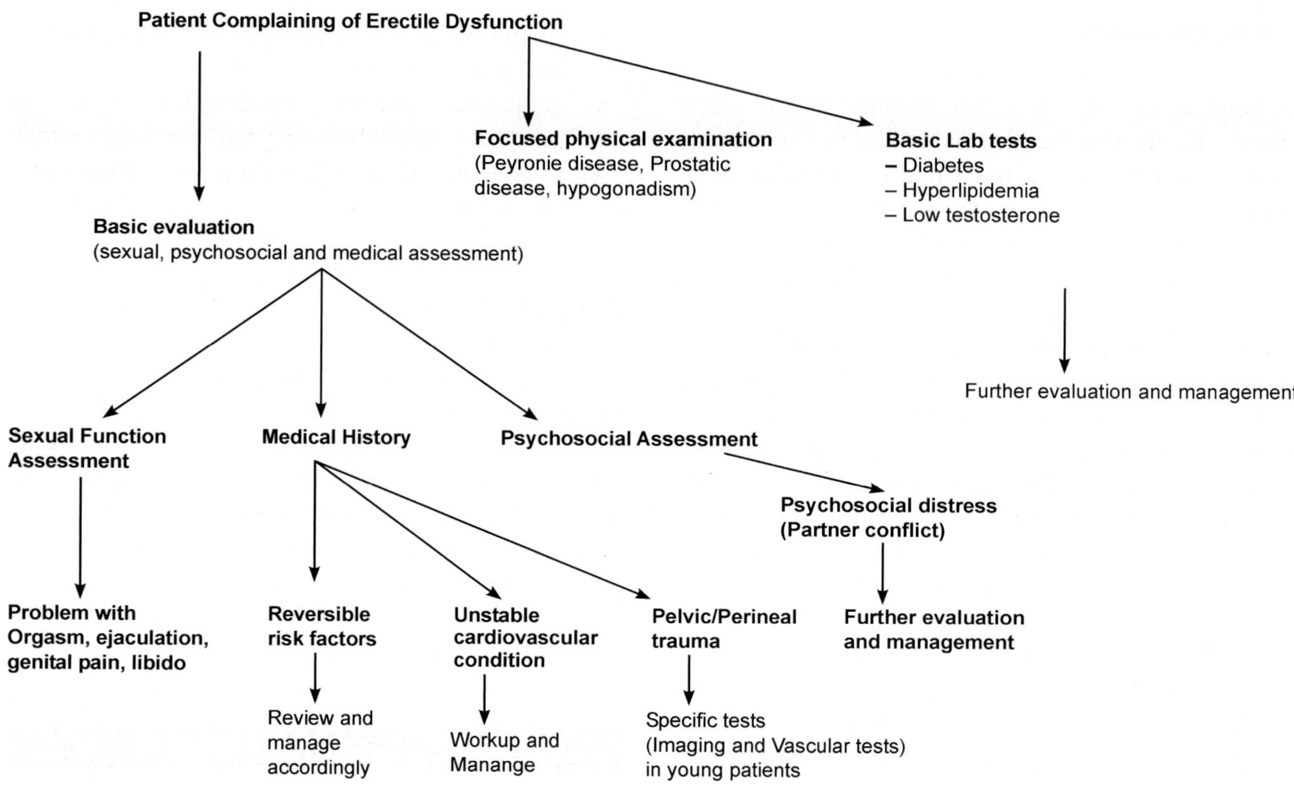

Fig. 44.3 Algorithm for sexual, psychosocial and medical assessment of erectile dysfunctions.

It is very practical to begin every evaluation of male sexual dysfunction with a good medical history to determine the patient's risks for organic ED, which includes hypertension, atherosclerotic coronary and peripheral vascular disease, diabetes mellitus, smoking and medications. A comprehensive sexual history is essential to confirm the diagnosis, as well as to evaluate the patient's overall sexual function. Because ED may have multiple causes, a detailed history and physical examination may help determine the etiology: anatomic, psychogenic, endocrinologic, neurologic or vascular. Most importantly, a history can reveal specific contraindications for drug therapy. Additional risk factors include smoking, pelvic, perineal, or penile trauma or surgery, neurologic disease, endocrinopathy, obesity, pelvic radiation therapy, Peyronie's disease, and prescription or recreational drug use. Other critical elements are alterations of sexual desire, ejaculation and orgasm, presence of genital pain, and lifestyle factors, such as sexual orientation, presence of spouse or partner and quality of relationship with the partner. Finally, a history of the partner's sexual function may be helpful. Attention is given to defining the problem, clearly distinguishing ED from complaints about ejaculation and/or orgasm, and establishing the chronology and severity of symptoms. An assessment of patient/partner needs and expectations of therapy is equally important.[17]

Physical Examination (AUA Guideline 2005)

Careful physical examination with particular attention to sexual and genital development may occasionally reveal an obvious cause (e.g., micropenis, chordee, Peyronie's plaque). The First International Consultation on ED recommends examination of every patient with assessment of body habits, secondary sexual characteristics and cardiovascular and neurologic systems, focusing on penile, testicular, rectal examinations and checking blood pressure. Prostate-specific antigen measurement and rectal examination should be

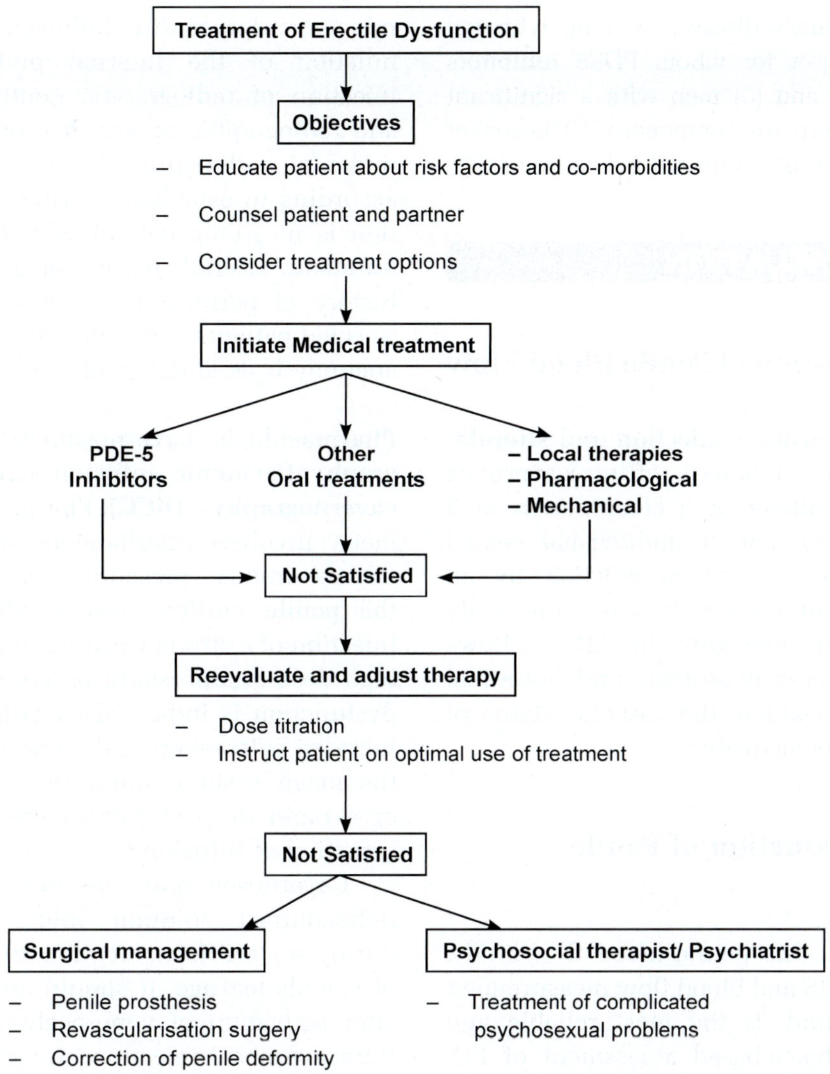

Fig. 44.4 Algorithm for the Treatment Strategy of Erectile Dysfunctions.

done to rule out prostate cancer when considering the use of testosterone in the management of male sexual dysfunctions.

Laboratory Testing

The laboratory testing is divided into three categories: recommended, optional and specialized. The recommended tests are used to identify the pathologic processes of diabetes mellitus, hyperlipidemia and the hypothalamic-pituitary-gonadal axis (fasting glucose or glycosylated hemoglobin, lipid profile and testosterone).

Shared Decision-Making and Treatment Planning

In accordance with the principle of patient-centred medicine, after the initial diagnostic evaluation, patients should be given a detailed description of the available treatment options.

Evaluation of Complex ED

Patients with complex ED include (1) those with penile/pelvic/perineal trauma; (2) young men with primary ED (present since age of sexual maturity);

(3) men with Peyronie's disease; (4) men who fail oral PDE inhibitors or for whom PDE5 inhibitors are contraindicated; and (5) men with a significant psychological or psychiatric component.[16] The goal of specialized evaluation is to find out the cause of ED.

VASCULAR EVALUATION

First-Line Evaluation of Penile Blood Flow

Combined intracavernosal injection and stimulation (CIS): The CIS test consists of intracavernous injection of a vasodilator or a combination of 2 or 3 vasodilators, genital or audiovisual sexual stimulation, and assessment of erection by an observer. This screening test is the most commonly performed diagnostic procedure for ED. It allows the clinician to bypass neurologic and hormonal influences and to evaluate the vascular status of penis directly and objectively.[16]

Second-Line Evaluation of Penile Blood Flow

Duplex ultrasound: The penile blood flow study, which consists of CIS and blood flow measurement by duplex ultrasound, is the most reliable and least invasive evidence-based assessment of ED. In the Mayo Clinic series, peak systolic velocity (PSV) of the cavernosal artery less than 25 cm/sec had a sensitivity of 100% and a specificity of 95% in selection patients with abnormal pudendal arteriography. When the Doppler spectral waveform continues to exhibit high systolic flow (>25 cm/PSV) and persistent end-diastolic flow velocity (EDV) of >5 cm/s accompanied by quick detumescence after self-stimulation, the patient is considered to have venogenic impotence.[19]

Third-Line Evaluation of Penile Blood Flow

Pharmacologic arteriography: Arteriography is performed by intracavernosal injection of a vasodilator agent (papaverine, papaverine + phentolamine, or alprostadil), followed by selective cannulation of the internal pudental artery and injection of radiographic contrast. The anatomy and radiographic appearance of the iliac, internal pudental and penile arteries are then evaluated according to established criteria. The best indication is in young patient with ED secondary to a traumatic arterial disruption or in patient with a history of perineal compression injury. In these selected patients, a detailed roadmap of the arterial anatomy is essential to plan reconstruction.[16]

Pharmacologic cavernosometry and cavernosography (Dynamic infusion cavernosometry and cavernography - DICC): Pharmacologic cavernosometry involves simultaneous saline infusion and intracavernous pressure monitoring to assess the penile outflow system after intracavernous injection of a strong vasodilating solution such as a high dose of alprostadil or Trimix. Veno-occlusive dysfunction is indicated by either the inability to increase intracavernosal pressure to the level of the mean systolic pressure with saline infusion or a rapid drop of intracavernosal pressure after cessation of infusion.[20]

Cavernosography involves the infusion of radiocontrast solution into corpora cavernosa during an artificial erection to visualize the site of venous leakage. It should always be performed after activation of veno-occlusive mechanism by intracavernosal injection of a vasodilator. Leakage sites to the glans, corpus spongiosum, superficial dorsal veins and DDVs, and cavernous and crural veins can then be detected. In a majority of patients, more than one site is visualized. DICC is reserved for young men who may be candidates for penile vascular operations, especially those with a history of pelvic trauma or lifelong ED.[21]

PSYCHOPHYSIOLOGICAL EVALUATION

Nocturnal Penile Tumescence and Rigidity (NPTR)

In 1985, the RigiScan was introduced; it was the first device to provide automated, portable recording of NPTR. The device combines monitoring of radial rigidity, tumescence, number and duration of erectile events with the convenience of a portable monitoring system that can be used at home.[22] Cilurzo and colleagues[23] recommend the following as normal NPTR criteria: four to five erectile episodes per night; mean duration greater than 30 minutes; an increase in circumference of greater than 3 cm at the base and greater than 2 cm at the tip; and greater than 70% maximal rigidity at both base and tip. The main advantages of NPTR testing are its relative freedom from psychologic influences and its ability to detect sleep-related abnormalities. The documented presence of a full erection indicates that the neurovascular axis is functionally intact and that the causes of ED are most likely psychogenic. The disadvantages of NPTR evaluation are that it is age-dependent and costly, because it is ideally done with a Rigiscan in a specially equipped sleep centre. Because of problems associated with various NPTR tests, this is not recommended as a routine part of ED evaluation.[24]

Neurologic Evaluation

Neurologic testing should assess peripheral, spinal and supraspinal centres and both somatic and autonomic pathways associated with all three types of erection and sexual arousal. But, the effect of a neurologic deficit on penile erection is a complicated phenomenon, and, with a few exceptions, neurologic testing will rarely change management.

1. **Sacral evoked response–Bulbocavernosus reflex (BCR) latency:** An abnormal BCR latency time, defined as a value greater than 3 standard deviations above the mean (30 to 40 msec), denotes a high probability of neuropathology.[25]
2. **Dorsal nerve conduction velocity:** Gerstenberg and Bradley have determined an average conduction velocity of 23.5 m/sec with a range of 21.4 to 29.1 m/sec in normal subjects.[26]

Hormonal Evaluation

For screening, a total testosterone determination is adequate. Circadian rhythm of testosterone levels should be considered in measuring serum testosterone, and blood should be drawn between 8 AM and 11 AM. The more commonly available option is measurement of total testosterone (240 to 950 ng/dl), free testosterone (9 to 30 ng/dl) and percentage of free testosterone (2% to 4.8%). If the results of total testosterone (in a patient younger than 50 years) or free testosterone in the elderly or obese patient are abnormal, repeat the testing in the early morning and obtain a free testosterone level and measure LH to differentiate primary from secondary hypogonadism. Only men with clearly documented hypogonadism are candidates for testosterone replacement therapy. In a small but significant number of patients, ED may be the initial clinical manifestation of a serious disease such as a prolactin-secreting tumor. Hyperprolactinemia may also be caused by certain drugs or medical conditions such as renal insufficiency and hypothyroidism, or may be idiopathic.[27] Many believe that the very low prevalence of significant hyperprolactinemia can hardly justify the routine determination of prolactin in men with ED, considering the frequency of ED and the cost of the determination.[24]

The investigations and evaluations required for the diagnosis of erectile dysfunction are summarized in Fig. 44.5. The flowchart for sexual, psychosocial and medical assessment is shown in **Fig. 44.3**.

NON-SURGICAL MANAGEMENT

Lifestyle Changes (AUA Guideline 2005)

Although it is difficult to prove its beneficial effect, a change of lifestyle should be encouraged (regular exercise, a healthy diet, smoking cessation, alcohol in moderation only). The pathophysiology of ED is intimately related to the pathophysiology of atherosclerotic coronary and peripheral vascular

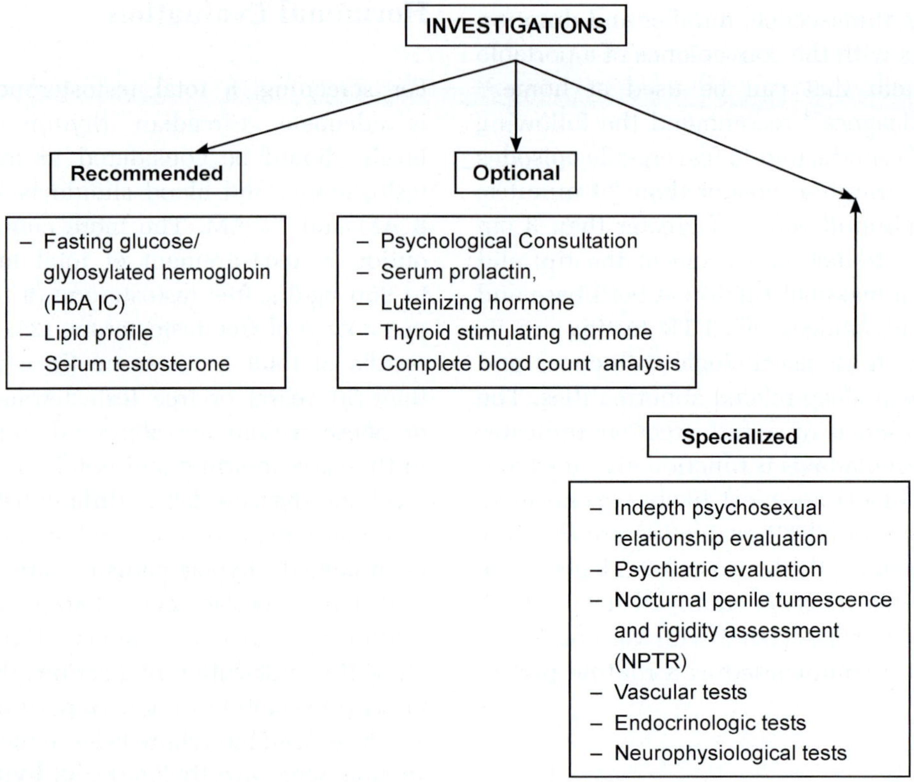

Fig. 44.5 Diagnosis and Evaluation of Erectile Dysfunctions.

diseases. Although the probability of complete ED was not statistically different between smokers and non-smokers in the MMAS (11% vs. 9.3%), cigarette smoking significantly increased impotence associated with cardiovascular disease, hypertension and medication usage. Since the risk of developing ED is increased in the presence of diabetes, heart disease and hypertension, it is logical to conclude that optimal management of these diseases may prevent the development of ED.[28-30] It is also logical to assume that lifestyle modifications to improve vascular function such as avoiding smoking, maintaining ideal body weight and engaging in regular exercise might either prevent or reverse ED; however, only minimal data exists today to support this supposition.[31,32] A syndrome of genital anesthesia and ED has been described among some long-distance bike riders. The detrimental effects of perineal compression on penile arteries may be lessened by changes in seat design and riding practices.

Changing Medications

Older antihypertensive drugs such as methyldopa and reserpine have a high incidence of sexual dysfunction because of their central suppressive effect. Thiazide diuretics are commonly associated with the complaint of ED, and spironolactone interferes with testosterone synthesis. Switching patients to newer agents such as calcium channel blockers and angiotensin-converting enzyme inhibitors may reverse ED in some patients.[27]

Pelvic Floor Muscle Exercises

Pelvic floor exercise is a realistic alternative to surgery in patients with mild venous leakage. Intensive phy-siotherapy consists of electrical stimulation of the isc-hiocavernosus muscle, graded pelvic floor exercises with muscle training, and a home exercise programme for lying, sitting and standing positions.[33,34]

Psychosexual Therapy

In some patients with mixed psychogenic and organic ED, psychosexual therapy may help relieve anxiety and remove unrealistic expectations associated with medical or surgical therapy.[35]

Managing ED in the Presence of Cardiovascular Disease (AUA Guideline 2005)

Cardiovascular disease and ED may share a common aetiology when endothelial dysfunction and athero-sclerosis affect both coronary arteries and penile vasculature.[36] Consequently, patients with ED frequently have concurrent cardiovascular disease.[37] Treatment of ED in patients with cardiovascular disease is complicated by a small increase in the risk of myocardial infarction (MI) related to sexual activity in these patients independent of the method of treatment. The major risk factors associated with cardiovascular disease are age, hypertension, diabetes mellitus, obesity, smoking, dyslipidemia and sedentary lifestyle. Patients with three or more of these risk factors[16] are considered to be at increased risk for MI during sexual activity. Guidelines for managing ED in patients with cardiovascular disease developed by the Princeton Consensus Panel[38] recommend assigning patients to one of three risk levels (high, intermediate and low) based on their cardiovascular risk factors. High-risk patients are defined as those with unstable or refractory angina; uncontrolled hypertension; congestive heart failure (MI) or a cardiovascular accident within the previous 2 weeks; high-risk arrhythmias; hypertrophic obstructive and other cardiomyopathies; or moderate-to-severe valvular disease. The document states that patients at high risk should not receive treatment for sexual dysfunction until their cardiac condition has stabilized. Patients at low risk may be considered for all first-line therapies. The majority of patients treated for ED are in the low-risk category defined as those who have asymptomatic coronary artery disease and less than three risk factors for coronary artery disease (excluding gender); controlled hypertension; mild, stable angina; a successful coronary revascularization; uncomplicated past MI; mild valvular disease; or CHF (left ventricular dysfunction). Patients whose risk is indeterminate should undergo further evaluation by a cardiologist before receiving therapies for sexual dysfunction.

Hormonal Therapy

In a patient with documented hypogonadism and ED, it is reasonable to initiate androgen therapy. Therapy should be continued for 2 to 3 months (Table 44.3). Our experience and that of others is that most patients experience improvement in libido, with far fewer noting increased erectile abilities.[39]

Table 44.3 Androgen Preparations

Drug	*Route*	*Dose (mg)*
Testosterone undecanuate	Oral	120–160; OD
Fluoxymesterone	Oral	5–20; OD
Enanthate (esterified testosterone)	IM	150–300; 2–4 weekly
Cypionate (esterified testosterone)	IM	14–300; 2–4 weekly
Transdermal patch		
– Testoderm	Scrotum	4–6; OD
– Endoderm	Skin	2.5–5; OD
– Testoderm T.T.S	Skin	5; OD
Transdermal cream Androgel 1%	Skin	25–50; OD

When taken orally, testosterone preparations are largely rendered metabolically inactive during the "first-pass" circulation through the liver. Metabolic inactivation requires oral dosing to exceed 200 mg/day to maintain normal serum levels. Large dosages of testosterone are toxic to the liver and can lead to hepatitis, cholestatic jaundice, hepatomas, hemorrhagic liver cysts and hepatocarcinoma.

Potential Adverse Effects

Supraphysiologic levels of testosterone will suppress LH and FSH production and result in infertility; breast tenderness and/or gynecomastia is not uncommon with parenteral testosterone dosing. Erythrocytosis is the most common laboratory alteration noted with long-term therapy. Cardiovascular risks are increased in some patients by increases in red cell mass; additionally, in young patients, abusing testosterone therapy moderately elevates low-density lipoprotein and decreases high-density lipoprotein. Increases in thromboxane A2 and platelet aggregation have also been attributed to testosterone therapy.[33] The presence of prostate or breast cancer is an absolute contraindication to androgen supplementation.

In patients with mild elevation of prolactin, other factors such as vascular or neurologic deficit may be the underlying cause of ED. If pituitary adenoma is identified (usually in patients with marked prolactin elevation, 10 times normal), the treatment of choice is bromocriptine or surgical ablation.

ORAL AGENTS

Peripheral initiators are agents that have their main site of action in the penis to activate biochemical events that lead to erection; this class includes the majority of available clinical options: injectable, intraurethral, topical and oral agents act this way. Peripheral conditioners are compounds that act mainly to improve local or systemic environment to enhance erection (e.g., l-arginine dosing or hormonal therapies). Central initiators are drugs with their primary activity in the CNS; they initiate neural events, resulting in enhanced signaling for erection (e.g., dopaminergics, apomorphine, 5-HT1 serotonergics). Central conditioners are agents that act mainly to improve the CNS environment to enable or enhance erection (hormonal therapies).[41]

CENTRALLY ACTING DRUGS

Yohimbine, an α_2-adrenergic antagonist, is obtained from the bark of the yohim tree. It acts centrally to promote sexual behaviour by blocking presynaptic autoreceptors and increasing adrenergic receptor activity, which also alters serotonin and dopamine transmission. Side effects of yohimbine include gastrointestinal intolerance, palpitations, headache, agitation, anxiety and increase in blood pressure (precautions are advised in men with cardiovascular disease). Yohimbine is not recommended in the treatment of erectile dysfunction.[42-44]

Serotonergic Drugs

A dual mechanism of (peripheral) α-adrenergic blocking and (central) inhibition of serotonin reuptake (increasing 5-HT_{1c}) is the proposed mechanism of action. It is probable that trazodone exerts both beneficial central initiator and peripheral conditioner effects on the neurophysiology of erection. Dosages ranging from 25 to 200 mg nightly have been used. Side effects are drowsiness, nausea, emesis, blood pressure changes (both hypotension and hypertension are reported), urinary retention and priapism (especially at therapeutic antidepressant levels). The use of trazodone in the treatment of erectile dysfunction is not recommended.[45]

Dopaminergic Agonist

Apomorphine is a D_1/D_2 dopaminergic agonist that stimulates proerectile signaling necessary for sexual arousal. The proprietary agent acts sublingually by buccal absorption, and erection efficacy is lost if the tablet is swallowed. The drug has a rapid onset of action, with mean time to erection of 12 minutes; the pharmacology permits a window of sexual opportunity of approximately 2 hours from ingestion. Maximal plasma concentrations are reached in 50 minutes. Eating before dosing had no effect on plasma concentrations. Adverse events described in clinical trials were nausea, 16.9%; dizziness, 8.3%; sweating, 5%; somnolence, 5.8%; yawning, 7.9%; and emesis, 3.7%.[46]

PERIPHERALLY ACTING DRUGS

Adrenoceptor Antagonists

Phentolamine is an α_1-adrenergic antagonist and has been used in combination with papaverine for ICI. Phentolamine is a non-specific α-adrenergic antagonist with equal affinity for blocking both α_1 and α_2 adrenoreceptors. Clinically direct intracorporeal injection of phentolamine results in penile tumescence but not rigidity.[47]

Phosphodiesterase Type 5 Inhibitors

Sildenafil (Viagra) was first approved by FDA in 1998 and has since been joined by vardenafil and tadalafil. Sildenafil citrate is a selective inhibitor of phosphodiesterase-5 (PDE5), the enzyme that breaks down the intracellular second messenger of erection, cGMP. When nitric oxide enters a vascular smooth muscle cell, it stimulates the enzyme guanylate cyclase to convert cGTP into cGMP. This intracellular second messenger cGMP triggers the mobilization of intracellular calcium by causing it to either be pumped out of the cell or sequestered into the sarcoplasmic reticulum; the result is smooth muscle relaxation. Improvement in erections were reported in 56%, 77% and 84% of subjects taking 25, 50, and 100 mg, respectively, and 25% in the placebo group. At the end of the U.S. flexible-dose study (6 months), 75% of subjects were on 100 mg, 23% on 50 mg, and 2% preferred the 25-mg dosage. Principal adverse events noted in clinical trials were headache, 15.8%; flushing, 10.5%; dyspepsia, 6.5%; nasal congestion, 4.2%; altered vision, 2.7%; diarrhoea, 2.6%; dizziness, 2.2%; and arthralgia, 2.0%. Table 44.4 gives the comparison between 3 PDE-5 inhibitors. Sildenafil is absolutely contraindicated for men using nitrates (oral, sublingual or topical), because sildenafil potentiates the hypotensive effects of all nitrates. A post-release product labeling update from the FDA also cautions use in several patient populations: men suffering myocardial infarction, stroke or life-threatening arrhythmia in the previous 6 months; men with resting blood pressure less than 90/50 or greater than 170/110 mm Hg; men with cardiac failure; men with unstable angina; and men with

Table 44.4 **Comparison of Currently Available PDE-5 Inhibitors**

	Sildenafil	*Tadalafil*	*Vardenafil*
Half-life	3-5 hr	17-5 hr	4-5 hr
Onset of action	15 min-2 hr	15 min-2 hr	15 min-1 hr
Reduced absorption with fatty food	Yes	No	Yes
Sideeffects			
• Backache, myalgia			
• Headache, facial flushing, dyspepsia			
• Blurred vision			
• Precaution with anti-arrhythmics			
• Contraindication with nitrates	Rare	Yes	Rare
	Yes	Yes	Yes
	Yes	Rare	Rare
	No	No	Yes
	Yes	Yes	Yes
Recommended dosage	25, 50, 100 mg	5, 10, 20 mg	5, 10, 20 mg

retinitis pigmentosa. The monitoring of patients receiving continuing PDE-5 inhibitor therapy should include a periodic follow-up of efficacy, side effects, and any significant change in health status including medications. Prior to proceeding to other therapies, patients reporting failure of PDE5 inhibitor therapy should be evaluated to determine whether the trial of PDE5 inhibition was adequate. Patients who have failed a trial with PDE5 inhibitor therapy should be informed of the benefits and risks of other therapies, including the use of a different PDE5 inhibitor, alprostadil intraurethral suppositories, intracavernous drug injection, vacuum constriction devices and penile prostheses.[48-51]

MISCELLANEOUS MEDICAL THERAPIES

Intraurethral Therapy: Medicated Urethral System for Erection

Alprostadil, the synthetic formulation of PGE1, is the only pharmacologic agent approved by the FDA for the management of ED by means of intracavernous and intraurethral routes. Alprostadil stimulates adenyl cyclase to increase intracellular levels of cAMP; lowering intracellular concentrations of calcium thus relaxes arterial and trabecular smooth muscle. Drug is transferred from urethra to corpus spongiosum to corpus cavernosum through venous channels (through circumflex and emissary veins perforating tunica albuginea). The medicated urethral system for erection (MUSE: VIVUS Inc,) consists of a very small semisolid pellet (3 × 1 mm) administered into the distal urethra (3 cm) by a proprietary applicator (MUSE). The alprostadil is rapidly absorbed by the urethral mucosa (residual urine in the urethra helps the pellet to dissolve). Sixty-six percent of men responded to an in-office trial; of these, 65% had successful intercourse at least once at home with MUSE, for a rate of 43%. Only 50.4% home administrations resulted in intercourse in those men who were office responders. With MUSE, rigidity can be enhanced by an elastic ring placed at the base of the penis (ACTIS: Vivus, Inc) to mechanically assist veno-occlusion.[52]

Transdermal Therapy

Topiglan (Macrochem) is a mixture of a PGE1 gel (0.5 to 2.5 mg) and a proprietary transdermal permeation enhancer (SEPA). The primary impediment to drug absorption is the relatively thick, bilayered tunica albuginea. The majority of these agents have been applied to the glans where transcutaneous administration should permit absorption into corpus spongiosum and then retrograde delivery to corpora cavernosa following the same route (across emissary veins) as transurethrally administered drugs. Unfortunately, efficacy has been limited, and hypotensive side effects are significant.[53]

Intracavernous Injection (ICI) (AUA Guideline 2005)

Physicians who prescribe intracavernous injection therapy should (1) inform patients of the potential occurrence of prolonged erections, (2) have a plan for urgent treatment of prolonged erections and (3) inform the patient of the plan. The initial trial dose of intracavernous injection therapy should be administered under healthcare provider supervision.

A healthcare provider should be present to instruct patients on the proper technique of intracavernous drug administration, to determine an effective dose and to monitor patients for side effects, especially prolonged erection.

Papaverine

Papaverine is an alkaloid isolated from the opium poppy. Its molecular mechanism of action is through its inhibitory effect on PDE, leading to increased cAMP and cGMP in penile erectile tissue. Papaverine also blocks voltage-dependent calcium channels, thus impairing calcium influx, and it may also impair calcium-activated potassium and chloride currents. All these actions relax cavernous smooth muscle and penile vessels. Papaverine is metabolized in the liver, and the plasma half-life is 1 to 2 hours. The advantages are its low cost and stability at room temperature. The major disadvantages are the higher incidence of priapism (0% to 35%) and corporeal fibrosis (1% to 33%), thought to be a result of low acidity (pH, 3 to 4)[54], and occasional elevation of liver enzymes. Systemic side effects include dizziness, pallor and cold sweats, which may be the result of vasovagal reflex or hypotension from its vasodilatory effect in patients with veno-occlusive dysfunction. The clinical dosages of papaverine monotherapy range from 20 to 80 mg.[54]

α-Adrenergic Antagonists

Phentolamine methylate (Regitine) is a competitive α-adrenoceptor antagonist with equal affinity for α_1 and α_2 receptors. Systemic hypotension, reflex tachycardia, nasal congestion and gastrointestinal upset are the most common systemic side effects. It has a short plasma half-life (30 minutes).

Alprostadil (PGE_1)

It causes smooth muscle relaxation, vasodilatation and inhibition of platelet aggregation through elevation of intracellular cAMP. After ICI, 96% of alprostadil (caverject) is locally metabolized within 60 minutes and no change in peripheral blood levels has been observed. The most frequent side effects were pain at the injection site or during erection (occurring in 16.8% of patients), hematoma/ ecchymosis (1.5%) and prolonged erection/ priapism (1.3%). In summary, alprostadil is an effective agent and should be considered the drug of first choice for the diagnosis and management of ED in the oral agent failure/contraindication group of patients.

Drug Combinations

Papaverine/phentolamine (Bimix) is an effective treatment and produces adequate erection in more than 70% of patients, with greater than 75% satisfaction rate among those who use this treatment. Prolonged erection has been reported in 1 to 23% and fibrosis in 1.4 to 16%.[55] In 1991, Bennett and coworkers introduced a three-drug mixture containing 2.5 ml papaverine (30 mg/ml), 0.5 ml phentolamine (5 mg/ml) and 0.05 ml alprostadil (500 μg/ml) for ICI. The triple-drug combination has been shown to be as effective as alprostadil alone but has a much lower incidence of painful erection. Generally Trimix is reserved for men who have failed PGE_1 monotherapy or who have significant penile pain at higher concentrations of PGE_1.

Dosage and Administration Patients must have the medical personnel and receive appropriate training and education before home injection. For alprostadil, an initial dose of 2.5 μg is recommended. If the response is inadequate, increases in 2.5 μg increments can be given until a full erection is achieved or a maximum of 60 μg is reached. One should start with a small dose (e.g., 7.5 mg of papaverine, 0.1 ml of combination drugs), especially in patients with non-vascular ED. The goal is to achieve an erection adequate for sexual intercourse but that lasts for less than 1 hour.

Contraindications The use of ICI therapy is contraindicated in patients with sickle-cell anemia, schizophrenia or a severe psychiatric disorder, or severe systemic disease.

Vacuum Constriction Device

It consists of a plastic cylinder connected directly or by tubing to a vacuum-generating source (manual or battery-operated pump). After the penis is engorged by negative pressure, a constricting ring is applied to the base to maintain erection. To avoid injury, the ring should not be left in place for longer than 30 minutes. In patients with severe proximal venous leakage or arterial insufficiency, fibrosis secondary to priapism or an infection from prosthesis, the device may not produce adequate erection. In these cases, combining ICI with the vacuum constriction device may enhance erection. The device can also be used successfully by men with a malfunctioning penile prosthesis in place and has been used after explantation. Derouet and coworkers[56] performed a retrospective review of their patients, finding that 20% rejected the device primarily and 30.9% after a period ranging to 16 weeks. They cite a primary drop-out rate of 50.9%

and a secondary drop-out rate of 7.3% after 10 months. Long-term users (41.8%) reported 98% satisfaction; partner satisfaction was 85%. The most common side effect was hematoma (9.8%).[56]

The treatment strategy algorithm for erectile dysfunction is shown in Fig. 44.4.

SURGERY

It is imperative that alternative non-surgical treatment modalities be fully explained to the potential patient. Decisions for management of impotence should be in the context of patient (and, when at all possible, the partner) goal-directed therapy. The choice of incision for erectile surgery varies markedly, and this should also be explained to the patient in preoperative counselling sessions.

Penile Prosthesis

Penile prostheses are basically of two broad categories: malleable or semi-rigid and inflatable devices. Selection of the appropriate device for the individual patient is largely based on three considerations: the patient's preference, the cost of the device and the surgeon's preference. No penile prosthesis will restore the full length previously achieved by the patient with his natural erection. A large part of the preparation of the patient is ensuring that he does have realistic expectations for the device and an understanding that any present erectile ability may be lost, particularly if the entire device ever has to be removed, and that future revision surgery may be necessary. Prosthetic surgery should not be performed in the presence of systemic, cutaneous or urinary tract infection.

Complications

A common intraoperative problem is crural perforation. This can be managed with a separate perineal direct closure of the tear after placement of the device or an artificial windsock repair.[57]

One of the most dreaded complications associated with penile prostheses is infection. The reported incidence is 0.6 to 8.9%. Most infections associated with penile prostheses occur in the first 3 months after surgery, but delayed infection or infection from hematogenous sources has been reported in literature. In those patients who have no previous history of genitourinary or prosthetic infection, a first-generation cephalosporin given as surgical prophylaxis is adequate. For others, a combination of an aminoglycoside and vancomycin surgical prophylaxis is recommended. The use of oral post-operative antibiotics is variable.[58] Antibiotics providing Gram-negative and Gram-positive coverage should be administered preoperatively.Based on the studies with other surgical procedures and implantable devices, broad-spectrum antibiotics providing both Gram-negative and Gram-positive coverage are administered prophylactically to promote implant survival.[59-60] These antibiotics are administered before the incision is made and usually are continued for 24 to 48 hours post-operatively.

The operative area is shaved immediately prior to surgery. If shaving is done earlier, small cuts in the skin may become infected.

Other surgical complications include problems with position, pain, cosmetics and size, encapsula-tion and pressure erosion. For patients who have primary placement of a modern penile prosthesis, reoperation for mechanical failure can be expected in 5% of cases when the device has been in place for 5 to 10 years. The chance of mechanical failure is greater in patients who have experienced previous prosthetic problems. These patients requiring secondary placement also have a more significant risk for infection, as well as those with other predisposing infection risk factors.

Patient and Partner Outcome

No major large prospective studies have been performed to determine actual patient and partner satisfaction. Most have relied on questionnaires sent to the patient after the device has been in place for a while, and response rate has varied from 56% to 85%. A common dissatisfaction expressed is inadequate length. In general, patient and partner satisfaction with penile prostheses ranges from 60 to 80%. The patient considering prosthesis implantation and, when possible, his partner should be informed of the following: types of prostheses available; possibility and consequences of infection and erosion, mechanical failure, and resulting reoperation; differences from the normal flaccid and erect penis, including penile shortening; and potential reduction of the effectiveness of other therapies if the device is subsequently removed.

Recent Developments

A study has been published evaluating the efficacy of a hydrophilic-coated device immersed in an antibiotic pre-operatively. At 1-year follow-up, the infection rate for non-coated prosthesis was 2.07% compared to 1.06% for the same prosthesis with hydrophilic coating.[61] Additional data are needed to confirm these initial findings.

Another design modification recently introduced by the Mentor Corporation was the addition of a lockout valve to prevent autoinflation. A study comparing the occurrence of autoinflation in 160 men implanted with the modified Mentor Alpha-1 prosthesis with that in 339 historical controls implanted with the Mentor Alpha-1 prosthesis with no lockout valve found rates of 1.3 and 11%, respectively.[62] Non-inflatable penile prostheses remain legitimate alternatives to inflatable devices with the advantages of lower cost, better mechanical reliability despite the design improvements of inflatable devices, and ease of use by the patient. Patient education about inflation and deflation techniques is not necessary. MRI may be utilized to evaluate the status of a penile implant or may be performed for other indications in a patient who has a penile prosthesis.[63]

In peyronie's disease, the injection of smooth muscle relaxants often demonstrates a degree of deformity and extent of erection. In patients with significant erectile failure associated with the disease, the most prudent treatment course may be the placement of a penile prosthesis with or without incision or excision of the penile plaque.[64]

Vascular Surgery

Vascular surgery for impotence can be divided into two major areas: penile revascularization and surgery for a veno-occlusive disorder.

Selection Criteria

Patients with discrete focal arterial lesions found on pudendal arteriography, particularly younger patients who have a history of trauma, who do not have insulin-dependent diabetes, who are not currently users of tobacco, and who do not have neurologic disease, are the best candidates for penile revascularization procedures.[65]

Criteria for recommending surgery for a veno-occlusive disorder consist of the following: (1) a patient complaint of short-duration erections or tumescence only with sexual stimulation, (2) failure to obtain or maintain an erection from the use of oral sildenafil and/or intracavernous injection on multiple trials with different agents with sexual stimulation, (3) normal cavernous arteries on colour duplex Doppler studies or second phase of DICC, (4) a faulty veno-occlusive mechanism as determined by infusion pump or gravity pharmacocavernosometry that is amenable to surgery (no massive venous leakage), (5) location of the site of venous leakage from corpora cavernosa on pharmacocavernosography, (6) no medical contraindication to surgery, (7) complete elimination of tobacco use, and (8) selection of presentation of alternative therapeutic choices in the presence of a long-term success rate of 40 to 50%.[66]

There is no single type of revascularization surgery that fits every case. The overall goal of penile revascularization surgery is the bypass of specific obstructive arterial lesions in the hypogastric- cavernosal arterial bed. Peno-occlusive surgery should consist of a thorough penile vein dissection and ligation.

Complications

Penile edema is common after vascular surgery of the penis. A lightly applied elastic dressing of the penis for 24 hours after surgery greatly aids in controlling this post-operative minor complication, and any mild to moderate edema after the removal of the dressing usually resolves without sequelae 2 to 3 weeks after surgery. Superficial ecchymosis and bruising of the penile shaft and scrotum is neither unusual nor debilitating; serious wound haematomas can be avoided by the use of the tubular fenestrated drain post-operatively for 24 to 48 hours.

Two significant complications of penile vascular surgery are penile numbness, or hypoesthesia, and penile shortening from scar entrapment, which is experienced in as many as 20% of patients. Penile sensation usually returns 12 to 18 months after surgery if no major penile sensory nerve has been significantly severed. Penile shortening from severe scar entrapment may require subsequent scar release surgery and the use of relaxing Z-plasty incisions or scrotal flap coverage.[65]

PEYRONIE'S DISEASE

The vast majority of patients with Peyronie's disease do not require surgery. Surgery, at best, can be viewed as palliation for the mechanical effects of Peyronie's disease and/or ED. The symptomatic incidence of Peyronie's disease has been estimated at 1%. In White men, the average age at onset of Peyronie's disease is 53 years. Peyronie's disease most likely begins with buckling trauma causing injury to the septal insertion of tunica albuginea.[67]

In most cases of Peyronie's disease, there are two phases. The first is an active phase, which often is associated with painful erections and changing deformity of the penis. It is followed by a quiescent secondary phase, which is characterized by stabilizing of the deformity, with disappearance of painful erections, if present, and, in general, stability of the process. Up to a third of patients, however, present with what appears to be a sudden development of painless deformity.

The presenting symptoms of Peyronie's disease include (1) in many patients, penile pain with erection; (2) penile deformity; (3) shortening with and without an erection; (4) notice of a plaque or indurated area in the penis; and (5) in many patients, ED. On physical examination, virtually all patients have either a well-defined plaque or an area of induration palpable. The plaque is usually located on the dorsal surface of the penis, intimately associated with the insertion of septal fibers. Patients not uncommonly can tolerate rather significant dorsal curvature (up to 45 degrees). Patients with lateral components or ventral Peyronie's disease tolerate deformity far less well.

The medical history should include the mode and time of onset (sudden vs. gradual). Because most patients with Peyronie's disease have an element, or at least the aura, of ED, the risk factors for ED should also be assessed. Detailed psychosexual history is imperative.

Medical Management

Any section on the medical management of Peyronie's disease must begin with the disclaimer that few medical methods of management have been subjected to double-blind drug testing. Vitamin E is inexpensive, safe and possibly effective. Potaba is poorly tolerated by some patients and is relatively costly. It is the recommendation of the consensus committee on penile curvatures that the use of intralesional corticosteroids be eliminated or at least initiated with extreme caution because of the rather significant local side effects, the inconsistent pattern of improvement in well-established curvature, and the lack of studies showing proven efficacy.[5]

Surgical Treatment

For a patient to be a surgical candidate, he must have stable and mature disease. Plication or corporoplasty techniques seem to preserve the patient's erectile function more effectively. However, excellent results can be achieved with incision or excision of plaque and grafting techniques. It is the consensus of the committee on Peyronie's disease at the World Health Organisation Second International Consultation on sexual dysfunctions that penile prosthesis is a reliable option for the older man with vascular impairment, erectile dysfunction and acquired deformity of the penis.[5]

REFERENCES

1. Dean RC , Lue TF .Physiology of penile erection and pathophysiology of erectile dysfunction. Urol Clin N Am, 2005; 32: 379-95.
2. Trigo-Rocha F, Hsu GL, Donatucci CF, et al. The role of cyclic adenosine monophosphate, cyclic guanosine monophosphate, endothelium and nonadrenergic, noncholinergic neurotransmission in canine penile erection. J Urol 1993; 149: 872-7.
3. Steers WD. Neural control of penile erection. Semin Urol 1990; 8: 66-70.
4. Johannes CB, Araujo AB, Feldman HA, et al.: Incidence of erectile dysfunction in men ages 40–69: Longitudinal results from the Massachusetts male aging study. J Urol 2000; 163: 460-3.
5. Lue TF , Basson R, Rosen R et al. Second International Consultation on Sexual Dysfunctions. Sexual Medicine: Sexual Dysfunctions in men and women . Paris, Health publications, 2004. www.jmh.sagepub.com.
6. Lizza EF, Rosen RC. Definition and classification of erectile dysfunction: Report of the Nomenclature Committee of the International Society of Impotence Research. Int J Impot Res 1999; 11: 141-3.
7. Catalona WJ, Bigg SW: Nerve-sparing radical prostatectomy: Evaluation of results after 250 patients. J Urol 1990; 143: 538-43.
8. Eardley I, Kirby RS. Neurogenic impotence. In Kirby RS, Carson CC, Webster GD (ed): Impotence: Diagnosis and Management of Male Erectile Dysfunction. Oxford, Butterworth-Heinemann, 1991, pp. 227-231.
9. Marson L, Platt KB, McKenna KE. Central nervous system innervation of the penis as revealed by the transneuronal transport of pseudorabies virus. Neuroscience 1993; 55: 263-80.
10. Mulligan T, Schmitt B. Testosterone for erectile failure. J Intern Med 1993; 8: 517-21.
11. Seftel AD, Vaziri ND, Ni Z, et al. Advanced glycation end products in human penis: Elevation in diabetic tissue, site of deposition, and possible effect through iNOS or eNOS. Urology 1997; 50: 1016-26.
12. Rosen MP, Greenfield AJ, Walker TG, et al. Arterio-genic impotence: Findings in 195 impotent men examined with selective internal pudendal angiography. Radiology 1990; 174: 1043-8.
13. Rosen MP, Greenfield AJ, Walker TG, et al. Cigarette smoking: An independent risk factor for atherosclerosis in the hypogastric-cavernous arterial bed of men with arteriogenic impotence. J Urol 1991; 145: 759-63.
14. Junemann KP, Lue TF, Luo JA, et al. The effect of cigarette smoking on penile erection. J Urol 1987; 138: 438-41.
15. Miller NS, Gold MS. The human sexual response and alcohol and drugs. J Subst Abuse Treat 1988; 5: 171-7.
16. Rosen, RC, Hatzichristou D, Broderick G, et al. Clinical evaluation and symptom scales: Sexual dysfunction assessment in men .In Lue TF, Basson R, Rosen R, et al. (eds): Sexual Medicine: Sexual Dysfunctions in Men and Women. Paris, Health Publications, 2004, 173-220.
17. Davis-Joseph B, Tiefer L, Melman A: Accuracy of the initial history and physical examination to establish the etiology of erectile dysfunction. Urology 1995; 45: 498-502.
18. Thompson, I., Carroll, P., Coley, C. et al., Prostate-specific antigen best practice policy. Oncology 2000; 14: 267-72.
19. Lewis RW, King BF. Dynamic colour Doppler sonography in the evaluation of penile erectile disorders. (Abstract). Int J Impot Res 1994; 6: A30.
20. Motiwala HG: Dynamic pharmacocavernosometry. A search for an ideal approach. Urol Int 1993; 51: 1-8.
21. Shabsigh R, Fishman IJ, Toombs BD, et al. Venous leaks: Anatomical and physiological observations. J Urol 1991; 146: 1260-5.
22. Bradley WE, Timm GW, Gallagher JM, et al. New method for continuous measurement of nocturnal penile tumescence and rigidity. Urology 1985; 26: 4-9.
23. Cilurzo P, Canale D, Turchi P, et al. [The Rigiscan system in the diagnosis of male sexual

impotence. Arch Ital Urol Nefrol Androl 1992; 64(Suppl 2): 81-5.
24. Shabsigh R, Alexandre L, Nielsen HB, et al.: Economical aspects of erectile dysfunction. In Jardin A, Wagner G, Khoury S, et al. (eds): Erectile Dysfunction: First International Consultation on Erectile Dysfunction—July 1–3, Paris, 1999. Plymouth, United Kingdom, Health Publication Ltd, 2000, pp 55-64.
25. Padma-Nathan H Neurophysiological studies of sexual dysfunction. In Singer C, Weiner WJ (eds): Sexual Dysfunction: A Neuro-Medical Approach. Armonk, NY, Futura, 1994, 101-15.
26. Gerstenberg TC, Bradley WE: Nerve conduction velocity measurement of dorsal nerve of penis in normal and impotent males. Urology 1983; 21: 90-2.
27. Meinhardt W, Kropman RF, Vermeij P, et al.: The influence of medication on erectile function. Int J Impot Res 1997; 9: 17-26.
28. Johannes, CB, Araujo AB, Feldman HA, et al. Incidence of erectile dysfunction in men 40 to 69 years old: longitudinal results from the Massachusetts male aging study. J Urol, 2000; 163: 460-3.
29. Baco C.G, Mittleman M.A, Kawachi I, et al. Sexual function in men older than 50 years of age: results from the health professionals' follow-up study. Ann Intern Med 2003; 139: 161-8.
30. U.S. Department of Health and Human Services. Physical Activity and Health: A report of the Surgeon General. Atlanta, GA: U.S. Department of Health and Human Services, Centers for Disease Control and Prevention, National Center for Chronic Disease Prevention and Health Promotion, 1996.
31. Esposito K, Giugliano F, Di Palo C, et al. Effect of lifestyle changes on erectile dysfunction in obese men: a randomized controlled trial. JAMA, 2004; 291: 2978-84.
32. Derby C.A, Mohr B.A, Goldstein I, et al. Modifiable risk factors and erectile dysfunction: can lifestyle change modify risk? Urology, 2000; 56: 302-6.
33. Nayal W, Schwarzer U, Klotz T, et al. Influences of gym exercises on the penile oxygen pressure. J Urol 1999; 161: A693.
34. Claes H, Baert L. Pelvic floor exercise versus surgery in the treatment of impotence. Br J Urol 1993; 71: 52-7.
35. Hengeveld MW: Erectile dysfunction: A sexological and psychiatric review. World J Urol 1983; 1: 227-32.
36. Kloner RA, Mulin S H, Shook T et al. Erectile dysfunction in the cardiac patient: how common and should we treat? J. Urol. 2003; 170: S46-50.
37. Feldman HA, Goldstein I, Hatzichristou DG, et al. Impotence and its medical and psychosocial correlates: results of the Massachusetts Male Aging Study. J Urol, 1994; 151: 54-61.
38. Jackson G, Rosen R C, Kloner R A et al. The second Princeton consensus on sexual dysfunction and cardiac risk: new guidelines, new challenges J Sex-Med 2006; 3: 28-36.
39. Nieschlag E, Behre HM. Pharmacological and clinical uses of testosterone. In Nieschlag E, Behre HM (eds): Testosterone: Action, Deficiency, Substitution, 2nd ed. Berlin, Springer-Verlag, 1998, pp 294-321.
40. Ajayi AA, Mathur R, Halushka PV. Testosterone increases human platelet thromboxane A2 receptor density and aggregation responses. Circulation 1995; 91: 2742-7.
41. Foreman MM, Wernicke JF. Approaches for the development of oral drug therapies for erectile dysfunction. Semin Urol 1990; 8: 107-12.
42. Montorsi F, Strambi LF, Guazzoni G, et al. Effect of yohimbine-trazodone on psychogenic impotence: A randomized, double-blind, placebo-controlled study. Urology 1994; 44: 732-6.
43. Weiner N. Drugs that inhibit adrenergic nerves and block adrenergic receptors, 7th ed. New York: Macmillan Company, 1985.
44. Lebret T, Herve JM, Gorny P, et al. Efficacy and safety of a novel combination of L-arginine glutamate and yohimbine hydrochloride: a new oral therapy for erectile dysfunction. Eur Urol 2002; 41: 608-13.
45. Fink HA, MacDonald R, Rutks IR, et al. Trazodone for erectile dysfunction: a systematic review and meta-analysis Br J Urol 2003; 92: 441-6.

46. Heaton JP, Morales A, Adams MA, et al. Recovery of erectile function by the oral administration of apomorphine. Urology 1995; 45: 200-6.
47. Zorgniotti AW. Experience with buccal phentolamine mesylate for impotence. Int J Impot Res 1994; 6: 37-41.
48. Ballard SA, Gingell CJ, Tang K, et al. Effects of sildenafil on the relaxation of human corpus cavernosum tissue in vitro and on the activities of cyclic nucleotide phosphodiesterase isozymes. J Urol 1998; 159: 2164-71.
49. Kloner RA, Hutter AM, Emmick JT, et al. Time course of the interaction between tadalafil and nitrates. J Am Coll Cardiol, 2003; 42: 1855-60.
50. Goldstein I, Lue TF, Padma-Nathan H, et al. Oral sildenafil in the treatment of erectile dysfunction. Sildenafil Study Group. N Engl J Med 1998; 338: 1397-1404.
51. Carson CC, Lue TF. Great drug classes: Phosphodiesterase type 5 inhibitors for erectile dysfunction . BJU Int 2005; 96: 257-80.
52. Padma-Nathan H, Hellstrom WJ, Kaiser FE, et al. Treatment of men with erectile dysfunction with transurethral alprostadil. Medicated Urethral System for Erection (MUSE) Study Group. N Engl J Med 1997; 336: 1-7.
53. Canale D, Cilurzo P, Giorgi PM, et al. Transdermal therapy of erectile insufficiency. Arch Ital Urol Nefrol Androl 1992; 64: 263-6.
54. Barada JH, McKimmy RM. Vasoactive pharmacotherapy. In Bennett AH (ed): Impotence: Diagnosis and Management of Erectile Dysfunction. Philadelphia, WB Saunders, 1994.
55. Armstrong DK, Convery A, Dinsmore WW. Intracavernosal papaverine and phentolamine for the medical management of erectile dysfunction in a genitourinary clinic. Int J STDs AIDS 1993; 4: 214-6.
56. Derouet H, Caspari D, Rohde V, et al. Treatment of erectile dysfunction with external vacuum devices. Andrologia 1999; 31(Suppl 1): 89-94.
57. Mulcahy JJ. A technique of maintaining penile prosthesis position to prevent proximal migration. J Urol 1987; 137: 294-6.
58. Carson CC. Management of penile prosthesis infection. Probl Urol 1993; 7: 368-80.
59. D'Amico DF, Parimbelli P, Ruffolo C. Antibiotic prophylaxis in clean surgery: breast surgery and hernia repair. J Chemother, 2001; 13: 108-11.
60. Zibari GB, Gadallah MF, Landreneau M, et al. Preoperative vancomycin prophylaxis decreases incidence of postoperative hemodialysis vascular access infections. Am J Kidney Dis 1997; 30: 343-8.
61. Hill C, Flamant R, Mazas F, Evrard J. Prophylactic cefazolin versus placebo in total hip replacement: report of a multicentre double-blind randomised trial. Lancet 1981; 11: 795-6.
62. Carson CC. Efficacy of antibiotic impregnation of inflatable penile prostheses in decreasing infection in original implants. J Urol 2004; 171: 1611-4.
63. Wolter CE, Hellstrom JG. The hydrophilic-coated penile prosthesis: 1-year experience. J Sex Med 2004; 1: 221-4.
64. Thiel, Broderick and Bridges M. Utility of magnetic resonance imaging in evalua-ting inflatable penile prosthesis malfunction and complaints. Int J Impot Res 2003; 15: S155-61.
65. Marzi M, Zucchi A, Lombi R, et al.: Implant surgery in Peyronie's disease. Urol Int 1997; 58: 113-6.
66. Hatzichristou D, Goldstein I. Penile microvascular and arterial bypass surgery. Urol Clin North Am 1993; 1: 39-60.
67. Sasso F, Gulino G, Wein J, et al. Patient selection criteria in the surgical treatment of veno-occlusive dysfunction. J Urol 1999; 161: 1145-7.
68. Iacono F, Barra S, DeRosa G, et al. Microstructural disorders of tunica albuginea in patients affected by Peyronie's disease with or without erection dysfunction. J Urol 1993; 150: 1806-9.
69. Tornehl CK, Carson CC. Surgical alternatives for treating Peyronie's disease. BJU Int 2004; 94: 774-83.

Part 10

General Guidelines in Clinical Approach to STDs

45 | CLINICAL APPROACH TO GENITAL ULCER DISEASE

Vinod K Sharma, Uttam Kumar

In this chapter

- Diagnosis of Genital Ulcer
- Diagnosis of GUD
- Treatment

INTRODUCTION

Genital ulcers are defined as breach in the continuity of genital mucosa and/or skin. Genital ulcer disease (GUD) may be due to STDs like syphilis, chancroid, donovanosis, lymphpogranuloma venereum (LGV), herpes genitalis, or non-STDs like traumatic ulcer, Behcet's disease, lichen planus, erythema multifome, lichen sclerosus et atrophicus, bullous diseases, Fournier's gangrene, squamous cell carcinoma, etc. (Table 45.1).

Table 45.1 Etiological Classification of GUD[1]

Venereal	*Non-venereal*
Herpes simplex	Trauma
Syphilis	Adverse drug reactions (SJS, FDE)
Chancroid	Vesiculobullous skin diseases
Lymphogranuloma venereum	Behcet's disease
Granuloma inguinale	Reiter's disease
	Crohn's disease
	Other infections (pyogenic, yeast, non-specific spirochaetes)
	Neoplasms (BCC, SCC)
	Premalignant conditions (Paget's disease, Bowen's disease, erythroplasia of Queyrat)
	Non-specific & Others

GUD is a commonly encountered STD accounting for 1-70% of STDs in different parts of the world, with the lowest incidence in America.[2] The incidence of GUD differs from place to place because of the regional variation in the prevalence of aetiological agents, sexual behaviour and sociocultural factors. Syphilis and chancroid are more prevalent in minority, Blacks and Hispanics; similarly herpetic ulcers are more common in the Whites. The civilization and economy has an influence in different STDs, e.g. developed countries have a higher incidence of herpes genitalis than in a developing country. Chancroid is common in the developing world, whereas syphilis is common in both developing and industrialized countries. Donovanosis is encountered in some parts of Asia,[3] especially in South India. Studies from several cities in India have shown a steady increase in herpes genitalis, and in some studies its prevalence has overtaken that of chancroid and syphilis.[4,5,6]

Genital ulcers are more frequently reported in men because these can be easily detected in men as compared to women. Symptomatic genital ulcers like herpes genitals have the same incidence in both sexes. The non-tender GUD of cervix in female often remains unnoticed and is under-reported. In some communities where female prostitution is prevalent, there is increased incidence of GUD in male because they act as the reservoir of infection constantly infecting the male population.

The clinical diagnosis may be misleading because of the increasing HIV coinfection, and mixed infection often alters the morphology of ulcer and the textbook description of the GUD may not be present.[7] The painful ulcer of chancroid can be easily confused with herpes genitalis. Primary chancre of syphilis if secondarily infected can mimic chancroid, and even coinfection of chancroid with herpes simplex, which occurs in around 10% of cases, may confuse the diagnosis. The ulcers do not remain confined to the genitalia and may be seen in extragenital sites due to changing sexual behavioural pattern. It has also been observed that the clinical diagnosis is incorrect in about 40% of GUD patients in comparison to laboratory tests.[2]

The clinical sensitivity of the diagnosis of GUD like herpes genitalis is up to 67%,[8] chancroid 33-52.6%,[7,9] syphilis 55% and herpes genitalis 22% in a study at Johannesburg, and subsequently similar results were observed in other cities of South Africa.[8,10] In practice, the documentation of a aetiological agent of the GUD remains difficult. The appropriate diagnostic tests are often not available or not properly utilized. The aetiological agent may not be demonstrated due to self-medication by the patient, or the ulcers are contaminated. However, the bedside and laboratory tests are fairly sensitive and specific in early lesions. The dark-ground illumination and Tzanck test are up to 80% positive in primary chancre and herpes genitalis.[3,10] The culture for herpes is approximately 100% sensitive at the vesicular stage and lower at the ulcerative stage.[11,12]

In the past few years the epidemic of HIV has shown an impact on the course, treatment and transmission of GUD, and there is possible impact of GUD on the spread and course of HIV. Enormous evidence is available indicating that both ulcerative and non-ulcerative STDs increase the risk of HIV infection. The reciprocal relationship between HIV infection and other STDs has been termed as epidemiological synergy whereby each may alter the transmission and manifestation of other STDs,[13] promote HIV transmission by facilitating HIV shedding in the genital tract, causing disruption of normal epithelial barrier and deploying and activating HIV susceptible cells at that site to promote HIV replication.[14] HIV has various effects on the course of STDs in the form of (a) modification of the natural course of disease, (b) unusual clinical presentation, (c) therapeutic challenge due to increased failure rates with conventional regimes, (d) diagnostic difficulties with altered serological tests and histopathology and (e) reactivation of latent infections.

The common organisms causing genital ulcers are *Treponema pallidum* (syphilis), *Haemophilus ducreyi* (chancroid), *Herpes simplex virus (HSV)-2* and *HSV-1* (herpes genitalis), *Calymmatobacterium granulomatis* (donovanosis) and *Chlamydia trachomatis* sero type L1-L3 (LGV).

DIAGNOSIS OF GENITAL ULCER

The approach to genital ulcer should include detailed history-taking, thorough examination, bedside tests and laboratory investigations in all cases.

History

History-taking is an important step in GUD, which includes recording of age, sex, occupation and address for follow-up after treatment. The history of sexual contact (single or multiple) with exact date to estimate approximate incubation period. Whether the sexual act was under the influence of alcohol or drugs? Because a forceful sexual act under the influence of alcohol or drugs can give rise to immediate injury at frenulum. The history of sexual partner, whether male or female? Was it a vaginal, anal or oral intercourse? Promiscuity of the patient and the partner and drug abuse history is essential. History of present or past genital ulcer in the partner, if there was vesicle formation, duration of ulcer, if it has healed, how long did it take to heal, are required in all cases of GUD. In female patients, history of abortion or stillbirth, and in children history suggestive of sexual abuse needs to be elicited. In all patients, history of associated STDs need to be enquired. As GUD patients have the higher incidence of HIV infection, one should also ask about associated symptoms of significant weight loss, frequent diarrhoea, persistent fever and chronic cough for more than one month to know about the immune status of the individual. History of treatment taken in the past, topical or systemic, partial or complete should also be sought in detail as it may alter the clinical features and course of the disease.

The healing time of genital ulcer may suggest the diagnosis. For example, spontaneous healing time for the primary chancre is about 3-8 weeks, primary herpes genitalis is 14-21 days and recurrent herpes genitalis is about 10 days. LGV ulcers heal in 2-5 days and often it remains unnoticed by the patient, whereas donovanosis and chancroid rarely show tendency for spontaneous healing.[1] Incubation period and healing time are summarized in Table 45.2 and clinical features in Table 45.3.

Examination

The examination of all suspected GUD patients should be carried out wearing gloves. Complete evaluation should include examination of skin, oral cavity, lymphnode, liver and spleen, chest, cardiovascular system and neurological examination. In the examination of lymphnodes, the group involved, tenderness, consistency, overlying skin and attachment to the surrounding structure is important. Genital examination is followed by the examination of the perianal area.

Table 45.2 **Incubation Period and Healing Time in GUD**

STD	*Incubation Period*	*Spontaneous Healing Time*	*On Treatment*
Primary chancre	9-90 days (mean 21 days)	3-8 weeks, never exceeds 3 months	1-2 weeks
Chancroid	5-8 days (one to several weeks)	Self-limiting but may persist for years	1-2 weeks
Herpes genitalis (primary)	5-7 days	14-21 days	6-12 days
LGV	10 days (5-30 days)	2-5 days (transient)	–
Donovanosis	9-50 days (probably)	No tendency for healing	3-4 weeks

Inspection

Look for number, site, size, depth, presence of necrotic slough or granulation tissue on the floor of ulcer margins and extension of erythema surrounding the ulcer. The primary chancre is usually solitary, whereas chancroid and herpetic ulcers are multiple. The classical ulcers of herpes and LGV are superficial, whereas chancroid ulcers are relatively deep. Beefy granulation tissue on the surface of the ulcer is characteristic of donovanosis, whereas chancroid ulcer is covered with necrotic slough and primary chancre is usually clean.

Palpation

In palpation, the presence of tenderness, induration, bleeding on manipulation, attachment to the surrounding structure and per-rectal examination findings are of help in diagnosis. Phimosis may cause difficulty in examining the lesion; efforts should be made to retract the prepuce or palpate through the preputial skin. If it is still not possible to examine, the patient is advised frequent saline irrigation and examination of the lesion may be possible the next day. If prepuce is not retractable after saline irrigation, dorsal slitting has been suggested but it is rarely needed. Tenderness is a feature of genital herpes and chancroid, whereas the primary chancre, donovanosis and LGV ulcers are relatively non-tender. Primary chancre usually has a button-like induration but other GUD are non-indurated. Donovanosis bleeds on manipulation. The comparative features of different genital ulcers are summarized in Table 45.4. In mixed infection, the picture is atypical and the combination of diseases responsible for it, e.g. primary chancre and chancroid, may result in indurated ulcer with an inflammatory bubo. Palpation of inguinal lymph nodes may also aid in the diagnosis. Lymph nodes are bilateral in herpes simplex and syphilis while mostly unilateral in chancroid and LGV. These are painful, firm, tender and non-suppurative in genital herpes; painless, discrete, firm, shotty, non-tender in syphilis; painful, very tender, suppurative and unilocular in chancroid; and tender, suppurative, soft/firm, multilocular in LGV.

Table 45.3 **Clinical Features of Common GUD**

Characteristics	*Syphilis*	*Herpes*	*Chancroid*	*LGV*	*Donovanosis*
Primary lesions	Papule	Vesicle	Pustule	Papule, pustule or vesicle	Papule
Number of lesions	Usually one, but in 1/3 cases >1	Multiple and may coalesce	Usually multiple and may coalesce	Usually one	Variable
Diameter	5-15 mm	1-2 mm	Variable	2-10 mm	Variable
Edges	Sharply demarcated, elevated, round or oval	Erythematous polycyclic	Undermined, ragged, irregular	Elevated, round or oval	Elevated irregular
Depth	Superficial or deep	Superficial	Excavated	Superficial or deep	Elevated
Base	Smooth, non-purulent covered with serous exudate	Erythematous	Purulent, bleeds easily	Variable	Red and velvety, bleeds readily
Induration	Button-like	None	Soft	Occasionally firm	Firm
Pain	Uncommon, but tender on firm pressure	Frequently tender	Usually very tender	Variable	Uncommon
Lymphadenopathy	Firm, nontender, bilateral, and 1/3 cases it may be tender	Firm, tender often bilateral with initial episode	Tender, may suppurate, loculated, usually unilateral, occasional cord like lymphangitis	Tender, may suppurate, loculated, usually unilateral	None, pseudobuboes (maybe)
Recurrence	No	Yes, in 80%	No	No	No

In a female patient, examination of external genitalia is followed by speculum and per-vaginal examination. The appropriate samples are also collected for investigations. An effort is made to look for other STDs that may be simultaneously present.

Investigations

Dark-ground illumination, Tzanck smear, tissue smear and smear for Gram stain are mandatory for all genital ulcers. All the patients with GUD should be serologically tested for syphilis, HIV and preferably for hepatitis B and C. Other tests for chlamydial serology, culture for HSV, *H. ducreyi* and chlamydia are performed subject to availability.

The biopsy of ulcer is helpful in the diagnosis of donovanosis and ruling out premalignant and malignant diseases of the genitals.

DIAGNOSIS OF GUD

Primary Chancre

Definitive diagnosis of syphilis depends on the demonstration of *T. pallidum* by dark-ground illumination (DGI) or fluorescence microscope examination. DGI is positive for *T. pallidum* in up to 80% of primary chancre.[3] The DGI is conventionally recommended to be repeated for 3 consecutive days prior to giving negative result or starting treatment. In our experience, compliance for three-day DGI test is poor; we prefer to repeat DGI twice in the first day itself and start the treatment. Non-treponemal tests like VDRL, rapid plasma reagen (RPR) or toludine red unheated serum test (TRUST) are 75-85% sensitive in primary chancre.[2] And if non-treponemal tests are positive, it should be confirmed by specific treponemal tests like FTA-Abs (fluorescence treponemal antibody absorbent) or MHA-TP (micro-haemaggulutination assay for antibody to *T. pallidum*). This specific and non-treponemal test in combination gives 69-85% positivity in patients with primary chancre.[2] VDRL test is mandatory during follow-up. The test is done on the first visit; if negative, repeated after 4-6 weeks of appearance of the ulcer. Recently polymerase chain reaction (PCR) has been used in the detection of *T. pallidum* and the results were found to be similar to direct fluorescent antibody (DFA) test.[15] It is helpful to differentiate *T. pallidum* from the saprophytic spirochetes of oral cavity, but it is not available in most laboratories.

Herpes Genitalis

The history of appearance of multiple vesicles prior to ulcer formation is definitive of the diagnosis of herpes. The Tzanck test is sensitive up to 80% and specificity is about 94%.[12] Immunofluorescence staining is more sensitive than Tzanck test. For this, fluorescein-labeled monoclonal antibody specific to HSV1 or HSV2 is added to the slide. This culture is the most sensitive and it is about 100% positive; the results are highly positive from vesicular lesion and least from ulcerative lesion.[11,12] The viral culture is specific and shows cytopathic changes within 1-3 days.[2] Antigen detection test for HSV is positive even in healing ulcer and is an alternative test.[15] The PCR is more helpful as it can detect HSV DNA from the healing lesion.[16]

Direct testing of the lesion with culture or antigen detection should always be done first to establish HSV as the aetiologic agent.[17] If these tests yield negative results or are unavailable or if there is no lesion amenable to testing, HSV-2 serological tests can assist in the diagnosis of a suspected symptomatic herpes virus infection.

Antibodies to HSV 2 and 1 are not diagnostic as they may reflect previous infection, and DNA hybridization and PCR are usually not available. Non-type-specific serological tests should not be used, because they cannot distinguish between HSV-1 and HSV-2.[18]

Currently available type-specific serological tests detect the majority of primary infections by 12 weeks and have a sensitivity of 93–99% and a specificity of 94–98%.[19] Type-specific HSV antibody tests are based on type-specific proteins, gG1 and gG2, and can distinguish between HSV-1 and HSV-2 infection.

In clinical practice, the diagnosis is made on clinical grounds and Tzanck smear. Culture, serology, immunofluorescence, and PCR are available only in research centers.

Chancroid

There is uncertainty in the accuracy of different laboratory tests, and clinical diagnosis continues to be the mainstay of treatment. Gram stain sensitivity and specificity is variable from negligible to as high as 62% sensitive and 99% specific.[20] The other tests are fluorescein-labelled monoclonal antibody for *H. ducreyi*, blot radioimmunoassay and DNA hybridization. Culture for *H. ducreyi* is positive in 0-80% of suspected cases of chancroid.[21] DNA probe and PCR are not available in most laboratories.

Lymphogranuloma Venereum (LGV)

Serology test and positive serology >1:64 with clinical features supports the diagnosis, but it is not specific of LGV. Infection by other chlamydial species can also give the similar titre. The other sensitive tests are direct fluorescence antibody staining, ELISA for chlamydial antigen and IgG antibody to chlamydia (>1:256). Culture for chlamydia, immunotyping, microimmunofluorescence serology, PCR, prove assay, chemiluminescence enhanced test, ligase chain reaction test (LCR) and sero-specific monoclonal antibody may be used.[22] A real-time multiplex PCR (M-PCR) assay has been developed for the diagnosis of Chlamydia infection and it simultaneously detects and differentiates LGV from non-LGV strains using swab specimen. It offers a relatively rapid and sensitive alternative to conventional genotyping method for diagnosis of LGV infection and a useful tool for screening.[23]

Donovanosis

Biopsy and tissue smear for the demonstration of Donovan bodies are diagnostic. There is no serological test, and the organism cannot be cultured in laboratory. In developing countries like India, specific tests are often not available for confirmation except in research or referral laboratories, and most patients are treated on the basis of clinical diagnosis.

Confirmation of donovanosis is done by either culture in human peripheral blood monocytes and Hep2 cells or polymerase chain reaction. It is clear from the above description that specific tests for aetiological agent for GUD are frequently not available and there is coexistence of multiple organisms in a single ulcer. The use of multiplex PCR (M-PCR) amplification assay can detect the simultaneous presence of multiple organisms from a single specimen. Morse *et al.* observed the resolved sensitivity of M-PCR for *H. duceryi* and herpes simplex virus culture to be 95% and 93% respectively, whereas the culture sensitivity of these organisms was 75% and 60%. The use of M-PCR reduces indeterminate laboratory diagnosis from 35 to 6% and the chances for detection of multiple agents from a single ulcer increases from 4 to 18%.[24]A study from Pune with multiplex PCR showed poor results in patients with suspected chancroid.[25]

The laboratory diagnosis of GUD is summarized in Table 45.4.

Table 45.4 Lab Diagnosis of Genital Ulcers

Lab Test	*Syphilis*	*Chancroid*	*Herpes*	*LGV*	*Donovanosis*
Microscopy	Darkfield direct immuno-flourence	Gram stain, fluorescent-labeled monoclobal antibody detection	Antigen detection by DFA. Immunoper-oxide staining and ELISA	Direct immuno-staining ELISA rapid assays like (1) Sure cell Chlamydia test, (2) Clear view Chlamydia test, (3) Test pack Chlamydia, Direct fluorescence for antibody to LGV, Immuno dot and microimmuno-fluorescence by ELISA	Giemsa stain tissue smears/ sections

(*Contd.*)

Lab Test	*Syphilis*	*Chancroid*	*Herpes*	*LGV*	*Donovanosis*
Culture	Not available	Enriched Mueller-Hinton (MH) chocolate agar, enriched gonococcal agar	Cell culture (vero cells/human diploid fibroblast, MCRC-5), baby hamster kidney cells, rabbit kidney cells	Cell culture (HeLa-229, McCoy cells, Baby hamster kidney cell, BHK-21)	No
Collection/ transport media	Not available	Thioyoglycolate hemin medium containing L glutamin and bovine albumin at 4°C	Swab-wire shaft with cotton tip. Viral transport media at 4°C; if time required for inoculation is >48 hours, freeze at 70°C	Swab-plastic shaft with Rayon swab and Cytobrush with plastic shaft	
Serology	Non-treponemal tests-VDRL/ RPR/Treponemal test ELISA, FTA-Abs, TPHA, MHA-TP, HATTS/Anti-treponemal 1gM detection	ELISA, immuno dot technique	Monoclonal antibodies to HSV 1 and 2, ELISA, DNA hybridization	CFT and immuno-flurescent antibody test	Experimental
Molecular techniques	PCR	PCR	PCR	PCR, LCR, Prove assay chemilumine-scence enhanced test in LGV. Immunotyping by PCR	Not available
Histopatho-logy	Perivascular infiltrate of lymphocyte, plasma cells accompanied by endarteritis obliterans	Surface zone - narrow consisting of neutrophils, fibrin, erythrocytes, necrotic tissue. Middle zone - wide newly formed blood vessels with marked proliferation of their endothelial cells. Deeper zone - dense inflammation of plasma cells and lymphoid cells	Degeneration of keratinocytes, resulting in acantholysis; 2 types of degeneration • Ballooning • Reticular	Small area of necrosis with proliferating epitheloid and endothelial cell with stellate abscess	Acanthosis/ pseudocarcino-matous hyperplasia at edge of ulcer Dermis-dense inflammation of histiocytes plasma cells with absence of lymphocytes, small neutrophilic abscess, Donovan bodies

TREATMENT

Often the immediate laboratory tests are unrewarding, and serology VDRL and HIV may be sent. The treatment administered is for the most likely clinical diagnosis and side lab investigations and the patient is reviewed after 7 days. Symptomatic improvement is usually evident in 3 days but donovanosis may take 5-7 days to respond. If the symptoms worsen, the patient is re-evaluated. If VDRL and HIV tests are negative during the follow-up, the test is repeated after 1 and 3 months. In case of HIV-negative report, the test has to be repeated after 6 months and 12 months of last exposure. Patients with positive VDRL test having meningeal symptoms should be evaluated for CSF VDRL, and in HIV-positive patients with positive VDRL, CSF VDRL is mandatory. The syndromic treatment (Appendix V) is often used, which includes treatment for syphilis and chancroid. In case of HIV-positive patients there is no consensus regarding the change of treatment regimen for STDs. However, the treatment recommendations are similar to the CDC guideline in most GUD. It is also mandatory that sex partners of the STD patient be examined, investigated and treated promptly.

Follow-Up

Primary chancre: Post-treatment VDRL is repeated at 3 month, 6 month and at one year.[26] In HIV positive patients with primary chancre, VDRL is repeated every month for the first 3 months and 3 monthly thereafter.[27]

Acknowledgement

The authors acknowledge the contribution of Dr. C.S. Sirka who was a co-author of the chapter in the first edition.

REFERENCES

1. Engelkens HJ, Stolz E. Genital ulcer disease. Int J Dermatol 1993; 32: 169-76.
2. Hoffman IF, Schmitz JL. Genital ulcer disease-Management in the HIV era. Post Grad Med 1995; 98: 67-82.
3. Schmid GP. Approach to the patient with genital ulcer disease. Med Clin North Am 1990; 74: 1559-72.
4. Kumar B, Handa S, Malhotra S. Changing trends in sexually transmitted diseases. Indian J Sex Transm Dis 1995; 16: 24-7.
5. Khanna N, Pandhi RK, Lakhanpal S. Changing trends in sexually transmitted diseases: A hospital based study. Indian J Sex Transm Dis 1996; 17: 79-81.
6. Sahni AK, Prasad VV, Seth P. Genomic diversity of human immunodeficiency virus type-1 in India. Int J STDs AIDS. 2002; 13: 115-8.
7. Chapel TA, Brown WJ, Jeffres C, et al. How reliable is the morphological diagnosis of penile ulceration? Sex Transm Dis 1977; 4: 150-2.
8. O'Farrell N, Hoosen AA, Coetzee KD, et al. Genital ulcer disease: accuracy of clinical diagnosis and strategies to improve control in Durban, South Africa. Genitourin Med 1994; 70: 7-11.
9. Sturm AW, Stolting GJ, Cormane RH, et al. Clinical and microbiological evaluation of 46 episodes of genital ulceration. Genitourin Med 1987; 63: 98-101.
10. Dangor Y, Ballard RC, Exposto F, et al. Accuracy of clinical diagnosis of genital ulcer disease. Sex Transm Dis 1990; 17: 184-9.
11. Mosley RC, Corey L, Benjamin D, et al. Comparison of viral isolation, direct immunofluorescence and direct immunoperoxidase

techniques for detection of genital herpes simplex virus infection. J Clin Microbiol 1981; 13: 913-8.
12. Solomon AR, Rasmussen JE, Varani J, et al. The Tzanck smear in the diagnosis of cutaneous herpes simplex. JAMA 1984; 251: 633-6.
13. Wasserheit JN. Epidemiological synergy. Interrelationships between human immunodeficiency virus infection and other sexually transmitted diseases. Sex Transm Dis. 1992; 19: 61-77.
14. Risbud A. Human immunodeficiency virus (HIV) & sexually transmitted diseases (STDs). Indian J Med Res. 2005; 121: 369-76.
15. Cone RW, Swenson PD, Hobson AC, et al. Herpes simplex virus detection from genitalia lesion: a comparative study using antigen detection (Herp Check) and culture. J Clin Microbiol 1993; 31: 1774-6.
16. Dyck EV, Meheus AZ, Piot P. Genital Herpes: Laboratory diagnosis of Sexually Transmitted Diseases.WHO. Geneva 1999; p 50-6.
17. Ashley RL. Genital herpes: review of the epidemic and potential use of type-specific serology.Clin Microbiol Rev. 1999; 12: 1-8.
18. Ashley RL. Sorting out the new HSV type specific antibody tests. Sex Transm Infect 2001; 77: 232-7.
19. Guerry SL, Bauer HM, Klausner JD et al. Recommendations for the selective use of herpes simplex virus type 2 serological tests. Clin Infect Dis. 2005; 40: 38-45.
20. Taylor DN, Duangmani C, Suvongse C, et al. The role of Haemophilus ducreyi in penile ulcers in Bangkok, Thailand. Sex Transm Dis 1984; 11: 148-51.
21. Dyck EV, Meheus AZ, Piot P. Chancroid Laboratory diagnosis of Sexually Transmitted Diseases.WHO, Geneva 1999; p 57-66.
22. Dyck EV, Meheus AZ, Piot P. *Chlamydia trachomatis* infection: Laboratory diagnosis of Sexually Transmitted Diseases.WHO, Geneva 1999; p 22-35.
23. Chen CY, Chi KH, Alexander S, et al. The molecular diagnosis of lymphogranuloma venerum: Evaluation of a real-time multiplex polymerase chain reaction test using rectal and urethral specimens. Sex Transm Dis 2007; 34: 451-5.
24. Morse SA, Trees DL, Htun Ye. Comparison of clinical diagnosis and standard laboratory and molecular methods for the diagnosis of genital ulcer disease in Lesotho: Association with human immunodeficiency virus infection. J Infect Dis 1997; 175: 583-9.
25. Risbud A, Chan-Tack K, Gadkari D, et al. The aetiology of genital ulcer disease by multiplex polymerase chain reaction and relationship to HIV infection among patients attending STDs clinics in Pune, India. Sex Trans Dis 1999; 26: 63-5.
26. Thappa DM. Current status of HIV modified Syphilis in Indian scenario. Indian J Sex Transm Dis 2002; 23: 1-13.
27. Siddappa K, Ravindra K. Syphilis and non venereal treponematosis. In: Valia RG, Valia AR, eds. IADVL Textbook and Atlas of Dermatology. Mumbai: Bhalani Publishing House; 2001. p. 1390-1422.

46 CLINICAL APPROACH TO VAGINAL/URETHRAL DISCHARGE

A J Kanwar

In this chapter

- Vaginal Discharge
- Candidiasis
- Trichomoniasis
- Bacterial Vaginosis
- Approach to a Patient with Abnormal Vaginal Discharge
- Urethral Discharge
- Approach to a Patient with Urethral Discharge

VAGINAL DISCHARGE

Vaginal discharge is one of the commonest presenting complaints in women attending gynaecology and STD clinics, general practitioners and reproductive health clinics. For ages, the term vaginal discharge has been used synonymously with leucorrhoea. A whitish discharge is usually not associated with menstruation.

The symptoms and signs of vaginal discharge are observed in several physiological and pathological conditions, which may be both local and systemic. Vaginal discharge should be considered as abnormal when anyone of the following feature is present.

1. Hypervaginal secretion not associated with menstruation
2. Offensive or malodorous discharge
3. Yellowish discharge

Prevalence

It has been estimated that upto one-third of females attending gynaecology clinics have complaints of vaginal discharge. Abnormal vaginal discharge can occur in women of all ages; however, it is quite common during pregnancy and more than 70% of pregnant women manifest abnormal vaginal discharge due to lower genital tract infections.

The commonest causative organisms of abnormal vaginal discharge in females of reproductive age group are *Neisseria gonorrhoeae, Chlamydia trachomatis, Gardnerella vaginalis, Trichomonas vaginalis* and *Candida*. Mixed infections are quite common.

In a study of 240 women of reproductive age with abnormal vaginal discharge, the prevalence of various causative conditions have been found to be 37.9% for bacterial vaginosis, 33.7% for mucopurulent cervicitis, 29.1% for non-infective leucorrhoea and 22% for vaginal candidiasis. Among these 240 women, 15.8% had infection with two organisms and 0.4% with more than two organisms.

Normal Vaginal Discharge

The normal vaginal discharge is whitish, non-malodorous and floccular in consistency. Its amount varies considerably between individuals. It may result in only minimal staining of the undergarments to profuse discharge. The normal pH is acidic and ranges from 3.5 to 4.5 due to the activity of Doderlein's lactobacilli. These bacilli convert glycogen into lactic acid. The cellular contents of the discharge are composed of sloughed cells of cervical columnar and vaginal squamous epithelium. The bulk of discharge consists of serous vaginal transudate and cervical mucous.[1,2] In addition to cellular debris, water and electrolytes, facultative microorganisms and organic compounds such as fatty acids, proteins and carbohydrates constitute vaginal secretion. The uterus and fallopian tube contribute little to vaginal discharge.

Normal Vaginal Flora

In healthy women, the vaginal flora consists of lactobacillus, anaerobic Gram-negative bacilli, *Bacteroides urealyticus*, β-hemolytic and non-hemolytic streptococci, *Candida albicans*, diptheroids, enterococci, *Escherechia coli, Fusobacterium nucleatum, Mobilincus spp., Mycoplasma hominis, Micrococcus pyogenes, Peptostreptococcus spp., Prevotella bivia disiens, Staphylococcus epidermidis* and *Ureaplasma urealyticum*. The vaginal ecosystem is a complex one, consisting of inter-relationships among endogenous microflora, host oestrogen and pH. Vaginal inflammation and infection occur when the vaginal ecosystem is altered.

Etiology of Vaginal Discharge

The symptoms and signs of abnormal vaginal discharge are attributable to vaginal infection. Increased profuse vaginal discharge is associated with trichomoniasis, bacterial vaginosis, vulvovaginal candidiasis (VVC), and in cases where there is coincidental sexual acquisition of cervical infection with *N. gonorrhoeae* and *C. trachomatis*.[3]

It has been shown in several studies that there is no association of cervical infection with symptoms or signs of abnormally increased amount or abnormal odour of vaginal discharge.

The various causes of abnormal vaginal discharge can be broadly divided into physiological and pathological. The physiological causes are either age-dependent (neonates, prepuberty and child-bearing) or due to excessive secretion (pregnancy, sexual arousal). Table 46.1 lists the various pathological causes of abnormal vaginal discharge.

The infective causes of abnormal vaginal discharge are described below and cervical infections associated with abnormal vaginal discharge are discussed elsewhere in this book.

Table 46.1 Pathological Causes of Abnormal Vaginal Discharge in Adolescents and Adult Women[4]

(a) **Infective**
Vaginitis
- Bacterial vaginosis
- Vaginal candidiasis
- Vaginal trichomoniasis

Cervicitis
- Mucopurulent cervicitis (MPC) due to *N. gonorrhoeae* and *C. trachomatis*

(b) **Non-infective**
Foreign bodies
- Intrauterine contraceptive device (IUCD)
- Tampons and other materials

Chemical irritants
- Antiseptics
- Deodorants
- Bath additives
- Detergent spermicide
- Douches
- Perfumed soaps

Gynaecological conditions
- Endocervical polyp
- Fistulae
- Radiation effects
- Post-operative
- Tumours
- Medication and nutrition

CANDIDIASIS

Vulvovaginal candiasis (VVC) is a frequent cause, affecting 15 to 30% of women attending a gynaecology clinic for complaints of vaginal discharge. Majority of yeast strains (85-90%) isolated from the vagina are *Candida albicans*. The rest are non-albicans species, the chief among them being *Candida glabrata*. Recently there has been an increased incidence of vaginitis caused by non-albicans species.[5,6]

C. albicans has an affinity to adhere to vaginal epithelial cells, although no epithelial cell receptor for candida has been identified. Only the germinative forms of *C. albicans* are able to produce VVC.

Pathogenic candida species secrete aspartyl proteinase.[7] This proteinase has been identified in vaginal secretion in women with symptomatic vaginitis only. Iron binding by candida organisms facilitates their virulence.[8] The ready availability of erythrocytes and haemoglobin in the vagina creates an ideal situation for yeast-possessing erythrocyte-binding surface receptors.

Pathogenesis and Predisposing Factors

Candida organisms gain access to vaginal epithelium and secretions predominantly from adjacent perianal area. The mechanisms whereby asymptomatic colonization of the vagina changes to symptomatic VVC is not exactly clear.

Spontaneous phenotypic stretching occurs in colony morphology of most candida species when they are grown on amino acid-rich agar in vitro at 24°C.[8] These variant phenotypes have a capacity to form mycelia spontaneously, to express virulence factors, adherence and the capacity to invade and survive in diverse body sites as well as to cause disease. It is possible that such spontaneous phenotypic switching transforms asymptomatic colonization to symptomatic vaginitis. Various predisposing factors for VVC are listed in Table 46.2. Epidemiological evidence for the role of sexual intercourse in the transmission of VVC is lacking.

Table 46.2 Predisposing Factors Associated with Vulvovaginal Candidiasis[5]

- Pregnancy
- Uncontrolled diabetes mellitus
- Corticosteroid therapy
- Tight-fitting synthetic underclothing
- Antimicrobial therapy
- Oestrogen therapy
- Contraceptives
  IUD
  Sponge
  Nonoxynol-9
  Diaphragm
  High-dose oestrogen oral contraceptive
- HIV infection
- Idiopathic

Sources of Infection

Persistent gastrointestinal tract carriage is a source of vaginal reinfection, as majority of candida strains isolated from rectum and vagina are identical.[9] However, women prone to recurrent VVC are not known to suffer form perianal or rectal candidiasis. As already mentioned, the role of sexual spread of candidiasis is limited. It has been shown that vaginal relapse is responsible for recurrent VVC. Small numbers of candida organisms possibly survive temporarily within cervical or vaginal epithelial cells only to re-emerge some weeks or months later. Fidel et al. have shown that systemic cell-mediated immunity (CMI) has only a minor role in providing a normal defense function at the level of vaginal mucosa. There is probably a local vaginal acquired defect in CMI predisposing to recurrent VVC.[8]

Probably the most important defense against both candidial colonization and symptomatic inflammation is the normal natural bacterial flora.

Candida organism in order to survive and persist must initially adhere to epithelial cells and then grow, proliferate and germinate, in order to colonize the vaginal mucosa successfully. Animal studies suggest that lactobacilli and candida frequently survive side by side.

Clinical Manifestations

Clinical spectrum of VVC varies from an acute florid exudative form with thick white vaginal discharge and large number of germinated yeast cells to other extremes of absent or minimal discharge, fewer organisms and pruritus. By and large, a quantitative relationship exists between signs and symptoms of VVC and the extent of yeast colonization.

The usual clinical presentation is acute pruritus and vaginal discharge. The discharge is classically described as typically cottage-cheese like in character. It may however at times be watery and homogenously thick. Odour is minimal and inoffensive. The patient complains of vaginal soreness, irritation, vulvar burning, dyspareunia and dysuria. Partners of patients with VVC may occasionally develop extensive balanoposthitis. More frequent, however, is a transient rash, erythema and a burning sensation. All these symptoms are self-limiting.

Diagnosis

A 10% KOH preparation would identify germinated yeast. A large number of WBC is usually absent in VVC and, if present, indicates mixed infection. The normal vaginal pH is 4.0 to 4.5. If pH is more than 5, it indicates either bacterial vaginosis, trichomoniasis or a mixed infection. If direct microscopy is positive, no culture is necessary. However, if it is negative and signs and symptoms suggest VVC, vaginal culture should be performed. Although vaginal culture is the most sensitive method for detection of candida, a positive culture does not necessarily indicate that the yeast is responsible for the vaginal symptoms.[8]

There is no reliable serologic test for the diagnosis of VVC.

A latex agglutination slide technique which employs polyclonal antibodies reactive with multiple species of candida is commercially available. It has a reported sensitivity of 81% with a specificity of 98.5%.[8]

Treatment

The treatment modalities of VVC are given in Appendix IV.

TRICHOMONIASIS

Trichomonas vaginalis is a flagellate pathogenic protozoan transmitted primarily by sexual contact. It causes vaginitis in women and urethritis in men. In addition to abnormal vaginal discharge, it is associated with increased incidence of preterm labour, premature rupture of membranes and post-abortion or post-caesarean infections. *T. vaginalis* is oval or fusiform in shape with a mean length of 15 μm. It has four anterior flagella which arise from an anterior kinetosomal complex. The cytoplasm is rich in glycogen granules, ribosomes and large chromatin granules which are known as hydrogenosomes. The reproduction is by mitotic division and longitudinal fission. It occurs every 8 to 12 hours under optimal conditions (temperature between 35°C and 37°C and pH between 4.9 and 7.5).[10] *T. vaginalis* exists only in trophozoite form. It is capable of phagocytosis and is an aerotolerant anaerobe. At high oxygen tension, its growth is inhibited as it lacks catalase.[11] Numerous host macromolecules like alpha-1 antitrypsin, fibronectin lipoproteins and lipids coat the cell surface of *T. vaginalis*.[12] These molecules are important for the survival of the parasite in vivo and contribute to metabolism and pathogenicity of trichomoniasis.

Cellular, humoral and secretory immune responses are elicited after infection with *T. vaginalis*. These, however, do not protect against repeated infection. The C3 component of the complement binds to receptor sites on the surface of *T. vaginalis* and leads to the death of the protozoan. The alternative complement pathway is involved.[13] It has been observed that symptoms of trichomoniasis are exacerbated shortly after menstruation, the time at which high levels of complement are found in vagina. *T. vaginalis* elicits predominantly a humoral response and the antibodies are directed against high molecular weight protein immunogen p270 as well as to cysteine proteinases.[10,14] For detailed information, refer Chapter 29.

Clinical Presentation

T. vaginalis primarily infects the vaginal epithelium. Less commonly it is isolated from the cervix, urethra, Bartholin's and Skene's glands. Extravaginal sites are rarely infected. These include fallopian tubes, perinephric spaces and cerebrospinal fluid.

The clinical manifestations vary from asymptomatic carriage to severe vaginitis. Patients with vaginitis complain of vulvar itching and purulent yellow-green discharge. The vulva may appear erythematous and oedematous with excoriations. As already mentioned, discharge may be absent in a few cases. The cervix has small punctate haemorrhages with ulcerations. This is referred to as 'strawberry' cervix.

Diagnosis

Diagnosis based solely on clinical signs and symptoms are unreliable as the spectrum of infection is broad and other sexually transmitted pathogens may cause similar signs and symptoms.

Laboratory Diagnosis

Direct Microscopic Examination

A purulent yellow-green vaginal discharge is characteristic of trichomoniasis. As the discharge is absent in a varying percentage of cases, diagnosis of trichomoniasis depends on the identification of *T. vaginalis* by wet mount, stains, culture, immunological and molecular methods.

Vaginal fluid or discharge is obtained during speculum examination using a cotton swab or wire loop. One drop of saline is placed on a microscopic slide and the vaginal sample is mixed directly in the saline on the slide. Slightly warming the saline enhances the motility of *T. vaginalis*. The motility is best observed by using phase contrast microscopy. For this, either the condenser is brought down or the diaphragm closed to increase the contrast. For diagnosis, it requires the identification of motile trichomonas with characteristic motility, size and morphology. In most cases, increased numbers of polymorphonuclear leucocytes are also present.

The identification of the protozoan on wet mount is better than staining methods which include staining with Gram, Giemsa, neutral red and other stains.[16,17] Wet mount preparations are also superior to Papanicolaou-stained smears which can detect *T. vaginalis* in asymptomatic women during routine cytologic examination.[18] However, there is a high percentage of false positive and false negative results.[10]

If the wet mount examination is negative, culture is the 'gold standard' for the diagnosis of trichomoniasis. Of the various media available, the modified Diamond medium is the best as it allows more prolific growth.

Several serological techniques have also been described to diagnose trichomoniasis, but these are less sensitive than culture or even wet mount examination. Other tests are antigen detection immunoassays using monoclonal antibodies and nuclear-acid based tests.

Treatment

Metronidazole and related drugs are highly effective for treatment of trichomoniasis. The various treatment options are given in Appendix IV.

Simultaneous treatment of sex partners is recommended.

Other Therapies

Topical therapy should be reserved for clinical situations in which systemic metronidazole is contraindicated.

Topical preparation of metronidazole gel has low efficacy. Clotrimazole applied intravaginally for 6 days may have a role in the first trimester when metronidazole is not recommended. Although a vaccine for active immunization against trichomoniasis is commercially available, it has not been evaluated in well-controlled double-blind-prospective studies.

BACTERIAL VAGINOSIS

Bacterial vaginosis (BV) is an important cause of abnormal vaginal discharge and affects about 30-45% of women in the reproductive age group. It is a polymicrobial condition and the culture of vaginal fluid reveals mixed flora which includes genital mycoplasmas, *Gardnerella vaginalis*, anaerobic bacteria and *Mobilincus species*.[19] There is a decrease in lactobacilli and increase in the total bacterial count from the normal of 10^5–10^6 cells/gm of secretion to 10^9–10^{11} organism/gm of secretion in patients of BV.

Clinical Features

Women with BV may be asymptomatic or may complain of increased vaginal discharge which is sticky and homogenous. It tends to adhere to the vaginal wall. The discharge has usually a fishy odour which is more noticeable after sexual intercourse. Pruritus is of only mild to moderate degree.

Diagnosis

In a patient suspected of BV, diagnosis can be made using Amsel's criteria[3] which are as follows:

1. Nonviscous homogenous white uniformly adherent vaginal discharge.
2. High pH – Vaginal pH of more than 4.7 has high sensitivity and negative predictive value, but of low specificity.
3. Clue cells – Vaginal squamous cells covered by bacterial rods which blur the border of squamous cells.
4. Whiff test – Adding 10% KOH to vaginal secretions produces an amine odour. It is due to the production of cadaverine, putrescine and trimethylamine by enzymatic action of decarboxylases.

   If any three of the above criteria are present, a diagnosis of BV can be made.

The other details of BV and its management are discussed in Chapter 24.

DEALING WITH ABNORMAL VAGINAL DISCHARGE

Symptoms and signs of abnormal vaginal discharge are mostly attributable to vaginal infection. Although in some studies an association between abnormal vaginal discharge and cervical infection has been found, by and large, there is no association of cervical infection with symptoms or signs of abnormal vaginal discharge.

As in other patients with STDs, the initial assessment in patients with abnormal vaginal discharge begins with history. In history, the following points should be specifically enquired:

1. Is there an abnormal increase in the amount of vaginal discharge?
2. Is there an abnormal or unpleasant odour of vaginal discharge?
3. Is the colour of the discharge unusually yellow?
4. Are there ulcers or painful lesions over genitalia?
5. Has the patient noticed any lumps or swellings?
6. Enquire specific details about the previous diagnosis, earlier treatments and their effects.
7. Ask about recent change of sex partner or multiple sex partners, history of STDs in partner.

After history, one should proceed to examination. General and physical examination should precede pelvic examination. Antiseptics should not be applied on external genitalia before pelvic examination to avoid vaginal contamination.

Speculum Examination

Warm water provides sufficient lubrication for speculum insertion. Following insertion, all aspects of vagina especially posterior fornix and cervix are assessed to see the presence or absence of mucopurulent cervicitis, ulceration, erythema and vesicular lesions of vulva or vagina. The amount, consistency and location of discharge within the vagina should be noted. Per-speculum examination should be followed by per-vaginal examination to look for cervical motion tenderness and tenderness in the posterior fornix.

Collection of Samples

The collection of vaginal discharge is done with a swab from the vaginal wall during speculum examination. In cases of cervical discharge, wipe the ectocervix with a large cotton swab and then collect the endocervical mucous on cotton-tipped swab. Vaginal secretions can be taken in prepubertal girls simply with swabs moistened with saline. A total of two samples from the cervix (for *N. gonorrhoeae* and Chlamydia) and three samples from the vagina (for candidiasis, bacterial vaginosis and trichomoniasis) must be taken. Cervical samples are taken initially and tested for gonococcus by Gram's stain, and Chlamydia by Giemsa stain. Vaginal discharge must be tested for candida by KOH test, bacterial vaginosis by Gram's stain and trichomoniasis by wet mount. The sample for wet mount is taken last so that motile trichomonas can be seen. Separate swabsticks must be used for culture and smear. It is preferable to use special swabsticks for certain organisms like:

- Gonococcus - non-cotton swab sticks (calcium alginate, rayon, dacron)
- Chlamydia - cotton top swabs with a plastic or metal shaft instead of wooden shaft, cytobrush
- Mycoplasma/ureaplasma-rayon swab
- Candida - polyester swab

Appearance of Vaginal Discharge

The vaginal discharge is then examined with special attention to the amount, consistency, colour, odour and location of discharge within the vagina. The character of vaginal discharge can be classified as floccular, granular, homogenous (milky) and curdy. Normal vaginal discharge is floccular or granular. The differential diagnosis of vaginal discharge is given in Table 46.3.

Table 46.3 Differential Diagnosis of Vaginal Discharge

Profile	*Normal Vaginal Discharge*	*Candidal Vulvovaginitis*	*Trichomonal Vaginitis*	*Bacterial Vaginosis*
Aetiology	Lactobacillus predominant	*Candida* spp. and other yeasts	*Trichomonas vaginalis*	Associated with *G. vaginalis*, anaerobic bacteria, and *Mycoplasma hominis*
Symptoms	None	Vulval pruritus and/or irritation; external dysuria, increased vaginal discharge	Profuse discharge, often malodourous; external dysuria and genital irritation often present	Malodourous, increased discharge (commonly present at introitus)
Discharge				
• Amount	• Variable; usually scanty	• Scant to moderate	• Profuse	• Moderate to profuse
• Colour	• Clear or white	• White	• White, yellow or green	• White or gray
• Consistency	• Non-homogenous flocculant	• Clumped, "cheesy" adherent exudative plaques	• Homogenous, watery, often frothy	• Homogenous, uniformly coating the vaginal walls
pH	Usually<4.5	<4.5	Usually>5.0	Usually>4.5
Amine odour with 10% KOH	None	None	Usually present	Present
Associated inflammatory signs	None	Erythema, oedema and/or erosions of vagina or external genitalia; vulval dermatitis common	Erythema of vaginal mucosa, introitus; occational cervical petechiae; vulval dermatitis	None
Microscopy of discharge	Normal epithelial cells; lactobacilli predominate	Leukocytes, epithelial cells; yeast, mycelia, seen	Leukocytes, motile trichomonads seen	Clue cells; rare leukocytes; lactobacilli outnumbered by mixed flora

Laboratory Evaluation

The colour of vaginal discharge should be noted againast the white colour of the swab.

The pH of the discharge is determined by directly rolling the swab containing the specimen on a pH indicator paper. The pH indicator paper should show colour variation with pH above and below 4.5. An additional specimen is first mixed with a drop of saline and then with a drop of 10% KOH on a microscopic slide. An abnormal fishy or amine odour released on mixing of the specimen with KOH provides the usual basis for a clinical diagnosis of BV. Separate cover slips are placed on both saline and KOH wet mounts for microscopic examination to detect the

(a) Presence and quantity of normal epithelial cells
(b) Clue cells
(c) Neutrophils
(d) Trichomonads – motile trophozoite forms
(e) Candidal hyphae and spores
(f) Gram stain of the vaginal fluid

In many patients, the symptoms and signs combined with risk assessment and with pH and amine tests and microscopic wet mount findings correspond to a consistent pattern, and further studies may be unnecessary. However, when the diagnosis cannot be established, further microbiological studies are indicated. The nature and choice of the study depends on the clinical findings. These may include

(a) Culture for *C. albicans* and non-albicans species
(b) Culture for *T. vaginalis*
(c) Culture for mycoplasma and ureaplasma

It is important to differentiate between normal flora and flora characteristic of bacterial vaginosis. Here one should note that in patients with prominent vaginal complaints but no abnormal findings,[20] all the three additional microbiological tests are indicated as at times the complaints may be functional. The endocervical mucous should be separately examined apart from the vaginal discharge. The characteristics of endocervical secretion can be classified into mucoid, cloudy and mucopurulent. Yellowish colour on white-cotton tipped swab is considered mucopus.

Endocervical Smear Stain

The swab is rolled onto an area of 1-2 square centimeters on a glass slide. The smeared secretion should be distributed in separate heterogeneous islands.

The smear is heated dry and stained with
(a) Gram stain
(b) Methylene blue/Giemsa

Emulsion oil is added and the microscopic slide is scanned to evaluate the presence of cervical mucous to look for contaminated squamous cells and microorganisms and to identify areas of mucous that contain inflammatory cells. Usually polymorphonuclear leucocytes are not uniformly distributed in the cervical mucous. Therefore, a representative area containing dense concentration of such leucocytes is selected. The presence of 10 or more PMN leukocytes per field (1000x) on a smear-stained specimen of endocervical mucous at least in five separate areas is classified as mucopus. The demonstration of intracellular diplococci at least 3 pairs or more is strongly suggestive of *N. gonorrhoeae* infection. If there are only few leucocytes, it suggests physiological endocervical discharge.

The various causes of mucopurulent cervicits like *C. trachomatis* and *N. gonorrhoeae*, which can be associated with vaginal discharge, are discussed elsewhere in this book.

Partner Evaluation

It is important to examine all recent partner(s) for similar symptoms and other STDs. According to WHO (2004), the partners of patients with gonorrhoea and trichomoniasis should be empirically treated. Bacterial vaginosis is an endogenous reproductive tract infection and treatment of male partners alone has not proved to be beneficial. Isolated episode of candidiasis is not sexually transmitted. Treatment of asymptomatic partners is not recommended. In case of recurrent vulvovaginal candidiasis or the male partner having balanitis/balanoposthitis, treatment should be given to the partner. In cases where syndromic management is followed, then the partner is also treated as the patient. According to NACO (2007), the partner is treated only if he is symptomatic or there is no improvement in the patient after initial treatment.

Condom

Barrier protection must be used till the infection subsides.

URETHRAL DISCHARGE

Urethritis or inflammation of the urethra is characterized by the discharge of a mucopurulent or purulent material associated with a burning sensation during micturition or urethral pruritus. Asymptomatic infections are common. The only bacterial pathogens of proven clinical importance in men who have urethritis are *N. gonorrhoeae* and *C. trachomatis*. Accordingly urethritis is termed as gonococcal when *N. gonorrhoeae* is detected in urethral smears, and non-gonococcal (NGU) when this organism cannot be visualized microscopically.

Aetiopathogenesis

Urethral discharge is prevalest in 15 to 20% of patients attending STD clinics in India. Urethritis due to *N. gonorrhoeae* is the most common cause of urethral discharge in developing countries. It accounts for about 50% of patients presenting with urethral discharge. NGU is diagnosed if Gram negative intracellular organisms cannot be identified on Gram stains. *C. trachomatis* is the most frequent cause (15-55%) of NGU; however, the prevalence varies by age group, with lower prevalence among older men. The proportion of NGU cases caused by Chlamydia has been declining gradually. Other pathogens are *Mycoplasma genitalium* and *Ureaplasma urealyticum*. *Trichomonas vaginalis*, HSV and adenovirus might also cause NGU.[21-23] Primary genital herpes is associated with urethritis in significant proportion of patients. Diagnostic and treatment procedures for these uncommon organisms are reserved for situations in which these infections are suspected (e.g. contact with trichomoniasis and genital lesions or severe dysuria and meatitis, which might suggest genital herpes) or when NGU is not responsive to treatment. Enteric bacteria have been identified as an uncommon cause of NGU and may be associated with insertive anal sex. Candida can be isolated in less than 1% of patients, although its significance is unknown. Rarely urethral discharge can be caused by other organisms. The causes are discussed in Chapter 22.

DEALING WITH URETHRAL DISCHARGE

Urethritis can be diagnosed on the basis of any of the following signs or laboratory tests:

1. Mucopurulent or purulent discharge.
2. Gram stain of urethral secretions demonstrating ≥5 WBC per oil immersion field. The Gram stain is highly sensitive and specific for documenting both urethritis and the presence or absence of gonococcal infections.
3. Positive leukocyte esterase test or microscopic examination of first- void urine sediment demonstrating ≥10 WBC per high-power field.

It is difficult to differentiate between gonococcal and NGU on clinical grounds. Both conditions present with urethral discharge, dysuria or urethral itching.[24] There are some differences, however. These are listed in Table 46.4.

Table 46.4 Clinical Features of Gonococcal and Non-Gonococcal Urethritis

Symptoms	*Gonorrhoea*	*NGU*
Discharge	Profuse, purulent and yellowish green	Scanty, mucoid or mucopurulent
Dysuria	Intense burning sensation	'Smarting' feeling in urethra on passing urine
Incubation period	2–5 days	2–3 weeks
Constitutional symptoms	Fever, malaise	Absent

(a) In many patients with NGU, the discharge many be absent while some may notice it only in the morning.
(b) It is not possible to differentiate between *C. trachomatis* positive and *C. trachomatis* negative NGU. In *C. trachomatis* negative urethritis, the discharge may be more profuse and purulent.[25]
(c) *U. urealyticum* infection may be associated in some cases with only dysuria and no discharge.[25]
(d) Some patients may present with other manifestations of NGU. These include
    (i) Chlamydial conjunctivitis
    (ii) Epididymitis
    (iii) Prostatitits
    (iv) Reiter's syndrome

Laboratory Approach to Urethral Discharge

Collection of Sample

Urethral material is obtained with meatal or intraurethral swabs; the choice depends on the type of organisms and the amount of urethral discharge. In males, the detection of urethral discharge can be enhanced by milking the penis from the base to the glans. Meatal discharge is an appropriate specimen for the detection of *N. gonorrhoeae*. If there is no meatal exudate, an intraurethral swab should be used. It is important that the patient should not have passed urine for at least 2 hours. The swab is introduced slowly for about 2–3 cm, rotated and then withdrawn gradually.[26]

In patients with no discharge, early morning urine sample or urine voided at least after 4 hours of retention should be collected and centrifuged for at least 10 minutes. The superficial part is decanted and the sediment is used as the specimen.

Gram Stain

The swab is rolled onto the slide which is then air-fixed or passed through a flame. It is then stained with Grams' stain. The slide is examined under 100× magnification. The area that shows maximum number of polymorphonuclear leucocytes (PMNL) is then examined under oil immersion (1000×). The presence or absence of diplococci and the number of PMNL in each field is noted.

1. Interpretation of the slide: The detection of Gram negative diplococci inside PMNL is diagnostic of gonococcal urethritis. In the presence of only extracellular Gram-negative diplococci, the diagnosis of gonorrhoea should be confirmed by culture.
2. The presence of greater than or equal to 5 WBC per oil immersion field in the absence of Gram negative diplococci is diagnostic of NGU.[27]
3. When the results of smear are equivocal with finding of only extracellular or atypical diplococci, it is imperative to do cultures.[25,27]
4. Cultures of *C. trachomatis* and *U. urealyticum* are not universally available. The cultivation of *C. trachomatis* in tissue culture requires the support of a well-equipped laboratory.
5. Positive leucocyte esterase test or microscopic examination of first void urine demonstrating greater than or equal to 10 WBC per HPF is diagnostic of NGU.[28] Various culture media used and other diagnostic tests employed for gonorrhoea and NGU are discussed elsewhere in this book.

Treatment Guidelines

Refer to Appendix IV for treatment guidelines by CDC, WHO and NACO. Refer Chapter 47 and Appendix V for syndromic management of urethral and vaginal discharge.

REFERENCES

1. Salerno LJ. Leukorrhoea. In: Sciarra JJ, Mc Elin TW, eds. Gynaecology and Obstetrics. Hagerstown: Harper and ROW Publishers; 1981. p. 1-5.
2. Siemmens JP, Wegner G. Estrogen deprivation and vaginal function in post menopausal women. JAMA 1982; 2481: 445-8.
3. Holmes KK, Stamm WE, et al. Lower genital tract infection syndrome in women. In: Holmes KK, Sparling PF, Mardh PA, et al. 3rd ed. Sexually Transmitted Diseases. McGraw Hill, New York: 1999; p 761-781.
4. Blackwell A. Management of vaginal discharge. Med Digest Asia 1983; 1: 12-20.
5. Sobel JD. Epidemiology and pathogenesis of recurrent vulvo-vaginal candidiasis. Am J Obstet Gynaecol 1985; 152: 926-9.
6. Morton RS, Rashid S. Candidal vaginitis: Natural history, predisposing factors and prevention. Proc R Soc Physc 1977; 70 (suppl 4): 3-6.
7. De Bernardis F. Evidence for a role for secreted aspartate proteinase of *Candida albicans*, in vulvo-vaginal candidiasis. J Infect Dis 1990; 161: 1276-8.
8. Sobel JD. Vulvovaginal candidiasis. In: Holmes KK, Sparling PF, Mardh PA, et al., eds. 3rd ed. Sexually Transmitted Diseases. New York: McGraw Hill; 1999. p. 629-39.
9. Meinhof WL. Demonstration of typical features of individual *C. albicans* strains as a means of studying sources of infection. Chemotherapy 1982; 28: 51-5.
10. Krieger JN, Aldrete JF. *Trichomonas vaginalis* and Trichomoniasis. In: Holmes KK, Sparling PF, Mardh PA, et al. eds. 3rd ed. Sexually Transmitted Diseases. New York: McGraw Hill, 1999. p. 587-604.
11. Honigberg BM. Trichomonads, Parasitic in humans. London, Springer Verlag 1989: p. 24.
12. Peterson KM, Aldrete JF. Host plasma proteins on the surface of pathogenic *Trichomonas vaginalis*. Infect Immun 1982; 37: 755-62.
13. Gillin F, Sher H. Activation of alternate complement pathway by *Trichomonas vaginalis*. Infect Immun 1981; 34: 268-72.
14. Aldrete JF. Alternating phenotypic expression of two classes of *Trichomonas vaginalis* surfaces markers. Rev Infect Dis 1988; 10 S: 408-12.
15. Wasserheit JN. Epidemiological synergy: Inter relationship between human immunodeficiency virus infection and other sexually transmitted diseases. Sex Trans Dis 1992; 19: 61-5.
16. Quinn TC, Krieger JN. Trichomoniasis. In: KS Warren, AAF Mahmoud eds Tropical and Geographic medicine. 2nd ed. New York: McGraw Hill: 1990; p. 358-65.
17. Nielsen R. *Trichomonas vaginalis*: II Lab investigations in trichomoniasis. Br J Vener Dis 1973; 49: 531-4.
18. Weinberger MW, Harger JH. Accuracy of Papanicolaou smear in the diagnosis of asymptomatic infection with *Trichomonas vaginalis*. Obstet Gyanecol 1993; 82: 425-8.
19. Hill GB. The microbiology of bacterial vaginosis. Am J Obstet Gyanecol 1993; 169: 450-4.
20. Hillier S, Holmes KK. Bacterial vaginosis In: Holmes KK, Sparling PF, Mardh PA, et al. eds. 3rd ed. Sexually Transmitted diseases. New York: McGraw Hill; 1999: p. 563-86.
21. Schwebke JR, Hook EW. High rates of *Trichomonas vaginalis* among men attending a sexually transmitted diseases clinic: Implications for screening and urethritis management. J Infect Dis 2003; 188: 465- 8.
22. Madeb R, Nativ O, Benilevi D, et al. Need for diagnostic screening of herpes simplex virus in patients with nongonococcal urethritis. Clin Infect Dis 2000; 30: 982-3.
23. Bradshaw CS, Tabrizi SN, Read TR, et al. Etiologies of nongonococcal urethritis: bacteria, viruses, and the association with orogenital exposure. J Infect Dis 2006; 193: 336- 45.
24. Munday PE, Attman DG, Taylor RD. Urinary abnormalities in non-gonococcal urethritis. Br J Vener Dis 1981; 57: 387-90.
25. Martin DH, Bowie WR. Urethritis in males. In: Holmes KK, Sparling PF, Mardh PA, et al. 3rd ed. Sexually transmitted diseases. McGraw Hill, New York 1999: p 833-45.

26. Dyck K EV, Meheus AZ, Piot P. In: Laboratory diagnosis of sexually transmitted diseases. Geneva WHO: 1999. p. 1-2
27. Jacobs NF, Kraus SJ. Gonococcal and non gonococcal urethritis in men. Clinical and laboratory differentiation. Ann Intern Med 1975; 82: 7-14.
28. Patrick DM, Rekart ML, Knowles L. Unsatisfactory performance of leukocyte esterase test of first voided urine for rapid diagosis of urethritis. Genitourin Med 1994; 70: 187-90.

47 CRITICAL EVALUATION OF SYNDROMIC MANAGEMENT OF SEXUALLY TRANSMITTED DISEASES

Vinod K Sharma, Uttam Kumar

In this chapter

- STI Associated Syndromes
- NACO 2007 Guidelines for Syndromic Management of STD
- STI Among Special Populations: FSW and MSM
- Critical Evaluation of Syndromic Approach

INTRODUCTION

An STI is a public health problem having social stigma, and it significantly increases the risk of HIV transmission. Most STIs are curable after adequate treatment, and this forms an important component of control and prevention of STIs. Early diagnosis and appropriate treatment of STI will definitely reduce the transmission of HIV/AIDS. WHO recognizes that "The control of sexually transmitted diseases is an intervention which improves the health status of the population and prevents HIV transmission". To achieve this, the concept of syndromic approach to STI management came into effect. In settings where lab tests are not available, the health care provider can easily treat patients based on their symptoms and clinical findings. Syndromic approach is a useful tool for patients with symptoms and signs related to STIs. However, if the patient is asymptomatic, the only way to exclude STI is by carrying out laboratory tests.

The STI case management should provide treatment for cure. It should also entertain bringing the partners for treatment and preventing the risk-taking behaviour.

There are three approaches to diagnosing and treating STIs:

(a) Aetiological diagnosis
(b) Clinical diagnosis
(c) Syndromic approach

Problems with Aetiological Diagnosis

Aetiological diagnosis is based on identifying the causative agent by laboratory tests.

- Skilled personnel and sophisticated equipment are needed to identify the causative agents of STIs.
- Laboratory tests are expensive and time-consuming.
- Treatment does not begin until the results are obtained.
- Testing facilities are not available at the primary health care level where most people with STIs seek care.

Problems with Clinical Diagnosis

Clinical diagnosis is based on identifying the STI based on clinician's experience. It is well known that even experienced STI clinicians may miss concurrent infections. Studies have shown that clinicians correctly identified only one-third of cases of chancroid and syphilis and less than 10% of mixed infections. Clinical diagnosis is only accurate for 50% of STI cases, and accuracy is especially lower in case of female patients. Mistreated and untreated infections can lead to complications and continued transmission.

Criticisms over the Syndromic Approach

- The syndromic approach is not a scientific procedure.
- Syndromic diagnosis is too simple for a physician to use, and the approach does not use a provider's clinical skills and experience.
- Some physicians prefer to treat according to clinical diagnosis in the absence of lab facilities and then, if symptoms do not improve, treating for another cause.
- The syndromic approach wastes a lot of drugs.
- It may promote the development of antibiotic resistance.
- Simple laboratory tests should be included.

STI-ASSOCIATED SYNDROMES[1,2]

The syndromic approach is based on treating the patient on the basis of a group of symptoms or syndromes as given in Table 47.1.

Table 47.1 STI-Associated Syndromes

STI Syndrome	*Possible Causes*
Urethral discharge	*N. gonorrhoeae* *C. trachomatis* D to K *Trichomonas vaginalis*
Scrotal swelling	*N. gonorrhoeae* *C. trachomatis* D to K

(*Contd.*)

Inguinal bubo	*Haemophilus ducreyi* *C. trachomatis* (L1, L2, L3)
Genital ulcer disease	*Treponema pallidum* *Haemophilus ducreyi* *C. trachomatis* (L1, L2, L3) *Klebsiella granulomatis* *Herpes simplex virus*
Vaginal discharge	*N. gonorrhoeae* *C. trachomatis* D to K *Trichomonas vaginalis* *Herpes simplex* *Candida albicans* *Gardenerella vaginalis* *Mycoplasma*
Lower abdominal pain	*N. gonorrhoeae* *C. trachomatis* *Mycoplasma* *Gardenerella vaginalis* *Anaerobes*
Oral and anal STI	*N. gonorrhoeae* *C. trachomatis* *Treponema pallidum* *Haemophilus ducreyi* *Klebsiella granulomatis* *Herpes simplex virus*

Diagnosing the Syndrome[1,2]

Simple flowcharts by WHO and NACO provide the information to institute treatment based on symptoms and signs. These flowcharts are prepared based on STI prevalence and drug availability and susceptibility to the organisms in that area. These are displayed as posters or as pamphlets for easy reference of the provider.

Syndromic management flowcharts **(Appendix V)** are designed to follow a diagnostic logic close to the provider's own thought processes. "This is, in fact, the approach that many doctors follow naturally and subconsciously," says Dr. Johannes van Dam of the Joint United Nations Programme on AIDS (UNAIDS), who further says that, "It simply provides a rational basis for a diagnosis or for a therapeutic decision by offering correct information based on the latest possible data".

In syndromic case management, the provider is less dependent on laboratory tests. The newer NACO guidelines suggest that simple lab tests should be done in every case as and when available. At the same time these tests are not a must to diagnose the syndrome and starting treatment; so in case of lack of facilities the health care provider can very well go ahead and start treatment on clinical findings, using the appropriate flowchart. The simplified procedure of the syndromic approach gives a readymade tool to health workers, and it enlarges the number of providers for STI care. The services will be available on a wider scale, and aim to reduce the prevalence of STIs in a short time period.

"Patients like the idea of being treated at first visit, and because syndromic management is more efficient, the waiting time for clinic visits is much shorter", says Dr. Alfred Brathwaite of the Jamaican Ministry of Health, which has implemented syndromic management in many of the country's STI clinics.

This approach includes treatment and return visit to ensure treatment compliance. It also emphasizes on prevention education and couselling, which includes change of high-risk behaviour, correct and consistent condom use, improvement in health-seeking behaviour, referring all patients for voluntary counselling and testing for HIV, syphilis and hepatitis B, partner management whereever indicated and management of special situations like STI with pregnancy. Through this approach cure rates of STIs are high, and infection spread is curtailed by reducing the length of illness. It also prevents STI-related complications and acquisition of HIV infection.

Validity of the Syndromic Approach

The validity of the syndromic approach depends on:

- The efficacy of drugs chosen against STI pathogens.
- The pathogens causing the diseases included in the syndrome.
- Diagnostic validity.
- Assessing the cure rate and compliance of treatment.

Challenges

- Syndromic algorithms must incorporate local data on STI prevalence.
- Affordable drugs must be prescribed on the flowchart.
- May need modification based on new treatment strategies.
- Development of algorithms for different situations and locations.
- Asymptomatic patients—Health workers must be trained to identify such cases.

NACO 2007 GUIDELINES FOR SYNDROMIC MANAGEMENT OF STD

Treatment of Urethral Discharge in Males

As dual infection is common, the treatment for urethral discharge should adequately cover therapy for both gonorrhoea and chlamydial infections.

Recommended Regimen for Uncomplicated Gonorrhoea + Chlamydia

Uncomplicated infections indicate that the disease is limited to the anogenital region (anterior urethritis and proctitis).

- Tab. Cefixime 400 mg orally, single dose Plus Tab Azithromycin 1 g orally single dose under supervision
- Advise the client to return after 7 days of start of therapy

When symptoms persist or recur after adequate treatment for gonorrhoea and chlamydia in the index client and partner(s), they should be treated for *Trichomonas vaginalis*.

If discharge or only dysuria persists after 7 days,

- Tab. Secnidazole 2 gm orally, single dose (to treat for *T. vaginalis*).

If symptoms still persist,

- Refer to a higher centre as early as possible

If individuals are allergic to azithromycin, give erythromycin 500 mg four times a day for 7 days

Management of Pregnant Partner

Pregnant partners of male clients with urethral discharge should be examined per speculum as well as per vaginal and should be treated for gonococcal chlamydial infections.

- Cephalosporins to cover gonococcal infection are safe and effective in pregnancy
- Tab. Cefixime 400 mg orally, single dose **or**
  Ceftriaxone 125 mg by intramuscular injection
  plus
  Tab. Erythromycin 500 mg orally four times a day for seven days **or**
  Cap. Amoxicillin 500 mg orally, three times a day for seven days to cover chlamydial infection
- Quinolones (like ofloxacin, ciprofloxacin) and doxycycline are contraindicated in pregnant women.

Syndrome-Specific Guidelines for Partner Management

- Treat all recent partners.
- Treat female partners (for gonorrhoea and chlamydia) on same lines after ruling out pregnancy and history of allergies.
- Advise sexual abstinence during the course of treatment.
- Provide condoms, educate about correct and consistent use.
- Refer for voluntary counselling and testing for HIV, syphilis and Hepatitis B.
- Schedule return visit after 7 days.

Follow-Up

After seven days

- To see reports of tests done for HIV, syphilis and Hepatitis B.
- If symptoms persist, to assess whether it is due to treatment failure or reinfection.

- For prompt referral, if required.

Treatment of Scrotal Swelling

Treat for both gonococcal and chlamydial infections

- Tab. Cefixime 400 mg orally BD for 7 days
  Plus
  Cap. Doxycycline 100 mg orally, twice daily for 14 days and refer to a higher centre as early as possible since complicated gonococcal infection needs parenteral and longer duration of treatment
- Supportive therapy to reduce pain (bed rest, scrotal elevation with T bandage and analgesics)

Note: If quick and effective therapy is not given, damage and scarring of testicular tissues may cause sub-fertility.

Syndrome-Specific Guidelines for Partner Management

The partner needs to be treated depending on the clinical findings.

Management Protocol in Case the Partner is Pregnant

- Depending on the clinical findings in pregnant partner (whether vaginal discharge or endocervical discharge or PID is present), the drug regimens should be used.
- Doxycycline is contraindicated in pregnancy.
- Erythromycin base/amoxicillin can be used in pregnancy. (Erythromycin estolate is contraindicated in pregnancy due to hepatotoxicity. Hence erythromycin base or erythromycin ethyl succinate should be given.)

Treatment of Inguinal Bubo

- Start Cap. Doxycycline 100 mg orally twice daily for 21 days (to cover LGV)
  Plus
  Tab. Azithromycin 1 g orally single dose **or** Tab. Ciprofloxacin 500 mg orally, twice a day for three days to cover chancroid
- Refer to a higher centre as early as possible.

Note:

- A bubo should never be incised and drained at the primary health centre, even if it is fluctuant, as there is a high risk of fistula formation and chronicity. If bubo becomes fluctuant, always refer for aspiration to a higher centre.
- In severe cases with vulval edema in females, surgical intervention may be required for which they should be referred to a higher centre.

Syndrome-specific Guidelines for Partner Management

- Treat all partners who are in contact with the client in the last 3 months.
- Partners should be treated for chancroid and LGV as given below:
- Tab. Azithromycin 1 g orally single dose to cover chancroid
  plus
- Cap. Doxycycline 100 mg orally, twice daily for 21 days to cover LGV
- Advise sexual abstinence during the course of treatment.
- Provide condoms, educate on correct and consistent use.
- Refer for voluntary counselling and testing for HIV, syphilis and hepatitis B.
- Schedule return visit after 7 days and 21 days.

Management of Pregnant Partner

- Quinolones (like ofloxacin, ciprofloxacin), doxycycline, and sulfonamides are contraindicated in pregnant women.
- Pregnant and lactating women should be treated with erythromycin regimen, and consideration should be given to the addition of a parenteral aminoglycoside (e.g., gentamicin)
- Tab. Erythromycin base, 500 mg orally, 4 times daily for 21 days and refer to a higher centre. (Erythromycin estolate is contraindicated in pregnancy due to hepatotoxicity. Hence erythromycin base or erythromycin ethyl succinate should be given.)

Treatment of Genital UlcersTo cover syphilis

- If vesicles or multiple painful ulcers are present, treat for herpes with Tab. Acyclovir 400 mg orally, three times a day for 7 days.
- If vesicles are not seen and only ulcer is seen, treat for syphilis and chancroid and counsel on herpes genitalis.

To cover syphilis

- Inj. Benzathine penicillin 2.4 million IU IM after a test dose in two divided doses (with emergency tray ready). In individuals allergic or intolerant to penicillin, doxycycline 100 mg orally, twice daily for 14 days.
  Plus
- Tab. Azithromycin 1 g orally single dose **or** Tab. Ciprofloxacin 500 mg orally, twice a day for three days to cover chancroid
  Treatment should be extended beyond 7 days if ulcers have not epithelialized, i.e. formed a new layer of skin over the sore.

Refer to a higher centre

- If not responding to treatment
- Genital ulcers coexistent with HIV
- Recurrent lesion

Syndrome-specific Guidelines for Partner Management

- Treat all partners who are in contact with the client in last 3 months.
- Partners should be treated for syphilis and chancroid.
- Advise sexual abstinence during the course of treatment.
- Provide condoms, educate about correct and consistent use.
- Refer for voluntary counselling and testing for HIV, syphilis and Hepatitis B.
- Schedule return visit after 7 days.

Management of Pregnant Women

- Quinolones (like ofloxacin, ciprofloxacin), doxycycline, and sulfonamides are contraindicated in pregnant women.
- Pregnant women who test positive for RPR should be considered infected unless adequate treatment is documented in the medical records and sequential serologic antibody titers have declined.
- Inj. Benzathine penicillin 2.4 million IU IM after a test dose (with emergency tray ready).
- A second dose of benzathine penicillin 2.4 million units IM should be administered 1 week after the initial dose for women who have primary, secondary or early latent syphilis.
- Pregnant women who are allergic to penicillin should be treated with erythromycin 500 mg orally four times a day for 15 days, and the neonate should be treated for syphilis after delivery. (Erythromycin estolate is contraindicated in pregnancy because of drug-related hepatotoxicity. Hence only erythromycin base or erythromycin ethyl succinate should be used in pregnancy.)
- All pregnant women should be asked history of genital herpes and examined carefully for herpetic lesions.
- Women without symptoms or signs of genital herpes or its prodrome can deliver vaginally.

- Women with genital herpetic lesions at the onset of labour should be delivered by caesarean section to prevent neonatal herpes.
- Acyclovir may be administered orally to pregnant women with the first episode of genital herpes or severe recurrent herpes.

Treatment of Vaginal Discharge in Females

Vaginitis (TV+BV+Candida)

- Tab. Secnidazole 2 gm orally, single dose **or** Tab. Tinidazole 500 mg orally, twice daily for 5 days
- Tab. Metoclopropramide taken 30 minutes before Tab. Secnidazole to prevent gastric intolerance
- Treat for candidiasis with Tab. Fluconazole 150 mg orally single dose or local Clotrimazole 500 mg vaginal pessaries once

Treatment for Cervical Infection (Chlamydia and Gonorrhoea)

- Tab. cefixim 400 mg orally, single dose
  Plus Azithromycin 1 g, 1 hour before lunch. If vomiting within 1 hour, give antiemetic and repeat
- If vaginitis and cervicitis are present treat for both
- Instruct the client to avoid douching
- Pregnancy, diabetes and HIV may also be influencing factors and should be considered in recurrent infections
- Follow-up after one week

Management in Pregnant Women

Per-speculum examination should be done to rule out pregnancy complications like abortion, premature rupture of membranes.

- Treatment for vaginitis (TV+BV+Candida) in first trimester of pregnancy – local treatment with Clotrimazole vaginal pessary/cream only for candidiasis. Oral Flucanozole is contraindicated in pregnancy. Metronidazole pessaries or cream intravaginally if trichomoniasis or BV is suspected.
- In second and third trimesters oral metronidazole can be given. Tab. Secnidazole 2 gm orally, single dose or Tab. Tinidazole 500 mg orally, twice daily for 5 days. Tab. Metoclopropramide taken 30 minutes before Tab. Metronidazole to prevent gastric intolerance.

Specific Guidelines for Partner Management

- Treat current partner only if no improvement after initial treatment.
- If partner is symptomatic, treat client and partner using the above protocols.
- Advise sexual abstinence during the course of treatment.
- Provide condoms, educate about correct and consistent use
- Schedule return visit after 7 days

Treatment of Lower Abdominal Pain in Females

Out-Client Treatment

In mild or moderate PID (in the absence of tubo ovarian abscess), out-client treatment can be given. Therapy is required to cover *Neisseria gonorrheae, Chlamydia trachomatis* and anaerobes.

- Tab. Cefixim 400 mg orally BD for 7 days + Tab. Metronidazole 400 mg orally, twice daily for 14 days
  Plus
- Doxycycline, 100 mg orally, twice a day for 2 weeks (to treat chlamydial infection)
- Tab. Ibuprofen 400 mg orally, three times a day for 3 to 5 days
- Tab. Ranitidine 150 mg orally, twice daily to prevent gastritis
- Remove intrauterine device, if present, under antibiotic cover of 24-48 hours

- Advise abstinence during the course of treatment and educate on correct and consistent use of condoms
- Observe for 3 days. If no improvement (i.e. absence of fever, reduction in abdominal tenderness, reduction in cervical movement, adnexal and uterine tenderness), or if symptoms worsen, refer for in-client treatment

Caution: PID can be a serious condition. Refer the client to a hospital if she does not respond to treatment within 3 days and even earlier if her condition worsens.

Syndrome-Specific Guidelines for Partner Management

- Treat all partners in the past 2 months.
- Treat male partners for urethral discharge (gonorrhoea and chlamydia).
- Advise sexual abstinence during the course of treatment.
- Provide condoms, educate on correct and consistent use.
- Refer for voluntary counselling and testing for HIV, syphilis and Hepatitis B.
- Inform about complications if left untreated and sequelae.
- Schedule return visit after 3 days, 7 days and 14 days to ensure compliance.

Management of Pregnant Women

Although PID is rare in pregnancy,

- Any pregnant woman suspected to have PID should be referred to a district hospital for hospitalization and treated with a parenteral regimen that is safe in pregnancy.
- Doxycycline is contraindicated in pregnancy.
- Metronidazole is generally not recommended during the first three months of pregnancy. However, it should not be withheld for a severely acute PID, which represents an emergency.

Hospitalization of clients with acute PID should be seriously considered when:

- Diagnosis is uncertain.
- Surgical emergencies, e.g. appendicitis or ectopic pregnancy, cannot be excluded.
- A pelvic abscess is suspected.
- Severe illness precludes the management on an out-client basis.
- The woman is pregnant.
- The client is unable to follow or tolerate an out-client regimen.
- The client has failed to respond to out-client therapy.

All clients requiring hospitalization should be referred to a district hospital.

STIs AMONG SPECIAL POPULATIONS: FSW AND MSM[1]

In some groups with high-risk practices such as female sex workers (FSW), men having sex with men (MSM) and intravenous drug users (IVDUs), the prevalence of STIs and HIV is higher than that in general population. Treating these clients early and appropriately will reduce risk of HIV infection. If already infected, they can be advised to seek available services at the integrated counselling and testing centre (ICTC) for knowing their HIV status and further follow-up action. It is desirable that all clients with risky behaviour be tested.

Effective prevention and treatment of STIs among FSW and MSM requires the attention to both symptomatic and asymptomatic infections. NACO suggests that symptomatic patients be treated using syndromic approach flowcharts, whereas asymptomatic patients in these high-risk groups be treated presumptively. The rationale for presumptively treating them although asymtomatic is that they are frequently exposed to STIs and they often do not show signs and symptoms. The appropriate flowcharts **(Appendix V)** for treatment of asymptomatic infections for FSW and MSM have been included in National Guidelines 2007 by NACO.

For screening and treatment of asymptomatic infections among FSW, the following Guidelines are advised:

1. Periodic history-taking, clinical examination and simple laboratory tests (where available).
2. Periodic presumptive treatment for asymptomatic gonococcal and chlamydial infections (in areas with high STI rates and minimal STI services).
3. Semi-annual serologic screening for syphilis.

As STI prevalence falls, periodic presumptive treatment of asymptomatic STI treatment among sex workers will be tapered to first visit asymptomatic treatment under the following conditions:

- Evidence of low gonococcal and chlamydial infections (10% and below)
- High condom use among sex workers (>70%)
- High-quality STI services for sex workers have been established, with almost 80% of them having access to STI services (80% provided with asymptomatic treatment at least once and are coming to clinics for regular STI screening)

CRITICAL EVALUATION OF SYNDROMIC APPROACH

Since the introduction of the syndromic approach in 1991 by the WHO, most centers across the world have been using this approach. However, there has been some controversy regarding the use of this approach. The operational performances of syndromic approach, its usefulness in the diagnosis, treatment and prevention of various STIs, and the sensitivity of syndromic approach have been studied in various centers.

Campbell and Plumb[3] from Canada have undertaken a Medline-based study to understand the use of syndromic approach in managing STIs in low-income countries, and to determine if evidence supports its continued use. In resource-poor countries, the use of syndromic approach is appropriate for high-risk groups and for symptomatic individuals. However, it is still a poor screening approach when applied to asymptomatic cases, particularly in women.

Syndromic approach has failed in women with vaginal discharge. It has resulted in over treatment in 90% of women with vaginal discharge.[4] So it is not suitable for treating women where prevalence of STIs is low.[5]

Risk scoring and simple laboratory tests help increase the algorithmic sensitivity of syndromic approach. Until inexpensive, simple and accurate STI diagnostic tests are developed and made available for use in low-income countries, a modified syndromic approach is the most feasible method of STI management.

In a report from South Africa, the sensitivity of a syndromic management approach in detecting STIs in patients at a public health clinic was evaluated.[6] All new patients attending the STI clinic were sampled systematically by gender over a 6-week period. All the patients were examined thoroughly and specimens were collected for laboratory tests. In a retrospective simulation, clinicians' syndromic diagnoses were validated against laboratory findings or for genital ulcer syndrome against the findings of research physicians. There were 170 men and 161 women. Syndromic diagnostic procedures achieved reasonable levels of sensitivity in detecting *N. gonorrhoea* and *C. trachomatis* in men and women and in detecting *Trichomonas vaginalis* and bacterial vaginosis in women. However, the sensitivity of detecting genital ulcers in women was only 36.4% and *Candida albicans* 0-12.3%. With syndromic approach 8.2% of men and 32.9% of women would leave the clinic with at least one infection inadequately treated. The study suggested that a proportion of STIs and genital tract infections are not being detected and treated owing to the high prevalence of multiple syndromes and mixed infections, both symptomatic and asymptomatic.

In a study by Hanson et al. from Zambia, the algorithms for the treatment of STI syndromes were evaluated.[7] A total of 436 patients were followed up. The cure rate for discharge syndrome was 97-98% for both sexes and for genital ulcer diseases, 83% for female and 69% for male patients. The large proportions of treatment failures especially in males were possibly related to decreased susceptibility of *Haemophilus ducreyi* to cotrimoxazole.

In a report of operational performance of a STI control programme in Tanzania by Grosskurth et al., during a 2-year period, 12,895 STI syndromes were treated at 25 intervention health units.[8] The most common syndromes were urethral discharge (67%) and genital ulcers (26%) in men and vaginal discharge (50%) in women. Based on various approaches, the utilization of improved health units by symptomatic STI patients in these communities was estimated at between 50% and 75%. During the first 6 months of intervention, attendance at intervention units increased by 53%. Thereafter, the average attendance rate was about 25% higher than in comparison communities. Home visits to 367 non-returners revealed that 89% had been free of symptoms after treatment, but 28% became symptomatic again within 3 months of treatment. 100% of these patients reported they had received treatment, but only 74% had been examined; only 57% had been given health education, and only 30% were offered condoms. Patients did not fully recall which treatment they had been given, but possibly only 63% had been treated exactly according to guidelines. The authors suggested that the syndromic approach to STI control should be supported by at least one reference clinic and laboratory per country to ensure monitoring of prevalent etiologies of the development of bacterial resistance and of the effectiveness of syndromic algorithms in use.[8]

At present only physicians are allowed to treat with syndromic approach.

Training pharmacists, chemists and other health workers to provide syndromic STI treatment may be one strategy to reduce STI morbidity and HIV transmission. Efforts are being made to encourage such strategies.[9,10]

Daly et al. in their report from Malawi compared the actual cost of observed antibiotic treatment for 144 patients receiving same day treatment for two STI syndromes with that of the syndromic approach for the management of STIs.[11] The costs of drug treatment in both categories were similar. The authors have concluded that syndromic management of STIs would result in more effective treatment of STIs at no additional cost.

Syndromic approach has been found to be more cost effective in male STD patients with urethral discharge symptoms and genital ulcer disease in various studies.[12-14]

In a study from rural India, it was found that 75% of symptomatic men presented with dhat and only 5.5% tested for positive gonorrhoea or chlamydia.[15] So syndromic management in such settings can result in over-diagnosis and over-treatment.

In a study of observations of STI consultation in India by Mertens et al., structured observations of consultation for STIs in health care facilities were undertaken.[16] With STI treatment, adequacy scored against the national guidelines. History-taking, examination and treatment were satisfactory in 76 out of 108 (70%) observed consultation. However, scoring with respect to syndromic approach towards selected STIs (male urethritis and non-herpetic genital ulcer in both sexes), only 8 out of 81 (10%) patients had satisfactory management. This suggests that further improvement is required in the form of simplifying the existing treatment guidelines and periodic assessment and feedback on the quality of STI care.

Syndromic Approach and HIV

Syndromic approach has failed to reduce HIV prevalence in female sex workers despite the high reported condom use in clients. This may be related to the fact that a large number of asymptomatic cases of STI is missed.[17,18]

Moreover, there is no reduction in genital shedding of HIV virus by syndromic treatment of genital discharge syndrome and genital ulcer syndrome.[19]

Recommedations for Future

- It is essential that health authorities regularly monitor and detect the relative prevalence of pathogens responsible for STIs syndromes in the local settings and the emergence of resistance to medicines for the treatment of STIs, so that treatment guidelines and national lists of essential medicines can be kept up-to-date.

- There is need for making recommendations for management programmes in areas of low STI prevalence and low income countries to overcome problems due to over-diagnosis and over-treatment.[20]
- The performance of syndromic approach is poor in sex workers as asymptomatic cases are missed.[17]
- It has been suggested to add treatment of herpes genitalis in the treatment of genital ulcer disease (GUD) as it is the commonest GUD especially in women.[21,22]
- There is need to train chemists, pharmacists and other health workers in delivering the syndromic approach.
- To change the strategies of syndromic approach with respect to change in the trends of STIs as there has been increase in viral STIs especially genital herpes as a cause of GUD and decrease in bacterial STIs.[23]

Acknowledgement

The authors acknowledge the contribution of Dr. B. Loganathan who was the author of this chapter in the previous edition.

REFERENCES

1. WHO. Guidelines for the management of sexually transmitted infection 2001. WHO/RHR/01.10.
2. National guidelines on prevention, management and control of reproductive tract infections including sexually transmitted infections, Maternal Health Division, NACO, Ministry of Health and Family Welfare, Government of India, August 2007.
3. Campbell RL, Plumb J. The syndromic approach to treatment of sexually transmitted diseases in low-income countries. issues, challenges, and future direcions. J Obstet Gynaecol Can 2002; 24: 417-24.
4. George R, Thomas K, Thyagarajan SP, et al. Genital syndromes and syndromic management of vaginal discharge in a community setting. Int J STDs AIDS 2004; 15: 367-70.
5. Wang Q, Yang P, Zhong M, et al. Validation of diagnostic algorithms for syndromic management of sexually transmitted diseases. Chin Med J (Engl) 2003; 116: 181-6.
6. Mathews C, van Rensburg A, Coetzee N. The sensitivity of a syndromic management approach in detecting sexually transmitted diseases in patients at a public health clinic in Cape Town. S Afr Med J 1998; 88: 1337-40.
7. Hanson S, Sunkutu RM, Kamanga J et al. STDs care in Zambia: an evaluation of the guidelines for case management through a syndromic approach. Int J STDs AIDS 1996; 7: 324-32.
8. Gorsskurth H, Mwijarubi E, Todd J, et al. Operational performance of an STDs control programme in Mwanza Region, Tanzania. Sex Transm Infect 2000; 76: 426-36.
9. Ward K, Butler N, Mugabo P, et al. Provision of syndromic treatment of sexually transmitted infections by community pharmacists: a potentially underutilized HIV prevention strategy. Sex Transm Dis 2003; 30: 609-13.
10. Adams EJ, Garcia PJ, Garnett GP, et al. The cost-effectiveness of syndromic management in pharmacies in Lima, Peru. Sex Transm Dis 2003; 30: 379-87.
11. Daly CC, Franco L, Chilongozi DA, et al. A cost comparison of approaches to sexually transmitted disease treatment in Malawi. Health Policy Plan 1998; 13: 87-93.
12. Tsai CH, Lee TC, Chang HL, et al. The cost-effectiveness of syndromic management for male STDs patients with urethral discharge symptoms and genital ulcer disease in Taiwan. Sex Transm Infect 2008. [Epub ahead of print]

13. Price MA, Stewart SR, Miller WC, et al. The cost-effectiveness of treating male trichomoniasis to avert HIV transmission in men seeking sexually transmitted disease care in Malawi. J Acquir Immune Defic Syndr 2006; 43: 202-9.
14. Liu H, Jamison D, Li X, et al. Is syndromic management better than the current approach for treatment of STDs in China? Evaluation of the cost-effectiveness of syndromic management for male STDs patients. Sex Transm Dis 2003; 30: 327-30.
15. Gautham M, Singh R, Weiss H, et al. Socio-cultural, psychosexual and biomedical factors associated with genital symptoms experienced by men in rural India. Trop Med Int Health 2008; 13: 384-95.
16. Mertens TE, Smith GD, Kantharaj K, et al. Observation of sexually transmitted disease consultations in India. Public Health 1998; 112: 123-28.
17. Desai VK, Kosambiya JK, Thakor HG, et al. Prevalence of sexually transmitted infections and performance of STI syndromes against aetiological diagnosis, in female sex workers of red light area in Surat, India. Sex Transm Infect 2003; 79: 111-5.
18. Kamali A, Quigley M, Nakiyingi J, et al. Syndromic management of sexually-transmitted infections and behaviour change interventions on transmission of HIV-1 in rural Uganda: a community randomised trial. Lancet 2003; 361: 645-52.
19. Wolday D, Gebremariam Z, Mohammed Z, et al. The impact of syndromic treatment of sexually transmitted diseases on genital shedding of HIV-1. AIDS 2004; 18: 781-5.
20. Hawkes S, Morison L, Foster S, et al. Reproductive-tract infections in women in low-income, low-prevalence situations: assessment of syndromic management in Matlab, Bangladesh. Lancet 1999; 354: 1776-81.
21. Pickering JM, Whitworth JA,Hughes P, et al. Aetiology of sexually transmitted infections and response to syndromic treatment in southwest Uganda. Sex Transm Infect 2005; 81: 488-93.
22. Ray K, Bala M, Bhattacharya M, et al. Prevalence of RTI/STI agents and HIV infection in symptomatic and asymptomatic women attending peripheral health set-ups in Delhi, India. Epidemiol Infect 2007 Dec 17:1-9. [Epub ahead of print]
23. Paz-Bailey G, Rahman M, Chen C, et al. Changes in etiology of sexually transmitted diseases in Botswana between 1993 and 2002: implications for the clinical management of genital ulcer disease. Clin Infect Dis 2006; 42: 888-9.

48 CLINICAL APPROACH TO THE HOMOSEXUALS WITH SEXUALLY TRANSMITTED DISEASES

Yogesh S Marfatia, Megha Modi

In this chapter

- Differences in Homosexual and Heterosexual Behaviour
- STDs in Homosexuals: The Epidemic Before the Epidemic
- Approach to Homosexuals with STDs
- Prevention of STDs Among Homosexuals

INTRODUCTION

Homosexuality is the "sexual desire or behaviour directed towards a person or persons of one's own sex." Homosexuality has a number of causal factors that influence its ultimate origin in individuals.[1] It has a variety of effects on individuals and society at large. Sexual relationships between members of the same sex expose gays, lesbians and bisexuals to extreme risks of STIs including HIV, physical injuries, mental disorders and even a shortened life span. Criminalizing homosexuals due to their unnatural sexual activities (under Section 377 of the Indian Penal Code)[2] is debated.

In the United States, as much as 4% of men and 1 to 2% of women are homosexual. The Center for Disease Control further estimates that approximately 2.5 million US men are exclusively homosexual (or 1% of the total US population, currently at 250 million), with an additional 2.5 to 7.5 million men engaging in occasional homosexual relations.[3] Obtaining the exact prevalence of homosexuality is difficult in India because of its associated taboo. Sexual behavioural studies in India have classified homosexual as anything from 1% of sexually active male population to nearly 28% of 'occasionally homosexual behavioural males'.[4]

DIFFERENCES IN HOMOSEXUAL AND HETEROSEXUAL BEHAVIOUR

Promiscuity: Instability and promiscuity typically characterize a homosexual relationship. Studies indicate that an average male homosexual has hundreds of sex partners in his lifetime. From 1994 to 1997, the percentage of homosexual men reporting multiple partners and unprotected anal sex increased from 23.6% to 33.3%, with the largest increase among men under 25.[5] Even in those homosexual relationships in which the partners consider themselves to be in a committed relationship, the meaning of "committed" typically means something radically different from marriage. An average male homosexual live-in relationship lasts between 2 and 3 years.[6]

Promiscuity among women having sex with women (WSW) is less extreme but is still higher than heterosexual women. In one study, 93% women who identified themselves as lesbians reported a history of sex with men.[7]

Bisexuals act as the bridge population between high-risk multipartner homosexuals having unprotected intercourse and married women who are immobile, have no negotiation powers, and generally do not have multipartner sex. The bridge population of bisexual men is not only into high-risk unprotected sex; it is also mobile, extremely diverse and reaches across every social status and age group.

Physical health: Men having sex with men (MSM) leads to greater health risks than men having sex with women not only because of promiscuity but also because of the nature of sex among men. Male homosexual behaviour is not simply either 'active' or 'passive,' since the involvement of penile-anal, penile-oral and hand-anal sexual contact is usual, and mouth-anal contact is not infrequent. Mouth-anal contact is the reason for the relatively high incidence of bowel pathogens in male homosexuals. Anal intercourse is the *sine qua non* of sex for many gay men.

Human physiology makes it clear that the body is not designed to accommodate this activity. The rectum is significantly different from the vagina with regard to the suitability for penetration by penis. The vagina has natural lubricants and is supported by a network of muscles. It is composed of a mucus membrane with a multi-layer stratified squamous epithelium that allows it to endure friction without damage and to resist immunological actions caused by semen and sperm. In comparison, the anus is a delicate mechanism of small muscles that comprise an "exit-only" passage. With repeated trauma, friction and stretching, the sphincter loses its tone and its ability to maintain a tight seal. Consequently, anal intercourse leads to the leakage of fecal material that can easily become chronic. The potential for injury is exacerbated by the fact that the intestine has only a single layer of cells separating it from the highly vascular tissue. Therefore, any organisms that are introduced into the rectum establish a foothold for infection than they would in a vagina. The single-layer tissue cannot withstand the friction associated with penile penetration, resulting in traumas that expose both participants to blood, organisms in faeces, and mixing of body fluids. The end result is that the fragility of the anus and rectum, along with the immunosuppressive effect of the ejaculate, make anogenital intercourse a most efficient manner of transmitting HIV and other infections.[7]

Fisting, the practice of insertion of a hand or forearm into the rectum, is far more damaging than anal intercourse. Anal tears and incompetence of the sphincter can occur. The result can include infection, inflammation and enhanced susceptibility to future STDs.

Asymptomatic, hidden infections and infections at atypical sites are more common in homosexuals.

Mental health: Psychiatric illness including depression, drug abuse and suicide attempts are common among homosexuals.[7]

STDs IN HOMOSEXUALS: THE EPIDEMIC BEFORE THE EPIDEMIC

Even before the first AIDS cases among homosexual men were diagnosed, the homosexual community was already in the midst of an epidemic of STDs like syphilis and gonorrhoea. Data suggest that an increasing number of MSM engage in sexual behaviours that place them at risk for STDs and HIV infection. Several factors may be contributing to this change, including the availability of highly active antiretroviral therapy (HAART) for HIV infection.

Most nationally notifiable STD surveillance data reported to CDC (Center for Disease Control and Prevention) do not include information regarding sexual behaviours; therefore, national trends in STDs among MSM in the United States are not currently available. Data from enhanced surveillance projects reported that, in 2006, median urethral gonorrhoea positivity in MSM was 10%, rectal and pharyngel 7% each, and median urethral chlamydia positivity 6%.[8] Overall, median seroreactivity among MSM tested for syphilis was 10%. Median HIV prevalence among MSM, including persons previously known to be HIV-positive and persons testing HIV-positive at their current visit, was 12% (range: 10-16%).

Only limited data are available about STD prevalence among MSM in India. A preliminary analysis of STDs among 85 MSM attending an STD clinic in Mumbai found that 4 had clinical rectal gonorrhoea, 4 had perianal warts, and 3 had gonococcal urethritis. The point prevalence of HIV in this population was 15% and VDRL was reactive in 16%.[4] In a 2001 study from Chennai, the analysis of 51 MSM who attended a community-based clinic over a period of three months showed 26% MSM were clinically diagnosed to have one or more STDs.[4]

Syphilis: Homosexuals acquire syphilis at a rate 10 times higher than that of heterosexuals.[6] Approximately 64% of all adult primary and secondary syphilis cases in 2006 in the United States were among MSM.[9]

Apart from usual manifestations of syphilis, homosexuals may increasingly suffer from anorectal syphilis. Primary anorectal syphilis is usually asymptomatic in homosexuals, but when symptoms are present they include mild anal pain, constipation, rectal bleeding, and occasionally a rectal discharge. It may appear as perianal kissing chancres. Inguinal adenopathy may help in the diagnosis. In secondary syphilis, condylomata may be found near or within the anal canal. These are smooth warty masses often pruritic and produce a foul discharge which is highly infectious. Constitutional symptoms, skin rash and mucous patches can also occur. Diagnosis of anorectal syphilis is based on serology, perianal and digital rectal examination, and anoscopy. Dark-field examination is useful for the evaluation of perianal and anal lesions but may be less specific for rectal examination. Benzathine penicillin, in a single dose of 2.4 million units intramuscularly, remains the treatment of choice for early syphilis.

Gonorrhoea: Although urethral gonorrhoea is com-monest, rectum is a frequent site of infection in homosexual men due to direct inoculation through receptive rectal intercourse. The symptoms may range from mild anal pruritus, painless mucopurulent discharge or scant rectal bleeding, to symptoms of overt proctitis including severe rectal pain, tenesmus and constipation. External inspection of the anus occasionally shows erythema and abnormal discharge, but anoscopy commonly reveals mucoid or purulent exudates, erythema, edema, friability or other inflammatory mucosal changes.

Pharyngeal infection occurs in upto 10-25% of homosexually active men.[10] Gonococcal infection is transmitted to the pharynx by orogenital sexual contact. It may cause acute pharyngitis or tonsillitis and is occasionally associated with fever or cervical adenopathy, but over 90% of pharyngeal infections are asymptomatic.[10] Pharyngeal infection may be a source of urethral gonorrhoea in homosexual males. Diagnosis is made by Gram stain and culture of material obtained by pharyngeal or rectal swabbing. A single dose of ceftriaxone 250 mg intramuscularly or cefixime 400 mg is preferred. Fluoroquinolones are no longer recommended due to increasing resistance.[11]

Chlamydia trachomatis infection: Primary anal or rectal infections with Chlamydia have been described in homosexual men practicing anal intercourse. In the pre-AIDS era, *C. trachomatis* appeared to be responsible for upto 15% of proctitis seen in homosexual males.[12] In these infections, rectal involvement is initially characterized by severe anorectal pain, a bloody mucopurulent discharge and tenesmus. Inguinal adenopathy, which is characteristic of genital lymphogranuloma venereum (LGV), is often present. Strictures and fistula may become prominent. Several groups have isolated non-LGV serovars from male homosexuals with proctocolitis.[13]

Of 1221 patients screened for urethral infection in a STD clinic, 5 and 14% of homosexual and heterosexual men, respectively, had positive urethral cultures for *C. trachomatis*.[14] Pharyngeal infection with *C. trachomatis* has been demonstrated in 3-6% of men and women attending STD clinics and correlated with a history of orogenital contact.[14] The diagnosis of chlamydial proctitis is best made by the isolation of *C. trachomatis* from the rectum together with response to appropriate therapy. Azithromycin, doxycycline or tetracyclines are the drugs of choice for infection with *C. trachomatis*.

Condylomata acuminata: Warts due to human papilloma virus (HPV) may occur anywhere in the anal or genital area but are particularly common in the anus in homosexual men practicing anal intercourse. Perianal condylomata acuminata appear as raised pink-to-brown papules usually in clusters, and occasionally as large cauliflower-like masses. Topical podophyllin, imiquimod and cryotherapy are effective in treating anogenital warts. Laser beam therapy and surgical excision have been used in refractory cases.

There has been an increase in the number of cases of anal intraepithelial neoplasia, and the role of HPV is suggested. High-grade intraepithelial neoplasia has been found in 0.5-5.4% of HIV-seronegative homosexual men as compared with 4-15.2% of HIV-seropositive men.[15]

Herpes simplex virus infection[15]: HSV is the most common cause of nongonococcal proctitis in sexually active male. Anorectal herpes is usually acquired by anal intercourse, although oral-anal contact with an individual who has HSV type 1 infection of the mouth or lips could lead to anorectal infection with HSV-1. The occurrence of constipation, anorectal pain and urinary retention in a homosexual man strongly suggests herpetic proctitis. Clinically many infected individuals will not have any visible ulcerative perianal lesions but instead will present with ulcerative findings deep in the anal canal or rectal mucosa. HIV coinfection may lead to chronic progressive disease leading to large, destructive perianal ulcers. Diagnosis can often be made on clinical presentation on the basis of typical herpetic lesions externally, proctitis with focal ulcerative changes of distal rectum, inguinal adenopathy, constitutional symptoms and urinary retention. For confirmation of diagnosis, culture and serology can be useful. Treatment includes analgesics and sitz bath. Oral acyclovir may be efficacious in shortening the duration of symptoms and viral shedding of anorectal herpes.

Hepatitis: Hepatitis A virus is transmitted through oral-anal contact among homosexual men. Outbreaks of Hepatitis A among homosexuals are a recurring problem in many large cities in the industrialized world. Hepatitis B can spread by saliva, semen or urine through mouth-to-mouth contact or anal-genital sexual contact. The male homosexual population represents a pool of individuals within which Hepatitis B virus is readily transmitted, particularly subclinical infections. Insertive, not receptive, anal intercourse was the major risk factor for Hepatitis B virus seroconversion suggesting that transurethral exposure is an important mode of transmission.[16] Although less than Hepatitis A and B, MSM who engage in unsafe sexual practices remain at increased risk for contracting Hepatitis C, which may lead to chronic liver disease.

Gay bowel syndrome: Gay bowel syndrome is a clinical pattern of anorectal and colon diseases which occur with unusual frequency in homosexual patients (the diseases are not exclusive to male homosexuals) increasing the risk of acquiring HIV greatly.[17] These include STDs such as gonorrhoea, Chlamydia, syphilis, herpes, infectious diarrhoeal diseases caused by bacteria and parasites, and injuries caused by anal-sexual activity. Other possibilities include bacteria such as *Shigella sonnei*, *Shigella flexneri*, *Campylobacter enteritis*, *Campylobacter jejuni* or *Salmonella enteritis*; intestinal parasites such as *Giardia lamblia*, *Entamoeba histolytica*, Cryptosporidia and *Entamoeba coli*. Most of these infections could be traced to exposure to faecal material either through oral/anal sexual acts, or through oral/genital sexual act occurring after anal/genital sexual acts. Bowel injury may occur during foreign body insertion, anal-rectal sex or anal manual sex. These can result in abscesses, fistula and haemorrhoids.

HIV: The gastrointestinal mucosa is the body surface through which HIV-1 enters the host in homosexuals. It is the largest lymphoid organ in the body containing the largest number of lymphocytes and macrophages of any body organ.[18] Consequently, the enteric mucosa may be an important reservoir for HIV-1 infected mononuclear cells. Risk of HIV transmission is higher in unprotected receptive anal intercourse (0.24-2.76%) as compared to unprotected receptive vaginal intercourse (0.05-0.15%).[19] AIDS-related Kaposi's sarcoma occurs overwhelmingly in MSM.

HIV prevalence among male homosexuals is about 6.4% in India which is nearly 10 times that of antenatal population.[20] MSM in India are at significant risk of HIV infection because of frequent anal sex (45-55% of MSM in India practice anal sex), infrequent use of condom during anal sex (5-20%), large number of partners (between 11-28 casual partners per month) and poor health-seeking behaviour with only 20-30% of MSM going for STI check-up.[21]

Bacterial vaginosis, Hepatitis B, Hepatitis C, intravenous drug use and prostitution were present in much higher proportion among female homosexual practitioners.[7]

APPROACH TO HOMOSEXUALS WITH STDs

The clinical setting must ensure privacy and reinforce confidentiality. The doctor's behaviour should be friendly, polite and confident. Questions should be phrased in a language the patient can understand; the use of technical words should be avoided. The choice of words is extremely important. At times direct questions are more likely to achieve a truthful answer. No patient should be subjected to intimate questions about their sexual lifestyle more than once. Moreover, a judgmental and moralistic attitude towards the patient should be avoided.

A detailed sexual history should be taken including the number and types of sexual contacts (viz. genital-genital, oral-genital, anal-genital, oral-anal) with dates, partners (whether regular or casual), and use of condoms or other forms of contraception.

Clinicians should routinely look for symptoms and signs consistent with common STDs including urethral discharge, dysuria, genital ulcers, regional lymphadenopathy and skin rash. In homosexuals, he should specifically ask for pharyngeal symptoms or anorectal symptoms consistent with proctitis. Complete oropharyngeal examination should be carried out to look for any ulcer or pharyngitis. A rectal examination/proctoscopy should be performed in patients with rectal symptoms and those who practice anoreceptive intercourse.

Routine laboratory screening for common STDs is indicated for all sexually active MSM. These tests should be performed at least annually for sexually active MSM, including men with or without established HIV infection:[22]

- HIV serology, if not tested within the previous year
- Syphilis serology
- Urethral swabs for Gram staining, gonococcal culture and chlamydia testing in men who have had insertive intercourse during the preceding year
- Rectal swabs for Gram staining and culture for *N. gonorrhoeae* and *C. trachomatis* in men who report receptive anal sex with men during the preceding year
- Throat swab for culture for *N. gonorrhoeae* in MSM and in men who report receptive oral sex with a person with anogenital gonorrhoea.

Additional investigations when appropriate are:

- Blood for hepatitis B and C serology
- Swabs for HSV and *Haemophilus ducreyi* from clinically suspicious lesions in special media
- Smears and swabs from the subpreputial area in men with balanoposthitis
- Stools for detection of giardia, entamoeba, salmonella and shigella from MSM

More frequent STD screening (i.e., at 3–6 month intervals) is indicated for MSM who have multiple or anonymous partners, have sex in conjunction with illicit drug use, or whose sex partners participate in these activities.[22]

PREVENTION OF STDs AMONG HOMOSEXUALS

STD prevention counselling should be an integral part of management. All patients should be counseled about STDs, safe sex and use of condoms. Counselling should be tailored to the patient's needs and expectations, e.g. sexual abstinence or monogamy is the ideal protective strategy but may be unacceptable for many patients. Clinicians should be familiar with local community resources available to assist MSM at high risk in facilitating behavioural change. Vaccination against Hepatitis A and B is recommended for all MSM in whom previous infection or immunization cannot be documented. Vaccinating persons who are immune to HAV or HBV infection because of previous infection or vaccination does not increase the risk for vaccine-related adverse events.[22] It was long-held consensus that thicker condoms should be recommended to gay men for anal intercourse. But in a study by Golombok et al., it was found that failure rates for standard and thicker condoms in homosexuals were comparable with appropriate use.[23] Post-exposure prophylaxis after sexual exposure (PEPSE) may be recommended after an unprotected receptive anal intercourse as it is the riskiest sexual activity for acquiring HIV.[19] Currently, rectal microbicides are in development that could be available in the form of a cream, gel, douche or enema and may be used to reduce a person's risk for HIV infection from anal intercourse without a condom, or provide additional protection with condoms.[24]

REFERENCES

1. Homosexuality (cited on 30/03/08). Available from http://www.conservapedia.com/Homosexuality
2. Reddy KSN. Sexual offences. Reddy KSN. In: The essentials of forensic medicine and toxicology. 25th ed. Published by K. Sugunadevi. Hyderabad
3. Prevalence of homosexuality, bisexuality (cited on 3/5/08). Available from http://www.cliffsnotes.com/WileyCDA/CliffsReviewTopic/Prevalence-of-Homosexuality-Bisexuality.topicArticleId-26957,articleId-26902.html
4. Shivananda Khan. MSM and HIV/AIDS in India. Naz Foundation International. January 2004 (cited on 3/5/08). Available from http://

www.nfi.net/NFI%20Publications/Essays/2004/MSM,%20HIV%20and%20India.pdf

5. Increases in Unsafe Sex and Rectal gonorrhoea among Men Who Have Sex with Men — San Francisco, California, 1994-1997 (cited on 30/03/08). Mortality and Morbidity Weekly Report, CDC, 48(03): 45-48, p. 45 (January 29, 1999). Available from http://www.cdc.gov/mmwr/PDF/wk/mm4803.pdf
6. Timothy JD. The Negative Health Effects of Homosexuality (cited on 30/03/08); Christian coalition International (Canada) inc. Available from http://www.ccicinc.org/policy-research/072103.html
7. DIGGS JR. The Health Risks of Gay Sex (cited on 30/03/08). Catholic Education Resource Center. Available from http://www.catholiceducation.org/articles/homosexuality/ho0075.html
8. STDs surveillance 2006. Special focus profiles – Men who have sex with men (cited on 3/5/08). Available from http://www.cdc.gov/STD/STATS/msm.htm
9. New CDC Data Show Syphilis Increasing in Men, CDC Media Relations Press Release, November 8, 2005 (cited on 30/03/08). Available from http://www.cdc.gov/od/oc/media/pressrel/r051108.htm
10. Hook EW, Handsfield HH. Gonococcal infections in the adult. Holmes KK, Sparling PF, Mardh PA, et al. eds. In: Textbook of Sexually Transmitted Diseases. 3rd edition. Mc Graw Hill Companies; 1999. United States of America: p. 455-56.
11. CDC Changes Recommendations for gonorrhoea Treatment Due to Drug Resistance (cited on 30/03/08). Press release (April 12, 2007). Available from http://www.cdc.gov/od/oc/media/pressrel/2007/r070412a.htm
12. Shahmanesh M, Pandit PG, Round R. Urethral lymphocyte isolation in non-gonococcal urethritis. Genitourin Med 1996; 72: 362-64.
13. Perine PL, Stamm WE. Lymphogranuloma venereum. Holmes KK, Sparling PF, Mardh PA, et al. eds. In: Textbook of Sexually Transmitted Diseases. 3rd edition. Mc Graw Hill Companies; 1999. United States of America: p 426.
14. Stamm WE. *Chlamydia trachomatis* infections of the adult. Holmes KK, Sparling PF, Mardh PA, et al. eds. In: Textbook of Sexually Transmitted Diseases. 3rd edition. Mc Graw Hill Companies; 1999. United States of America: p 407.
15. Verley JR, Quinn TC. Sexually transmitted intestinal syndromes. Holmes KK, Sparling PF, Mardh PA, et al. eds. In: Textbook of Sexually Transmitted Diseases. 3rd edition. Mc Graw Hill Companies; 1999. United States of America: p 939-51.
16. Kingsley LA, Rinaldo CR, Lyter DW et al. Sexual transmission efficiency of hepatitis B virus and human immunodeficiency virus among homosexual men. JAMA July 1990; Vol. 264 (2): Available from http://jama.ama-assn.org/cgi/content/abstract/264/2/230.
17. Gay bowel syndrome (cited on 30/03/08). Available from http://www.conservapedia.com/Gay_Bowel_Syndrome.
18. Smith PD, Meng G, Sellers MT et al. Biological parameters of HIV-1 infection in primary intestinal lymphocytes and macrophages (cited on 7/4/08). Available from http://www.jleukbio.org/cgi/reprint/68/3/360.
19. Lorenzen T, Graefe K. Post exposure prophylaxis. Hoffmann C, Rockstroh JK, Kamps BS eds. In: HIV Medicine 2006. Flying publishers; 15th edition. Paris: p 698, 700.
20. HIV sentinel surveillance and HIV estimation, 2006. NACO (cited on 8/3/08). Available from http://www.nacoonline.org/upload/NACO%20PDF/Note%20on%20HIV%20Sentinel%20Surveillance%20and%20HIV%20Estimation_01%20Feb%2008.pdf
21. Kavi AR. Criminalising high risk groups such as MSM (cited on 30/03/08). Available from http://www.infochangeindia.org/agenda10_08.jsp
22. Sexually transmitted diseases treatment guidelines 2006; special populations: MSM (cited on 30/03/08). Available from http://www.cdc.gov/std/treatment/2006/specialpops.htm
23. Golombok S, Harding R, Sheldon J. An evaluation of a thicker versus a standard condom with gay men, AIDS 2001; 15(2): 245-250. Available from http://www.aidsonline.com/pt/re/aids/abstract.00002030-200101260-00015.htm;jsessionid=H6TSLKZJLyxV7CtSBVVJSyxZPcRcYBWKHc1vr6QlG5q7zMlk3Xcm!132671813!181195628!8091!-1
24. International rectal microbicide advocates (IRMA) (cited on 07/04/08). Available from http://www.aidschicago.org/rectalmicrobicides/news.php

Part 11

Appendices

APPENDIX

I HISTORY TAKING AND EXAMINATION OF PATIENT IN STD CLINIC

V S Dorairaj, K P Narendar

In this chapter

INTRODUCTION

The history taking and examination of patient with sexually transmitted disease is an art and discipline that is gradually learnt. The doctor is required to be non-judgemental and convey no sense of surprise or disapproval to any description related to sexual activity or general behaviour by the patient. The history needs to be taken in privacy and patient may be encouraged to describe the events as they took place. Special emphasis is placed on eliciting sequence and duration of different symptoms, incubation period of disease, sexual orientation-heterosexual or homosexual, whether risk of transmission to spouse or regular partner, treatment taken and response etc. The steps of history taking and examination are explained below:

I. PRESENTING COMPLAINTS

Presenting complaints can be broadly divided into two components

- Complaints related to the genitalia & related areas
- Complaints related to their sexual activity
  - (a) Erosion or ulcer in the genitalia and related areas
  - (b) Discharge—urethral or vaginal
  - (c) Problems related to the act of micturition-dysuria, dribbling of urine, increased frequency of micturition
  - (d) Swelling in the inguinal region-lymphadenopathy
  - (e) Skin and mucous membrane lesions
  - (f) Growth in the genitalia-genital warts, molluscum contagiosum, malignant tumour
  - (g) Bone and joint-arthralgia, arthritis
  - (h) Scrotal swelling-epididymitis, epididymo orchitis, elephantoid changes of the scrotum
  - (i) Elephantoid changes of the female genitalia

II. COMPLAINTS RELATED TO SEXUAL ACTIVITY

Disinclination towards sexual intercourse

(a) Impotency, frigidity
(b) Loss of libido
(c) Premature ejaculation
(d) Dyspareunia
(e) Infertility
(f) Venerophobia/HIV phobia

III. HISTORY TAKING

The important points are

(a) History of marital status of the patient
  - (i) Whether married or unmarried (single).
  - (ii) If married, the number of legal spouses, as well as any other regular sex partners.
  - (iii) Even in the unmarried, history of having a regular sex partner is to be elicited (this history is important since partner treatment is essential in the control of STDs)

(b) History of presenting complaint with duration

(c) History of treatment taken for the present complaint, under which the following is to be elicited, namely
  - (i) Nature of medicine
  - (ii) Route of administration (topical, parenteral, oral)
  - (iii) Duration of treatment

(d) History of sexual contact (exposure) is to be elicited, namely
  - (i) Nature of contact -marital or extramarital
  - (ii) Genitogenital, orogenital, anogenital
  - (iii) Date of contact (for calculation of incubation period)
  - (iv) Whether the patient has used any protective mechanism like condom

(e) History of previous STDs and the treatment taken. This is important because the lesion for which the patient has come may be due to the past contact. There are certain STDs like syphilis which has got various stages like primary, secondary and late and the primary and secondary lesions have got the tendency to heal on its own with or without proper diagnosis and medication and pass on to later stage. The other example being genital herpes, which has got a tendency to recur without a fresh exposure.

EXAMINATION

The patients should be explained and counseled regarding the steps of examination. The clinical examination should be conducted in a well-lit room with privacy. It is advisable to have an assistant of the same sex as the client, present during examination of clients of sex opposite to the doctors. Before proceeding to genital examination, the skin and other relevant systems should be examined with gloves. As far as possible, complete body examination of the client should be carried out so that none of the skin & mucosal lesions or lymph nodes is missed.

Skin

Generalized rashes, which occur in secondary syphilis, acute HIV seroconversion syndrome, acute hepatitis B, infectious mononucleosis should be looked for. In disseminated gonococccal infection, pustular lesions are seen mainly on the limbs particularly around the joints. Psoriasiform plaques are found in Reiter's disease. Burrows, excoriated papules and pustules in the web spaces of the hands and shaft of the penis are features of scabies. Special attention should be given to the palms and soles. Keratoderma blenorrhagicum of Reiter's disease is classically seen in the palm & soles. Hyperpigmentation of palms and soles is seen in secondary syphilis. Cutaneous features of HIV infection like atypical viral, bacterial and fungal infections, generalized erythematous rash, and Kaposi's sarcoma may be seen.

Oral Mucosa

Extragenital primary syphilitic chancre and oral warts can be seen in patients experiencing oral sex. Syphilitic chancre may be present on the lips, buccal mucosa or tongue. Mucous patches and snail track ulcers of secondary syphilis are seen in the oral mucosa. In late syphilis, patients can have leucoplakia, chronic superficial glossitis and gummatous perforation of the palate. Rhagades and Hutchinson's teeth are features of congenital syphilis. Oral manifestations of HIV infection include oral hairy leucoplakia, oral thrush, aphthous ulcers, gingivitis and herpes labialis.

Lymph Nodes

Generalized lymphadenopathy is usually seen in secondary syphilis and HIV infection.

Eyes

Patients with congenital syphilis can have iritis, interstitial keratitis and chorioretinitis. Argyll-Robertson pupil is a feature of neurosyphilis. Conjunctivitis can be seen in chlamydial, gonococcal and herpetic infections and also in Reiter's disease. Iridocyclitis may be seen in Reiter's disease, secondary & late syphilis, Behcet's disease and HIV infection. Retinal exudate and haemorrhage is seen in HIV infection.

Bones and Joints

In secondary syphilis, osteolgia and gummatous lesion (saber tibia) in late benign syphilis may be seen. Painful joint swellings are seen in disseminated gonococcal infection and Reiter's disease. Charcot's joints are painless, deformed and hypermobile joints which are seen in tabes dorsalis. Clutton's joints are bilateral painless joint with effusions seen in congenital syphilis.

Abdomen

Abdomen should be examined for evidence of pelvic inflammatory disease (PID) due to gonococcal and non-gonococcal infections. Organomegaly may be seen in secondary syphilis and HIV infection.

Other Systems

Respiratory, cardiovascular and nervous systems should be examined.

Pubic Region and Groin

Pubic region should be examined for pediculosis (pubic louse and nits) and pearly white umbilicated papules of molluscum contagiosum.

Groin should be examined for lymphadenopathy. Tender suppurative lymphadenopathy is usually seen in LGV, chancroid and herpes genitalis. 'Sign of groove'-inguinal lymphadenopathy both above and below the inguinal ligament is suggestive of LGV. Syphilis usually gives rise to discrete painless rubbery nodes. Lymphnodes are not involved in donovanosis but pseudobubo due to subcutaneous granulomas can occur. True lymphadenopathy in donovanosis suggests secondary infection or malignant transformation. Anal, penile and vulvar carcinoma can give rise to hard lymphadenopathy.

Examination of Male Genitalia

Penis and scrotum are examined for any congenital abnormalities like hypospadias and other lesions. The presence of urethral discharge should be looked for. If there is urethral discharge, note whether it is mucoid or mucopurulent or thick pus. Urethral discharge may occur either due to urethritis or secondary to sexually transmitted ulcerative lesions or non STDs ulcerative lesions in the under surface of the prepuce or on the glans penis. In uncircumcised males, retract the prepuce by gently withdrawing it over the glans penis and determine whether the discharge is due to STDs related urethritis or ulcer or non-STDs. If there is scanty urethral discharge, then milking of urethra should be done from the root of the penis towards urethral orifice.

If there are genital ulcers, one should examine whether they are elevated or depressed ulcers. Elevated ulcers are seen in syphilis and donovanosis. Syphilitic ulcer is usually a single small, painless indurated, button like ulcer seen in the coronal sulcus. Donovanosis has large granulomatous destructive ulcers. Depressed ulcers are seen in herpes genitalis, chancroid and LGV. The classical herpetic ulcers are painful superficial polycyclic erosions and in chancroid the ulcers are multiple, deep, tender and circular with necrotic slough. In LGV, the ulcers are herpetiform but are rarely seen. Traumatic ulcers are usually seen on the frenulum of the penis.

The penis is examined for any growth like condyloma acuminata or malignancy. Lesions of Bowenoid papulosis are usually seen on the shaft of the penis. Uniform inflammation of the glans penis and the undersurface of the prepuce with pustular lesions are seen in candidal balanoposthitis. Linear fissuring of the prepuce is characteristic of candidal balanoposthitis. Circinate balanitis of Reiter's disease manifests as erythematous eroded lesions with polycyclic edge.

Scabeitic excoriated papules and burrows are usually seen on the shaft of the penis. In Peyronie's disease there may be induration or fibrotic lump inside the penile shaft. Urethral meatus should be examined carefully for syphilitic chancre or any other ulcers, discharge, narrowing and warts.

One should be aware of some of the physiological conditions, which might pose diagnostic dilemma. Pearly penile papules otherwise known as hirsute papillomas are tiny regular papules arranged in rows around the coronal sulcus. These may be mistaken for warts. Multiple small yellow or white submucous ectopic sebaceous glands, which are known as Fordyce's spots may be seen on the inner surface of the prepuce.

Scrotum should be examined for swelling, erythema and ulcers. Ulcers are most often due to Behcet's disease. However, it can also result from syphilitic gumma or fungating testicular cancer. Tiny dark red papules are seen in angiokeratoma, whereas firm whitish nodules are seen in sebaceous cysts. Erythematous pruritic nodules are seen in scabies.

Testes and Epididymis

Testes and epididymis should be examined. The normal testes are equal in size varying between 3.5 and 4 cm in length. Presence of any tenderness, swelling or nodularity of the testis and testicular sensations are examined. The epididymis has head and tail ends. The head end is present at the upper pole of the testes on its posterior aspect and is a soft nodular structures about 1 cm in length. The tail is found on the posterolateral aspect of the inferior pole of the testes. It is a soft-coiled tubular structure. Tender enlargement is seen in acute gonococcal and chlamydial infections.

Genital examination is incomplete without anorectal examination. It should be done in both homosexual and heterosexual men. The patient should lie down in the left lateral position with the knee drawn up or in the knee-elbow position. 'Funnel' shaped and lax anus is suggestive of homosexuals. One should look for ulceration, warty growth, fissures and tags. Syphilitic chancre and herpetic infection can be confused with an anal fissure. Anal tags may resemble that of warts or condylomata lata of secondary syphilis.

Digital rectal examination is performed if symptoms are suggestive of prostatic disease. However, it should not be carried out if the client has painful perianal disease such as herpetic ulcers, fissures, or haemorrhoids.

Proctoscopic examination is indicated if there is unprotected anal intercourse to examine rectal mucosa for rectal discharge, ulceration, warty lesions or any other inflammation after inserting the proctoscope lubricated with KY jelly or liquid paraffin.

Examination of Female Genitalia

Women should be examined with their consent and in the presence of a female attendant. The best position is lithotomy. The perineum, vulva, labia majora and labia minora are examined for discharge, redness, swelling, excoriation, ulcers, warts and any other skin lesions. The approach to the genital ulcer is same as in men. Swelling of the vulva, erythema and excoriation are suggestive of either candidiasis or trichomoniasis.

Separate the labia and look for any discharge, wipe away any excessive discharge and insert a bivalve Cusco speculum after moistening with water. Look for evidence of vaginitis. If there is vaginal discharge, note the colour, consistency, and odour of the discharge. Curdy white discharge is suggestive of candidiasis. Frothy greenish yellow and malodorous discharge is characteristic of trichomoniasis. In bacterial vaginosis, the discharge is non-inflammatory and whitish. Also look for any other lesions. After careful examination of the vagina, one should examine the cervix. Wipe the cervix with a cotton swab and look for any discharge from the os, ulcers/erosion, warts and cervicitis. For cervical cytology smear can be taken from the cervix. Once the examination is over then remove the speculum and see the urethral orifice for inflammation, discharge or warts. If there is no obvious discharge, milk the urethra gently forward.

Examination of the anal and perianal region is done as in men.

Bimanual pelvic examination is performed to detect PID or abnormalities of the upper genital tract. It is customary to use the fingers of the right hand in the vagina and to place the left hand on the abdomen. In virgins and children only a rectal examination should be performed. For per vaginal examination, separate the labia with the left hand to expose the vestibule and insert the examining finger of the right hand. The cervix is palpated and any hardness or irregularity is noted. The examining left hand is placed over the abdomen just below the umbilicus and the fingers of both hands are then used to palpate the uterus. The size, shape, position, mobility and tenderness of the uterus are noted. The tips of the vaginal fingers are then placed into each lateral fornix and the adnexae are examined on either side. Tender uterus, fallopian tubes and positive cervical motion tenderness is suggestive of PID.

Speculum examination in women is helpful for diagnosis of STDs. The patient is advised to pass urine before speculum examination. You must be sure the speculum has been properly disinfected before you use it. The following signs should be looked for during speculum examination. The vaginal discharge and redness of the vaginal walls are common signs of vaginitis. The colour, smell and characteristics of any vaginal discharge have to be noted. When the discharge is white and curd-like, candidiasis is likely. Presence of foreign body or IUD thread, ulcers, warts, sores or blisters, redness of cervical & vaginal epithelium, cervical erosion, discharge or bleeding from the cervix have to be noted. A strawberry appearance of the cervix may be due to trichomoniasis. A uniform bluish discolouration of the cervix may indicate pregnancy, which needs to be kept in mind. PAP smear can be obtained during speculum examination.

The various lab diagnostic procedures including collection of samples for urethral and vaginal discharge are discussed in a separate chapter.

REFERENCES

1. Genitalia and sexually transmitted diseases. In: Swash M, edr. Hutchison's Clinical Methods. 21st edn. London: ELBS; 2002. p. 407-419.
2. The Gynaecological history and examnation. In: Campbell S, Monga A, eds. Gynaecology by ten teachers. 17th edn, London: ELST; 2000. p. 1-5.

APPENDIX

IIa TREATMENT OF OPPORTUNISTIC INFECTIONS IN HIV/AIDS (NACO 2007)

Komal Aggarwal

Etiology	*Management and Treatment*	*Unique Features*
RESPIRATORY SYSTEM ***M. tuberculosis***	The management and treatment of TB is as per RNTCP guidelines following the DOTS regimen.	More common with HIV and worsens HIV disease. Atypical presentation, if there is severe immunosuppression. Pulmonary TB at any CD4 level; disseminated TB usually at CD4 <200 cells/mm3.
Streptococcus pneumoniae	Cefotaxime 2 g IV q6h Ceftriaxone 2 gm/day IV Amoxicillin 750 mg PO tid; Fluoroquinolone: Levofloxacin 500 mg PO/IV qd; gatifloxacin 400 mg PO/IV qd; moxifloxacin 400 mg PO/day. Alternative treatment: Macrolides (azithromycin clarithromycin, erythromycin), vancomycin.	Pneumonia in HIV positive patients is more frequently associated with bloodstream infections and is not an uncommon cause of early death in HIV infected patients in developing countries. Treat an acute respiratory illness accompanied by fever and chills in an HIV-infected person as an emergency.
Haemophilus influenzae	Cefuroxime. Alternative regimens: TMP–SMX, cephalosporins (2nd and 3rd-generation) or fluoroquinolones.	
Staphylococcus aureus		Often other signs of staphylococcal infection, including pyomyositis, abscess.
Toxoplasmosis gondii		Consider *Toxoplasma* pneumonitis where induced sputum fails to demonstrate PCP.
***Pneumocystis jiroveci* (PCP)**	TMP–SMX containing 15 mg/kg/day of trimethoprim PO or IV × 21 days + if PO2 <70 mm Hg or a gradient >35 mm Hg: prednisone 40 mg bid × 5 days, then 40 mg/day × 5 days, then 20 mg/day to completion of treatment. Alternative treatments: TMP 15 mg/kg/day PO + dapsone 100 mg/day × 21 days; Pentamidine 4 mg/kg/day IV × 21 days; Clindamycin 600 mg IV q8h or 300–400 mg PO q6h + primaquine 15–30 mg base/day × 21 days; Atovaquone 750 mg PO bid with meal × 21 days.	PCP is the most frequently identified serious OI in HIV disease. Treatment is effective, but early recognition and treatment are important because of acute morbidity and mortality. More common in those with CD4 counts <200 cells/mm3; Chronic maintenance therapy (secondary prophylaxis) should be discontinued if CD4+ T lymphocyte count increases in response to ART from <200 to >200 cells mm3 for >6 months.
Penicillium marneffei		Skin involvement occurs in patients with disseminated disease. The typical appearance is one of multiple, papular lesions, often with central umbilication or ulceration, resembling molluscum contagiosum.

Etiology	*Management and Treatment*	*Unique Features*
		The lesions are typically on the face, scalp and upper trunk. The condition must be differentiated from TB and disseminated cryptococcal disease. If there are no skin lesions, the diagnosis is difficult, CD4 <50 cells/mm3.
ORAL CAVITY **Oral hairy leukoplakia (OHL)**		This condition is caused by EBV. It is neither dangerous nor painful and does not require any treatment. It is a sign of immune suppression and heralds a poor prognosis.
Candida albicans	Oral thrush: Nystatin (1 tablet of 500 000 IU) gargled 4–5 times/day × 7–14 days; Clotrimazole troche 10 mg 5 times/day (7–14 d); Fluconazole 100 mg/day PO × 7–14 days, Fluconazole 200 mg/day × 14–21 days. 2nd choice — Itraconazole (100 mg bid, doses can be increased to a maximum of 400 mg a day × 14–21days) Use intermittent therapy for as long as possible to delay the emergence of resistant candidiasis.	Oral candidiasis is a rare condition in a healthy person, but is frequently the first indication of immune impairment in HIV-infected patients. It is often used as an indicator disease for TMP–SMX prophylaxis. The diagnosis of oral candidiasis in an HIV positive patient classifies the patient as being in WHO stage III. Recurrent episodes of oral candidiasis usually occur in patients with CD4 counts <300 cells/mm3. Suppressive therapy generally not recommended unless patients have frequent severe recurrences of oropharyngeal candidiasis. Oesophageal candidiasis will develop in 10–20% of AIDS patients with CD4 counts <100 cells/mm3 and is the most common cause of dysphagia (inability or difficulty in swallowing) This indicates the patient is in WHO stage IV.
GASTROINTESTINAL SYSTEM **CMV oesophagitis**	If treatment of suspected oesophageal candidiasis does not improve symptoms after seven days, the patient may have CMV or HSV infection or infection with another species of Candida. Increase fluconazole to 200 mg/day and add acyclovir 800 mg thrice daily for 10 days. If not resolving, and ganciclovir is not available to treat CMV, consider prednisone 1 mg/kg/day in the morning to relieve pain.	The most frequent clinical manifestation of CMV disease is retinitis, followed by gastrointestinal symptoms Clinically, if it cannot be distinguished from candidal oesophagitis, consider CMV infection in patients with oesophageal symptoms that do not respond to empirical antifungal therapy. Most oesophageal ulcers result from CMV infection, the other main cause being aphthous ulcers. In the presence of fever, CMV infection is more likely than aphthous lesions

Etiology	*Management and Treatment*	*Unique Features*
Necrotizing gingivitis		Caused by bacteria of the oral cavity
Herpes simplex virus (HSV) (stomatitis and oesophagitis		HSV oesophagitis is a rare cause of viral oesophagitis in AIDS patients. Without biopsy and tissue culture, it is difficult to make a differential diagnosis between HSV and CMV ulcerative oesophagitis. Often there is bacterial and fungal secondary infection. Empirical antifungal treatment may improve symptoms.
Epstein–Barr virus infection (EBV)	Primarily symptomatic	Often the patient has OHL
Kaposi's sarcoma	Ganciclovir, foscarnet, cidofovir	
Aphthous ulcers and aphthous oesophagitis	Topical treatment 2– 4 times/day: lidocaine, triamicinolone, oral and intralesional prednisolone, colchicine, dapsone, thalidomide.	Of unknown origin. Herpes simplex and CMV should be excluded. After CMV infection, oesophageal ulcers are most often due to aphthous ulcers. May be very debilitating. CMV is more likely in the presence of fever.
Salmonella	In case of signs of sepsis, IV therapy is necessary Ciprofloxacin 500 mg bid or ofloxacin 400 mg bid or ceftriaxone 2 g IV for 7–10 days. Many patients often relapse after treatment, and chronic maintenance therapy (TMP–SMX 1 double strength tablet daily) is sometimes necessary.	Salmonellosis is a frequent cause of bacteraemia in people living with HIV/AIDS (PLHA).
Shigella	TMP–SMX (160/800) mg bid × 5 days or amoxicillin 500 mg tid × 5 days. If resistant to the above, give ciprofloxacin 500 mg bid, or norfloxacin 400 mg bid × 5 days or nalidixic acid 1 g qid × 10 days.	In many developing countries, resistance of Shigella (and Salmonella) to TMP–SMX has increased.
Cryptosporidium	Rehydration (IV and/or ORS), Paramomycin 500 mg qid for 2–3 weeks; maintenance with 500 mg bid often required. Codeine phosphate 30–60 mg tid until under control (or other antidiarrhoeal agents such as loperamide 2–4 mg tid or qid—maximum of 32 mg in 24 hours). ARV is protective against cryptosporidiosis	Cryptosporidia are highly infectious and transmitted through water, food, animal-to-human and human-to human contact. Special precautions should be taken to prevent exposure. People with HIV infection and a CD4 count <200 cells/mm3 should boil tap water for at least one minute to reduce risk of ingestion of oocysts in potentially contaminated drinking water.

Etiology	Management and Treatment	Unique Features
Entamoeba histolytica	Metronidazole 400 mg tid × 7 days	*E. histolytica* may be common in the general population in developing countries, but may be recurrent or more severe in HIV infected patients.
Giardia lamblia	Metronidazole 200 mg PO tid × 10 days	Common cause of diarrhoea in general population, but may be recurrent or more severe in HIV-infected.
Isospora belli	Most cases are readily treated with TMP–SMX (160/800 mg qid for 10 days) followed by 1 double-strength tablet (160/800 mg bid for 3 weeks), then chronic suppression with TMP–SMX (160/800 mg) daily. High dose of pyrimethamine with calcium folinate required to prevent myelosuppression. Long-term maintenance therapy may be necessary to prevent relapse.	
Microsporidium	Disseminated disease: Itraconazole 400 mg PO od and albendazole 400 mg PO bid.	Chronic maintenance therapy may be discontinued if patients remain asymptomatic; sustained CD4+ T lymphocyte counts >200 cells/mm3 for >6 months on ART.
Strongyloides stercoralis	Ivermectin 12 mg daily for 3 days. This is also the drug of choice for the treatment of systemic strongyloidiasis An alternative treatment is albendazole 400 mg bid × 5 days. Maintenance therapy once a month is necessary to suppress symptomatic infection (albendazole 400 mg or ivermectin 6 mg once a month).	In immunocompromised patients, *Strongyloides* can cause overwhelming infection. This serious complication is called *Strongyloides* hyperinfection syndrome and has a high case fatality rate.
CENTRAL NERVOUS SYSTEM ***Toxoplasma gondii*** **(toxoplasmosis)**	Treatment for acute phase: >6 weeks Pyrimethamine 100–200 mg loading dose, then 50–100 mg/day PO + folinic (or folic) acid 10 mg/day PO + sulfadiazine 1–2 g qid (Dexamethasone 4 mg PO or IV q 6 h for mass effect) OR TMP/SMX 5/25mg/kg daily OR Clindamycin (600 mg tid) + pyrimethamine 100 mg daily loading dose followed by 50 mg daily + folinic acid 10 mg daily.	Usually occurs when CD4 count <100 cells/mm3. Clinical response in 1 week and MRI reponse expected in 2 weeks. Check blood picture regularly as the relatively high doses of drugs can lead to toxicities. Leukopenia, the thrombocytopenia and rash are common. Folinic acid reduces the risk of myelosuppresion. During treatment, advise patients to maintain a high fluid intake and urine output. Secondary *prophylaxis* may be discontinued if free of *Toxoplasma* encephalitis; and

Etiology	*Management and Treatment*	*Unique Features*
	For maintenance, preferred regimen: suppressive therapy required after a patient has had toxoplasmosis: Pyrimethamine 25–75 mg PO qid + folinic acid 10 mg qid + sulfadiazine 0.5–1.0 g PO qid (50% of acute dose) If allergic to sulfa, give dapsone PO 100 mg once daily or clindamycin IV (or oral) 600 mg qid or atovaquine 750 mg PO qid Eptoin 50–100 mg bid or tid or tegretol 100–200 mg bid or tid (to be started only if the patient has convulsions).	sustained CD4+ T lymphocyte count of >200 cells/mm3 for >6 months of ART of the neurological system.
Mycobacterial infection – *M. tuberculosis* (TB meningitis)		**Mycobacterial infection – *M. tuberculosis* (TB meningitis)** show involvement of the meninges. This results from rupture of a cerebral tuberculoma or is blood-borne. Always exclude cryptococcal meningitis by CSF microscopy (India ink stain).
***Streptotoccus pneumoniae, Neisseria meningitidis* (Bacterial meningitis)**	Penicillin (24 million units daily in divided doses every 2–3 hours) or ampicillin (12 g daily in divided doses every 2–3 hours) or chloramphenicol (4–6 g IV/day). Treatment should be continued for 10–14 days Crystalline penicillin 2–3 mega units and chloramphenicol 500–750 mg 6 hourly for 10–14 days.	Often encountered during late stages of HIV disease. Prompt diagnosis and aggressive management and treatment ensure a quick recovery.
***Cryptococcus neoformans* (cryptococcal meningitis)**	Preferred regimen: Amphotericin B 0.7 mg/kg/day IV + flucytosine 100 mg/kg/day PO × 14 days, followed by fluconazole 400 mg/day × 8–10 weeks. Finally, maintenance therapy with fluconazole 200 mg/day for life. Alternate regimen: Amphotericin B 0.7 mg/kg/day IV + flucytosine 100 mg/kg/day PO × 14 days followed by itraconazole 200 mg bid for 8 weeks Fluconazole 400 mg/day PO × 8 weeks, followed by 200 mg once daily. Itraconazole 200 mg PO tid × 3 days, then 200 mg PO bid × 8 weeks after initial treatment with amphotericin. Fluconazole 400 mg/day PO + flucytosine 100 mg/kg/day PO	If untreated, it is slowly progressive and ultimately fatal. It occurs most often in patients with a CD4 count <100 cells/mm3. Headache is secondary to fungal accumulation, so the headache increases gradually over time, goes away and then comes back and is harder to get rid of. Then it becomes continuous, and this is what the patient reports. Repeated LP might be indicated as adjunctive therapy among patients with increased intracranial pressure. Discontinuation of antifungal therapy can be considered among patients who remain asymptomatic, with CD4+ T-lymphocyte count >100–200 cells/mm3 for >6 months

Etiology	*Management and Treatment*	*Unique Features*
Cytomegalovirus (CMV)	Foscarnet 60 mg/kg IV q8h or 90 mg/kg IV q12h × 14–21 days; ganciclovir 5 mg/kg IV bid × 14–21 days, then valganciclovir 900 mg PO qid. Patients without immune recovery will need to be on maintenance therapy lifelong for retinitis. Extraocular: ganciclovir and/or foscarnet.	Evolution: <2 weeks CD4 count <100 cells/mm3. Although any part of the retina may be involved, there is a predilection for the posterior pole; involvement of the optic nerve head and macular region is common. Treatment is very expensive and usually not available. CMV management needs special care. Therefore, early referral is essential.
Progressive multifocal leukoencephalopathy (PML)	There is no treatment for this illness. ART can improve symptoms and prolong life.	An end-stage complication of HIV, caused by JC virus. PML is rare in the general community, but relatively common in HIV infection (affecting 4% of all AIDS patients). Routine testing for HIV should be considered for any patient with PML. Evolution: weeks to months Usually occurs when CD4 count <100 cells/mm3.
Primary CNS lymphoma	There is no cytotoxic chemotherapy for this disease. Irradiation can help some patients, but is considered palliative. Corticosteroids can also help some patients deficits (confusion, hemiplegia, seizures). Mental status change (60%), personality or behavioural changes, seizures (15%).	Primary CNS lymphoma is rare in the general community, but affects about 2% of AIDS patients. Survival after diagnosis is usually limited (a few months only). Typical end-stage complication of HIV disease. Evolution: 2–8 weeks. Usually occurs when CD4 count <100 cells/mm3.
AIDS dementia complex (ADC) (HIV-associated dementia [HAD])	Possible benefit from antiretroviral regimens with agents that penetrate the CNS (AZT, d4T, ABC, nevirapine) Benefit of AZT at higher dose for mild or moderately severe cases is established; monitor therapy with neurocognitive tests. Anecdotal experience indicates response to ART, if started early. Sedation for those who are agitated and aggressive—use smaller doses initially to avoid oversedation Close monitoring: to prevent self-harm, to ensure adequate nutrition, to diagnose and treat.	Prevalence increases with improvement in general management of various OIs because patients live long enough to develop severe immune suppression. Patients present with a demeanour similar to Parkinson disease and may even be misdiagnosed.

Source: www.nacoonline.org/upload/publication/Treatment Accessed on June 1, 2008

APPENDIX

IIb TREATMENT OF OPPORTUNISTIC INFECTIONS IN HIV/ AIDS (CDC 2004)

Sushruta Dash

Disease	*Drug/ Dose*	*Secondary prophylaxis (chronic maintenance therapy)*	*When to stop secondary prophylaxis*	*When to reintroduce secondary prophylaxis*
Pneumocystis jiroveci Pneumonia	TMP-SMZ for 21 days. If room air pO2 <70 mm/Hg or arterial-alveolar O2 gradient >35 mm/Hg: add prednisone 40 mg by mouth twice a day for days 1–5, 40 mg daily for days 6–10, and 20 mg daily for days 11–21 within 72 hours after starting specific PCP therapy. Alternative regimes: dapsone and TMP, primaquine plus clindamycin, intravenous pentamidine, atovaquone suspension, trimetrexate with leucovorin.	TMP-SMZ	Continue for life if no immune reconstitution occurs, or continue till CD4+ has increased from <200 cells/μL to >200 cells/μL for at least 3 months as a result of ART.	CD4 decreases to <200 cells/μL or if PCP recurs at a CD4+ T lymphocyte count of >200 cells/μL.
***Toxoplasma gondii* Encephalitis**	Pyrimethamine plus sulfadiazine plus leucovorin. Alternative regimen: pyrimethamine plus clindamycin plus leucovorin. Acute therapy should be continued for at least 6 weeks if there is clinical and radiologic improvement. Longer courses might be appropriate if clinical or radiologic disease is extensive or response is incomplete at 6 weeks. Adjunctive corticosteroids (e.g. dexamethasone) should be administered only for treatment of a mass effect associated with focal lesions or associated edema. Anticonvulsants should be added with a history of seizures during acute therapy but not prophylactically to all patients.		Continue lifelong if no immune restoration occurs on ART or till sustained (>6 months) increase in CD4+ counts to >200 cells/μL on ART.	CD4+ <200 cells/μL.
Cryptosporidiosis	ART with immune restoration (an increase of CD4+ T lymphocyte count to >100 cells/μL) is associated with complete resolution of cryptosporidiosis. No consistently effective pharmacologic or immunologic therapy directed specifically against *C. parvum* exists. Symptomatic treatment of diarrhea should be given.			

Disease	*Drug/ Dose*	*Secondary prophylaxis (chronic maintenance therapy)*	*When to stop secondary prophylaxis*	*When to reintroduce secondary prophylaxis*
Microsporidiosis	ART with immune restoration (an increase of CD4+ T lymphocyte count to >100 cells/μL) is associated with resolution of symptoms of enteric microsporidiosis. No specific therapeutic agent is active against *E. bieneusi* infection. Albendazole is recommended for initial therapy of intestinal and disseminated (not ocular) microsporidiosis caused by microsporidia other than *E. bieneusi*. Itraconazole also might be useful in disseminated disease when combined with albendazole especially in infections caused by *Trachipleistophora* or *Brachiola*.	Treatment for ocular microsporidiosis should be continued indefinitely because recurrence or relapse might follow treatment discontinuation.	Patients remain asymptomatic with regard to signs and symptoms of microsporidiosis and have a sustained (e.g. >6 months) increase in their CD4+ T lymphocyte counts to levels >200 cells/μL after ART.	
M. tuberculosis	DOTS similar to that for non-HIV patients	Not required		
Disseminated Mycobacterium avium Complex Disease	Clarithromycin/ azithromycin with ethambutol +/- rifabutin.	Lifelong secondary prophylaxis (chronic maintenance therapy), unless immune reconstitution occurs as a result of ART.	In those who have completed >12 months of treatment for MAC, and remain asymptomatic with respect to MAC signs and symptoms, and have a sustained increase (e.g., >6 months) in their CD4+ T lymphocyte counts to >100 cells/μL after ART.	CD4+ T lymphocyte count decreases to <100 cells/μL.
Bartonellosis	Erythromycin and doxycycline for atleast 3months are first-line treatment for bacillary angiomatosis, peliosis hepatica, bacteremia, and osteomyelitis. Doxycyline is the treatment of choice for central nervous system bartonellosis.	No firm recommendation.		

Disease	Drug/ Dose	Secondary prophylaxis (chronic maintenance therapy)	When to stop secondary prophylaxis	When to reintroduce secondary prophylaxis
Syphilis	Similar to non-HIV patient	Not recommended		
Mucocutaneous Candidiasis	Oropharyngeal candidiasis: topical clotrimazole or nystatin, oral fluconazole or itraconazole solution. Esophageal candidiasis: 14–21-day course of either fluconazole or itraconazole solution. Ketoconazole and itraconazole capsules are less effective than fluconazole because of variable absorption. Uncomplicated vulvovaginal candidiasis: short-course oral or topical treatment with any of several therapies including single-dose regimens: topical azoles (clotrimazole, butaconazole, miconazole, ticonazole, or terconazole) for 3–7 days; topical nystatin 100,000 units daily for 14 days; itraconazole oral solution 200 mg twice a day for 1 day or 200 mg daily for 3 days; or oral fluconazole 150 mg for 1 dose. Complicated vaginitis (prolonged or refractory episodes): antimycotic therapy for >7 days.	Not recommended		
Cryptococcosis	Amphotericin B, usually combined with flucytosine, for a 2-week duration followed by fluconazole alone for an additional 8 weeks. Flucytosine decreases the risk for relapse. Lipid formulations of amphotericin B appear effective. The optimal dose of lipid formulations of amphotericin B has not been determined, but AmBisome has been effective at doses of 4 mg/kg body weight/daily.	Fluconazole is superior to itraconazole for preventing relapse and is the preferred drug.	Lifelong unless immune reconstitution occurs as a consequence of ART.	CD4+ T lymphocyte count decreases to <100–200 cells/μL.

Disease	*Drug/ Dose*	*Secondary prophylaxis (chronic maintenance therapy)*	*When to stop secondary prophylaxis*	*When to reintroduce secondary prophylaxis*
Histoplasmosis	Severe disseminated histoplasmosis who meet one or more selected criteria (temperature >102°F [>39°C], systolic blood pressure <90 mm Hg, pO2 <70 torr, weight loss >5%, Karnofsky performance score <70, hemoglobin <10 g/dL, neutrophil count <1000 cells/μL, platelet count <100,000 cells/μL, aspartate aminotransferase >2.5 times normal, bilirubin or creatinine >2 times normal, albumin <3.5 g/dL, coagulopathy, presence of other organ system dysfunction, or confirmed meningitis) should be treated with intravenous amphotericin B, either the deoxycholate formulation or liposomal amphotericin B, for the first 3–10 days until they clinically improve followed by oral therapy with itraconazole capsules to complete 12 weeks of treatment. Confirmed meningitis, amphotericin B should be continued for 12–16 weeks, followed by maintenance therapy. Acute pulmonary histoplasmosis in an HIV-1 infected patient with intact immunity, as indicated by a CD4+ T lymphocyte count >500 cells/μL, might not require therapy and should be managed in a similar way to infection in an otherwise noncompromised host.	itraconazole 200 mg twice daily.	Lifelong, no recommendation to stop with immune restoration.	
Coccidioidomycosis	Nonmeningeal pulmonary or disseminated disease: amphotericin B. Coccidioidal meningitis: fluconazole.	Fluconazole 400 mg daily or itraconazole 200 mg twice daily.	Lifelong suppressive therapy, no recommendation for stopping after immune restoration.	

Disease	*Drug/ Dose*	*Secondary prophylaxis (chronic maintenance therapy)*	*When to stop secondary prophylaxis*	*When to reintroduce secondary prophylaxis*
Aspergillosis	Invasive aspergillosis: voriconazole. Amphotericin B, either conventional or lipid formulations, in doses equivalent to 1 mg/kg body weight/daily of standard amphotericin B is an alternative regimen.	No data available to base a recommendation.		
Cytomegalovirus Disease	CMV retinitis: Oral valganciclovir, intravenous ganciclovir, intravenous ganciclovir followed by oral valganciclovir, intravenous foscarnet, intravenous cidofovir, and the ganciclovir intraocular implant coupled with valganciclovir. Certain HIV specialists recommend the intraocular implant plus valganciclovir as the preferred initial therapy, particularly for patients with immediately sight-threatening lesions (adjacent to the optic nerve or fovea). CMV colitis or esophagitis: intravenous ganciclovir or foscarnet (or with oral valganciclovir if symptoms are not severe enough to interfere with oral absorption) for 21–28 days or until signs and symptoms have resolved. Neurological disease: combination treatment with ganciclovir and foscarnet might be preferred as initial therapy to stabilize disease and maximize response.	Parenteral or oral ganciclovir, parenteral foscarnet, combined parenteral ganciclovir and foscarnet, parenteral cidofovir, and (for retinitis only), ganciclovir administration through intraocular implant or repetitive intravitreous injections of fomivirsen, oral valganciclovir. Chronic maintenance therapy is not routinely recommended for gastrointestinal disease but should be considered if relapses occur.	Lifelong unless immune reconstitution occurs as a result of ART, sustained (> 6 months) increase in CD4+ T lymphocyte counts >100–150 cells/μL in response to ART.	CD4+ T lymphocyte count has decreased to <100–150 cells/μL.
Herpes Simplex Virus Disease	Orolabial: oral famciclovir, valacyclovir, or acyclovir for 7 days. Moderate-tosevere mucocutaneous HSV: intravenous acyclovir. Patients may be switched to oral therapy after the lesions have begun to regress. Therapy should be continued until the	Daily suppressive therapy with oral acyclovir, oral famciclovir, or oral valacyclovir.		

Disease	*Drug/ Dose*	*Secondary prophylaxis (chronic maintenance therapy)*	*When to stop secondary prophylaxis*	*When to reintroduce secondary prophylaxis*
	lesions have completely healed. Initial or recurrent genital HSV: oral famciclovir, valacyclovir, or acyclovir for 7–14 days Herpes keratitis: Trifluridine is the treatment of choice for, one drop onto the cornea every 2 hours, not to exceed 9 drops/day; it is not recommended for longer than 21 days. HSV encephalitis: intravenous acyclovir, 10 mg/kg body weight every 8 hours for 14–21 days.			
Varicella Zoster	Famciclovir or valacyclovir for 7–10 days, If cutaneous lesions are extensive or if clinical evidence of visceral involvement is observed, intravenous acyclovir should be initiated Intravenous acyclovir for 7–10 days is the recommended initial treatment for immunocompromised adults and adolescents with chickenpox.	No drug has been proven to prevent the recurrence of zoster (shingles) among HIV-1 infected persons.		
Human Herpes virus-8 Disease	Larger and more definitive studies are needed to determine whether antiviral therapy has a useful role in managing HHV-8 associated diseases. Potent ART that suppresses HIV-1 replication reduces the frequency of occurrence of Kaposi sarcoma among HIV-1–infected persons and should be considered for all persons who qualify for such therapy.	Effective suppression of HIV-1 replication with ART.		
Human Papilloma virus Disease	Patient-applied treatments for uncomplicated external lesions: Podofilox to be applied topically to wart lesions as a 0.5% solution or a 0.5% gel; twice daily applications for 3 consecutive days can be repeated weekly for up to 4 weeks.	No indication exists for secondary prophylaxis.		

Disease	Drug/ Dose	Secondary prophylaxis (chronic maintenance therapy)	When to stop secondary prophylaxis	When to reintroduce secondary prophylaxis
	Imiquimod 5% cream applied to lesions at bedtime and removed in the morning by washing. The drug should be applied on three nonconsecutive nights/week for up to 16 weeks. Provider-applied treatments recommended for complex or multicentric lesions or those lesions inaccessible to patient-applied treatments: Cryotherapy with liquid nitrogen can be repeated every 1–2 weeks up to 3–4 times. Trichloroacetic or bichloroacetic acids 80%– 95% aqueous solution and applied to each lesion. The treatment can be repeated weekly for 3–6 weeks. Surgical treatments like excision by scissor, shave, or curette or by electrosurgery. Laser surgery Topical cidofovir Podophyllin resin 10%–25% suspension in tincture of benzoin. It is applied by the provider to all lesions (up to 10 cm2 of skin area) and then removed by washing a few hours later. Applications can be repeated weekly for 3–6 weeks. Intralesional interferon is not generally recommended because of its high cost, difficult administration, and potential for systemic side effects (i.e., fever, fatigue, myalgias, and leukopenia). The overall efficacy of interferon is no better than other therapies, and it has not been specifically studied for genital warts among HIV-1 infected persons.			
Penicilliosis	Amphotericin B in a dose of 0.6 mg/kg body weight/day administered intravenously for	Oral itraconazole in a dose of 200 mg/day		

Disease	*Drug/ Dose*	*Secondary prophylaxis (chronic maintenance therapy)*	*When to stop secondary prophylaxis*	*When to reintroduce secondary prophylaxis*
	2 weeks, followed by oral itraconazole solution in a dose of 400 mg/day for a subsequent duration of 10 weeks.			
Leishmaniasis	Pentavalent antimony, 20 mg/kg body weight/day, administered by intravenous or intramuscular routes for 3-4 weeks, is the initial treatment of choice for leishmaniasis both for cutaneous or visceral.	Pentavalent antimony, amphotericin B, or pentamidine, administered at least every 2-4 weeks, is recommended, particularly for those with CD4+ T lymphocyte counts <200 cell/μL.	After a sustained (i.e., >3–6 months) increase in the CD4+ lymphocyte count to levels >350 cells/μL after initiation of ART.	
Paracoccidioidomycosis	Amphotericin B, TMP-SMX, itraconazole, 100–200 mg daily, ketoconazole 200–400 mg, sulfonamides, fluconazole.	AIDS and CD4+ T lymphocyte counts of <200 cells/ μL, although no data indicate appropriate regimens in this setting.		

APPENDIX

IIc PROPHYLAXIS FOR OPPORTUNISTIC INFECTIONS IN HIV/AIDS

Sushruta Dash

Disease	*Initiating primary prophylaxis*	*Regime*	*Stop primary prophylaxis*	*Restarting primary prophylaxis*
PCP CDC 2002	CD4 < 200/μl or history of oropharyngeal candidiasis	TMP-SMZ 1 DS (160/800) tab OD	CD4 >200/μl for ≥ 3months	CD4 <200/μl
NACO 2007	CD4 <200/μl or presence of other AIDS-defining illness	TMP-SMZ 1 DS (160/800) tab OD	CD4 >200 cells/mm3 on 2 consecutive occasions over 6 months.	
Toxoplasmic encephalitis CDC 2002	CD4 < 100/μl	TMP-SMZ 1 DS (160/800) tab OD	CD4 >200 cells/μL for >3 months	CD4+ <100–200 cells/μL
NACO 2007	CD4 < 100/μl	TMP-SMZ 1 DS (160/800) tab OD		
Tuberculosis CDC 2002	HIV patients with positive TST (≥5mm of induration) but no evidence of active TB and no history of treatment for active or latent TB should be treated for latent TB infection	Isoniazid daily or twice weekly for 9 months; rifampin or rifabutin daily for 4 months or 2 months of therapy with either rifampin and pyrazinamide or rifabutin and pyrazinamide		
NACO 2007	No prophylaxis			
MAC CDC 2002	CD4+ count <50 cells/μL	Clarithromycin or azithromycin.	CD4+ >100 cells/μL for >3 months	CD4+ <50–100 cells/μL
NACO 2007	CD4 count <75 cells/mm3. Routine prophylaxis presently not recommended in India.	Azithromycin once weekly or Clarithromycin OD		
Bacterial pneumonias CDC 2007	CD4 >200 cells/μL	Single dose of 23-valent polysaccharide pneumococcal vaccine (PPV) if not received during the previous five years		

Disease	*Initiating primary prophylaxis*	*Regime*	*Stop primary prophylaxis*	*Restarting primary prophylaxis*
NACO 2007	CD4 counts ≤200 cells/mm3	Single dose of 23-valent polysaccharide pneumococcal vaccine if not received during the preceding five years.		
Histoplasmosis CDC 2002	May be considered in patients with CD4+ <100 cells/μL who are at high risk because of occupational exposure or who live in a community with a hyperendemic rate of histoplasmosis (>10 cases/100 patient-years)			
NACO 2007	No specific recommendation			
CMV CDC 2002	CMV-seropositive and who have a CD4+ <50 cells/μL	Ganciclovir		
NACO 2007	No specific recommendation			

Routine prophylaxis not recommended by CDC or NACO

- Bacterial intestinal infections
- Candidiasis
- Cryptococcosis
- Coccidiodomycosis
- Herpes simplex
- Varicella zoster
- Kaposi's sarcoma

Data Insufficient/ No Exact Recommendations

Cryptosporidiosis

CDC 2002

Wash hands after contact with human feces (e.g., diaper changing), after handling pets, and after gardening or other contact with soil.
Avoid sexual practices that might result in oral exposure to feces (e.g., oral-anal contact).
Boil water for 1 minute.
Use submicron personal-use water filters (home/office types) or bottled water.

NACO 2007

Avoid contaminated drinking water.
Drink bottled or boiled water.

Fruits and vegetables should be peeled and washed thoroughly in boiled water.
Routine methods of water purification are ineffective against *Cryptosporidium* because the organisms are not filtered by municipal water systems and are resistant to chlorine and ozone.

The risk of contracting cryptosporidial infection can be minimized by using microstraining filters (0.1–1 μm), boiling water for 1 min, or using high-quality bottled water.

APPENDIX

IId TREATMENT OF SKIN DISEASES IN HIV/AIDS (NACO 2007)

Sushruta Dash

Skin Disease	Management and Treatment	Unique Features
Skin abscess or pyomyositis	Surgical drainage and care of the lesion. Antibiotics: Cloxacillin 500 mg qid for 10 days or Cloxacillin 1–2 g IV qid for 10 days Vancomycin in case of severe sepsis.	
Furunculosis or folliculitis	Local lesion care. Antibiotics: cloxacillin 500 mg PO qid for 10 days.	Usually caused by staphylococci. Needs careful Management because life-threatening disseminated infections may occur. WHO stage II.
Syphilis	Benzathine penicillin 2.4 million units IM single dose. Follow-up VDRL q 6 months until negative.	It is recommended that syphilis testing be offered to all clients presenting for voluntary counselling and testing (VCT) in high-prevalence areas because it is treatable in the early stages, and has an accelerated course in HIV infection.
Bacillary angiomatosis (BA)	Erythromycin 500 mg PO qid or Doxycycline 100 mg PO or IV × >3 months. Alternative: Azithromycin 600 mg qid.	Clinical response is slow and relapse is common.
Impetigo	As impetigo is highly contagious, maintain good hygiene and handwashing techniques to prevent spread to others. In severe cases, give cloxacillin or erythromycin 50 mg/kg/day qid for 5 days.	
Dermatophytosis	Use a broad-spectrum antifungal topically, such as clotrimazole cream 1% daily bid for 2–4 weeks. Widespread dermatophytosis may necessitate systemic treatment with terbinafine 250 mg qid × 2–4 weeks or itraconazole 100–200 mg qid × 2–4 weeks for skin lesions and up to 12 weeks for lesions of the nails.	Onychomycosis requires long-term therapy, and not all patients with dystrophic nails have a fungal infection, therefore, it is necessary to make the correct diagnosis. Direct microscopy of a KOH preparation is sufficient to confirm diagnosis.
Seborrhoeic dermatitis or generalized erythroderma	Topical steroids: Triamicinolone 1% with or without ketoconazole 2% cream twice daily for the duration of the flare. Shampoos: Tar-based or selenium sulfide or ketoconazole based twice weekly.	A very common complaint and one of the earliest clinical markers of HIV infection.

Skin Disease	*Management and Treatment*	*Unique Features*
Cutaneous candidiasis	Topical antifungal drug, such as clotrimazole 1% cream or ketoconazole. In severe cases, or if there still is no response to therapy, fluconazole 100– 200 mg PO bid × 10 days may be required.	
Chronic mucocutaneous herpes simplex (HSV)	Acyclovir 400 mg tid daily for 7 days (14 days if disseminated mucocutaneous herpes simplex infection). Treat local lesion by using local antiseptics such as gentian violet or cleaning the ulcerative vesicles with salt water and keeping them dry.	Recurrences occur frequently (more than 6/year) in some patients: administer chemosuppression with oral acyclovir 400 mg bid or famciclovir 250 mg bid. WHO stage IV.
Herpes zoster	For extensive lesions present for less than 48 hours, use famciclovir 500 mg tid or acyclovir 800 mg × 5 times × 7–10 days to avoid postherpetic pain. Local application of lidocaine gel 2% may help relieve pain in some patients. Calamine lotion is cheap, soothes the skin, reduces intense pruritus and accelerates the drying up process.	Herpes zoster in a young person is highly predictive of HIV infection. If the ophthalmic branch of the trigeminal nerve is involved, the cornea may get involved leading to corneal scarring with loss of vision in that eye. WHO stage II. Post-herpetic neuralgia should be treated with pain modifying agents: phenytoin 100 mg slowly increasing to 250–300 mg daily or carbamazepine 100 mg daily, increasing to 400 mg daily in 10 days
Molluscum contagiosum	Prick each lesion with a needle dipped in phenol; follow by expression of the central core Alternatively, where available, cryotherapy with liquid nitrogen or curettage is recommended. The recurrence rate is high.	Differential diagnosis: disseminated cryptococcosis, histoplasmosis and penicilliosis These systemic mycoses are usually associated with fever, pulmonary or meningeal involvement. Remission following treatment with ARVs.
Condylomata acuminata (genital warts)	Treat with podophyllin 20% solution twice weekly until cleared. Podophyllin 20% can be corrosive to the surrounding unaffected skin It should only be applied to the tips of the warts and washed away no later than 6 hours after application. For warts on the genital mucosa and mouth, a lower concentration of podophyllin (10%) may be applied. Alternatively, glacial trichloracetic acid may be applied 1–2 times a	The recurrence rate is high.

Skin Disease	*Management and Treatment*	*Unique Features*
	week until the lesion has cleared. Where available, cryotherapy with liquid nitrogen is recommended.	
Scabies	Topical permethrin cream (5%) applied to total body, neck down, and washed off 8–14 hours later. Re-treat after 1–2 weeks. All household contacts must be treated. Avoid contact with the eyes.	
Kaposi sarcoma	Discrete, solitary or few lesions are best left alone. Lesions of the face or exposed parts of the body may be treated locally with cryotherapy (topical liquid nitrogen), intralesional therapy with either vinblastine (0.2–0.4 mg at two-week intervals) or alpha interferon, and surgical excision. In single lesions, the results with any of the treatment choices mentioned are promising. If lesions are disseminated or extensive and if treatment is envisaged, do a biopsy. Radiotherapy: for localized intraoral or pharyngeal KS, painful cutaneous KS, and lymphoedema of the face and extremities.	Remission reported with ARVs.

http:www.nacoonline.org/upload/Publication/Treatment%20Care%20and%20support/Guidelines%20for%20Prevention%20and%20Management%20of%20common%20opportunistic%20infections.pdf

APPENDIX

III POST EXPOSURE PROPHYLAXIS GUIDELINES (NACO 2007)

Komal Aggarwal

The average risk of acquiring HIV infection after different types of occupational exposure is low compared to risk of infection with HBV or HCV. In terms of occupational exposure, the important routes are needle stick exposure (0.3% risk for HIV, 9-30% for HBV and 1-10% for HCV) and mucous membrane exposure (0.90% for HIV).

HIV Transmission Risk of Different Routes

Exposure route	*HIV*
Blood transfusion	90-95%
Perinatal	20-40%
Sexual intercourse	0.1 to 10%
Vaginal	0.05-0.1%
Anal	0.065-0.5%
Oral	0.005-0.01%
Injecting drugs use	0.67%
Needle stick exposure	0.3%
Mucous membrane splash to eye, oro-nasal	0.09%

Step 1: Management of Exposure Site-First Aid

If the skin is broken after a needle-stick or sharp instrument:

- Immediately wash the wound and surrounding skin with water and soap, and rinse. Do not scrub.
- Do not use antiseptics or skin washes (bleach, chlorine, alcohol, betadine)

After a splash of blood or body fluids:

- To unbroken skin:
  Wash the area immediately
  Do not use antiseptics
- For the eye:
  Irrigate exposed eye immediately with water or normal saline
  Sit in a chair, tilt head back and ask a colleague to gently pour water or normal saline over the eye.
  If wearing contact lens, leave them in place while irrigating, as they form a barrier over the eye and will help protect it. Once the eye is cleaned, remove the contact lens and clean them in the normal manner. This will make them safe to wear again.
  Do not use soap or disinfectant on the eye.
- For mouth:
  Spit fluid out immediately
  Rinse the mouth thoroughly, using water or saline and spit again. Repeat this process several times
  Do not use soap or disinfectant in the mouth
  Consult the designated physician of the institution for management of the exposure immediately.

Steps for Managing Occupational Exposure

Establish eligibility for PEP

0 hr 0 min	As soon as possible		Ideally within 2 hr, but certainly within 72 hr		6 m
Step 1	Step 2	Step 3	Step 4	Step 5	Step 6
Manage exposure site	Establish eligibility for PEP	Counsel for PEP	Prescribe PEP	Lab evaluation	Follow up and monitoring and adherence
Wash wound and surrounding skin with water and soap or Irrigate exposed eye immediately with water or Normal saline or rinse the mouth thoroughly using water or saline spit again Refer to physician	Exposure within 72 hrs ↓ Assess exposed individual ↓ Assess exposure source ↓ Assess type of exposure ↓ Determine risk of transmission ↓ Determine eligibility for PEP	Provide information on HIV and PEP ↓ Obtain consent for PEP ↓ Offer special leave from work	Assess source Patient's ARV status ↓ Check pregnancy if female ↓ Explain side effects of ARVs ↓ Explain post exposure measures against HBV and HBC	Provide HIV pre Check immunization status for hepatitis B ↓ Offer HIV, HBV, HBC test ↓ Draw blood to include CBC, LFT, pregnancy tests if applicable ↓ Provide post test HIV counselling	Record keeping

www.nacoonline.org/National_AIDS_Conrol_Programme/PEP_full/Accessed on June 1, 2008

Summary of Do's and Don't

Do	*Do Not*
Remove gloves, if appropriate	Do not panic
Wash the exposed site thoroughly with running water	Do not put the pricked finger in mouth
Irrigate with water or saline if eyes or mouth have been exposed	Do not squeeze the wound to bleed it
Wash the skin with soap and water	Do not use bleach, chlorine, alcohol, betadine, iodine or other antiseptics/detergents on the wound

** Do consult the designated physician immediately as per institutional guidelines for management of the occupational exposure

Step 2: Categories of Exposure

Category	*Definition and example*
Mild exposure:	Mucous membrane/non-intact skin with small volumes e.g. a superficial wound (erosion of the epidermis) with a plain or low caliber needle, or contact with the eyes or mucous membranes, subcutaneous injections following small-bore needles
Moderate exposure:	Mucous membrane/non intact skin with large volumes OR percutaneous superficial exposure with solid needle e.g.: a cut or needle stick injury penetrating gloves
Severe exposure:	Percutaneous with large volume e.g: • An accident with a high caliber needle (>18G) visibly contaminated with blood • A deep wound (haemorrhagic wound and/or very painful); • Transmission of a significant volume of blood. • An accident with material that has previously been used intravenously or intra-arterially.

Step 3: Categories of Situations Depending on Results of the Source

Source HIV Status	*Definition of risk in source*
HIV negative	Source is not HIV infected but consider HBV and HCV
Low risk	HIV positive and clinically asymptomatic
High risk	HIV positive and clinically symptomatic (see WHO clinical staging)
Unknown	Status of the patient is unknown, and neither the patient nor his/her blood is available for testing (e.g. injury during medical waste management the source patient might be unknown). The risk assessment will be based only upon the exposure (HIV prevalence in the locality can be considered)

Step 4: Key Information to Provide Informed Consent to the Client after Occupational Exposure

Key information to exposed person (client)	*Specific Details include*
The risk of acquiring HIV infection from the specific exposure	Ask client for understanding of HIV transmission risk after exposure
	The risk of getting HIV infection from a person known to be HIV positive is estimated to be - sharps injury: 3 in 1000 exposures (0.3%) - Mucous membrane splash: 1 in 1000 exposures (0.1%)

(*Contd.*)

Key information to exposed person (client)	*Specific Details include*
	- The risk in increased with large exposure e.g. needle stick from hollow bore needles with visible blood, from artery or vein and from source patients with high viral load (usually very sick persons with Ois)
What is known about PEP efficacy	• Ask client's understanding of PEP • PEP is provided to prevent potential transmission of the HIV virus • PEP is not 100% effective and should be given within 72 hours (ideally as soon as possible, if eligible). • Balance risk and benefits of PEP:PEP may prevent HIV transmission, versus possible risk of side effects.

Step 5: Deciding on PEP Regimen

There are two types of regimens:

- Basic regimen: 2-drug combination
- Expanded regimen: 3 drug combination

The decision to initiate the type of regimen depends on the type of exposure and HIV serostatus of the source person

Exposure	*Status of source*		
	HIV+ and asymptomatic	**HIV+ and Clinically symptomatic**	**HIV status unknown**
Mild	Consider 2-drug PEP	Start 2- drug PEP	Usually no PEP or consider 2-drug PEP
Moderate	Start 2-drug PEP	Start 3-drug PEP	Usually no PEP or consider 2-drug PEP
Severe	Start 3-drug PEP	Start 3-drug PEP	Usually no PEP or consider 2- drug PEP

- HIV testing of the source patient should not delay the decision about whether or not to start PEP. Start 2-drugs first if required, then send for consultation or refer.
- In the case of a high risk exposure from a source patient who has been exposed to or is taking antiretroviral medications, consult an expert to choose the PEP regimen, as the risk of drug resistance is high. Refer/consult expert physician. Start 2 drug regimen first.

Initiate HIV Chemoprophylaxis

Because post-exposure prophylaxis (PEP) has its greatest effect if begun within 2 hours of exposure, it is essential to act immediately. There is little benefit if >72 hours later. The prophylaxis needs to be continued for 4 weeks.

- Report exposure immediately to appropriate authority.
- Fill in the medical form (see annex 11.)

- Never delay start of the therapy due to debate over regimen. Begin with basic 2-drug regimen, and once expert advice is obtained, change as required.
- The 3rd drug can be added after consultation with an expert.

Dosages of the Drugs for PEP

Medication	*2-drug regimen*	*3-drug regimen*
Zidovudine (AZT)	300 mg twice a day	300 mg twice a day
Stavudine (d4T)	30 mg twice a day	30 mg twice a day
Lamivudine (3TC)	150 mg twice a day	150 mg twice a day 1st choice: Lopinavir/ritonavir (LPV/r)400/100 mg twice a day or 800/200 mg once daily with meals 2nd choice: Indinavir (IND) 800 mg every 8 hours and drink 8-10 glassess (>1.5 litres) of water daily)

Step 6: Recommended Baseline Laboratory Evaluation

Timing	*In persons taking PEP (standard regimen)*	*In persons not taking PEP*
Baseline (within 8 days after AEB)	HIV, HCV, anti-HBs* Complete blood count Transaminases	HIV, HCV, anti-HBs*

* HIV, HBV and HCV testing of exposed staff within 8 days of an AEB is required (baseline serostatus). Offer an HIV test in case of an AEB, as a positive HIV status may indicate the need to discontinue PEP. The decision on whether to test for HIV or not should be based on informed consent of the exposed person

Step 7: Recommended Follow-up Laboratory Tests

Timing	*In persons taking PEP (standard regimen)*	*In persons not taking PEP*
Weeks 2 and 4	Transaminases* Comploete blood counts	Clinical monitoring for hepatitis
Week 6	HIV-Ab	HIV-A-b
Month 3	HIV-Ab, anti-HCV,HBs Ag Transaminases*	HIV-Ab, anti-HCV, HBsAg
Month 6	HIV-Ab, anti-HCV, HbsAg Transaminases*	HIV-Ab, anti-HCV, HbsAg

* Transaminases should be checked at week 2 and 4 detect hepatitis in case the exposed person contracted HBV from the AEB For persons started on AZT containing PEP regimens

APPENDIX

IV

COMPARATIVE (WHO/CDC/NACO) TREATMENT OF SEXUALLY TRANSMITTED DISEASES

Komal Aggarwal, Vinod K Sharma

Disease	*WHO 2003*	*CDC 2006*	*NACO 2004*
Chancroid	**Ciprofloxacin**, 500 mg BD × 3 d or **Erythromycin base**, 500 mg orally QID × 7 d or **Azithromycin** 1 g single dose or **Ceftriaxone**, 250 mg by IM single dose	**Azithromycin** 1 g single dose or **Ceftriaxone** 250 mg IM single dose or **Ciprofloxacin** 500 mg orally BD × 3 d or **Erythromycin base** 500 mg TDS × 7 d Ciprofloxacin is contraindicated for pregnant and lactating women. Saftey of Azithromycin is not established in pregnanacy	**Erythromycin stearate/erythromycin base**, 500 mg QID × 7 d **Erythromycin ethyl succinate**, 800 mg QID × 7 days or **Ciprofloxacin**, 500 mg BD × 3-5 days or **Ceftriaxone**, 250 mg IM single dose or **Azithromycin**, 1 g single dose or **Doxycycline**, 100 mg BD × 7 days or **Trimethoprim** (80 mg) + **Sulphamethoxazole** (400 mg), 2 tabs BD × 14 d Hot fomentation. Buboes should not be incised, but aspirated with a wide bore needle. Aspiration should be done through the surrounding normal skin, from the non-dependent area.
Genital herpes	***First Clinical Episode*** **Acyclovir**, 200 mg, 5 times daily 7 d or **Acyclovir** 400 mg, 3 times daily for 7 days or **Valaciclovir**, 1 g BD × 7 days or **Famciclovir**, 250 mg, TDS × 7 days ***For severe disease*** **Acyclovir**, 5–10 mg/kg IV, every 8 hours for 5–7 days or until clinical resolution is attained	***First Clinical Episode*** **Acyclovir** 400 mg TDS 7–10 d or **Acyclovir** 200 mg five times a day × 7–10 d or **Famciclovir** 250 mg TDS × 7–10 d or **Valacyclovir** 1 g BD 7–10 d **NIL**	***First Clinical Episode*** **Acyclovir** 200 mg 5 times a day for 7 days or **Acyclovir** 400 mg TDS × 7d ***Severe For disease*** **Acyclovir**, 5-10 mg/kg IV every 8 hours for 5 to 7 days

Disease	*WHO 2003*	*CDC 2006*	*NACO 2004*
	Episodic treatment in recurrent infections **Acyclovir**, 200 mg, 5 times daily for 5 days or **Acyclovir**, 400 mg, 3 times daily for 5 days or **Acyclovir**, 800 mg twice daily for 5 days or **Valaciclovir**, 500 mg orally, BD × 5 d or **Valaciclovir**, 1000 mg once daily for 5 days or **Famciclovir**, 125 mg orally, BD for 5 days	***Episodic treatment in recurrent infections*** **Acyclovir** 400 mg TDS × 5 d or **Acyclovir** 800 mg BD × 5 d or **Acyclovir** 800 mg TDS × 2 d or **Famciclovir** 125 mg BD × 5 d or **Famciclovir** 1000 mg BD × 1 d	***Episodic treatment in recurrent infections*** **Acyclovir**, 200 mg 5 times daily for 7 days or **Acyclovir** 400 mg TDS × 7 days or **Acyclovir**, 800 mg BD × 7 days
	Suppressive therapy **Acyclovir** 400 mg BD or **Valaciclovir**, 500 mg OD or **Valaciclovir**, 1000 mg OD or **Famciclovir**, 250 mg BD	***Suppressive Therapy*** **Acyclovir** 400 mg BD or **Famiciclovir** 250 mg BD or **Valacyclovir** 500 mg OD or **Valacyclovir** 1 g OD	***Suppressive Therapy*** **Acyclovir**, 400 mg BD continuously for at least one year recurrence rate should than be re-assessed after the stoppage of acyclovir.
	Severe herpes simplex lesions with coinfection with HIV **Acyclovir**, 400 mg orally, 3–5 times daily until clinical resolution is attained	***Episodic Infection in HIV Infected*** **Acyclovir** 400 mg TDS × 5–10 d or **Famiciclovir** 500 mg BD × 5–10 d or **Valacyclovir** 1 g BD × 5–10 d ***Suppressive Therapy in HIV Infected*** **Acyclovir** 400–800 mg BD-TDS or **Famciclovir** 500 mg BD or **Valacyclovir** 500 mg BD	***Herpes And HIV Co – Infection*** **Acyclovir**, 400 mg orally 3–5 times daily until complete clinical healing of lesions

Disease	*WHO 2003*	*CDC 2006*	*NACO 2004*
Granuloma inguinale	**Azithromycin**, 1 g orally on first day, then 500 mg orally, once a day or **Doxycycline**, 100 mg orally, twice daily or **Erythromycin**, 500 mg orally, 4 times daily or **Tetracycline**, 500 mg orally, 4 times daily or **Trimethoprim 80 mg/ sulfamethoxazole 400 mg,** 2 tablets orally, twice daily for a minimum of 14 days	**Doxycycline** 100 mg BD at least 3 weeks and until all lesions have completely healed or **Azithromycin** 1 g once per week for at least 3 weeks or **Ciprofloxacin** 750 mg BD for at least 3 weeks or **Erythromycin base** 500 mg orally four times a day for at least 3 weeks or **Trimethoprim-sulfamethoxazole** one double-strength (160 mg/800 mg) tablet BD for 3 weeks *All drugs to be continued until all lesions have completely healed **Pregnant and lactating women should be treated with the erythromycin regimen, and consideration should be given to the addition of a parenteral aminoglycoside (e.g., gentamicin).	**Doxycycline**, 100 mg BD × 14 days or **Tertracycline HCL**, 500 mg QID × 14 days or **Erythromycin stearate or base** 500 mg QID × 14 days or **Trimethoprim (80 mg) + Sulphamethoxazole** (400 mg), 2 tabs twice a day orally for 14 days or until lesions have completely healed Lesions should be kept clean.
Lympho-granuloma venerum	**Doxycycline**, 100 mg BD × 14 d or **Erythromycin**, 500 mg QID × 14 d or **Tetracycline**, 500 mg QID × 14 d	**Doxycycline** 100 mg BD × 21 d or **Erythromycin** base 500 mg QID × 21 d or **Azithromycin** 1 g once a week × 3 weeks (May be used)	**Doxycycline**, 100 mg BD × 21 days or **Tetracycline**, 500 mg QID × 21 days or **Trimethoprim (80 mg) + sulphamethoxazole** (400 mg) 2 tabs BD × 21 days or **Erythromycin stearate or base**, 500 mg orally QID × 2 weeks * In pregnant and lactating females, erythomycine base/ stearate, 500 mg orally 4 time a day for 21 days

Disease	WHO 2003	CDC 2006	NACO 2004
Primary and Secondary Syphilis, Early Latent Syphilis	**Benzathine benzylpenicillin** 2.4 million IU IM at a single session, given as two injections at separate sites or **Procaine benzylpenicillin** 1.2 million IU IM daily for 10 days	**Benzathine penicillin G** 2.4 million units IM in a single dose	**Benzathine benzylpenicillin**, 2.4 million IU deep IM in a single session (two equally divided doses in each buttock) after doing intradermal sensitivity test for penicillin or **Procaine benzylpenicillin**, 1.2 million IU (3 vials, each having combination of 1 lakh units of benzyl penicillin G sodium +3 lakh units of procaine benzylpenicillin), IM once daily for 10 days
	For penicillin allergic non-pregnant patients **Doxycycline** 100 mg orally BD × 14 d or **Tetracycline** 500 mg QID × 14 days	***For penicillin allergic non-pregnant patients*** **Doxycycline** 100 mg orally BD × 14 d or **Tetracycline** 500 mg QID × 14 days	***For penicillin hyper-sensitive, non pregnant patients*** **Doxcycline** 100 mg BD × 15 days or **Minocycline**, 100 mg BD × 15 days or **Erythromycin base/stearate** 500 mg QID × 15 days or **Tetracycline HCl** 500 mg QID × 15 days
	For penicillin allergic pregnant patients **Erythromycin**, 500 mg orally, QID × 14 days	***For penicillin allergic pregnant patients*** Desensitise and treat with penicillin	***For penicillin allergic pregnant patients*** Erythromycin base/stearate 500 mg QID × 15 days
Late Latent Syphilis	**Benzathine benzylpenicillin** 2.4 million IU by intramuscular injection, once weekly for 3 consecutive wks **Procaine benzylpenicillin**, 1.2 million IU by IM once daily for 20 consecutive days	**Benzathine penicillin G** 7.2 million units total, administered as 3 doses of 2.4 million units IM each at 1 week intervals	**Benzathine benzylpenicillin** 2.4 million IU deep IM weekly for 3 consecutive weeks or **Procaine benzylpenicillin** 1.2 million IU IM once daily for 20 consecutive days
	For penicillin-allergic non-pregnant patients **Doxycycline**, 100 mg BD × 30 d	***For penicillin-allergic non-pregnant patients*** **Doxycycline** 100 mg BD × 28 d	***For penicillin allergic, nonpregnant patients*** **Doxycycline**, 100 mg orally twice daily for 30 days

Disease	*WHO 2003*	*CDC 2006*	*NACO 2004*
or Latent Syphilis of unknown duration and Begin Tertiary Syphilis	or **Tetracycline**, 500 mg QID × 30 days	or **Tetracycline**, 500 mg QID × 28 days	or **Tetracycline HCL**, 500 mg orally 4 times daily for 30 days or **Erythromycin base/stearate**, 500 mg orally 4 times a day for 30 days.
	For penicillin-allergic pregnant patients **Erythromycin**, 500 mg 4 times X 14 d	***For penicillin-allergic pregnant patients*** Desensitise and treat with penicillin	***For penicillin-allergic pregnant patients*** **Erythromycin base/stearate**, 500 mg orally 4 times a day for 30 days
Cardiovascular syphilis	No specific recommendation except: Management of patients with cardiovascular syphilis should include consultation with a cardiologist. All patients with cardiovascular syphilis and neurosyphilis should be monitored for many years. The follow-up should include clinical, serological, CSF and, based on the clinician's assessment of the individual patient's condition, radiological examinations.	Some providers treat all patients who have cardiovascular syphilis with a neurosyphilis regimen. The complete management of patients who have cardiovascular or gummatous syphilis is beyond the scope of these guidelines. These patients should be managed in consultation with an infectious diseases specialist.	**Procaine benzylpenicillin**, 1.2 million IU IM, daily for 20 consecutive days. ***For penicillin allergic, non pregnant patients*** **Doxycycline**, 100 mg BD × 30 days. **Tetracycline HCl**, 500 mg QID × 30 days. **Erythromycin base/stearate**, 500 mg orally 4 times a day for 30 days NB. To prevent complications of Jarisch-Herxheimer reaction in cardiovascular syphilis, 3 tablets of prednisolone (5 mg each) in a single oral dose should be given daily in the morning, after food, for two days prior to treatment, and 3 days after. Cardiologists should be associated while treating cardiovascular syphilis.
	Aqueous benzylpenicillin 12–24 million IU IV administered daily in doses of 2–4 million IU, every 4 hours for 14 days or **Procaine benzylpenicillin**, 1.2 million IU IM once daily, and probenecid, 500 mg orally, 4 times daily, both for 10–14 days	**Aqueous crystalline penicillin G** 18–24 million units per day, administered as 3–4 million units IV every 4 hours or continuous infusion, for 10–14 days or **Procaine penicillin** 2.4 million units IM once daily ***PLUS***	**Aqueous benzylpenicillin**, 12-24 million IU daily intravenously administered as 2-4 million IU 4 hourly for 14 days or **Procaine benzylpenicillin**, 1.2 million IU IM once daily for 4 weeks or

Disease	*WHO 2003*	*CDC 2006*	*NACO 2004*
Neurosyphilis		**Probenecid** 500 mg orally four times a day, both for 10–14 days	**Procaine benzylpenicillin**, 1.2 million IU IM once daily + probenecid, 500 mg orally 4 times daily for 4 weeks
	For penicillin-allergic non-pregnant patients **Doxycycline**, 200 mg orally, twice daily for 30 days or **Tetracycline**, 500 mg orally, 4 times daily for 30 days	***For penicillin-allergic non-pregnant patients*** Desensitise and treat with penicillin	***For pencillin hyper-sensitive patients*** **Doxycycline**, 100 mg BD × 30 days or **Tetracycline** HCl 500 mg QID × 30 days or **Erythromycin base/stearate**, 500 mg QID × 30 days
	For penicillin-allergic pregnant patients NIL	***For penicillin-allergic pregnant patients*** Desensitise and treat with penicillin	***For pencillin hyper sensitive pregnant patients*** **Erythromyein base/stearate**, 500 mg QID × 30 days
Pregnancy **Early congenital syphilis**	**Aqueous benzylpenicillin** 100 000–150 000 IU/kg/day administered as 50 000 IU/kg/dose IV every 12 hours, during the first 7 days of life and every 8 hours thereafter for a total of 10 days or **Procaine benzylpenicillin** 50 000 IU/kg IM as a single daily dose for 10 days	**Benzathine penicillin G** 50,000 units/kg IM, up to the adult dose of 2.4 million units in a single dose	**Aqueous benzylpenicillin**, 100,000 ~ 150,000 IU/kg/day IV in two divided doses daily for 10 days or **Procaine benzylpenicillin**, 50,000 IU/kg IM in a single daily dose for 10 days In infants with normal cerebro-spinal fluid, the following can be recommended: **Benzathine benzylpenicillin**, 500,000 units/kg IM in a single dose ***For penicillin hypersensitive patients (after the first month of life)*** **Erythromycin base/stearate,** 7.5-12.5 mg/kg/day orally 4 times a day for 30 days
	Aqueous benzylpenicillin 200 000–300 000 IU/kg/day by IV or IM, administered as 50 000 IU/kg/dose every 4–6 hours for 10–14 days	**Benzathine penicillin G** 50,000 units/kg IM, up to the adult dose of 2.4 million units, administered as 3 doses at 1-week intervals (total 150,000 units/kg up to the adult total dose of 7.2 million units	**Aqueous benzylpenicillin** 2 to 3 lakh units/kg/day IV or IM in divided doses for 14 days or **Erythromycin base/stearate**, 7.5-12.5 mg/kg/day orally 4 times a day for 30 days

Disease	*WHO 2003*	*CDC 2006*	*NACO 2004*
	For penicillin-allergic patients after the first month of life **Erythromycin**, 7.5–12.5 mg/kg orally, 4 times daily for 30 days	***For penicillin-allergic patients*** Desensitise and treat with penicillin	***For penicillin-allergic patients*** **Erythromycin base/stearate**, 7.5-12.5 mg/kg/day orally 4 times a day for 30 days
Congenital syphilis of 2 or more years **Non gonococcal urethritis/ cervicitis/ chlamydia infection**	**Doxycycline**, 100 mg BD × 7 d or **Azithromycin**, 1 g single dose or **Amoxycillin**, 500 mg orally, TDS × 7 d or **Erythromycin** 500 mg QID × 7 d or **Ofloxacin** 300 mg BD × 7 d or **Tetracycline** 500 mg QID × 7 d ***In pregnancy*** **Erythromycin**, 500 mg QID × 7 d or **Amoxycillin**, 500 mg TDS × 7 d	**Azithromycin** 1 g single dose or **Doxycycline** 100 mg BD × 7 d **Erythromycin** base 500 mg QID x 7d or **Erythromycin ethylsuccinate** 800 mg QID × 7 d or **Ofloxacin** 300 mg BD × 7 d or **Levofloxacin** 500 mg OD × 7 d	**Azithromycin**, 2g single dose or **Doxycycline**, 100 mg BD × 7 d or **Erythromycin base/ erythromycin stearate**, 500 mg orally for 7 days * Will treat both gonococcal and chlamydial infections. NB. Doxycycline is contra-indicated during pregnancy. ***Regimens in pregnancy*** **Erythromycin base/stearate**, 500 mg orally 4 times a day for 7 days; erythromycin should not be taken on empty stomach or **Amoxycillin**, 500 mg orally three times a day for 7 days on empty stomach or **Azithromycin**, 2 g orally as a single dose on empty stomach *Azithromycin has not been adequately evaluated during pregnancy
	NIL	**Metronidazole** 2 g orally in a single dose or **Tinidazole** 2 g orally in a single dose ***PLUS*** **Azithromycin** 1 g orally in a single dose (if not used for initial episode) ***In pregnancy*** **Azithromycin** 1 g orally in a single dose	NIL

Disease	*WHO 2003*	*CDC 2006*	*NACO 2004*
Recurrent and Persistent Urethritis		or **Amoxicillin** 500 mg orally TDS × 7 d or **Erythromycin base** 500 mg QID × 7d or **Erythromycin base** 250 mg QID × 14d or **Erythromycin ethylsuccinate** 800 mg QID × 7 d or **Erythromycin ethylsuccinate** 400 mg QID × 14 d *Erythromycin estolate is contraindicated during pregnancy	
	Should be treated for both *N. gonorrhoeae* and *C. trachomatis* **Erythromycin** syrup, 50 mg/kg per day orally, in 4 divided doses for 14 days or **Trimethoprim** 40 mg with **sulfamethoxazole** 200 mg orally, BD × 14 d	**Erythromycin base or ethylsuccinate** 50 mg/kg/day orally divided into 4 doses daily for 14 days	**Erythromycin** syrup, 50 mg/kg per day orally in four divided doses for 2 weeks In case of non-availability of erythromycin syrup trimethroprim, 40 mg with sulfamethoxazole 200 mg orally twice daily for 14 days
Ophthalmia neonatorum due to Chlamydiae	**Erythromycin** syrup, 50 mg/kg per day (given orally in four doses) for 14 days	**Erythromycin base** or **ethylsuccinate** 50 mg/kg/day orally divided into 4 doses daily for 14 days	**Erthromycin base/stearate** syrup, 50 mg/kg per day orally in 4 divided doses for 3 weeks. In case of non-availability of erythromycin syrup, **Co-trimoxazole** (trimethoprim, 40 mg plus sulphamethoxazole, 200 mg) to be given orally, twice daily for 3 weeks
Infant penumonia	**Ciprofloxacin**, 500 mg single dose or **Ceftriaxone**, 125 mg IM as a single dose or	**Ceftriaxone** 125 mg IM single dose or **Cefixime** 400 mg orally single dose or	**Azithromycin**, 2g orally as a single dose* or **Cefixime**, 400 mg orally as a single dose or

Disease	*WHO 2003*	*CDC 2006*	*NACO 2004*
Uncomplicated Gonococcal Infections of the Cervix, Urethra, and Rectum	**Cefixime**, 400 mg single dose or **Spectinomycin**, 2 g IM single dose ***Ciprofloxacin** is contraindicated in pregnancy	**Ciprofloxacin** 500 mg orally single dose or **Ofloxacin** 400 mg orally in a single dose* or **Levofloxacin** 250 mg orally single dose ***PLUS*** Treatment for chlamydia if chlamydial infection is not ruled out * **Heterosexuals with a history of recent travel** **Ceftriaxone** 125 mg IM in a single dose or **Cefixime** 400 mg orally in a single dose ***PLUS*** Treatment for chlamydia if chlamydial infection is not ruled out	**Ceftriaxone**, 250 mg intramuscular (IM) as a single injection *Will treat both gonococcal and chlamydial infections.
Uncomplicated gonococcal pharynx infection	**Ciprofloxacin**, 500 mg orally, as a single dose or **Ceftriaxone**, 125 mg by intramuscular injection, as a single dose or **Cefixime**, 400 mg orally, as a single dose or **Spectinomycin**, 2 g by intramuscular injection, as a single dose *Ciprofloxacin is contraindicated in pregnancy, and is not recommended for use in children and adolescents. There are variations in the anti-gonococcal activity of individual quinolones, and it is important to use only the most active.	**Ceftriaxone** 125 mg IM in a single dose or **Ciprofloxacin** 500 mg orally in a single dose ***PLUS*** Treatment for chlamydia if chlamydial infection is not ruled out ****MSM or Heterosexuals with a History of Recent Travel*** **Ceftriaxone** 125 mg IM in a single dose ***PLUS*** Treatment for chlamydia if chlamydial infection is not ruled out	**Ceftriaxone**, 500 mg/1g IM as a single dose

Disease	WHO 2003	CDC 2006	NACO 2004
Gonococcal conjunctivitis	***Recommended regimen*** **Ceftriaxone**, 125 mg by intramuscular injection, as a single dose or **Spectinomycin**, 2 g by intramuscular injection, as a single dose or **Ciprofloxacin**, 500 mg orally, as a single dose ***Alternative regimen*** **Kanamycin**, 2 g by intramuscular injection, as a single dose	**Ceftriaxone** 1 g IM in a single dose	**Ceftriaxone**, 500 mg IM as a single dose or **Kanamycin**, 2g IM as a single dose. Local cleaning of eyes by irrigation with saline or tap water is essential. Proper hand washing with soap and water of the patient's attendant is essential.
Disseminated Gonococcal Infections (DGI)	**Ceftriaxone**, 1 g IM/IV OD for 7 days (alternative third-generation cephalosporins may be required where ceftriaxone is not available, but more frequent administrations will be needed) or **Spectinomycin**, 2 g IM BD for 7 days.	**Ceftriaxone** 1 g IM or IV every 24 hrs or **Cefotaxime** 1 g IV every 8 hrs or **Ceftizoxime** 1 g IV every 8 hrs or **Ciprofloxacin** 400 mg IV every 12 hrs or **Ofloxacin** 400 mg IV every 12 hrs or **Levofloxacin** 250 mg IV daily* or **Spectinomycin** 2 g IM every 12 hours All of the preceding regimens should be continued for 24–48 hrs after improvement begins, at which time therapy may be switched to one of the following regimens to complete at least 1 week of antimicrobial therapy. **Cefixime** 400 mg orally twice daily or	**Ceftriaxone**, 1g IM or IV once daily for 7 days (An alternative third generation cephalosporin may be required if ceftriaxone is not available, but more frequent daily dosage will be needed) **Cefixime**, 400 mg twice daily orally for 7 days

Disease	WHO 2003	CDC 2006	NACO 2004
		Ciprofloxacin 500 mg orally twice daily or **Ofloxacin** 400 mg orally twice daily or **Levofloxacin** 500 mg orally once dail *Quinolones should not be used for infections in MSM and history of recent foreign travel or partners' travel	
Gonococcal Meningitis and Endocarditis	As for disseminated gonococcal infection for menigitis but in endocarditis the duration of therapy will need to be increased to 4 weeks	**Ceftriaxone** 1–2 g IV every 12 hours For meningitis should be continued for 10–14 d therapy for endocarditis should be continued for at least 4 weeks.	As for disseminated gonococcal infection but the duration of intravenous therapy will be increased to two weeks for meningitis and four weeks for endocarditis.
	Ceftriaxone, 50 mg/kg by IM single dose, to a maximum of 125 mg **Where ceftriaxone is not available** **kanamycin**, 25 mg/kg by IM as a single dose, to a maximum of 75 mg or **Spectinomycin**, 25 mg/kg by IM as a single dose, to a maximum of 75 mg	**Ceftriaxone** 25–50 mg/kg IV or IM in a single dose, not to exceed 125 mg	**Ceftriaxone**, 50 mg/kg IM as a single dose to a maximum of 125 mg/kg or **Kanamycin**, 25 mg/kg IM as a single dose to a maximum of 75 mg/kg In case of discharge from the eyes, these can be gently cleaned with distilled water.
Ophthalmia Neonatorum caused by *N. gonorroheae*	NIL	**Ceftriaxone** 25–50 mg/kg/day IV or IM in a single daily dose for 7 days, with a duration of 10–14 days, if meningitis is documented or **Cefotaxime** 25 mg/kg IV or IM every 12 hours for 7 days, with a duration of 10–14 days, if meningitis is documented	NIL
	Metronidazole, 400 mg or 500 mg orally, twice daily for 7 days or	**Metronidazole** 500 mg orally BD for 7 days or	**Metronidazole**, 400 mg orally twice daily for 7 days **Metronidazole**, 2 g orally as a single dose

Disease	*WHO 2003*	*CDC 2006*	*NACO 2004*
DGI and Gonococcal Scalp Abscesses in Newborns **Bacterial Vaginosis**	**Metronidazole**, 2 g orally, as a single dose or **Clindamycin** 2% vaginal cream, 5 g intravaginally, at bedtime for 7 days or **Metronidazole** 0.75% gel, 5 g intravaginally, twice daily for 5 days or **Clindamycin**, 300 mg orally, twice daily for 7 days **For pregnant women** **Metronidazole**, 200 or 250 mg orally, TDS × 7 d after first trimester **Metronidazole** 2 g orally, as a single dose, if treatment is imperative during the first trimester of pregnancy	**Metronidazole gel**, 0.75%, one full applicator (5 g) intravaginally, once a day for 5 days or **Clindamycin cream**, 2%, one full applicator (5 g) intravaginally at bedtime for 7 days or **Clindamycin** 300 mg orally twice a day for 7 days or **Clindamycin** ovules 100 mg intravaginally once at bedtime for 3 days ****For Pregnant Women*** **Metronidazole** 500 mg orally twice a day for 7 days or **Metronidazole** 250 mg orally three times a day for 7 days or **Clindamycin** 300 mg orally twice a day for 7 days	or ii. **Tinidazole**, 2 gm orally as a single dose However, in symptomatic women, in the first trimester and those intolerant to metronidazole tinidazole, imidazole pessaries cream may be given for 7 days ***Pregnancy*** **Metronidazole** is contra-indicated during the first trimester of pregnancy, but may be used, if necessary, during the second and third trimesters. There is some evidence that bacterial vaginosis may increase the incidence of premature rupture of the membranes. It should, therefore be treated when diagnosed in third trimester
	Metronidazole, 2 g orally in a single dose or **Tinidazole** 2 g orally, in a single dose or **Metronidazole**, 400 mg or 500 mg orally, BD × 7 d or **Tinidazole** 500 mg BD × 5 days	**Metronidazole** 2 g orally in a single dose or **Tinidazole** 2 g orally in a single dose or **Metronidazole** 500 mg orally twice a day for 7 days	**Metronidazole**, 2 g orally in a single dose or **Metronidazole**, 400 mg orally twice daily for 7 days or **Tinidazole** 2g orally in a single dose
Trichomonia-sis	**Miconazole or clotrimazole**, 200 mg intravaginally, daily for 3 days or **Clotrimazole**, 500 mg intravaginally, as a single dose or	*Intravaginal Agents:* **Butoconazole** 2% cream 5 g intravaginally for 3 days* or **Butoconazole** 2% cream 5 g (Butaconazole1-sustained release), single intravaginal application	**Miconazole** or **clotrimazole**, 100 mg intravaginally daily for 6 days or **Clotrimazole**, 500 mg intra-vaginally as a single dose or **Fluconazole**, 150 mg orally as a single dose

Disease	*WHO 2003*	*CDC 2006*	*NACO 2004*
Vulvovaginal Candidiasis	**Fluconazole**, 150 mg orally, as a single dose or **Nystatin**, 100 000 IU intravaginally, daily for 14 days	or **Clotrimazole** 1% cream 5 g intravaginally for 7–14 days* or **Clotrimazole** 100 mg vaginal tablet for 7 days or **Clotrimazole** 100 mg vaginal tablet, two tablets for 3 days or **Miconazole** 2% cream 5 g intravaginally for **Miconazole** 100 mg vaginal suppository, one suppository for 7 days* or **Miconazole** 200 mg vaginal suppository, one suppository for 3 days* or **Miconazole** 1,200 mg vaginal suppository, one suppository for 1 day* or **Nystatin** 100,000-unit vaginal tablet, one tablet for 14 days or **Tioconazole** 6.5% ointment 5 g intravaginally in a single application* or **Terconazole** 0.4% cream 5 g intravaginally for 7 days or **Terconazole** 0.8% cream 5 g intravaginally for 3 days or **Terconazole** 80 mg vaginal suppository, one suppository for 3 days ***Oral Agent:*** **Fluconazole** 150 mg oral tablet, one tablet in single dose	

Disease	*WHO 2003*	*CDC 2006*	*NACO 2004*
Pelvic inflammatory disease	***Outpatient therapy*** **Ceftriaxone**, 125 mg IM as a single dose **PLUS** • **Doxycycline**, 100 mg orally, twice daily, or **Tetracycline**, 500 mg orally, 4 times daily for 14 days **PLUS** • **Metronidazole**, 400–500 mg orally, twice daily for 14 days ***Note*** • Patients taking metronidazole should be cautioned to avoid alcohol. • Tetracyclines are contraindicated in pregnancy. Adjuncts to therapy: removal of intrauterine device (IUD) If PID should occur with an IUD in place, treat the PID using appropriate antibiotics. There is no evidence that removal of the IUD provides any additional benefit. Thus, if the individual should wish to continue its use, it need not be removed. If she does not want to keep the IUD, removal of the IUD is recommended after antimicrobial therapy has been commenced. When the IUD is removed, contraceptive counselling is necessary. ***Follow-up*** Outpatients with PID should be followed up after 72 hours and admitted if their condition has not improved.	***Oral treatment*** ***Recommended Regimen A*** **Levofloxacin** 500 mg orally once daily for 14 days* or **Ofloxacin** 400 mg orally twice daily for 14 days* **WITH or WITHOUT** **Metronidazole** 500 mg orally twice a day for 14 days ***Regimen B*** **Ceftriaxone** 250 mg IM in a single dose ***PLUS*** **Doxycycline** 100 mg orally twice a day for 14 days **WITH or WITHOUT** **Metronidazole** 500 mg orally twice a day for 14 days or **Cefoxitin** 2 g IM in a single dose and Probenecid, 1 g orally administered concurrently in a single dose ***PLUS*** **Doxycycline** 100 mg orally twice a day for 14 days **WITH or WITHOUT** **Metronidazole** 500 mg orally twice a day for 14 days or Other parenteral third-generation **cephalosporin** (e.g., **ceftizoxime** or **cefotaxime**) ***PLUS*** **Doxycycline** 100 mg orally twice a day for 14 days **WITH or WITHOUT** **Metronidazole** 500 mg orally twice a day for 14 days ***Recommended Parenteral Regimen A*** **Cefotetan** 2 g IV every 12 hours	***Out Patient Therapy*** ***Recommended regimen*** i. **Azithromycin**, 2 g orally single dose under supervision (to treat both gonococcal and chlamydial infections) PLUS ii. **Metronidazole**, 400 mg orally twice a day for 2 weeks (to treat anaerobic bacteria) **Alternative regimen** i. **Cefixime**, 400 mg orally single dose under supervision (to treat gonococcal infection) PLUS ***Doxycycline**, 100 mg orally, twice a day for 2 weeks (to treat chlamydial infection) PLUS **Metronidazole**, 400 mg orally twice a day for 2 weeks (to treat anaerobic bacteria) ii. **Ceftriaxone**, 250 mg I.M. single dose (to treat gonococcal infection) PLUS ***Doxycycline**, 100 mg orally, twice a day for 2 weeks (to treat chlamydial infection) PLUS **Metronidazole**, 400 mg orally twice a day for 2 weeks (to treat anaerobic bacteria) * In individuals allergic/intolerant to doxycycline and in all pregnant women, erythromycin base/stearate, 500 mg orally 4 times day for 14 days

Disease	*WHO 2003*	*CDC 2006*	*NACO 2004*
		or **Cefoxitin** 2 g IV every 6 hours ***PLUS*** **Doxycycline** 100 mg orally or IV every 12 hours	
	Inpatient Therapy ***Recommended syndromic treatment options for PID*** 1. **Ceftriaxone**, 250 mg by intramuscular injection, once daily **PLUS** • **Doxycycline**, 100 mg orally or by intravenous injection, twice daily, or tetracycline, 500 mg orally 4 times daily **PLUS** • **Metronidazole**, 400–500 mg orally or by intravenous injection, twice daily, or chloramphenicol, 500 mg orally or by intravenous injection, 4 times daily 2. **Clindamycin**, 900 mg by intravenous injection, every 8 hours **PLUS** • **Gentamicin**, 1.5 mg/kg by intravenous injection every 8 hours 3. **Ciprofloxacin**, 500 mg orally, twice daily, or spectinomycin 1 g by intramuscular injection, 4 times daily **PLUS** • **Doxycycline**, 100 mg orally or by intravenous injection, twice daily, or tetracycline, 500 mg orally, 4 times daily **PLUS** • **Metronidazole**, 400–500 mg orally or by intravenous injection, twice daily, or chloramphenicol, 500 mg orally or by intravenous injection, 4 times daily	***Recommmended Parenteral Regimen B*** **Clindamycin** 900 mg IV every 8 hours ***PLUS*** **Gentamicin** loading dose IV or IM (2 mg/kg of body weight), followed by a maintenance dose (1.5 mg/kg) every 8 hours. Single daily dosing ***Alternative parentral regimens*** **Levofloxacin** 500 mg IV once daily* **WITH or WITHOUT** **Metronidazole** 500 mg IV every 8 hours or **Ofloxacin** 400 mg IV every 12 hours* **WITH or WITHOUT** **Metronidazole** 500 mg IV every 8 hours or **Ampicillin/Sulbactam** 3 g IV every 6 hours ***PLUS*** **Doxycycline** 100 mg orally or IV every 12 hours	***Inpatient Therapy*** Out patients with PID should be followed up for 72 hours and admitted if there is no improvement in their condition. ***Recommended Regimens*** i. **Ceftriaxone**, 250 mg IM injection once daily PLUS **Doxycycline**, 100 mg orally twice daily or tetracycline HCl, 500 mg orally 4 times daily PLUS **Metronidazole**, 400 mg orally or by IV twice daily ii. **Ciprofloxacin**, 500 mg orally or by IV twice daily or **Spectinomycin**, 2g IM twice daily PLUS **Doxycycline**, 100 mg orally twice daily or tetracycline HCl, 500 mg orally 4 times daily PLUS **Metronidazole**, 400 mg orally or by IV twice daily NB. Therapy in both the above mentioned regimens

Disease	*WHO 2003*	*CDC 2006*	*NACO 2004*
	Note For all three regimen, therapy should be continued until at least two days after the patient has improved and should then be followed by either doxycycline, 100 mg orally, twice daily for 14 days, or tetracycline, 500 mg orally, 4 times daily, for 14 days. • Patients taking metronidazole should be cautioned to avoid alcohol. • **Tetracyclines** are contraindicated in pregnancy.		
Epididymitis	No recommendations for Epididymitis, only for **DISSEMINATED GONOCOCCAL INFECTION** **Recommended regimen** • **Ceftriaxone**, 1 g by intramuscular or intravenous injection, once daily for 7 days (alternative third-generation cephalosporins may be required where ceftriaxone is not available, but more frequent administrations will be needed) or • **Spectinomycin**, 2 g by intramuscular injection, twice daily for 7 days. There are some data to suggest that therapy for 3 days is adequate **Note** • For gonococcal meningitis and endocarditis the same dosages apply but for endocarditis the duration of therapy will need to be increased to 4 weeks.	***For acute epididymitis most likely caused by gonococcal or chlamydial infection:*** **Ceftriaxone** 250 mg IM in a single dose ***PLUS*** **Doxycycline** 100 mg orally twice a day for 10 days ***For acute epididymitis most likely caused by enteric organisms or for patients allergic to cephalosporins and/or tetracyclines:*** **Ofloxacin** 300 mg orally twice a day for 10 days or **Levofloxacin** 500 mg orally once daily for 10 days	**Complicated and disseminated gonococcal infection** This includes posterior urethritis, prostatitis, **epididymo-orchitis**, tysonitis, cowperitis and bartholinitis. The patient should, if necessary, be admitted to a hospital. **Recommended regimen** i. ***Ceftriaxone**, 1g IM or IV once daily for 7 days (An alternative third generation cephalosporin may be required if ceftriaxone is not available, but more frequent daily dosage will be needed) ii. **Cefixime**, 400 mg twice daily orally for 7 days *For gonococcal meningitis and endocarditis the same dosages apply, but the duration of intravenous therapy will be increased to two weeks for meningitis and four weeks for endocarditis. N B. Appropriate supportive treatment like scrotal support, analgesics and sedatives are to be added, if required

APPENDIX

V

FLOWCHARTS FOR MANAGEMENT OF RTI/STI SYNDROMES (NACO 2007)

Flowchart 5.1: Management of Urethral Discharge/Burning Micturition in Males

SYNDROME: URETHRAL DISCHARGE IN MALES

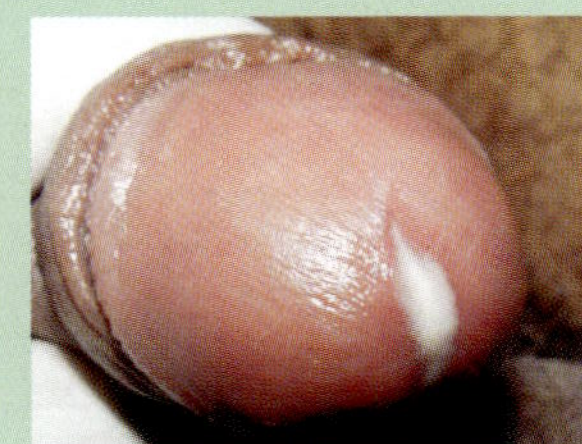

RTIs/STIs: Gonorrhoea, Chlamydial Infection, Trichomoniasis

Causative Organisms

- *Neisseria gonorrhoeae*
- *Chlamydia trachomatis*
- *Trichomonas vaginalis*

History of

- Urethral discharge
- Pain or burning while passing urine, increased frequency of urination
- Sexual exposure of either partner to high risk practices including oro-genital sex

→

Examination

Look for

- The urethral meatus for redness and swelling
- If urethral discharge is not seen, then gently massage the urethra from the ventral part of the penis towards the meatus and look for thick, creamy greenish-yellow or mucoid discharge

→

Laboratory Investigations (if available)

- Gram stain examination of the urethral smear will show gram-negative intrac-ellular diplococci in case of gonorrhoea,
- In non-gonococcal urethritis more than 5 neutrophils per oil immersion field (I000X) in the urethral smear or more than 10 neutrophils per high power field in the sediment of the first void urine are observed

Treatment

As dual infection is common, the treatment for urethral discharge should adequately cover therapy for both, gonorrhoea and chlamydial infections.

Recommended regimen for uncomplicated gonorrhoea + chlamydia

Uncomplicated infections indicate that the disease is limited to the anogenital region (anterior urethritis and proctitis).

- Tab. Cefixime 400 mg orally, single dose Plus
  Tab Azithromycin 1 gram orally single dose under supervision
- Advise the client to return after 7 days of start of therapy

When symptoms persist or recur after adequate treatment for gonorrhoea and chlamydia in the index client and partner(s), they should be treated for *Trichomonas vaginalis*.

If discharge or only dysuria persists after 7 days

- Tab. Secnidazole 2gm orally, single dose (to treat for *T. vaginalis*)

If the symptoms still persists

- Refer to higher centre as early as possible

If individuals are allergic to Azithromycin, give Erythromycin 500 mg four times a day for 7 days

Syndrome specific guidelines for partner management

- Treat all recent partners
- Treat female partners (for gonorrhoea and chlamydia) on same lines after ruling out pregnancy and history of allergies
- Advise sexual abstinence during the course of treatment
- Provide condoms, educate about correct and consistent use
- Refer for voluntary counselling and testing for HIV, Syphilis and Hepatitis B
- Schedule return visit after 7 days

Follow up

After seven days

- To see reports of tests done for HIV, syphilis and Hepatitis B
- If symptoms persist, to assess whether it is due to treatment failure or re-infection
- For prompt referral if required

Management of pregnant partner

Pregnant partners of male clients with urethral discharge should be examined by doing a per speculum as well as per vaginal examination and should be treated for gonococcal as well as chlamydial infections.

- Cephalosporins to cover gonococcal infection are safe and effective in pregnancy
  - Tab. Cefixime 400 mg orally, single dose or
  - Ceftriaxone 125 mg by intramuscular injection

    +
  - Tab. Erythromycin 500 mg orally four times a day for seven days or
  - Cap Amoxicillin 500 mg orally, three times a day for seven days to cover chlamydial infection
  - Quinolones (like ofloxacin, ciprofloxacin), doxycyclin are contraindicated in pregnant women.

Flowchart 5.2: Management of Scrotal Swelling

Syndrome: Scrotal Swelling

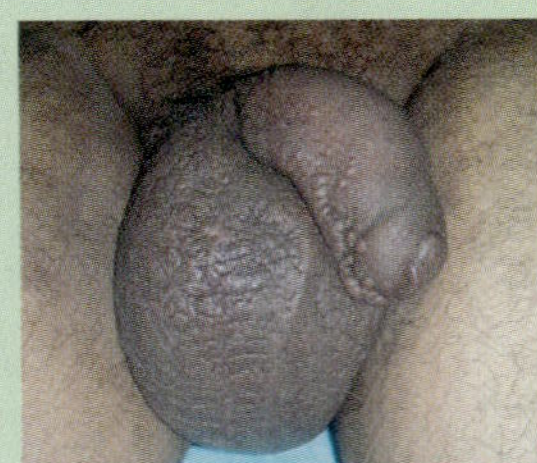

RTIs/STIs : Gonorrhoea, Chlamydial Infection

Causative Organisms

- *Neisseria gonorrhoeae*
- *Chlamydia trachomatis*

History of

- Swelling and pain in scrotal region
- Pain or burning while passing urine
- Systemic symptoms like malaise, fever
- Sexual exposure of either partner to high risk practices including oro-genital sex

→

Examination

Look for

- Scrotal swelling
- Redness and edema of the overlying skin
- Tenderness of the epididymis and vas deferens
- Associated urethral discharge/genital ulcer/inguinal lymph nodes and if present refer to the respective flowchart
- A transillumination test to rule out

→

Laboratory Investigations

(*If available*)

- Gram stain examination of the urethral smear will show gram-negative intra-cellular diplococci in case of complicated gonococcal infection
- In non-gonococcal urethritis more than 5 neutrophils per oil immersion field in the urethral smear or more than 10 neutrophils per high power field in the sediment of the first void urine are observed

Differential diagnosis (non RTIs/STIs)

Infections causing scrotal swelling:

Tuberculosis, filariasis, coliforms, pseudomonas, mumps virus infection.

Non infectious causes:

Trauma, Hernia, Hydrocoele, Testicular torsion, and Testicular tumors

↓

Treatment

- Treat for both gonococcal and chlamydial infections
  Tab Cefixime 400 mg orally BD for 7 days Plus
  Cap. Doxycycline 100 mg orally, twice daily for 14 days and refer to higher centre as early as possible since complicated gonococcal infection needs parental and longer duration of treatment
- Supportive therapy to reduce pain (bed rest, scrotal elevation with T-bandage and analgesics)

Note

If quick and effective therapy is not given, damage and scarring of testicular tissues may result causing subfertility

↓

Syndrome specific guidelines for partner management

Partner needs to be treated depending on the clinical findings

Management protocol in case the partner is pregnant

- Depending on the clinical findings in the pregnant partner (whether vaginal discharge or endocervical discharge or PID is present) the drug regimens should be used.
- Doxycycline is contraindicated in pregnancy
- Erythromycin base/Amoxicillin can be used in pregnancy.

(Erythromycin estolate is contraindicated in pregnancy due to hepatotoxicity. Erythromycin base or erythromycin ethyl succinate should be given)

Flowchart 5.3: Management of Inguinal Bubo

SYNDROME: INGUINAL BUBO

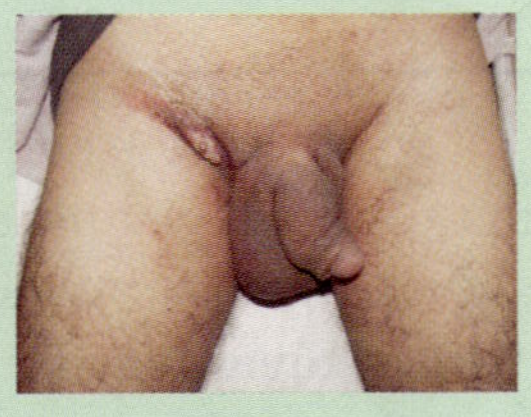

RTIs/STIs: LGV, CHANCROID

Causative Organisms

- *Chlamydia trachomatis* serovars LI, L2, L3, causative agent of lymphogranuloma venerum (LGV)
- *Haemophilus ducreyi* causative agent of chancroid

History

- Swelling in inguinal region which may be painful
- Preceding history of genital ulcer or discharge
- Sexual exposure of either partner to high risk practices including orogenital sex
- Systemic symptoms like malaise, fever

Examination

Look for

- Localized enlargement of lymph nodes in groin which may be tender and fluctuant
- Inflammation of skin over the swelling
- Presence of multiple sinuses
- Edema of genitals and lower limbs
- Presence of genital ulcer or urethral discharge and if present refer to respective flowchart

Laboratory Investigations

Diagnosis is on clinical grounds

Differential diagnosis

- Mycobacterium tuberculosis, filariasis
- Any acute infection of skin of pubic area, genitals, buttocks, anus and lower limbs can also cause inguinal swelling If malignancy or tuberculosis is suspected refer to higher centre for biopsy.

Treatment

- Start Cap. Doxycycline 100mg orally twice daily for 21 days (to cover LGV)
  Plus
- Tab Azithromycin ig orally single dose OR
- Tab. Ciprofloxacin 500 mg orally, twice a day for three days to cover chancroid
- Refer to higher centre as early as possible.

Note:

- *A bubo should never be incised and drained at the primary health centre, even if it is fluctuant, as there is a high risk of a fistula formation and chronicity. If bubo becomes fluctuant always refer for aspiration to higher centre.*
- *In severe cases with vulval edema in females, surgical intervention may be required for which they should be referred to higher centre.*

Syndrome specific guidelines for partner management

- Treat all partners who are in contact with client in last 3 months
- Partners should be treated for chancroid and LGV
- Tab Azithromycin 1 g orally single dose to cover chancroid
  +
  Cap Doxycycline 100 mg orally, twice daily for 21 days to cover LGV
- Advise sexual abstinence during the course of treatment
- Provide condoms, educate on correct and consistent use
- Refer for voluntary counselling and testing for HIV, syphilis and Hepatitis B
- Schedule return visit after 7 days and 21 days

Management of pregnant partner

- Quinolones (like ofloxacin, ciprofloxacin), doxycycline, sulfonamides are contraindicated in pregnant women.
- Pregnant and lactating women should be treated with the erythromycin regimen, and consideration should be given to the addition of a parenteral aminoglycoside (e.g., gentamicin)

Tab. Erythromycin base, 500 mg orally, 4 times daily for 21 days and refer to higher centre.

(Erythromycin estolate is contraindicated in pregnancy due to hepatotoxicity. Erythromycin base or erythromycin ethyl succinate should be given)

Flowchart 5.4: Management of Genital Ulcers

SYNDROME: GENITAL ULCERS

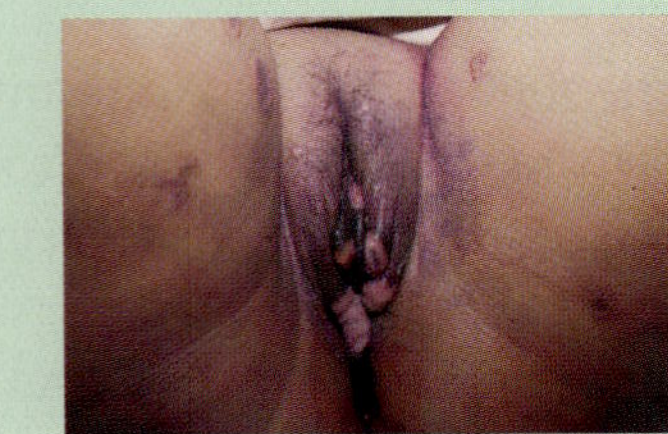

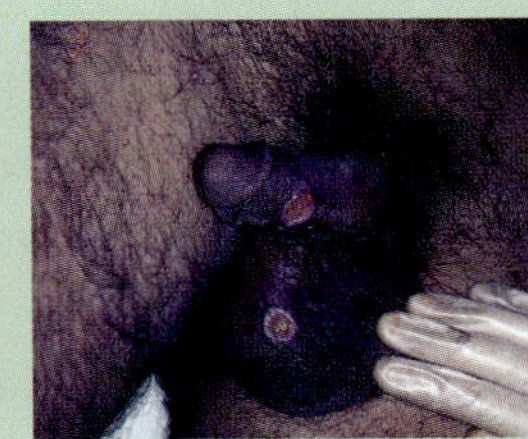

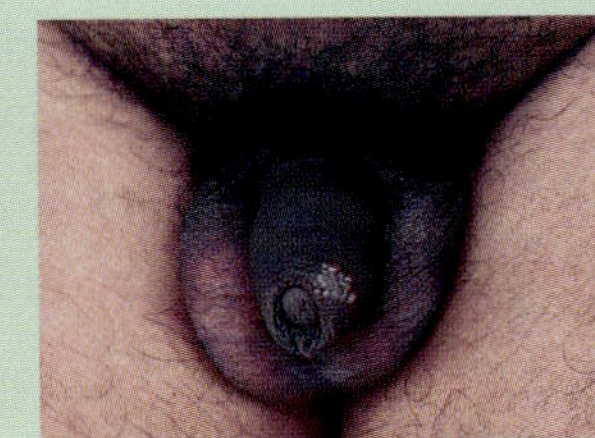

RTIs/STIs: **Syphilis** **Chancroid** **Genital Herpes**

Causative Organisms

- *Treponema pallidum* (syphilis)
- *Haemophilus ducreyi* (chancroid)
- *Klebsiella granulomatis* (granuloma inguinale)
- *Chlamydia trachomatis* (lymphogranuloma venerum)
- *Herpes simplex* (genital herpes)

History

- Genital ulcer/vesicles
- Burning sensation in the genital region
- Sexual exposure of either partner to high risk practices including orogenital sex

→

Examination

- Presence of vesicles
- Presence of genital ulcer- single or multiple
- Associated inguinal lymph node swelling and if present refer to respective flowchart

Ulcer characteristics:

- Painful vesicles/ulcers, single or multiple - Herpes simplex
- Painless ulcer with shotty lymph node - Syphilis
- Painless ulcer, No inguinal lymph node - Granuloma inguinale
- Painful ulcer usually single sometimes - Chancroid associated with painful bubo

→

Laboratory Investigations

- RPR test for syphilis
- For further investigations refer to higher centre

Treatment

- if vesicles or multiple painful ulcers are present treat for herpes with Tab. Acyclovir 400 mg orally, three times a day for 7 days
- If vesicles are not seen and only ulcer is seen, treat for syphilis and chancroid and counsel on herpes genitalis

To cover syphilis give

Inj Benzathine penicillin 2.4 million IU IM after test dose in two divided doses (with emergency tray ready)
(In individuals allergic or intolerant to penicillin, Doxycycline 100mg orally, twice daily for 14 days)
+
Tab Azithromycin 1g orally single dose or
Tab. Ciprofloxacin 500 mg orally, twice a day for three days to cover chancroid
Treatment should be extended beyond 7 days if ulcers have not epithelialized i.e. formed a new layer of skin over the sore)

Refer to higher centre

- If not responding to treatment
- Genital ulcers co-existent with HIV
- Recurrent lesion

Syndrome specific guidelines for partner management

- Treat all partners who are in contact with client in last 3 months
- Partners should be treated for syphilis and chancroid
- Advise sexual abstinence during the course of treatment
- Provide condoms, educate about correct and consistent use
- Refer for voluntary counselling and testing for HIV, Syphilis and Hepatitis B
- Schedule return visit after 7 days

Management of Pregnant Women

- Quinolones (like ofloxacin, ciprofloxacin), doxycycine, sulfonamides are contraindicated in pregnant women.
- Pregnant women who test positive for RPR should be considered infected unless adequate treatment is documented in the medical records and sequential serologic antibody titers have declined.
- Inj Benzathine penicillin 2.4 million IU IM after test dose (with emergency tray ready)
- A second dose of benzathine penicillin 2.4 million units IM should be administered 1 week after the initial dose for women who have primary, secondary, or early latent syphilis.
- Pregnant women who are allergic to penicillin should be treated with erythromycin and the neonate should be treated for syphilis after delivery.
- Tab. Erythromycin 500 mg orally four times a day for 15 days
- (Note: Erythromycin estolate is contraindicated in pregnancy because of drug related hepatotoxicity. Only Erythromycin base or erythromycin ethyl succinate should be used in pregnancy)
- All pregnant women should be asked history of genital herpes and examined carefully for herpetic lesions.
- Women without symptoms or signs of genital herpes or its prodrome can deliver vaginally.
- Women with genital herpetic lesions at the onset of labour should be delivered by caesarean section to prevent neonatal herpes.
- Acyclovir may be administered orally to pregnant women with first episode genital herpes or severe recurrent herpes.

Flowchart 5.5: Management of Vaginal Discharge in Females

SYNDROME: VAGINAL DISCHARGE

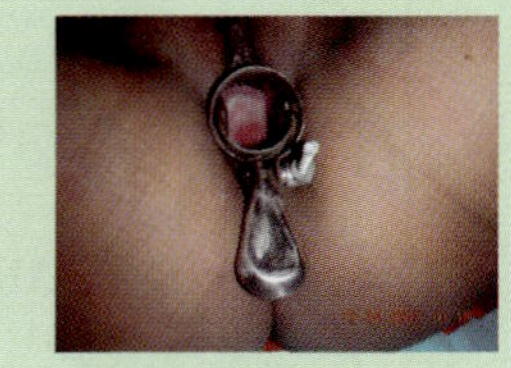

VAGINITIS

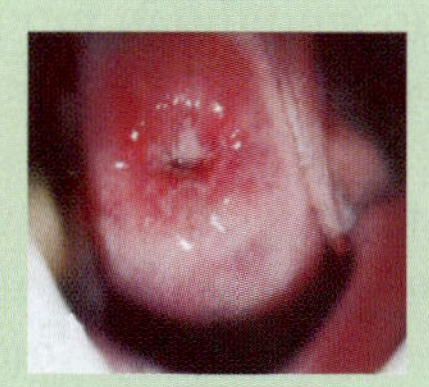

CHALAMYDIAL CERVICITIS

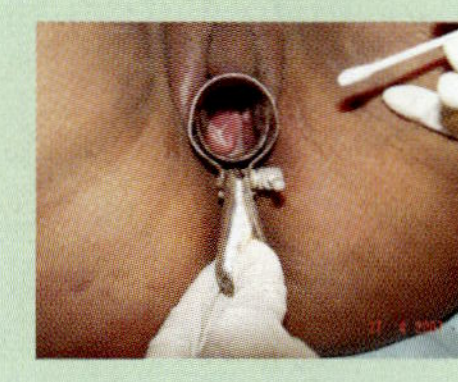

GONOCOCCAL CERVICITIS

Causative Organisms
Vaginitis

- *Trichomonas vaginalis* (TV)
- *Candida albicans*
- *Gardnerella vaginalis*, *Mycoplasma* causing bacterial vagiosis (BV)

Causative Organisms
Cervicitis

- *Neisseria gonorrhoeae*
- *Chlamydia trachomatis*
- *Trichomonas vaginalis*
- *Herpes simplex virus*

History

- Menstrual history to rule out pregnancy
- Nature and type of discharge (amount, smell, x, consistency)
- Genital itching
- Burning while passing urine, increased frequency
- Presence of any ulcer, swelling on the vulval or inguinal region
- Genital complaints in sexual partners
- Low backache

→

Examination

- Per speculum examination to differentiate between vaginitis and cervicitis.

  (a) Vaginitis:
  Trichomoniasis - greenish frothy discharge
  Candidiasis - curdy white discharge
  Bacterial vaginosis – adherent discharge
  Mixed infections may present with atypical discharge

  (b) Cervicitis:
- Cervical erosion /cervical ulcer/mucopurulent cervical discharge
- Bimanual pelvic examination to rule out pelvic inflammatory disease
- If Speculum examination is not possible or client is hesitant, treat both for vaginitis and cervicitis

→

Laboratory Investigations
(*if available*)

- Wet mount microscopy of the discharge for *Trichomonas vaginalis* and clue cells
- 10% KOH preparation for *Candida albicans*
- Gram stain of vaginal smear for clue cells seen in bacterial vaginosis
- Gram stain of endocervical smear to detect gonococci

Treatment

Vaginitis (TV+BV+Candida)

- Tab. Secnidazole 2 gm orally, single dose or
  Tab. Tinidazole 500 mg orally, twice daily for 5 days
  Tab. Metoclopropramide taken 30 minutes before Tab. Secnidazole, to prevent gastric intolerance
- Treat for candidiasis with Tab Fluconazole 150 mg orally single dose or local Clotrimazole 500 mg vaginal pessaries Once

Treatment for cervical infection (chlamydia and gonorrhoea)

- Tab cefixime 400 mg orally, single dose
  Plus Azithromycin 1 gram, 1 hour before lunch. If vomiting within 1 hour, give anti-emetic and repeat
- If vaginitis and cervicitis are present treat for both
- Instruct client to avoid douching
- Pregnancy, diabetes, HIV may also be influencing factors and should be considered in recurrent infections
- Follow-up after one week

Management in pregnant women

Per speculum examination should be done to rule out pregnancy complications like abortion, premature rupture of membranes

Treatment for vaginitis (TV+BV+Candida)

In first trimester of pregnancy

- Local treatment with Clotrimazole vaginal pessary/cream only for candidiasis. Oral Flucanozole is contraindicated in pregnancy.
- Metronidazole pessaries or cream intravaginally if trichomoniasis or BV is suspected.

In second and third trimester oral metronidazole can be given

- Tab. Secnidazole 2 gm orally, single dose or
  Tab. Tinidazole 500 mg orally, twice daily for 5 days
- Tab. Metodopropramide taken 30 minutes before Tab. Metronidazole, to prevent gastric intolerance

Specific guidelines for partner management

- Treat current partner only if no improvement after initial treatment
- If partner is symptomatic, treat client and partner using above protocols
- Advise sexual abstinence during the course of treatment
- Provide condoms, educate about correct and consistent use
- Schedule return visit after 7 days

Flowchart 5.6: Management of Lower Abdominal Pain in Females

SYNDROME: LOWER ABDOMINAL PAIN

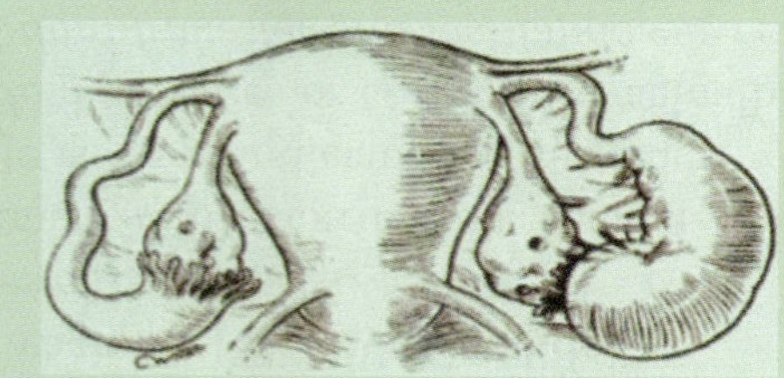

Pelvic inflammatory disease

Causative Organisms

- *Neisseria gonorrhoeae*
- *Chlamydia trachomatis*
- *Mycoplasma,Gardnerella*, Anaerobic bacteria (Bacteroides sp,gram positive cocci)

History

- Lower abdominal pain
- Fever
- Vaginal discharge
- Menstrual irregularities like heavy, irregular vaginal bleeding
- Dysmenorrhoea
- Dyspareunia
- Dysuria, tenesmus
- Low backache
- Contraceptive use like IUD

Examination

- General examination: temperature, pulse, blood pressure
- Per speculum examination: vaginal/ cervical discharge, congestion or ulcers
- Per abdominal examination: lower abdominal tenderness or guarding
- Pelvic examination: Uterine/adnexal tenderness, cervical movement tenderness,

Note: A urine pregnancy test should be done in all women suspected of having PID to rule out ectopic pregnancy.

Laboratory Investigations

If available

- Wet smear examination
- Gram stain for gonorrhoea
- Complete blood count and ESR
- Urine microscopy for pus cells

Differential diagnosis

- Ectopic pregnancy
- Twisted ovarian cyst
- Ovarian tumor
- Appendicitis
- Abdominal tuberculosis

Treatment (Out Client treatment)

In mild or moderate PID (in the absence of tubo ovarian abscess), out Client treatment can be given. Therapy is required to cover *Neisseria gonorrhoeae*, *Chlamydia trachomatis* and anaerobes.

- Tab. Cefixim 400 mg orally BD for 7 days + Tab. Metronidazole 400 mg orally, twice daily for 14 days
  +
- Doxycycline, 100 mg orally, twice a day for 2 weeks (to treat chlamydial infection)
- Tab. Ibuprofen 400 mg orally, three times a day for 3-5 days
- Tab. Ranitidine 150 mg orally, twice daily to prevent gastritis
- Remove intra uterine device, if present, under antibiotic cover of 24-48 hours
- Advise abstinence during the course of treatment and educate on correct and consistent use of condoms
- Observe for 3 days. If no improvement (i.e. absence of fever, reduction in abdominal tenderness, reduction in cervical movement, adnexal and uterine tenderness) or if symptoms worsen, refer for in Client treatment.

Caution: PID can be a serious condition. Refer the client to the hospital if she does not respond to treatment within 3 days and even earlier if her condition worsens.

Syndrome specific guidelines for partner management

- Treat all partners in past 2 months
- Treat male partners for urethral discharge (gonorrhoea and chlamydia)
- Advise sexual abstinence during the course of treatment
- Provide condoms, educate on correct and consistent use
- Refer for voluntary counselling and testing for HIV, Syphilis and Hepatitis B
- Inform about the complications if left untreated and sequelae
- Schedule return visit after 3 days, 7 days and 14 days to ensure compliance

Management of Pregnant Women

Though PID is rare in pregnancy,

- Any pregnant woman suspected to have PID should be referred to district hospital for hospitalization and treated with a parenteral regimen which would be safe in pregnancy.
- Doxycycline is contraindicatcd in pregnancy.
- Note: Metronidazole is generally not recommended during the first three months of pregnancy. However, it should not be withheld for a severely acute PID, which represents an emergency.

Hospitalization of clients with acute PID should be seriously considered when:

- The diagnosis is uncertain
- Surgical emergencies e.g. appendicitis or ectopic pregnancy cannot be excluded
- A pelvic abscess is suspected
- Severe illness precludes management on an out Client basis
- The woman is pregnant
- The client is unable to follow or tolerate an out Client regimen
- The client has failed to respond to outClient therapy

Note: All Clients requiring hospitalization should be referred to the district hospital

Flowchart 5.7: Management of Oral & Anal STIs

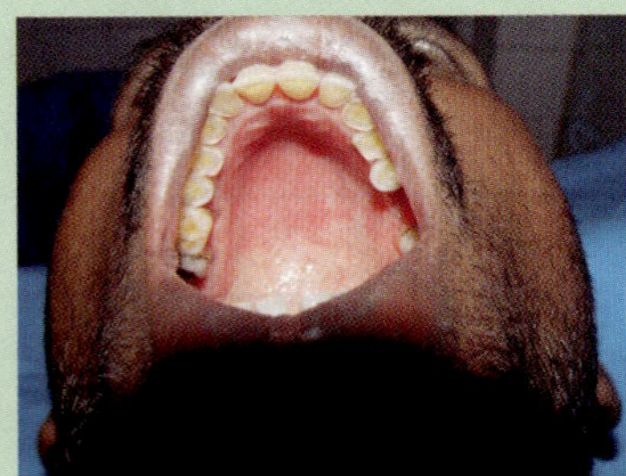

→

Causative Organisms

- *Neisseria gonorrhoeae*
- *Chlamydia trachomatis*
- *Treponema pallidum* (syphilis)
- *Haemophilus ducreyi* (chancroid)
- *Klebsiella granulomatis* (granuloma inguinale)
- Herpes simplex (genital herpes)

History of

- Unprotected oral sex with pharyngitis.
- Unprotected anal sex with anal discharge or tenesmus, diarrhoea, blood in stool, abdominal cramping, nausea, bloating

→

Examination

Look for

- Oral ulceration, redness, pharyngeal inflammation
- Genital or anorectal ulcers – single or multiple
- Presence of vesicles
- Rectal pus
- Any other STI syndrome (Do proctoscopy for rectal examination if available)

→

Laboratory Investigations

- RPR/VDRL for syphilis
- Gram stain examination of rectal swab will show gram negative intracellular diplococcic in case of gonorrhoea.

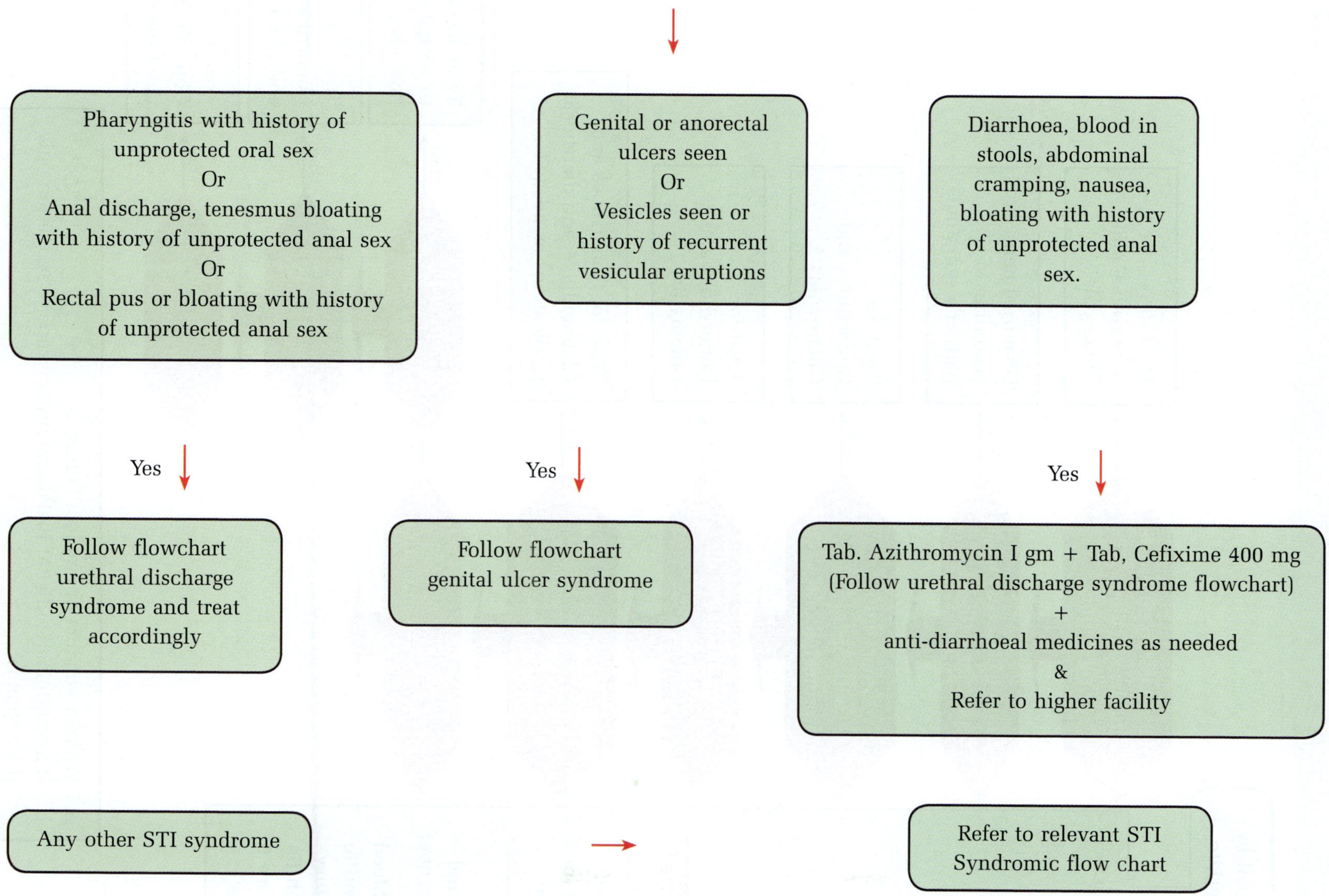
Pharyngitis with history of unprotected oral sex
Or
Anal discharge, tenesmus bloating with history of unprotected anal sex
Or
Rectal pus or bloating with history of unprotected anal sex
Genital or anorectal ulcers seen
Or
Vesicles seen or history of recurrent vesicular eruptions
Diarrhoea, blood in stools, abdominal cramping, nausea, bloating with history of unprotected anal sex.
Yes
Yes
Yes
Follow flowchart urethral discharge syndrome and treat accordingly
Follow flowchart genital ulcer syndrome
Tab. Azithromycin I gm + Tab, Cefixime 400 mg (Follow urethral discharge syndrome flowchart)
+
anti-diarrhoeal medicines as needed
&
Refer to higher facility
Any other STI syndrome
Refer to relevant STI Syndromic flow chart

Management of STI/RTI During Routine Visit of a Male or Transgender Sex Worker

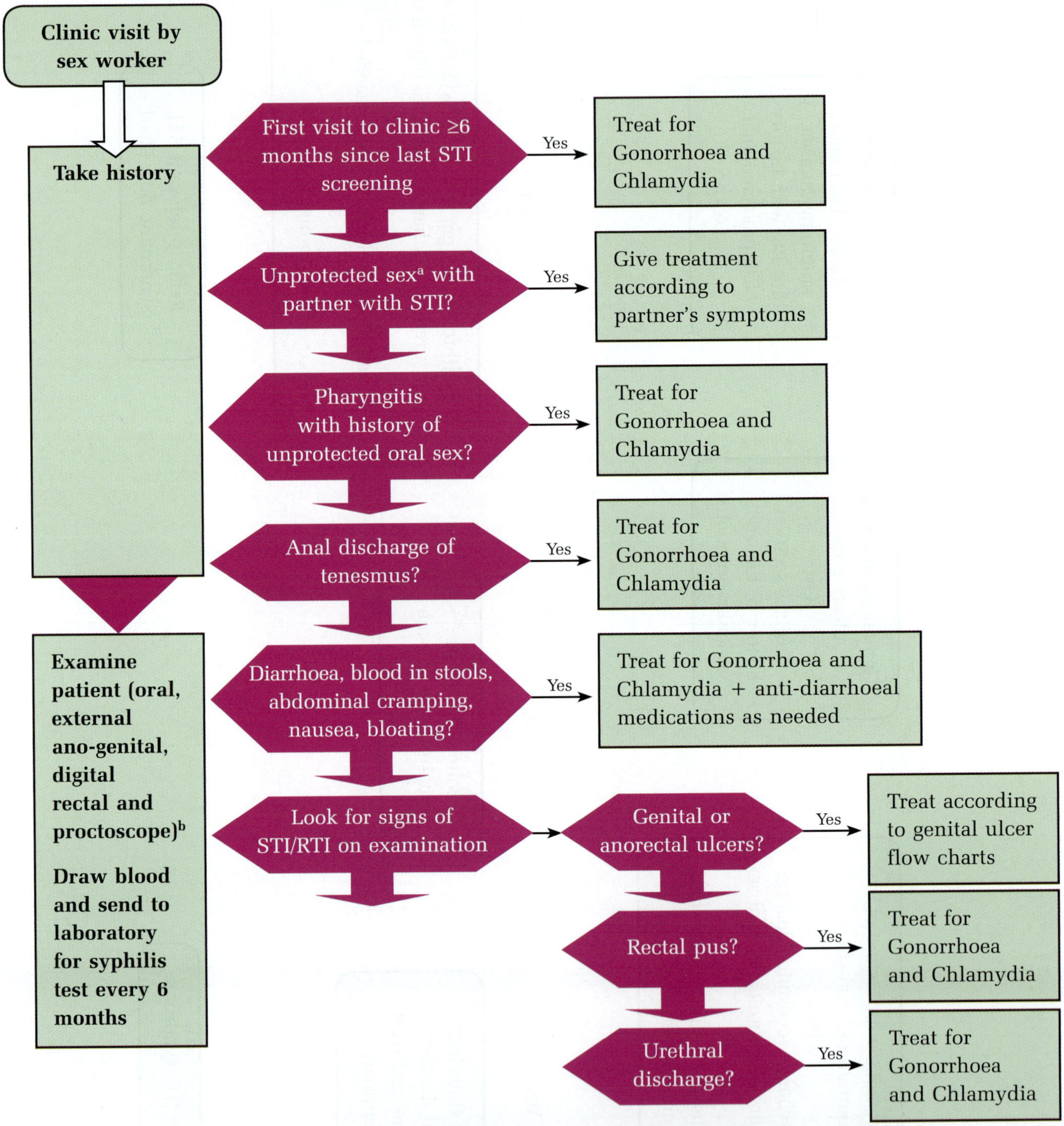

a. Without condom or condom failure.
b. If asymptomatic, digital rectal and proctoscope examination only if acceptable.

INDEX

D

E

H

I

J

K

L

M

T

U